Primer on the Metabolic Bone Diseases and Disorders of Mineral Metabolism

Fourth Edition

An Official Publication of the American Society for Bone and Mineral Research

Primer on the Metabolic Bone Diseases and Disorders of Mineral Metabolism

Fourth Edition

EDITOR

Murray J. Favus, M.D.
Department of Medicine
The University of Chicago Medical Center
Chicago, Illinois

ASSOCIATE EDITORS

Sylvia Christakos, Ph.D.
University of Medicine and Dentistry of New
  Jersey
New Jersey Medical School
Newark, New Jersey

Pamela Gehron Robey, Ph.D.
National Institute of Dental Research
National Institutes of Health
Bethesda, Maryland

Steven R. Goldring, M.D.
Beth Israel Deaconess Medical Center
Boston, Massachusetts

Michael F. Holick, Ph.D., M.D.
Boston University School of Medicine
Boston, Massachusetts

Frederick S. Kaplan, M.D.
University of Pennsylvania School of Medicine
Philadelphia, Pennsylvania

Sundeep Khosla, M.D.
Mayo Clinic and Mayo Medical School
Rochester, Minnesota

Michael Kleerekoper, M.D., F.A.C.E.
Wayne State University
Detroit, Michigan

Craig B. Langman, M.D.
Northwestern University Medical School
Children's Memorial Hospital
Chicago, Illinois

Jane B. Lian, Ph.D.
University of Massachusetts Medical School
Worcester, Massachusetts

Elizabeth Shane, M.D.
Columbia University
College of Physicians and Surgeons
New York, New York

Dolores M. Shoback, M.D.
Veterans Affairs Medical Center
University of California
San Francisco, California

Andrew F. Stewart, M.D.
University of Pittsburgh School of Medicine
Pittsburgh, Pennsylvania

Michael P. Whyte, M.D.
Washington University School of Medicine
St. Louis, Missouri

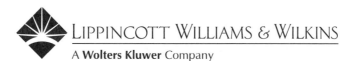

LIPPINCOTT WILLIAMS & WILKINS
A **Wolters Kluwer** Company
Philadelphia · Baltimore · New York · London
Buenos Aires · Hong Kong · Sydney · Tokyo

Acquisitions Editor: Kathey Alexander
Associate Editor: Anne Sydor
Assistant Developmental Editor: Anjou Dargar
Production Editor: Elaine Verriest
Manufacturing Manager: Tim Reynolds
Cover Designer: Patricia Gast
Compositor: PRD Group
Printer: Edwards Bros.

Library of Congress Cataloging-in-Publication Data

Primer on the metabolic bone diseases and disorders of mineral
  metabolism / editor, Murray J. Favus ; associate editors, Sylvia
Christakos ... [et al.]. — 4th ed.
     p. cm.
   ''An official publication of the American Society for Bone and
Mineral Research''—P. preceeding t.p.
   Includes bibliographical references and index.
   ISBN 0-7817-2038-9
   1. Bones—Metabolism—Disorders. 2. Mineral metabolism—
Disorders. I. Favus, Murray J. II. American Society for Bone and
Mineral Research.
   [DNLM: 1. Bone Diseases, Metabolic. 2. Minerals—metabolism.
3. Bone and Bones—metabolism. WE 250 P953 1999]
RC931.M45P75 1999
616.7'16—dc21
DNLM/DLC
for Library of Congress   99-12660
                                  CIP

10 9 8 7 6 5 4

Contents

Section I. Anatomy and Biology of Bone Matrix and Cellular Elements
(Section Editors: Jane B. Lian and Steven R. Goldring)

Section II. Skeletal Physiology
(Section Editors: Elizabeth Shane and Michael Kleerekoper)

Section III. Mineral Homeostasis
(Section Editors: Sylvia Christakos and Michael F. Holick)

Section IV. Clinical Evaluation of Bone and Mineral Disorders
(Section Editors: Craig B. Langman and Dolores M. Shoback)

Section V. Disorders of Serum Minerals
(Section Editors: Elizabeth Shane and Andrew F. Stewart)

Section VI. Metabolic Bone Diseases
(Section Editors: Michael Kleerekoper and Sundeep Khosla)

Contributing Authors

John S. Adams, M.D.
Professor of Medicine, Department of Medicine, University of California, Los Angeles School of Medicine; and Director, Division of Endocrinology and Metabolism, Burns and Allen Research Institute, Cedars-Sinai Medical Center, 8700 Beverly Boulevard, Los Angeles, California 90048

Daniel T. Baran, M.D.
Professor, Departments of Orthopedics and Medicine, University of Massachusetts Medical School, University of Massachusetts Memorial Health Care, 55 Lake Avenue North, Worcester, Massachusetts 01655

Roland Baron, D.D.S., Ph.D.
Professor, Departments of Cell Biology and Orthopaedics, Yale University School of Medicine, 333 Cedar Street, SHM IE-55, New Haven, Connecticut 06520-8044

Daniel D. Bikle, M.D., Ph.D.
Professor, Departments of Medicine and Dermatology, University of California, San Francisco, 3rd and Parnassus, San Francisco, California 94143; and Co-Director Special Diagnostic and Treatment Unit, Department of Medicine, Veterans Affairs Medical Center, 4150 Clement Street (111N), San Francisco, California 94121

John P. Bilezikian, M.D.
Professor of Medicine and Pharmacology; Chief, Division of Endocrinology, College of Physicians and Surgeons; and Attending Physician, Department of Medicine, Columbia Presbyterian Medical Center, 630 West 168th Street, PH8W, New York, New York 10032

Eberhard Blind, M.D.
Department of Medicine, Endocrinology, University of Würzburg, Josef-Schneider Strasse 2, D 97080 Würzburg, Germany

Sydney L. Bonnick, M.D., F.A.C.P.
Research Professor, Center for Research on Women's Health, Texas Woman's University, P.O. Box 425876, Denton, Texas 76204

Adele L. Boskey, Ph.D.
Professor, Program in Cell Biology and Genetics and Biochemistry, Department of Biochemistry/Graduate School of Medical Sciences, Cornell University Medical College, 525 East 68th Street; and Director of Research, Research Division, Hospital for Special Surgery, 535 East 70th Street, New York, New York 10021

Alan Boyde, Ph.D.
Department of Anatomy and Developmental Biology, University College London, Gower Street, London, WC1E 6BT, England

Arthur E. Broadus, M.D., Ph.D.
Professor, Department of Internal Medicine, Yale University School of Medicine, 333 Cedar Street, New Haven, Connecticut 06520-8020

Edward M. Brown, M.D.
Professor of Medicine, Department of Medicine, Harvard Medical School; and Chief, Calcium Section, Endocrine-Hypertension Division, Department of Medicine, Brigham and Women's Hospital, 221 Longwood Avenue, Boston, Massachusetts 02115

David A. Bushinsky, M.D.
Professor of Medicine and of Pharmacology and Physiology, University of Rochester School of Medicine; and Chief, Nephrology Unit, Strong Memorial Hospital, 601 Elmwood Avenue, Box 675, Rochester, New York 14642

Ernesto Canalis, M.D.
Professor, Department of Medicine, University of Connecticut School of Medicine, Farmington, Connecticut 06030; and Director, Department of Research, Saint Francis Hospital and Medical Center, 114 Woodland Street, Hartford, Connecticut 06105-1299

Thomas O. Carpenter, M.D.
Associate Professor, Department of Pediatrics, Yale University School of Medicine, 333 Cedar Street, P.O. Box 208064, New Haven, Connecticut 06520-8064; and Attending Physician, Department of Pediatrics, Yale-New Haven Hospital, 20 York Street, New Haven, Connecticut 06504

Russell W. Chesney, M.D.
Professor and Chair, Department of Pediatrics, University of Tennessee; and Chief, Department of Pediatrics, Le Bonheur Children's Medical Center, 50 North Dunlap Street, Memphis, Tennessee 38103-4909

Sylvia Christakos, Ph.D.
Professor of Biochemistry and Molecular Biology, Department of Biochemistry and Molecular Biology, University of Medicine and Dentistry of New Jersey, New Jersey Medical School, 185 South Orange Avenue, Newark, New Jersey 07103

Thomas L. Clemens, Ph.D.
Professor of Medicine and Molecular and Cellular Physiology, University of Cincinnati College of Medicine, 231 Bethesda Avenue, MSB 5564, Cincinnati, Ohio 45267-0547

Jack W. Coburn, M.D.
Professor of Medicine, University of California, Los Angeles School of Medicine, Staff Physician, Nephrology Section (111L), West Los Angeles Veterans Affairs Medical Center, 11301 Wilshire Boulevard, Los Angeles, California 90073

Fredric L. Coe, M.D.
Professor of Medicine and Physiology, Section Chief: Nephrology, The University of Chicago, 5841 South Maryland Avenue, MC 5100, Chicago, Illinois 60637-1470

David E. C. Cole, M.D., Ph.D., F.R.C.P.C.
Associate Professor of Laboratory Medicine and Pathobiology, University of Toronto, 100 College Street; and Director, Genetic Repository, The Toronto Hospital, Toronto, Ontario, Canada M5G 1L5

Gary J. R. Cook, M.B.B.S., M.Sc., M.R.C.P., F.R.C.R.
Clinical Lecturer, Department of Radiological Sciences, Guy's, King's College, St. Thomas' School of Medicine; and Honorary Consultant, Nuclear Medicine, Guy's Hospital, St. Thomas Street, London, SEI 9RT, England

Felicia Cosman, M.D.
Medical Director, Clinical Research Center; and Associate Professor of Clinical Medicine, Columbia University, CRC, Helen Hayes Hospital, Route 9W, West Haverstraw, New York 10993

Gilbert J. Cote, Ph.D.
Associate Professor, Section of Endocrine Neoplasia and Hormonal Disorders, University of Texas M. D. Anderson Cancer Center, 1515 Holcombe Boulevard, Box 15, Houston, Texas 77030

Bess Dawson-Hughes, M.D.
Professor of Medicine, Division of Endocrinology, New England Medical Center at Tufts, 75 Kneeland Street, 12th Floor; and Chief, Calcium and Bone Metabolism Laboratory, U.S.D.A. Human Nutrition Research Center on Aging at Tufts University, 711 Washington Street, Boston, Massachusetts 02111

Leonard J. Deftos, M.D., J.D.
Professor, Department of Medicine, University of California, San Diego; and Staff Physician and Head, Endocrine Research Laboratory, 3350 La Jolla Village Drive; and Veterans Affairs San Diego Healthcare System, San Diego, California 92161

Marc K. Drezner, M.D.
Professor, Department of Medicine, Duke University Medical Center, Box 3285, Durham, North Carolina 27710

Richard Eastell, M.D., F.R.C.P.
Professor, Division of Clinical Sciences, University of Sheffield, Northern General Hospital; and Honorary Consultant Physician, Department of Medicine, Northern General Hospital, Herries Road, Sheffield, 557 AU, England

Thomas A. Einhorn, M.D.
Professor and Chairman, Department of Orthopaedic Surgery, Boston University School of Medicine, Doctors Office Building, 720 Harrison Avenue; and Chief, Orthopaedic Surgery, Boston Medical Center, Boston, Massachusetts 02118-2393

Murray J. Favus, M.D.
Professor, Department of Medicine, University of Chicago; and Director, Bone Program, University of Chicago Hospitals, 5841 South Maryland Avenue, MC 5100, Chicago, Illinois 60637

Ignac Fogelman, B.Sc., M.D., F.R.C.P.
Professor, Department of Radiological Sciences, Guy's, King's College and St. Thomas' Hospital Medical School; and Honorary Consultant, Department of Nuclear Medicine, Guy's Hospital, St. Thomas Street, London, SE1 9RT, England

Robert F. Gagel, M.D.
Professor of Medicine, Section of Endocrine Neoplasia and Hormonal Disorders; and Chairman/Chief, Department of Internal Medicine Specialties, Section of Endocrine Neoplasia and Hormonal Disorders, University of Texas M. D. Anderson Cancer Center, 1515 Holcombe Boulevard, Box 47, Houston, Texas 77030

Pamela Gehron Robey, Ph.D.
Chief, Craniofacial and Skeletal Diseases Branch, National Institute of Dental and Craniofacial Research, National Institutes of Health, 30 Convent Drive, MSC 4320, Bethesda, Maryland 20892

Harry K. Genant, M.D.
Professor of Radiology, Medicine, Epidemiology, and Orthopedic Surgery; and Executive Director, Osteoporosis and Arthritis Research Group, University of California, San Francisco, 505 Parnassus Avenue, San Francisco, California 94143-0628

Joseph M. Gertner, M.B., M.R.C.P.
Lecturer, Department of Pediatrics, Harvard Medical School; and Physician, Department of Endocrinology, Boston Children's Hospital, 330 Longwood Avenue, Boston, Massachusetts 02115

Francis H. Glorieux, M.D., Ph.D.
Professor, Departments of Surgery and Pediatrics, McGill University, Montreal, Quebec; and Director of Research, Shriners Hospital, 1529 Cedar Avenue, Montreal, Quebec, Canada H3G 1A6

Steven R. Goldring, M.D.
Chief of Rheumatology, Beth Israel Deaconess Medical Center, Harvard Medical School, 110 Francis Street, Boston, Massachusetts 02215

David Goltzman, M.D.
Professor and Chair, Department of Medicine, McGill University; and Physician-in-Chief, Department of Medicine, McGill University Health Centre, Royal Victoria Hospital, 687 Pine Avenue West, Montreal, Quebec, Canada H3A 1A1

William G. Goodman, M.D.
Professor of Medicine, University of California, Los Angeles School of Medicine, Department of Medicine, Division of Nephrology, 7-155 Factor Building, Los Angeles, California 90095-1689

Theresa A. Guise, M.D.
Associate Professor, Department of Medicine, Division of Endocrinology, The University of Texas Health Science Center at San Antonio, 7703 Floyd Curl Drive, San Antonio, Texas 78284-7877

Robert P. Heaney, M.D., F.A.C.P., F.A.I.N.
John A. Creighton University Professor, Creighton University, 601 North 30th Street, Omaha, Nebraska 68131

Hunter Heath III, M.D.
Director, Endocrine Medical Affairs, U.S. Medical Division, Ely Lilly and Company, Lilly Corporate Center, Indianapolis, Indiana 46285; and Volunteer Attending, Department of Internal Medicine, The Wishard Hospital, Iupui Medical Center, Indianapolis, Indiana

Maurine R. Hobbs, Ph.D.
Research Assistant Professor, Department of Internal Medicine, Division of Endocrinology, University of Utah, 50 North Medical Drive, Salt Lake City, Utah 84132

Michael F. Holick, Ph.D., M.D.
Professor of Medicine, Dermatology, and Physiology, Department of Medicine; and Chief, Section of Endocrinology, Nutrition, and Diabetes, Boston University Medical Center, 1 Boston Medical Center Place, M1013, Boston, Massachusetts 02118

Jeffrey O. Hollinger, D.D.S., Ph.D.
Professor of Surgery, Anatomy, and Developmental Biology, Department of Surgery, Division of Plastic and Reconstructive Surgery, Oregon Health Sciences University, 3181 Southwest Sam Jackson Park Road, L352A, Portland, Oregon 97201-3098

Bruce W. Hollis, Ph.D.
Professor, Departments of Pediatrics, Biochemistry, and Molecular Biology, Medical University South Carolina, 171 Ashley Avenue, Charleston, South Carolina 29425

Keith A. Hruska, M.D.
Professor of Medicine, Renal Division, Barnes-Jewish Hospital, 216 South Kingshighway, St. Louis, Missouri 63010

Olafur S. Indridason, M.D., M.H.Sc.
Associate in Medicine, Department of Medicine, Division of Nephrology, Duke University Medical Center, Box 3014, Durham, North Carolina 27710

Marjorie K. Jeffcoat, D.M.D.
James Rosen Professor of Dental Research and Chair, Department of Periodontics, The University of Alabama at Birmingham School of Dentistry, 1919 7th Avenue South, SDB 412, Birmingham, Alabama 35294-0007

Michael D. Jergas, M.D.
Associate Professor, Department of Radiology, Ruhr-University Bochum, D-44801; and Department of Radiology, St. Josef-Hospital, Gudrunstrasse 56, D-44791, Bochum, Germany

Sheila J. Jones, Ph.D.
Professor, Department of Anatomy and Developmental Biology, University College London, Gower Street, London, WC1E 6BT, England

Harald Jüppner, M.D.
Associate Professor of Pediatrics, Department of Pediatrics, Harvard Medical School; and Associate Biologist, Department of Medicine, Endocrine Unit, Massachusetts General Hospital, 50 Blossom Street, Boston, Massachusetts 02114-2698

Frederick S. Kaplan, M.D.
Isaac and Rose Nassan Professor of Orthopaedic Molecular Medicine, The University of Pennsylvania School of Medicine; and Chief, Division of Molecular Orthopaedics and Metabolic Bone Diseases, Department of Orthopaedics, The University of Pennsylvania Medical Center, Silverstein 2, 3400 Spruce Street, Philadelphia, Pennsylvania 19104-4283

Sundeep Khosla, M.D.
Associate Professor, Department of Medicine, Mayo Medical School; and Chair, Metabolic Bone Group, Division of Endocrinology, Mayo Clinic, 200 First Street Southwest, Rochester, Minnesota 55905

Douglas P. Kiel, M.D., M.P.H.
Assistant Professor of Medicine, Division on Aging, Harvard Medical School; and Associate Director, Medical Research, Research and Training Institute, Hebrew Rehabilitation Center for Aged, 1200 Centre Street, Boston, Massachusetts 02131-1097

Michael Kleerekoper, M.D., F.A.C.E.
Professor, Departments of Medicine, Obstetrics and Gynecology, and Pathology, Wayne State University, UHC-4H, 4201 St. Antoine, Detroit, Michigan 48201

Gordon L. Klein, M.D., M.P.H.
Professor, Departments of Pediatrics and Preventive Medicine, University of Texas Medical Branch, 301 University Boulevard, Galveston, Texas 77555-0352

Christopher S. Kovacs, M.D., F.R.C.P.C.
Assistant Professor of Medicine (Endocrinology), Obstetrics and Gynecology, Nuclear Medicine, and Basic Medical Sciences, Department of Medicine–Endocrinology, Health Sciences Centre, Memorial University of Newfoundland, 300 Prince Philip Drive, St. John's, Newfoundland, Canada A1B 3V6

Paul H. Krebsbach, D.D.S., Ph.D.
Assistant Professor, Department of Oral Medicine/ Pathology/Oncology, University of Michigan School of Dentistry, 1011 N. University Avenue, Ann Arbor, Michigan 48109-1078

Henry M. Kronenberg, M.D.
Professor, Department of Medicine, Harvard Medical School; and Chief, Endocrine Unit, Department of Medicine, Massachusetts General Hospital, 50 Blossom Street, WEL501, Boston, Massachusetts 02114-2698

Craig B. Langman, M.D.
Professor of Pediatrics, Department of Pediatrics, Northwestern University Medical School, 303 East Chicago Avenue, Chicago, Illinois 60611; and Division Head, Nephrology and Mineral Metabolism Department, Children's Memorial Hospital, 2300 Children's Plaza, MS 37, Chicago, Illinois 60614

Eleanor D. Lederer, M.D., Ph.D.
Associated Professor of Medicine, Department of Medicine/Nephrology, University of Louisville, 615 South Preston Street, Louisville, KY 40202-1718; and Renal Department, University of Louisville Affiliated Hospitals

Jacob Lemann, Jr., M.D.
Clinical Professor of Medicine, Nephrology Section, Department of Medicine, Tulane University School of Medicine, SL45, 1430 Tulane Avenue, New Orleans, Louisiana 70112-2669; and Staff, Department of Medicine, New Orleans Veterans Affairs Medical Center, 1601 Perdido Street, New Orleans, Louisiana 70112-9922

Michael A. Levine, M.D.
Professor of Pediatrics, Medicine, and Pathology; and Director, Pediatric Endocrinology, The Johns Hopkins University School of Medicine, 863 Ross Research Building, 720 Rutland Avenue, Baltimore, Maryland 21205

Jane B. Lian, Ph.D.
Professor, Department of Cell Biology, University of Massachusetts Medical School, 55 Lake Avenue North, Worcester, Massachusetts 01655-0106

Uri A. Liberman, M.D., Ph.D.
Professor of Physiology and Medicine; and Head, Division of Endocrinology and Metabolism, Rabin Medical Center, Metabolic Diseases, Beilinson Campus, Sackler Faculty of Medicine, Tel Aviv University, 49100 Petah-Tikva, Israel

Robert Lindsay, Ph.D., M.B.Ch.B., F.R.C.P.
Chief, Internal Medicine, Helen Hayes Hospital; and Professor of Clinical Medicine, Columbia University, Helen Hayes Hospital, Route 9W, West Haverstraw, New York 10993

James E. Lingeman, M.D.
Director of Research, Methodist Hospital Institute for Kidney Stone Disease, 1801 North Senate Boulevard, Indianapolis, Indiana 46202

Marjorie M. Luckey, M.D.
Associate Clinical Professor, Mount Sinai Medical Center, 1 Gustav-Levy Place, New York, New York 10029; and Medical Director, Osteoporosis and Metabolic Bone Disease Center, Saint Barnabas Medical Center, 200 South Orange Avenue, Livingston, New Jersey 07039

Barbara P. Lukert, M.D., F.A.C.P.
Professor of Medicine, Department of Medicine, University of Kansas School of Medicine; and Director of Osteoporosis Clinic, Department of Medicine, University of Kansas Hospital, 3901 Cambridge, Kansas City, Kansas 66160-7318

Robert Marcus, M.D.
Professor of Medicine, Stanford University, Director, Aging Study Unit, Geriatrics Research, Education and Clinical Center, Veterans Affairs Medical Center, GRECC 182-B, 3801 Miranda Avenue, Palo Alto, California 94304

Stephen J. Marx, M.D.
Chief, Genetics and Endocrinology Section, National Institute of Diabetes and Digestive and Kidney Diseases, National Institutes of Health, Building 10, Bethesda, Maryland 20892-1802

Paul D. Miller, M.D.
Clinical Professor, Department of Medicine, University of Colorado Health Sciences Center, 4200 East 9th Avenue, Denver, Colorado 80262; and Medical Director, Colorado Center for Bone Research, 3190 South Wadsworth, Lakewood, Colorado 80227

Gregory R. Mundy, M.D.
Professor and Head, Heyser Professor of Bone and Mineral Metabolism, Department of Medicine, Division of Endocrinology and Metabolism, The University of Texas Health Science Center, 7703 Floyd Curl Drive, San Antonio, Texas 78284-7877

Robert A. Nissenson, Ph.D.
Professor, Department of Medicine and Physiology, University of California, San Francisco, California 94143; and Career Scientist, Endocrine Research Unit, Veterans Affairs Medical Center, 4150 Clement Street, San Francisco, California 94121

Michael E. Norman, M.D.
Clinical Professor, Department of Pediatrics, University of North Carolina, CB#7220, 509 Burnett-Womack Building, Chapel Hill, North Carolina 27599-7220; and Chairman and Residency Program Director, Department of Pediatrics, Carolinas Medical Center, P.O. Box 32861, Charlotte, North Carolina 28232-2861

Edward L. Oates, Ph.D.
Investigator, Geriatric Research, Education, and Clinical Center, Veterans Affairs Medical Center, 1201 Northwest 16th Street, Miami, Florida 33125

Bjorn R. Olsen, M.D., Ph.D.
Hersey Professor of Cell Biology, Department of Cell Biology, Harvard Medical School; and Harvard-Forsyth Professor of Oral Biology, Harvard-Forsyth Department of Oral Biology, Harvard School of Dental Medicine, 240 Longwood Avenue, Boston, Massachusetts 02115

Eric S. Orwoll, M.D.
Professor of Medicine, Department of Medicine, Oregon Health Sciences University, 3181 Southwest Sam Jackson Park Road, Portland, Oregon 97201-3098

Joan H. Parks, M.B.A.
Assistant Professor, Administrator, Kidney Stone Program, The University of Chicago, Department of Medicine, Section of Nephrology, 5841 South Maryland Avenue, MC 5100, Chicago, Illinois 60637

Peter J. Polverini, D.D.S., D.M.Sc.
Donald H. Kerr Professor and Chair, Department of Oral Medicine/Pathology/Oncology, University of Michigan School of Dentistry, 1011 North University, Ann Arbor, Michigan 48103-1078

Anthony A. Portale, M.D.
Professor of Pediatrics and Medicine; and Chief, Division of Pediatric Nephrology, University of California, San Francisco, 533 Parnassus Avenue, San Francisco, California 94143-0126

Andrew K. Poznanski, M.D.
Professor, Department of Radiology, Northwestern University Medical School; and Radiologist-in-Chief, Children's Memorial Hospital, 2300 Children's Plaza, #9, Chicago, Illinois 60614-3394

L. Darryl Quarles, M.D.
Associate Professor of Medicine, Department of Medicine, Division of Nephrology, Duke University Medical Center, Box 3036, Durham, North Carolina 27710

Robert R. Recker, M.D., F.A.C.P., F.A.C.E.
Professor, Department of Medicine, Creighton University School of Medicine; Chief, Section of Endocrinology, Creighton University Medical Center; Senior Active Staff, St. Joseph Hospital; Director, Osteoporosis Research Center, 601 North 30th Street, Omaha, Nebraska 68131; and Attending Physician, Omaha Veterans Affairs Hospital

Ian R. Reid, M.D., F.R.A.C.P.
Professor, Department of Medicine, University of Auckland, Private Bag 92019; and Endocrinologist, Department of Endocrinology, Auckland Hospital, Park Avenue, Auckland, New Zealand

Michelle M. Roberts, M.D.
Associate Professor, Department of Medicine, University of Pittsburgh, E1140 Biomedical Science Tower, Pittsburgh, Pennsylvania 15261

Bernard A. Roos, M.D.
Professor of Medicine and Neurology, Divisions of Endocrinology and Gerontology and Geriatric Medicine, University of Miami School of Medicine; and Geriatric Research, Education, and Clinical Center, Veterans Affairs Medical Center, 1201 Northwest 16th Street, Miami, Florida 33125

Clifford J. Rosen, M.D.
Professor of Nutrition, Department of Nutrition, University of Maine, Orono, Maine; and Director, Maine Center for Osteoporosis Research and Education, St. Joseph Hospital, 360 Broadway, Bangor, Maine 04401

Clinton T. Rubin, Ph.D.
Professor and Director, Center for Biotechnology, State University of New York at Stony Brook, Life Sciences Center, 130, Stony Brook, New York 11794-5208

Janet Rubin, M.D.
Associate Professor, Department of Medicine, Emory University School of Medicine; and Endocrinologist, Department of Medicine, Veterans Affairs Medical Center, 1670 Clairmont Road, Atlanta, Georgia 30033

Robert K. Rude, M.D.
Professor, Department of Medicine, University of Southern California, 2025 Zonal Avenue, Los Angeles, California 90033

Isidro B. Salusky, M.D.
Professor of Pediatrics, Division of Pediatric Nephrology, University of California, Los Angeles School of Medicine, 10833 Le Conte Avenue, Box 951752, Los Angeles, California 90095-1752

K. C. Saw, M.A., F.R.C.S.
Fellow in Endourology and Urolithiasis, Methodist Hospital Institute for Kidney Stone Disease, 1801 North Senate Boulevard, Indianapolis, Indiana 46202

Elizabeth Shane, M.D.
Professor, Department of Medicine, Columbia University College of Physicians and Surgeons; and Attending Physician, Department of Medicine, New York Presbyterian Hospital, 630 West 168th Street, New York, New York 10032

Dolores M. Shoback, M.D.
Staff Physician, Department of Medicine, Department of Endocrine-111N, Veterans Affairs Medical Center, 4150 Clement Street, San Francisco, California 94127; and Associate Professor, Department of Medicine, University of California, San Francisco, California 94143

Eileen M. Shore, Ph.D.
Research Assistant and Professor, Department of Orthopaedic Surgery, The University of Pennsylvania School of Medicine, Stemmler Hall, 36th and Hamilton Walk, Philadelphia, Pennsylvania 19104

Richard M. Shore, M.D.
Assistant Professor, Department of Radiology, Northwestern University Medical School, 303 East Chicago Avenue, Chicago, Illinois 60611-3008; and Attending Radiologist, Children's Memorial Hospital, 2300 Children's Plaza, Number 9, Chicago, Illinois 60614-3394

Ethel S. Siris, M.D.
Madeline C. Stabile Professor of Clinical Medicine, Department of Medicine, Columbia University College of Physicians and Surgeons, 630 West 168th Street, New York, New York 10032; and Director, Toni Stabile Center for the Prevention and Treatment of Osteoporosis, Metabolic Bone Diseases Program, Columbia-Presbyterian Medical Center, 180 Fort Washington Avenue, New York, New York 10032

Peter M. Sklarin, M.D.
Menlo Medical Clinic, 1300 Crane Street, Menlo Park, California 94025

Eduardo Slatopolsky, M.D.
Joseph Friedman Professor of Renal Diseases in Medicine, Department of Medicine, Washington University School of Medicine, 660 South Euclid Avenue, Box 8126; and Physician/Renal Consultant, Barnes-Jewish Hospital, One Barnes Hospital Plaza Drive, St. Louis, Missouri 63110

Martha J. Somerman, D.D.S., Ph.D.
William K. and Mary Anne Najjar Professor and Chair, Department of Periodontics/Prevention/Geriatrics, University of Michigan School of Dentistry; and Professor and Chair of the Department of Pharmacology, University of Michigan School of Medicine, 1011 North University, Ann Arbor, Michigan 48109-1078

Thomas C. Spelsberg, Ph.D.
George M. Eisenberg Professor, Department of Biochemistry and Molecular Biology, Mayo Graduate and Medical Schools, Mayo Clinic, 200 First Street, Southwest, Guggenheim Building, Rochester, Minnesota 55905

Gary S. Stein, Ph.D.
Professor and Chair, Department of Cell Biology, University of Massachusetts Medical School, 55 Lake Avenue North, Worcester, Massachusetts 01655

Andrew F. Stewart, M.D.
Professor of Medicine, Department of Medicine, University of Pittsburgh School of Medicine; and Chief, Division of Endocrinology, Department of Medicine, University of Pittsburgh Medical Center, E1140 Biomedical Science Tower, 3550 Terrace Street, Pittsburgh, Pennsylvania 15213

Gordon J. Strewler, M.D.
Professor, Department of Medicine, Harvard Medical School, 25 Shattuck Street, Boston, Massachusetts 02115; and Chief, Department of Medicine, Boston Healthcare System, West Roxbury Campus Veterans Affairs Medical Center, 1400 VFW Parkway (111), West Roxbury, Massachusetts 02132

Richard D. Wasnich, M.D., F.A.C.P.
Clinical Professor, Department of Medicine, University of Hawaii; and Medical Director, Radiant Research-Honolulu, 401 Kamakee Street, Honolulu, HI 96814

Katrina M. Waters, Ph.D.
Endocrine, Reproductive, and Developmental Toxicology, Chemical Industry Institute of Toxicology, 6 Davis Drive, Research Triangle Park, North Carolina 27709

Nelson B. Watts, M.D.
Professor of Medicine, Emory University School of Medicine; and Director, Osteoporosis and Metabolic Bone Diseases Program, The Emory Clinic, 1365 Clifton Road, Northeast, Atlanta, Georgia 30322

Michael P. Whyte, M.D.
Professor of Medicine, Pediatrics, and Genetics, Division of Bone and Mineral Diseases, Washington University School of Medicine at Barnes–Jewish Hospital, 216 South Kingshighway, St. Louis, Missouri 63110; and Medical Director, Metabolic Research Unit, Shriners Hospital for Children, 2001 South Lindbergh Boulevard, St. Louis, Missouri 63131

Toshiyuki Yoneda, Ph.D., D.D.S.
Professor, Department of Medicine, Division of Endocrinology, The University of Texas Health Science Center, 7703 Floyd Curl Drive, San Antonio, Texas 78284-7877

The American Society for Bone and Mineral Research

Now over twenty years old, the American Society for Bone and Mineral Research (ASBMR) has become truly international and the leading organization for professionals in its field. The Society's mission includes fostering research and education in bone and mineral metabolism. The annual meeting regularly attracts several thousand participants. In 1998, over 2,000 presentations in clinical and basic research were made.

The Society's *Journal of Bone and Mineral Research* publishes advances in the field and is both a research and educational resource.

The *Primer on the Metabolic Bone Diseases and Disorders of Mineral Metabolism,* now in its fourth edition, is the Society's most important educational instrument. Widely used in medical school curricula and by graduate students, post-graduate trainees, clinicians, and researchers, it is "up-to-the-minute" at the time of publication. The information it contains reflects the remarkable growth of the field and the broadening interface between basic and clinical sciences in bone and mineral metabolism. A product of members of ASBMR, experts in their respective areas, we hope this excellent book will help practitioners and investigators, and attract those on the threshold of their careers to this rapidly evolving field.

Michael Rosenblatt, M.D.
Past President, ASBMR

Preface to the First Edition

Our understanding of the scientific basis for clinical bone and mineral disorders has grown rapidly since the founding of the American Society for Bone and Mineral Research (ASBMR) in 1977. The number of basic scientists and clinicians involved in either research or patient care in bone and mineral metabolism has grown dramatically, attracting the interest of medical students, house officers, and practitioners. While textbooks of Medicine, Pediatrics, Endocrinology, Nephrology, Radiology, and Orthopedic Surgery devote chapters or sections to metabolic bone disease, none provide a comprehensive description of the clinical manifestations of the diseases and the basic science necessary to understand pathophysiology. Three years ago the Education Committee of the ASBMR undertook the task of creating a comprehensive educational source, and this *Primer* is the result of our efforts.

The primary purpose of the *Primer* is to provide a comprehensive, yet concise description of the clinical manifestations, pathophysiology, diagnostic approaches, and therapeutics of diseases that come under the rubric of "bone and mineral disorders."

The organization of the *Primer* into twelve sections reflects the several basic science and clinical disciplines that contribute to the field. The first three sections contain the basic science core material that provides the underpinning of our understanding of normal bone and mineral structure and biology. Section I contains a thorough description of the gross anatomy and ultrastructure of bone, the physiology of skeletal growth, development and remodeling, the biochemistry of the bone matrix, and the unique structural features and functions of the cellular elements of bone. Section II provides a dynamic view of the biologic importance of the major elements of bone (usually referred to as the minerals) and their body distribution and balance, including the processes of accumulation and elimination across epithelial barriers in the intestine and kidney. Section III focuses on the details of the synthesis, secretion, metabolism, and biologic actions of the key hormones (parathyroid hormone, vitamin D, and calcitonin) that regulate skeletal growth and remodeling, calcium homeostasis, and the assimilation of minerals to support these processes.

The clinical portion of the *Primer* begins with the eleven chapters in Section IV. Laboratory assays, radiographic and imaging techniques, and bone histomorphometry used to evaluate patients suspected of having bone or mineral disorders are described. Section V contains 26 chapters that describe the many clinical entities that may present to the clinician with disordered levels of serum minerals including hyper- and hypo- calcemia, -phosphatemia, and -magnesemia. Chapters in Section VI describe the several genetic and acquired causes of the classic metabolic bone diseases of rickets, osteomalacia, osteoporosis, and the many presentations of renal osteodystrophy.

Section VII contains the genetic and developmental disorders that primarily affect bone. These conditions may present in infancy, childhood, or adulthood as abnormal radiographs, fractures, growth retardation, or skeletal pain. Section VIII includes vascular, tumoral and degenerative processes that may cause bone pain, skeletal deformity, and fracture. Section IX is devoted solely to Paget's disease of bone, a common and important entity with many presentations.

Diseases characterized by pathologic calcification of soft tissue are presented in Section X, and Section XI contains the metabolic disorders in which pathologic crystalization is selective for the urinary tract.

Section XII is the Appendix, composed of seven subsections containing information useful to the practitioner, including growth charts, ossification center tables, normal values for commonly used biochemical analyses, instructions on how to conduct and interpret dynamic tests of calciotropic hormone secretion, recommended daily mineral and vitamin D intake for all ages, and a drug formulary.

The full credit for any educational benefit that the *Primer* may offer goes to the many scientists and clinicians who have captured their knowledge and experience on the pages of their chapters. The high quality of their contributions and their cooperation are deeply appreciated. I am also deeply indebted to the seven Associate Editors of the *Primer*: Sylvia Christakos, Robert F. Gagel, Michael Kleerekoper, Craig B. Langman, Elizabeth Shane, Andrew F. Stewart, and Michael P. Whyte for their hard work and devotion to the project. Their ability to enlist the participation of over seventy authors, continued enthusiasm and critical editing served to forge the *Primer* into its final form. I also express my deepest appreciation to the presidents of ASBMR who held office during the development of the *Primer*—Norman Bell, Gideon Rodan, John Haddad, and Armen Tashjian. They were most generous in devoting time and effort to find the resources necessary to bring the *Primer* to publication.

I would also express my sincere appreciation to the people at Byrd Press for their guidance and assistance in the preparation and publication of the *Primer*. Finally, I would like to gratefully acknowledge Shirley Hohl, ASBMR Executive Secretary, and John Hohl for their much valued assistance in preparing the *Primer* for publication and distribution.

Murray J. Favus, M.D.
The University of Chicago
Pritzker School of Medicine

Preface to the Fourth Edition

The subject of the Fourth Edition of the *Primer* is the core knowledge of bone biology, mineral metabolism, action of hormones on bone and mineral metabolism, and the clinical disorders that involve these complex systems. The study of bone structure and function is important because of the insight it provides into the pathogenesis of the many disorders that affect bone and mineral, and because new knowledge of the basic science of bone offers our best opportunity to develop novel approaches to treat and reverse these disorders.

The diseases referred to as metabolic bone diseases and mineral disorders are a collection of rare and unusual diseases admixed with very common conditions. The recent, rapid expansion of osteoporosis research has resulted in many new insights into its pathogenesis, has led to new diagnostic assays and procedures, and has yielded new therapies that may benefit the millions of people affected. Many other bone and mineral diseases that affect people of all ages have also experienced important advances in recent years.

This new knowledge is incorporated into the revised chapters that appeared in previous editions as well as twenty-five chapters that are new to the Fourth Edition. The new chapters have significantly expanded the basic science sections, which now include chapters on bone morphogenesis and embryological development as well as on bone biomechanics. The substantial problem of osteoporosis is reflected in the large number of chapters on this topic included in the clinical sections of the *Primer*. New therapies for osteoporosis have led to new chapters on treatment. Because of important scientific advances in oral biology and the significance of dental manifestations of systemic mineral disorders, the *Primer* now contains four new chapters in these areas of dental science.

The *Primer* offers a concise yet thorough discussion of the basic information needed to become familiar with the diseases, the underlying pathophysiology, and the basic sciences that provide an understanding for the basis of the disorders. The book is directed to clinicians, basic scientists, students, and residents in a variety of disciplines including general practice, internal medicine, pediatrics, gynecology, orthopaedic surgery, radiology, and nuclear medicine. A number of subspecialty groups will be particularly interested in the *Primer*, including those in endocrinology, genetics, rheumatology, nephrology, nutrition, gastroenterology, and geriatrics. Basic scientists interested in bone and in mineral metabolism will find the *Primer* to be useful at all levels of inquiry including molecular biology, cell biology, biochemistry, physiology, genetics, pathology, immunology, and nutrition.

Because research in this field continues to expand at a rapid rate, and direct benefits are being appreciated in the clinical sciences, the *Primer* continues to be a work in evolution. Therefore, I welcome readers' comments and suggestions as to how to present this field in the most useful and informative way.

Murray J. Favus, M.D.
University of Chicago

Acknowledgments

The editorial board's efforts to bring out the Fourth Edition of the *Primer* faced challenges similar to that of any far-flung group attempting to work together. With a strong dependence upon new communication systems, the Fourth Edition is truly a product of the computer age. Talk between and among editors, authors, and the staff at Lippincott Williams & Wilkins was largely conducted by e-mail and via the Lippincott Williams & Wilkins website. The ease of communication permitted more detailed reviews of each chapter and a better overall integration of information. The successful communication was ably directed by Associate Editor Anne Sydor. The editorial board is deeply appreciative of her organizational and interpersonal skills and for her commitment to the project. Throughout her work, Anne was ably assisted by Anjou Dargar. We are also grateful to Executive Vice President Kathey Alexander, who was with us from start to finish on this edition. She provided an environment at the publisher that made our collaboration possible.

Of course, it was the collaborative work of the editorial board that once again resulted in a successful edition. I thank Sylvia Christakos, Steven R. Goldring, Michael F. Holick, Frederick S. Kaplan, Sundeep Khosla, Michael Kleerekoper, Craig B. Langman, Jane B. Lian, Pamela Gehron Robey, Elizabeth Shane, Dolores M. Shoback, Andrew F. Stewart, and Michael P. Whyte for their enthusiasm, dedication, and selfless work.

Murray J. Favus

SECTION I

Anatomy and Biology of Bone Matrix and Cellular Elements

1. Anatomy and Ultrastructure of Bone

Roland Baron, D.D.S., Ph.D.

Departments of Cell Biology and Orthopaedics, Yale University School of Medicine, New Haven, Connecticut

Bone is a specialized connective tissue that makes up, together with cartilage, the skeletal system. These tissues serve three functions: (a) mechanical, support and site of muscle attachment for locomotion; (b) protective, for vital organs and bone marrow; and (c) metabolic, as a reserve of ions, especially calcium and phosphate, for the maintenance of serum homeostasis, which is essential to life.

In bone, as in all connective tissues, the fundamental constituents are the cells and the extracellular matrix. The latter is particularly abundant in this tissue and is composed of collagen fibers and noncollagenous proteins. In bone, cartilage, and the tissues forming the teeth, however, unlike those in other connective tissues, the matrices have the unique ability to become calcified (or else have lost the ability to prevent calcification).

BONE AS AN ORGAN: MACROSCOPIC ORGANIZATION

Anatomically, two types of bones can be distinguished in the skeleton: flat bones (skull bones, scapula, mandible, and ilium) and long bones (tibia, femur, humerus, etc.). These two types are derived by two distinct types of development, intramembranous and endochondral, respectively (see later section, Bone Development and Growth), although the development and growth of long bones actually involve both types of processes.

External examination of a long bone (Fig. 1) shows two wider extremities (the epiphyses), a more or less cylindrical tube in the middle (the midshaft or diaphysis), and a developmental zone between them (the metaphysis). In a growing long bone, the epiphysis and the metaphysis, which originate from two independent ossification centers, are separated by a layer of cartilage, the *epiphyseal cartilage* (also called growth plate). This layer of proliferative cells and expanding cartilage matrix is responsible for the longitudinal growth of bones; it becomes entirely calcified and remodeled and replaced by bone by the end of the growth period (see later section, Bone Development and Growth). The external part of the bones is formed by a thick and dense layer of calcified tissue, the *cortex* (compact bone), which in the diaphysis, encloses the medullary cavity where the hematopoietic bone marrow is housed. Toward the metaphysis and the epiphysis, the cortex becomes progressively thinner, and the internal space is filled with a network of thin, calcified trabeculae; this is the *cancellous* bone, also named spongy or *trabecular* bone. The spaces enclosed by these thin trabeculae also are filled with hematopoietic bone marrow and are in continuity with the medullary cavity of the diaphysis. The bone surfaces at the epiphyses that take part in the joint are covered with a layer of articular cartilage that does not calcify.

There are consequently two bone surfaces at which the bone is in contact with the soft tissues (Fig. 1): an external surface (the periosteal surface) and an internal surface (the endosteal surface). These surfaces are lined with osteogenic

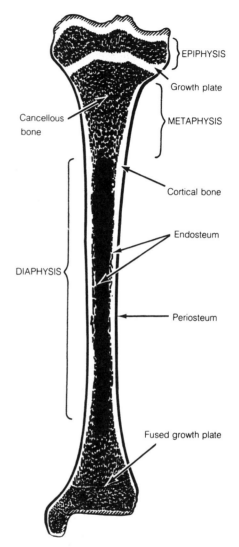

FIG. 1. Schematic view of a longitudinal section through a growing long bone. (From: Jee WSS. The skeletal tissues. In: Weiss L, ed. *Histology, cell and tissue biology.* New York: Elsevier Biomedical, 1983:200–255.)

cells organized in layers, the *periosteum* and the *endosteum*. Cortical and trabecular bone are constituted of the same cells and the same matrix elements, but there are structural and functional differences. The primary structural difference is quantitative: 80% to 90% of the volume of compact bone is calcified, whereas only 15% to 25% of the trabecular bone is calcified (the remainder being occupied by bone marrow, blood vessels, and connective tissue). The result is that 70% to 85% of the interface with soft tissues is at the endosteal bone surface, which leads to the functional difference: the cortical bone fulfills mainly a mechanical and protective function, and the trabecular bone, a metabolic function.

BONE AS A TISSUE

Microscopic Organization

Bone Matrix and Mineral

Bone is formed by *collagen fibers* (type I, 90% of the total protein), usually oriented in a preferential direction, and noncollagenous proteins. Spindle- or plate-shaped crystals of hydroxyapatite $[3Ca_3(PO_4)_2]\cdot(OH)_2$ are found on the collagen fibers, within them, and in the ground substance. They tend to be oriented in the same direction as the collagen fibers. The ground substance is primarily composed of glycoproteins and proteoglycans. These highly anionic complexes have a high ion-binding capacity and are thought to play an important part in the calcification process and the fixation of hydroxyapatite crystals to the collagen fibers.

Numerous noncollagenous proteins present in bone matrix have recently been purified and sequenced (see Chapter 4), but their role has been only partially characterized. Most of these proteins are synthesized by bone-forming cells, but not all: a number of plasma proteins are preferentially absorbed by the bone matrix, such as α_2-HS-glycoprotein, which is synthesized in the liver.

The preferential orientation of the collagen fibers alternates in adult bone from layer to layer, giving to this bone a typical *lamellar* structure, best seen under polarized light or by electron microscopy. This fiber organization allows the highest density of collagen per unit volume of tissue. The lamellae can be parallel to each other if deposited along a flat surface (trabecular bone and periosteum), or concentric if deposited on a surface surrounding a channel centered on a blood vessel (haversian system, Fig. 2). However, when bone is being formed very rapidly (during development and fracture healing, or in tumors and some metabolic bone diseases), there is no preferential organization of the collagen fibers. They are then not so tightly packed and found in somewhat randomly oriented bundles: this type of bone is

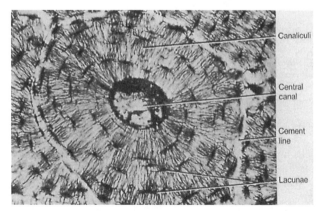

FIG. 2. Cross-sectional view of a haversian system in cortical bone, showing the lamellar organization of collagen in mature bone, and the structure and canalicular organization of osteocytes. (From: Jee WSS. The skeletal tissues. In: Weiss L, ed. *Histology, cell and tissue biology.* New York: Elsevier Biomedical, 1983:200–255.)

called *woven* bone (see later section, Bone Development and Growth), as opposed to lamellar bone.

Cellular Organizations within the Bone Matrix: Osteocytes

The calcified bone matrix is not metabolically inert, and cells (osteocytes) are found embedded deep within the bone in small osteocytic lacunae ($25,000/mm^3$ of bone; Figs. 2 and 3). They were originally bone-forming cells (osteoblasts), which became trapped in the bone matrix that they produced and which later became calcified. They nevertheless express some specific membrane proteins. These cells have numerous and long cell processes rich in microfilaments, which are in contact with cell processes from other osteocytes (there are frequent *gap junctions*), or with processes from the cells lining the bone surface (osteoblasts or flat lining cells in the endosteum or periosteum). These processes are organized during the formation of the matrix and before its calcification; they form a network of thin canaliculi permeating the entire bone matrix (Fig. 2).

Between the osteocyte's plasma membrane and the bone matrix itself is the *periosteocytic space.* This space exists both in the lacunae and in the canaliculi, and it is filled with extracellular fluid (ECF).

The physiological significance of this system is readily demonstrated by some numbers. The total bone surface area of the canaliculae and lacunae is 1000 to 5000 m^2 in an adult (compared with a surface area of 140 m^2 for lung capillaries); the volume of bone ECF is 1.0 to 1.5 L; and the surface calcium contained on bone mineral crystals is approximately 5 to 20 g, which accounts for a significant percentage of the total exchangeable bone calcium. The fact that the calcium concentration in the bone ECF (0.5 mmol/L) is lower than in plasma (1.5 mmol/L) suggests that there is a constant flow of calcium ions out of the bone.

The morphology of the osteocytes varies according to their age and functional activity. A young osteocyte has most of the ultrastructural characteristics of the osteoblast from which it was derived, except that there has been a decrease in cell volume and in the importance of the organelles involved in protein synthesis (rough endoplasmic reticulum, Golgi). An older osteocyte, located deeper within the calcified bone, shows these decreases further accentuated, and there is an accumulation of glycogen in the cytoplasm. These cells have been shown to be able to synthesize new bone matrix at the surface of the osteocytic lacunae, which can subsequently calcify. Although historically they have been considered able to resorb calcified bone from the same surface, this point has recently been disputed. The fate of the osteocytes is to be phagocytized and digested, together with the other components of bone, during osteoclastic bone resorption. These cells also may play a role in local activation of bone turnover (remodeling).

The Bone Surface

Most of the bone-tissue turnover occurs at the bone surfaces, mainly at the endosteal surface where it interfaces with bone marrow. This surface is morphologically heteroge-

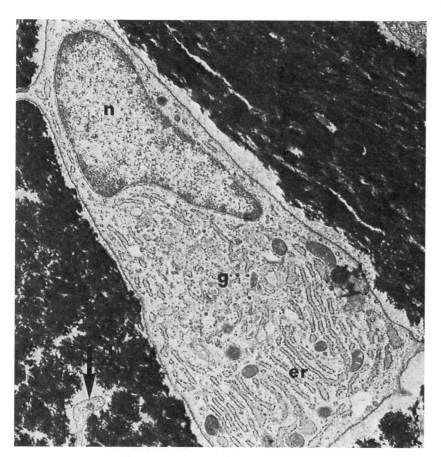

FIG. 3. Osteocyte. Electron micrograph of an osteocyte embedded in calcified bone matrix (black, hydroxyapatite crystals). The cell has a basal nucleus *(n)*, a large Golgi complex *(g)*, and a relatively well developed endoplasmic reticulum *(er)*. Cytoplasmic extensions can be seen in the matrix *(arrow)* in their canaliculi. Approximate magnification, ×5000.

neous, reflecting the various specific cellular activities involved in remodeling and turnover.

The Osteoblast and Bone Formation

The osteoblast is the bone-lining cell responsible for the production of the matrix constituents (collagen and ground substance) (Fig. 4). It originates from a local mesenchymal stem cell (bone marrow stromal stem cell or connective tissue mesenchymal stem cell). These precursors, with the right stimulation, undergo proliferation and differentiate into preosteoblasts and then into mature osteoblasts. Osteoblasts never appear or function individually but are always found in clusters of cuboidal cells along the bone surface (~100 to 400 cells per bone-forming site). At the light-microscope level, the osteoblast is characterized by a round nucleus at the base of the cell (opposite the bone surface), a strongly basophilic cytoplasm, and a prominent Golgi complex located between the nucleus and the apex of the cell. Osteoblasts are always found lining the layer of bone matrix that they are producing, before it is calcified (called, at this point, *osteoid tissue*). Osteoid tissue exists because of a time lag between matrix formation and its subsequent calcification (the osteoid maturation period), which is approximately 10 days. Behind the osteoblast can usually be found one or two layers of cells: activated mesenchymal cells and preosteoblasts. At the ultrastructural level, the osteoblast is characterized by (a) the presence of an extremely well-developed rough endoplasmic reticulum with dilated cisternae and a dense granular content, and (b) the presence of a large circular Golgi complex comprising multiple Golgi stacks. Cytoplasmic processes on the secreting side of the cell extend deep into the osteoid matrix and are in contact with the osteocyte processes in their canaliculi. Junctional complexes (gap junctions) are often found between the osteoblasts. The plasma membrane of the osteoblast is characteristically rich in alkaline phosphatase (the concentration of which in the serum is used as an index of bone formation) and has been shown to have receptors for parathyroid hormone but not for calcitonin. Osteoblasts also express steroid receptors for estrogens and vitamin D_3 in their nuclei, as well as several adhesion molecules (integrins) and receptors for cytokines. Toward the end of the secreting period, the osteoblast becomes either a flat lining cell or an osteocyte.

The Osteoclast and Bone Resorption

The osteoclast is the bone-lining cell responsible for bone resorption (Fig. 5).

Morphology

The osteoclast is a giant multinucleated cell, containing four to 20 nuclei. It is usually found in contact with a calcified bone surface and within a lacuna (Howship's lacunae) that is the result of its own resorptive activity. It is possible to

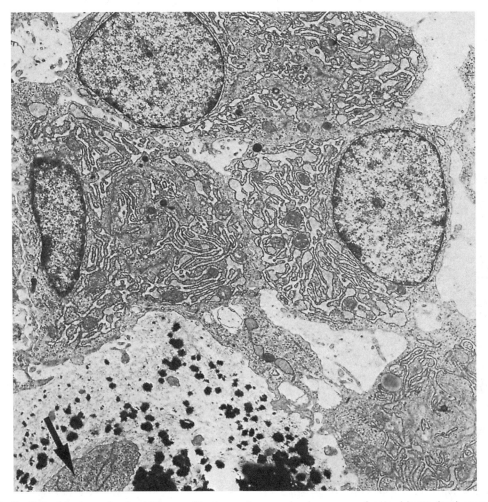

FIG. 4. Osteoblasts and osteoid tissue. Electron micrograph of a group of osteoblasts *(top)* covering a layer of mineralizing osteoid tissue *(bottom)* with a newly embedded osteocyte *(arrow)*. Basal nuclei, prominent Golgi and endoplasmic reticulum, and characteristics of active osteoblasts. Approximate magnification, ×3000.

find up to four or five osteoclasts in the same resorptive site, but there usually are only one or two. Under the light microscope, the nuclei appear to vary within the same cell: some are round and euchromatic, and some are irregular in contour and heterochromatic, possibly reflecting the asynchronous fusion of mononuclear precursors. The cytoplasm is ''foamy'' with many vacuoles. The zone of contact with the bone is characterized by the presence of a ruffled border with dense patches on each side (the sealing zone).

Characteristic ultrastructural features of this cell are the abundant Golgi complexes characteristically disposed around each nucleus, the mitochondria, and the transport vesicles loaded with lysosomal enzymes. The most prominent features of the osteoclast are, however, the deep foldings of the plasma membrane in the area facing the bone matrix: the ruffled border in the center is surrounded by a ring of contractile proteins (sealing zone) that serve to attach the cell to the bone surface, thus sealing off the subosteoclastic bone-resorbing compartment. The attachment of the cell to the matrix is performed by integrin receptors, which bind to specific sequences in matrix proteins. The plasma membrane in the ruffled border area contains proteins that also are found at the limiting membrane of lysosomes and related organelles, and a specific type of electrogenic proton adenosine triphosphatase (ATPase) involved in acidification. The basolateral plasma membrane of the osteoclast is highly and specifically enriched in (Na^+, K^+) ATPase (sodium–potassium pumps), HCO_3^-/Cl^- exchangers, and Na^+/H^+ exchangers.

Mechanisms of Bone Resorption

Lysosomal enzymes (tartrate resistant acid phosphatase, cathepsin K, etc.) are actively synthesized by the osteoclast and are found in the endoplasmic reticulum, Golgi, and many transport vesicles. The enzymes are secreted, through the ruffled border, into the extracellular bone-resorbing compartment; they reach a sufficiently high extracellular concentration because this compartment is sealed off. The transport and targeting of these enzymes for secretion at the apical pole of the osteoclast involves mannose-6-phosphate receptors.

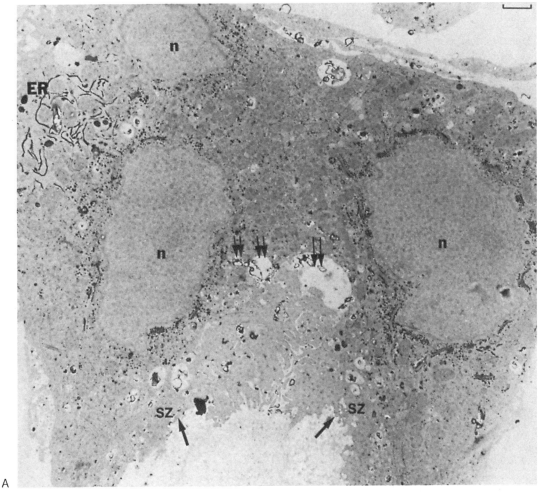

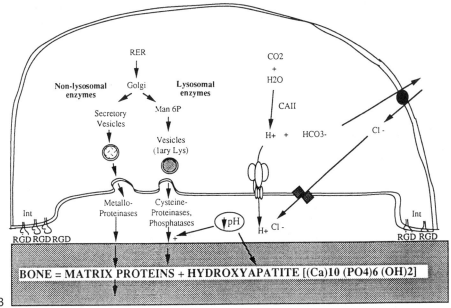

FIG. 5. Osteoclast. **A:** Section of an osteoclast stained for the lysosomal enzyme arylsulfatase. The osteoclast contains multiple nuclei *(n)*, an endoplasmic reticulum where lysosomal enzymes are synthesized *(ER)*, and prominent Golgi stacks around each nucleus. The cell is attached to bone matrix *(bottom)* and forms a separate compartment underneath itself, limited by the sealing zone (SZ) *(single arrows)*. The plasma membrane of the cell facing this compartment is extensively folded and forms the ruffled border, with pockets of extracellular space between the folds *(double arrows)*. Multiple small vesicles for transporting enzymes toward the bone matrix can be seen in the cytoplasm. Approximate magnification, ×9000. **B:** Schematic representation of enzyme-secretion and ion transport polarity in osteoclasts. (From: Baron R, Ravesloot J-H, Neff L, Chakraborty M, Chatterjee D, Lomri A, Horne WC. Cellular and molecular biology of the osteoclast. In: Noda M, ed. *Cellular and molecular biology of bone.* Orlando, Florida: Academic Press Inc., 1993:446–495.)

Furthermore, the cell secretes several metalloproteinase such as collagenase and gelatinase.

The osteoclast acidifies the extracellular compartment by secreting protons across the ruffled-border membrane (by proton pumps). Recent evidence suggests the presence of an electrogenic proton-pump ATPase, related to but different from that of the kidney-tubule–acidifying cells. The protons are provided to the pumps by the enzyme carbonic anhydrase, and they are highly concentrated in the cytosol of the osteoclast; ATP and CO_2 are provided by the mitochondria. The basolateral membrane activity exchanges bicarbonate for chloride, thereby avoiding an alkalinization of the cytosol. The basolateral sodium pumps might be involved in secondary active transport of calcium and/or protons in association with a Na^+/Ca^{2+} exchanger and/or a Na^+/H^+ antiport. This cell could therefore function in a manner similar to that of kidney tubule or gastric parietal cells, which also acidify lumens.

The extracellular bone-resorbing compartment is therefore the functional equivalent of a secondary lysosome, with (a) a low pH, (b) lysosomal enzymes, and (c) the substrate. The low pH dissolves the crystals, exposing the matrix. The enzymes, now at optimal pH, degrade the matrix components; the residues from this extracellular digestion are either internalized, or they are transported across the cell (by transcytosis) and released at the basolateral domain, or they are released during periods of relapse of the sealing zone, possibly induced by a calcium sensor responding to the increase of extracellular calcium in the bone-resorbing compartment.

First, the hydroxyapatite crystals are mobilized by digestion of their link to collagen (the noncollagenous proteins) and dissolved by the acid environment. Then the residual collagen fibers are digested either by the activation of latent collagenase or by the action of cathepsins at low pH.

Clinically this explains why (a) bone resorption helps to maintain calcium and inorganic phosphate levels in the plasma, and (b) the concentrations of hydroxyproline and N-terminal collagen peptides in the urine are used as indirect measurements of bone resorption in humans (collagen type I is highly enriched in hydroxyproline and pyridinoline links).

Origin and Fate of the Osteoclast. The work of Walker on osteopetrotic mice established the hematogenous origin of the osteoclast. The osteoclast derives from cells in the mononuclear/phagocytic lineage. Although this differentiation may occur at the early promonocyte stage, monocytes and macrophages already committed to their own lineage might still be able to form osteoclasts under the right circumstances.

Despite its mononuclear/phagocytic origin, the osteoclast membrane expresses distinct markers: it is devoid of Fc and C_3 receptors, as well as of several other macrophage markers; like mononuclear phagocytes, however, the osteoclast is rich in nonspecific esterases, synthesizes lysozyme, and expresses colony-stimulating factor 1 (CSF-1) receptors. Monoclonal antibodies have been produced that recognize osteoclasts but not macrophages. The osteoclast, unlike macrophages, also expresses millions of copies of the calcitonin and vitronectin (integrin $\alpha_v\beta_3$) receptors. Whether it expresses receptors for parathyroid hormone, estrogen, or vitamin D is still controversial. Recent evidence suggest that the osteoclast undergoes apoptosis after a cycle of resorption.

BONE REMODELING

The previously described activity of bone cells is performed along the surfaces of bone, mainly the endosteal surface, and it results in bone remodeling, a process involved in bone growth and turnover. Bone formation and bone resorption do not, however, occur along the bone surface at random: they are either part of the process of bone development and growth or part of the turnover mechanism by which old bone is replaced by new bone. In the normal adult skeleton, (i.e., after the period of development and growth), bone formation occurs only where bone resorption has previously occurred. The sequence of events at the remodeling site (Fig. 6; see Chapter 4) is the activation–resorption–formation (ARF) sequence. During the intermediate phase between resorption and formation (the reversal phase), some macrophage-like, uncharacterized mononuclear cells are observed at the site of the remodeling, and a cement line is formed that marks the limit of resorption and acts to cement together the old and the new bone. The duration of these various phases has been measured (Fig. 7: the complete remodeling cycle at each microscopic site takes about 3 to 6 months. Although cortical bone is anatomically different, its remodeling follows the same biological principles (Fig. 8). Lamellar bone being formed within such a system gives the characteristic structure of a haversian system when seen in cross section (see Fig. 2).

BONE DEVELOPMENT AND GROWTH

There are two types of processes involved in bone development: intramembranous ossification (flat bones) and endo-

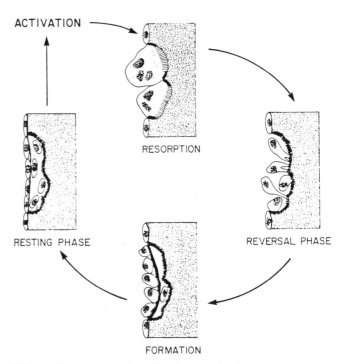

FIG. 6. Bone remodeling. The bone-remodeling sequence as it occurs in trabecular bone. (The same principles apply to haversian remodeling; see text.)

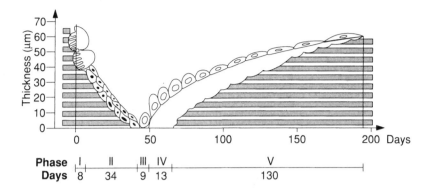

FIG. 7. Duration and depth of the various phases of the normal cancellous bone–remodeling sequence, calculated from histomorphometric analysis of bone biopsy samples obtained from young individuals. Note the balance between the erosion depth and the mean wall thickness. (From Eriksen EF, Axelrod DW, Melsen F. *Bone histomorphometry.* New York: Raven Press, 1994, pp 13–20.)

chondral ossification (long bones). The main difference between them is the presence of a cartilaginous phase in the latter.

Intramembranous Ossification

In intramembranous ossification, a group of mesenchymal cells within a highly vascularized area of the embryonic connective tissue proliferates and differentiates directly into preosteoblasts and then into osteoblasts. These cells synthesize a bone matrix with the following characteristics: (a) the collagen fibers are not preferentially oriented but appear as irregular bundles, (b) the osteocytes are large and extremely numerous, and (c) calcification is delayed and does not proceed in an orderly fashion but in irregularly distributed patches. This type of bone is called woven bone. At the periphery, mesenchymal cells continue to differentiate, by following the same steps. Blood vessels incorporated between the woven bone trabeculae will form the hematopoietic bone marrow. Later, this woven bone is remodeled by following the ARF sequence, and it is progressively replaced by mature lamellar bone.

Endochondral Ossification

Formation of a Cartilage Model

Mesenchymal cells proliferate and differentiate into prechondroblasts and then into chondroblasts. These cells secrete the cartilaginous matrix. Like the osteoblasts, the chondroblasts become progressively embedded within their own matrix, where they lie within lacunae; they are then called chondrocytes. Unlike the osteocytes, they continue to proliferate for some time, this being allowed in part by the gel-like consistency of cartilage. At the periphery of this cartilage (the perichondrium), the mesenchymal cells continue to proliferate and differentiate. This is called appositional growth. Another type of growth is observed in the cartilage by synthesis of new matrix between the chondrocytes (interstitial growth). In the growth plate, the cells appear in regular columns called isogenous groups. Later on, the chondrocytes enlarge progressively, become hypertrophic, and undergo programed cell death (apoptosis).

Vascular Invasion and Longitudinal Growth (Remodeling)

The embryonic cartilage is avascular. During its early development, a ring of woven bone is formed by intramembranous ossification in the future midshaft area under the perichondrium (which is then a periosteum). Just after the calcification of this woven bone, blood vessels (preceded by osteoclasts) penetrate the cartilage, bringing the blood supply that will form the hematopoietic bone marrow.

The growth plate in a growing long bone shows, from the epiphyseal area to the diaphyseal area, the following cellular events (Fig. 9). In a proliferative zone, chondroblasts divide actively, forming isogenous groups and actively synthesizing the matrix. These cells become progressively larger, enlarging their lacunae in the hypertrophic zone, and

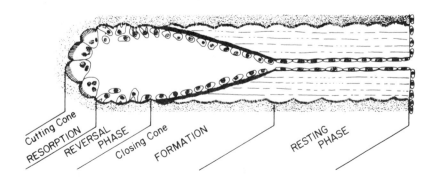

FIG. 8. The bone-remodeling activity in cortical bone as seen in longitudinal sequence. Osteoclasts dig out a tunnel, creating a "cutting cone." Subsequently new bone is formed in the area of the "closing cone," leading to the creation of a new bone structural unit (i.e., the haversian system).

then they undergo apoptosis. At this level of the epiphyseal plate, the matrix of the longitudinal cartilage septa selectively calcifies (zone of provisional calcification). Once calcified, the cartilage matrix is resorbed, but only partially, by osteoclasts, and then blood vessels appear in the zone of invasion. After resorption, osteoblasts differentiate and form a layer of woven bone on top of the cartilaginous remnants of the longitudinal septa.

Thus the first ARF sequence is complete: the cartilage has been remodeled and replaced by woven bone. The resulting trabeculae are called the primary spongiosa. Still lower in the growth plate, this woven bone is subjected to further remodeling (a second ARF sequence), in which the woven bone and the cartilaginous remnants are replaced with lamellar bone, resulting in the mature state of trabecular bone called secondary spongiosa (Fig. 10).

Growth in Diameter and Shape Modification (Modeling)

Growth in the diameter of the shaft is the result of a deposition of new membranous bone beneath the periosteum that will continue throughout life. In this case, resorption

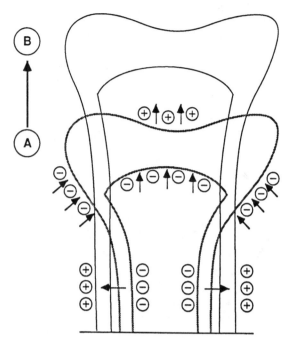

FIG. 10. Resorption (−) and formation (+) activities during the longitudinal growth of bones. During growth from A to B, the cortex in the diaphysis must be resorbed inside and reformed outside *(bottom)*. The growth plate moves upward (see Fig. 9), and the wider parts of the bone must be reshaped into a diaphysis. (From Jee WSS. The skeletal tissues. In: Weiss L, ed. *Histology, cell and tissue biology.* New York: Elsevier Biomedical, 1983:200–255.)

does not immediately precede formation. The midshaft is narrower than the metaphysis, and the growth of a long bone progressively destroys the lower part of the metaphysis and transforms it into a diaphysis, accomplished by continuous resorption by osteoclasts beneath the periosteum (Fig. 10).

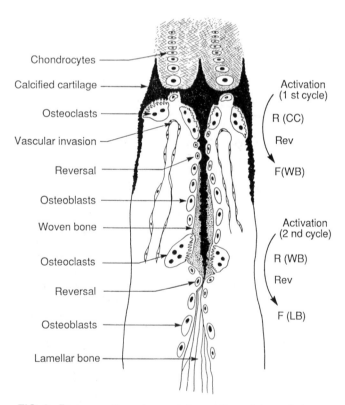

Chondrocytes

Calcified cartilage

Osteoclasts

Vascular invasion

Reversal

Osteoblasts

Woven bone

Osteoclasts

Reversal

Osteoblasts

Lamellar bone

Activation (1 st cycle)

R (CC)

Rev

F(WB)

Activation (2 nd cycle)

R (WB)

Rev

F (LB)

FIG. 9. Bone growth and remodeling at the epiphyseal plate. Schematic representation of the cellular events occurring at the growth plate in long bones. R, resorption; Rev, reversal; F, formation; CC, calcified cartilage; WB, woven bone; LB, lamellar bone.

SUGGESTED READINGS

1. Baron R, Chakraborty M, Chatterjee D, Horne W, Lomri A, Ravesloot J-H. Biology of the osteoclast. In: Mundy GR, Martin TJ, eds. *Physiology and pharmacology of bone.* New York: Springer-Verlag, 1993:111–147.
2. Eriksen EF, Axelrod DW, Melsen F. *Bone histomorphometry.* New York: Raven Press, 1994.
3. Jee WSS. The skeletal tissues. In: Weiss L, ed. *Histology, cell and tissue biology.* New York: Elsevier Biomedical, 1983:200–255.
4. Nijweide P, Burger EH, Feyen JHM. Cells of bone: proliferation, differentiation and hormonal regulation. *Physiol Rev* 1986;66:855–886.
5. Suda T, Takahashi N, Martin TJ. Modulation of osteoclast differentiation. *Endocr Rev* 1992;13:66–80.
6. Marks SC Jr, Hermey DC. The structure and development of bone. In: Bilezikian JP, Raisz LG, Rodan GA, eds. *Principles of bone biology.* San Diego, California: Academic Press, 1996:3–14.
7. Aubin JE, Fina L. The osteoblast lineage. In: Bilezikian JP, Raisz LG, Rodan GA, eds. *Principles of bone biology* California: Academic Press, 1996:51–68.
8. Roodman GD. Advances in bone biology: the osteoclast. *Endocr Rev* 1996;17:308–332.

2. Bone Morphogenesis and Embryologic Development

Bjorn R. Olsen, M.D., Ph.D.

Department of Cell Biology, Harvard Medical School and Harvard-Forsyth Department of Oral Biology, Harvard School of Dental Medicine, Boston, Massachusetts

The cells that make up the vertebrate skeleton are derived from three lineages. *Neural crest cells* give rise to the branchial arch derivative of the craniofacial skeleton; the *sclerotome division of the somites* forms most of the axial skeleton; and cells in the *lateral plate mesoderm* contribute to the skeleton of the limbs. In areas where bones are formed, mesenchymal cells from these sources condense and form regions of high cell density that represent outlines of future skeletal elements. During this condensation process, important changes take place in the extracellular matrix between the cells, allowing cells to establish contact with each other and to activate signaling pathways that regulate cell differentiation. Classic experiments demonstrated that by the time mesenchymal condensations appear, the cells within them have already acquired properties that give them positional identity. Mechanisms that ensure the development of a complex skeleton with elements of unique size, shape, and anatomic identity can therefore be traced back to molecular and cellular events in precondensed mesenchyme.

CARTILAGE MODELS OF DEVELOPING BONES

As mesenchymal cells within condensations differentiate, they can follow one of two paths. They can either differentiate into bone-forming cells, *osteoblasts*, or they can differentiate into *chondrocytes* and secrete the characteristic extracellular matrix of hyaline cartilage. Differentiation into osteoblasts occurs in areas of *membranous ossification*, such as in the calvarium of the skull, the maxilla and the mandible, and in the subperiosteal bone-forming layer of long bones. Differentiation into chondrocytes occurs in the remaining skeleton where cartilage models of the future bones are formed. These models, frequently described by their German term *anlagen*, are subsequently replaced by bone in a process called *endochondral ossification*. The differentiation of chondrocytes and the formation of cartilage starts with cells becoming large and round in the center of mesenchymal condensations. They develop organelles for high-level synthesis and secretion of proteins (endoplasmic reticulum and Golgi complex) and switch from production of an extracellular matrix containing collagens I and III to a matrix containing the cartilage-specific collagens II, IX, and XI. The cartilage anlagen grow by interstitial and appositional growth so that they over time come to resemble the future bones in shape and size. Although they normally are replaced by bone through endochondral ossification, they can grow into shapes that resemble the final bones, even in the absence of bone formation. This is dramatically seen in mice that carry two inactivated alleles of the gene for the transcription factor CBFA1 (1,2). This factor is required for osteoblast differentiation (3), and in mice without CBFA1, no osteoblasts are formed. The cartilaginous anlagen are not ossified, yet they form a nearly complete "skeleton" of the correctly shaped elements, consisting entirely of cartilage. The pat-

terning of the endochondral skeleton therefore depends on processes that regulate the spatial differentiation and growth of cartilage.

REGULATION OF MESENCHYMAL CONDENSATION AND CHONDROCYTE DIFFERENTIATION IN THE AXIAL SKELETON

During the fourth week of human development, cells of the so-called *paraxial mesoderm* condense to the segmented structures called *somites* on either side of the neural tube and the notochord (Fig. 1). Within the somites, cells undergo transition from a mesenchymal to an epithelial phenotype, and this is followed by migration of cells in the most ventral region of the somites into an area surrounding the notochord (Fig. 1). These cells form the *sclerotomes*.

Sclerotome cells differentiate into chondrocytes that form the anlagen of *vertebral bodies*. The notochord subsequently disappears within the vertebral bodies but remains as the *nucleus pulposus* within intervertebral discs. The *neural arches* of the vertebrae are formed by sclerotome cells that migrate dorsally around the neural tube, whereas sclerotome cells that migrate laterally form the rib anlagen in the thoracic region. In the anterior body wall, mesenchymal cell condensations on each side of the midline form the sternal anlagen. Cells within these condensations form two cartilaginous bars that later fuse into the *sternum*. Condensations above the sternum give rise to the *manubrium* and pairs of lateral condensations form the anterior cartilaginous portions of the ribs that are connected with the sternum.

The condensation, segmentation, and mesenchymal–epithelial transformation of paraxial mesoderm cells to somites is controlled in part by signaling between neighboring cells involving the cell-surface receptor *Notch1* and ligands that bind to it (4,5). Notch1 is a large transmembrane protein with several repeated amino acid sequence domains. The ligands that bind to Notch1 and activate signaling pathways that are downstream of Notch1 are themselves transmembrane molecules with signaling potential (6). The interactions between Notch1 and its ligands therefore require cell–cell contact. In mice carrying inactivated alleles for a mouse homologue of the *Drosophila Notch* ligand *Delta* (7) and in mice with inactivated Notch1 genes (5), early defects in the condensation and patterning of somites lead to defects in the vertebral column. Genes that control the expression of Notch1 or are controlled by Notch1 have been shown to be important for early stages of vertebral column development (8,9).

Differentiation of cells within sclerotomes to cartilage-producing chondrocytes also is under complex regulation. A master regulator of sclerotome cell differentiation and therefore of vertebral column formation is the secreted cytokine *sonic hedgehog* (10). Sonic hedgehog is produced by the notochord as a protein that undergoes proteolytic self-

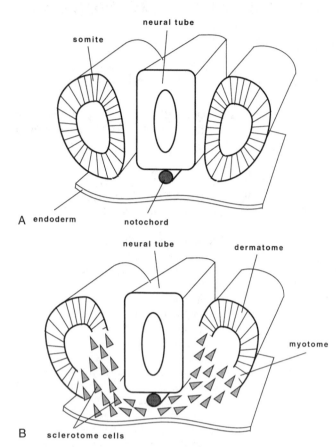

FIG. 1. Differentiation of somites in the trunk region of the embryo. The ectoderm has been removed to reveal the somites adjacent to the neural tube **(A)**. At this stage, the cells of the somites have an epithelial organization. Later **(B)**, cells from the medial region of the somites migrate toward the notochord and form the sclerotomes. The remainder differentiate into dermatome (skin) and myotome (striated muscle). (Modified from Hogan B, Beddington R, Costantini F, Lacy E. *Manipulating the mouse embryo: a laboratory manual.* 2nd ed. Cold Spring Harbor, NY: Cold Spring Harbor Laboratory Press, 1994:77.)

cleavage and has a cholesterol residue attached before it becomes an active cytokine (11,12). That its signaling activity is absolutely required for sclerotome differentiation is evident from the phenotype of mice that carry inactivated sonic hedgehog alleles (13). Such mice develop without a vertebral column and the posterior portions of the ribs. They do, however, form a sternum and the anterior portions of ribs, the shoulder, and pelvic girdles, showing that the anlagen for those portions of the skeleton are not controlled by sonic hedgehog. Another important regulator is the transcription factor *PAX1,* which is, at least in part, induced by sonic hedgehog. A mutation in PAX1 in humans causes a neural tube defect (14), and mutations in mice lead to defective sclerotome differentiation and abnormalities in the vertebral column (15).

SKELETAL MORPHOGENESIS IN THE LIMB

Skeletal development in the limb starts with formation of *limb buds,* outgrowths of the lateral body wall, appearing

early in the second month of human development as a result of proliferation of mesenchymal cells from the lateral plate mesoderm. A group of tall, specialized epithelial cells, called the *apical ectodermal ridge* (AER), caps the limb bud. As the limb bud grows and cartilage anlagen of future bones develop within it, the developing limb is patterned along three axes (Fig. 2): A proximal-to-distal axis, a dorsal-to-ventral axis, and a posterior-to-anterior axis.

Patterning along the proximal-to-distal axis is largely controlled by factors produced by the AER (16). These include *fibroblast growth factors* that are important for stimulating proliferation and patterning of the underlying mesenchyme (17,18). They are therefore essential for normal limb outgrowth. As the limb grows out, mesenchymal cells condense in the center to form the cartilage anlagen of the limb bones. The anlagen develop in a proximal-to-distal direction, and their development can be described as a series of bifurcations and segmentations that follow an axis along the humerus, through the ulna and the distal carpal (or tarsal in the foot) anlagen (Fig. 3) (19).

In the lower arm (leg) and hands (feet), the patterning of the anlagen from one side to the other is regulated by a cascade of signaling molecules and transcription factors. The most important of these include sonic hedgehog, secreted by a small group of cells (called the *zone of polarizing activity*) located at the posterior (ulnar) aspect of the developing limb bud, *homeobox transcription factors,* and members of the *transforming growth factor-β* (TGF-β) *superfamily* of signaling molecules (20). How all these and many other molecules work together as an orchestrated system to generate the normal limb skeletal pattern is not known in detail, but recent studies are rapidly filling in the missing pieces.

Mutations in many of these genes result in striking abnor-

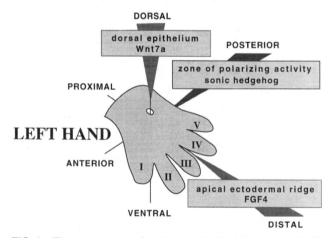

FIG. 2. The three axes of patterning for the developing (left) hand. Key regulatory molecules that play important roles in these patterning processes are indicated in the boxed-in areas under their cellular sources. Thus the secreted molecule Wnt7a produced by dorsal epithelial cells is important for dorsal–ventral patterning; sonic hedgehog, produced by cells in the zone of polarizing activity, is important for establishing the pattern along the posterior–anterior axis; FGF4 is one of the fibroblast growth factors produced by cells of the apical ectodermal ridge that control limb outgrowth and proximal–distal patterning.

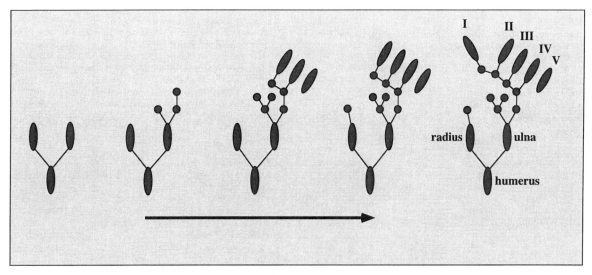

FIG. 3. Branching and segmentation of mesenchymal condensations during limb development. As the limb bud grows *(indicated by the horizontal arrow from left to right)*, the condensations develop in a distinct sequence to form the cartilage anlagen of the future bones [humerus, radius, ulna, carpal bones and metacarpal bones for the five fingers (I to V)]. (Based on Shubin NH, Alberch P. A morphogenetic approach to the origin and basic organization of the tetrapod limb. *Evol Biol* 1986;20:319–387.)

malities in the limb skeleton. For example, mutations involving expansions of a polyalanine stretch in the transcription factor *HOXD13* cause *polysyndactyly* (extra fingers) in humans (21); other polysyndactyly syndromes have been shown to be caused by mutations in an intracellular, downstream target of sonic hedgehog signaling, a transcription factor called *GLI3* (22,23). Mutations in a TGF-β-homologue (*CDMP1*) cause abnormal shortening of distal limb bones, perhaps as a result of a defect in formation of joints between bones (24).

Several studies are beginning to provide insights into mechanisms that ensure patterning along the dorsal–ventral axis. As a consequence of such studies, the basis for the *nail–patella syndrome* in humans, characterized by dysplasia of nails and absent or hypoplastic patellae, has been found to be mutations in a transcription factor called *LMX-1* (25).

CHONDROCYTE PROLIFERATION AND DIFFERENTIATION IN GROWTH PLATES

During endochondral ossification, the cartilage anlagen are replaced by bone marrow and bone. In this process (see Chapter 1), epiphyseal growth plates are formed. A sequence of chondrocyte proliferation, differentiation to hypertrophy, and cell death within growth plates results in longitudinal bone growth and thus the final steps in bone morphogenesis. Proliferation and differentiation of growth-plate chondrocytes are controlled in several ways. An important brake on chondrocyte proliferation is local signaling through fibroblast growth factor (FGF) interaction with the cell-surface tyrosine kinase receptor *FGFR3*. Activating mutations in FGFR3 cause decreased bone growth in *achondroplasia* and *hypochondroplasia* in humans (26,27). The cytokine parathyroid hormone-related peptide (PTHrP) has an inhibitory effect on chondrocyte differentiation to hypertrophy (28),

and activating mutations in the PTHrP receptor (a cell-surface G protein–coupled receptor) cause decreased bone growth and a distinct form of dwarfism because of inhibition of chondrocyte hypertrophy in growth plates (29). Signaling from the PTHrP receptor appears to involve an inhibitory effect on the expression of a secreted signaling molecule called *Indian hedgehog* (28). Indian hedgehog is homologous to sonic hedgehog and acts on cells through the same type of receptor as does sonic hedgehog. Indian hedgehog induces expression of PTHrP, so the two molecules appear to be involved in a self-regulating feedback loop within growth plates (28).

Chondrocyte hypertrophy leads to the synthesis of an extracellular matrix that is significantly different from that of the rest of growth-plate cartilage. This hypertrophic matrix is readily degraded and permits ingrowth of blood vessels and osteoblasts from the underlying bone marrow. Loss-of-function mutations in collagen X, a unique extracellular matrix component made by hypertrophic chondrocytes (30), cause a distinct form of dwarfism, Schmid-type metaphyseal chondrodysplasia, in humans (31).

REFERENCES

1. Otto F, Thornell AP, Crompton T, et al. CBFA1, a candidate gene for the cleidocranial dysplasia syndrome, is essential for osteoblast formation and bone development. *Cell* 1997;89:765–771.
2. Komori T, Yagi H, Nomura S, et al. Targeted disruption of Cbfa1 results in a complete lack of bone formation owing to maturational arrest of osteoblasts. *Cell* 1997;89:755–764.
3. Ducy P, Zhang R, Geoffroy V, Ridall AL, Karsenty G. Osf2/Cbfa1: a transcriptional activator of osteoblast differentiation. *Cell* 1997;89:747–754.
4. Gossler A, Hrabe de Angelis M. Somitogenesis. *Curr Top Dev Biol* 1998;38:225–287.
5. Conlon RA, Reaume AG, Rossant J. Notch1 is required for the coordinate segmentation of somites. *Development* 1995;121:1533–1545.

6. Lendahl U. A growing family of Notch ligands. *Bioessays* 1998;20:103–107.
7. Kusumi K, Sun ES, Kerrebrock AW, et al. The mouse pudgy mutation disrupts Delta homologue Dll3 and initiation of early somite boundaries. *Nat Genet* 1998;19:274–278.
8. Wong PC, Zheng H, Chen H, et al. Presenilin 1 is required for Notch1 and DI1 expression in the paraxial mesoderm. *Nature* 1997;387:288–292.
9. Saga Y, Hata N, Koseki H, Taketo MM. Mesp2: a novel mouse gene expressed in the presegmented mesoderm and essential for segmentation initiation. *Genes Dev* 1997;11:1827–1839.
10. Johnson RL, Laufer E, Riddle RD, Tabin C. Ectopic expression of Sonic hedgehog alters dorsal-ventral patterning of somites. *Cell* 1994;79:1165–1173.
11. Porter JA, von Kessler DP, Ekker SC, et al. The product of hedgehog autoproteolytic cleavage active in local and long-range signalling. *Nature* 1995;374:363–366.
12. Porter JA, Young KE, Beachy PA. Cholesterol modification of hedgehog signaling proteins in animal development. *Science* 1996;274:255–259.
13. Chiang C, Litingtung Y, Lee E, et al. Cyclopia and defective axial patterning in mice lacking Sonic hedgehog gene function. *Nature* 1996;383:407–413.
14. Hol FA, Geurds MP, Chatkupt S, et al. PAX genes and human neural tube defects: an amino acid substitution in PAX1 in a patient with spina bifida. *J Med Genet* 1996;33:655–660.
15. Wilm B, Dahl E, Peters H, Balling R, Imai K. Targeted disruption of Pax1 defines its null phenotype and proves haploinsufficiency. *Proc Natl Acad Sci USA* 1998;95:8692–8697.
16. Robertson KE, Tickle C. Recent molecular advances in understanding vertebrate limb development. *Br J Plast Surg* 1997;50:109–115.
17. Niswander L, Jeffrey S, Martin GR, Tickle C. A positive feedback loop coordinates growth and patterning in the vertebrate limb. *Nature* 1994;317:609–612.
18. Crossley PH, Minowada G, MacArthur CA, Martin GR. Roles for FGF8 in the induction, initiation, and maintenance of chick limb development. *Cell* 1996;84:127–136.
19. Shubin NH, Alberch P. A morphogenetic approach to the origin and basic organization of the tetrapod limb. *Evol Biol* 1986;20:319–387.
20. Johnson RL, Tabin CJ. Molecular models for vertebrate limb development. *Cell* 1997;90:979–990.
21. Muragaki Y, Mundlos S, Upton J, Olsen BR. Altered growth and branching patterns in synpolydactyly caused by mutations in HOXD13. *Science* 1996;272:548–551.
22. Wild A, Kalff-Suske M, Vortkamp A, Bornholdt D, Konig R, Grzeschik KH. Point mutations in human GLI3 cause Greig syndrome. *Hum Mol Genet* 1997;6:1979–1984.
23. Kang S, Graham JM Jr, Olney AH, Biesecker LG. GLI3 frameshift mutations cause autosomal dominant Pallister-Hall syndrome. *Nat Genet* 1997;15:266–268.
24. Polinkovsky A, Robin NH, Thomas JT, et al. Mutations in CDMP1 cause autosomal dominant brachydactyly type C [Letter]. *Nat Genet* 1997;17:18–19.
25. Dreyer SD, Zhou G, Baldini A, et al. Mutations in LMX1B cause abnormal skeletal patterning and renal dysplasia in nail patella syndrome. *Nat Genet* 1998;19:47–50.
26. Shiang R, Thompson LM, Zhu YZ, et al. Mutations in the transmembrane domain of FGFR3 cause the most common genetic form of dwarfism, achondroplasia. *Cell* 1994;78:335–342.
27. Bellus GA, McIntosh I, Smith EA, et al. A recurrent mutation in the tyrosine kinase domain of fibroblast growth factor receptor 3 causes hypochondroplasia. *Nat Genet* 1995;10:357–359.
28. Vortkamp A, Lee K, Lanske B, Segre GV, Kronenberg HM, Tabin CJ. Regulation of rate of cartilage differentiation by Indian hedgehog and PTH-related protein. *Science* 1996;273:613–622.
29. Schipani E, Langman CB, Parfitt AM, et al. Constitutively activated receptors for parathyroid hormone and parathyroid hormone-related peptide in Jansen's metaphyseal chondrodysplasia. *N Engl J Med* 1996;335:708–714.
30. Linsenmayer TF, Eavey RD, Schmid TM. Type X collagen: a hypertrophic cartilage-specific molecule. *Pathol Immunopathol Res* 1988;7:14–19.
31. Warman ML, Abbott MH, Apte SS, et al. A type X collagen mutation causes Schmid metaphyseal chondrodysplasia. *Nat Genet* 1993;5:79–82.

3. Bone Formation: Osteoblast Lineage Cells, Growth Factors, Matrix Proteins, and the Mineralization Process

Jane B. Lian, Ph.D., Gary S. Stein, Ph.D., *Ernesto Canalis, M.D., †Pamela Gehron Robey, Ph.D., and ‡Adele L. Boskey, Ph.D.

*Department of Cell Biology, University of Massachusetts Medical School, Worcester, Massachusetts; *Department of Medicine, University of Connecticut School of Medicine, Farmington, Connecticut and Department of Research, St. Francis Hospital and Medical Center, Hartford, Connecticut; †Craniofacial and Skeletal Diseases Branch, National Institute of Dental and Craniofacial Research, National Institutes of Health, Bethesda, Maryland; and ‡Department of Biochemistry/Graduate School of Medical Sciences, Cornell University Medical College and Research Division, Hospital for Special Surgery, New York, New York*

Bone is a dynamic connective tissue, comprising an exquisite assembly of functionally distinct cell populations that are required to support both the structural, biochemical, and mechanical integrity of this connective mineralized tissue and its central role in mineral homeostasis. The responsiveness of bone to mechanical forces and metabolic regulatory signals that accommodate requirements for maintaining the organ and connective tissue functions of bone are operative throughout life. Bone tissue undergoes remodeling, a continual process of resorption and renewal. The principal cells that mediate the bone-forming processes of the mammalian skeleton are *stromal osteoprogenitor cells* that contribute to maintaining the osteoblast population and bone mass; *osteoblasts* that synthesize the bone matrix on bone-forming surfaces; *osteocytes,* organized throughout the mineralized bone matrix, that support bone structure; and the protective bone-surface *lining cells* (Fig. 1). The fidelity of bone-tissue structure and metabolic functions necessitates exchange of regulatory signals among these cell populations. Current concepts for understanding molecular and cellular mechanisms regulating the progression of osteoblast differentiation and functional activities of distinct cell populations

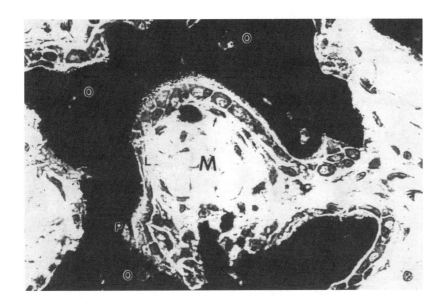

FIG. 1. Tissue organization of bone-forming cells. Mineralized section of trabecular bone in surrounding marrow *(M)* shows osteocytes *(O)* in their lacunae, a preosteocyte *(P)* at the mineralizing front of the osteoid, and plump-active surface osteoblasts laying down matrix. A few preosteoblasts *(arrows)* are observed and flattened lining cells *(L).*

are outlined. In this context, a basis can be provided for improved diagnosis of skeletal disease and treatment that is targeted to specific cells in bone tissue.

OSTEOPROGENITORS

Different regions of the skeleton arise from distinct embryonic lineages reflecting origins from specific primordial structures (see Chapter 2). Considering the different embryonic developmental programs of the mesoderm to form membranous bone (e.g., calvarium) and subtypes of endochondral bone (e.g., limbs and vertebrae), an early osteoprogenitor may divert from a stem cell at these skeletal sites. It has been well documented that osteoblasts from axial and appendicular bone exhibit selective responsiveness to hormones [see for example (1)]. It remains to be determined whether this reflects the tissue environment or inherent properties of the cells selected at an early stage during osteoblast differentiation.

Progenitors of the bone-forming cells are largely of mesenchymal origin derived from the mesodermal germ cell layer. The progression of the most primitive pluripotent cell to the undifferentiated multipotential mesenchymal cell is not understood. The stem cells that give rise to progeny for bone formation and tissue renewal can be identified only by biologic consequences. The most direct assay of stem cell activity is competency for an undifferentiated cell to proliferate and subsequently acquire, as well as sustain, phenotype-restricted structural and functional properties after transplantation in intact animals (2). The periosteum and bone marrow are important sources of mesenchymal progenitor cells (inducible osteoprogenitor) and osteoprogenitor cells. The marrow and its stromal bedding give rise to stem cells of the hematopoietic lineage, origin of osteoclasts, and cells of nonhematopoietic lineages from which many tissue-specific cells are derived (e.g., osteoblasts, chondrocytes, myoblasts, and adipocytes). Stages of development of the osteoblast phenotype and characteristic features of the dis-

tinct osteoblast subpopulation are presented in Fig. 2. The pluripotent mesenchymal/stromal cell and osteoprogenitor appear to have limited self-renewal capacity and also, in contrast to the stem cell, have a capacity for extensive proliferation (3). By using characterization of hematopoietic stem cells as a paradigm, several groups developed antibodies to marrow stromal cell-surface proteins. These reagents permit both recognition and purification of presumptive skeletal mesenchymal stem cells and determine osteoprogenitor populations (4–12).

Cytokines, growth factors, and hormones mediating commitment of stem cells to osteoblast lineage cells, as well as influencing osteoprogenitor growth and differentiation, are indicated in Fig. 2. Fibroblast growth factor (FGF) and transforming growth factor-β1 (TGF-β1) are potent mitogens for periosteal osteoprogenitors and marrow stromal cells and are synthesized by osteoblast lineage cells. The osteoinductive effects of the various bone morphogenetic proteins (BMPs) are complex [recently reviewed in (13)]. Activities are dependent on concentration and the progenitor cell phenotype. BMP-2, BMP-4, and BMP-7 (also designated OP-1) are potent inducers of osteogenesis *in vivo* and *in vitro*. Parathyroid hormone (PTH) stimulates growth of osteoprogenitor populations, whereas parathyroid hormone-related peptide (PTHrP) functions as a local cytokine regulating cell growth for differentiation during development [reviewed in (14)]. Glucocorticoids promote the differentiation of human and rat marrow mesenchymal cells to osteoblasts *in vitro* but can have negative effects on bone formation. A detailed discussion of these signaling molecules that regulate both osteoblast and osteoclast activities is presented later in this chapter and in Chapter 4.

The progression of osteoblast maturation requires the sequential activation and suppression of genes that encode phenotypic and regulatory proteins (Fig. 3). Signaling molecules like BMPs and TGFs indirectly mediate a cascade of gene expression. Transcription factors and regulatory proteins that directly engage in protein–DNA as well as in protein–protein interactions also are important for the development of bone-tissue and osteoblast differentiation. Tran-

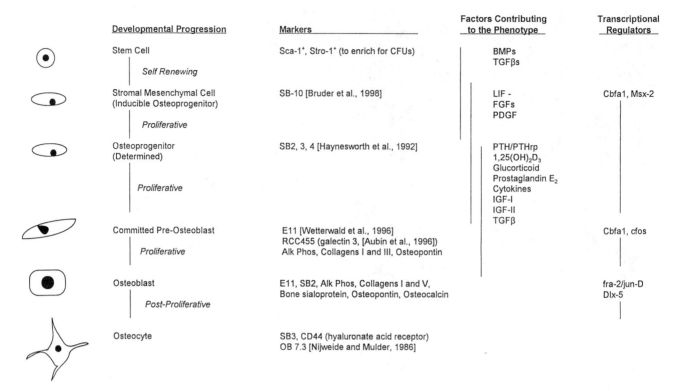

Developmental Progression	Markers	Factors Contributing to the Phenotype	Transcriptional Regulators
Stem Cell	Sca-1⁺, Stro-1⁺ (to enrich for CFUs)	BMPs TGFβs	
Self Renewing			
Stromal Mesenchymal Cell (Inducible Osteoprogenitor)	SB-10 [Bruder et al., 1998]	LIF - FGFs PDGF	Cbfa1, Msx-2
Proliferative			
Osteoprogenitor (Determined)	SB2, 3, 4 [Haynesworth et al., 1992]	PTH/PTHrp 1,25(OH)₂D₃ Glucorticoid Prostaglandin E₂ Cytokines IGF-I IGF-II TGFβ	
Proliferative			
Committed Pre-Osteoblast	E11 [Wetterwald et al., 1996] RCC455 (galectin 3, [Aubin et al., 1996]) Alk Phos, Collagens I and III, Osteopontin		Cbfa1, cfos
Proliferative			
Osteoblast	E11, SB2, Alk Phos, Collagens I and V, Bone sialoprotein, Osteopontin, Osteocalcin		fra-2/jun-D Dlx-5
Post-Proliferative			
Osteocyte	SB3, CD44 (hyaluronate acid receptor) OB 7.3 [Nijweide and Mulder, 1986]		

FIG. 2. Regulation of osteoblast growth and differentiation. The properties of osteoblast lineage cells are indicated. Column 1 illustrates the morphologic features of differentiating osteoblasts at each stage from stem cell to osteocyte, the final stage of maturation. The mature osteoblast on the quiescent bone surface, the bone-lining cell, is not shown. Column 2 describes either cell-surface markers or proteins that are highly expressed at the indicated stage of maturation. Column 3 lists those factors that promote differentiation of the precursor cell populations. In column 4, those transcription factors that have been identified as key regulators of bone formation or expression of osteoblast-specific genes are indicated.

scription factors playing key roles in the differentiation of mesenchymal stem cells to osteoblasts have been identified by several approaches, including characterization of bone tissue–specific transcription factors, transgenic mouse models overexpressing proteins, and the knockout of specific genes that revealed skeletal defects (3,14). The bone-specific osteocalcin gene promoter has provided a blueprint for characterization of regulatory factors that control osteoblast differentiation (15). Key regulatory factors necessary for expression of bone phenotypic genes are steroid receptors, fos and jun family proteins that form complexes that interact with AP-1 regulatory sequences, the helix–loop–helix (HLH) proteins (Twist, Id, Scleraxis), leucine zipper proteins (hXBP-1), zinc-finger proteins (zif268), homeodomain proteins (Msx-2, Dlx-5), and most recently, *runt* domain transcription factors (Cbfa/AML/PEBP2α). Requirements for Cbfa1 in bone formation have been demonstrated by the inhibition of bone-tissue formation in a null mutation mouse model (16) and Cbfa1 antisense inhibition of osteoblast differentiation *in vitro* (17). The developmental representation of transcription factors during osteoblast maturation reflect their roles as key determinants of osteoblast differentiation (Figs. 2 and 3). Id and Twist expression must be downregulated for osteoblast differentiation to proceed (18); overexpression of these factors inhibits osteogenesis *in vitro* (19). During bone formation *in vivo* and osteoblast differentiation *in vitro*, Msx-2 is expressed maximally in the mesenchymal/

osteoprogenitor population and subsequently downregulated in the mature bone-forming cells (20). *In vitro* Dlx-5 appears in the postproliferative osteoblast and increases during mineralization (21). C-*fos* is expressed in osteoprogenitor cells and periosteal tissues, but not in the mature osteoblasts (22), where fra-2 is abundant and regulates expression of bone-specific genes (23).

OSTEOBLASTS

Committed preosteoblasts in a nondividing state are recognizable in bone by their proximity to surface osteoblasts and by histochemically detectable levels of alkaline phosphatase enzyme activity, one of the earliest markers of the osteoblast phenotype. The final stages of osteoblast differentiation are defined by the biosynthesis and organization of the bone extracellular matrix (ECM). When the preosteoblast ceases to proliferate, a key signaling event occurs for development of the large cuboidal osteoblast on the bone surface from the spindle-shaped osteoprogenitor (Fig. 3). The morphologic and ultrastructural properties of the active osteoblast are typical of a cell engaged in secretion of a connective tissue matrix, having a large nucleus, enlarged Golgi, and extensive endoplasmic reticulum (see Chapter 1). On quiescent bone surfaces, a single layer of flattened osteoblasts or bone-lining cells, which form the endosteum against the

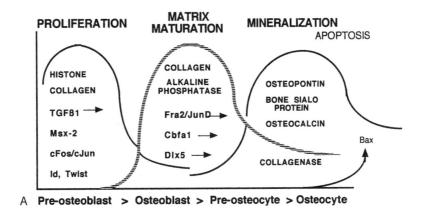

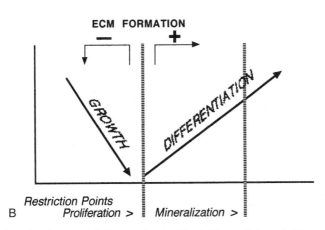

FIG. 3. In vitro developmental stages of osteoblast differentiation. **A:** Temporal expression of cell growth and osteoblast phenotype-related genes during 35 days of culture of primary fetal rat calvarium–derived osteoblasts as they synthesize a mineralizing matrix. Peak expression levels of each gene, which were determined in total cellular RNA prepared at 3-day intervals, define the growth period, the postproliferative matrix-maturation stage, and the mineralization stage. Experimental conditions and origin of the probes are detailed in Stein et al. (14). During the proliferation period, (H4) histone, growth factors (TGF-β1), adhesion proteins (fibronectin), collagen, and low levels of osteopontin (not shown) are expressed. Peak levels of alkaline phosphatase mRNA (AP) characterize the matrix-maturation period. In the mineralization period, an increase in mRNA transcripts of osteocalcin, osteopontin, and bone sialoprotein reflect calcium (Ca^{2+}) deposition. Increased levels of collagenase are related to remodeling or editing of the extracellular matrix. Apoptotic cells are observed during the mineralization period associated with the bone-forming nodule. The expression of transcription factors during osteoblast differentiation is based on either mRNA levels (Msx-2, Dlx-5, Id, Twist) or functional protein levels determined by Western blot or DNA binding activity of nuclear extracts in gel-shift analyses (c-*fos*, c-*jun*, *fra*-2, jun D, Cbfa1). See text for references. **B:** Signaling events during osteoblast differentiation. Arrows show the reciprocal relation between cell growth and differentiation-related gene expression in mature osteoblasts. Two experimentally established transition points, designated by vertical lines, exhibited by normal diploid osteoblasts during sequential acquisition of bone-cell phenotype are indicated: (1) at completion of proliferation when genes associated with extracellular matrix development and maturation of the phenotype are upregulated, and (2) at onset of extracellular matrix mineralization. Formation of the extracellular matrix contributes to cessation of cell growth (−) and induction of genes (+) rendering the matrix competent for mineralization.

marrow and underlying the periosteum lie directly on the mineralized surfaces.

The active osteoblast is highly enriched in alkaline phosphatase and vectorially secretes type I collagen and specialized bone-matrix proteins as osteoid toward the mineralizing front of the tissue. The osteoid seam width is in the range of 10 μm, and the mineral apposition rate is approximately 0.55 μm/day in adults (24). The collagen fibers must mature to support mineral deposition. Cell–matrix and cell–cell interactions, facilitated by integrins and cadherins, are important for osteoblast differentiation and mineralization of the osteoid matrix. Signaling pathways from the ECM through the cytoskeleton and finally to the nucleus mediate responsiveness of bone tissue to systemic factors and mechanical forces. These responses allow the expression and regulation of bone-specific and bone-related genes.

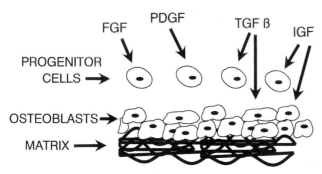

FIG. 4. Regulation of bone formation by polypeptide growth factors.

The temporal expression of proteins involved in cell adhesion, ECM biosynthesis, and matrix mineralization provides a panel of markers that reflect stages of osteoblast differentiation (Fig. 3). The growth stage is downregulated by the accumulated ECM. Cessation of cell growth leads to the matrix-maturation stage when induced expression of alkaline phosphatase and specialized bone proteins (detailed below) renders the ECM competent for mineral deposition. The mineralization stage leads to expression of markers of the mature osteoblast (for example, osteocalcin and bone sialoprotein), which may function in regulating the ordered deposition of mineral. This developmental sequence of gene expression can be visualized at the single-cell level in bone tissue by in situ methods. Variations in levels of gene products are dependent on location of the osteoblast in bone tissue. Subtle yet important differences may reflect selective responses of osteoblasts that relate to either homeostatic functions or to the establishment and maintenance of bone structure (24,25). Many of the bone phenotypic markers (alkaline phosphatase, osteocalcin) can be monitored in serum and are useful markers of bone function.

OSTEOCYTES

The osteocyte is the terminal differentiation stage of the osteoblast-supporting bone structure. Osteocytes develop as the mineralizing osteoid envelopes the surface osteoblasts (Fig. 1). A distinguishing feature of osteocytes is the numerous cellular extensions of the osteocyte plasma membrane that lie in the canaliculi (see Chapter 1). The osteocyte, when isolated directly from bone tissue, does not reinitiate proliferation, retaining its morphologic features *in vitro* (26). Osteocytes have the capacity to synthesize certain matrix molecules as abundantly as osteoblasts, visualized by in situ studies. The detection of osteocalcin, for example, is particularly robust. In aging bone, empty lacunae are observed, suggesting that osteocytes may undergo apoptosis. Osteoblasts recruited to bone-forming surfaces that do not eventually mature to osteocytes may be removed by apoptosis (27).

Osteocytes within the mineralized matrix are in direct communication with surface osteoblasts through their cellular processes. Thus the osteocytes and surface-lining cells form a continuum or syncytium by connection of their cell processes through gap junctions. Osteoblasts and osteocytes are metabolically and electrically coupled through different gap-junction proteins called connexins (28). Rapid fluxes of bone calcium across these junctions are thought to facilitate transmission of information between osteoblasts on the bone surface and osteocytes within the structure of bone itself (29). This structural organization and the direct contact of active osteoblast or surface-lining cells with the osteocytes are consistent with the concept that bone cells, responding to varying physiological signals, can communicate their responses.

FUNCTIONAL ACTIVITIES OF OSTEOBLAST LINEAGE CELLS

The functional properties and regulated activity of bone cells evolve during progression of osteoblast differentiation. As described earlier, they form the structural components of bone, producing a mineralized matrix and a cellular syncytium to respond to physiological and mechanical demands on the skeleton. An equally important function of osteoblasts, as well as the preosteoblasts that lie in close proximity, and osteocytes is their responsiveness to endocrine factors and the production of paracrine and autocrine factors for the recruitment of osteoprogenitors, the growth of preosteoblasts, and the regulation of osteoclastic resorption of the mineralized bone matrix. The bone microenvironment appears to be essential for two components of osteoclastogenesis: (a) maturation and fusion of the mononuclear precursor to the multinucleated osteoclast, and (b) activation and regulation of the activity of the functional osteoclast. The protective bone-lining cell must retract from the surface to allow osteoclast attachment for bone resorption.

The requirement for stromal osteoprogenitors or osteoblasts in mediating osteoclast differentiation is linked to the role of osteotrophic hormones and cytokines in regulating development of preosteoclasts and the multinucleated phenotype. Osteoblasts and osteocytes have receptors for cytokines; PTH; 1,25-dihydroxyvitamin D_3 [1,25 $(OH)_2$ D_3]; and estrogen, which are key regulators of bone turnover. Stromal osteoblastic cells are the major source of the colony-stimulating factors (CSFs) and the interleukin-6 (IL-6) family of cytokines, which also are potent stimulators of bone resorption and participate in osteoclastogenesis at early and later stages. Recently an osteoclast-differentiating factor produced by osteoblasts was identified as a ligand that binds an inhibitor of osteoclastogenesis, called osteoprotegerin (OPG) (30). The osteoblast ligand is identical to the known RANK (receptor activation of NF-$\kappa\beta$) and TRANCE (TNF-related activation-induced cytokine) ligand (31). Expression of the OPG/RANK/TRANCE ligand in osteoblasts is upregulated by 1,25 $(OH)_2$ D_3, IL-11, and prostaglandin E_2 (PGE_2), stimulators of bone resorption (32). The ligand thus promotes osteoclast formation. All these features of the osteoblast provide mechanisms for coupling of osteoblasts to the formation of osteoclast activity (see Chapter 4 for additional detail).

POLYPEPTIDE GROWTH FACTORS

Bone remodeling is a complex process involving a number of cellular functions directed toward the coordinated resorp-

TABLE 1. *Polypeptide skeletal growth factors*

Insulin-like growth factors (IGFs)
Transforming growth factor-β (TGF-β) family of peptides, including bone morphogenetic proteins (BMPs)
Fibroblast growth factors (FGFs), or heparin-binding growth factors
Platelet-derived growth factors (PDGFs)
Selected cytokines of the interleukin (IL), tumor necrosis factor (TNF), and colony-stimulating factor (CSF) families

tion and formation of new bone. Bone remodeling is regulated by systemic hormones and by local factors, which affect cells of the osteoclast or osteoblast lineage and exert their effects on (a) the replication and differentiation of undifferentiated cells, (b) the recruitment of cells, and (c) the differentiated function of cells. The end product of remodeling is the maintenance of a mineralized bone matrix, and the major organic component of this matrix is collagen. The local factors synthesized by skeletal cells include growth factors, cytokines, and prostaglandins (Table 1). Growth factors are polypeptides that regulate the replication and differentiated function of cells. Bone is a rich source of growth factors with important actions in the regulation of bone formation and bone resorption (Table 1; Fig. 4). Frequently these local factors are synthesized by bone-forming cells, although some cytokines are secreted by stromal cells and by cells of the immune or hematologic system, and as such, they are present in the bone microenvironment (33,34). Therefore, growth factors have effects on cells of the same class (autocrine factors) or on cells of another class within the tissue (paracrine factors). Growth factors also are present in the circulation and may act as systemic regulators of skeletal metabolism. Locally their activity can be modulated by changes in synthesis, activation, receptor binding, and binding proteins.

Insulin-like Growth Factors

Insulin-like growth factors (IGFs) are polypeptides with a relative molecular mass (M_r) of 7600 (35). Two IGFs have been characterized, IGF-I and IGF-II. These peptides are present in the systemic circulation and are synthesized by multiple tissues, including bone, where they act as local regulators of cell metabolism. Systemic IGF-I is secreted by the liver, and its synthesis is growth-hormone dependent, whereas the synthesis of IGF-I in peripheral tissues is regulated by diverse hormones (35,36). In the circulation, IGFs are bound to IGF-binding proteins (IGFBPs) and to an acid-labile subunit (35). The most abundant IGFBP in serum is IGFBP-3, which also is growth-hormone dependent. IGF-I and IGF-II have similar biologic activities, although in bone, IGF-I is more potent than IGF-II. *In vitro,* IGFs enhance bone collagen and matrix synthesis and stimulate the replication of cells of the osteoblastic lineage (37). The effect of IGFs on matrix synthesis is in part dependent on an increased number of cells, but IGFs directly modulate the differentiated function of the osteoblast. IGFs increase type I collagen transcription and decrease the transcription of collagenase 3 or matrix metalloproteinase (MMP)-13, a collagen-degrading protease

(38). As a consequence of a decrease in collagenase levels, IGFs inhibit bone-collagen degradation. This dual effect, an increase in collagen synthesis and a decrease in its degradation, is central to the maintenance of bone matrix and bone mass. Infusions of IGF-I to humans cause a generalized anabolic effect and an increase in bone remodeling (39). IGFs can be modified by changes in their synthesis, receptor binding, and IGFBPs. The synthesis of skeletal IGF-I is regulated by hormones and growth factors, whereas the synthesis of IGF-II is regulated by growth factors and not by hormones (36,40). PTH and other agents that stimulate cyclic adenosine monophosphate (cAMP) in bone cells are major stimulators of IGF-I synthesis (36). In contrast, growth hormone plays a modest role in enhancing IGF-I production in bone. Glucocorticoids inhibit skeletal IGF-I synthesis, and this may be important in the mechanism of glucocorticoid action in bone (41). Skeletal growth factors with mitogenic properties, such as fibroblast growth factor (FGF)2 and platelet-derived growth factor (PDGF), inhibit the synthesis of IGF-I and IGF-II by the osteoblast (36,40). This effect correlates with a decrease in the differentiated function of the osteoblast. Bone cells also secrete the six known IGFBPs, termed IGFBP-1 through -6. The precise role of the IGFBPs is under study; they may prolong the half-life of IGF, neutralize or enhance its biologic activity, or be involved in the transport of IGF to its target cells. Some binding proteins, like IGFBP-4, have inhibitory activity. Others, like IGFBP-5, can be stimulatory (35). The regulation of IGFBP synthesis in bone cells is complex. Selected IGFBPs, such as IGFBP-3, -4, and -5, are under cAMP control, and others are under IGF-I and IGF-II control. The expression of IGFBP-5 is to an extent coordinated with that of IGF-I and, like IGF-I, it is inhibited by glucocorticoids and mitogenic growth factors (41). IGFBPs are degraded by specific and nonspecific proteases secreted by skeletal cells, including serine proteases and MMPs.

Transforming Growth Factor-β Family

Transforming growth factor (TGF)β is a polypeptide with an M_r of 25,000. Three forms of TGF-β, which have similar biologic activities, are expressed by mammalian cells, including those of bone. They are TGF-β1, TGF, and TGF-β3 (33). TGF stimulates the replication of precursor cells of the osteoblast lineage, and it has a direct stimulatory effect on bone-collagen synthesis (42). Therefore, TGF modulates bone-matrix synthesis by various mechanisms, including an increase in the number of cells capable of expressing the osteoblast phenotype, as well as by direct actions on the differentiated function of the osteoblast. TGF also decreases bone resorption by inducing apoptosis of osteoclasts (42). The levels of TGF can be modified by changes in its synthesis and activity. The gene elements responsible for the control of TGF-β1, TGF, and TGF-β3 expression are different (33). Consequently, different hormones and factors regulate the synthesis of the three forms of TGF-β. This factor is released in an inactive form bound to a precursor and to a binding protein. Hormones capable of inducing bone resorption, such as PTH, activate and increase the release of TGF-β from bone. The available TGF-β could be instrumental in suppressing bone resorption and initiating the bone-forming phase of remodeling. TGF-β binds to two signal-transducing receptors, termed TGF-β receptors I and II, and to the non–signal transducing betaglycan. Changes in the expression of betaglycan can regulate the amount of biologically available TGF-β (41).

A number of additional polypeptides share amino acid sequence homology with TGF-β. These include a large family of BMPs or osteogenic proteins (43). BMPs are osteoinductive factors that induce normal endochondral bone formation, and they share some activities with TGF-β. However, they have specific receptors and induce the differentiation of cells of the osteoblast lineage. Because of their ability to increase the formation of new bone, BMPs may be important in the treatment of fractures.

Fibroblast Growth Factors

Acidic and basic FGF, or heparin-binding growth factors 1 and 2, are polypeptides with an M_r of 17,000 (44). FGFs are members of a large family of related genes. FGFs have angiogenic properties and are considered important for neovascularization and wound healing. Acidic and basic FGF stimulate bone cell replication, which results in an increased bone cell population capable of synthesizing bone collagen (45). Basic FGF is more potent than acidic FGF. Bones treated with FGF synthesize higher amounts of collagenous matrix because they contain a greater number of collagen-synthesizing cells, but not because of a direct effect of FGF on the differentiated function of the osteoblast. In fact, basic FGF inhibits type I collagen transcription in osteoblasts. The stimulatory effects of FGFs on neovascularization, in association with those on bone cell replication, suggest that they are important in the process of healing and bone repair, particularly, because their release from cells may occur after cell injury or death. Neither acidic nor basic FGF modifies bone resorption, but basic FGF increases the expression of MMP-13, indicating a possible function in bone-collagen degradation and remodeling. The systemic administration of basic FGF causes an early increase in the number of preosteoblasts, followed by a recruitment of osteoblasts and an increase in bone formation (46). Systemically, basic FGF has been known to accelerate the healing of fractures. Studies on the synthesis of FGF in osteoblasts have been limited, but TGF and basic FGF increase FGF expression in osteoblast cell lines (33). There are four related FGF receptor (FGFR) genes, termed FGFR-1 to FGFR-4. Their expression in bone cells has not been studied, but in other cells, FGFR-1, -2, and -3 mediate the mitogenic response to FGF. Recent studies demonstrated diverse skeletal abnormalities in patients with mutations of FGFR-1, -2, and -3. These abnormalities vary with the mutated receptor and include achondroplasia, a common cause of dwarfism and early closure of cranial sutures (47).

Platelet-Derived Growth Factor

PDGF, a polypeptide with an M_r of 30,000, was initially isolated from blood platelets and was considered important in the early phases of wound repair (48). Normal and neoplastic tissues also synthesize PDGF, indicating that it may act as a systemic or local regulator of tissue growth. PDGF is a dimer of the products of two genes, PDGF-A and -B, so that mature peptides can exist as PDGF-AA or -BB homodimers or as PDGF-AB heterodimers. PDGF-AB and -BB are the predominant isoforms present in the systemic circulation. Normal osteoblasts and osteosarcoma cells express both the PDGF-A and -B genes and have the potential to synthesize all PDGF isoforms (49). PDGF has activities similar to those described for FGF. It stimulates bone cell replication, and as a consequence of an increased number of cells, PDGF stimulates bone-collagen synthesis. However, PDGF does not stimulate the differentiated function of the osteoblast, and it acutely inhibits bone-matrix apposition rates (50). PDGF-BB also stimulates bone resorption by increasing the number of osteoclasts, and it induces the expression of MMP-13 by the osteoblast. The synthesis of the locally produced PDGF is regulated by growth factors (49). PDGF-A expression is enhanced by TGF-β and PDGF itself, but not by systemic hormones. PDGF-B expression is stimulated by TGF-β. There are two PDGF receptors, α and β, and the activity of PDGF can be regulated by changes in receptor binding. There are no specific binding proteins for PDGF, but PDGF-B chains bind to osteonectin (SPARC), which modifies the activity of PDGF by decreasing its binding to specific receptors. PDGF may act primarily as a systemic agent and, when released by the aggregating platelet, it may increase cells critical for the process of fracture and wound repair.

Other Cytokines

A number of cytokines, such as IL-1, -4, -6, and -11, macrophage and granulocyte/macrophage (GM) colony-stimulating factors (CSFs), and tumor necrosis factors (TNFs), have important effects in bone remodeling. They stimulate bone resorption, most likely by enhancing the recruitment of osteoclasts, the bone-resorbing cells (34). IL-1 seems relevant in the mechanism of hypercalcemia in certain hematologic malignancies, and increased IL-1 levels are found in selected cases of osteoporosis. IL-1 increases the synthesis of IL-6 by stromal cells, and IL-6 stimulates bone resorption by increasing the recruitment of cells of the osteoclast lineage. The synthesis of IL-1 and IL-6 is diminished by estrogens (34). It is postulated that the two cytokines are responsible for the increased bone resorption observed after estrogen discontinuation, such as in postmenopausal osteoporosis. TNF-α, or cachectin, is a cytokine known for its cytostatic, cytolytic, and antiviral actions. TNF-α stimulates bone resorption and bone cell replication. CSFs play a role in the maturation of osteoclasts, and GM-CSF-1 deficiency causes osteopetrosis.

In summary, bone-associated factors play a role in the maintenance of normal bone remodeling, have a function in wound and fracture healing, and play a role in the pathogenesis of specific bone diseases and hypercalcemia.

THE EXTRACELLULAR MATRIX PROTEINS OF BONE

Bone composes the largest proportion of the body's connective tissue mass. Unlike most other connective tissue

TABLE 2. *Characteristics of collagen-related genes and proteins found in bone matrix*

Protein	Gene	Function
Type I		
$[\alpha 1(I)_2\alpha 2(I)]$	COL1A1 17q21.3-22 18 kb, 51 exons 7.2 and 5.9 kb mRNA	Most abundant protein in bone matrix (90% of organic matrix)
$[\alpha 1(I)_3]$	COL1A2 7q21.3-22 35 kb, 52 exons 6.5 and 5.5 kb mRNA	Serves as scaffolding
		May bind and orient other proteins that nucleate hydroxyapatite deposition
Type X		
$[\alpha 1(x)]_3$	COL10A1 6q21-22.3	Present in hypertrophic cartilage but does not appear to regulate matrix mineralization
		Matrix organization and template for type I collagen
Others:		
Type III		
$[\alpha 1(III)]_3$	COL3A1 2q24.3-q31	Present in bone in trace amounts
		May regulate collagen fibril diameter
Type V	COL5A1 9q34.2-34.3	Their paucity in bone may explain the large-diameter size of bone collagen fibrils
$[\alpha 1(V)_2\alpha 2(V)]$	COL5A2 2q24.3-q31	
$[\alpha 1(V)\alpha 2(V)\alpha 3(V)]$	COL5A3 9q34.2-34.3	

matrices, bone matrix is physiologically mineralized and is unique in that it is constantly regenerated throughout life as a consequence of bone turnover. Information on the gene and protein structure and potential function of bone ECM constituents has exploded during the last 2 decades. This information was described in great detail in several recent reviews (51,52), to which the reader is referred for specific references, which are too numerous to be listed adequately here. This chapter summarizes salient features of the classes of bone-matrix proteins, and the tables list specific details of the individual components of bone matrix.

Collagen

The basic building block of the bone-matrix fiber network is *type I collagen,* which is a triple-helical molecule containing two identical $\alpha 1(I)$ chains and a structurally similar, but genetically different $\alpha 2(I)$ chain [reviewed in (53); (Table 2)]. Collagen α chains are characterized by a Gly-X-Y repeating triplet (where X is usually proline), and by several posttranslational modifications including (a) hydroxylation of certain prolyl and lysyl residues, (b) glycosylation of certain lysyl or hydroxylysyl residues with glucose or galactose residues or both, and (c) formation of intra- and intermolecular covalent cross-links that differ from that in soft connective tissues. Measurement of these bone-collagen cross-links in urine have proved to be good measures of bone resorption (54). Bone consists predominantly of type I collagen; however, trace amounts of type III, V, X, and FACIT collagens may be present during certain stages of bone formation and may regulate collagen fibril diameter (Table 2).

Noncollagenous Proteins

Noncollagenous proteins (NCPs) compose 10% to 15% of the total bone protein content. Approximately one fourth of bone NCP is exogenously derived. This fraction is largely composed of serum-derived proteins, such as *albumin* and

α_2-*HS-glycoprotein* (Table 3), which are acidic in character and bind to bone matrix because of their affinity to hydroxyapatite. Although these proteins are not endogenously synthesized, they may exert effects on matrix mineralization, and α_2-HS-glycoprotein, which is the human analogue of fetuin, also may regulate bone cell proliferation. The remainder of this exogenous fraction is composed of growth factors and a large variety of other molecules present in trace amounts, which also may influence local bone cell activity [see (51) for review].

Of the endogenously synthesized molecules, bone cells synthesize and secrete as many molecules of NCP as of collagen, on a mole-to-mole basis. These molecules can be broken down into four general (and sometimes overlapping) groups: (a) proteoglycans, (b) glycosylated proteins, (c) glycosylated proteins with potential cell-attachment activities, and (d) τ-carboxylated (gla) proteins. The physiological roles for individual bone-protein constituents are not well defined; however, they may participate not only in forming the structure of mineralized matrix, but also in the control of osteoblastic and osteoclastic metabolism.

Proteoglycans and Hyaluronan

Proteoglycans are macromolecules that contain acidic polysaccharide side chains (glycosaminoglycans) attached to a central core protein, and bone matrix contains several members of this family (55). During initial stages of bone formation, the large dermatan sulfate proteoglycan, *versican,* and the glycosaminoglycan, *hyaluronan* (which is not attached to a protein core), are produced and may delineate areas that will become bone (Table 4). With continued osteogenesis, versican is replaced by two small chondroitin sulfate proteoglycans, *decorin* and *biglycan,* composed of tandem repeats of a leucine-rich repeat sequence. Decorin has been implicated in the regulation of collagen fibrillogenesis and is distributed predominantly in the ECM space of connective tissues and in bone, whereas biglycan tends to be found in pericellular locales. Although their exact

TABLE 3. *Gene and protein characteristics of serum proteins found in bone matrix*

Protein	Gene	Function
Albumin	4q11-13	Transports proteins
69 kDa	17kb, 15 exons	Inhibits hydroxyapatite crystal growth, 60% of
Nonglycosylated		serum
One sulfhydryl and 17 disulfide bonds		
High-affinity hydrophobic binding pocket		
α-2HS glycoprotein	3q27-29	Promotes endocytosis
Precursor protein cleaved to form A and B chains that	two RFLPs	Has opsonic properties
are disulfide linked	1.5 kb mRNA	Chemoattractant for monocytic cells
Ala-Ala and Pro-Pro repeat sequences		Bovine analog (fetuin) is a growth factor
N-linked oligosaccharides		Mineralization inhibitor
Cystatin-like domains		

physiological functions are not known, they are assumed to be important for the integrity of most connective tissue matrices. One function might rise from their ability to bind and modulate the activity of the TGF-β family in the extracellular space, thereby influencing cell proliferation and differentiation. Recently it was determined that deletion of the biglycan gene in transgenic animals leads to a significant decrease in the development of trabecular bone, indicating that it is a positive regulator of bone formation (56). Other proteoglycans, such as *fibromodulin, osteoglycin,* and *osteoadherin* (57) (some of which are also leucine-rich repeat

proteins), are found in bone matrix but at lower levels than decorin and biglycan, and may function in other aspects of bone metabolism (Table 4).

Glycoproteins

One of the hallmarks of bone formation is the synthesis of high levels of *alkaline phosphatase* (Table 5). This enzyme, primarily bound to the cell surface via a phosphoinositol linkage, and can be cleaved from the cell surface and found

TABLE 4. *Gene and protein characteristics of glycosaminoglycan-containing molecules in bone matrix*

Protein	Gene	Function
Versican	5q12-14	May "capture" space that is destined to
~1×10^6 intact protein	90 kb, 15 exons	become bone
~360 kDa core	One-splice variant	
~12 CS chains of 45 kDa	10, 9, 8 kb mRNAs	
G1 and G3 globular domains with		
hyaluronan binding sites		
EGF- and CRP-like sequences		
Decorin	12q21-23	Binds to collagen and may regulate fibril diameter
~130 kDa intact protein	>45 kb, 9 exons	
~38–45 kDa core with 10 leucine-rich	Alternative promoters, 1.6 and	Binds to TGF-β
repeat sequences	1.9 kb mRNA	May modulate activity, inhibits cell attachment
1 CS chain of 40 kDa		to fibronectin
Biglycan	Xq27	May bind to collagen
~270 kDa intact protein	7 kb, 8 exons, 2.1 and 2.6 kb	May bind to TGF-β
~38–45 kDa core protein with 10	mRNA	Pericellular environment
leucine-rich repeat sequences		Regulates mineralization in vitro
2 CS chains of 40 kDa		
Fibromodulin	1q32	Binds to collagen
59 kDa intact protein	8.5 kb, 3 exons	May regulate fibril formation
42 kDa core protein with 10 leucine-rich		Binds to TGF-β
repeat sequences		
One N-linked KS chain		
Osteoadherin	Gene not yet isolated	May mediate cell attachment
85 kDa intact protein		
47 kDa core protein		
11 leucine-rich repeat sequences (5)		
RGD sequence		
Hyaluronan	Multigene complex	May work with versican-like molecule to capture space destined to become bone
Not bound to a protein core		
Synthesized by multiple proteins associated outside of the cell		
Structure unknown		

TABLE 5. *Gene and protein characteristics of glycoproteins in bone matrix*

Protein	Gene	Function

Alkaline phosphatase (bone-liver-kidney isozyme)
  Two identical subunits of ~80 kDa
  Disulfide bonded
  Tissue-specific posttranslational modifications
	1p34-36.1
	50 kb, 12 exons
	Alternative promoters, one RFLP
	2.5, 4.1, 4.7 kb mRNA
		A phosphotransferase
		Potential Ca^{2+} carrier
		Hydrolyzes inhibitors of mineral deposition such as pyrophosphates

Osteonectin
  ~35–45 kDa
  Intramolecular disulfide bonds, a helical amino terminus with multiple low-affinity Ca^{2+} binding sites
  Two EF hand high-affinity Ca^{2+} sites
  Ovomucoid homology
  Glycosylated and phosphorylated tissue-specific modifications
	5q31-33
	20 kb, 10 exons, One RFLP
	2.2, 3.0 kb mRNA
		May mediate deposition of hydroxyapatite
		Binds to growth factors
		May influence cell-cycle antiadhesive protein

Tetranectin
  21-kDa protein
  Composed of four identical subunits of 5.8 kDa
  Sequence homologies with asialoprotein receptor and G3 domain of aggrecan
	Two genes
	12 kb, 3 exons
	1 kb mRNA
		Binds to plasminogen
		May regulate matrix mineralization

Tenascin-C
  Hexameric structure
  Six identical chains of 320 kDa
  Cys rich
  EGF-like repeats
  FN type III repeats
	8–9 kb mRNA	Interferes with cell–FN interactions

within mineralized matrix. The function of alkaline phosphatase in bone cell biology has been the matter of much speculation, and remains undefined (58). The most abundant NCP produced by bone cells is *osteonectin,* a phosphorylated glycoprotein accounting for ~2% of the total protein of developing bone in most animal species. Osteonectin is transiently produced in nonbone tissues that are rapidly proliferating, remodeling, or undergoing profound changes in tissue architecture and is found constitutively in certain types of epithelial cells, cells associated with the skeleton, and in platelets. Its function(s) in bone may be multiple, with potential association with osteoblast growth, proliferation, or both, as well as with matrix mineralization (51,59). A transgenic mouse deficient in osteonectin has not been reported to exhibit any skeletal defect (60). *Tetranectin* and *tenascin* also have been found in bone matrix, but their function is not yet known.

RGD-Containing Glycoproteins

All connective tissue cells interact with their extracellular environment in response to stimuli that direct or coordinate (or both) specific cell functions, such as migration, proliferation, and differentiation (Table 6). These particular interactions involve cell attachment via transient or stable focal adhesions to extracellular macromolecules, which are mediated by cell-surface receptors that subsequently transduce intracellular signals. Bone cells synthesize at least nine proteins that may mediate cell attachment: *type I collagen, fibronectin, thrombospondin(s)* (there are three different genes, but it is not known which are expressed in bone),

vitronectin, fibrillin, osteopontin, bone sialoprotein (BSP), BAG-75 (52,55,61), and *DMP-1* (dentin matrix phosphoprotein-1) (62). All of these proteins contain RGD (Arg-Gly-Asn), the cell-attachment consensus sequence that binds to the integrin class of cell-surface molecules. However, in some cases, cell attachment appears to be independent of RGD, indicating the presence of other sequences or mechanisms of cell attachment. Thrombospondin(s), fibronectin, vitronectin, fibrillin, and osteopontin are expressed in many tissue systems, whereas BSP is virtually specific to the skeleton, and its appearance is tightly correlated with the appearance of mineral. Both osteopontin and BSP are known to anchor osteoclasts to bone, and in addition to supporting cell attachment, bind Ca^{2+} with extremely high affinity by polyacidic amino acid sequences. However, their function in bone is still not well defined because transgenic animals null for either of these proteins have not yet been reported to have skeletal abnormalities (63). It is not immediately clear why there are such a plethora of RGD-containing proteins in bone; however, the pattern of expression varies from one RGD protein to another, as does the pattern of expression of the different integrins that bind to these proteins. This variability indicates that cell–matrix interactions change as a function of maturational stage, suggesting that they also may play a role in osteoblastic maturation (51,64).

γ-Carboxylic Acid (Gla)-Containing Proteins

Three bone-matrix NCPs, *matrix-gla-protein (MGP), osteocalcin* [bone gla-protein (BGP), both of which are made by bone cells], and *protein S* (made primarily in the liver

TABLE 6. *Gene and protein characteristics of glycoproteins in bone matrix—continued RGD-containing glycoproteins*

Protein	Gene	Function
Thrombospondins (I, II, III, IV)	15q15-I	Cell attachment (but usually not
~450-kDa molecule	6q27-II	spreading)
Three identical disulfide-linked subunits of	1q21-24-III	Binds to heparin, platelets, types I and
~150–180 kDa	IV-not known	V collagens, thrombin, fibrinogen,
Homologies to fibrinogen, properdin, EGF, colla-		laminin, plasminogen and plasmino-
gen, von Willebrand, *P. falciparum,* and cal-	All very similar	gen activator inhibitor, histidine-rich
modulin	>16 kb, 22 exons	glycoprotein
RGD at the C terminal globular domain	6.1 kb kmRNA	
Fibronectin	2q34	Binds to cells, fibrin heparin, gelatin,
~400 kDa	50 kb in chicken, 50 exons,	collagen
Two nonidentical protein subunits of ~200 kDa	multiple splice forms, 6	
Composed of types I, II, and III repeats	RFLPs, 7.5 kb mRNA	
RGD in the 11th type III repeat 2/3 from N ter-		
minus		
Vitronectin	17q11	Cell-attachment protein
~70 kDa	4.5 kb, 8 exons,	Binds to collagen, plasminogen and
RGD close to N terminus	1.7 kb mRNA	plasminogen activator inhibitor, and
Homology to somatomedin B		to heparin
Rich in cysteines, sulfated and phosphorylated		
Fibrillin	15q21.1	May regulate elastic fiber formation mu-
350 kDa	110 kb, 65 exons,	tations found in Marfan's syndrome
EGF-like domains	10 kb mRNA	
RGD		
Cysteine motifs		
Osteopontin	4q21	Binds to cells
~60–75 kDa	8.2 kb, 7 exons, multiple al-	Inhibits mineralization
Polyaspartyl stretches no disulfide bonds	leles, one RFLP, one	May regulate proliferation
Glycosylated and phosphorylated	splice variant, several al-	Inhibits nitric oxide synthase
RGD located 2/3 from the N-terminal	leles	May regulate resistance to viral in-
	1.6 kb mRNA	fection
		May regulate tissue repair
Bone sialoprotein	4q21	Binds to cells, binds Ca²⁺ with high af-
60–75 kDa	15 kb, 7 exons, 2.0 mRNA	finity
Polyglutamyl stretches		May initiate mineralization
No disulfide bonds		Associated with cancers that metasta-
50% carbohydrate, tyrosine-sulfated phosphor-		size to bone
ylated		
RGD near the C terminus		
BAG-75	Gene not yet isolated,	Binds to Ca²⁺
~75 kDa	mRNA not yet cloned	May act as a cell-attachment protein
7% sialic acid		(RGD sequence not yet confirmed)
8% phosphate		May regulate bone resorption
Sequence homologies to phosphophoryn, osteo-		Found only in woven bone
pontin, DMP-1, and bone sialoprotein		Self-associates into large complexes
Dentin matrix acidic phosphoprotein (DMP-1)	4q21	Function unknown
513 amino acids (predicted from cDNA) acidic,	3.0 kb mRNA, 6 exons	
RGD 2/3 from N-terminus		

but also made by osteogenic cells), are posttranslationally modified by the action of vitamin K–dependent γ-carboxyl-ases (51,65) (Table 7). The production of dicarboxylic gluta-myl (gla) residues enhances calcium binding. MGP is found in many connective tissues, whereas osteocalcin is somewhat bone specific, although messenger RNA (mRNA) has been found in platelets and megakaryocytes. The physiological role of both of these proteins is still somewhat unclear; however, they may function in the inhibition of mineral deposition. MGP-deficient mice develop calcification in ex-traskeletal sites such as in the aorta (66). Osteocalcin-deficient mice are reported to have increased bone mineral density compared with normal (67). In human bone, it is concentrated in osteocytes, and its release may be a signal in the bone-turnover cascade. Osteocalcin measurements in serum have proved valuable as a marker of bone turnover in metabolic disease states.

BONE MINERALIZATION

The composition of bone enables it to perform its unique mechanical, protective, and homeostatic functions. Although this composition varies with age, anatomic location, diet, and health status, in general, mineral accounts for 50% to 70% of adult mammalian bone, the organic matrix for 20%

TABLE 7. *Gene and protein characteristics of γ-carboxy glutamic acid–containing proteins in bone matrix*

Protein	Gene	Function
Matrix Gla protein ~15 kDa Five gla residues One disulfide bridge Phosphoserine residues	12p 3.9 kb, 4 exons	May function in cartilage metabolism May inhibit mineralization
Osteocalcin (bone Gla protein: BGP) ~5 kDa One disulfide bridge Gla residues located in a helical region	1q25-31 1.2 kb, 4 exons	May regulate activity of osteoclasts and their precursors May mark the turning point between bone formation and re-sorption Regulates mineral maturation
Protein S ~73 kDa	3p11.1-q11.2 3.3 kb mRNA	Protein S deficiency may result in osteopenia

to 40%, water for 5% to 10%, and lipids for <3%. The mineral, an analogue of the geologic mineral, hydroxyapatite $[Ca_{10}(PO_4)_6(OH)_2]$, provides mechanical rigidity and load-bearing strength to the bone composite. In contrast to large geologic hydroxyapatite crystals, bone mineral crystals are extremely small (~200Å in their largest dimension). Bone mineral contains numerous impurities (carbonate, magnesium, acid phosphate) and vacancies (missing OH^-), and is usually referred to as a poorly crystalline, carbonate-substituted apatite (68). These small imperfect crystals are more soluble than geologic apatite, allowing bone to act as a reservoir for calcium, phosphate, and magnesium ions.

The organic matrix, predominantly type I collagen, provides elasticity and flexibility to bone and also determines its structural organization. Both the collagen and the noncollagenous proteins associated with the collagen influence the way bone mineralization occurs. The cells responsible for bone formation, repair, and remodeling respond to hormonal, mechanical, and other signals. Lipids, found in the membranes of these cells, control the flux of ions and also are directly involved mineralization. Water, found within the cells and in the ECM, is important for maintenance of tissue properties and nutrition.

Bone mineral is initially deposited at discrete sites in the collagenous matrix (68). As bone matures, the mineral crystals become larger and more perfect (containing fewer impurities). The increase in crystal dimension is due both to the actual addition of ions to the crystals (crystal growth) and to aggregation of the crystals (69). The initial sites of mineralization are the "hole" zones between the collagen fibrils (68). There is still debate as to whether bone mineral forms concurrently in the protected environment of membrane-bound bodies known as ECM vesicles, as it does in calcifying cartilage and mineralizing turkey tendons (51). Because the body fluids are undersaturated with respect to apatite (i.e., apatite will not precipitate spontaneously), the bone matrix must contain one or more components that facilitate apatite deposition.

Initial Mineral Deposition

The membrane-bound extracellular bodies released from chondrocytes (and osteoblasts) known as ECM vesicles, can facilitate initial mineral deposition by accumulating calcium and phosphate ions in a protected environment. Additionally, they provide enzymes that can degrade inhibitors of mineralization [e.g., adenosine triphosphate (ATP), pyrophosphate, proteoglycans], which are found in the surrounding matrix. They also contain a nucleational core, consisting of proteins and a complex of acidic phospholipids, calcium, and inorganic phosphate, which can induce apatite formation (51). Because these matrix vesicles are not directly associated with the collagen fibrils, the question of how mineral crystals form at discrete sites on the collagen fibrils remains. It is thought that there may be some association of vesicle mineral with the mineral in the collagen matrix, or that the matrix vesicle mineral may serve as a source of calcium and phosphate ions to support initial collagen-based mineralization.

In general, crystals form when the component ions of the crystal lattice, or clusters of those ions, come together with the right orientation and with sufficient energy to generate the first stable crystal ("critical nucleus"). The formation of this miniature crystal, perhaps only one or two unit cells in size, is the most energy-demanding step of crystallization. Nucleation is then followed by the addition of ions and ion clusters to the critical nucleus as the crystal grows. Growth may occur in one or more dimensions, or additional crystals may start to form at "kink" sites on the crystal, in a fashion analogous to glycogen branching. This so-called "secondary nucleation" allows exponential proliferation of crystals.

Macromolecules may facilitate the formation of the critical nucleus; sequester ions, increasing the local concentrations; or bind one or more ions, creating a structure on which "heterogeneous nucleation" occurs. As crystals proliferate, the macromolecules may bind to crystal surfaces, blocking growth in one or more directions, thereby regulating the size, shape, or (if secondary nucleation is blocked) the number of crystals.

Several possible promoters (nucleators) of bone mineral formation have been identified, based on solution studies. Originally collagen was thought to be the bone mineral nucleator (70), but more recent studies demonstrated that removal of noncollagenous proteins from bone-collagen matrices prevented these matrices from causing apatite formation (71). Removal of protein phosphate from demineralized bones reduced their nucleational ability in a concentration-dependent fashion (72), implying that one of the bone mineral nucleators was a phosphoprotein.

TABLE 8. *Bone-matrix proteins that affect* in vitro *and* in vivo *mineralization*

In vitro action	In vivo action	
	Disease model	Bone features
Apatite nucleators		
Collagen (I)	Osteogenesis imperfecta (m) oim mouse (m) mov 14 mouse (m)	Bones mechanically weak; mineral crystals small; some mineral outside collagen
Proteolipid (matrix vesicle nucleational core)	—	
Mineralization inhibitors		
Aggrecan	Brachymorphic mouse (m)	Accelerated growth-plate calcification
α_2-HS glycoprotein (fetuin)	Knockout mouse ($\downarrow$)	Adult ectopic calcification
Matrix gla protein (MGP)	Knockout mouse ($\downarrow$)	Excessive cartilage calcification
	Tiptoe-walking Yoshimura mouse ($\uparrow$)	Osteochondral lesions
Osteocalcin	Knockout mouse ($\downarrow$)	Thickened bones; decreased crystal size; increased mineral content
	Osteopetrotic mouse ($\downarrow$)	
Osteopontin	Knockout mouse ($\downarrow$)	Slightly decreased crystal size; slightly increased mineral content
Dual function (nucleate and inhibit)		
Biglycan	Knockout mouse ($\downarrow$)	Thin bones, decreased mineral content, increased crystal size
	Turner's syndrome ($\downarrow$)	Short stature, thin bones
	Kleinfelder's disease ($\uparrow$)	Excessive height
Osteonectin	Knockout mouse ($\downarrow$)	Normal to 6 mo
Decorin	Knockout mouse ($\downarrow$)	No bone phenotype
BAG-75	—	—
Thrombospondin	Knockout mouse ($\downarrow$)	Large collagen fibrils, thickened bones
Type X collagen	Transgenic mouse (m)	Altered mineral distribution in growth plate
Enzymes important for mineralization		
Alkaline phosphatase	Hypophosphatasia (a $\downarrow$)	Growth impaired; decreased mineralization
	TNAP knockout mouse ($\downarrow$)	
Gelatinase	Knockout mouse ($\downarrow$)	Delayed bone formation
Casein kinase II	Hypophosphatemic (hyp) mouse (a $\downarrow$)	Decreased crystal size

$\downarrow$, decreased expression; $\uparrow$, increased expression; m, altered expression due to mutation; a $\downarrow$, decreased enzyme activity.

The phosphoproteins of bone include collagen itself, osteopontin, BSP, and bone acidic glycoprotein-75 (BAG-75) (51). Of these, only BSP has been shown to act as an apatite nucleator in solution (73). Both osteopontin (74) and BSP (74,75) inhibit apatite proliferation and growth in solution. Table 8 lists the bone-matrix proteins that have been shown to affect apatite formation and growth in solution. As can be seen from this table, most of these macromolecules are anionic, and thus can bind Ca^{2+} in solution or on the apatite crystal surface. The table also indicates animal and human models in which the alteration or deficiency of the protein affects bone properties.

Several enzymes that regulate phosphoprotein phosphorylation and dephosphorylation also have been associated with the mineralization process (51). Of these, the phosphoprotein kinases, which regulate phosphoprotein phosphorylation, and alkaline phosphatase, and other phosphoprotein phosphatases, seem to be most important. Alkaline phosphatase hydrolyzes phosphate esters, increasing the local phosphate concentration, enhancing the rate and extent of mineralization. Blocking phosphoprotein phosphorylation in culture decreases rates of mineralization, and cells that lack alkaline phosphatase do not mineralize in certain culture systems unless transfected with that enzyme. Patients with hypophosphatasia, a deficiency of alkaline phosphatase, also show abnormal bone mineralization. Whether the function of alkaline phosphatase is simply to increase local phosphate concentrations; to remove phosphate containing inhibitors of apatite growth (such as ATP); or to modify phosphoproteins, thereby controlling their ability to act as nucleators, is still undetermined.

Growth, Proliferation, and Maturation of Mineral Crystals

The growth of bone mineral crystals is governed in part by the constraints of the collagen matrix on which the mineral is deposited. Noncollagenous proteins that bind to the mineral crystals can also regulate their size and shapes. These proteins also are important in recruiting bone-resorbing cells (osteoclasts) to the apatite crystal surface (51). As bone apatite crystals grow and mature, species other than proteins and lipids can affect their fates. These species may be introduced through the diet, given therapeutically, or accumulate from dialysis fluids. For example, of the dietary cations, both Mg^{2+} and Sr^{2+} can be incorporated directly into the bone mineral, substituting for Ca^{2+} in the crystal lattice, and yielding mineral crystals that are smaller and less perfect than those formed in their absence. Carbonate (CO_3^-), part of the body fluids, is a common constituent impurity of bone mineral, substituting for both OH^- and PO_4^{-3}, as well as adsorbing onto the crystal surface. Citrate is another impurity that adsorbs onto the surface of bone mineral. With age the total amount of carbonate increases, but the surface (labile) carbonate decreases with maturation of the mineral (76).

Whereas each of these impurities tends to make the crystals smaller, more imperfect, and more soluble, fluoride incorporation increases the size and therefore decreases the solubility of the apatite crystals (77,78). This in part is the basis for fluoride supplementation in osteoporosis therapy, as larger crystals are more resistant to osteoclastic turnover. Another type of antiresorptive agent used in osteoporosis, the bisphosphonates bind to the surface of apatite crystals and thereby block dissolution. Thus although bisphosphonate-treated crystals are not apparently altered in size (79), they tend to accumulate, increasing the bone mineral content. Tetracycline and other fluorescent compounds used to measure bone-formation rates are Ca-chelators that bind with high affinity to the surface of the most recently formed mineral. Because the newest formed crystals are small, their surface-to-volume ratios are very high, and the amount of label bound is similarly high.

Effects of Mineral Alteration on Bone Properties

Whereas the inclusion of "foreign" ions into the bone-apatite lattice can influence the properties of bone, cellular activities also can influence mineral properties. For example, where mineral deposition is retarded (e.g., hypophosphatemic rickets), crystals tend to be larger than normal (80). Crystals are smaller in osteopetrotic bone (81) where resorption is impaired, and the small crystals persist rather than being resorbed. In osteoporosis, where bone formation may be impaired and resorption accelerated, it is the larger crystals that persist (82). In skeletal fluorosis, and, in general, as bone-fluoride content increases, mineral content is increased, and crystals are increased in size (78).

The size and distribution of mineral crystals in the bone matrix can influence bone mechanical properties (83). Bone strength is dependent on bone architecture, as well as numerous other factors. Although the mechanical strength of bone has been correlated with bone mineral density (84), a measurement that describes the amount of bone in a given area without providing information on architecture, mineral content, or crystal properties, few studies have related mechanical properties to mineral characteristics. It should be clear from the diseases mentioned earlier that if there are too few crystals, or crystals are too small, the mechanical strength will be compromised. Similarly, if there are too many crystals, or crystals are excessively large, as in the case of skeletal fluorosis, bones many become brittle. Thus there is an optimal crystal size distribution, as well as an optimal amount of mineral.

Mineral Formation in Cell Culture

Osteoblasts *in vitro* synthesize an ECM that mineralizes in the presence of an exogenous phosphate source. Cell-culture studies have been used to determine mineralization mechanisms, focusing on the sequence of expression of matrix proteins. Only a few these studies (e.g., 85–89), however, demonstrated that the mineral formed was bone-like apatite. Numerous methods can be used to prove that apatite is present. The least rigorous are the histochemical stains (von Kossa for phosphate or alizarin red for calcium). Because the von Kossa silver stain gives positive reactions with anions that complex silver and all phosphate-containing materials, it cannot distinguish apatite from membranes. The alizarin red stain, specific for calcium, similarly cannot distinguish calcium complexed to the organic matrix from calcium bound to phosphate. Even when these two stains are colocalized, this does not prove that apatite is present. Similarly, more sophisticated electron-microscopic methods, such as microprobe analyses, or chemical analyses of Ca and PO_4 contents, cannot conclusively establish the presence of apatite. The uncertainly of the analytic methods is reflected in the range of Ca/PO_4 mole ratios measured for bone mineral ($1:3$ to $2:1$), distinct from the predicted $1.67:1$. The wide range of ratios is attributed to the presence of impurities and to the inclusion of nonmineral phosphate or calcium or both in the assays. Electron micrographs showing the presence of thin plates or needles associated with collagen fibrils provide more convincing evidence of the presence of apatite, but structure can be confusing, and calcium phosphates can take on other shapes (apatite in Greek means "deceiving"). Thus the electron micrographs must be accompanied by electron-diffraction analyses, which provide definite structure verification, or by other diffraction methods (x-ray, synchrotron, or neutron) which provide unambiguous proof that the mineral phase examined is apatite. Unambiguous identification of apatite also can be provided by nuclear magnetic resonance (NMR) and infrared methods (68). The infrared spectra also reveal the relative proportions and properties of the organic matrix, data not obtainable from diffraction methods.

Table 8 includes those bone-matrix proteins that have been demonstrated to affect mineral deposition in culture, as well as in solution, and lists animal models and human diseases in which the absence, modification, or overexpression of these proteins affects bone-mineral properties. It thus should be apparent that the bone cells, the bone matrix, and the extracellular environment can influence mineralization, and in turn, because the mineral properties affect mechanical strength, the properties of bone.

ACKNOWLEDGMENT

Dr. Boskey's work described in this study was supported by NIH grants DE04141, AR 37661, and AR 41325.

REFERENCES

1. Suwanwalaikorn S, van Auken M, Kang MI, Alex S, Braverman LE, Baran DT. Site selectivity of osteoblast gene expression response to thyroid hormone localized by in situ hybridization. *Am J Physiol* 1997;272:E212–E217.
2. Dunbar CE, Tisdale J, Yu JM, et al. Transduction of hematopoietic stem cells in humans and in nonhuman primates [Review]. *Stem Cells* 1997;15:135–139.

3. Aubin JE, Liu F. The osteoblast lineage. In: Bilezikian JP, Raisz LG, Rodan GA, eds. *Principles of bone biology.* San Diego: Academic Press, 1996:51–68.

4. Bruder SP, Ricalton NS, Boynton RE, et al. Mesenchymal stem cell surface antigen SB-10 corresponds to activated leukocyte cell adhesion molecule and is involved in osteogenic differentiation. *J Bone Miner Res* 1998;13:655–663.

5. Gronthos S, Graves SE, Ohta S, Simmons PJ. The STRO-1- fraction of adult human bone marrow contains the osteogenic precursors. *Blood* 1994;84:4164–4173.

6. Haynesworth SE, Baber MA, Caplan AI. Cell surface antigens on human marrow-derived mesenchymal cells are detected by monoclonal antibodies. *Bone* 1992;13:69–80.

7. Wetterwald A, Hoffstetter W, Cecchini MG, et al. Characterization and cloning of the E11 antigen, a marker expressed by rat osteoblasts and osteocytes. *Bone* 1996;18:125–132.

8. Joyner CJ, Bennett A, Triffitt JT. Identification and enrichment of human osteoprogenitor cells by using differentiation stage-specific monoclonal antibodies. *Bone* 1997;21:1–6.

9. Nijweide PJ, Mulder RJ. Identification of osteocytes in osteoblast-like cell cultures using a monoclonal antibody specifically directed against osteocytes. *Histochemistry* 1986;84:342–347.

10. Hughes DE, Salter DM, Simpson R. CD44 expression in human bone: a novel marker of osteocytic differentiation. *J Bone Miner Res* 1994;9:39–44.

11. Aubin JE, Gupta AK, Bhargava U, Turksen K. Expression and regulation of galectin 3 in rat osteoblastic cells. *J Cell Physiol* 1996;169:468–480.

12. Onishi T, Ishidou Y, Nagamine T, et al. Distinct and overlapping patterns of localization of bone morphogenetic protein (BMP) family members and a BMP type II receptor during fracture healing in rats. *Bone* 1998;22:605–612.

13. Moseley JM, Martin TJ. Parathyroid hormone-related protein: physiological actions. In: Bilezikian JP, Raisz LG, Rodan GA, eds. *Principles of bone biology.* San Diego: Academic Press, 1996:363–376.

14. Stein GS, Lian JB, Stein JL, van Wijnen AJ, Frenkel B, Montecino M. Mechanisms regulating osteoblast proliferation and differentiation. In: Bilezikian JP, Raisz LG, Rodan GA, eds. *Principles of Bone Biology.* San Diego: Academic Press, 1996;69–86.

15. Komori T, Yagi H, Nomura S, et al. Targeted disruption of Cbfa1 results in a complete lack of bone formation owing to maturational arrest of osteoblasts. *Cell* 1997;89:755–764.

16. Otto F, Thornell AP, Crompton T, et al. Cbfa1, a candidate gene for cleidocranial dysplasia syndrome, is essential for osteoblast differentiation and bone development. *Cell* 1997;89:765–771.

17. Banerjee C, McCabe LR, Choi J-Y, et al. Runt homology domain proteins in osteoblast differentiation: AML-3/CBFA1 is a major component of a bone specific complex. *J Cell Biochem* 1997;66:1–8.

18. Ogata T, Noda M. Expression of Id, a negative regulator of helix-loop-helix DNA binding proteins, is down-regulated at confluence and enhanced by dexamethasone in a mouse osteoblastic cell line, MC3T3E1. *Biochem Biophys Res Commun* 1991;181:1194–1199.

19. Glackin CA, Lee M, Lowe G, Morales S, Wergedal J, Strong D. Overexpressing human TWIST in high SaOS (HSaOS) cells results in major differences in cellular morphology, proliferation rates, and ALP activities: knocking out human Id-2 greatly reduces the expression of all TWIST family members, indicating that Id-2 may regulate TWIST during osteoblast differentiation [Abstract]. *J Bone Miner Res* 1997;12:S154.

20. Sumoy L, Wang CK, Lichtler AC, Pierro LJ, Kosher RA, Upholt WB. Identification of a spatially specific enhancer element in the chicken Msx-2 gene that regulates its expression in the apical ectodermal ridge of the developing limb buds of transgenic mice. *Dev Biol* 1995;170:230–242.

21. Ryoo H-M, Hoffmann HM, Beumer TL, et al. Stage-specific expression of Dlx-5 during osteoblast differentiation: involvement in regulation of osteocalcin gene expression. *Mol Endocrinol* 1997;11:1681–1694.

22. Machwate M, Jullienne A, Moukhtar M, Marie PJ. Temporal variation of c-*fos* proto-oncogene expression during osteoblast differentiation and osteogenesis in developing bone. *J Cell Biochem* 1995;57:62–70.

23. McCabe LR, Banerjee C, Kundu R, et al. Developmental expression and activities of specific fos and jun proteins are functionally related to osteoblast maturation: role of fra-2 and jun D during differentiation. *Endocrinology* 1996;137:4398–4408.

24. Parfitt AM, Han ZH, Palnitkar S, Rao DS, Shih MS, Nelson D. Effects of ethnicity and age or menopause on osteoblast function, bone mineralization, and osteoid accumulation in iliac bone. *J Bone Miner Res* 1997;12:1864–1873.

25. Bodine PVN, Henderson RA, Green J, et al. Estrogen receptor-α is developmentally regulated during osteoblast differentiation and contributes to selective responsiveness of gene expression. *Endocrinology* 1998;139:2048–2057.

26. van der Plas A, Aarden EM, Feijen JH, et al. Characteristics and properties of osteocytes in culture. *J Bone Miner Res* 1994;9:1697–1704.

27. Lynch MP, Capparelli C, Stein JL, Stein GS, Lian JB. Apoptosis during bone-like tissue development in vitro. *J Cell Biochem* 1998;68:31–49.

28. Civitelli R, Beyer EC, Warlow PM, Robertson AJ, Geist ST, Steinberg TH. Connexin43 mediates direct intercellular communication in human osteoblastic cell networks. *J Clin Invest* 1993;91:1888–1896.

29. Rubin CT, Lanyon LE. Osteoregulatory nature of mechanical stimuli: function as a determinant for adaptive bone remodeling. *J Orthop Res* 1987;5:300–310.

30. Simonet WS, Lacey DL, Dunstan CR, et al. Osteoprotegerin: a novel secreted protein involved in the regulation of bone density [Comments]. *Cell* 1997;89:309–319.

31. Wong BR, Josien R, Lee SY, et al. TRANCE (tumor necrosis factor [TNF]-related activation-induced cytokine): a new TNF family member predominantly expressed in T cells, is a dendritic cell-specific survival factor. *J Exp Med* 1997;186:2075–2080.

32. Yasuda H, Shima N, Nakagawa N, et al. Identity of osteoclastogenesis inhibitory factor (OCIF) and osteoprotegerin (OPG): a mechanism by which OPG/OCIF inhibits osteoclastogenesis in vitro. *Endocrinology* 1998;139:1329–1337.

33. Canalis E, Pash J, Varghese S. Skeletal growth factors. *Crit Rev Eukaryot Gene Expr* 1993;3:155–166.

34. Manolagas SC, Jilka R. Bone marrow, cytokines, and bone remodeling: emerging insights into the pathophysiology of osteoporosis. *N Engl J Med* 1995;232:305–311.

35. Jones JI, Clemmons DR. Insulin-like growth factors and their binding proteins: biological actions. *Endocr Rev* 1995;16:3–34.

36. Delany AM, Pash JM, Canalis E. Cellular and clinical perspectives on skeletal insulin-like growth factor I. *J Cell Biochem* 1994;55:328–333.

37. Hock JM, Centrella M, Canalis E. Insulin-like growth factor I (IGF-I) has independent effects on bone matrix formation and cell replication. *Endocrinology* 1988;122:254–260.

38. Canalis E, Rydziel S, Delany A, Varghese S, Jeffrey J. Insulin-like growth factors inhibit interstitial collagenase synthesis in bone cell cultures. *Endocrinology* 1995;136:1348–1354.

39. Ebeling PR, Jones JD, O'Fallon WM, Janes CH, Riggs BL. Short-term effects of recombinant human insulin-like growth factor I on bone turnover in normal women. *J Clin Endocrinol Metab* 1993;77:1384–1387.

40. Gangji V, Rydziel S, Gabbitas B, Canalis E. Insulin-like growth factor II promoter expression in cultured rodent osteoblasts and adult rat bone. *Endocrinology* 1998;139:2287–2292.

41. Canalis E. Mechanisms of glucocorticoid action in bone: implications to glucocorticoid-induced osteoporosis. *J Clin Endocrinol Metab* 1996;81:3441–3447.

42. Centrella M, McCarthy TL, Canalis E. Transforming growth factor-beta and remodeling of bone. *J Bone Joint Surg Am* 1991;73:1418–1428.

43. Wozney JM, Rosen V, Celeste AJ, et al. Novel regulators of bone formation: molecular clones and activities. *Science* 1988;242:1528–1534.

44. Burgess WH, Maciag T. The heparin-binding (fibroblast) growth factor family of proteins. *Annu Rev Biochem* 1989;58:575–606.

45. Canalis E, Centrella M, McCarthy T. Effects of basic fibroblast growth factor on bone formation in vitro. *J Clin Invest* 1988;81:1572–1577.

46. Nakamura T, Hanada K, Tamura M, et al. Stimulation of endosteal bone formation by systemic injections of recombinant basic fibroblast growth factor in rats. *Endocrinology* 1995;136:1276–1284.

47. Shiang R, Thompson LM, Zhu YZ, et al. Mutations in the transmembrane domain of FGFR3 cause the most common genetic form of dwarfism, achondroplasia. *Cell* 1994;78:335–342.

48. Heldin CH, Westermark B. PDGF-like growth factors in autocrine stimulation of growth. *J Cell Physiol* 1987;5:31–34.

49. Rydziel S, Shaikh S, Canalis E. Platelet-derived growth factors AA and BB enhance the synthesis of platelet-derived growth factor AA in bone cell cultures. *Endocrinology* 1994;134:2541–2546.

50. Hock JM, Canalis E. Platelet-derived growth factor enhances bone cell replication but not differentiated function of osteoblasts. *Endocrinology* 1994;134:1423–1428.

51. Gehron Robey P, Boskey AL. The biochemistry of bone. In: Marcus R, Feldman D, eds. *Osteoporosis.* New York: Raven Press, 1996:95–184.

52. Gorski JP. Is all bone the same? Distinctive distributions and properties of non-collagenous matrix proteins in lamellar vs. woven bone imply the existence of different underlying osteogenic mechanisms. *Crit Rev Oral Biol Med* 1998;9:201–223.

53. Rossert J, de Crombrugghe B. Type I collagen: structure, synthesis and regulation. In: Bilezikian JP, Raisz LG, Rodan GA, eds. *Principles of bone biology.* San Diego: Academic Press, 1996:127–142.

54. Eyre DR. Biochemical basis of collagen metabolites as bone turnover markers. In: Bilezikian JP, Raisz LG, Rodan GA, eds. *Principles of bone biology.* San Diego: Academic Press, 1996:143–154.

55. Gehron Robey P. Bone matrix proteoglycans and glycoproteins. In: Bilezikian JP, Raisz LG, Rodan GA, eds. *Principles of bone biology.* San Diego: Academic Press, 1996:155–165.

56. Xu T, Bianco P, Fisher LW, et al. Targeted disruption of the biglycan gene leads to an osteoporosis-like phenotype in mice. *Nat Genet* 1998; 20:78–82.

57. Wendel M, Sommarin Y, Heinegard D. Bone matrix proteins: isolation and characterization of a novel cell-binding keratan sulfate proteoglycan (osteoadherin) from bovine bone. *J Cell Biol* 1998;141:839–847.

58. Henthorn PS. Alkaline phosphatase. In: Bilezikian JP, Raisz LG, Rodan GA, eds. *Principles of bone biology.* San Diego: Academic Press, 1996: 197–206.

59. Lane TF, Sage EH. The biology of SPARC, a protein that modulates cell-matrix interactions. *FASEB J* 1994;8:163–173.

60. Gilmour DT, Lyon GJ, Carlton MB, et al. Mice deficient for the secreted glycoprotein SPARC/osteonectin/BM40 develop normally but show severe age-onset cataract formation and disruption of the lens. *EMBO J* 1998;17:1860–1870.

61. Butler WT, Ridall AL, McKee MD. Osteopontin. In: Bilezikian JP, Raisz LG, Rodan GA, eds. *Principles of bone biology.* San Diego: Academic Press, 1996:167–182.

62. D'Souza RN, Cavender A, Sunavala G, et al. Gene expression patteof murine dentin matrix protein 1 (Dmp1) and dentin sialophosphorprotein (DSPP) suggest distinct developmental functions in vivo. *J Bone Miner Res* 1997;12:2040–2049.

63. Liaw L, Birk DE, Ballas CB, Whitsitt JS, Davidson JM, Hogan BL. Altered wound healing in mice lacking a functional osteopontin gene. *J Clin Invest* 1998;101(Supp 1):1468–1478.

64. Gehron Robey P, Bianco P, Termine JD. The cell biology and molecular biochemistry of bone formation. In: Favus MJ, Coe FL, eds. *Disorders of mineral metabolism.* New York: Raven Press, 1992:241–263.

65. Ducy P, Karsenty G. Skeletal gla proteins: gene structure, regulation of expression and function. In: Bilezikian JP, Raisz LG, Rodan GA, eds. *Principles of bone biology.* San Diego: Academic Press, 1996:183–196.

66. Luo G, Ducy P, McKee MD, et al. Spontaneous calcification of arteries and cartilage in mice lacking matrix GLA protein. *Nature* 1997; 386:78–81.

67. Ducy P, Desbois C, Boyce B, et al. Increased bone formation in osteocalcin-deficient mice. *Nature* 1996;382:448–452.

68. Glimcher MJ. The nature of the mineral phase in bone: biological and clinical implications. In: Avioli LV, Krane SM, eds. *Metabolic bone disease and clinically related disorders.* 3rd ed. San Diego, 1998: 23–51.

69. Landis WJ. The strength of a calcified tissue depends in part on the molecular structure and organization of its constituent mineral crystals in their organic matrix. *Bone* 1995;16:533–544.

70. Glimcher MJ. Molecular biology of mineralized tissues with particular reference to bone. *Rev Mod Physics* 1959;31:359–393.

71. Termine JD, Belcourt AB, Conn KM, Kleinman HK. Mineral and collagen-binding proteins of fetal calf bone. *J Biol Chem* 1981; 256:10403–10408.

72. Glimcher MJ. Mechanisms of calcification in bone: role of collafibrils and collagen-phosphoprotein complexes in vitro and in vivo. *Anat Rec* 1989;224:139–153.

73. Hunter GK, Goldberg HA. Nucleation of hydroxyapatite by bone sialoprotein. *Proc Natl Acad Sci U S A* 1993;90:8562–8565.

74. Boskey AL. Osteopontin and related phosphorylated sialoproteins: effects on mineralization. *Ann N Y Acad Sci* 1995;760:249–256.

75. Stubbs JT III, Mintz KP, Eanes ED, Torchia DA, Fisher LW. Characterization of native and recombinant bone sialoprotein: delineation of the mineral-binding and cell adhesion domains and structural analysis of the RGD domain. *J Bone Miner Res* 1997;12:1210–1222.

76. Rey C, Renugopalakrishnan V, Shimizu M, Collins B, Glimcher MJ. A resolution-enhanced Fourier transform infrared spectroscopic study of the environment of the $CO_3(2-)$ ion in the mineral phase of enamel during its formation and maturation. *Calcif Tissue Int* 1991;49: 259–268.

77. Posner AS. Significance of calcium phosphate crystallographic studies to orthopedics. *Bull Hosp Joint Dis* 1970;31:14–26.

78. Grynpas MD. Fluoride effects on bone crystals. *J Bone Miner Res Suppl* 1990;1:S169–S175.

79. Fratzl P, Schreiber S, Roschger P, Lafage MH, Rodan G, Klaushofer K. Effects of sodium fluoride and alendronate on the bone mineral in minipigs: a small-angle x-ray scattering and backscattered electron imaging study. *J Bone Miner Res* 1996;11:248–253.

80. Boskey AL, Gilder H, Neufeld E, Ecarot B, Glorieux FH. Phospholipid changes in the bones of the hypophosphatemic mouse. *Bone* 1991; 12:345–351.

81. Boskey AL, Marks SC Jr. Mineral and matrix alterations in the bones of incisors-absent (ia/ia) osteopetrotic rats. *Calcif Tissue Int* 1985; 37:287–292.

82. Paschalis EP, Betts F, DiCarlo E, Mendelsohn R, Boskey AL. Fmicrospectroscopic analysis of human iliac crest biopsies from untreated osteoporotic bone. *Calcif Tissue Int* 1997;61:487–492.

83. Martin RB. Aging and strength of bone as a structural material. *Calcif Tissue Int* 1993;53:34–40.

84. Currey JD, Brear K, Zioupos P. The effects of ageing and changes in mineral content in degrading the toughness of human femora. *J Biomech* 1996;29:257–260.

85. Ecarot-Charrier B, Glorieux FH, van der Rest M, Pereira G. Osteoblasts isolated from mouse calvaria initiate matrix mineralization in culture. *J Cell Biol* 1983;96:639–643.

86. Gerstenfeld LC, Chipman SD, Kelly CM, Hodgens KJ, Lee DD, Landis WJ. Collagen expression, ultrastructural assembly, and mineralization in cultures. *J Cell Biol* 1988;106:979–989.

87. Rey C, Kim HM, Gerstenfeld L, Glimcher MJ. Characterization of the apatite crystals of bone and their maturation in osteoblast cell culture: comparison with native bone crystals. *Connect Tissue Res* 1996;35: 343–349.

88. Nagata T, Bellows CG, Kasugai S, Butler WT, Sodek J. Biosynthesis of bone proteins [SPP-1 (secreted phosphoprotein-1, osteopontin), BSP (bone sialoprotein) and SPARC (osteonectin)] in association with mineralized-tissue formation by fetal-rat calvarial cells in culture. *Biochem J* 1991;274:513–520.

89. Boskey AL, Stiner D, Binderman I, Doty SB. Effects of proteoglycan modification on mineral formation in a differentiating chick limb-bud mesenchymal cell culture system. *J Cell Biochem* 1997;64:632–643.

4. Bone Remodeling

Gregory R. Mundy, M.D.

Department of Medicine, Division of Endocrinology and Metabolism,
University of Texas Health Science Center, San Antonio, Texas

The adult skeleton is in a dynamic state, being continually broken down and reformed by the coordinated actions of osteoclasts and osteoblasts on trabecular (also called cancellous) bone surfaces and in haversian systems. This turnover or remodeling of bone occurs in focal and discrete packets throughout the skeleton. The remodeling of each packet takes a finite period (estimated to be about 3 to 4 months, but differing in cortical and cancellous bone, and probably longer in cancellous bone). The remodeling that occurs in each packet [called a bone-remodeling unit by Frost, who gave the first modern description of this sequence over 30 years ago (1)] is geographically and chronologically separated from other packets of remodeling. This suggests that activation of the sequence of cellular events responsible for remodeling is locally controlled, most likely by local mechanisms in the bone microenvironment. The sequence is always the same: activation of osteoclast precursors, and then osteoclastic bone resorption, followed by osteoblastic bone formation to repair the defect. A diagram of the cellular events involved in bone remodeling is shown in Fig. 1. The new bone that is formed is called a bone structural unit (BSU) (1).

In this chapter, a review of the cellular events involved in remodeling, the disturbances in remodeling that occur in bone diseases, and the hypotheses that have been proposed for coordination of these cellular events are outlined.

REMODELING IN DIFFERENT PARTS OF THE SKELETON

The bones of the adult skeleton consist either of cortical (or compact) bone and cancellous (or trabecular) bone. Current evidence indicates that cortical bone and cancellous bone do not change with age in exactly the same way, and so they probably should be considered as two separate

functional entities. The proportions of cortical and cancellous bone differ at the different sites in the skeleton where osteoporotic fractures frequently occur (Fig. 2). Cancellous bone is relatively prominent in the vertebral column, the most common site of fracture associated with osteoporosis. In the lumbar spine, cancellous bone composes >66% of the total bone. In the intertrochanteric area of the femur, bone is composed of 50% cortical and 50% cancellous. In the neck of the femur, the bone is 75% cortical and 25% cancellous. In contrast, in the midradius, >95% of the bone is cortical bone. The differences in behavior of bone at these different sites are most likely the result of the different environments of the bone cells in cortical or cancellous bone. Bone-remodeling cells on cancellous bone surfaces are in intimate contact with the cells of the marrow cavity, which produce a variety of potent osteotropic cytokines. It is likely that the cells in cortical bone, which are more distant from the influences of these cytokines, are controlled more by the systemic osteotropic hormones, such as parathyroid hormone and 1,25-dihydroxyvitamin D_3. Osteoclasts and osteoblasts on cancellous bone surfaces may be controlled primarily by factors produced by adjacent bone marrow cells. Similar cells that are present in haversian systems of cortical bone are not in such close contact with the myriad osteotropic cytokines produced by marrow mononuclear cells.

REMODELING OF CORTICAL BONE

Cortical bone is dense or compact bone. It composes 85% of the total bone in the body and is relatively most abundant in the long-bone shafts of the appendicular skeleton. The volume of cortical bone is regulated by the formation of periosteal bone, by remodeling within haversian systems, and by endosteal bone resorption. Cortical bone is removed primarily by endosteal resorption and resorption within the

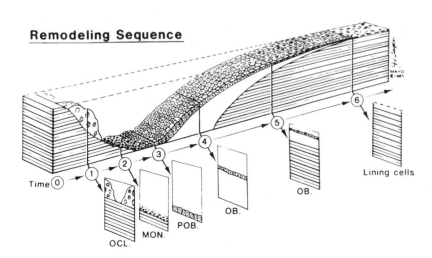

Remodeling Sequence

Time 0 1 2 3 4 5 6
OCL. MON. POB. OB. OB. Lining cells

FIG. 1. Bone remodeling in cancellous bone as seen in longitudinal sequence and cross sections. Five different phases can be distinguished over time: (1) osteoclastic resorption, (2) reversal, (3) preosteoblastic migration and differentiation into osteoblasts, (4) osteoblastic matrix (osteoid) formation, and (5) mineralization. The end product of remodeling in cancellous bone is the completed cancellous bone structural unit (BSU) covered by lining cells (6). (From Eriksen EF, Axelrod DW, Melsen F. *Bone histomorphometry.* New York: Raven Press, 1994: 3–12.)

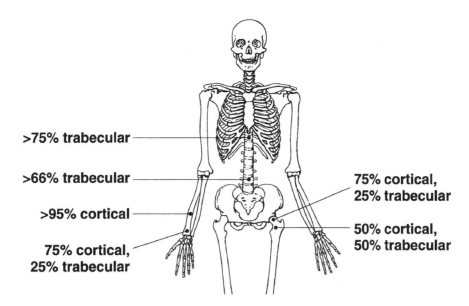

FIG. 2. Relative proportions of cortical (compact) and trabecular (cancellous) bone in different parts of the skeleton.

haversian canals. The latter leads to increased porosity of cortical bone. However, periosteal bone formation continues to increase the diameter of cortical bone throughout life. Cortical bone loss probably begins to occur after age 40 years (according to most studies), and an acceleration of cortical bone loss occurs for 5 to 10 years after the menopause. This accelerated phase of cortical bone loss continues for 15 years and then gradually slows. There is irrefutable evidence that estrogen-replacement therapy after the menopause preserves cortical bone. In later life, women with osteoporosis lose cortical bone at rates similar to those of premenopausal women. Loss of cortical bone is the major predisposing factor for fractures that occur at the hip and around the wrist. Cortical bone is particularly prone to increased resorption in patients with primary hyperparathyroidism.

REMODELING OF CANCELLOUS BONE

Although cancellous bone composes only 15% of the skeleton, the changes that occur in this type of bone after age 30 years largely determine whether spinal osteoporotic fractures will occur. Depending on the technique used, decline in cancellous bone mass begins in early adult life, occurring earlier than the decline in cortical bone mass (2). Other studies disagreed with these findings and suggested that the decline in cancellous bone mass begins later, after ovarian function ceases (3). Riggs and Melton (4) suggested that acceleration in cancellous bone loss occurring at the time of the menopause is not so prominent as the accelerated loss of cortical bone mass that occurs at this time.

Cancellous bone is the type of bone lost predominantly in patients with osteolytic bone disease due to malignancy. In this situation, the malignant cells lodge in the marrow cavity and produce local factors that stimulate adjacent osteoclasts on trabecular plates and on endosteal surfaces of

cortical bone (5,6). The loss of cancellous bone that occurs with aging is not due simply to a generalized thinning of the bone plates, but is rather due to complete perforation and fragmentation of trabeculae (7,8). Because cancellous bone has a broad surface area, resorption may be modulated by focal osteoclastic resorption regulated by local hormonal factors produced by cells in the bone-marrow microenvironment, including marrow cells as well as other types of bone cells.

Osteoclast activation is the initial step in the remodeling sequence. Osteoclasts are activated in specific focal sites by mechanisms that are still not understood. The rate of bone remodeling is to a large degree dependent on the activation frequency of osteoclasts. The mechanism responsible for the initiation of bone remodeling is unknown. One possibility is that osteoclast precursors recognize a change in the mechanical properties of aging bone, which requires replacement with new bone for optimal structural integrity. This theoretic possibility could occur because other cells, such as immune cells or osteocytes, recognize a change in the bone surface and send signals to osteoclasts to activate them. However, the initial trigger for such activation of immune cells is unknown. The eventual activation of the osteoclast may occur because of interactions that occur between integral membrane proteins (integrins) on osteoclast cell membranes with proteins in bone matrix that contain RGD (arginine-glycine-asparagine) amino acid sequences (such as osteopontin) (9). The resorptive phase of the remodeling process has been estimated to last 10 days (Fig. 1). This period is followed by repair of the defect by a team of osteoblasts, which are attracted to the site of the resorption defect and then presumably proceed to make new bone. This part of the process takes approximately 3 months. The initial events in the formation phase are possibly unidirectional migration (chemotaxis) of osteoblast precursors to the site of the defect, followed by enhanced cell proliferation. The complete sequence of cellular events that occur at the bone surface during the remodeling process was described in detail by Baron et al. (10) from studies on the alveolar bone of the rat and from Boyce et al. (11,12) from the calvarial bone of the mouse. The cellular events that occur in these models are similar to those in adult human bone.

BONE REMODELING AND DISEASE

All of the diseases of bone are superimposed on this normal cellular-remodeling sequence. In diseases such as primary hyperparathyroidism, hyperthyroidism, and Paget's disease, in which osteoclasts are activated, there is a compensatory and (relatively) balanced increase in the formation of new bone. However, there are also a number of well-described conditions in which osteoblast activity does not completely repair and replace the defect left by previous resorption. One example is myeloma, usually characterized by punched-out lytic bone lesions with little new bone formation (13). In myeloma, there appears to be a specific defect in osteoblast maturation (14). There are probably increased numbers of osteoblasts around the edges of the lytic lesions, but the osteoblasts fail (in the great majority of patients) to synthesize more than thin osteoid seams. In solid tumors associated with malignancy, there is a failure of bone formation to repair resorptive defects, especially in patients dying of their malignancy (15). In elderly patients with osteoporosis, there is a decrease in mean wall thickness, presumably reflecting the inability of osteoblasts to repair adequately the resorptive defects made during normal osteoclastic resorption (16). It also should be stressed that progressive bone loss, beginning at about 35 years of age (depending on the bone) occurs in all humans, and is indicative of a ''physiologic'' imbalance between resorption and formation.

Although bone formation usually occurs on sites of previous osteoclastic resorption in normal adult humans, there are several special situations in which osteoblasts may lay down new bone on surfaces not previously resorbed. Two examples are osteoblastic metastases associated with tumors such as carcinoma of the prostate and breast and during prolonged exposure to pharmacologic doses of fluoride therapy.

COUPLING

In most physiologic and pathologic circumstances, the coupling of bone formation to previous bone resorption occurs faithfully. Packets of bone removed during resorption are replaced during formation. The cellular and humoral mechanisms responsible for mediating the coupling process (or disrupting it, as in the diseases described earlier) are still not clear. Several theories have been proposed to account for coupling. Almost 20 years ago, Rasmussen and Bordier (17) suggested that the osteoclast, once it finishes the resorptive phase of the remodeling sequence, undergoes fission to form mononuclear cells that are the precursors of osteoblasts. However, it is now widely accepted that osteoclasts and osteoblasts have different origins. Osteoclasts arise from hematopoietic stem cells or at least stem cells in the marrow environment that have the capacity to circulate. Osteoblasts,

in contrast, arise from stromal mesenchymal cells. Many workers have favored the notion that coupling is humorally mediated, that an osteoblast-stimulating factor [such as insulin-like growth factor (IGF)-I, IGF-II, or transforming growth factor-β (TGF-β)] is released from bone matrix during the process of osteoclastic bone resorption, and the stimulation of osteoblast activity leads to new bone formation (18). A variation on this humoral concept is that the factor that stimulates resorption also acts directly (but more slowly) on osteoblasts to cause their activation and subsequent new bone formation (19). This notion suggests that coupling does not involve sequential signals released during the process of bone remodeling, but rather that factors that work through the GP-130 signal-transduction mechanism are responsible for simultaneous stimulation of osteoclast and osteoblast lineages. Mesenchymal stem cells in the bone microenvironment have been emphasized as important regulators of the entire process. An alternative to the humoral hypothesis for coupling is that because osteoblasts normally line bone surfaces, once the phase of osteoclastic resorption is over and osteoclasts disappear from the resorption site, osteoblasts and their precursors repopulate the resorption site and merely reline the bone surface. Possibly through cell-surface molecules, they recognize the resorption site, and this stimulates their differentiation into mature bone-forming cells. They may thus repair the resorptive defect without the necessity for involvement of a humoral mediator that is specifically generated as a consequence of resorption.

Obviously, understanding this sequence of cellular events may lead to clarification of the mechanisms responsible for the decreased osteoblast activity that occurs in age-related bone loss, and possibly the pathophysiology of osteoporosis, as well as the specific defects in osteoblast function that occur in malignancies such as myeloma, breast cancer, and prostate cancer.

CELLULAR EVENTS INVOLVED IN THE RESORPTION PHASE

Osteoclast Origin and Cell Lineage

The first event during bone remodeling is osteoclast activation, followed by osteoclast formation, polarization, formation of a ruffled border, resorption, and ultimately apoptosis. Apoptosis occurring at the conclusion of the resorbing phase of the bone-remodeling process is a recently observed phenomenon (20). The morphologic characteristics of osteoclast apoptosis are condensation of the nuclear chromatin, darker staining of the osteoclast cytoplasm, loss of ruffled border and detachment from the mineralized bone matrix, and cessation of bone resorption. Observations by Hughes and Boyce (21) suggested that osteoclast apoptosis is a common occurrence at reversal sites and may be precipitated by resorption inhibitors such as estrogen and bisphosphonates and also by TGF-β (21). Regulation of the process of osteoclast apoptosis may potentially be important during bone resorption, because this represents a step by which bone resorption could be regulated.

Regulation of Osteoclast Activity

Osteoclasts lie on bone surfaces in a bed of elliptic or fusiform spindle-shaped cells called lining cells, which are probably members of the osteoblast lineage. When exposed to a bone-resorbing agent, the first response is that these lining cells retract, and the osteoclasts insinuate an arm into the retracted area, a ruffled border forms, and bone is resorbed at the exposed surface (22). The molecular mechanisms by which these complicated processes are controlled are unknown. Why lining cells retract at specific sites and how the osteoclast is activated is still not clear. It appears most likely that the osteoclast is activated by a soluble signal released from the lining cell (23,24), and the recently discovered RANK ligand (also called TRANCE and ODIF) is a likely candidate (25).

Many hormones and factors have been shown to stimulate osteoclast activity. Their mechanisms of action differ. Osteoclastic resorption may be stimulated by factors that enhance proliferation of osteoclast progenitors, which cause differentiation of committed precursors into mature cells or activation of the mature multinucleated cell to resorb bone (26). Similarly, osteoclasts could be inhibited by agents that block proliferation of precursors, which inhibit differentiation or fusion, or which inactivate the mature multinucleated resorbing cell. Current evidence indicates that most factors that stimulate or inhibit osteoclasts act on at least two of these steps.

Systemic Hormones

The systemic hormones, parathyroid hormone, 1,25-dihydroxyvitamin D [1,25 (OH)$_2$ D], and calcitonin, all influence osteoclast activity.

Parathyroid Hormone

Parathyroid Hormone (PTH) stimulates differentiation of committed progenitors to fuse to form mature multinucleated osteoclasts. It also activates preformed osteoclasts to resorb bone. However, it does not increase granulocyte/macrophage–colony-forming unit (GM-CFU), the earliest detectable cells in the osteoclast lineage. The activation of osteoclasts is probably indirect, likely mediated through cells in the osteoblast lineage such as the lining cells (27). The mechanisms by which osteoblasts send the second signal to the multinucleated osteoclasts in response to PTH is not known.

Parathyroid hormone-related protein (PTHrP) has effects identical to those of PTH on osteoclasts.

1,25-Dihydroxyvitamin D

1,25-Dihydroxyvitamin D is a potent stimulator of osteoclastic bone resorption. Like PTH, it stimulates osteoclast progenitors to differentiate and fuse (28). It has a similar effect on macrophage polykaryons that are not osteoclasts. It also activates mature preformed osteoclasts, possibly by a mechanism similar to that of PTH. 1,25 (OH)$_2$ D also has other indirect effects on bone resorption. It is a potent immunoregulatory molecule (29). It inhibits T-cell proliferation and the production of the cytokine interleukin-2. Under some circumstances, it can enhance interleukin-1 production from cells with monocyte characteristics. Thus the overall effects of 1,25 (OH)$_2$ D on bone resorption are multiple and complex.

Calcitonin

Calcitonin is a polypeptide hormone that is a potent inhibitor of osteoclastic bone resorption, but its effects are only transient. Osteoclasts escape from the inhibitory effects of calcitonin after continued exposure (30). Thus patients treated for hypercalcemia with calcitonin will respond for only a limited period before hypercalcemia recurs (usually 48 to 72 hours). Even in pagetic patients, the beneficial effects of calcitonin may eventually be lost with continued treatment. The "escape" phenomenon is likely due to down-regulation of messenger RNA (mRNA) for the receptor (31). Calcitonin causes cytoplasmic contraction of the osteoclast cell membrane, which has been correlated with its capacity to inhibit bone resorption (32). It also causes the dissolution of mature osteoclasts into mononuclear cells. However, it also inhibits osteoclast formation, inhibiting both proliferation of the progenitors and differentiation of the committed precursors. The effects of calcitonin on osteoclasts are mediated by cyclic adenosine monophosphate (cAMP).

Local Hormones

Local hormones may be more important than systemic hormones for the initiation of physiologic bone resorption and for the normal bone-remodeling sequence. Because bone remodeling occurs in discrete and distinct packets throughout the skeleton, it seems probable that the cellular events are controlled by factors generated in the microenvironment of bone. Recently a number of potent local stimulators and inhibitors of osteoclast activity were identified.

Interleukin-1

There are two interleukin-1 molecules, interleukin-1α and -1β. Their effects on bone appear to be the same and are mediated through the same receptor. Interleukin-1 is released by activated monocytes but also by other types of cells including osteoblasts and tumor cells. It is a potent stimulator of osteoclasts. It works at all phases in the formation and activation of osteoclasts. It stimulates proliferation of the progenitors and differentiation of committed precursors into mature cells (33). It also activates the mature multinucleated osteoclast indirectly through another cell (possibly a bone-lining cell) (34).

Interleukin-1 also stimulates osteoclastic bone resorption when infused *in vivo* and causes a substantial increase in the plasma calcium (35,36). At least part of its effects may be mediated by prostaglandin generation. It was recently implicated as a potential mediator of bone resorption and increased bone turnover in osteoporosis (37). It may be responsible for the increase in bone resorption seen in some malignancies, as well as the localized bone resorption associated with collections of chronic inflammatory cells in diseases such as rheumatoid arthritis.

Lymphotoxin and Tumor Necrosis Factor

Lymphotoxin and tumor necrosis factor (TNF) are molecules that are related functionally to interleukin-1. Many of their biologic properties overlap with those of interleukin-1. They share the same receptor with each other, which is distinct from that of interleukin-1. Their effects on bone are synergistic with those of interleukin-1. Lymphotoxin is released by activated T lymphocytes, and TNF, by activated macrophages. TNF is one of the mediators of the systemic effects of endotoxic shock. It also causes wasting (cachexia) and suppresses erythropoiesis or red blood cell formation. Lymphotoxin and TNF stimulate proliferation of osteoclast progenitors, cause fusion of committed precursors to form multinucleated cells, and activate multinucleated cells (through cells in the osteoblast lineage) to resorb bone (38–40). Lymphotoxin may be an important mediator of bone resorption in myeloma (41). Lymphotoxin and TNF cause osteoclastic bone resorption and hypercalcemia when infused or injected *in vivo* (39,41,42).

Colony-Stimulating Factor-1

Colony stimulating factor-1 (CSF-1), also called monocyte–macrophage CSF or M-CSF, which was once thought to be specific for the monocyte–macrophage lineage, was recently shown to be required for normal osteoclast formation in rodents during the neonatal period. In the op/op variant of osteopetrosis, there is impaired production of CSF-1, and the consequence is osteopetrosis due to decreased normal osteoclast formation (see earlier). The disease can be cured by treatment with CSF-1 (43). CSF-1 is produced by stromal cells in the osteoclast microenvironment. Presumably cells in the osteoclast lineage contain the CSF-1 receptor (a receptor tyrosine kinase), and this is the mechanism by which CSF-1 mediates osteoclast formation.

Interleukin-18

The cytokine interleukin-18 is an inhibitor of osteoclast formation, its effects dependent on the release of granulocyte/macrophage–colony-stimulating factor by T cells, but independent of the cytokine interferon-γ (44).

ODIF/RANK Ligand

A member of the TNF-receptor superfamily, osteoclastogenesis inhibitory factor (OCIF) or osteoprotegerin (OPG) has recently been identified. OCIF inhibits bone resorption independent of the stimulus (45,46). This protein represents a peptide that is a soluble secreted form of the TNF receptor and acts as an antagonist to osteoclastic bone resorption both *in vitro* and *in vivo*. Even more recently, the ligand for this endogenous antagonist was identified as the putative

osteoclastogenesis differentiation–inducing factor (ODIF), which acts directly on osteoclasts. It appears to be identical or at the very least related to RANK ligand (also called TRANCE) (25). This peptide, which has a membrane-bound form, is also a ligand for OPG/OCID (47) and has been shown to stimulate osteoclastic bone resorption in marrow cultures by acting directly on cells in the osteoclast lineage. This has led to the concept that osteoprotegerin or OCIF inhibits bone resorption by binding directly to TRANCE/ODIF, the final common mediator of osteoclastic bone resorption.

Interleukin-6

Interleukin-6 is a pleiotropic cytokine with important effects on bone. It is expressed and secreted by normal bone cells in response to osteotropic hormones such as PTH; 1,25 $(OH)_2$ D; and interleukin-1 (48). The osteoclast is the most prodigious cell source of interleukin-6 so far described. Interleukin-6 is a fairly weak stimulator of osteoclast formation and less powerful than other cytokines such as interleukin-1, TNF, and lymphotoxin (49,50). It was recently implicated in the bone loss associated with estrogen withdrawal (ovariectomy) in the mouse (51). It is probable that related cytokines such as interleukin-11 and leukemia inhibitory factor work through similar mechanisms.

Interferon-γ

Interferon-γ is a multifunctional lymphokine produced by activated T lymphocytes. In contrast to the other immune cell products, it inhibits osteoclastic bone resorption (52,53). Its major effect appears to be to inhibit differentiation of committed precursors to mature cells (54). It also has effects on osteoclast-precursor proliferation but is less potent. Unlike calcitonin, it does not cause cytoplasmic contraction of isolated osteoclasts.

Transforming Growth Factor-β

TGF-β is a multifunctional polypeptide produced by immune cells but also is released from the bone matrix during resorption. TGF-β has unique effects on osteoclasts. In most systems, it inhibits osteoclast formation by inhibiting both proliferation and differentiation of osteoclast precursors (33,55). In addition, it directly inhibits the activity of mature osteoclasts by decreasing superoxide production and inhibits accumulation of tartrate-resistant acid phosphatase in osteoclasts. Because TGF-β has a powerful effect on osteoblasts (stimulates proliferation and synthesis of differentiated proteins, increases mineralized bone formation) (56), it may be a pivotal factor in the bone-remodeling process. For example, it could be released during this resorption process and then be available as a natural endogenous inhibitor of continued osteoclast activity. At the same time, working in conjunction with other bone factors, it may lead to osteoblast stimulation and the eventual formation of new bone. However, the effects of TGF-β are complex and may differ in different species. In one system, neonatal mouse calvariae, it stimulates prostaglandin generation, which in turn leads to bone resorption, the effect opposite that seen in the rat or human systems (57).

Other Factors

A number of other factors have precise roles in physiologic and pathologic bone resorption still to be delineated.

Retinoids. Vitamin A is the only fully characterized factor that has a direct stimulatory effect on osteoclasts (58). Vitamin A excess eventually leads to increased bone resorption *in vivo* and hypercalcemia. It is unknown whether the effects of vitamin A on osteoclasts have physiological significance.

Transforming Growth Factor-β. TGF-β, like the related compound epidermal growth factor (EGF), is a powerful stimulator of osteoclastic bone resorption (57,59–61). TGF-β is produced by many tumors and is likely involved in increased bone resorption associated with cancer. It is probably produced normally during embryonic life. It stimulates the proliferation of osteoclast progenitors and probably also acts on immature multinucleated cells. Its actions on osteoclasts are comparable to those of the colony-stimulating factors on other hematopoietic cells (62). The effects of TGF-β on bone cells are mediated through the EGF receptor, although it is more potent than EGF on bone resorption. Injections or infusions of TGF-β increase the plasma calcium *in vivo* (42).

Neutral Phosphate and Calcium. Neutral phosphate inhibits osteoclast activity in organ cultures (63). The precise mode of action is not clear. Phosphate is a useful form of therapy in patients with increased bone resorption and diseases such as cancer or primary hyperparathyroidism, although it may have other effects in addition to those of inhibiting bone resorption, such as impairment of calcium absorption from the gut.

High extracellular calcium concentrations also lead to decreased osteoclast activity associated with an increase in intracellular calcium concentrations. This suggests another mechanism by which continued osteoclast activity to resorb bone may be regulated by increased local calcium concentrations.

Prostaglandins. Prostaglandins have complex and multiple effects on osteoclasts, depending on the species. Prostaglandins have been linked to the hypercalcemia and increased bone resorption associated with malignancy and chronic inflammation (64). However, the effects of prostaglandins are confusing. Prostaglandins of the E series stimulate osteoclastic bone resorption in organ culture. Moreover, some bone-resorbing factors, and particularly growth factors, appear to mediate their effects through the production of prostaglandins in mouse bones. Prostaglandins inhibit the formation of human osteoclasts and cause cytoplasmic contraction of isolated osteoclasts in much the same way as calcitonin. However, prostaglandins stimulate the formation of mouse multinucleated osteoclasts from marrow progenitors. The overall significance of prostaglandins depends on the species studied. Their overall effects on bone resorption in humans are still a mystery.

Leukotrienes. Leukotrienes, like prostaglandins, are arachidonic acid metabolites that have been linked to osteoclastic bone resorption (65). They are produced by the metabolism of arachidonic acid by a 5-lipoxygenase enzyme. Several of these leukotrienes have been shown to activate osteoclasts *in vitro* and may be related to the bone resorption seen in giant-cell tumors of bone. These arachidonic acid metabolites have different effects on osteoclasts from prostaglandins of the E series, which stimulate osteoclastic bone resorption in organ culture and cause transient inhibition of the activity of isolated osteoclasts. In contrast, the leukotrienes stimulate osteoclastic bone resorption in organ culture but also enhance the capacity of isolated osteoclasts to form resorption pits. Null mutant mice in which the 5-lipoxygenase gene is nonfunctional have increased amounts of cortical bone (66).

Thyroid Hormones. The thyroid hormones thyroxine and triiodothyronine stimulate osteoclastic bone resorption in organ cultures (67). Some patients with hyperthyroidism have increased bone loss, increased osteoclast activity, and hypercalcemia. Thyroid hormones act directly on osteoclastic bone resorption, but their precise mode of action is unknown.

Glucocorticoids. Glucocorticoids inhibit osteoclast formation *in vitro* and inhibit osteoclastic bone resorption in organ cultures. Their efficacy depends on the stimulus to bone resorption. They are less effective in inhibiting bone resorption stimulated by PTH than they are in inhibiting bone resorption stimulated by cytokines such as interleukin-1 (68).

In vivo, glucocorticoid administration is associated with increased bone resorption. This is an indirect effect, and is due to the effects of glucocorticoids to inhibit calcium absorption from the gut. As a consequence, parathyroid gland activity is stimulated, and secondary hyperparathyroidism leads to a generalized increase in osteoclastic bone resorption.

Estrogens and Androgens. Estrogen lack is associated with increased osteoclastic bone resorption in the 10 years after the menopause (69). The mechanisms are not clear. Recent separate reports suggested that estrogens may affect osteoclasts directly (70), but in addition, estrogens may mediate their effects on osteoclasts indirectly by suppressing the production of bone-resorbing cytokines such as interleukin-1 and interleukin-6 (37,51,71). These notions suggested that estrogen withdrawal, for example, at the menopause, then leads to enhanced bone resorption.

Pharmacologic Agents. A number of pharmacologic agents have been used as inhibitors of bone resorption and are useful therapies in patients with diseases such as malignancy associated with hypercalcemia. These include plicamycin (mithramycin), gallium nitrate, and the bisphosphonates (26). All of these agents inhibit osteoclastic activity, although their specific mechanism of action is unknown or controversial. In the case of the cytotoxic drugs plicamycin and gallium nitrate, it is possible that their actions are mediated through cytotoxic effects on osteoclasts or inhibition of proliferation of the osteoclast progenitors.

Bisphosphonates are very important inhibitors of osteoclastic bone resorption *in vivo* and are achieving increased use in diseases associated with increased bone resorption, and particularly in osteoporosis, hypercalcemia of malignancy, Paget's disease of bone, and osteolytic bone disease. Their molecular mechanism of action is still debated. Some investigators suggested that they work primarily by coating bone surfaces and rendering mineralized bone surfaces toxic to resorbing osteoclasts (72), whereas others postulated a cellular effect in bone cells in the osteoclast lineage during their formation (73), or in osteoblastic cells, which control osteoclastic bone resorption (74). Whatever their target, it was recently shown that the result is osteoclast apoptosis (75).

Sex hormone deficiency increases osteoclastic bone resorption. The mechanism is still unclear. Thus estrogens or androgens may be used as therapy in postmenopausal women or hypogonadal men, respectively. Estrogens and androgens cause increases in all cells at all stages in the osteoclast lineage. Although relatively small numbers of estrogen receptors are present in osteoclasts (70), it is likely that the main primary cellular target is not the osteoclast, and that inhibitory effects on osteoclasts are mediated through accessory cells for bone resorption. Several cytokines have been implicated in the increased bone resorption associated with estrogen withdrawal, including interleukin-1, interleukin-6, TGF-β, and prostaglandins of the E series. As indicated earlier, evidence from *in vivo* studies suggested that both interleukin-1 and interleukin-6 may be involved (37,51). Because the majority of patients will not take estrogens, attempts are now being made to develop drugs that have estrogen-like effects on bone and the cardiovascular system, but not the deleterious effects of estrogens on the breast and endometrium of the uterus. One member of this group of estrogen agonists/antagonists is raloxifene (76).

CELLULAR EVENTS INVOLVED IN THE FORMATION PHASE OF THE REMODELING SEQUENCE

The specific cellular events that occur at sites of osteoclastic resorption are osteoclast apoptosis, followed by a series of sequential changes in cells in the osteoblast lineage, including osteoblast chemotaxis, proliferation, and differentiation, which in turn is followed by formation of mineralized bone and cessation of osteoblast activity. The osteoblast changes are preceded by osteoclast apoptosis, which may be dependent on active TGF-β released from the resorbed bone (21). This is followed by chemotactic attraction of osteoblasts or their precursors to the sites of the resorption defect. Chemotactic attraction of osteoblast precursors also is likely mediated by other local factors produced during the resorption process, because resorbing bone releases chemotactic factors for cells with osteoblast characteristics *in vitro* (77,78). Structural proteins such as collagen or osteocalcin also could be involved, because type 1 collagen and osteocalcin and their fragments cause the same chemotactic effects (77,78). TGF-β, which is enriched in the bone matrix and released in active form as a consequence of bone resorption, also is chemotactic for bone cells (79). Platelet-derived growth factor is chemotactic for some mesenchymal cells (80–83), and it is possible that a combination of chemotactic factors is responsible for attraction of osteoblast precursors to resorption sites.

Proliferation of osteoblast precursors is an important event at the remodeling site. This also is likely to be enhanced by local osteoblast growth factors released during the resorption process. Likely candidates include members of the TGF-β superfamily (TGF-βs 1 and 2) and PDGF, which also causes proliferation of cells with osteoblast characteristics. The IGFs I and II and the heparin-binding fibroblast growth factors also stimulate osteoblast proliferation. All of these factors are stored in the bone matrix.

The next sequential event during the formation phase is the differentiation of the osteoblast precursor into the mature cell. Several of the bone-derived growth factors can cause the appearance of markers of the differentiated osteoblast phenotype, including expression of alkaline phosphatase activity, Type I collagen and osteocalcin synthesis. Most prominent of these are IGF-I and BMP-2. Active TGF-β inhibits osteoblast differentiation *in vitro*, which suggests its role may be to "trigger" the process of bone formation by attracting a pool of committed and proliferating precursors to the right sites, after which it is removed or becomes inactivated, allowing this increased pool of precursors to undergo differentiation.

The final phase of the formation process is cessation of osteoblast activity. The resorption lacunae are usually repaired either completely or almost completely. It is not known how this level of time regulation is achieved. One possibility is that factors produced during osteoblast differentiation decrease osteoblast activity. One such factor could be TGF-β because active TGF-β decreases differentiated function in osteoblasts and, as noted earlier, is expressed by osteoblasts as they differentiate (84).

OSTEOBLASTOTROPIC FACTORS THAT MAY BE INVOLVED IN THE COUPLING PROCESS

Osteotropic factors that could be involved in the coupling phenomenon are TGF-β, BMPs, IGF-I and II, platelet-derived growth factor, and heparin-binding fibroblast growth factors. This area also was reviewed by Canalis et al. (85,86). These factors are likely to be released locally from bone as it resorbs, or by bone cells activated as a consequence of the resorption process. They may then act in a sequential manner to regulate all of the cellular events required for the formation of bone.

The TGF-β superfamily may be particularly important in the coupling that links bone formation to prior bone resorption (Fig. 3). Prolonged primary cultures of fetal rat calvarial osteoblasts show that the BMPs are expressed as these cells differentiate to form new bone, in parallel with other differentiation markers such as osteocalcin and alkaline phosphatase. Transient exposure of these cells to TGF-β stimulates proliferation of the osteoblasts (continued exposure inhibits the formation of mineralized bone expression of differentiation markers). Addition of BMPs to the culture leads to increased numbers of mature osteoblasts and mineralized bone nodules.

The potential interactions between these factors are extraordinarily complex, possibly even as complex as the interactions between the colony-stimulating factors during hematopoiesis, but it will be essential to unravel them to understand the local controls responsible for bone formation. It is likely that the complicated interactions between these

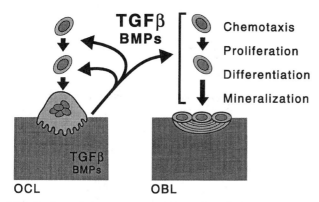

FIG. 3. Growth-factor concept of coupling. This concept suggests that coupling of osteoblast (OBL) differentiation and bone formation is due to growth factors such as TGF-β and related family members and other growth factors such as IGF-1 and the FGFs being released from bone in active form as a consequence of osteoclastic (OCL) resorption.

factors released locally in active form, as a consequence of the resorption process, are responsible for the carefully coordinated formation of new bone that occurs at these sites.

REFERENCES

1. Frost HM. *Bone biodynamics.* Boston: Little, Brown, 1964:315.
2. Riggs BL, Wahner HW, Melton LJ III, et al. Rates of bone loss in the axial and appendicular skeletons of women: evidence of substantial vertebral bone loss prior to menopause. *J Clin Invest* 1986:77:1487–1491.
3. Genant HK, Cann CE, Ettinger B, et al. Quantitative computed tomography of vertebral spongiosa: a sensitive method for detecting early bone loss after oophorectomy. *Ann Intern Med* 1982:97:699–705.
4. Riggs BL, Melton LJ III. Involutional osteoporosis. *N Engl J Med* 1986;14:1676–1686.
5. Mundy GR, Luben RA, Raisz LG, et al. Bone-resorbing activity in supernatants from lymphoid cell lines. *N Engl J Med* 1974:290:867–871.
6. Mundy GR, Raisz LG, Cooper RA, et al. Evidence for the secretion of an osteoclast stimulating factor in myeloma. *N Engl J Med* 1974;291:1041–1046.
7. Parfitt AM, Mathews CHE, Villanueva AR, et al. Relationships between surface, volume, and thickness of iliac trabecular bone in aging and in osteoporosis. *J Clin Invest* 1983;72:1396–1409.
8. Kleerekoper M, Villanueva AR, Stanciu J, et al. The role of three dimensional trabecular microstructure in the pathogenesis of vertebral compression fractures. *Calcif Tissue Int* 1985;37:594–597.
9. Miyauchi A, Alvarez J, Greenfield EM, et al. Recognition of osteopontin and related peptides by an $\alpha_v \beta 3$ integrin stimulates immediate cell signals in osteoclasts. *J Biol Chem* 1991;266:20369–20374.
10. Baron R, Vignery A, Horowitz M. Lymphocytes, macrophages and the regulation of bone remodeling. In: Peck WA, ed. *Bone and mineral research.* Amsterdam: Elsevier, 1984:175–243.
11. Boyce BF, Aufdemorte TB, Garrett IR, et al. Effects of interleukin-1 on bone turnover in normal mice. *Endocrinology* 1989;125:1142–1150.
12. Boyce BF, Yates AJP, Mundy GR. Bolus injections of recombinant human interleukin-1 cause transient hypocalcemia in normal mice. *Endocrinology* 1989;125:2780–2783.
13. Snapper I, Kahn A. *Myelomatosis.* Basel: Karger, 1971.
14. Valentin-Opran A, Charhon SA, Meunier PJ, et al. Quantitative histology of myeloma induced bone changes. *Br J Haematol* 1982;52:601–610.
15. Stewart AF, Vignery A, Silvergate A, et al. Quantitative bone histomorphometry in humoral hypercalcemia of malignancy: uncoupling of bone cell activity. *J Clin Endocrinol Metab* 1982;55:219–227.
16. Darby AJ, Meunier PJ. Mean wall thickness and formation periods of trabecular bone packets in idiopathic osteoporosis. *Calcif Tissue Int* 1981;33:199–204.
17. Rasmussen H, Bordier P. *The physiological and cellular basis of metabolic bone disease.* Baltimore: Williams & Wilkins, 1974.
18. Howard GA, Bottemiller BL, Turner RT, et al. Parathyroid hormone stimulates bone formation and resorption in organ culture: evidence for a coupling mechanism. *Proc Natl Acad Sci U S A* 1981;78:3204–3208.
19. Manolagas SC, Jilka RL. Mechanisms of disease: bone marrow, cytokines, and bone remodeling: emerging insights into the pathophysiology of osteoporosis. *N Engl J Med* 1995;332:305–311.
20. Hughes DE, Wright KR, Uy HL, et al. Bisphosphonates promote apoptosis in murine osteoclasts in vitro and in vivo. *J Bone Miner Res* 1995;10:1478–1487.
21. Hughes DE, Dai A, Tiffee JC, et al. Estrogen promotes apoptosis of murine osteoclasts mediated by TGF-beta. *Nat Med* 1996;2:1132–1136.
22. Jones SJ, Boyde A, Ali NN, et al. A review of bone cell substratum interactions. *Scanning* 1985;7:5–24.
23. Rodan GA, Martin TJ. Role of osteoblasts in hormonal control of bone resorption: a hypothesis. *Calcif Tissue Int* 1981;33:349–351.
24. McSheehy PMJ, Chambers TJ. Osteoblastic cells mediate osteoclastic responsiveness to parathyroid hormone. *Endocrinology* 1986;118:824–828.
25. Wong BR, Josien R, Lee SY, et al. TRANCE (tumor necrosis factor (TNF)-related activation-induced cytokine), a new TNF family member predominantly expressed in T cells, is a dendritic cell-specific survival factor. *J Exp Med* 1997;186:2075–2080.
26. Mundy GR, Roodman GD. Osteoclast ontogeny and function. In: Peck W, ed. *Bone and mineral research.* Amsterdam: Elsevier, 1987:209–280.
27. McSheehy PMJ, Chambers TJ. Osteoblastic cells mediate osteoclastic responsiveness to parathyroid hormone. *Endocrinology* 1986;118:824–828.
28. Roodman GD, Ibbotson KJ, MacDonald BR, Kuehl TJ, Mundy GR. 1,25-Dihydroxyvitamin D_3 causes formation of multinucleated cells with several osteoclast characteristics in cultures of primate marrow. *Proc Natl Acad Sci USA* 1985;82:8213–8217.
29. Tsoukas CD, Provvedini DM, Manolagas SC. 1,25-dihydroxyvitamin D_3: a novel immunoregulatory hormone. *Science* 1984;224:1438–1440.
30. Wener JA, Gorton SJ, Raisz LG. Escape from inhibition of resorption in cultures of fetal bone treated with calcitonin and parathyroid hormone. *Endocrinology* 1972;90:752–759.
31. Takahashi S, Goldring S, Katz M, Hilsenbeck S, Williams R, Roodman GD. Downregulation of calcitonin receptor mRNA expression by calcitonin during human osteoclast-like cell differentiation. *J Clin Invest* 1995;95:167–171.
32. Chambers TJ, Magnus CJ. Calcitonin alters the behavior of isolated osteoclasts. *J Pathol* 1982;136:27–40.
33. Pfeilschifter JP, Seyedin S, Mundy GR. Transformed growth factor β inhibits bone resorption in fetal rat long bone cultures. *J Clin Invest* 1988;82:680–685.
34. Thomson BM, Saklatvala J, Chambers TJ. Osteoblasts mediate interleukin-1 stimulation of bone resorption by rat osteoclasts. *J Exp Med* 1986;164:104–112.
35. Sabatini M, Boyce B, Aufdemorte T, Bonewald L, Mundy GR. Infusions of recombinant human interleukins 1 alpha and 1 beta cause hypercalcemia in normal mice. *Proc Natl Acad Sci USA* 1988;85:5235–5239.
36. Boyce BF, Aufdemorte TB, Garrett IR, Yates AJP, Mundy GR. Effects of interleukin-1 on bone turnover in normal mice. *Endocrinology* 1989;123:1142–1150.
37. Pacifici R, Rifas L, McCracken R, et al. Ovarian steroid treatment blocks a postmenopausal increase in blood monocyte interleukin 1 release. *Proc Natl Acad Sci USA* 1989;86:2398–2402.
38. Bertolini DR, Nedwin GE, Bringman TS, Mundy GR. Stimulation of bone resorption and inhibition of bone formation in vitro by human tumour necrosis factors. *Nature* 1986;319:516–518.
39. Johnson RA, Boyce BF, Mundy GR, Roodman GD. Tumors producing human TNF induce hypercalcemia and osteoclastic bone resorption in nude mice. *Endocrinology* 1989;124:1424–1427.
40. Thomson BM, Mundy GR, Chambers TJ. Tumor necrosis factors alpha and beta induce osteoblastic cells to stimulate osteoclastic bone resorption. *J Immunol* 1987;138:775–779.
41. Garrett IR, Durie BGM, Nedwin GE, et al. Production of the bone

resorbing cytokine lymphotoxin by cultured human myeloma cells. *N Engl J Med* 1987;317:526–532.

42. Tashjian AH Jr, Voelkel EF, Lazzaro M, et al. Tumor necrosis factor-alpha (cachectin) stimulates bone resorption in mouse calvaria via a prostaglandin-mediated mechanism. *Endocrinology* 1987;120:2029–2036.

43. Felix R, Cecchini MG, Fleisch H. Macrophage colony stimulating factor restores in vivo bone resorption in the op/op osteopetrotic mouse. *Endocrinology* 1990;127:2592–2594.

44. Horwood NJ, Udagawa N, Elliott J, et al. Interleukin 18 inhibits osteoclast formation via T cell production of granulocyte macrophage colony-stimulating factor. *J Clin Invest* 1998;101:595–603.

45. Simonet WS, Lacey DL, Dunstan CR, et al. Osteoprotegerin: a novel secreted protein involved in the regulation of bone density. *Cell* 1997;89:309–310.

46. Tsuda E, Goto M, Mochizuki S, et al. Isolation of a novel cytokine from human fibroblasts that specifically inhibits osteoclastogenesis. *Biochem Biophys Res Commun* 1997;234:137–142.

47. Yasuda H, Shima N, Nakagawa N, et al. Osteoclast differentiation factor is a ligand for osteoprotegerin/osteoclastogenesis-inhibitory factor and is identical to TRANCE/RANKL. *Proc Natl Acad Sci USA* 1998;95:3597–3602.

48. Feyen JHM, Elford P, Dipadova FE, Trechsel U. Interleukin-6 is produced by bone and modulated by parathyroid hormone. *J Bone Miner Res* 1989;4:633–638.

49. Black K, Garrett IR, Mundy GR. Chinese hamster ovarian cells transfected with the murine interleukin-6 gene cause hypercalcemia as well as cachexia, leukocytosis and thrombocytosis in tumor-bearing nude mice. *Endocrinology* 1991;128:2657–2659.

50. Ishimi Y, Miyaura C, Jin CH, et al. IL-6 is produced by osteoblasts and induces bone resorption. *J Immunol* 1990;145:3297–3303.

51. Jilka RL, Hangoc G, Girasole G, et al. Increased osteoclast development after estrogen loss: mediation by interleukin-6. *Science* 1992;257:88–91.

52. Gowen M, Mundy GR. Actions of recombinant interleukin-1, interleukin-2 and interferon gamma on bone resorption in vitro. *J Immunol* 1986;136:2478–2482.

53. Gowen M, Nedwin G, Mundy GR. Preferential inhibition of cytokine stimulated bone resorption by recombinant interferon gamma. *J Bone Miner Res* 1986;1:469–474.

54. Takahashi N, Mundy GR, Kuehl TJ, Roodman GD. Osteoclast like formation in fetal and newborn long term baboon marrow cultures is more sensitive to 1,25-dihydroxyvitamin D₃ than adult long term marrow cultures. *J Bone Miner Res* 1987;2:311–317.

55. Chenu C, Pfeilschifter J, Mundy GR, Roodman GD. Transforming growth factor β inhibits formation of osteoclast-like cells in long-term human marrow cultures. *Proc Natl Acad Sci USA* 1988;85:5683–5687.

56. Noda M, Camilliere JJ. In vivo stimulation of bone formation by transforming growth factor-beta. *Endocrinology* 1989;124:2991–2994.

57. Tashjian AH Jr, Voelkel EF, Lloyd W, et al. Actions of growth factors on plasma calcium: epidermal growth factor and human transforming growth factor-alpha cause elevation of plasma calcium in mice. *J Clin Invest* 78:1405–1409.

58. Fell HB, Mellanby E. The effect of hypervitaminosis A on embryonic limb bones cultured in vitro. *J Physiol* 1952;116:320–349.

59. Ibbotson KJ, D'Souza SM, Smith DD, Carpenter G, Mundy GR. EGF receptor antiserum inhibits bone resorbing activity produced by a rat Leydig cell tumor associated with the humoral hypercalcemia of malignancy. *Endocrinology* 1985;116:469–471.

60. Ibbotson KJ, Harrod J, Gowen M. Human recombinant transforming growth factor alpha stimulates bone resorption and inhibits formation in vitro. *Proc Natl Acad Sci USA* 1986;83:2228–2232.

61. Stern PH, Krieger NS, Nissenson RA, et al. Human transforming growth factor alpha stimulates bone resorption in vitro. *J Clin Invest* 1985;76:2016–2020.

62. Takahashi N, MacDonald BR, Hon J, et al. Recombinant human transforming growth factor alpha stimulates the formation of osteoclast-like cells in long term human marrow cultures. *J Clin Invest* 1986;78:894–898.

63. Raisz LG, Niemann I. Effect of phosphate, calcium and magnesium on bone resorption and hormonal responses in tissue culture. *Endocrinology* 1969;85:446–452.

64. Tashjian AH, Voelkel EF, Levine L, et al. Evidence that the bone resorption-stimulating factor produced by mouse fibrosarcoma cells is prostaglandin E₂: a new model for the hypercalcemia of cancer. *J Exp Med* 1972;136:1329–1343.

65. Gallwitz WE, Mundy GR, Oreffo ROC, Gaskell SJ, Bonewald LF. Purification of osteoclastotropic factors produced by stromal cells: identification of 5-lipoxygenase metabolites. *J Bone Miner Res* 1991;6(Suppl):457.

66. Flynn MA, Holt S, Bonewald LF. Lipopolysaccharide (LPS) induces osteoclast formation through 5-lipoxygenase (5LO). *J Bone Miner Res* (submitted).

67. Mundy GR, Shapiro JL, Bandelin JG, Canalis EM, Raisz LG. Direct stimulation of bone resorption by thyroid hormones. *J Clin Invest* 1976;58:529–534.

68. Mundy GR, Rick ME, Turcotte R, Kowalski MA. Pathogenesis of hypercalcemia in lymphosarcoma cell leukemia: role of an osteoclast activating factor-like substance and mechanism of action for glucocorticoid therapy. *Am J Med* 1978;65:600–606.

69. Lindsay R, Hart DM, Forrest C, et al. Prevention of spinal osteoporosis in oophorectomised women. *Lancet* 1980;2:1151–1153.

70. Oursler MJ, Osdoby P, Pyfferoen J, Riggs BL, Spelsberg TC. Avian osteoclasts as estrogen target cells. *Proc Natl Acad Sci USA* 1991;88:6613–6617.

71. Girasole G, Jilka RL, Passeri G, et al. 17 beta-Estradiol inhibits interleukin-6 production by bone marrow-derived stromal cells and osteoblasts in vitro: a potential mechanism for the antiosteoporotic effect of estrogens. *J Clin Invest* 1992;89:883–891.

72. Sato M, Grasser W, Endo N, et al. Bisphosphonate action: alendronate localization in rat bone and effects on osteoclast ultrastructure. *J Clin Invest* 1991;88:2095–2105.

73. Hughes DE, MacDonald BR, Russell RGG, Gowen M. Inhibition of osteoclast-like cell formation by bisphosphonates in long-term cultures of human bone marrow. *J Clin Invest* 1989;83:1930–1935.

74. Sahni M, Guenther HL, Fleisch H, Collin P, Martin TJ. Bisphosphonates act on rat bone resorption through the mediation of osteoblasts. *J Clin Invest* 1993;91:2004–2011.

75. Hughes DE, Wright KR, Uy HL, et al. Bisphosphonates promote apoptosis in murine osteoclasts in vitro and in vivo. *J Bone Miner Res* (in press).

76. Black LJ, Sato M, Rowley ER, et al. Raloxifene (LY139481 HCI) prevents bone loss and reduces serum cholesterol without causing uterine hypertrophy in ovariectomized rats. *J Clin Invest* 1994;93:63–69.

77. Mundy GR, Rodan SB, Majeska RJ, et al. Unidirectional migration of osteosarcoma cells with osteoblast characteristics in response to products of bone resorption. *Calcif Tissue Int* 1982;34:542–546.

78. Mundy GR, Poser JW. Chemotactic activity of the gamma-carboxyglutamic acid containing protein in bone. *Calcif Tissue Int* 1983;35:164–168.

79. Pfeilschifter J, Bonewald L, Mundy GR. Characterization of the latent transforming growth factor complex in bone. *J Bone Miner Res* 1990;5:49–58.

80. Deuel TF, Senior RM, Huang JS, et al. Chemotaxis of monocytes and neutrophils to platelet-derived growth factor. *J Clin Invest* 1982;69:1046–1049.

81. Grotendorst GR, Seppa HEJ, Kleinman HK, et al. Attachment of smooth muscle cells to collagen and their migration toward platelet-derived growth factor. *Proc Natl Acad Sci USA* 1981;78:3669–3672.

82. Seppa H, Grotendorst G, Seppa S, et al. Platelet-derived growth factor is chemotactic for fibroblasts. *J Cell Biol* 1982;92:584–588.

83. Senior RM, Griffin GL, Huang JS, et al. Chemotactic activity of platelet alpha granule proteins for fibroblasts. *J Cell Biol* 1983;96:382–385.

84. Dallas SL, Park-Snyder S, Miyazono K, et al. Characterization and autoregulation of latent TGFβ complexes in osteoblast-like cell lines: production of a latent complex lacking the latent TGFβ-binding protein (LTBP). *J Biol Chem* 1994;269:6815–6821.

85. Canalis E, Centrella M, Burch W, et al. Insulin-like growth factor I mediates selective anabolic effects of parathyroid hormone in bone cultures. *J Clin Invest* 1989;83:60–65.

86. Canalis E, McCarthy T, Centrella M. Growth factors and the regulation of bone remodeling. *J Clin Invest* 1989;81:277–281.

5. Biomechanics of Bone

Clinton T. Rubin, Ph.D. and *Janet Rubin, M.D.

*Center for Biotechnology, State University of New York at Stony Brook, Stony Brook, New York; and *Department of Medicine, Emory University School of Medicine and Veterans Affairs Medical Center, Atlanta, Georgia*

The primary responsibility of the skeleton is to provide structural support for the body. In this role, the skeleton is the basis of posture, opposes muscular contraction resulting in motion, withstands functional load bearing, and protects internal organs. The skeleton's structural success can be jeopardized by genetic disorders such as osteogenesis imperfecta, metabolic diseases such as Paget's, or even the bone loss that parallels the aging process (i.e., osteopenia). To appreciate the structural risks that accompany metabolic bone diseases, it is essential that several interdependent concepts of the biomechanical properties of bone be considered.

STRAIN

When a force (newton = N = force that will cause a 1 Kg mass to accelerate at 1 ms^{-2}; essentially, the force of a 100 g apple in Earth's gravitational pull) is applied to any material, such as bone, it deforms. The amount of deformation in the material, relative to its original length, is the strain. Strain is a dimensionless unit formally defined as the change in length divided by its original length ($\varepsilon = \Delta L/L$). When a material is pulled, it gets longer (tensile strain). When pushed together, the material shortens (compressive strain). Shear strain is the angle, measured in radians, through which a material has been deformed by forces acting parallel, rather than opposed, to the material. Shear strain arises when layers of a material slide against another, as might occur with torsion or bending (1). Peak compressive strains in bone during vigorous activity can reach as high as 3500 microstrain ($\mu\varepsilon$) in compression (0.35% strain), 1000 $\mu\varepsilon$ in tension, and 1500 $\mu\varepsilon$ in shear (Fig. 1). Interestingly, these peak strains are very similar across a spectrum of vertebrates, despite a wide variety of activity (2).

STRESS

To determine the material properties of bone, a machined sample is subjected to a known tensile or compressive load. To aid in comparing this specific test with other materials or studies from other laboratories, it is preferable to report the magnitude of the force in terms of the cross-sectional area of the material on which it is acting (3). The force per unit area is the stress (σ = Force/Area), and is reported in newtons per square meter (Nm^{-2}), or pascals (Pa). To put this in perspective, a pascal is essentially the stress caused by the weight of one apple acting on a square meter tabletop. The compressive stress caused in the third metacarpal of a thoroughbred racehorse during a gallop is on the order of 63,000,000 pascals, or 63 MPa (4). Now imagine 63 × 10^6 apples on that same table.

MODULUS

The degree to which a material deforms depends not only on the magnitude of the forces and moments (turning, twisting, or rotational effect of a force; M = Nm) applied to the structure, but also on the stiffness of the constituent materials (5). In the case of bone, stiffness is determined by the relative proportions of the hydroxyapatite crystals and the collagen fibers that make up the composite (6). During the initial stages of a test to define a bone's material properties, there

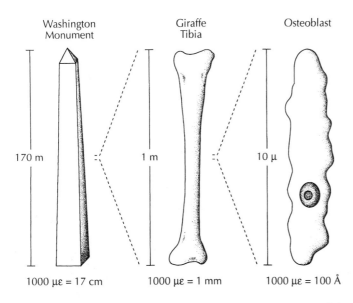

FIG. 1. Strain is defined as a (load-induced) change in length relative to the structure's original length. 1000 microstrain, or 0.1% strain, reflects the amount of strain experienced by bone tissue during an activity such as walking. For a structure such as the 170-m Washington monument, 1000 microstrain would represent a 17-cm change in length over the unloaded length of the entire structure. In a giraffe tibia, 1000 microstrain would reflect a 1-mm change in the bone's original 1000-mm length. At the level of a 10 μm bone-lining cell resting on the periosteum of that giraffe tibia, the 1000 microstrain induced by walking would relate to a 100-angstrom change in the cell's original length. The mechanisms responsible for perceiving and responding to such small biomechanical signals, whatever they may be, must be extremely sensitive. (From Rubin CT, Gross TS, Donahue HJ, Guilak F, McLeod KJ. Physical and environmental influences on bone formation. In: Brighton CT, Friedlaender G, Lane J. *Bone formation and repair*. 1st ed. Rosemont, IL: American Academy of Orthopaedic Surgeons, 1994:61–78, with permission.)

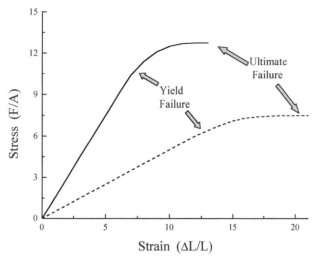

FIG. 2. The stress–strain curve of two different materials is given. In material A *(solid line)*, the material is stiffer, as depicted by the steeper slope of the line ($E = \sigma/\varepsilon$). Thus for a given stress, there is less strain. However, the yield strain of material A is lower than that of material B *(dashed line)*, as depicted by the point where the relation between stress and strain is no longer linear (Yield Failure). As well, the ultimate strain of material A is lower than that of material B, as depicted by the point where there is catastrophic failure of the material [i.e., there is no longer any stress necessary to cause strain (Ultimate Failure)]. Material A is more brittle than material B. The area beneath the curves reflects the toughness of the materials.

is a linear increase in strain as the stress increases (Fig. 2). This is known as the elastic region. Should the load be removed during this phase of the test, the specimen will return to its original size and shape almost immediately, without incurring permanent damage. The linear relation between strain and stress is called Hooke's Law ($E = \sigma/\varepsilon$; where E is the elastic modulus). *Ut tensio, sic vis:* as the extension, so the force (7).

The slope of the elastic region of the stress–strain curve reflects the stiffness of the material, otherwise known as the modulus of elasticity. The stiffer the material, the steeper the slope of the line. One hundred Newtons pulling on a tendon will result in far greater strain than the same force pulling on a sample of bone of the same dimensions (8). Whereas the stress is identical, the modulus of the bone is much higher than the tendon (the slope of the stress–strain curve is much steeper), and thus the bone deforms much less.

An isotropic material, like steel, has equivalent material property values in all directions. A material like bone, which has distinct mechanical properties in different directions, is anisotropic. The modulus of mature cortical bone is on the order of 18 gigaPascals (GPa) in the longitudinal direction, 12 GPa in the transverse direction, and 3.3 GPa in shear (9). The material properties of cancellous bone are even more complex, as trabecular orientation, connectivity, and density greatly influence the stiffness (10). Depending on location, the modulus of trabecular bone can range from 0.1 to 3.5 GPa (11). The degree of mineralization (e.g., immature or woven bone) or porosity (e.g., old bone) will compromise the stiffness of the bone and thereby lower the elastic modulus.

YIELD FAILURE

When the increase in strain is no longer proportional to the stress, the elastic region ends, and with it the ability of the material to resume its original shape (Fig. 2). The bone specimen has moved into the plastic region where permanent damage has begun to accrue. In terms of bone, yield failure arises through ultrastructural microcracks within the hydroxyapatite and the disruption of the collagen fibrils. The yield strain of cortical bone is on the order of 6800 $\mu\varepsilon$ (12), suggesting that a safety factor of 2 exists between peak strains caused by normal functional activity and the point where damage is inevitable. The yield stress is approximately 130 MPa. In other words, by the time there are 130×10^6 apples on the table, the table surface begins to crack.

ULTIMATE FAILURE

As loading continues in the plastic region, the material will eventually reach ultimate failure, at which point the specimen fails catastrophically (13). The point at which the bone breaks can be viewed as either the ultimate strain (15,000 $\mu\varepsilon$ in tension) or the ultimate stress (140 MPa in tension, 200 MPa in compression, and 65 MPa in shear). Because of this disparity, it should become clear that the cause of fracture in "normal" bone material is most likely due to tensile or shear failure.

The amount of postyield strain that occurs before ultimate failure is a measure of the material's ductility, reflecting its ability to resist the propagation of cracks (3). A ductile material is one that can change form without breaking; a tendon is more ductile than bone. A material that manages little postyield behavior before ultimate failure is considered brittle (e.g., glass or ceramic). Whereas osteoporosis is often referred to as the brittle-bone disease, in reality, little experimental evidence supports an actual reduction in the ductility of bone material examined from patients with this disease (14). There is just less bone to resist a given force (stress during functional activity is just that much closer to yield stress). Perhaps a better example of brittle bone is provided by osteogenesis imperfecta, in which a qualitative or quantitative deficiency in type I collagen in the material (15) reduces its ductility, condemning it to ultimate failure soon after the material has begun to yield.

TOUGHNESS

The stress–strain curve yields another important property of the material. The area under the curve reflects the amount of work, or energy per unit volume, possessed by the material at any given point on the curve. At ultimate failure, the area under the curve defines the energy required to break the object, or toughness. A major contributor to the toughness of bone is its composite nature of haversian, circumferential, and interstitial lamellae. The analogy of a bundle of straws versus a plastic stick illustrates how the architecture of a composite, anisotropic structure outperforms a single, uniform isotropic material in resisting loads and avoiding yield and ultimate strain. The plastic stick breaks with relatively little bending because high strains are generated within the periphery of the material. A bundle of straws composed of the same mass and subjected to the same bending conditions will continue to strain rather than break, as each independent element slips relative to adjacent bundles.

Bone, as an organ, has a requirement to be both stiff and tough. There is, however, an inevitable trade-off between these two attributes, as they must be attained by a balance between the resistance to crack propagation provided by collagen and the resistance to deformation provided by the mineral. Comparatively small changes in the mineral content of bone tissue can have significant effects on its properties as a material, as demonstrated by Curry (16) in his determination of the mechanical properties of bones' with diverse functional responsibilities. By comparing the bovine femur, the deer antler, and the whale tympanic bulla, he illustrated that the mineral content changed to accommodate a specific functional responsibility. In the extreme, the mineral content ranged from 86% in the bulla, which requires high acoustic impedance, to 59% in the antler, which must resist high impact loads. The consequence of this high mineral content is revealed by comparing the relative toughness of these bones; the bulla is only 3% as tough as the antler.

BONE AS A COMPOSITE MATERIAL

The composite structure of bone allows it to withstand compressive and tensile stresses, as well as bending and torsional moments. The inorganic phase of bone, with hydroxyapatite crystals arrayed in a protein matrix, provides the ability to resist compression. Individual calcium phosphate crystals of multiple sizes are imbedded in and around the fibrils of the collagen type I lattice (17). Hydroxyapatite crystal, although effectively resisting compressive loads, has a poor ability to withstand tensile loads. As in concrete, a material that excels at resisting compression but is poor in resisting tension, tensile elements (e.g., steel reinforcing rods) are added to create a composite material that can cope with complex loading environments. In the case of bone, this tensile strength arises from collagen fibrils organized into lamellae.

The collagen orientation between adjacent lamellae can rotate by as much as 90 degrees, permitting the tissue to resist forces and moments acting from several different directions, much like the added strength in plywood realized by the distinct orientation of the fibers in each specific ply (18). Whereas the ultrastructural organization is, to a certain extent, defined by the genome, the functional environment also contributes to the distribution of lamellae as well to the osteons that house them (19). This directed deposition of collagen adds to the anisotropy of the bone. Given that >80% of functional strains are due to bending (and thus a high percentage of strain is tensile), the structural quality of the bone may ultimately be determined by the quality of the collagen and the organization of the microarchitecture. Recent studies have shown that collagen itself deteriorates with age and undoubtedly contributes to the declining material properties of the skeleton (20).

Alterations in either the organic (e.g., collagen) or inorganic (e.g., hydroxyapatite) matrix components can bring about changes in bone strength. Mutations in the collagen gene give rise to several genetic skeletal problems, some of which increase fracture risk. In some forms of osteogenesis imperfecta, mutations in the primary structure of type I procollagen lead to brittle bone (21). Another disorder of collagen resulting in excessively fragile bone is fibrogenesis imperfecta ossium (22), a rare disease in which remodeling results in a disorganized, collagen-deficient tissue. Although the number of hydroxyapatite crystals contributes to the ability to resist compression, density is not everything. Fluoroapatite, which incorporates into the mineral phase of bone during fluoride poisoning, is denser than hydroxyapatite, but is brittle and shatters easily (23).

AREAL PROPERTIES OF BONE

Areal properties, which define the overall mass and pattern of the structure, are as important as material properties to the ultimate success of the skeleton. Size, density, and architecture effectively describe areal properties at the gross level. Other, more subtle properties also are key contributors to the structural efficacy of bone, including the long-bone curvature, the girth and geometry of the cross-sectional area, and the trabecular organization (e.g., connectivity).

Axial loading results in very little strain for a given load: imagine how strong a pencil is when you press straight down on the long axis of the shaft. At the same time, it is important to consider how easily the pencil is snapped when it is subject to bending. Consider now the neck of the femur while climbing a flight of stairs: the functional demands on bones, as opposed to pencils, are very complex, and subject not only to axial conditions, but also to bending and torsional moments (1). With the diversity of the functional environment, it is clear that a strategy of minimal mass will not serve as a successful structure. Instead, the structure of the bone must be designed to resist a wide assortment of loading conditions, perhaps to control and regulate the loading environment rather than to minimize the strain (24).

Even the simplest of loading cases create complex strain and stress environments in a material, including bone. Axial loads applied to a slightly curved beam will cause tensile strain on the convex side, and compressive strain on the concave side. The strains are greatest at these extremes and decrease to zero in the middle of the beam. This area is called the neutral axis, where strain approaches zero. The flexural rigidity of the material, EI, represents the amount of force per unit cross-sectional area required to deform the material a given amount, where E is elastic modulus (see earlier), and I is the second moment of area (25). The second moment, or moment of inertia, reflects the contribution of each bit of material to the stiffness in each position in the cross-section of the beam ($I = \Sigma y^2 dA$, where y is the distance of each element of area A from the neutral axis). Therefore the further the material is relative to the neutral axis, the better placed it will be to resist bending (Fig. 3). This areal property is a powerful means of rapidly increasing flexural rigidity for a small investment of material. For example, in the elderly, it was shown that the subtle increases in the

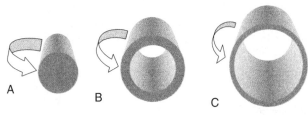

FIG. 3. The cross-sectional areas of these three cylinders are identical ($A_A = A_B = A_C$). The elastic modulus of the material that makes up these cylinders also is identical ($E_A = E_B = E_C$). Therefore for an axial force (i.e., pushing or pulling the ends of the bar), the stress is identical ($\sigma_A = \sigma_B = \sigma_C$). However, because the geometry of the cross sections is different, the ability of each of these cylinders to resist bending and/or torsion is strongly dependent on the distance of the material relative to the center of the cylinder. The relative resistance to bending of these cylinders is $I_A =$ 100%, $I_B = 400\%$, and $I_C = 700\%$. Subtle changes in a bone's cross-sectional geometry will contribute heavily to the bone's structural properties.

second moment of area, which are achieved through periosteal expansion, may to a certain degree structurally compensate for the bone loss and cortical thinning that parallels the aging process (26).

An appreciation of the biomechanical attributes of bone is critical to an improved understanding of both the pathogenesis of metabolic bone disease and the emerging possibility of controlling bone mass and structure *through* mechanical stimuli. As important as inherent mechanical properties may be, it also is essential to appreciate that bone is extremely sensitive to its mechanical environment, and to a large extent, it is this functional milieu that defines skeletal structure and ultrastructural organization. This ''form follows function'' aspect of skeletal tissue is known as Wolff's Law and helps us to understand how mechanically based prophylaxes such as exercise serve as an anabolic agent to bone, and how disuse, cast immobilization, and bed rest put the skeleton at risk (24). Clinicians must be aware that the most devastating complication of bone disease is the structural collapse of the skeleton. There is every reason to believe that mechanical strategies can retard, prevent, or even reverse the structural demise of the skeleton, and that therapeutic options such as these should be actively pursued. As important, scientists beginning to generate bone with molecular triggers must assure that the new bone is adequate to the functional demands placed on it. Skeletal science must strive to incorporate an understanding of the biomechanical functions of the skeleton and consider not only the engineering basis of the bone material, but also the biologic response of the bone tissue to the potent mechanical stimuli that arise from function.

REFERENCES

1. Mow VC, Hayes WC. *Basic orthopaedic biomechanics*. New York: Raven Press, 1991:93–142.
2. Rubin CT, Lanyon LE. Dynamic strain similarity in vertebrates; an alternative to allometric limb bone scaling. *J Theor Biol* 1984;107:321–327.
3. Carter DR, Hayes WC. Bone compressive strength: the influence of density and strain rate. *Science* 1976;194:1174–1176.
4. Gross TS, McLeod KJ, Rubin CT. Characterizing bone strain distributions in vivo using three triple rosette strain gages. *J Biomech* 1992;25:1081–1087.
5. Einhorn TA. Biomechanics of bone. In: Bilezikian L, Raisz L, Rodan G, eds. *Principles of bone biology*. San Diego, CA: Academic Press, 1996:25–37.
6. Martin RB, Burr DB. *Structure, function, and adaptation of compact bone*. New York: Raven Press, 1989:18–56.
7. Vincent JFV. *Structural biomaterials*. London: Macmillan Press, 1982:1–33.
8. Wainwright SA, Biggs WD, Currey JD, Gosline JM. *Mechanical design in organisms*. New York: Wiley, 1976:64–109.
9. Reilly DT, Burstein AH. The elastic and ultimate properties of compact bone tissue. *J Biomech* 1975;8:393–405.
10. Goldstein SA. The mechanical properties of trabecular bone: dependence on anatomic location and function. *J Biomech* 1987;20:1055–1061.
11. Cowin S. *Bone mechanics*. Boca Raton, FL: CRC Press, 1989:129–157.
12. Carter DR. Mechanical loading histories and cortical bone remodeling. *Calcif Tissue Int* 1984;36:S19–S24.
13. Carter DR, Harris WH, Vasu R, Caler E. The mechanical and biological response of cortical bone to in vivo strain histories. American Society of Mechanical Engineers publication *AMD* 1981;45:81.
14. Turner CH, Burr DB. Basic biomechanical measurements of bone: a tutorial. *Bone* 1993;14:595–608.
15. Prockop KJ. Mutations that alter the primary structure of type I collagen. *J Biol Chem* 1990;265:15349–15352.
16. Currey JD. Mechanical properties of bone tissues with greatly differing functions. *J Biomech* 1979;12:313–319.
17. Weiner S, Traub W. Bone structure: from angstroms to microns. *FASEB J* 1992;6:879–885.
18. Alexander M. *Bones: the unity of form and function*. New York, NY: Macmillan, 1994:25–57.
19. Skedros JG, Mason MW, Nelson MC, Bloebaum RD. Evidence of structural and material adaptation to specific strain features in cortical bone. *Anat Rec* 1996;246:47–63.
20. Oxlund H, Mosekilde L, Ortoft G. Reduced concentration of collagen reducible cross links in human trabecular bone with respect to age and osteoporosis. *Bone* 1996;19:479–484.
21. Misof K, Landis WJ, Klaushofer K, Frati P. Collagen from the osteogenesis imperfecta mouse model (oim) shows reduced resistance against tensile stress. *J Clin Invest* 1997;100:40–45.
22. Carr AJ, Smith R, Athanasou N, Woods CG. Fibrogenesis imperfecta ossium. *J Bone Joint Surg Br* 1995;77:820–829.
23. Kroger H, Alhava E, Honkanen R, Tuppurainen M, Saarikoski S. The effect of fluoridated drinking water on axial bone mineral density: a population-based study. *Bone Miner* 1994;27:33–41.
24. Rubin CT, Gross TS, Donahue HJ, Guilak F, McLeod KJ. Physical and environmental influences on bone formation. In: Brighton CT, Friedlaender G, Lane J. *Bone formation and repair*. 1st ed. Rosemont, IL: American Academy of Orthopaedic Surgeons, 1994:61–78.
25. Wainwright SA. *Axis and circumference: the cylindrical shape of plants and animals*. Cambridge, MA: Harvard University Press, 1988.
26. Ruff CB, Hayes WC. Subperiosteal expansion and cortical remodeling of the human femur and tibia with aging. *Science* 1982;217:945–948.

SECTION II

Skeletal Physiology

6. Childhood and Adolescence

Joseph M. Gertner, M.B., M.R.C.P.

Department of Pediatrics, Harvard Medical School and Department of Endocrinology, Boston Children's Hospital,
Boston, Massachusetts

INTRODUCTION

From birth to the end of the pubertal period of growth, the healthy child increases in length by about threefold, undergoes sharp changes in the relative proportions of limb, body, and head size, and accumulates large quantities of calcium and phosphate within the skeleton. This chapter covers the normal course of these changes and examines the mechanisms that control them and the methods used to assess their progress.

THE STRUCTURE OF THE EPIPHYSEAL GROWTH PLATE

Proliferation, Differentiation, and Fusion in the Growth Plate

Skeletal growth in long bones depends on the proliferation of cartilage cells in the epiphyseal growth plate. As the columns of chondrocytes grow outward from the growth plate, they mature and eventually die, while their surrounding matrix mineralizes. A zone of each growth plate is constantly in the process of maturation, with mineralization of the surrounding matrix. Under the influence of hormones and local factors, the balance between proliferation and maturation eventually shifts in the direction of maturation, with reduction in the width of the zone of proliferating chondrocytes until the epiphysis fuses and the growth plate is eliminated. This event occurs in a defined sequence, permitting assessment of skeletal maturity by observation of the sites at which fusion has occurred. Although the growth hormone (GH)/insulin-like growth factor (IGF-I) axis and androgens appear to promote proliferation, thyroid hormone and estrogens (1) are major factors in the induction of epiphyseal fusion, and estrogen can be used to limit the height of pathologically tall adolescents (2). Local factors that operate to promote epiphyseal fusion include the basic fibroblast growth factors (FGFs; 3) and retinoic acid–receptor agonists (4). Clinically, the participation of these systems can be appreciated by reference to the epiphyseal distortion that occurs in achondroplasia (due to an activating mutation in the FGF3 receptor) and to the premature epiphyseal fusion described after excessive exposure to retinoids such as etretinate (5).

SKELETAL GROWTH IN CHILDHOOD AND ADOLESCENCE

The assessment of linear growth in children is a technically sophisticated procedure that demands accurate and reproducible measurement techniques. Suitable growth databases drawn from a representative reference population also are required. The major such database in the United States is that of the National Health, Education, and Nutrition Survey (NHANES), which is analyzing results of its fourth survey. Most growth charts used in the United States and disseminated by health care organizations and commercial firms are derived from earlier NHANES data (6).

Because the rate or "velocity" of growth also is often of interest in clinical situations, curves of percentiles for this parameter also have been developed. These data are inherently less reliable and standardized than height information. The period over which the growth-rate information is measured (e.g., 6 months vs. 1 year) significantly affects the values, as does the choice of longitudinal versus cross-sectional input data. In addition, small measurement errors are more likely to increase the variability of height-velocity data than are similar errors in the measurement of stature (or height "distance"). These topics are well discussed, along with the presentation of U.S. longitudinal data, by Tanner and Davies (7).

Knemometry (8) is a research method designed to make very accurate measurements of the length of single bones, which can then be used to observe the short-term effects of local or systemic interventions that might affect growth. The limb containing the bone in question is fixed in a metal frame while the ends of the measuring device are accurately placed against bony landmarks, and the distance between them measured with a micrometer. Although theoretically attractive, this approach has few adherents and is little used.

Body Proportion and Its Changes through the Growth Period

The newborn infant has a relatively large head and limbs, which are, by adult standards, disproportionately short relative to the rest of the body. Accurate measurement of the proportions of the skeleton and the availability of tables of normal values throughout childhood permit the detection of abnormal patterns of growth and help in the diagnosis of their cause. Conventionally, the upper segment of the skeleton is defined as the region between the vertex of the skull and the upper margin of the symphysis pubis, whereas the lower segment runs from the symphysis to the base of the heel (tarsus).

Zero to 3 Years

Infancy is the period of most rapid skeletal growth, not only in relative terms but also in absolute terms. Table 1 shows the normal occipitofrontal skull circumference, length, upper/lower segment ratio, and annualized growth rate from birth to 3 years at 6-month intervals.

Prepuberty

From about age 3 years until the onset of puberty, children of both sexes grow at a slowly decelerating rate with no

TABLE 1. *Normal occipitofrontal skull circumference, length, upper/lower segment ratio, and annualized growth rate from birth to 3 years at 6-month intervals*

Age (mo)	Occipitofrontal skull circumference (cm)	Length (cm)	Upper/lower segment ratio	Growth velocity (cm/yr)
0	34.0	50.0	1.68	—
6	42.8	66.1	1.61	32.2
12	45.8	74.6	1.55	17.0
18	47.2	81.0	1.46	12.8
24	48.0	86.7	1.37	11.4
30	48.5	91.6	1.32	9.8
36	49.0	95.9	1.28	8.6

major systematic fluctuations (see Fig. 1), although there may be a small growth spurt at around age 8 years and a distinct deceleration immediately before puberty.

Puberty and the Sexual Dimorphism of Skeletal Growth

During puberty, both sexes show a sharp increase in growth rate followed by epiphyseal fusion and the complete cessation of growth. The average age for the start and peak of the pubertal growth spurt, as for all manifestations of puberty, is younger in girls than in boys. The peak velocity and duration of the growth spurt also are less in girls than in boys, resulting in the 13-cm mean difference in adult height between men and women. It is the high degree of variability observed in the magnitude and duration of the pubertal growth spurt that renders prediction of adult height so inaccurate.

HORMONAL CONTROL OF SKELETAL GROWTH

The major hormonal systems directly affecting skeletal growth are the GH–IGF-1 axis, the gonadal axis, and the pituitary–thyroid axis. Although glucocorticoid excess (Cushing's syndrome) severely limits skeletal growth, there is little evidence that deficiencies in the production of cortisol lead to significant growth failure.

Growth Hormone

As its name implies, GH, or somatotropin, is a major stimulant of postnatal somatic growth. Fetal growth, on the other hand, is much less, if at all dependent on the GH–IGF-I axis. GH is a pleiotropic 191-amino acid peptide hormone secreted by the somatotrophs of the anterior pituitary. Secretory bursts are driven by growth hormone–releasing hormone (GHRH) from the medial hypothalamus and influenced by the inhibitory action of somatostatin and possibly by another stimulatory system acting on the GHR secretagogue (GHRS) receptors.

GH interacts with a specific receptor that forms part of the cytokine superfamily (9). A major action of GH at many of the sites at which it operates, including the skeletal growth plate, is to induce the release of IGF-I, formerly called somatomedin-C. This substance, which resembles proinsulin structurally and acts through receptors homologous with the insulin receptor, may act as both an endocrine and a paracrine hormone. The products of the GH–IGF-I system induce proliferation without marked maturation of the epiphyseal growth plate and thus induce linear skeletal growth that lasts until sex hormone–mediated epiphyseal closure. The relative extent to which these actions are a function of locally produced versus circulating IGF-I and the nature of any direct action of GH at that site remain topics for research (10).

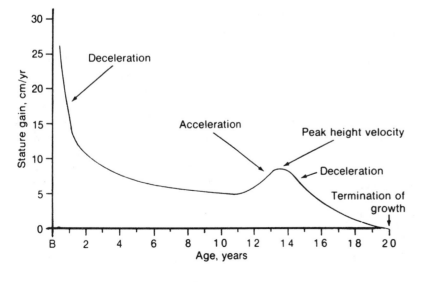

FIG. 1. The age-dependent phases of childhood skeletal growth velocity. (From Malina RM. *Growth and development: the first 20 years in man.* Minneapolis: Burgess Publishing Company, 1975.)

As in the case of GH, important evidence for the participation of the thyroid hormones, thyroxine (T_4) and triiodothyronine (T_3) in skeletal growth comes from observation of states of hormone deficiency. T_3, the active metabolite, enters its target cells and signals via a nuclear receptor of the steroid hormone–retinoic acid receptor class. It appears to be necessary for both proliferation and maturation of the growth plate.

The third class of hormones influencing skeletal growth is that of the sex hormones testosterone and estradiol and their derivatives. Present in very low quantities between infancy and puberty, these are produced in abundance during and after puberty and promote both proliferation and maturation in the epiphyseal growth plate. The ''pure'' actions of the individual sex hormones on the skeleton are hard to define because of the increased activity of the GH–IGF-I axis and of insulin during puberty and because of the convertibility by aromatization of testosterone to estrogens. Because epiphyseal proliferation and fusion are active during puberty in both sexes, the process was considered to involve both male and female gonadal hormones. Recently, however, it was observed that male subjects who lack aromatase (11) or functional estrogen receptors (1) manifest delayed epiphyseal fusion. These observations suggest that even in male subjects, it is estrogenic hormones that play a key role in epiphyseal maturation and fusion and the ultimate limitation of the adolescent growth spurt.

THE CONTROL OF MINERAL ACCRETION DURING SKELETAL GROWTH

The full-grown fetus at term contains about 21 g (range, 13 to 33 g) of calcium (12). During growth, this increases steadily to the 1000 g seen in the typical adult. The factors that control the accumulation of calcium into the skeleton during the growth period have been examined by calcium-balance techniques, by the use of nonradioactive isotopic calcium tracers (13), and by longitudinal and cross-sectional imaging of bone mineral density (14).

The consensus emerging from these observations is that calcium accumulation is particularly intense during puberty. The precise role of the hormonal changes of puberty in promoting the influx and retention of calcium is unclear, but a pubertal increase in calcitriol levels has been well described (Fig. 2) and presumably contributes to the process. As discussed later under biochemical markers, the activity of enzymes involved in mineralization and the turnover and accumulation of bone matrix also increases sharply during puberty.

QUANTITATIVE IMAGING DURING SKELETAL GROWTH

Radiology provides powerful tools for tracking skeletal development. These have developed in tandem with progress in technology and the availability of standardized age and sex-related norms.

The Assessment of Skeletal Maturity

As the epiphyseal growth plate matures, its shape and width change in a predictable fashion, with eventual fusion of the epiphysis with elimination of the radiologically visible ''gap'' between the epiphysis and its corresponding metaphysis. The peripheral small limb bones mature from cartilage in a similar manner but, lacking a shaft, undergo mineralization and maturation without epiphyseal fusion.

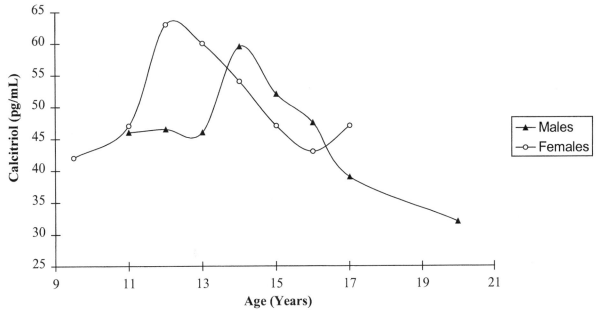

FIG. 2. Changes in calcitriol levels during growth. Note the resemblance of this curve to the growth velocity/age curve in Fig. 1. (From Aksnes L, Aarskog D. Plasma concentrations of vitamin D metabolites in puberty: effect of sexual maturation and implications for growth. *J Clin Endocrinol Metab* 1982;55:94–101.)

By radiologic observation of the bones of the hand and wrist in a large number of normal children, Greulich and Pyle (15) and Tanner et al. (16) were able to define specific developmental stages for each observed bone and to assign a sex-specific mean age at which each stage was reached. The clinician can assign a skeletal maturational age by averaging the maturational stage of a child's hand and wrist bones. This overall skeletal age or ''bone age'' provides a remarkable degree of insight into the child's skeletal development. Although the process of reading bone ages requires skill and patience, it is widely used to assess an individual's prognosis for growth and eventual adult height and as part of the evaluation of hormonal and metabolic disorders that may affect the skeleton.

The Measurement of Bone Mineral Content

The two methods that can provide usable data on bone density in children are dual-energy densitometry (DXA) and quantitative computed tomography (qCT). Because it is inexpensive, delivers a low radiation dose, and there is an increasing body of normative data for children, DXA is the most widely used method.

Dual-Energy X-Ray Absorptiometry

DXA is the most convenient method of assessing bone mineral content with reasonable accuracy. The low radiation doses administered have permitted study of normal children with the publication of normative data from a number of surveys (17). The big drawback of DXA bone densitometry in children is that the method actually measures the attenuation of an x-ray beam across a projected cross section of bone. This attenuation depends not only on the actual density

of skeletal mineral but also on the dimensions of the bone along the axis of the x-ray beam. These dimensions change through childhood so that corrections based on the child's size have to be applied to the machine's output (18).

Quantitative Computed Tomography

Quantitative computed tomography gives a true bone density (mass/unit volume). However, both cost and radiation dose preclude the study of large number of child subjects by using techniques devised for detailed imaging, so much fewer normative data are available. Low-radiation methods for qCT in children do exist, and this method still has potential importance. Recent studies by Gilsanz et al. (19) used qCT to assess the changes in skeletal mineral content during puberty and to look at intraethnic differences in bone mineral content (20).

BIOCHEMICAL MARKERS OF SKELETAL GROWTH

Histomorphometric studies show that children's bones are active by adult standards not only in the epiphyses but also in the cortical and trabecular regions of the established bone. As a corollary of this activity, all well-established markers of bone formation and resorption are increased in childhood, the graph of activity against age often bearing a striking similarity to the growth-velocity curve. This phenomenon was first observed in the longer-established markers such as alkaline phosphatase and urinary hydroxyproline excretion and has since been extended to osteocalcin (Fig. 3), serum markers of collagen formation and breakdown, and urinary pyridinium cross-links and N-terminal type I collagen telo-

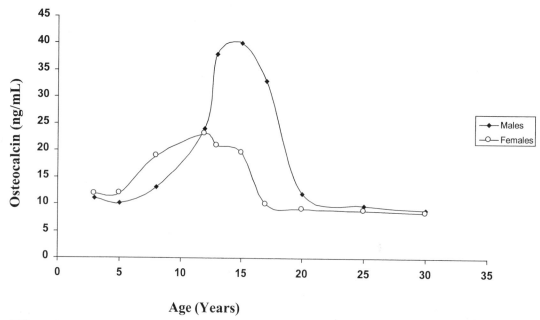

FIG. 3. Changes in serum osteocalcin levels during growth. Note the resemblance of this curve to the growth velocity/age curve in Fig. 1. (From Hauschka PV, Lian JB, Cole DE, Gundberg CM. Osteocalcin and matrix Gla protein: vitamin K-dependent proteins in bone. *Physiol Rev* 1989;69:990–1047.)

peptide. It is always important to bear in mind when investigating children with suspected bone disease that very high levels, relative to adults, of such markers are quite normal in pediatric samples (21).

ABNORMAL PATTERNS OF SKELETAL GROWTH AND DEVELOPMENT

Abnormalities of growth form a major part of the clinical practice of pediatric endocrinology and have given insights into the normal mechanisms whereby skeletal growth is promoted and controlled. Before the causes of growth failure were well understood, the various disorders were divided into proportionate and disproportionate growth failure, a classification that remains useful both in the clinic and for an appreciation of the underlying pathophysiology.

Proportionate Growth Failure

This term refers to shortness in which the body proportions, specifically the upper/lower segment or the arm span/height ratio, are close to normal. The commonest causes of this type of shortness are the polygenic influences that lead to familial shortness and constitutional delay of growth and maturation. However, disordered secretion or action of GH, thyroxine, or sex hormones may similarly retard skeletal growth.

Disproportionate Growth Failure

A classification and nomenclature of the specific inherited epiphyseal, metaphyseal, diaphyseal, and vertebral disorders that can lead to disproportionate growth is beyond the scope of this chapter. The theoretic importance of these diseases lies in the information they can provide concerning the roles of structural and signaling protein components of bone matrix (22).

Similarly, much has been learned from genetic investigations of a range of inherited disorders that interfere with the physiology of bone mineralization by altering the metabolism and availability of phosphate (23), calcium, or calcitriol (24). Such disorders all cause disproportionate short stature through the long-term effect of rickets on lower-limb development.

REFERENCES

1. Smith EP, Williams TC, Lubahn D, et al. Estrogen resistance caused by a mutation in the estrogen-receptor gene in a man. *N Engl J Med* 1994;331:1056–1061.
2. Binder G, Grauer ML, Wehner AV, Wehner F, Ranke MB. Outcome in tall stature: final height and psychological aspects in 220 patients with and without treatment. *Eur J Pediatr* 1997;156:905–910.
3. Baron J, Klein KO, Yanovski JA, et al. Induction of growth plate cartilage ossification by basic fibroblast growth factor. *Endocrinology* 1994;135:2790–2793.
4. Wu LN, Ishikawa Y, Nie D, Genge BR, Wuthier RE. Retinoic acid stimulates matrix calcification and initiates type I collagen synthesis in primary cultures of avian weight-bearing growth plate chondrocytes. *J Cell Biochem* 1997;65:209–230.
5. Prendiville J, Bingham EA, Burrows D. Premature epiphyseal closure: a complication of etretinate therapy in children. *J Am Acad Dermatol* 1986;15:1259–1262.
6. Hamill PV, Drizd TA, Johnson CL, Reed RB, Roche AF, Moore WM. Physical growth: National Center for Health Statistics percentiles. *Am J Clin Nutr* 1979;32:607–629.
7. Tanner JM, Davies PSW. Clinical longitudinal standards for height and height velocity in North American children. *J Pediatr* 1985;107:317–329.
8. Hermanussen M, Sippell WG, Valk IM. Knemometric monitoring of early effects of human growth hormone on leg length in children with growth hormone deficiency. *Lancet* 1985;1:1069–1071.
9. Postel-Vinay MC, Kelly PA. Growth hormone receptor signalling. *Baillieres Clin Endocrinol Metab* 1996;10:323–336.
10. Isaksson OG, Ohlsson C, Nilsson A, Isgaard J, Lindahl A. Regulation of cartilage growth by growth hormone and insulin-like growth factor I. *Pediatr Nephrol* 1991;5:451–453.
11. Morishima A, Grumbach MM, Simpson ER, Fisher C, Qin K. Aromatase deficiency in male and female siblings caused by a novel mutation and the physiological role of estrogens. *J Clin Endocrinol Metab* 1995;80:3689–3698.
12. Crowley S, Trivedi P, Risteli L, Risteli J, Hindmarsh PC, Brook CG. Collagen metabolism and growth in prepubertal children with asthma treated with inhaled steroids. *J Pediatr* 1998;132:409–413.
13. Abrams SA, O'Brien KO, Stuff JE. Changes in calcium kinetics associated with menarche. *J Clin Endocrinol Metab* 1996;8:2017–2020.
14. Gilsanz V. Bone density in children: a review of the available techniques and indications. *Eur J Radiol* 1998;26:177–182.
15. Greulich WW, Pyle SE. *Radiographic atlas of skeletal development of the hand and wrist.* 2nd ed. Stanford: Stanford University Press, 1959.
16. Tanner JM, Whitehouse RH, Marshall WA, et al. *Assessment of skeletal maturity and prediction of adult height.* London: Academic Press, 1975.
17. Glastre C, Braillon P, David L, Cochat P, Meunier PJ, Delmas PD. Measurement of bone mineral content of the lumbar spine by dual energy x-ray absorptiometry in normal children: correlations with growth parameters. *J Clin Endocrinol Metab* 1990;70:1330–1333.
18. Prentice A, Parsons TJ, Cole TJ. Uncritical use of bone mineral density in absorptiometry may lead to size-related artifacts in the identification of bone mineral determinants. *Am J Clin Nutr* 1994;60:837–842.
19. Mora S, Goodman WG, Loro ML, Roe TF, Sayre J, Gilsanz V. Age-related changes in cortical and cancellous vertebral bone density in girls: assessment with quantitative CT. *AJR Am J Roentgenol* 1994;162:405–409.
20. Gilsanz V, Roe TF, Mora S, Costin G, Goodman WG. Changes in vertebral bone density in black girls and white girls during childhood and puberty. *N Engl J Med* 1991;325:1597–1600.
21. Bollen AM, Eyre DR. Bone resorption rates in children monitored by the urinary assay of collagen type I cross-linked peptides. *Bone* 1994;15:31–34.
22. Horton WA. Molecular genetic basis of the human chondrodysplasias. *Endocrinol Metab Clin North Am* 1996;25:683–697.
23. Carpenter TO. New perspectives on the biology and treatment of X-linked hypophosphatemic rickets. *Pediatr Clin North Am* 1997;44:443–466.
24. Kitanaka S, Takeyama K, Murayama A, et al. Inactivating mutations in the 25-hydroxyvitamin D_3-1-alpha-hydroxylase gene in patients with pseudovitamin D-deficiency rickets. *N Engl J Med* 1998;338:653–661.

7. Pregnancy and Lactation

Christopher S. Kovacs, M.D. and *Henry M. Kronenberg, M.D.

*Department of Medicine–Endocrinology, Health Sciences Centre, Memorial University of Newfoundland, St. John's, Newfoundland, Canada; and *Department of Medicine, Harvard Medical School and Endocrine Unit, Massachusetts General Hospital, Boston, Massachusetts*

Normal pregnancy places a demand on the calcium homeostatic mechanisms of the human female, as the fetus and placenta draw calcium from the maternal circulation to mineralize the fetal skeleton. Similar demands are placed on the lactating woman to supply sufficient calcium to the breast milk to enable continued skeletal growth in a nursing infant. Despite a similar magnitude of calcium demand in pregnant and lactating women, the adjustments made in each of these reproductive periods differ significantly (Fig. 1). These hormone-mediated adjustments normally satisfy the daily calcium needs of the fetus and infant without long-term consequences to the maternal skeleton (1).

PREGNANCY

In total, up to 33 g of calcium is accumulated by the developing fetal skeleton, and about 80% of the accretion occurs during the third trimester when the fetal skeleton is rapidly mineralizing. This calcium demand appears to be largely met by a doubling of maternal intestinal calcium absorption, mediated by 1,25-dihydroxyvitamin D [1,25 $(OH)_2$ D] and other factors.

Mineral Ions and Calcitropic Hormones

Normal pregnancy results in altered levels of calcium and the calcitropic hormones, as schematically depicted in Fig. 2 (1). The total serum calcium decreases early in pregnancy because of a decrease in the serum albumin. This decrease should not be mistaken for true hypocalcemia, because the ionized calcium (the physiologically important fraction) remains constant. Serum phosphate levels also are normal during pregnancy.

The serum parathyroid hormone (PTH) level, when measured with a two-site immunoradiometric assay (IRMA), decreases to the low-normal range (i.e., <50% of the mean nonpregnant value) during the first trimester but increases steadily to the midnormal range by term. Free and bound 1,25 $(OH)_2$ D levels double early in pregnancy and maintain this increase until term. The increase in 1,25 $(OH)_2$ D may be largely independent of changes in PTH, because PTH levels are typically low or normal at the time of the increase in 1,25 $(OH)_2$ D.

Serum calcitonin levels also are increased during pregnancy. It has been speculated that this increased level of calcitonin reflects its postulated role in protecting the maternal skeleton from excessive resorption of calcium, but this hypothesis remains unproved.

PTH-related protein (PTHrP) levels are increased during pregnancy, as determined by assays that detect PTHrP fragments encompassing amino acids 1 to 86. Because PTHrP is produced by many tissues in the fetus and mother (including the placenta, amnion, decidua, umbilical cord, fetal parathyroids, and breast), it is not clear which source(s) contribute to the increase detected in the maternal circulation. PTHrP may contribute to the increases in 1,25 $(OH)_2$ D and suppression of PTH that are noted during pregnancy. PTHrP may have other roles during pregnancy, such as regulating placental calcium transport in the fetus (1,2). PTHrP also may have a role in protecting the maternal skeleton during pregnancy, because the carboxyl-terminal portion of PTHrP (''osteostatin'') has been shown to inhibit osteoclastic bone resorption (3).

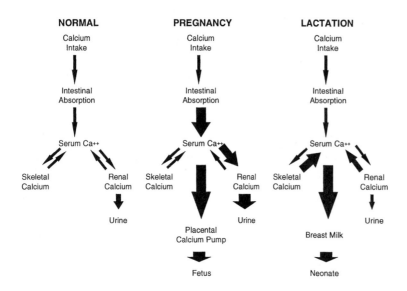

FIG. 1. Calcium homeostasis in human pregnancy and lactation as compared with normal. The thickness of arrows indicates a relative increase or decrease with respect to the normal, nonpregnant state. (From Kovacs CS, Kronenberg HM. Maternal-fetal calcium and bone metabolism during pregnancy, puerperium and lactation. *Endocr Rev* 1997;18:832–872, with permission of The Endocrine Society.)

Pregnancy induces an increase in the levels of other hormones, including the sex steroids, prolactin, and placental lactogen. The possibility that each of these, in turn, may have direct or indirect effects on calcium and bone metabolism during pregnancy has been largely unexplored.

Intestinal Absorption of Calcium

Intestinal absorption of calcium is doubled during pregnancy from as early as 12 weeks of gestation (the earliest time point studied); this appears to be a major maternal adaptation to meet the fetal need for calcium. This increase may be largely the result of a 1,25 $(OH)_2$ D–mediated increase in intestinal calbindin$_{9K}$-D and other proteins; prolactin and placental lactogen (and possibly other factors) also may mediate part of the increase in intestinal calcium absorption. The increased absorption of calcium early in pregnancy may allow the maternal skeleton to store calcium in advance of the peak fetal demands.

Renal Handling of Calcium

The 24-hour urine calcium excretion is increased as early as week 12 of gestation (the earliest time point studied) and averages 300 ± 61 mg in the third trimester (levels in the hypercalciuric range are not uncommon). Because fasting urine calcium values are normal or low, the increase in 24-hour urine calcium likely reflects the increased intestinal absorption of calcium (absorptive hypercalciuria).

Skeletal Calcium Metabolism

Animal models indicate that histomorphometric parameters of bone turnover are increased during pregnancy, but comparable histomorphometric data are not available for human pregnancy. Instead, markers of bone formation and resorption have been assessed (1). Several markers of bone resorption (tartrate-resistant alkaline phosphatase, deoxypyridinoline/creatinine, pyridinoline/creatinine, and hydroxyproline/creatinine) are low in the first trimester but peak at values up to twice normal in the last trimester. Among the bone-formation markers, osteocalcin is low or undetectable early in gestation but may increase to normal levels by term. Procollagen I carboxypeptides and bone specific alkaline phosphatase also are low in the first trimester, but may increase to normal or above in the last trimester. Total alkaline phosphatase increases early in pregnancy largely because of contributions from the placental fraction; it is not a useful marker of bone formation in pregnancy.

These findings indicate that bone turnover is probably decreased in the first half of pregnancy but may be increased in the third trimester. The third-trimester increase in bone turnover corresponds to time of the peak rate of calcium transfer to the fetus and may reflect mobilization of skeletal calcium stores (which contain 99% of the body's stores of calcium) to help supply the fetus.

Because of concerns about fetal radiation exposure, few studies of maternal bone density during pregnancy have been done, and all used outdated techniques. By using single- or

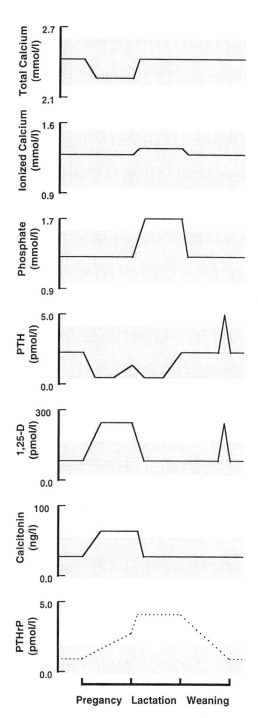

FIG. 2. The longitudinal changes in calcium, phosphate, and calcitropic hormone levels that occur during pregnancy and lactation. Normal adult ranges are indicated by the shaded areas. The progression in PTHrP levels is depicted by a dashed line to reflect that the data are less complete; the implied comparison of PTHrP levels in late pregnancy and lactation are uncertain extrapolations because no reports followed up patients serially. In both situations, PTHrP levels are increased. (Adapted from Kovacs CS, Kronenberg HM. Maternal-fetal calcium and bone metabolism during pregnancy, puerperium and lactation. *Endocr Rev* 1997;18:832–872, with permission of The Endocrine Society.)

dual-photon absorptiometry (SDA, DPA) or both, prospective studies did not find a significant change in cortical or trabecular bone density during pregnancy (1). Most recently, longitudinal studies found a progressive decrease during pregnancy in indices thought to correlate with bone mineral density, as determined by ultrasonographic measurements of the os calcis.

Retrospective, epidemiologic studies of pre- and postmenopausal women generally indicated that parity has no association with bone density or fracture risk (1,4). Although many of these studies could not separate the effects of parity from those of lactation, it may be reasonable to conclude that if parity has any effect on bone density or fracture risk, it must be only a very modest effect.

Osteoporosis in Pregnancy

Occasionally, a woman may be seen with fragility fractures and low bone mineral density during pregnancy. Some cases may be confounded by other recognizable causes of secondary osteoporosis, such as chronic heparin, anticonvulsant, or corticosteroid therapy. Some of these rare cases may result from excessive resorption of calcium from the maternal skeleton, perhaps in the setting of inadequate dietary calcium, low stores of 25-hydroxyvitamin D, or an excessive increase of PTHrP in the maternal circulation. It is also possible that these rare cases may simply represent idiopathic osteoporosis occurring in pregnant women by mere chance.

Focal, transient osteoporosis of the hip is also a rare form of pregnancy-associated osteoporosis. These patients have unilateral or bilateral hip pain, limp, or hip fracture or a combination of these in the third trimester and have objective evidence of reduced bone density of the symptomatic femoral head and neck. The condition is self-limited: the decreased bone mineral density typically resolves within 2 to 6 months after delivery. As yet, the etiology remains unclear; its association with pregnancy also may be by mere chance. In any case, this focal or localized disorder is likely not a manifestation of altered calcitropic hormone levels or mineral balance during pregnancy.

Primary Hyperparathyroidism

Although probably a rare condition (there are no data available on its prevalence), primary hyperparathyroidism in pregnancy has been associated in the literature with an alarming rate of adverse outcomes in the fetus and neonate, including a 30% rate of spontaneous abortion or stillbirth (5). The adverse postnatal outcomes are thought to result from suppression of the fetal and neonatal parathyroid glands; this suppression may occasionally be prolonged after birth for months. To prevent these adverse outcomes, surgical correction of primary hyperparathyroidism during the second trimester has been almost universally recommended. Several case series have found elective surgery to be well tolerated and to reduce dramatically the rate of adverse events when compared with the earlier cases reported in the literature. However, many of the women in those early cases had a relatively severe form of primary hyperparathyroidism

that is not often seen today (symptomatic, with nephrocalcinosis and renal insufficiency). Whether the milder, asymptomatic form of primary hyperparathyroidism commonly seen today has the same risk of adverse fetal or neonatal outcomes has not been determined.

Familial Hypocalciuric Hypercalcemia

Although familial hypocalciuric hypercalcemia (FHH; see Chapter 32) has not been reported to affect adversely the mother during pregnancy, maternal hypercalcemia can cause fetal and neonatal parathyroid suppression with subsequent tetany.

Hypoparathyroidism and Pseudohypoparathyroidism

Early in pregnancy, hypoparathyroid women may have fewer hypocalcemic symptoms and require less supplemental calcium. This is consistent with a limited role for PTH in the pregnant woman and suggests that an increase in $1,25 (OH)_2 D$ or increased intestinal calcium absorption or both will occur in the absence of PTH. However, it is clear from other case reports that some pregnant hypoparathyroid women may require increased calcitriol replacement to avoid worsening hypocalcemia. It is important to maintain a normal ionized calcium level in pregnant women because maternal hypocalcemia has been associated with the development of intrauterine fetal hyperparathyroidism and fetal death. Late in pregnancy, hypercalcemia may occur in hypoparathyroid women unless the calcitriol dosage is substantially reduced or discontinued. This effect may be mediated by the increasing levels of PTHrP in the maternal circulation in late pregnancy.

In limited case reports of pseudohypoparathyroidism, pregnancy was noted to normalize the serum calcium level, reduce the PTH level by half, and increase the $1,25 (OH)_2 D$ level two- to threefold (6). The mechanism by which pseudohypoparathyroidism is improved in pregnancy remains unclear.

LACTATION

The typical daily loss of calcium in breast milk has been estimated to range from 280 to 400 mg, although daily losses as great as 1000 mg calcium have been reported. A temporary demineralization of the skeleton appears to be the main mechanism by which lactating humans meet these calcium requirements. This demineralization does not appear to be mediated by PTH or $1,25 (OH)_2 D$, but may be mediated by PTHrP and the decrease in estrogen levels.

Mineral Ions and Calcitropic Hormones

The normal lactational changes in maternal calcium, phosphate, and calcitropic hormone levels are schematically depicted in Fig. 2 (1). The mean ionized calcium level of exclusively lactating women is increased. Serum phosphate levels also are higher during lactation, and the level may exceed the normal range. Because reabsorption of phosphate by the kidneys appears to be increased, the increased serum phosphate levels may, therefore, reflect the combined effects of increased flux of phosphate into the blood from diet, from skeletal resorption, and from decreased renal phosphate excretion.

Intact PTH, as determined by a two-site IRMA assay, was found to be reduced 50% or more in lactating women. It increases to normal at weaning, but may increase above normal after weaning. In contrast to the high 1,25 $(OH)_2$ D levels of pregnancy, maternal free and bound 1,25 $(OH)_2$ D levels decrease to normal within days of parturition and remain there throughout lactation. Calcitonin levels decrease to normal after the first 6 weeks after delivery.

PTHrP levels, as measured by two-site IRMA assays, are significantly higher in lactating women than in nonpregnant controls. The source of PTHrP may be the breast, because PTHrP was detected in breast milk at concentrations exceeding 10,000 times the level found in the blood of patients with hypercalcemia of malignancy or normal human controls. Indeed, a small increase in the maternal level of PTHrP can be demonstrated after suckling (7,8). The primary role of PTHrP in the breast or breast milk is not clear. Studies in animals suggest that PTHrP may have a primary role in the breast to regulate mammary development and mammary blood flow. In addition, PTHrP may reach the maternal circulation from the lactating breast to cause resorption of calcium from the maternal skeleton, renal tubular reabsorption of calcium, and (indirectly) suppression of PTH. In support of this hypothesis, PTHrP levels were found to correlate negatively with PTH levels and positively with the ionized calcium levels of lactating women (7,9). PTHrP levels also correlate with the loss of bone mineral density during lactation in humans (10).

Intestinal Absorption of Calcium

Intestinal calcium absorption is not increased during lactation, despite calcium requirements similar to those in pregnancy. The decrease in intestinal calcium absorption from the higher levels of pregnancy coincides with the decrease in 1,25 $(OH)_2$ D levels to normal.

Renal Handling of Calcium

In humans, the glomerular filtration rate decreases during lactation, and the renal excretion of calcium is typically reduced to levels as low as 50 mg/24 h. The low urine calcium with high calcium in the blood suggests that tubular reabsorption of calcium might be increased to account for the reduction in calcium excretion.

Skeletal Calcium Metabolism

Although histomorphometric data from animals consistently show increased bone turnover during lactation, definitive histomorphometric data are lacking for humans. Markers of bone resorption are increased twofold to threefold during lactation and are higher than the levels attained in the third trimester. Markers of bone formation are generally high

during lactation and increased over the levels attained during the third trimester. Total alkaline phosphatase decreases immediately after delivery because of loss of the placental fraction but may still remain above normal because of the increase in the bone-specific fraction. These findings suggest that bone turnover is significantly increased during lactation.

Serial measurements of bone density during lactation [by SPA, DPA, or dual-energy x-ray absorptiometry (DXA)] showed a decrease of 3% to 8% in bone mineral content after 2 to 6 months of lactation at trabecular sites (lumbar spine, hip, femur, and distal radius), with smaller losses at cortical sites (1,4). Loss of bone mineral from the maternal skeleton appears to be a normal consequence of lactation and may not be preventable by increasing the calcium intake above the recommended dietary allowance. For example, in a randomized clinical intervention trial that studied the effect of consuming dietary calcium in excess of the recommended daily allowance (2.4 g daily), lactating women still lost 6.3% of bone mineral density at the lumbar spine and up to 8% from the radius and ulna, as determined by DXA (11). In a preliminary report, the lactational decrease in lumbar spine bone mineral density was not influenced by maternal calcium intake but was negatively and significantly correlated with the breast-milk output (12).

It is not clear whether this loss of bone mineral content is simply due to relative estrogen deficiency of lactation or a more complex, possibly humorally mediated mechanism. No published study has adequately addressed the relative role of estrogen withdrawal during lactation in a definitive way, because no study manipulated estrogen independent of lactation. It is evident from studying the effects of acute estrogen deficiency induced by gonadotropin-releasing hormone (GnRH)-agonist therapy in young women that estrogen deficiency alone is unlikely to account for all of the changes in skeletal calcium metabolism seen during lactation (1). Therefore, in lactation, the greater losses of bone mineral density (at both trabecular and cortical sites), the normal 1,25 $(OH)_2$ D levels, and the reduced urinary calcium excretion may be due to the effects of other factors (such as PTHrP) in addition to the effects of estrogen withdrawal alone (Fig. 3).

The bone-density losses of lactation appear to be substantially reversed during weaning (1,4). In the long term, the consequences of lactation-induced depletion of bone mineral content appear clinically unimportant. The vast majority of epidemiologic studies of pre- and postmenopausal women found no adverse effect, or a protective effect, of a history of lactation on peak bone mass, bone density, or hip-fracture risk.

Osteoporosis of Lactation

Rarely osteoporosis is seen during lactation; like osteoporosis in pregnancy, this may be a coincidental, unrelated disease. Alternatively, it may be a continuum of a condition that may be seen in pregnancy and an exacerbation of the normal degree of skeletal demineralization that occurs during lactation. It is possible that excessive PTHrP release from the lactating breast into the maternal circulation could cause excessive bone resorption, osteoporosis, and fractures

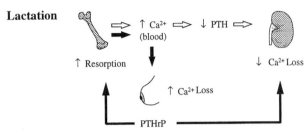

FIG. 3. Acute estrogen deficiency (e.g., gonadotropin hormone–releasing hormone analogue therapy) increases skeletal resorption and increases the blood calcium; in turn, parathyroid hormone is suppressed, and renal calcium losses are increased. During lactation, the combined effects of parathyroid hormone–related peptide (secreted by the breast) and estrogen deficiency increase skeletal resorption, reduce renal calcium losses, and increase the blood calcium, but calcium is directed into breast milk. (From Kovacs CS, Kronenberg HM. Maternal-fetal calcium and bone metabolism during pregnancy, puerperium and lactation. *Endocr Rev* 1997;18:832–872, with permission of The Endocrine Society.)

in some of these cases. PTHrP levels were high in one case of lactational osteoporosis and were found to remain high for months after weaning (13). However, the extent to which PTHrP contributes to the reduction of bone density during lactation has yet to be established.

Hypoparathyroidism and Pseudohypoparathyroidism

Calcitriol requirements of hypoparathyroid women decrease early in the postpartum period, especially if the woman breastfeeds, and hypercalcemia may occur if the calcitriol dosage is not substantially reduced (14). This is consistent with PTHrP reaching the maternal circulation in amounts sufficient to allow stimulation of 1,25 (OH)$_2$ D synthesis and maintenance of normal (or slightly increased) maternal serum calcium (15).

The management of pseudohypoparathyroidism has been less well documented. Because these patients are likely resis-

tant to the renal actions of PTHrP, and the placental sources of 1,25 (OH)$_2$ D are lost at parturition, the calcitriol requirements might well increase and may require further adjustments during lactation.

REFERENCES

1. Kovacs CS, Kronenberg HM. Maternal-fetal calcium and bone metabolism during pregnancy, puerperium and lactation. *Endocr Rev* 1997;18: 832–872.
2. Kovacs CS, Lanske B, Hunzelman JL, Guo J, Karaplis AC, Kronenberg HM. Parathyroid hormone-related peptide (PTHrP) regulates fetal-placental calcium transport through a receptor distinct from the PTH/PTHrP receptor. *Proc Natl Acad Sci U S A* 1996;93:15233–15238.
3. Cornish J, Callon KE, Nicholson GC, Reid IR. Parathyroid hormone-related protein-(107-139) inhibits bone resorption in vivo. *Endocrinology* 1997;138:1299–1304.
4. Sowers M. Pregnancy and lactation as risk factors for subsequent bone loss and osteoporosis. *J Bone Miner Res* 1996;11:1052–1060.
5. Shangold MM, Dor N, Welt SI, Fleischman AR, Crenshaw MC Jr. Hyperparathyroidism and pregnancy: a review. *Obstet Gynecol Surv* 1982;37:217–228.
6. Breslau NA, Zerwekh JE. Relationship of estrogen and pregnancy to calcium homeostasis in pseudohypoparathyroidism. *J Clin Endocrinol Metab* 1986;62:45–51.
7. Dobnig H, Kainer F, Stepan V, et al. Elevated parathyroid hormone-related peptide levels after human gestation: relationship to changes in bone and mineral metabolism. *J Clin Endocrinol Metab* 1995;80: 3699–3707.
8. Lippuner K, Zehnder HJ, Casez JP, Takkinen R, Jaeger P. Effects of PTH-related protein (PTH-rP) on calcium-phosphate metabolism in nursing mothers [Abstract]. *Bone* 1995;16(Suppl 1):209S.
9. Kovacs CS, Chik CL. Hyperprolactinemia caused by lactation and pituitary adenomas is associated with altered serum calcium, phosphate, parathyroid hormone (PTH), and PTH-related peptide levels. *J Clin Endocrinol Metab* 1995;80:3036–3042.
10. Sowers MF, Hollis BW, Shapiro B, et al. Elevated parathyroid hormone-related peptide associated with lactation and bone density loss. *JAMA* 1996;276:549–554.
11. Cross NA, Hillman LS, Allen SH, Krause GF. Changes in bone mineral density and markers of bone remodeling during lactation and postweaning in women consuming high amounts of calcium. *J Bone Miner Res* 1995;10:1312–1320.
12. Laskey MA, Prentice A, Jarjou LM, Beavan S. Lactational changes in bone mineral of the lumbar spine are influenced by breast-milk output but not calcium intake, breast-milk calcium concentration, or vitamin-D receptor genotype [Abstract]. *J Bone Miner Res* 1996;11: 1815.
13. Reid IR, Wattie DJ, Evans MC, Budayr AA. Post-pregnancy osteoporosis associated with hypercalcaemia. *Clin Endocrinol (Oxf)* 1992;37: 298–303.
14. Caplan RH, Beguin EA. Hypercalcemia in a calcitriol-treated hypoparathyroid woman during lactation. *Obstet Gynecol* 1990;76:485–489.
15. Mather KJ, Chik CL, Corenblum B. Maintenance of serum calcium by parathyroid hormone-related peptide during lactation in a hypoparathyroid patient. *J Clin Endocrinol Metab* 1999;84:424–427.

8. Menopause

Ian R. Reid, M.D., F.R.A.C.P.

Department of Medicine, University of Auckland and Department of Endocrinology, Auckland Hospital, Auckland, New Zealand

Menopause refers to the cessation of menstruation, which occurs at about age 48 to 50 years in healthy women. The decline in ovarian hormone production, however, is gradual and starts several years before the last period. Changes in bone mass and calcium metabolism are evident during this perimenopausal transition. Estrogen is the ovarian product that has the greatest impact on mineral metabolism, although both progesterone and ovarian androgens may have some influence. Menopause ushers in a period of bone loss that extends until the end of life and that is the central contributor to the development of osteoporotic fractures in older women.

EFFECTS ON BONE

Before the menopause, there is virtually no bone loss, and fracture rates are stable in most regions of the skeleton. The most obvious effect of menopause on bone is an increase in the incidence of fractures, which, for the forearms and vertebrae, is clearly apparent within the first postmenopausal decade. This is attributable to the rapid decline in bone mass that occurs in the perimenopausal years. This bone loss is more marked in trabecular than in cortical bone because the former has a far greater surface area over which bone resorption can take place. Thus the fractures that occur early in the menopause are in trabecular-rich regions of the skeleton such as the distal forearm and vertebrae. The loss of bone and the increase in fracture rates are both preventable with estrogen replacement (1).

The perimenopausal increase in bone loss is associated with increased bone resorption. Bone biopsies in normal postmenopausal women show an increase in the fraction of bone surfaces at which resorption is taking place and an increase in the depth of resorption pits. Similar findings emerge from studies of biochemical markers of bone cell function. After the menopause, indices of bone resorption are twice the levels found in premenopausal women (2). There also is an increase in markers of bone formation, but these are only about 50% above premenopausal levels (2). These histomorphometric and marker changes can be returned to premenopausal levels with estrogen-replacement therapy.

The changes in bone turnover that accompany the menopause are at least in part accounted for by the direct actions of estrogen on bone cells. Estrogen receptors are present in both osteoblasts and osteoclasts. Studies of the effects of estrogen on isolated osteoblasts have not produced entirely consistent results, although increases in production of a number of osteoblast proteins (e.g., insulin-like growth factor-1, type I procollagen, transforming growth factor-β [TGF-β], bone morphogenetic protein-6) have been reported. These findings suggest that estrogen tends to have an anabolic effect on the isolated osteoblast, and it may be important in maintaining osteocyte function also (3). *In vivo,* however, there is a reduction in osteoblast numbers and activity associated with postmenopausal estrogen-replacement therapy (4). This is accounted for by the tight coupling of osteoblast activity to that of osteoclasts and the overriding effect of estrogen directly to reduce bone resorption by osteoclasts, in part by promoting osteoclast apoptosis (5). The reduction in bone resorption also may be contributed to by the effect of estrogen to increase levels of nitric oxide and TGF-β, which (in addition to having effects on osteoblast growth) are potent inhibitors of osteoclastic differentiation and bone resorption (6).

Recent studies suggest that bone marrow stromal and mononuclear cells are possibly the most important target cells for sex hormones in bone. These cells produce cytokines such as interleukin-1 (IL-1), interleukin-6 (IL-6), and tumor necrosis factor-α (TNF), which are potent stimulators of osteoclast recruitment or activity or both (7). Estrogen decreases production of each of these cytokines, and a number of studies indicated that this is important to the effects of estrogen on bone. The increase in osteoclast numbers or bone loss after ovariectomy is reduced by blockers of either IL-6, IL-1, or TNF (8), and mice not expressing the IL-6 gene do not lose bone after ovariectomy. IL-1 and TNF may act in part by regulating stromal cell production of IL-6 and macrophage colony-stimulating factor (9). Thus effects on production of cytokines and growth factors within the bone marrow may act together with direct effects of estrogen on bone cells to modulate both bone resorption and bone formation. There may be a further contribution from the regulation of the release of systemic factors, such as growth hormone, by estrogen.

EFFECTS ON CALCIUM METABOLISM

The loss of bone that follows the menopause is accompanied by negative changes in external calcium balance, which are approximately equally contributed to by decreases in intestinal calcium absorption and by increases in urinary calcium loss (10). The reduction in intestinal calcium absorption is accompanied by reduced circulating concentrations of total but not free 1,25-dihydroxyvitamin D [1,25 (OH)$_2$ D], suggesting that the principal effect of estrogen in this regard is on synthesis of the protein that carries 1,25 (OH)$_2$ D in plasma. Thus oral administration of estrogen to postmenopausal women increases total 1,25 (OH)$_2$ D concentrations, but use of transdermal estrogen, which bypasses the liver where vitamin D–binding protein is synthesized, does not. However, estrogen may directly regulate intestinal calcium absorption independent of vitamin D.

In the kidney, it is clear that tubular reabsorption of calcium is higher in the presence of estrogen. Some studies found higher parathyroid hormone (PTH) concentrations in the presence of estrogen and inferred that this was the mechanism of the renal calcium conservation. However, higher PTH levels have not been the finding in a number of other studies (11). Thus it is likely that estrogen directly modulates

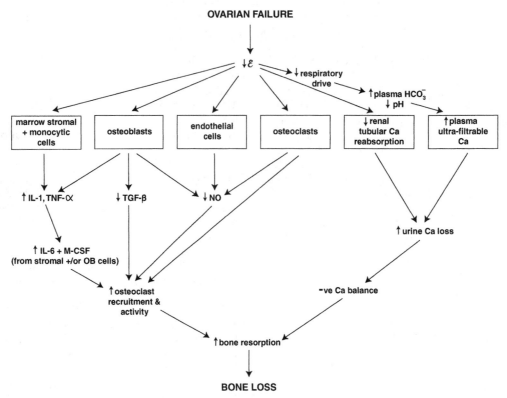

FIG. 1. The potential pathways by which menopause leads to bone loss. For simplicity, the figure does not show a contribution from loss of any anabolic effect of estrogen on the osteoblast. E, estrogen; NO, nitric oxide; =ve, negative; other abbreviations as in text. (Copyright 1998 I. Reid, used with permission.)

renal tubular calcium absorption by its own receptor, which is present in the kidney.

The changes in the handling of calcium by the gut and kidney could each be a cause of postmenopausal bone loss, or they could represent homeostatic responses to it. If the former were the case, then PTH concentrations would be increased in postmenopausal women to maintain plasma calcium concentrations in the face of intestinal and renal losses. This, in turn, would cause bone loss. If, on the other hand, bone loss were the primary event, then suppression of PTH would be expected, leading to secondary declines in intestinal and renal calcium absorption. The effect of menopause on PTH concentrations has been addressed many times without any consistent pattern emerging. This suggests that the situation is more complicated than this simple formulation allows. Possibly estrogen has direct effects on bone, kidney, and gut, and the opposing effects on PTH secretion of these actions leads to inconsistent changes in PTH levels in clinical studies. Further, estrogen may directly modulate PTH secretion.

There are small but consistently demonstrable effects of menopause on circulating concentrations of calcium. Total calcium is 0.05 mmol/L higher after the menopause. This is partly attributable to a contraction of the plasma volume and resulting increase in albumin concentrations that occurs in the absence of estrogen and partly to an increase in plasma bicarbonate, which leads to an increase in the complexed fraction of plasma calcium. The higher bicarbonate levels

in postmenopausal women are attributable to a respiratory acidosis that results from the loss of the respiratory stimulatory effects of progesterone on the central nervous system, an action potentiated by estrogen (12). Despite changes in protein-bound and complexed calcium fractions, ionized calcium concentrations are usually found to be the same in pre- and postmenopausal women.

SUMMARY

The effects of the menopause on skeletal physiology are summarized in Fig. 1. The major effect is an increase in bone turnover, which is predominantly an increase in bone resorption. This results in bone loss, which may be contributed to by reductions in both intestinal and renal tubular absorption of calcium. Bone loss persists throughout the entire postmenopausal period and results in a high risk of fractures in those women whose peak bone mass was in the lower part of the normal range.

REFERENCES

1. Lindsay R, Hart DM, Forrest C, Baird C. Prevention of spinal osteoporosis in oophorectomised women. *Lancet* 1980;2:1151–1153.
2. Garnero P, Sornayrendu E, Chapuy MC, Delmas PD. Increased bone turnover in late postmenopausal women is a major determinant of osteoporosis. *J Bone Miner Res* 1996;11:337–349.

3. Tomkinson A, Reeve J, Shaw RW, Noble BS. The death of osteocytes via apoptosis accompanies estrogen withdrawal in human bone. *J Clin Endocrinol Metab* 1997;82:3128–3135.

4. Vedi S, Compston JE. The effects of long-term hormone replacement therapy on bone remodeling in postmenopausal women. *Bone* 1996;19:535–539.

5. Kameda T, Mano H, Yuasa T, et al. Estrogen inhibits bone resorption by directly inducing apoptosis of the bone-resorbing osteoclasts. *J Exp Med* 1997;186:489–495.

6. Ralston SH. The Michael-Mason-Prize essay 1997: nitric oxide and bone: what a gas. *Br J Rheumatol* 1997;36:831–838.

7. Manolagas SC, Jilka RL. Mechanisms of disease: bone marrow, cytokines, and bone remodeling: emerging insights into the pathophysiology of osteoporosis. *N Engl J Med* 1995;332:305–311.

8. Kimble RB, Matayoshi AB, Vannice JL, Kung VT, Williams C, Pacifici R. Simultaneous block of interleukin-1 and tumor necrosis factor is required to completely prevent bone loss in the early postovariectomy period. *Endocrinology* 1995;136:3054–3061.

9. Kimble RB, Srivastava S, Ross FP, Matayoshi A, Pacifici R. Estrogen deficiency increases the ability of stromal cells to support murine osteoclastogenesis via an interleukin-1 and tumor necrosis factor-mediated stimulation of macrophage colony-stimulating factor production. *J Biol Chem* 1996;271:28890–28897.

10. Heaney RP, Recker RR, Saville PD. Menopausal changes in calcium balance performance. *J Lab Clin Med* 1978;92:953–963.

11. Prince RL. Counterpoint: estrogen effects on calcitropic hormones and calcium homeostasis. *Endocr Rev* 1994;15:301–309.

12. Bayliss DA, Millhorn DE. Central neural mechanisms of progesterone action: application to the respiratory system. *J Appl Physiol* 1992;73:393–404.

9. The Aging Skeleton

Clifford J. Rosen, M.D. and *Douglas P. Kiel, M.P.H., M.D.

*Department of Nutrition, University of Maine, Orono, Maine and Maine Center for Osteoporosis Research and Education, St. Joseph Hospital, Bangor, Maine; and *Division on Aging, Harvard Medical School, and Research and Training Institute, Hebrew Rehabilitation Center for Aged, Boston, Massachusetts*

BONE MASS AND AGE

Elderly individuals are at very high risk for hip and spine fractures for a host of reasons. These include low bone mineral density (BMD), falls, changes in the geometry of bone, life-style factors and the rate of bone remodeling. In addition, older men and women are likely to have greater morbidity from those fractures than do younger individuals. Thus prevention is a critical paradigm in osteoporosis medicine for all people including the very oldest. Advanced age is a relatively strong risk factor for an osteoporotic fracture, but low BMD increases the risk of a fracture independent of the risk associated with advancing age (1,2). Both appendicular and axial measurements of bone mass reveal that women at highest risk for fracture are those with a BMD >1.0 standard deviation below a preset value for young normals or in relation to an age-matched population. This risk increases linearly with progressively lower BMD with no threshold effect evident, even at the lowest values (1–3). Site-specific measurements predict fracture at one location better than measurements at another do for that same location (3). For example, a 1-standard deviation decline in femoral BMD is associated with a 2.5-fold greater risk of a hip fracture between 1.5 and 2.0. Although a single BMD measurement at any site is the sum of several variables (i.e., peak bone mass, menopausal bone loss, hormonal alterations, and age-associated changes), advanced age is almost uniformly associated with low BMD at all sites, whether measured by dual-energy x-ray absorptiometry, calcaneal ultrasound, or radioabsorptiometry. The reasons for this are noted later. Still, there appears to be an additive effect of age on BMD in relation to the factor of risk, so that an 80-year-old woman with a femoral BMD of 0.700 g/cm^2 is at much higher risk for an osteoporotic fracture than a 50-year-old with the same absolute femoral BMD measurement.

BONE REMODELING IN THE ELDERLY

Over a life span, women lose approximately 42% of their spinal and 58% of their femoral bone mass (1). Surprisingly, rates of bone loss in decades 8 and 9 of life may exceed those found in the immediate perimenopausal period, in part because there is uncoupling in the remodeling cycle (2,4). Changes in bone turnover in the elderly can be detected by biochemical markers of bone turnover, which include bone-resorption indices (e.g., urinary N-telopeptide, C-telopeptide, free and total deoxypyridinoline) and bone-formation markers (e.g., osteocalcin, procollagen peptide, bone-specific alkaline phosphatase). Bone-turnover markers are significantly higher in older than in younger postmenopausal women, and these indices are inversely related to bone density (5). For example, in the prospective EPIDOS trial of elderly women, the highest levels of osteocalcin, N-telopeptide, C-telopeptide, and bone-specific alkaline phosphatase were found among those in the lowest tertile of femoral BMD (6). Increased bone-resorption indices also were associated with a greater fracture risk independent of bone density (6). For those women in EPIDOS with low bone density and a high bone-resorption rate, there was a nearly fivefold greater risk of a hip fracture.

In contrast to a consistent pattern of high bone-resorption indices, bone-formation markers in the elderly are variable. Serum osteocalcin levels are high in elderly individuals, but this may be indicative of an increase in bone turnover rather than reflecting a true increase in bone formation (6). On the other hand, bone-specific alkaline phosphatase and procollagen peptides levels were reported to be high, normal, or low in elders (7). Bone histomorphometric indices in elders also are quite variable. Thus although there is strong evidence for an age-associated increase in bone resorption, changes in bone formation are inconsistent. Still there is uncoupling of the remodeling unit, which leads to bone loss, altered skeletal architecture, and an increased propensity to fractures.

FACTORS THAT CONTRIBUTE TO AGE-RELATED BONE LOSS

Nutritional

By far the most common cause of increased bone resorption in older individuals is calcium deficiency. Low calcium intake is very common in the elderly and usually results in secondary hyperparathyroidism. Moreover, older men and women consume less vitamin D and cannot generate as much previtamin D in the skin in response to ultraviolet exposure as can younger individuals. This leads to a reduction in serum 25-hydroxyvitamin D [25 (OH) D] levels, which contributes to reduced calcium absorption (8,9). In addition, there is impaired renal conversion of 25 (OH) D to 1,25-dihydroxyvitamin D [1,25 (OH)$_2$ D], and there may be an element of intestinal resistance to 1,25 (OH)$_2$ D because of reduced numbers of vitamin D receptors (VDRs), impaired binding of vitamin D to the VDRs, or a postreceptor defect. In concert, all these factors can lead to an increase in PTH secretion among elderly individuals (8). Further evidence in support of the calcium-deficiency hypothesis comes from longitudinal trials of elderly men and women supplemented with both calcium and vitamin D. These studies demonstrated preservation of bone density, a decrease in bone resorption, and a reduction in osteoporotic fractures in elders administered calcium and vitamin D (9,10). Furthermore, these data have led the National Academy of Science to recommend an increase in the minimal daily requirement for calcium intake in people older than 65 years to 1500 mg/day (11).

Other nutritional factors may play a role in age-related osteoporosis. Vitamin D deficiency is found in upwards of 10% of the elderly population and may be important in the pathogenesis of some hip fractures (11). Malnutrition, also common in some older individuals, may lead to acceleration of bone resorption, possibly as a result of reduced protein intake. Vitamin K deficiency may contribute to an increased risk of osteoporotic fractures, although the pathogenesis of this condition has not been precisely delineated.

Hormonal

Estrogen deficiency has long been recognized as a major cause of bone loss in the first decade after menopause. More recently, investigators identified a strong relation of endogenous estrogen and bone mass in elderly men and women. In one prospective study, Slemenda et al. (12) noted that both estrogens and androgens were independent predictors of bone loss in older postmenopausal women. In the Rancho Bernardo cohort, bioavailable estradiol was very strongly related to bone mineral density at the spine, hip, and forearm (13).

Men also suffer from age-related bone loss, and recent evidence suggests that absolute estrogen levels rather than testosterone concentrations may be essential for maintenance of bone density. In the Rancho Bernardo cohort, serum estradiol levels in elderly men correlated closely with bone mass at several sites (13). Testosterone levels also decline with age at a rate of approximately 1.2% per year, whereas sex hormone–binding globulin (SHBG) levels increase. However, it is debatable whether changes in male hormone levels are causally related to bone loss in the elderly man.

Changes in the growth hormone (GH)–insulin-like growth factor (IGF-I) axis also may contribute to age-related bone loss. GH secretion declines 14% per decade and is the principal cause for low serum IGF-I concentrations in both elderly men and women (14). It is likely that part of the impairment in bone formation noted in elderly individuals is more closely related to alterations in several IGF-binding proteins than to IGF-I itself (4). Similarly, the adrenal androgens, dihydroepiandrosterone (DHEA) and DHEA sulfate (DHEA-S), also decline precipitously with age and are 10% to 20% of young adult serum levels (15). Some studies showed a positive correlation between DHEA levels and bone mass in the elderly, whereas others failed to show any relation.

As noted earlier, there is an age-associated increase in PTH. Part of this can be attributed to reduced calcium intake or absorption or both. However, it also is possible that other factors contribute to secondary hyperparathyroidism in the elderly. For example, many older individuals have impaired renal function, and this can lead to an increase in PTH secretion. Despite higher levels of circulating PTH, 1,25 (OH)$_2$ D levels are not increased. This would suggest that there may be renal resistance to PTH, thereby requiring higher levels of this hormone to maintain vitamin D and calcium homeostasis. It is likely also that age-related declines in GH and IGF-I contribute to the reduction in renal 1α-hydroxylase activity, thereby further accentuating the secondary increase in PTH. Finally, it is conceivable that with aging, there is an altered set point in the parathyroid gland to tonic inhibition by either calcium or 1,25 (OH)$_2$ D. This could result in a sustained increase in PTH and contribute to the secondary hyperparathyroidism of aging.

Heritable and Environmental Factors

Age-related bone loss can be very dramatic in certain individuals, and this decline cannot be attributed solely to hormonal or nutritional factors. Several investigators hypothesize that genetic programming, when triggered, may lead to bone loss. However, this concept is controversial because animal models have been unable to demonstrate a heritable component to age-related bone loss. Moreover, the multiplicity of environmental factors makes the determination of fracture heritability very complicated. On the other hand, environmental agents such as smoking, alcohol, glucocorticoids, and anticonvulsants may contribute to an excessive rate of bone loss in some elders.

REFERENCES

1. Riggs BL, Wahner W, Seeman E, et al. Changes in bone mineral density of the proximal femur and spine with aging: differences between the postmenopausal and senile osteoporosis syndromes. *J Clin Invest* 1982;70:716–723.
2. Ensrud KE, Palmero L, Black MD, et al. Hip and calcaneal bone loss increase with advancing age: longitudinal results from the study of osteoporotic fractures. *J Bone Miner Res* 1995;10:1778–1787.
3. Hui SL, Slemenda CW, Johnston CC. Baseline measurement of bone mass predicts fractures in white women. *Ann Intern Med* 1989;111:355–361.

4. Ross PD, Knowlton W. Rapid bone loss is associated with increased levels of biochemical markers. *J Bone Miner Res* 1998;13:297–302.

5. Dresner-Pollak R, Parker RA, Poku M, Thompson J, Seibel MJ, Greenspan SL. Biochemical markers of bone turnover reflect femoral bone loss in elderly women. *Calcif Tissue Int* 1996;59:328–333.

6. Garnero P, Hausherr E, Chapuy MC, et al. Markers of bone resorption predict hip fracture in elderly women: the EPIDOS prospective study. *J Bone Miner Res* 1996;11:1531–1538.

7. Bollen AM, Kiyak HA, Eyre DR. Longitudinal evaluation of a bone resorption marker in elderly subjects. *Osteoporos Int* 1997;7:544–549.

8. Chapuy MC, Schott AM, Garnero P, et al. Healthy elderly French women living at home have secondary hyperparathyroidism and high bone turnover in winter. *J Clin Endocrinol Metab* 1996;81:1129–1133.

9. Dawson-Hughes B, Harris SS, Krall EA, Dallal GE. Effect of calcium and vitamin D supplementation on bone density in men and women 65 years of age and older. *N Engl J Med* 1997;337:670–676.

10. Recker RR, Hinders S, Davies M, et al. Correcting calcium nutritional deficiency prevents spine fractures in elderly women. *J Bone Miner Res* 1996;11:1961–1966.

11. NIH Consensus Conference. Optimal calcium intake. *JAMA* 1995;272:1942–1948.

12. Slemenda CW, Longcope C, Zhou L, Hui S, Peacock M, Johnston CC. Sex steroids and bone mass in older men: positive associations with serum estrogens and negative associations with androgens. *J Clin Invest* 1997;100:1755–1759.

13. Greendale GA, Edelstein S, Barrett-Connor E. Endogenous sex steroids and bone mineral density in older women and men: the Rancho Bernardo Study. *J Bone Miner Res* 1997;12:1833–1843.

14. Rosen CJ, Donahue LR, Hunter SJ. IGFs and bone: the osteoporosis connection. *Proc Soc Exp Biol Med* 1994;206:83–102.

15. Barrett-Connor E, Kritz-Silverstein D, Edelstein SL. A prospective study of DHEAS and bone mineral density in older men and women. *Am J Epidemiol* 1993;137:201–206.

SECTION III

Mineral Homeostasis

10. The Intestinal Absorption of Calcium, Magnesium, and Phosphate

Jacob Lemann, Jr., M.D. and *Murray J. Favus, M.D.

*Nephrology Section, Department of Medicine, Tulane University School of Medicine and New Orleans Veterans Affairs Medical Center, New Orleans, Louisiana; and *Department of Medicine, University of Chicago and Bone Program, University of Chicago Hospitals, Chicago, Illinois*

Intestinal absorption of calcium (Ca), magnesium (Mg), and phosphate (PO_4) determines the supply of these minerals to meet the needs of increasing body mass, especially bone mineralization, during growth and the ongoing needs related to tissue turnover and bone remodeling in adults. The quantities of Ca, Mg, and PO_4 that are absorbed by the intestine are determined by the availability of these minerals in the diet and by the capacity of the intestine to absorb them. In general, intestinal mineral absorption represents the sum of two transport processes, saturable transcellular absorption, which is physiologically regulated, and nonsaturable paracellular absorption, which is dependent on mineral concentration within the lumen of the gut.

METHODS OF MEASURING ABSORPTION

Serum concentrations, urinary concentrations, and urinary excretion rates of Ca, Mg, or PO_4 are easily and routinely measured in the evaluation and care of patients with disorders of mineral metabolism and bone. However, quantitation of intestinal absorption of Ca, Mg, and PO_4 is difficult and has generally been assessed only in a research setting. Several techniques are available.

Metabolic Balance

Subjects are fed constant diets, and the diets are analyzed for Ca, Mg, and PO_4. The subjects must be adapted to the diet for 7 to 10 days, especially if the quantity of Ca, Mg, or PO_4 in the diet differs significantly from a given subject's customary intake. In addition, because defecation occurs at irregular intervals, the subjects are continuously fed a measured quantity of a nonabsorbable marker that can be easily and reliably quantitated in the feces to verify achievement of the steady state and to assign a time interval to the stool collections. Polyethylene glycol (PEG), chromium sesquioxide, or small segments of radiopaque tubing often are used as markers. After the adaptation period, feces are collected during a balance period of at least 6 days' duration and analyzed for Ca, Mg, and PO_4. Dietary intake minus average daily fecal excretion during the balance period provides an estimate of net intestinal absorption of Ca, Mg, or PO_4.

Absorption from a Single Meal after Intestinal Washout

After overnight fasting, subjects undergo intestinal lavage over a period of 4 hours with a solution that does not cause either net intestinal absorption or secretion of water and electrolytes. Four hours after completion of lavage, they are fed a meal together with a known amount of the nonabsorbable marker PEG. A duplicate meal is analyzed for Ca, Mg, and PO_4. Twelve hours after the meal, intestinal lavage is repeated for 3 hours. The rectal effluent is collected and, together with any stool passed after ingestion of the meal, analyzed for Ca, Mg, PO_4, and PEG. Intake in the meal minus effluent excretion, corrected for the recovery of PEG, provides an estimate of net intestinal absorption of Ca, Mg, or PO_4. The study also can be repeated on a separate day when the subjects ingest only PEG without food to measure the quantities of Ca, Mg, or PO_4 secreted into the intestine. Total intestinal Ca, Mg, or PO_4 absorption (true absorption) can then be calculated as the sum of net absorption from the meal plus the quantity appearing in the effluent during fasting.

Both the balance method and the intestinal washout method provide estimates of actual net mineral input to the body from the intestine.

Absorption of Isotopic Minerals

A measured quantity of ^{47}Ca is administered orally. The fraction of the dose absorbed can be estimated either by external counting of radioisotope in the arm at a fixed time after dosing, by counting of isotope in serial blood samples and expressing fractional absorption as percentage of dose per liter of plasma when counts peak, or by collecting and counting isotope excreted in the feces over a period of 4 to 6 days after dosing and subtracting isotope excreted from the dose. Alternatively and more precisely, a measured quantity of ^{45}Ca can be administered intravenously together with the oral dose of ^{47}Ca. Ca absorption can then be estimated from the ratio of isotope concentrations or specific activities in serum or urine, or absorption rate can be estimated by compartmental kinetic analysis by using multiple serum samples collected over a period of 4 to 6 hours after dosing. The stable isotopes ^{42}Ca and ^{44}Ca also have been used with measurement by mass spectrometry. Absorption of isotopic Mg and PO_4 have not been studied because ^{28}Mg has a half-life of only 21 hours and because of the unacceptably intense β-emission of ^{32}P.

Segmental Intestinal Absorption

Subjects fast overnight, and a triple-lumen tube is passed to the duodenum, jejunum, ileum, or colon. Perfusate, containing Ca, Mg, or PO_4, together with a nonabsorbable marker, is instilled via the proximal lumen and aspirated at a constant rate from both the middle lumen, where mixing of the perfusate with intestinal contents has been completed, and from the distal lumen, which is the end of the intestinal-study segment between the middle and distal lumens, usually

30 cm in length. Absorption of Ca, Mg, or PO_4 can then be estimated by the change in mineral concentration in the fluid aspirated distally relative to that aspirated at the end of the mixing segment, taking into account the simultaneous change in PEG concentration as a measure of perfusate absorption.

Indirect Assessment of Intestinal Mineral Absorption

After overnight fasting and collection of control urine and blood specimens, subjects are given 25 mmol Ca (1000 mg) orally, usually as calcium gluconate. Two subsequent 2-hour urines are collected, together with blood samples 1 and 3 hours after the load. Fasting $U_{Ca}V$/GFR, calculated as $([Ca]_{urine}*[creatinine]_{plasma}/[creatinine]_{urine}$, is normally <0.035 mmol/L GFR (<0.13 mg/100 ml GFR). Among subjects exhibiting normal rates of intestinal Ca absorption the increment in $U_{Ca}V$/GFR following the load is <0.05 mmol/L GFR (<0.20 mg/100 ml GFR). Greater increases in $UCaV$/GFR after the oral Ca load provide evidence for increased intestinal Ca absorption.

CALCIUM ABSORPTION

The relation between net intestinal Ca absorption/day (dietary Ca intake/day − fecal Ca excretion/day) and dietary Ca intake/day, derived from metabolic-balance studies of healthy adults, is illustrated in Fig. 1. On the average, net intestinal Ca absorption is less than zero (e.g., fecal Ca excretion/day exceeds dietary Ca intake/day) when dietary Ca intake/day is <5 mmol/day (<200 mg/day). Thus on the average, healthy adults require daily Ca intakes ≥10 mmol/day (≥400 mg/day) to maintain Ca balance, taking into account both the inability of the normal kidney to excrete urine that is essentially free of Ca (unlike Na, Mg, or PO_4) and ongoing minor skin losses of Ca. As dietary Ca intake/day increases from minimal intakes of 3 to 5 mmol/day (120

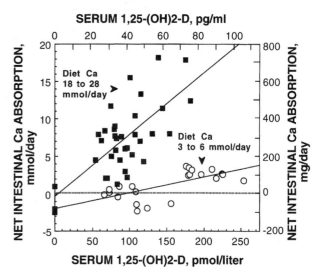

FIG. 2. Net intestinal Ca absorption in relation to serum 1,25 $(OH)_2$ D concentrations among healthy subjects fed normal-Ca diets and including anephric subjects (*solid symbols;* net intestinal Ca absorption, mmol/day = −0.4 + 0.082 × serum 1,25 $(OH)_2$ D, pmol/L; r = 0.71) or healthy subjects fed low-Ca diets or administered calcitriol (*open symbols;* net intestinal Ca absorption, mmol/day = −2.0 + 0.021 × serum 1,25 $(OH)_2$ D, pmol/L; r = 0.56).

to 200 mg/day), net intestinal Ca absorption/day increases but in progressively decreasing quantity, such that when Ca intake exceeds about 25 mmol/day (1000 mg/day), net intestinal Ca absorption tends, on the average, to plateau at an average value of about 7.5 mmol/day (300 mg/day). The curvilinear relation between net intestinal Ca absorption and dietary Ca intake reflects the sum of two absorptive mechanisms, active, saturable absorption and passive absorption dependent on the concentration gradient between intestinal lumen and blood. The wide variation of net intestinal Ca absorption among healthy adults at any given level of dietary intake that is seen in Fig. 1, especially when dietary Ca intake is >15 to 20 mmol/day (600 to 800 mg/day), is presumed primarily to reflect variation in active Ca absorption between subjects.

Currently 1,25-dihydroxyvitamin D [1,25 $(OH)_2$ D] is the only recognized hormonal stimulus of active intestinal Ca absorption that occurs principally in the duodenum and jejunum. Regardless of whether absorption is measured by the balance technique, by intestinal washout after a meal, or by isotopic methods and expressed as a percentage of dietary or meal intake or isotope administered, Ca absorption increases as plasma calcitriol increases by an average of about 0.2% Ca absorbed/pmol 1,25 $(OH)_2$ D/L or about 0.5% Ca absorbed/pg 1,25 $(OH)_2$ D/ml.

The interaction of dietary Ca intake and prevailing serum 1,25 $(OH)_2$ D concentrations as determinants of net intestinal Ca absorption is depicted in Fig. 2. When dietary Ca intake is very low (4 mmol/day; 160 mg/day), net intestinal Ca absorption reaches a maximum of about 3 mmol/day (120 mg/day) even when serum 1,25 $(OH)_2$ D levels are higher than the upper limit of the normal range (>135 pmol/L or >56 pg/ml). By contrast, when dietary Ca intake is normal,

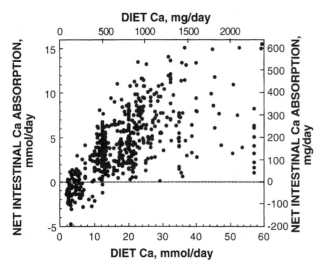

FIG. 1. Net intestinal Ca absorption as measured by the metabolic balance method in relation to dietary Ca intake among healthy adults.

TABLE 1. *Causes of increased and decreased intestinal Ca absorption*

Increased Ca absorption	Decreased Ca absorption
Increased renal 1,25 (OH)$_2$ D production	Decreased renal 1,25 (OH)$_2$ D production
Growth	Vitamin D deficiency
Pregnancy	Vitamin D–dependent rickets, type I
Lactation	
Primary hyperparathy- roidism	Chronic renal insuffi- ciency
Idiopathic hypercalciuria (some)	Hypoparathyroidism
	Aging
Increased extrarenal 1,25 (OH)$_2$ D production	Normal renal 1,25 (OH)$_2$ D production
Sarcoidosis	Glucocorticoid excess
Other granulomatous dis- orders	Thyroid hormone excess
B-cell lymphoma	Short-bowel syndrome

20 mmol/day (800 mg/day), net intestinal Ca absorption may exceed 10 mmol/day (400 mg/day), a value at the upper limit of the wide normal range shown in Fig. 1, when serum 1,25 (OH)$_2$ D levels average 120 pmol/L (50 pg/ml), a concentration that is within the upper limit of the normal range. Thus reduced net intestinal Ca absorption occurs when dietary Ca intake is limited, when serum 1,25 (OH)$_2$ D concentrations are low, or when the intestine is unresponsive to this hormone (Table 1). Increased intestinal Ca absorption occurs when serum 1,25 (OH)$_2$ D concentrations are high or, possibly, even only high-normal because of the effect of 1,25 (OH)$_2$ D to upregulate its own receptor. Very high Ca intakes also increase absorption, but such an increase in passive Ca absorption is accompanied by suppression of serum 1,25 (OH)$_2$ D, which would tend to blunt the increase in absorption. The major disorders reducing or enhancing intestinal Ca absorption are listed in Table 1.

The effect of the amount of Ca available to limit absorption was directly documented during perfusion studies of jejunal Ca absorption, as shown in Fig. 3. Ca absorption increases progressively as the jejunum is perfused with solutions containing 1.25, 5.0, or 10.0 mM Ca, tending to plateau at the highest Ca concentration. Ca absorption also was greater at any given perfusate Ca concentration among subjects who had been eating a low-Ca diet (7.5 mmol or 300 mg per day) for 1 month compared with subjects eating diets containing larger amounts of Ca (50 mmol or 2000 mg per day). The increase in the efficiency of absorption results from increased parathyroid hormone–stimulated 1,25 (OH)$_2$ D synthesis. The data also demonstrate the reduced capacity for Ca absorption among men and women older than 60 years, as compared with young adults, regardless of prior dietary Ca intake. Thus the intestinal adaptation to meet Ca requirements in young adults is lost with aging.

MAGNESIUM ABSORPTION

The relation between net intestinal Mg absorption/day (dietary Mg intake/day minus fecal Mg excretion/day) and dietary Mg intake/day, derived from metabolic balance studies of healthy adults, is illustrated in Fig. 4. Net intestinal Mg absorption is directly related to dietary Mg intake, on the average about 35% to 40% being absorbed when dietary Mg intake is in the normal range for adults of 7 to 30 mmol/day (168 to 720 mg/day). Because Mg is a constituent of all cells, and normal diets contain foods of cellular origin, dietary Mg intake is generally proportional to total caloric intake, thus assuring adequate intestinal Mg absorption. The data in Fig. 4 also include observations from studies of Mg balance with synthetic diets that are nearly Mg free. Net intestinal Mg absorption is less than zero (e.g., fecal Mg excretion/day exceeds dietary Mg intake/day) only when dietary Mg intake is <2 mmol/day (48 mg/day). The variation in net intestinal Mg absorption among healthy subjects

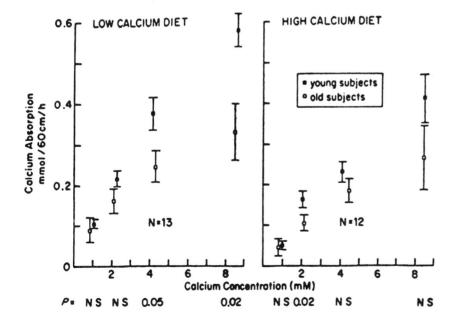

FIG. 3. Interaction of age and prior dietary Ca intake on jejunal Ca absorption by the perfusion technique by using 1.0, 2.5, 5.0, or 10.0 mM Ca solutions. Seven young and six older subjects were studied on a high-Ca intake. The *p* values are by grouped *t* test. (From Ireland P, Fordtran JS. Effect of dietary calcium and age on jejunal calcium absorption in humans studied by intestinal perfusion. *J Clin Invest* 1973;52:2672–2680, with permission.)

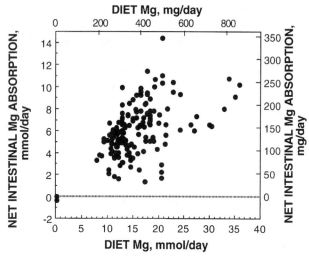

FIG. 4. Net intestinal Mg absorption in relation to dietary Mg intake among healthy adults.

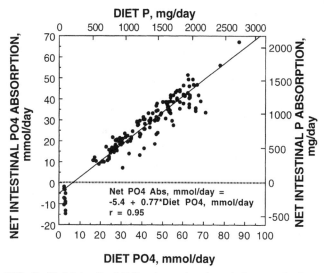

FIG. 5. Net intestinal PO_4 absorption in relation to dietary PO_4 intake among healthy adults. Net intestinal PO_4 in mmol/day = $-5.4 + 0.77 \times$ dietary PO_4, mmol/day; $r = 0.95$.

at any given normal level of dietary Mg intake appears to be related to other constituents of the diet, such as PO_4 content, that complex Mg within the intestinal lumen and limit absorption. In contrast to Ca absorption, Mg absorption is not increased as serum 1,25 $(OH)_2$ D concentrations vary from undetectable to high among adults. Dietary Mg intakes >35 mmol/day (840 mg/day) seldom occur spontaneously. Additional oral Mg often is taken as a cathartic [$Mg(OH)_2$, Mg-citrate], and although a small fraction of this Mg may be absorbed, such an effect is apt to lead to hypermagnesemia only in the presence of significant reductions in kidney function. Thus Mg-containing laxatives and antacids should not be given to patients with kidney disease. Reduced intestinal Mg absorption occurs with diffuse intestinal diseases causing malabsorption or as a consequence of laxative abuse.

PHOSPHATE ABSORPTION

Intestinal PO_4 absorption, like the absorption of Ca, is dependent on both passive PO_4 transport related to the luminal [PO_4] prevailing after a meal and on active PO_4 transport that is stimulated by 1,25 $(OH)_2$ D. The relation between net intestinal PO_4 absorption/day (dietary PO_4 intake/day minus fecal PO_4 excretion/day) and dietary PO_4 intake/day, derived from metabolic-balance studies in healthy adults, is shown in Fig. 5. As for Mg absorption in relation to dietary Mg intake, PO_4 absorption is directly related to dietary PO_4 intake. Because PO_4 is a major constituent of all cells, dietary PO_4 intake seldom is <20 mmol/day (<620 mg P/day) among healthy adults. Based on studies using synthetic diets providing only 2 to 3 mmol PO_4/day (62 to 93 mg P/day), there is net intestinal secretion of PO_4 when dietary PO_4 intake is less than about 10 mmol/day (<310 mg P/day), fecal PO_4 excretion exceeding dietary PO_4 intake. When dietary PO_4 intake varies over the usual normal range of 25 to 60 mmol/day (775 to 1860 mg P/day), 60% to 80% of dietary PO_4 is absorbed. Higher oral PO_4 intakes seldom occur spontaneously.

Intestinal PO_4 absorption is reduced in vitamin D deficiency, and the administration of 1,25 $(OH)_2$ D to patients with chronic renal failure who lack this hormone stimulates jejunal PO_4 absorption. However, experimental increases of serum 1,25 $(OH)_2$ D in healthy subjects do not further stimulate jejunal PO_4 absorption significantly and, as shown in Fig. 6, fractional PO_4 absorption estimated by the balance technique increases only slightly, although significantly, as serum 1,25 $(OH)_2$ D concentrations vary from normal to high among adults fed diets providing normal amounts of PO_4. Even in the presence of very low serum 1,25 $(OH)_2$ D

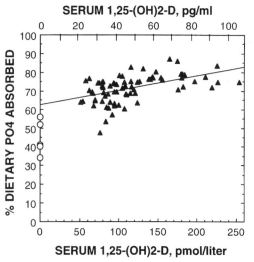

FIG. 6. Relation between percentage dietary PO_4 absorbed [(Net intestinal PO_4 absorption $\times$ 100)/(Dietary PO_4 intake)] and serum 1,25 $(OH)_2$ D concentrations in vitamin D–replete adults eating diets containing normal amounts of vitamin D alone or given calcitriol. Data for five anephric patients also taking aluminum hydroxide with undetectable serum 1,25 $(OH)_2$ D concentrations are shown.

levels, patients with chronic renal failure exhibit significant concentration-dependent jejunal PO_4 absorption. Thus the availability of PO_4 in the diet appears to be the major determinant of net PO_4 input to the body from the intestine. Continuing absorption of dietary PO_4 is a major factor in the pathogenesis of secondary hyperparathyroidism in patients with progressive kidney disease. Net intestinal PO_4 absorption among patients with chronic kidney disease is nearly identical to that among normal subjects, as dietary PO_4 intake varies over the range of 10 to 50 mmol/day (310 to 1550 mg P/day). Intestinal PO_4 absorption is also not apparently significantly reduced among patients with disorders associated with chronic hyperphosphatemia such as hypoparathyroidism and tumoral calcinosis. Because of the ability of Al^{3+} and of Ca^{2+} to form insoluble PO_4 salts and thus limit intestinal PO_4 absorption, aluminum hydroxide gel, aluminum carbonate, and, more recently in an attempt to prevent the potential toxicity of aluminum, calcium carbonate, calcium acetate, or calcium citrate, are routinely used in the care of patients with advanced renal failure. Chronic abuse of aluminum-containing antacids, by inhibiting absorption of dietary PO_4 and reabsorption of PO_4 entering the lumen of the gut in intestinal secretions, can rarely result in PO_4 depletion. PO_4 malabsorption also can occur with diffuse disease of the small intestine.

SELECTED READINGS

1. Albright F, Reifenstein EC Jr. *The parathyroid glands and metabolic bone disease.* Baltimore: Williams & Wilkins, 1948.
2. Malm OJ. Calcium requirement and adaptation in adult men. *Scand J Clin Lab Invest* 1958;Suppl 35:1–289.
3. Ireland P, Fordtran JS. Effect of dietary calcium and age on jejunal calcium absorption in humans studied by intestinal perfusion. *J Clin Invest* 1973;52:2672–2680.
4. Nordin BEC, ed. *Calcium, phosphate, and magnesium metabolism.* Edinburgh: Churchill Livingstone, 1976.
5. Favus MJ. Factors that influence absorption and secretion of calcium in the small intestine and colon. *Am J Physiol* 1985;248:G147–G157.
6. Bronner F, Pansu D, Stein WD. An analysis of intestinal calcium transport across the rat intestine. *Am J Physiol* 1986;250:G561–G569.
7. Sheikh MS, Ramirez A, Emmett N, Santa Ana C, Schiller LR, Fordtran JS. Role of vitamin D-dependent and vitamin D-independent mechanisms in absorption of food calcium. *J Clin Invest* 1988;81:126–132.
8. Nemere IA, Norman AW. Transport of calcium. In: Schultz SG, ed. *Handbook of physiology, section 6: the gastrointestinal system.* Bethesda, MD: American Physiological Society, 1991.
9. Klugman VA, Favus MJ. Intestinal absorption of calcium, magnesium, and phosphorus. In: Coe FL, Favus MJ, Pak CYC, Parks JH, Preminger GM, eds. *Kidney stones: medical and surgical management.* Philadelphia: Lippincott-Raven Press, 1996:201–221.
10. Marsh RN, Riley SE. Digestion and absorption of nutrients and minerals. In: Slesenger MH, Feldman M, Scharschmidt BG, eds. *Gastrointestinal and liver disease.* Philadelphia: WB Saunders, 1998.

11. Calcium, Magnesium, and Phosphorus: Renal Handling and Urinary Excretion

David A. Bushinsky, M.D.

Departments of Medicine, Pharmacology and Physiology, University of Rochester School of Medicine and Nephrology Unit, Strong Memorial Hospital, Rochester, New York

Adult, nonpregnant humans have no appreciable daily net gain or loss of body calcium, magnesium, or phosphorus. This remarkable homeostasis is due to the coordinated interaction of the intestine, the site of net absorption; the kidney, the site of net excretion; and the bone, the largest repository of these ions in the body (1,2). This neutral ionic balance requires that net intestinal mineral absorption must equal renal mineral excretion. In this chapter, we discuss renal filtration, reabsorption, and the factors that influence urinary excretion of these ions.

CALCIUM

Filtration

The concentration of serum calcium is maintained at between 9.0 and 10.4 mg/dL or 2.25 and 2.6 mmol/L (1,2). Approximately 40% of serum calcium is protein bound, especially to albumin and to a lesser extent globulins and

other proteins, and is not filtered by the glomerulus. Approximately 10% of calcium is complexed to phosphate, citrate, carbonate, and other anions, and the remaining 50% exists in the ionized form. The complexed and ionized calcium, which together are termed the ultrafilterable calcium, are freely filtered by the glomerulus, and this ultrafiltrate has a calcium concentration of approximately 1.5 mmol/L.

A typical 70-kg man with a normal glomerular filtration rate of 180 L/day will filter approximately 270 mmol of calcium per day (180 L/day × 1.5 mmol) (2). This quantity of calcium, >10 g, is far more than the calcium content of the entire extracellular fluid compartment and far more than the quantity of net calcium absorption, which is approximately 5 mmol/day. To maintain neutral calcium balance, approximately 98% of the filtered calcium must be reabsorbed along the renal tubule.

The process of massive filtration coupled to almost complete reabsorption of the filtrate intuitively seems energetically wasteful; however, one must consider that calcium is but one component of this ultrafiltrate. Many other substances, for example, creatinine and urea, undergo filtration and virtually no reabsorption, resulting in complete excretion. Thus substantial filtration followed by selective reabsorption allows precise control of excretion.

Reabsorption

Approximately 70% of filtered calcium is reabsorbed in the proximal tubule (Fig. 1). Proximal reabsorption is thought to be predominantly passive for two principal reasons: sodium and calcium are reabsorbed in parallel, and the proximal tubule epithelium is very "leaky," in that there is a large calcium flux from the bath to the lumen observed in micropuncture experiments (3). The mechanism of proximal calcium reabsorption appears to be predominantly paracellular, with salt and water carrying calcium from the lumen to the interstitium through the transport mechanism of solvent drag. Additionally, calcium reabsorption occurs as a result of a concentration and potential difference. There is clear evidence for a component of active transport of calcium in the latter portions of the proximal tubule. Here calcium enters the cytosol down an electrical and chemical gradient through calcium channels. The calcium is shuttled across the cell to the basolateral membrane, where it is transported against a large chemical gradient to the interstitium. Active transport is mediated by a magnesium-dependent calcium adenosine triphosphatase (ATPase) and by sodium for calcium exchange.

Approximately 20% of filtered calcium is reabsorbed in the loop of Henle (Fig. 2). There appears to be little calcium transport in the thin descending or thin ascending limbs of Henle's loop. However, in the thick ascending limb of the loop of Henle (TALH), the lumen-positive voltage, generated by the Na–K–2Cl transporter, provides a strong driving force for paracellular calcium reabsorption (4). In addition there appears to active calcium transport, especially near the kidney cortex. The loop diuretics, such as furosemide, impair calcium reabsorption in this segment by decreasing lumen-positive voltage (5).

The distal convoluted tubule is responsible for approximately 8% of calcium reabsorption and is the major site of regulation of urine calcium excretion (Fig. 3). In this segment, active calcium transport occurs against both electrical

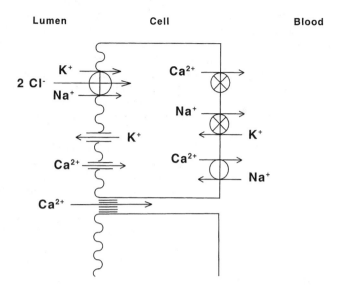

FIG. 2. Paracellular and transcellular calcium transport in the thick ascending limb of the loop of Henle.

and chemical gradients. Whereas transport of calcium generally follows sodium in this segment, reabsorption and subsequent excretion of the two ions can be dissociated, providing further evidence for the regulation of calcium reabsorption in the distal convoluted tubule. Calcium channels are clearly present in this segment, and the vitamin D–dependent calcium-binding protein, calbindin, has been localized to the distal convoluted tubule and the more distal tubule segments. This binding protein allows large amounts of calcium to be ferried across the cytosol without altering the free intracellular calcium concentration.

There appears to be reabsorption of <5% of filtered calcium in the collecting duct.

Factors Affecting Reabsorption

Sodium

Extracellular fluid volume expansion with saline infusion increases urinary sodium and calcium excretion, whereas extracellular fluid volume contraction decreases urinary sodium and calcium excretion (6). Volume expansion principally causes a decrease in proximal tubule sodium and calcium reabsorption, which is independent of alterations in

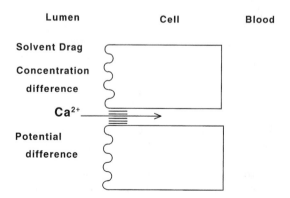

FIG. 1. Predominant mode of calcium transport in the proximal tubule: paracellular transport.

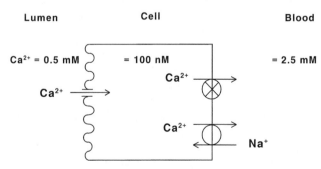

FIG. 3. Calcium transport in the distal convoluted tubule.

TABLE 1. *Factors influencing calcium excretion*

Glomerular filtration
  Increased
    Hypercalcemia
  Decreased
    Hypocalcemia
    Renal insufficiency
Tubular reabsorption
  Increased
    Extracellular fluid volume depletion
    Hypocalcemia
    Phosphate administration
    Metabolic alkalosis
    Parathyroid hormone
    Parathyroid hormone–related protein
    Thiazide diuretics
  Decreased
    Extracellular fluid volume expansion
    Hypercalcemia
    Phosphate depletion
    Metabolic acidosis
    Loop diuretics

PTH, although a decrease in distal calcium reabsorption also may occur (Table 1).

Calcium

Increases in dietary calcium result in an increase in urinary calcium; approximately 6% to 8% of an increase in dietary calcium appears in the urine (7). Hypercalcemia will increase both ionized and complexed calcium, resulting in an increase in the ultrafilterable calcium. However, this increase in serum calcium will be opposed by a decrease in the glomerular filtration rate, mediated through a decrease in the glomerular capillary ultrafiltration coefficient. Hypercalcemia results in a decline in reabsorption in the proximal tubule, in the loop of Henle, and in the distal tubule segments, resulting in greater urinary excretion of calcium than sodium. Hypocalcemia will result in a decrease in ultrafilterable calcium and an increase in the glomerular filtration rate. The hypocalcemia-induced increase in PTH will result in enhanced tubular calcium reabsorption and a decrease in urinary calcium excretion.

There are receptors for the recently identified calcium receptor on the basolateral membrane of the TALH (8). Increased serum calcium appears to stimulate the receptor, which decreases activity of the Na–K–2Cl pump. The positive lumen potential is lessened, leading to a decrease in tubular calcium reabsorption.

Phosphate

Phosphate administration, whether by the oral or intravenous route, reduces urine calcium excretion; micropuncture studies implicate an increase in distal calcium reabsorption. Several extrarenal mechanisms can contribute to the hypocalciuria of phosphate administration. An increase in phosphate will directly stimulate PTH secretion (9) and can reduce ionized calcium, also enhancing PTH secretion; the increased PTH will enhance calcium reabsorption. Phosphate will complex with calcium in the intestine, decreasing the amount of calcium available for absorption, and can complex with calcium in the bone and soft tissues, resulting in a decrease in the filtered load of calcium.

Phosphate depletion will result in hypercalciuria (10). Although a defect in proximal tubule calcium reabsorption is controversial, there appears to be a direct effect of phosphate to decrease calcium reabsorption in the distal nephron.

Protons

Acute and chronic metabolic acidosis lead to an increase in urine calcium excretion, whereas metabolic alkalosis leads to a decrease in calcium excretion (7). Micropuncture studies demonstrated that during acute metabolic acidosis, proximal tubule calcium reabsorption declines in parallel with a decrease in tubule bicarbonate concentration (11). During chronic metabolic acidosis, proximal tubule calcium reabsorption is unchanged, whereas there is a decrease in distal calcium reabsorption. The decreased calcium reabsorption is not mediated through changes in PTH or filtered load. Bone appears to be the source of the additional urinary calcium, as intestinal calcium absorption is not increased (12,13). Respiratory acidosis appears to cause a minimal increase in calcium excretion compared with isohydric metabolic acidosis.

On a daily basis, humans generate approximately 1 mEq/kg/24 h of protons (13). This endogenous acid production is related to the metabolism of sulfur-containing amino acids (especially cysteine and methionine), which are found in animal protein. A very mild, almost undetectable, metabolic acidosis results before the excretion of these acids (14). Any impairment of renal function, as occurs as part of the aging process, results in a greater degree of metabolic acidosis (15). When elderly patients are given potassium bicarbonate to neutralize their endogenous acid production, there is a decrease in urine calcium excretion (14). Compared with sodium bicarbonate, potassium bicarbonate results in a greater decrement in calcium excretion, perhaps because potassium administration does not result in extracellular fluid volume expansion.

Parathyroid Hormone and Parathyroid Hormone-Related Peptide

Parathyroid hormone (PTH) is a principal regulator of renal tubule calcium reabsorption, with increasing levels of PTH increasing renal tubule calcium reabsorption (1,16) (Fig. 4). PTH will reduce glomerular filtration, and thus the filtered load of calcium, by reducing the glomerular ultrafiltration coefficient. The effects of PTH on proximal renal tubule calcium reabsorption remain controversial. PTH appears to increase active calcium transport in the TALH. However, PTH clearly increases calcium reabsorption in the distal convoluted tubule, apparently through facilitating the opening of calcium channels. The actions of PTH are mimicked by cyclic adenosine monophosphate.

Although PTH clearly increases net renal tubule calcium reabsorption, patients with hyperparathyroidism are hypercalciuric (17). The PTH-induced increased tubule calcium reabsorption leads to hypercalcemia and an increased filtered

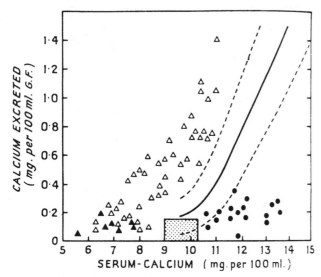

FIG. 4. Urinary excretion of calcium as a function of serum calcium concentration in normal subjects *(solid line)* and in patients with hypoparathyroidism *(triangles)* and hyperparathyroidism *(circles). Dashed lines,* ±2 SD; *shaded area,* the normal physiologic situation. (From Nordin BEC, Peacock M. Role of kidney in regulation of plasma-calcium. *Lancet* 1969:2:1280–1283.)

load of calcium, which leads to increased urinary calcium excretion. PTH also stimulates the conversion of 25 (OH) D_3 to 1,25-dihydroxyvitamin D_3 [1,25 (OH)$_2$ D_3] in the renal proximal tubule, resulting in enhanced intestinal calcium absorption, bone resorption, and an increase in the filtered load of calcium.

PTHrP is secreted by malignant cells and shares significant amino acid homology with PTH (1,8). Although it is not detected on standard PTH assays, this hormone mimics the actions of PTH on renal calcium reabsorption.

Dihydroxyvitamin D_3

The direct effects of 1,25 (OH)$_2$ D_3 on renal tubule calcium reabsorption are complex and not well understood. Vitamin D depletion will reduce renal tubule calcium reabsorption, irrespective of the presence of PTH, and repletion of vitamin D will increase calcium reabsorption. However, administration of 1,25 (OH)$_2$ D_3 to parathyroidectomized rats does not alter calcium reabsorption. Administration of vitamin D to humans results in hypercalciuria, although this effect may be mediated by the effects of vitamin D on the intestine or the bone or both. In mouse distal tubule cell culture, 1,25 (OH)$_2$ D_3 did not alter calcium absorption but enhanced the effects of PTH on calcium transport (18). Patients with excess 1,25 (OH)$_2$ D_3 are hypercalciuric because of the enhanced intestinal calcium absorption and a component of bone resorption.

Calcitonin and Others

Although calcitonin will increase calcium reabsorption in cultured distal convoluted cells, the in vivo effects of calcito-

nin are not straightforward. Physiologic doses of calcitonin are hypocalciuric, whereas supraphysiologic doses are hypercalciuric. Glucocorticoids, insulin, and glucagon have been reported to decrease tubular calcium reabsorption (19).

Thiazide

The acute administration of thiazide diuretics, including hydrochlorothiazide, chlorthalidone, or indapamide, results in an increase in urine sodium excretion with a small but variable change in urine calcium excretion. With prolonged thiazide administration, the increased sodium excretion continues; however, there is a marked increase in tubular calcium reabsorption and hypocalciuria. The dissociation of sodium and calcium excretion occurs in the distal convoluted tubule. Here thiazides inhibit sodium chloride transport, leading to a hyperpolarization of the cell membrane. Because cellular calcium entry is mediated by calcium channels in the luminal cell membrane, hyperpolarization of this membrane enhances calcium entry and leads to increased calcium reabsorption. Administration of sodium can reverse the hypocalciuria, suggesting that thiazides also increase proximal renal tubule calcium reabsorption, in part, through inducing volume depletion. Thiazide administration is integral in the treatment of calcium nephrolithiasis, as a reduction in urinary calcium excretion will reduce calcium supersaturation and stone formation (20).

Loop Diuretics

The acute administration of the loop diuretics, including furosemide, torosemide, or ethacrynic acid, results in a rather marked increase of urine calcium and sodium excretion. The loop diuretics inhibit the Na–K–2Cl transporter in the TALH, leading to a decrease in the positive lumen potential and a decline in calcium reabsorption at this site. As opposed to thiazide diuretics, which decrease sodium and increase calcium reabsorption, the loop diuretics cause a decrease in the reabsorption of both ions. As long as the lost urinary sodium is replaced, the hypercalciuria continues. Loop diuretic administration is useful in acute treatment of hypercalcemia (21).

Renal Function

During renal insufficiency, renal calcium filtration decreases in direct proportion to the decline in the glomerular filtration rate. In addition, there is enhanced calcium reabsorption resulting from the usual increase in PTH. The increase in PTH is multifactorial (2,22). It appears to be caused by the decrease in renal 1,25 (OH)$_2$ D_3 synthesis, resulting from a decrease in renal mass and from an increase in serum phosphorus due to a decrease in renal phosphorus excretion. The decrease in 1,25 (OH)$_2$ D_3 not only decreases intestinal calcium absorption, resulting in hypocalcemia and subsequent increased PTH secretion, but the decreased 1,25 (OH)$_2$ D_3 also leads to a direct increase in PTH secretion. The increase in phosphorus directly increases serum PTH.

MAGNESIUM

Filtration

In humans, the concentration of serum magnesium is maintained at a constant level between 1.8 and 2.2 mg/dL or 1.5 and 1.9 mEq/L (21). Of the total serum magnesium, approximately 30% is protein bound, 55% is ionized, and 15% is complexed; the ionized and complexed magnesium constitute the ultrafilterable magnesium. The concentration of free magnesium is influenced by pH, with a decrease in pH increasing the proportion of ionized magnesium.

A 70-kg man with a glomerular filtration rate of 180 L/day and a mean serum magnesium concentration of 1.8 mEq/L filters approximately 227 mEq of magnesium per day as approximately 70% of serum magnesium is ultrafilterable (180 L/day × 1.8 mEq/L × 0.7). Urine magnesium excretion averages about 12 mEq per day, indicating that approximately 95% of the glomerular filtrate is reabsorbed before excretion.

Reabsorption

Approximately 40% of filtered magnesium is reabsorbed in the proximal convoluted and straight tubules (3). Magnesium reabsorption follows that of sodium and water and appears to be a passive paracellular process, including solvent drag, dependent on sodium and water reabsorption and the luminal concentration of magnesium.

At least 50% of magnesium reabsorbed in the TALH is driven by the positive lumen potential generated by the Na–K–2Cl transporter. In addition, there may be a component of transcellular magnesium transport requiring a basolateral magnesium transporter.

Approximately 5% of magnesium is reabsorbed in the distal convoluted tubule through an active transport process that operates close to capacity and is therefore not fundamental to regulation of magnesium excretion. A small amount of magnesium is reabsorbed in more distal segments of the nephron. Distal tubular magnesium reabsorption normally operates near maximal capacity and is not capable of increasing reabsorption; thus any increased distal delivery of magnesium appears in the urine.

Factors Affecting Reabsorption

Sodium

Extracellular fluid volume expansion with sodium chloride decreases tubular magnesium reabsorption and increases urinary magnesium excretion. Decreased proximal magnesium reabsorption parallels the decline in sodium reabsorption. As the distal portions of the nephron are normally incapable of increased magnesium reabsorption, the increased delivery to the distal portions of the nephron appears in the urine (Table 2).

Magnesium

Hypermagnesemia increases urine magnesium excretion (23). An increased filtered load of magnesium, in spite of

TABLE 2. *Factors influencing magnesium reabsorption*

Glomerular filtration
  Increased
    Hypermagnesemia
  Decreased
    Hypomagnesemia
    Renal insufficiency
Tubular reabsorption
  Increased
    Extracellular fluid volume expansion
    Hypomagnesemia
    Hypocalcemia
    Metabolic alkalosis
    Parathyroid hormone
  Decreased
    Extracellular fluid volume depletion
    Hypermagnesemia
    Phosphate depletion
    Hypercalcemia
    Loop diuretics
    Aminoglycoside antibiotics
    Cisplatin
    Cyclosporine

some increased proximal tubular magnesium reabsorption, results in increased distal delivery. Magnesium reabsorption in the TALH appears to decline with the resultant increased distal delivery and excretion of magnesium. Hypomagnesemia results in a prompt decrease in urine magnesium excretion. There is little change in proximal reabsorption and an increase in magnesium reabsorption in the TALH.

Phosphate

Phosphate depletion results in an increase in magnesium excretion due to a defect in reabsorption in the TALH, which can result in significant hypomagesemia.

Calcium

Hypercalcemia leads to a prompt decline in overall magnesium reabsorption (3). There is decreased magnesium reabsorption in both the proximal tubule and the TALH. Hypocalcemia leads to an increase in overall tubule magnesium reabsorption.

Protons

Although metabolic alkalosis consistently decreases magnesium excretion, reports of the effects of metabolic acidosis on magnesium excretion are not consistent. Magnesium reabsorption in the distal nephron appears to be directly correlated with the level of luminal bicarbonate concentration.

Hormones

PTH itself increases magnesium reabsorption; however, the PTH-induced hypercalcemia opposes this increase in resorption.

Diuretics

The loop diuretics lead to a marked increase in magnesium excretion (21). In contrast to their effects on calcium excretion, the thiazide diuretics cause a minimal increase in magnesium excretion.

Other Medications

The aminoglycoside antibiotics, cisplatin and cyclosporine, have been shown to inhibit magnesium reabsorption in the TALH, leading to increased urinary magnesium excretion.

Renal Function

Any impairment of renal function will lead to a parallel decline in magnesium excretion. Continued dietary magnesium intake will result in marked hypermagnesemia. Patients with renal insufficiency must limit magnesium intake, which is often found in high concentrations in oral antacids and cathartics, to avoid hypermagnesemia (21).

PHOSPHORUS

Filtration

The concentration of serum phosphorus in adults ranges between 2.5 and 4.5 mg/dL or 0.81 to 1.45 mM (2,21). Serum phosphorus levels are highest in infants and decrease in childhood, reaching the normal adult levels in late adolescence. Approximately 70% of blood phosphorus is organic and contained in phospholipids, and 30% of the blood phosphorus is inorganic. Of the inorganic phosphorus, the majority, 85%, is free and circulates as monohydrogen or dihydrogen phosphate or complexed with sodium, magnesium, or calcium, whereas the minority, 15%, is protein bound.

A 70-kg man with a glomerular filtration rate of 180 L/day and a mean serum phosphorus concentration of 1.25 mM filters approximately 200 mmol of phosphorus per day as approximately 85% of serum phosphorus is ultrafilterable (180 L/day × 1.25 mmol/L × 0.85) (21). Urine phosphorus excretion averages about 25 mmol/day so that approximately 12.5% of the glomerular filtrate is excreted in the urine.

Reabsorption

The bulk of phosphorus reabsorption, 85%, occurs in the proximal tubule (Fig. 5). Proximal phosphorus transport oc-

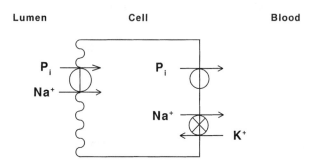

FIG. 5. Phosphorus transport in the proximal tubule.

curs against an electrochemical gradient (3). Reabsorption appears to be transcellular, absorptive, and dependent on the low concentration of intracellular sodium maintained by the basolateral Na–K–ATPase. An Na–P cotransporter in the brush border is responsible for phosphorus absorption (24). Once inside the cell, the absorbed phosphorus equilibrates with cytosolic phosphorus; elimination of luminal phosphorus leads to a marked decline in intracellular phosphorus. Phosphorus transport across the basolateral membrane occurs down a favorable electrochemical gradient by using an anion exchanger. It is tightly regulated to avoid depletion of intracellular phosphorus. In the presence of PTH, the bulk of proximal tubule phosphorus absorption occurs in the initial 25% of this segment. Transport appears more robust in the deeper juxtamedullary nephrons compared with the more cortical nephrons.

There appears to be little phosphorus transport in the loop of Henle. A small quantity of phosphorus is reabsorbed in the distal convoluted tubule, especially in the absence of PTH. Whether there is phosphorus reabsorption more distally is not clear.

The overall tubular maximum for the reabsorption of phosphorus is approximately equal to the normal amount of phosphorus filtered by the glomerulus. Thus any appreciable increase in the filtered load of phosphorus leads to an increase in urinary phosphorus excretion; decreases in filtration can be reabsorbed.

Factors Affecting Reabsorption

Phosphorus

A low phosphorus intake will stimulate tubular phosphorus reabsorption, whereas a high phosphorus intake will inhibit phosphorus reabsorption. Alterations in phosphorus intake alter renal phosphorus reabsorption, independent of changes in PTH, extracellular fluid volume, or the level of serum calcium. Variations in phosphorus intake lead to an inverse modulation in the maximal rate of transport of the proximal tubule Na–P cotransporter within hours and alter the level of phosphorus reabsorption (Table 3).

Calcium

Chronic hypercalcemia decreases, whereas chronic hypocalcemia increases, renal reabsorption of phosphorus (25). Acute changes in calcium have a number of effects on phosphorus filtration and reabsorption. An acute increase in serum calcium will decrease the glomerular filtration rate because of a decrease in the ultrafiltration coefficient and the renal blood flow. Increases in calcium lead to a release in red blood cell phosphorus and an increase in serum phosphorus; however, the phosphorus may bind to calcium and protein, forming an unfilterable complex. Calcium is a principal regulator of PTH, which is phosphaturic. In general, filtered phosphorus appears to increase with mild increases in serum calcium and decrease as the level of calcium increases.

Sodium

Extracellular fluid volume expansion decreases renal tubular phosphorus reabsorption, and volume concentration

TABLE 3. *Factors influencing phosphorus reabsorption*

Filtration
  Increased
    Hyperphosphatemia
    Mild hypercalcemia
  Decreased
    Hypophosphatemia
    Renal insufficiency
    Moderate hypercalcemia
Tubular reabsorption
  Increased
    Phosphorus depletion
    Hypercalcemia
    Extracellular fluid volume depletion
    Chronic metabolic alkalosis
  Decreased
    Phosphorus excess
    Hypocalcemia
    Extracellular fluid volume expansion
    Acute metabolic alkalosis
    Chronic metabolic acidosis
    Parathyroid hormone
    Parathyroid hormone–related protein
    $1,25 (OH)_2 D_3$
    Thiazide diuretics
    Loop diuretics

increases reabsorption (26). Volume expansion leads to a decrease in proximal sodium reabsorption, which dilutes proximal tubular phosphorus concentration, leading to a decline in reabsorption.

Protons

Although acute metabolic acidosis does not significantly alter renal tubular phosphorus reabsorption, acute metabolic alkalosis leads to a decline in phosphorus reabsorption. Chronic metabolic acidosis decreases tubular phosphorus reabsorption through an modulation of the Na–P cotransporter independent of changes in PTH, whereas chronic alkalosis increases reabsorption.

Parathyroid Hormone and Parathyroid Hormone-Related Peptide

PTH is a principal regulator of renal phosphorus reabsorption and excretion; the hormone is phosphaturic. PTH regulates phosphorus reabsorption, principally through regulation of the proximal Na–P cotransporter. PTH also appears to decrease distal tubular reabsorption. PTHrP mimics the action of PTH on renal tubular phosphorus reabsorption. The hypophosphaturia of phosphorus depletion overrides the hyperphosphaturia induced by PTH.

1,25-Dihydroxyvitamin D₃

Chronic excess of $1,25 (OH)_2 D_3$ results in a decrease in renal phosphorus reabsorption and causes phosphaturia. Vitamin D increases intestinal phosphorus absorption, resulting in hyperphosphatemia and an increased filtered load of phosphorus.

Other Hormones

Insulin increases whereas glucocorticoids and glucagon decrease renal phosphorus reabsorption. The effect of calcitonin on phosphorus reabsorption is unclear.

Diuretics

Both the loop and thiazide diuretics are phosphaturic.

Renal Function

During renal insufficiency, urine phosphorus excretion remains relatively constant until the glomerular filtration rate decreases to about 25% of normal (13). Phosphorus excretion is maintained in the presence of a decrease in glomerular filtration rate and the subsequent decline in the filtered load of phosphorus by the phosphaturic effect of increased PTH levels. Renal insufficiency and failure are principal causes of hyperphosphatemia, which has an integral role in the pathogenesis of renal osteodystrophy (27).

REFERENCES

1. Bushinsky DA, RD Monk. Calcium. *Lancet* 1998;352:306–311.
2. Bushinsky DA. Disorders of calcium and phosphorus homeostasis. In: Greenberg A, ed. *Primer on kidney diseases.* San Diego: Academic Press, 1997:106–113.
3. Suki WN, Rouse D. Renal transport of calcium, magnesium, and phosphate. In: Brenner BM, ed. *The kidney.* Philadelphia: WB Saunders, 1996:472–515.
4. Bourdeau JE, Burg MB. Voltage dependence of calcium transport in the thick ascending limb of Henle's loop. *Am J Physiol* 1979;236:F357.
5. Edwards BR, Baer PG, Sutton RAL, Dirks JH, eds. Micropuncture study of diuretic effects on sodium and calcium reabsorption in the dog nephron. *J Clin Invest* 1973;52:2418.
6. Blythe WB, Gitelman HJ, Welt LG. Effect of expansion of the extracellular space on the rate of urinary excretion of calcium. *Am J Physiol* 1968;14:52.
7. Lemann J Jr, Adams ND, Gray RW. Urinary calcium excretion in human beings. *N Engl J Med* 1979;301:535–541.
8. Brown EM, Pollock AS, Hebert SC. The extracellular calcium-sensing receptor: its role in health and disease. *Annu Rev Med* 1998;49:15–29.
9. Slatopolsky E, Finch J, Denda MC, et al. Phosphorus restriction prevents parathyroid gland growth: high phosphorus directly stimulates PTH secretion in vitro. *J Clin Invest* 1996;97:2534–2540.
10. Yangawa N, Lee DBN. Renal handling of calcium and phosphorus. In: Coe FL, Favus MJ, eds. *Disorders of bone and mineral metabolism.* New York: Raven Press, 1992:3–40.
11. Sutton RAL, Wong NLM, Dirks JH. Effects of metabolic acidosis and alkalosis on sodium and calcium transport in the dog kidney. *Kidney Int* 1979;15:520–533.
12. Lemann J Jr, Litzow JR, Lennon EJ. The effects of chronic acid loads in normal man: further evidence for the participation of bone mineral in the defense against chronic metabolic acidosis. *J Clin Invest* 1966;45:1608–1614.
13. Bushinsky DA. The contribution of acidosis to renal osteodystrophy. *Kidney Int* 1995;47:1816–1832.
14. Sebastian AST, Harris JH, Ottaway KM, Todd R, Morris RC Jr. Improved mineral balance and skeletal metabolism in postmenopausal women treated with potassium bicarbonate. *N Engl J Med* 1994:330:1776–1781.

15. Bushinsky DA. Acid-base imbalance and the skeleton. In: Burckhardt B, Dawson-Hughes B, Heaney RP, eds. *Nutritional aspects of osteoporosis.* Norwell, MA: Serono Symposia USA, 1998:208–217.
16. Nordin BEC, Peacock M. Role of kidney in regulation of plasma-calcium. *Lancet* 1969:2:1280–1283.
17. Monk RD, Bushinsky DA. Pathogenesis of idiopathic hypercalciuria. In: Coe F, Favus M, Pak J, Parks J, Preminger G, eds. *Kidney stones: medical and surgical management.* New York: Raven Press, 1996: 759–772.
18. Friedman PA, Gesek FA. Cellular calcium transport in renal epithelia: measurement, mechanisms and regulation. *Physiol Rev* 1995:75: 429–471.
19. Breslau NA. Calcium, magnesium, and phosphorus: renal handling and urinary excretion. In: Favus M, ed. *Primer on the metabolic bone diseases and disorders of mineral metabolism.* Philadelphia: Lippincott-Raven, 1996:49–57.
20. Bushinsky A. Renal lithiasis. In: Kelly WF, ed. *Kelly's textbook of medicine.* New York: JB Lippincott, 1996:1024–1028.
21. Monk RD, Bushinsky D. Treatment of calcium, phosphorus, and magnesium disorders. In: Halperin M, ed. *Therapy in nephrology and hypertension: a companion to Brenner and Rector's the kidney.* Philadelphia: WB Saunders, 1999:303–315.
22. Bushinsky DA. Bone disease in moderate renal failure: cause, nature and prevention. *Annu Rev Med* 1997;48:167–176.
23. Wen SF, Evanson RL, Dirks JH. Micropuncture study of renal magnesium transport in proximal and distal tubule of the dog. *Am J Physiol* 1970;219:570.
24. Magagnin SA, Werner D, Markovich V, et al. Expression cloning of human and rat renal cortex Na/P cotransport. *Proc Natl Acad Sci USA* 1993;90:5979–5983.
25. Bonjour JP, Fleisch H. Calcium supply and renal handling of phosphate. *Miner Electrolyte Metab* 1980;3:261.
26. Massry SG, Coburn JW, Kleeman CR. The influence of extracellular volume expansion on renal phosphate reabsorption in the dog. *J Clin Invest* 1969;48:1237.
27. Bushinsky DA. Renal osteodystrophy. In: Jamison R, Wilkinson B, eds. *Nephrology.* London: Chapman & Hall, 1997:369–382.

12. Mineral Balance and Homeostasis

Arthur E. Broadus, M.D., Ph.D.

Department of Internal Medicine, Yale University School of Medicine, New Haven, Connecticut

Life began in a primordial sea, rich in potassium and magnesium and poor in sodium and calcium, and it is thought that the present composition of the cytosol, also rich in potassium and magnesium and poor in sodium and calcium, reflects this ancient heritage. With time, geologic changes altered the composition of the seas to one rich in sodium and calcium, and primitive organisms adapted to this altered milieu by developing ion pumps to maintain the asymmetry of the concentrations of monovalent and divalent cations across their plasma membranes. The evolution of these pumps and channels may be viewed as one of the most fundamental developments in cell biology.

The progression to terrestrial life carried with it a complete dependence on minerals from the environment. With this came the evolution of the mineral-exchange mechanisms in intestine, kidney, and bone (which subserve systemic mineral needs), as well as the key systemic hormones, parathyroid hormone (PTH) and 1,25-dihydroxyvitamin D [1,25 (OH)$_2$ D], which regulate these exchange mechanisms. This integrated regulatory system has many checks and balances and is an elegant example of biologic control.

CALCIUM

An adult human contains approximately 1000 g of calcium (1). Some 99% of this calcium is in the skeleton in the form of hydroxyapatite, and 1% is contained in the extracellular fluids and soft tissues. The extracellular concentration of calcium ions (Ca^{2+}) is in the range of 10^{-3} M, whereas the concentration of Ca^{2+} in the cytosol is about 10^{-6} M.

Calcium plays two predominant physiologic roles in the organism. In bone, calcium salts provide the structural integrity of the skeleton. In the extracellular fluids and in the cytosol, the concentration of Ca^{2+} is critically important in the maintenance and control of a number of biochemical processes, and the concentrations of Ca^{2+} in both compartments are maintained with great constancy.

PHOSPHORUS

An adult human contains approximately 600 g of phosphorus. Some 85% of this phosphorus is present in crystalline form in the skeleton and plays a structural role. About 15% is present in the extracellular fluids, largely in the form of inorganic phosphate ions, and in soft tissues, almost totally in the form of phosphate esters. Intracellular phosphate esters and phosphorylated intermediates are involved in a number of important biochemical processes, including the generation and transfer of cellular energy. Intracellular and extracellular concentrations of phosphorus (as the phosphate divalent anion) are approximately 1×10^{-4} M and 2×10^{-4} M, respectively, and these concentrations are less rigidly maintained than are those of calcium and magnesium.

MAGNESIUM

An adult human contains approximately 25 g or 2000 mEq of magnesium. About two thirds is present in the skeleton and one third in soft tissues. The magnesium in bone is not an integral part of the hydroxyapatite lattice structure but appears to be located on the crystal surface. Only a minor fraction of the magnesium in bone is freely exchangeable with extracellular magnesium. Magnesium is the most abundant intracellular divalent cation, and cellular magnesium is important as a cofactor for a number of enzymatic reactions and in the regulation of neuromuscular excitability. Approximately 1% of total body magnesium is contained in the extracellular compartment, and its concentration in plasma does not provide a reliable index of either total body or soft-tissue magnesium content. The concentration of magnesium ions (Mg^{2+}) is about 5×10^{-4} M in the cytosol as well as in the extracellular fluids, and its concentration in both compartments is rigidly maintained.

EXTRACELLULAR MINERAL METABOLISM

Calcium

There are three definable fractions of calcium in serum: ionized calcium (about 50%), protein-bound calcium (about 40%), and calcium that is complexed, mostly to citrate and phosphate ions (about 10%) (1). Both the complexed and ionized fractions are ultrafilterable, so that about 60% of the total calcium in serum crosses semipermeable membranes. About 90% of the protein-bound calcium is bound to albumin, and the remainder, to globulins. Alterations in the serum albumin concentration have a major influence on the measured total serum calcium concentration. At pH 7.4, each gram per deciliter of albumin binds 0.8 mg/dL of calcium, and this simple relation can be used to "correct" the total serum calcium concentration when circulating albumin is abnormal (e.g., given measured albumin and calcium concentrations of 2.0 g/dL and 7.4 mg/dL, respectively, the corrected serum calcium concentration is 9.0 mg/dL, assuming a normal mean serum albumin concentration of 4.0 g/dL). Calcium is bound largely to the carboxyl groups in albumin, and this binding is highly pH dependent. Acute acidosis decreases binding and increases ionized calcium, and acute alkalosis increases binding with a consequent decrease in ionized calcium. These changes are not reflected in the total serum calcium concentration and can be appreciated only by actual measurement of ionized serum calcium at the ambient pH. Calcium concentrations are typically recorded in milligrams per deciliter (mg%); these concentrations can be converted to molar units simply by dividing by 4 (e.g., 10 mg/dL converts to 2.5 mM).

It is the ionized fraction of calcium (Ca^{2+}) that is physiologically important and that is rigidly maintained by the combined effects of PTH and 1,25 $(OH)_2$ D (2). Examples of the physiological functions of extracellular Ca^{2+} include (a) serving as a cofactor in the coagulation cascade (e.g., for factors VII, IX, X, and prothrombin), (b) maintenance of the normal mineral ion product required for skeletal mineralization, and (c) contributing stability to plasma membranes by binding to phospholipids in the lipid bilayer and also regulating the permeability of plasma membranes to sodium ions. A reduction in ionized calcium increases sodium permeability and enhances the excitability of all excitable tissues; an increase in ionized calcium has the opposite effect. For example, the pH dependency of calcium binding to carboxyl groups noted earlier is the explanation for the reduction in ionized calcium that is responsible for the neuromuscular symptoms that characterize the hyperventilation syndrome (which produces a respiratory alkalosis).

Phosphorus

Serum inorganic phosphate also exists as three fractions: ionized, protein-bound, and complexed. Protein binding is relatively insignificant for phosphate, representing some 10% of the total, but about 35% is complexed to sodium, calcium, and magnesium. Thus approximately 90% of the inorganic phosphate in serum is ultrafilterable. The major ionic species of phosphate in serum at pH 7.4 is the divalent anion (HPO_4^{2-}).

In contrast to the rigidly regulated concentration of calcium in serum, the serum phosphorus concentration varies quite widely throughout the day and is influenced by age, sex, diet, pH, and a variety of hormones. An adequate serum phosphate concentration is important in maintaining a sufficient ion product for normal mineralization.

Magnesium

About 55% of serum magnesium is ionized, with 30% being protein bound and 15% complexed. The protein-bound fraction interacts with the carboxyl groups of albumin and is influenced by pH in a fashion analogous to that of calcium. It is the ionized fraction of magnesium that is physiologically important (e.g., to plasma membrane excitability). The extracellular concentration of ionized magnesium is tightly controlled by the tubular maximum or threshold for magnesium in the nephron (3).

Only fasting measurements of serum calcium and phosphorus should be considered reliable.

CELLULAR MINERAL METABOLISM

A detailed summary of the numerous metabolic functions of calcium, magnesium, and phosphorus within cells is beyond the scope of this syllabus. This section attempts simply to highlight briefly some of the important roles of these ions in cellular physiology.

Calcium

The control of cellular calcium homeostasis is complex, and the regulation of the concentration of the calcium ion in the cytosol is as rigidly maintained as is its concentration in extracellular fluids (4). Cells are bathed in extracellular fluids containing approximately 10^{-3} M Ca^{2+}. The concentration of Ca^{2+} in the cytoplasm is approximately 10^{-6} M, or one thousandth that in extracellular fluids. Cytosolic calcium is to some extent buffered by binding to other cytoplasmic constituents, and certain cells contain a specific calcium-binding protein that may serve as a buffer or a calcium-transport protein or both within the cytosol. The mitochondria and microsomes contain 90% to 99% of the intracellular calcium, bound largely to organic and inorganic phosphates. The calcium content of these organelles is sufficient to replenish cytosolic calcium some 500 times.

The low Ca^{2+} concentration in the cytosol is maintained by three pump-leak transport systems: an external system located in the plasma membrane and two internal systems located in the microsomal membrane and the inner mitochondrial membrane, respectively. Calcium diffuses into the cytosol across these three membranes. Each of the three pumps is oriented in a direction of calcium egress from the cytosol; each requires energy, and each shares a high affinity for calcium (K_m, approximately $10^{-6} M$).

The importance of these three calcium-transport systems in regulating cellular calcium metabolism varies considerably from cell to cell, depending on the function of a particular cell type. Several examples illustrate how the details of cellular calcium homeostasis have been adapted to subserve the specific physiologic function of a given cell type.

Calcium ions constitute the coupling factor that links excitation and contraction in all forms of skeletal and cardiac muscle. In striated muscle, the microsomes are extensively developed as the sarcoplasmic reticulum, which serves as the principal storehouse of intracellular calcium in muscle and which is the most highly developed calcium-transport system known. Depolarization of the plasma membrane is accompanied by the entry of a small amount of extracellular calcium into the cell, and this acts as a trigger to release large quantities of calcium stored in the sarcoplasmic reticulum. The abrupt increase in cytosolic calcium interacts with troponin, a specific calcium-binding protein, leading to a conformational change and the actin—myosin interaction that constitutes muscle contraction. The reticulum vesicles are capable of reaccumulating the large quantity of cytosolic calcium with the extreme speed required by the relaxation process.

In most mammalian cells other than muscle, the principal internal calcium pump-leak system is that of the inner mitochondrial membrane. In a number of cells, calcium serves as a second messenger, mediating the effects of membrane signals on the release of secretory products (e.g., neurotransmitters, exocrine secretions such as amylase, and endocrine secretions such as insulin and aldosterone) (4). The calcium messenger system involves a flow of information along several pathways: (a) the calmodulin pathway and (b) the phosphoinositide C–kinase pathway. It is now recognized that in many cells, the several branches of the calcium messenger system and the cyclic adenosine monophosphate (cAMP) messenger system are intimately related, and that these systems are integrated in such a way that the net cellular response to a given stimulus is determined by a complex interplay (''cross-talk'') between these systems.

Phosphorus

The transport of phosphate ions across the plasma membrane and the membranes of intracellular organelles proceeds passively but is determined by the movement of cations, mostly calcium. The phosphate content in mitochondria is high, and it is largely in the form of calcium salts. The cytoplasmic concentration of free phosphate ions is estimated to be quite low, and the remaining portion of intracellular phosphate is either bound or in the form of organic phosphate esters. These phosphate esters play a variety of critically important roles in cellular metabolism: purine nucleotides provide the cell with stored energy; phosphorylated intermediates are concerned with energy conservation and transfer; and phospholipids are major constituents of cell membranes, and the phosphorylation of proteins is an important means of regulating their function.

Magnesium

Magnesium is the most abundant intracellular divalent cation and the second most abundant intracellular cation after potassium. Approximately 60% of cellular magnesium is contained in the mitochondria, and it is estimated that only 5% to 10% of intracellular magnesium exists as free ions in the cytoplasm. The transport mechanisms responsible for maintaining the asymmetric distribution of magnesium in intracellular compartments are less well studied than the corresponding calcium-transport systems, but it is clear that the cellular metabolisms of calcium and magnesium are regulated independently. Magnesium is an essential cofactor in the functioning of a wide variety of key enzymes, including essentially all enzymes concerned with the transfer of phosphate groups, all reactions that require adenosine triphosphate (ATP), and each of the steps concerned with the replication, transcription, and translation of genetic information.

MINERAL ION BALANCE AND MECHANISMS FOR MAINTAINING SYSTEMIC MINERAL HOMEOSTASIS

Mineral ion influx and efflux in the intestine, bone, and kidney, and the regulation of these processes by PTH and 1,25 (OH)$_2$ D are described in detail in other chapters (see also ref. 2). The information in the sections that follow attempts to integrate these processes at the level of the intact organism, and it describes the fine set of checks and balances that regulate mineral homeostasis *in vivo*.

The term *mineral ion balance* refers to the state of mineral homeostasis in the organism vis-à-vis the environment. In zero balance, mineral intake and accretion exactly match mineral losses. In positive balance, mineral intake and accretion exceed mineral losses. In negative balance, mineral losses exceed mineral intake and accretion. A growing child is in positive mineral balance, whereas an immobilized patient is in negative mineral balance. Formal balance studies are a relic of the past and are no longer performed, but the concept of balance is central to even a cursory understanding of systemic mineral ion homeostasis. Figure 1 is a schematic representation of calcium, phosphorus, and magnesium metabolism in a normal adult on an average diet who is in zero mineral ion balance.

Calcium

The total extracellular pool of calcium is approximately 900 mg. This pool is in dynamic equilibrium with calcium entering and exiting via the intestine, bone, and renal tubule. In zero balance, bone resorption and formation are equivalent at about 500 mg/day, and the net quantity of calcium absorbed by the intestine, approximately 175 mg/day, is quantitatively excreted into the urine. Thus under normal circum-

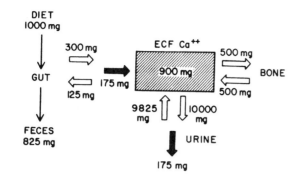

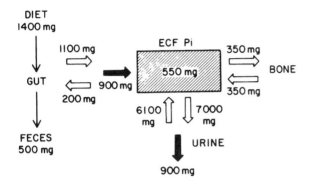

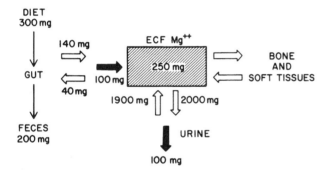

FIG. 1. Calcium, phosphorus, and magnesium fluxes in a normal adult in zero mineral ion balance. *Open arrows,* unidirectional mineral fluxes; *solid arrows,* net fluxes; all values are given in mg/day. (From Stewart AF, Broadus AE. Mineral metabolism. In: Felig P, Baxter JD, Broadus AE, Frohman LA, eds. *Endocrinology and metabolism.* 2nd ed. New York: McGraw-Hill, 1987:1317–1453.)

stances, net calcium absorption provides a surplus of calcium that considerably exceeds systemic requirements.

Several points illustrated in this schema merit some emphasis. The first is the quantitative importance of the kidney in the regulation of calcium homeostasis. The filtered load of calcium is a whopping 10,000 mg/day, and 10% of this, or 1000 mg/day, is under the control of PTH-regulated reabsorption in the distal nephron. The second is the elegance of biologic control that must underlie a system in which calcium absorption and excretion are matched on essentially a milligram-for-milligram basis.

Phosphorus

The extracellular pool of orthophosphate is approximately 550 mg (Fig. 1). This pool is in dynamic equilibrium with phosphate entry and exit via the intestine, bone, kidney, and soft tissues (not depicted in the figure). In zero balance, fractional net phosphorus absorption is about two thirds of phosphorus intake; this amount represents a vast excess over systemic requirements and is quantitatively excreted into the urine.

Again, several points merit emphasis. The first is that the absorption of phosphate in the intestine is far less rigidly regulated than is the absorption of calcium. The second is the dominant role of the kidney; in this case, the threshold for phosphate reabsorption in the proximal tubule [tubular maximum for phosphate/glomerular filtration rate (TmP/GFR)] is essentially the setpoint that defines the fasting serum phosphorus concentration, and it is the setpoint that is regulated by PTH (5).

Magnesium

The extracellular pool of magnesium is approximately 250 mg and is in bidirectional equilibrium with magnesium fluxes across the intestine, kidney, bone, and soft tissues (Fig. 1). In zero balance, the magnesium derived from net intestinal absorption, approximately 100 mg/day, represents a systemic surplus and is quantitatively excreted. The kidney is responsible for regulating the serum magnesium concentration by a setpoint or Tm-limited process that is reminiscent of the setpoint for phosphorus, except that the TmMg is not hormonally regulated (3).

Two key points are made in the preceding paragraphs: (a) normally, hormonal or intrinsic mechanisms (or both) of mineral ion absorption in the intestine provide the organism with a mineral supply that exceeds systemic mineral needs by a considerable measure, and (b) the renal tubule plays the dominant quantitative role in maintaining normal mineral homeostasis. Within this framework, minor fluctuations in systemic requirements are easily met by the surfeit of normal mineral absorption and do not require hormonal adjustments.

Systemic Calcium Homeostasis and Maintenance of a Normal Serum Calcium Concentration

The parathyroid chief cell is exquisitely sensitive to the ionized serum calcium concentration and is capable of responding to changes in this concentration so small that they are not measurable by human hands (2). The recently identified calcium receptor is the sensing device (see Chapter 13) that is at the core of the chief cell's sensitivity to the ambient calcium concentration (6).

The integrated actions of PTH on distal tubular calcium reabsorption, bone resorption, and 1,25 $(OH)_2$ D-mediated intestinal calcium absorption are responsible for the fine regulation of the serum ionized calcium concentration. The precision of this integrated control is such that, in a normal individual, serum ionized calcium probably fluctuates by no more than 0.1 mg/dL in either direction from its normal setpoint value throughout the day.

Distal tubular calcium reabsorption and osteoclastic bone resorption are the major control points in minute-to-minute serum calcium homeostasis; of these two processes, the effect of PTH on the distal tubule is quantitatively the more important. Indeed, the 1000 mg/day of calcium that is under PTH control as it passes through the distal nephron is clearly the centerpiece of the organism's ability to fine tune the serum calcium concentration. The effects of PTH on the acute phase of bone resorption and calcium reclamation in the distal tubule together constitute a classic "short-loop" feedback system, in that the calcium so provided feeds back directly in the parathyroid chief cell.

The parathyroid–renal (PTH–1,25 (OH)$_2$ D) axis is reminiscent of the pituitary–adrenal [adrenocorticotropic hormone (ACTH)–cortisol] axis, and use of the axis concept and terminology is encouraged. Whereas 1,25 (OH)$_2$ D does influence PTH secretion directly as a short-loop feedback, the essence of the PTH–1,25 (OH)$_2$ D axis in practice is a long-loop feedback system in which 1,25 (OH)$_2$ D-mediated calcium absorption provides the ultimate feedback on the parathyroid chief cell. This "long-loop" system is the only means by which the organism can regulate its capacity to obtain calcium from the environment, and it is therefore a crucial component of the organism's response to either a prolonged or a major hypocalcemic challenge. Maximal adjustments to the rate of calcium absorption in the intestine via the PTH-1,25 (OH)$_2$ D axis require 24 to 48 hours to become fully operative, so that this system has little to do with minute-to-minute regulation.

A 12- to 15-hour fast in a normal individual represents a minor physiologic hypocalcemic challenge that requires only subtle hormonal readjustments for correction. The total quantity of calcium lost into the urine during this time is in the range of 50 to 75 mg. An unmeasurable decrease in serum calcium occurs, leading to a slight increase in PTH secretion. The dip in serum calcium is corrected by an increased efficiency of calcium reclamation in the distal tubule and by the rapid resorptive response to PTH in bone; by 12 hours, only minor increases in 1,25 (OH)$_2$ D synthesis will have occurred.

An abrupt reduction in dietary calcium intake to <100 mg/day, or the administration of 80 mg of furosemide daily to a normal individual, represents a moderate hypocalcemic challenge; in each case, the initial deficit of calcium is in the range of 100 to 150 mg/day. A series of adjustments occurs, leading to a new steady state by 48 hours (Fig. 2). A moderate increase in the secretion rate of PTH results in (a) increased calcium reabsorption from the distal tubule, (b) increased mobilization of calcium and phosphorus from bone, and (c) increased synthesis of 1,25 (OH)$_2$ D, which participates with PTH in bone resorption and increases the efficiency of calcium and phosphorus absorption in the intestine. The increased circulating concentration of PTH resets the renal tubular phosphate threshold (TmP/GFR) at a lower level so that the increased amount of phosphorus mobilized from bone and absorbed from the intestine is quantitatively excreted into the urine. In the new steady state, serum calcium has returned to normal, serum phosphorus is unchanged or slightly reduced, and a state of mild secondary hyperparathyroidism and efficient intestinal mineral absorption exists. At this point, the initial requirement for calcium mobilization

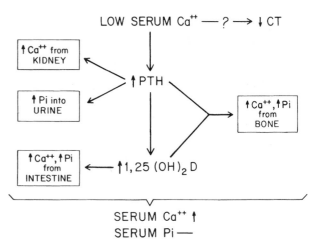

FIG. 2. The sequence of adjustments that are called into play in response to a moderate hypocalcemic challenge. (From Stewart AF, Broadus AE. Mineral metabolism. In: Felig P, Baxter JD, Broadus AE, Frohman LA, eds. *Endocrinology and metabolism.* 2nd ed. New York: McGraw-Hill, 1987:1317–1453.)

from the skeleton is largely replaced by the enhanced absorption of calcium in the intestine.

The systemic mechanisms for the prevention of hypercalcemia consist largely of a reversal of the sequence just described: an inhibition of PTH and 1,25 (OH)$_2$ D synthesis, with a reduction in calcium mobilization from bone, absorption from the intestine, and reclamation from the distal renal tubule. Whether the putative effects of calcitonin are of pathophysiologic importance in humans remains unclear. The bottleneck in the system's defense against hypercalcemia is the limited capacity of the kidneys to excrete calcium. In theory, normal kidneys can excrete a calcium load of 1000 or more mg/day. In practice, calcium-excretion rates in this range are rarely seen. Limitations in the theoretic ability of the kidney to combat hypercalcemia include (a) the fact that abnormalities in distal tubular reabsorption are actually involved in the genesis of hypercalcemia in a number of conditions (e.g., primary hyperparathyroidism), (b) the fact that a degree of renal impairment frequently accompanies many hypercalcemic conditions, and (c) the fact that an increased calcium concentration inhibits the ability of the renal tubule to conserve water, which may lead to a vicious cycle of dehydration, prerenal azotemia, and worsening hypercalcemia. One or more of these limitations can usually be demonstrated in any given patient with hypercalcemia.

A patient with advanced breast carcinoma metastatic to bone represents a severe hypercalcemic challenge. In such a patient, calcium is mobilized from bone, usually by local osteolytic mechanisms. Parathyroid function and 1,25 (OH)$_2$ D synthesis are appropriately suppressed, and the normal mechanisms of bone resorption, intestinal calcium absorption, and distal tubular calcium reabsorption are virtually eliminated. Initially, these adjustments may lead to a compensated steady state in which approximately 800 to 1000 mg/day of mobilized calcium is excreted, with a serum calcium that is high-normal or only slightly increased. With advancing disease or, as often occurs, with immobilization resulting from the basic disease process or an intercurrent illness, the quantity of mobilized calcium overwhelms the renal capacity for calcium excretion, and the spiral of hypercalcemia, dehydration, azotemia, and worsening hypercalcemia begins. In this circumstance, the serum calcium may climb from 10.5 to 15 mg/dL within 48 hours.

Systemic Phosphorus Homeostasis and Maintenance of a Normal Serum Phosphorus Concentration

The kidney plays the dominant role in systemic phosphorus homeostasis and maintains the serum phosphorus concentration at a value very close to the tubular phosphorus threshold or TmP/GFR (5). Because of the normal efficiency and lack of fine regulation of phosphorus absorption in the intestine, only in unusual circumstances (e.g., prolonged use of phosphate-binding antacids) is the systemic supply of phosphorus a limiting factor in phosphorus homeostasis. Thus most disorders associated with chronic hypophosphatemia or phosphorus depletion or both in humans result from either intrinsic (e.g., familial hypophosphatemic rickets) or extrinsic (e.g., primary hyperparathyroidism) alterations in TmP/GFR. Similarly, most conditions of chronic hyperphosphatemia result from either intrinsic (e.g., renal impairment) or extrinsic (e.g., hypoparathyroidism) abnormalities in the renal threshold for phosphorus. Acute hypophosphatemia most commonly results from the flux of extracellular phosphate ions into soft tissues. The PTH receptors in the proximal tubule that mediate regulation of TmP/GFR and those in the distal nephron that regulate Ca^{2+} reabsorption are coupled to different intracellular signal-transduction systems. This results in the use of Ca^{2+} as a second messenger in the case of the proximal tubular cell, whereas in the distal tubular cell, PTH regulates the reversible insertion of calcium channels into the luminal membrane, this being the means by which distal tubular calcium reabsorption is controlled. This is a particularly interesting example of specialized Ca^{2+} deployment/handling in the different cell types of the same organ (7).

The sequence of events initiated in the face of a hypophosphatemic challenge (Fig. 3) includes (a) stimulation of 1,25 $(OH)_2$ D synthesis in the kidney, (b) enhanced mobilization of phosphorus and calcium from bone, and (c) a hypophosphatemia-induced increase in TmP/GFR (the exact mechanism of which is unknown). The increased circulating concentration of 1,25 $(OH)_2$ D leads to increases in phosphorus and calcium absorption in the intestine and provides an additional stimulus for phosphorus and calcium mobilization from bone. The increased flow of calcium from bone and the intestine results in an inhibition of PTH secretion, which diverts the systemic flow of calcium into the urine and further increases TmP/GFR. The net result of this sequence of adjustments is a return of the serum phosphorus concentration to normal without change in the serum calcium concentration.

The defense against hyperphosphatemia consists largely of a reversal of the sequence of adjustments just described. The principal humoral factor that combats hyperphosphatemia is PTH, but its action is indirect. The product of the concentrations of calcium and phosphorus in serum is referred to as the mineral ion (Ca × P) product. This product

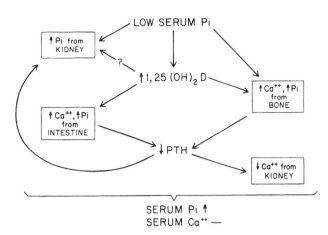

FIG. 3. The sequence of adjustments initiated in response to hypophosphatemia. (From Stewart AF, Broadus AE. Mineral metabolism. In: Felig P, Baxter JD, Broadus AE, Frohman LA, eds. *Endocrinology and metabolism.* 2nd ed. New York: McGraw-Hill, 1987:1317–1453.)

tends to be a biologic constant, in the sense that an increase in the concentration of one member leads to a reciprocal change in the concentration of the other. Thus an acute increase in the serum phosphorus concentration produces a transient decrease in the concentration of serum ionized calcium and a stimulation of PTH secretion, which reduces TmP/GFR and leads to a readjustment in serum phosphorus and calcium concentrations. A prolonged increase in the serum phosphorus concentration results in (a) an intrinsic downward adjustment in TmP/GFR that is independent of PTH, and (b) a persistent increase in PTH secretion that can ultimately lead to chief-cell hyperplasia. If hyperphosphatemia is prolonged and severe (e.g., as occurs in chronic renal insufficiency), the degree of secondary hyperparathyroidism is sufficient to lead to the typical findings of parathyroid bone disease.

Systemic Magnesium Homeostasis and Maintenance of a Normal Serum Magnesium Concentration

The understanding of systemic magnesium homeostasis remains at a relatively primitive state. Unlike calcium and phosphorus, there appears to be no important systemic or hormonal regulation of the magnesium concentration in the extracellular fluids. Instead, maintenance of the serum magnesium concentration seems to result from the combined fluxes of magnesium at the levels of the intestine, kidney, intracellular fluids, and perhaps the skeleton. The kidney is primarily responsible for the regulation of the serum magnesium concentration (3).

The fractional absorption of magnesium is approximately 30%. In conditions of dietary magnesium excess, a smaller proportion may be absorbed, and in conditions of dietary magnesium deficiency, a higher proportion may be absorbed. The cellular mechanisms mediating magnesium absorption in the small intestine are poorly defined but would appear to consist of both passive and facilitated (but not active) elements. These elements do not seem to be sensitive to

PTH, calcitonin, or 1,25 (OH)$_2$ D. Thus the net quantity of magnesium absorbed appears to be primarily a function of magnesium intake.

Of the approximately 2000 mg of magnesium filtered per day, 96% is reabsorbed along the nephron, and some 4% is excreted in the urine (fractional magnesium excretion). The mechanisms of magnesium reabsorption along the nephron at a cellular level are poorly understood, but, as is the case for calcium and phosphorus, it is possible to define a renal magnesium threshold or tubular maximum for magnesium (TmMg). The TmMg represents the net effects of magnesium reabsorption at different sites along the nephron. The TmMg is approximately 1.4 mg/dL when expressed as a function of the ultrafilterable serum magnesium concentration, or 2.0 mg/dL when expressed as a function of the total serum magnesium concentration (3). The tubular maximum functions essentially as a setpoint for reabsorption, such that magnesium filtered at a concentration greater than the TmMg is excreted and that filtered at a concentration less than the TmMg is retained. As in the intestine, renal tubular magnesium handling does not appear to be regulated by systemic or hormonal mechanisms in any important way.

In summary, systemic magnesium homeostasis does not seem to be hormonally regulated and therefore reflects largely the quantitative interplay of net magnesium absorption in the intestine and the fractional excretion of magnesium by the kidney. The fractional excretion of magnesium functions as a Tm-limited process and is primarily responsible for maintaining the serum magnesium concentration within rather narrow limits. The fine regulation of the serum magnesium concentration in the absence of hormonal controls provides an excellent example of the biologic power of a Tm-limited transport process.

ACKNOWLEDGMENT

Supported in part by National Institutes of Health grant RR125.

REFERENCES

1. Bringhurst FR. Calcium and phosphate distribution, turnover and metabolic actions. In: DeGroot LJ, ed. *Endocrinology*. 3rd ed. Philadelphia: Saunders, 1995:1015–1043.
2. Bilezikian JP, Marcus R, Levine MA, eds. *The parathyroids: basic and clinical concepts*. New York: Raven Press, 1994.
3. Rude RK, Singer FR. Magnesium deficiency and excess. *Annu Rev Med* 1981;32:245–253.
4. Rasmussen H, Isales CM, Calle R, et al. Diacylglycerol production, Ca^{2+} influx, and protein kinase C activation in sustained cellular responses. *Endocr Rev* 1995;16:649–681.
5. Bijvoet OLM. Relation of plasma phosphate concentration to renal tubular reabsorption of phosphate. *Clin Sci* 1969;37:23–36.
6. Brown EM, Pollak M, Hebert SC. The extracellular calcium-sensing receptor: its role in health and disease. *Annu Rev Med* 1998;49:15–29.
7. Friedman PA, Gesek FA. Cellular calcium transport in renal epithelia: measurement, mechanisms, and regulation. *Physiol Rev* 1995;75:429–471.

13. Parathyroid Hormone

Harald Jüppner, M.D., *Edward M. Brown, M.D., and †Henry M. Kronenberg, M.D.

*Departments of Pediatrics and *†Medicine, Harvard Medical School and †Department of Medicine, Endocrine Unit, Massachusetts General Hospital; and *Calcium Section, Endocrine-Hypertension Division, Department of Medicine, Brigham and Women's Hospital, Boston, Massachusetts*

Parathyroid hormone (PTH) and the active form of vitamin D, 1,25-dihydroxyvitamin D$_3$ [1,25 (OH)$_2$ D$_3$], are the principal regulators of calcium homeostasis for humans and most likely all terrestrial vertebrates (1,2) (Fig. 1). In bone, PTH stimulates the release of calcium and phosphate, and in the kidney, it stimulates the reabsorption of calcium and inhibits the reabsorption of phosphate. Furthermore, PTH stimulates the activity of the renal 1α-hydroxylase, thereby enhancing the synthesis of 1,25 (OH)$_2$ D$_3$, which in turn increases the intestinal absorption of calcium and phosphate. As a result of these PTH-dependent actions, blood calcium concentration increases and blood phosphate concentration decreases. The extracellular calcium concentration is the most important physiological regulator of the minute-to-minute secretion of PTH, but other factors, particularly 1,25 (OH)$_2$ D$_3$ and phosphate, can modulate its synthesis. These mutual regulatory interactions of PTH, calcium, 1,25 (OH)$_2$ D$_3$, and phosphate maintain blood calcium level constant, even in the presence of significant fluctuations in dietary calcium, bone metabolism, or renal function. In this chapter, we review the structure and biosynthesis of PTH, the regulation of its secretion, the physiologic actions of PTH, and then examine the cellular and subcellular mechanisms responsible for those actions.

PARATHYROID HORMONE

During evolution, the parathyroid glands first appear as discrete organs in amphibians (i.e., with the migration of vertebrates from an aquatic to a terrestrial existence) (3). In mammals, PTH is produced by the parathyroid glands, although small amounts of its messenger RNA (mRNA) also have been detected in the rat hypothalamus (4). PTH is a single-chain polypeptide that comprises in all investigated mammalian species 84 amino acids; chicken PTH, the only nonmammalian homologue isolated thus far, contains 88 residues (2) (Fig. 2). The amino-terminal region of PTH, which is associated with most of its known biologic actions, shows high homology among the different vertebrate species. The middle and carboxyl-terminal regions are more variable, and these portions of the PTH molecule may have distinct biologic properties (5–8).

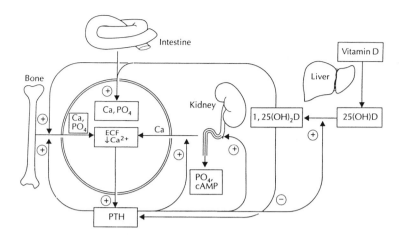

FIG. 1. Control of Ca_0^{2+} homeostasis. The *solid lines* and *arrows* denote the effects of PTH and 1,25 $(OH)_2 D_3$; the *dotted lines* and *arrows* demonstrate examples of direct actions of Ca_0^{2+} or phosphate ions. Ca, calcium; PO_4, phosphate; ECF, extracellular fluid; 1,25 $(OH)_2$ D, 1,25 dihydroxyvitamin D; 25 (OH) D, 25-hydroxyvitamin D; + signs, positive actions; − signs, inhibitory effects. (From Brown EM, Pollak M, Hebert SC. Cloning and characterization of extracellular Ca^{2+}-sensing receptors from parathyroid and kidney: molecular physiology and pathophysiology of Ca^{2+} sensing. *Endocrinologist* 1994;4:419–426, with permission.)

THE PARATHYROID CELL

Regulation of PTH Synthesis and Secretion, and Parathyroid Cell Proliferation

Although a large number of factors modulate parathyroid function *in vitro,* only a few regulators are known to be of physiological relevance *in vivo* [for review, see (9)]. The extracellular concentration of calcium (Ca_0^{2+}) is the most important determinant of the minute-to-minute secretory rate of the parathyroid gland; low Ca_0^{2+} stimulates, whereas increased Ca_0^{2+} inhibits PTH secretion. High calcium also suppresses PTH gene expression and parathyroid cellular proliferation. 1,25 $(OH)_2 D_3$ has similar inhibitory actions on PTH synthesis and parathyroid cell proliferation, whereas phosphate, the most recently recognized modulator of parathyroid function, independently stimulates PTH gene expression. Phosphate also stimulates, probably through effects on calcium, PTH secretion and the proliferation of parathyroid cells (1,9–12). The parathyroid cell has a temporal hierarchy of responses to changes in Ca_0^{2+}; those responses mount a progressively larger increase in PTH secretion in response to prolonged hypocalcemia (1,9,12). To meet acute hypocalcemic challenges, PTH is rapidly released from secretory vesicles by exocytosis (e.g., over a period of seconds to a few minutes). For the correction of prolonged hypocalcemia, parathyroid cells reduce the intracellular degradation of PTH

(over a period of minutes to an hour or so), increase PTH gene expression (over a period of several hours to a few days), and enhance the proliferative activity of parathyroid cells (over a period of days to weeks or longer). Many, if not all, of these processes are controlled by a G protein–coupled receptor that recognizes extracellular calcium ions as its principal physiological ligand. This calcium-sensing receptor (CaR) is expressed on the surface of parathyroid cells and several other cell types that are involved in regulating mineral ion homeostasis (13), including the calcitonin-secreting C-cells of the thyroid and renal tubular cells (see Fig. 3). The CaR also is expressed in bone cells and in intestinal epithelial cells that are involved in the absorption of dietary calcium, but its calcium-homeostatic role(s), if any, in these cells have not yet been established (12). A more detailed understanding of the CaR in the regulation of systemic Ca_0^{2+} homeostasis, particularly the roles of parathyroid and kidney in these processes, was obtained through the molecular definition of several human disorders and through the genetic manipulation of mice (14–19). Familial hypocalciuric hypercalcemia [FHH; also known as familial benign hypocalciuric hypercalcemia (FBHH)] is an autosomal dominant disorder now known to be caused by a large variety of heterozygous inactivating CaR mutations. Affected individuals show mild to moderate resistance of the parathyroids to Ca_0^{2+} (i.e., there is a modest increase in the parathyroid setpoint, and higher levels of Ca_0^{2+} are thus

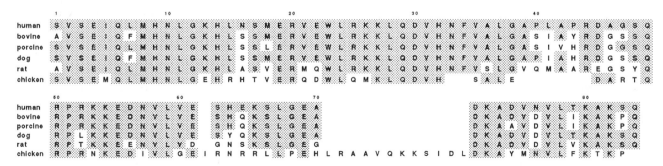

FIG. 2. Alignment of the amino acid sequences of all known vertebrate parathyroid hormone. Conserved residues are shaded; numbers indicate the positions of amino acids in the mammalian peptide sequences.

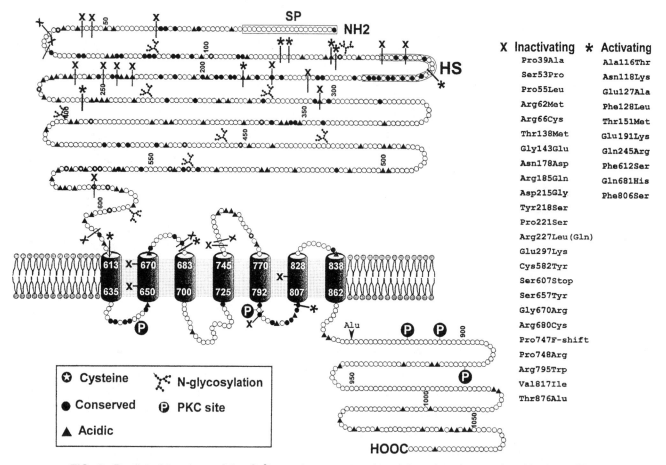

FIG. 3. Predicted topology of the Ca_o^{2+}-sensing receptor cloned from human parathyroid gland. SP, signal peptide; HS, hydrophobic segment. Also indicated are the positions of the described missense and nonsense mutations causing either benign hypocalciuric hypercalcemia (FHH) or autosomal dominant hypocalcemia (ADH); the latter are depicted by using the three-letter amino acid code. The normal amino acid is indicated before and the mutant amino acid after the number of the relevant codon. (From Brown EM, Bai M, Pollak MR. Familial benign hypocalciuric hypercalcemia and other syndromes of altered responsiveness to extracellular calcium. In: Krane S, Avioli LV, eds. *Metabolic bone diseases and clinically related disorders.* 3rd ed. San Diego: Academic Press, 1997:479–499, with permission.)

needed to achieve half-maximal inhibition of PTH release). Because of the expression of mutant CaRs in the kidney, patients with FHH show a reduced capacity to upregulate Ca^{2+} excretion despite persistent PTH-dependent hypercalcemia. Homozygous or compound heterozygous inactivating CaR mutations result in a much more severe resistance toward Ca_o^{2+} and cause the severe PTH-dependent hypercalcemia observed in neonatal severe hyperparathyroidism (NSHPT), an acutely life-threatening disorder (14,17,19). Mice in which one allele encoding the CaR had been deleted through homologous recombination show biochemical abnormalities similar to those observed in humans with FHH [i.e., apparently asymptomatic, mild hypercalcemia that is PTH dependent and is furthermore accompanied by relative hypocalciuria (e.g., urinary calcium excretion is inappropriately low for the level of serum calcium] (16). As in humans, mice that are homozygous for CaR gene ablation show severe hypercalcemia as the result of severe hyperparathyroidism, and consequently develop significant hyperparathyroid

bone disease and marked growth retardation; the animals typically die within the first few days to weeks of life. Inactivating CaR mutations in humans thus have similar consequences as disruption of the CaR gene in mice. Activating CaR mutations have been identified in patients with autosomal dominant hypocalcemia (ADH) (15,18,19). These mutations increase the responsiveness of the parathyroid glands to Ca_o^{2+} (e.g., lower levels of Ca_o^{2+} are needed to obtain half-maximal inhibition of glandular PTH release), and thus lead to inappropriately low normal levels of PTH and relative hypercalciuria. In patients with ADH, the changes in the regulation of Ca_o^{2+} are thus reciprocal to those observed in patients with FHH or NSHPT, and to those observed in mice with heterozygous or homozygous "knockout" of the CaR gene. These observations provide strong evidence for an important nonredundant role of the CaR in calcium homeostasis. Like other G protein–coupled receptors, the CaR is predicted to have seven membrane-spanning domains. It couples to different G proteins and thereby either activates various phospholipases or inhibits adenylate cyclase (12,13). It remains uncertain which of these second-messenger pathways is most important for Ca_o^{2+}-dependent regulation of PTH secretion and renal calcium conservation [for review, see (9)]. It also should be noted that the CaR is expressed in numerous other tissues (i.e., neurons and glia in the brain, lens epithelial cells), in which it may serve yet unknown biologic role(s) (e.g., controlling cell proliferation and differentiation), which are most likely unrelated to the systemic regulation of Ca_o^{2+} homeostasis (12).

Physiologic Regulation of PTH Secretion

Figure 4 illustrates the steep inverse sigmoidal relation between PTH levels and Ca_o^{2+} *in vivo* and *in vitro* (9,12). The steepness of this curve ensures large changes in PTH for small alterations in Ca_o^{2+} and contributes importantly to the near constancy with which Ca_o^{2+} is maintained in vivo. Parathyroid cells readily detect alterations in Ca_o^{2+} of only a few percentage points. The midpoint or setpoint of this parathyroid function curve is a key determinant of the level at which Ca_o^{2+} is "set" *in vivo*. The parathyroid cell responds to changes in Ca_o^{2+} within a matter of seconds and contains sufficient PTH to sustain a maximal secretory response for 60 to 90 minutes. Through actions on PTH synthesis, 1,25 $(OH)_2 D_3$ reduces PTH secretion (1,9,12), whereas increases in the extracellular phosphate concentration stimulate PTH secretion after several hours (11,20).

Regulation of Intracellular Degradation of PTH

The pool of stored, intracellular PTH is small, and the parathyroid cell must therefore have mechanisms to increase hormone synthesis and release in response to sustained hypocalcemia. One such adaptive mechanism is to reduce the intracellular degradation of the hormone, thereby increasing the net amount of intact, biologically active PTH that is available for secretion. During hypocalcemia, the bulk of the hormone that is released from the parathyroid cell is intact PTH(1–84). As the level of Ca_o^{2+} increases, a greater fraction of intracellular PTH is degraded, and with overt hypercalcemia, the majority of the secreted immunoreactive PTH consists of carboxyl-terminal fragments [for review, see (2,9)].

Physiologic Control of PTH Gene Expression

The second adaptive mechanism of the parathyroid cell to sustained reductions in Ca_o^{2+} is to increase the cellular levels of PTH mRNA, a response that takes several hours. A reduction in Ca_o^{2+} increases, whereas an increase in Ca_o^{2+} reduces the cellular levels of PTH mRNA by affecting both its stability and the transcriptional rate of its gene (1,9,12,21). Available data suggest that phosphate ions also directly regulate PTH gene expression. Hypo- and hyperphosphatemia in the rat decrease and increase, respectively, the levels of the mRNA for PTH through a mechanism of action that is independent of changes in Ca_o^{2+} or 1,25 $(OH)_2 D_3$ (1,10,21). This action of an increased extracellular phos-

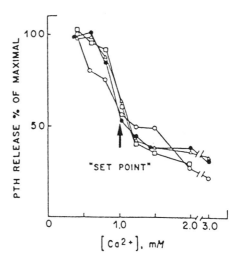

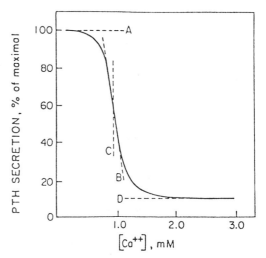

FIG. 4. Inverse sigmoidal relation between Ca_o^{2+} and parathyroid hormone (PTH) release and the four-parameter model that describes such curves. **Top:** Results that were obtained by using dispersed normal human parathyroid cells; they are expressed as percentage of the maximal rate of PTH release seen at 0.3 mM Ca_o^{2+}. The setpoint indicates the level of Ca_o^{2+} at which PTH release is half-maximally suppressed. **Bottom:** The four parameters that can be used to describe such sigmoidal curves. (From Brown EM. PTH secretion in vivo and in vitro: regulation by calcium and other secretagogues. *Miner Electrolyte Metab* 1982;8:130–150, with permission.)

phate concentration could potentially contribute importantly to the secondary hyperparathyroidism frequently encountered in end-stage renal failure with chronically high serum phosphate.

Metabolites of vitamin D, principally 1,25 $(OH)_2 D_3$, play an important role in the long-term regulation of parathyroid function and may act at several levels by affecting secretion of PTH and by affecting expression of its gene, by controlling expression of the CaR and the vitamin D receptor (VDR) gene, as well as the regulation of parathyroid cellular proliferation (1,9,12). 1,25 $(OH)_2 D_3$ is by far the most important vitamin D metabolite that modulates parathyroid function. It acts through a nuclear receptor (i.e., VDR), often in concert with other such receptors (i.e., those for retinoic acid or glucocorticoids), on DNA sequences upstream from the PTH gene (22,23). The 1,25 (OH)$_2$ D$_3$-induced upregulation of VDR expression in the parathyroid could potentiate its inhibitory action(s) on PTH synthesis and secretion (1,9,12). Recently developed, noncalcemic or less calcemic analogues of 1,25 (OH)$_2$ D (e.g., 22-oxacalcitriol and calcipotriol) inhibit PTH secretion while producing relatively little stimulation of intestinal calcium absorption and of bone resorption (24) and thus may be attractive candidates for treating the hyperparathyroidism of chronic renal insufficiency.

Physiologic Regulation of Parathyroid Cellular Proliferation

The final adaptive mechanism contributing to changes in overall secretory activity of the parathyroid gland is to adjust the rate of parathyroid cellular proliferation. Under normal conditions, there is little or no proliferative activity of parathyroid cells. The parathyroid glands, however, can enlarge greatly during states of chronic hypocalcemia, particularly in renal failure [probably because of a combination of hypocalcemia, hyperphosphatemia, and low levels of 1,25 (OH)$_2$ D$_3$ in the latter condition (9)].

PARATHYROID HORMONE ACTION

Receptors for PTH

PTH-dependent regulation of mineral ion homeostasis is largely mediated through the PTH/parathyroid hormone-related peptide (PTHrP) receptor, which is coupled to adenylate cyclase and to phospholipase C (25,26). This receptor belongs to a distinct family of G protein–coupled receptors and mediates with similar or indistinguishable efficacy biologic actions of both PTH and PTHrP. The latter peptide, first discovered as the most important cause of the syndrome of humoral hypercalcemia of malignancy (27–29), shares structural and functional similarities with PTH, and it is likely that both genes evolved through an early duplication event (30). The PTH/PTHrP receptor is most abundantly expressed in the target tissues for PTH actions (i.e., kidney and bone), but it is also found in a large variety of other fetal and adult tissues, and at particularly high concentrations in growth-plate chondrocytes (31,32). In tissues other than kidney and bone, the PTH/PTHrP receptor most likely mediates the para-/autocrine actions of PTHrP, rather than the endocrine actions of PTH. Of considerable importance is the receptor's role in cartilage and bone development, because it mediates in this tissue the PTHrP-dependent regulation of chondrocyte proliferation and differentiation; thus it has a major role in bone growth (33–36).

There is considerable pharmacologic evidence, however, for the existence of other receptors that are activated by either PTH or PTHrP, or by both peptides. These presumably novel receptors mediate biologic functions that are only partially characterized and may be unrelated to the control of calcium and phosphorus homeostasis [for review, see (2)].

So far, only cDNAs encoding the PTH-2 receptor, which is activated by PTH [and possibly a recently characterized hypothalamic peptide (37)], but not by PTHrP (38), have been isolated. Expression of the PTH-2 receptor is restricted to few tissues, and biologic function(s) mediated by this novel receptor are currently unknown.

Actions of PTH on Bone

PTH has complex and only partially understood actions on bone that require the presence of and often direct contact between several different specialized cell types, including osteoblasts, bone marrow stromal cells, hematopoietic precursors of osteoclasts, and mature osteoclasts (39). Administration of PTH leads to the release of calcium from a rapidly turning over pool of calcium near the surface of bone; after several hours, calcium is also released from an additional pool that turns over more slowly (40). Prolonged administration of PTH (or increased secretion of PTH associated with primary hyperparathyroidism) leads to an increase in osteoclast cell number and activity (41). The release of calcium is accompanied by the release of phosphate and matrix components, such as degradation products of collagen. Paradoxically, particularly when given intermittent, PTH administration leads to the formation of increased amounts of trabecular bone; these anabolic actions of PTH are currently being explored for the prevention and treatment of osteoporosis (42).

The osteoblast and its precursor, the marrow stromal cell, have central roles in directing both the catabolic (bone resorption) and anabolic (bone formation) actions of PTH. Although cell lines capable of differentiating into osteoclasts have been shown to express PTH/PTHrP receptors (43–48), these receptors are not needed for the stimulation of PTH-dependent osteoclastic development (49). Instead, PTH affects osteoclast maturation and function only indirectly by stimulating the expression of osteoclast-differentiating factor (ODF; also termed TRANCE, RANKL, or osteoprotegerin-ligand), a key osteoblastic protein related to tumor necrosis factor that activates osteoclast development and increases the activity of mature osteoclasts (50). ODF is anchored to the cell surface of osteoblasts, and on interaction with the ODF receptor (which is most likely RANK or a closely related protein) on preosteoclasts, these precursors differentiate into mature osteoclasts, if macrophage–colony-stimulating factor (M-CSF) also is present (50). PTH stimulates the expression of ODF on the cell surface of osteoblasts, and the same response is stimulated by other molecules [e.g., interleukin 11 (IL-11), prostaglandin E$_2$, and 1,25 (OH)$_2$ D$_3$], which were previously noted to stimulate the formation of osteoclasts (39,50–53). It remains to be determined whether PTH can stimulate ODF synthesis directly, or whether cytokines secreted in response to PTH are obligatory intermediaries.

The interaction between ODF and its preosteoclastic receptor is further controlled by a secreted protein, osteoprotegerin (OPG) which is a soluble decoy receptor with homology to the probable ODF receptor (53) and which causes hypocalcemia when injected into rats (54). Recent studies in mice that overexpressed OPG under the control of a liver-specific promoter, and in animals that lack both copies of its gene, suggested that OPG importantly modulates the communication between osteoblasts and osteoclasts (55–57).

Actions of PTH in Kidney

In kidney, PTH has three major biologic functions that are essential for the regulation of mineral ion homeostasis; these include stimulating the reabsorption of calcium, inhibiting the reabsorption of phosphate, and enhancing the synthesis of 1,25 $(OH)_2$ D_3.

Phosphate is normally reabsorbed from the glomerular filtrate in both the proximal and distal tubules, and at both these sites, reabsorption is inhibited by PTH (2,58). Best studied is its effect on proximal tubular cells where phosphate is transported into the cell through the actions of a membrane-anchored sodium–phosphate cotransporter, Npt2 (previously termed NaPi2) (59). PTH reduces the amount of Npt2 on the cell surface, primarily by increasing its internalization and subsequent lysosomal degradation (60), but also by decreasing its synthesis (61). The complete lack of Npt2 expression, recently accomplished in mice through the ablation of its gene, leads to severe renal phosphate wasting and other abnormalities that are similar to those observed in hereditary hypophosphatemic rickets with hypercalciuria (HHRH) (62). PTH is only one of several determinants of Npt2 activity, as dietary phosphate restriction leads, independent of changes in blood concentrations of PTH, to a markedly enhanced renal phosphate reabsorption and thus a virtual elimination of urinary phosphate losses (63). In the distal tubules, PTH also inhibits phosphate reabsorption; the transporter(s) that are involved in this process have not yet been identified.

Most calcium reabsorption occurs in the proximal tubule (64–66), but only the calcium reabsorption in the distal nephron is PTH dependent (63,65,66). Even though the kidneys reabsorb calcium more efficiently when stimulated by PTH, the absolute amount of calcium in the urine usually increases when the circulating concentrations of PTH are chronically increased to levels sufficient to produce hypercalcemia, as in patients with primary hyperparathyroidism. This increase in urinary calcium excretion is caused by the substantial increase in the filtered load of calcium (2,58). The calcium-sensing receptor plays, independent of PTH, an important role in directly regulating renal calcium reabsorption—inhibiting tubular reabsorption of calcium when the level of peritubular Ca_o^{2+} increases—as indicated by the effects of activating and inactivating mutations in different genetic disorders (see earlier).

PTH also activates the mitochondrial vitamin D 1α-hydroxylase in proximal tubular cells; this leads to an increase of the blood 1,25 $(OH)_2$ D_3 concentration (67,68), which, in turn, is a potent inducer of intestinal calcium absorption (as well as of bone resorption). This effect of PTH is not immediate, because the stimulation of 1,25 $(OH)_2$ D_3 production occurs over several hours and requires the synthesis of new protein (69,70). Along with its action on the 1α-hydroxylase, PTH decreases the activity of the renal vitamin D 24-hydroxylase, thus enhancing the effect on 1,25 $(OH)_2$ D_3 synthesis. Other factors, particularly a low blood phosphate concentration, also markedly increase the synthesis of this biologically active vitamin D metabolite, whereas hypercalcemia, as would be generated by sustained increases in PTH, suppresses the 1α-hydroxylase activity and thus limits the production of 1,25 $(OH)_2$ D_3 in a homeostatic manner (71,72).

Because of its effectiveness in increasing blood calcium concentration, 1,25 $(OH)_2$ D_3 is widely used, along with oral calcium supplementation, in the treatment of hypoparathyroidism (and pseudohypoparathyroidism). However, because 1,25 $(OH)_2$ D_3 cannot mimic the renal, calcium-sparing effects of PTH, urine calcium excretion can increase quickly as serum calcium approaches the normal range during therapy, particularly when the underlying hypoparathyroidism is caused by activating mutations in the calcium-sensing receptor, as in autosomal dominant hypocalcemia (see earlier). In these latter patients, blood calcium is best kept at or below the lower limit of normal, with periodic monitoring of 24-hour urinary calcium excretion, to avoid the long-term consequences of hypercalciuria.

Molecular Defects in the PTH/PTHrP Receptor

The endocrine actions of PTH, and the autocrine/paracrine actions of PTHrP, are mediated through the PTH/PTHrP receptor. A single G protein–coupled receptor is thus essential for the biologic roles of two distinct ligands, which are important for regulation of calcium homeostasis and for the regulation of chondrocyte proliferation and differentiation, respectively. The ablation of one allele encoding the PTH/PTHrP receptor gene in mice did not lead to discernible abnormality, whereas the ablation of both alleles resulted in fetal death during middle or late gestation and severe skeletal abnormalities (35). Based on these findings in mice, it appeared likely that activating or inactivating PTH/PTHrP-receptor mutations in humans would affect mineral ion homeostasis and bone development.

Mutations in the PTH/PTHrP receptor were initially suspected as a cause of pseudohypoparathyroidism type Ib (PHP-Ib), in which patients exhibit PTH-resistant hypocalcemia and hyperphosphatemia (73). However, these patients lack growth-plate abnormalities, indicating that the actions of PTHrP are appropriately mediated. It was therefore not surprising, at least in retrospect, that PTH/PTHrP-receptor mutations could not be identified in PHP-Ib patients (74,75). Recent studies with several large PHP-Ib kindreds indicated that the disease is linked to the telomeric end of chromosome 20q, a region that contains the gene encoding the alpha subunit of the G_s protein (76).

However, PTH/PTHrP-receptor mutations have been identified in two rare genetic disorders, Jansen's metaphyseal chondrodysplasia and Blomstrand's lethal chondrodysplasia. Activating mutations that lead to ligand-independent accumulation of cyclic adenosine monophosphate (cAMP) were identified as the cause of the autosomal dominant Jansen's disease, which is characterized by short-limbed dwarfism and severe hypercalcemia and hypophosphatemia, despite normal or undetectable levels of PTH and PTHrP in the circulation (77). Inactivating PTH/PTHrP-receptor mutations (homozygous or compound heterozygous) were identified in patients with Blomstrand's disease, who are typically born prematurely and die at birth or shortly thereafter. These patients have advanced bone maturation, accelerated chondrocyte differentiation, and, most likely, severe abnormalities in mineral ion homeostasis (78,79,80).

REFERENCES

1. Silver J, Kronenberg HM. Parathyroid hormone: molecular biology and regulation. In: Bilezikian JP, Raisz LG, Rodan GA, eds. *Principles of bone biology.* New York: Academic Press, 1996:325–346.
2. Potts JT Jr, Jüppner H. Parathyroid hormone and parathyroid hormone-related peptide in calcium homeostasis, bone metabolism, and bone development: the proteins, their genes, and receptors. In: Avioli LV, Krane SM, eds. *Metabolic bone disease.* 3rd ed. New York: Academic Press, 1997:51–94.
3. Wendelaar-Bonga SE, Pang PK. Control of calcium regulating hormones in the vertebrates: parathyroid hormone, calcitonin, prolactin, and stanniocalcin. *Int Rev Cytol* 1991;128:139–213.
4. Nutley MT, Parimi SA, Harvey S. Sequence analysis of hypothalamic parathyroid hormone messenger ribonucleic acid. *Endocrinology* 1995;136:5600–5607
5. Murray TM, Rao LG, Rizzoli RE. Interaction of parathyroid hormone, parathyroid hormone-related peptide, and their fragments with conventional and nonconventional receptor sites. In: Bilzikian JP, Levine MA, Marcus R, eds. *The parathyroids: basic and clinical concepts.* New York: Raven Press, 1994:185–211.
6. Kaji H, Sugimoto T, Kanatani M, et al. Carboxyl-terminal PTH fragments stimulate osteoclast-like cell formation and osteoclastic activity. *Endocrinology* 1994;134:1897–1904.
7. Inomata N, Akiyama M, Kubota N, Jüppner H. Characterization of a novel PTH-receptor with specificity for the carboxyl-terminal region of PTH(1-84). *Endocrinology* 1995;136:4732–4740.
8. Erdmann S, Muller W, Bahrami S, et al. Differential effects of parathyroid hormone fragments on collagen gene expression in chondrocytes. *J Cell Biol* 1996;135:1179–1191.
9. Diaz R, El-Hajj GF, Brown E. Regulation of parathyroid function. In: Fray FGS, ed. *Handbook of physiology, section 7: endocrinology, vol. III, hormonal regulation of water and electrolyte balance.* New York: Oxford University Press, 1999.
10. Naveh-Many T, Rahaminov R, Livini N, Silver J. Parathyroid cell proliferation in normal and chronic renal failure in rats: the effects of calcium, phosphate, and vitamin D. *J Clin Invest* 1995;96:1786–1793.
11. Slatopolsky E, Finch J, Denda M, et al. Phosphorus restriction prevents parathyroid gland growth: high phosphorus directly stimulates PTH secretion in vitro. *J Clin Invest* 1996;97:2534–2540.
12. Yamaguchi T, Chattopadhyay N, Brown E. G Protein-coupled extracellular $Ca^{2+}(Ca_0^{2+})$-sensing receptor (CaR): roles in cell signaling and control of diverse cellular functions. In: O'Malley B, ed. *Hormones and signalling.* San Diego: Academic Press, 1999.
13. Brown EM, Gamba G, Riccardi D, et al. Cloning and characterization of an extracellular Ca^{2+}-sensing receptor from bovine parathyroid. *Nature* 1993;366:575–580.
14. Pollak MR, Brown EM, WuChou YH, et al. Mutations in the human Ca^{2+}-sensing receptor gene cause familial hypocalciuric hypercalcemia and neonatal severe hyperparathyroidism. *Cell* 1993;75:1297–1303.
15. Pollak MR, Brown EM, Estep HL, et al. Autosomal dominant hypocalcaemia caused by a Ca^{2+}-sensing receptor gene mutation. *Nat Genet* 1994;8:303–307.
16. Ho C, Conner DA, Pollak M, et al. A mouse model for familial hypocalciuric hypercalcemia and neonatal severe hyperparathyroidism. *Nat Genet* 1995;11:389–394.
17. Heath H III, Odelberg S, Jackson CE, et al. Clustered inactivating mutations and benign polymorphisms of the calcium receptor gene in familial benign hypocalciuric hypercalcemia suggest receptor functional domains. *J Clin Endocrinol Metab* 1996;81:1312–1317.
18. Pearce SH, Williamson C, Kifor O, et al. A familial syndrome of hypocalcemia with hypercalciuria due to mutations in the calcium-sensing receptor. *N Engl J Med* 1997;335:1115–1122.
19. Brown EM, Pollak M, Bai M, Hebert SC. Disorders with increased or decreased responsiveness to extracellular Ca^{2+} owing to mutations in the Ca^{2+}-sensing receptor. In: Spiegel AM, ed. *G proteins, receptors, and disease.* Totowa, NJ: Humana Press, 1998:181–204.
20. Almaden Y, Canalejo A, Hernandez A, et al. Direct effect of phosphorus on PTH secretion from whole rat parathyroid glands in vitro. *J Bone Miner Res* 1996;11:970–976.
21. Moallem E, Kilav R, Silver J, Naveh-Many T. RNA-Protein binding and post-transcriptional regulation of parathyroid hormone gene expression by calcium and phosphate. *J Biol Chem* 1998;273:5253–5259.
22. Russell J, Sherwood L. The effects of 1,25-dihydroxyvitamin D_3 and high calcium on transcription of the pre-proparathyroid hormone glue are direct. *Trans Assoc Am Physicians* 1987;100:256–262.
23. Okazaki T, Igarashi T, Kronenberg HM. 5′-Flanking region of the parathyroid hormone gene mediates negative regulation by 1,25(OH)$_2$ vitamin D$_3$. *J Biol Chem* 1989;263:2203–2208.
24. Slatopolsky E, Finch J, Ritter C, et al. A new analog of calcitrol, 19-nor-1,25-(OH)$_2$D$_2$, suppress parathyroid hormone secretion in uremic rats in the absence of hypercalcemia. *Am J Kidney Dis* 1995;26:852–860.
25. Jüppner H, Abou-Samra AB, Freeman MW, et al. A G protein-linked receptor for parathyroid hormone and parathyroid hormone-related peptide. *Science* 1991;254:1024–1026.
26. Abou-Samra AB, Jüppner H, Force T, et al. Expression cloning of a common receptor for parathyroid hormone and parathyroid hormone-related peptide from rat osteoblast-like cells: a single receptor stimulates intracellular accumulation of both cAMP and inositol triphosphates and increases intracellular free calcium. *Proc Natl Acad Sci USA* 1992;89:2732–2736.
27. Suva LJ, Winslow GA, Wettenhall RE, et al. A parathyroid hormone-related protein implicated in malignant hypercalcemia: cloning and expression. *Science* 1987;237:893–896.
28. Strewler GJ, Stern PH, Jacobs JW, et al. Parathyroid hormone-like protein from human renal carcinoma cells: structural and functional homology with parathyroid hormone. *J Clin Invest* 1987;80:1803–1807.
29. Mangin M, Webb AC, Dreyer BE, et al. Identification of a cDNA encoding a parathyroid hormone-like peptide from a human tumor associated with humoral hypercalcemia of malignancy. *Proc Natl Acad Sci USA* 1988;85:597–601.
30. Yang KH, Stewart AF. Parathyroid hormone-related protein: the gene, its mRNA species, and protein products. In: Bilezikian JP, Raisz LG, Rodan GA, eds. *Principles of bone biology.* New York: Academic Press, 1996:347–362.
31. Segre GV. Receptors for parathyroid hormone and parathyroid hormone-related protein. In: Bilezikian JP, Raisz LG, Rodan GA, eds. *Principles of bone biology.* New York: Academic Press, 1996:377–403.
32. Lee K, Lanske B, Karaplis AC, et al. Parathyroid hormone-related peptide delays terminal differentiation of chondrocytes during endochondral bone development. *Endocrinology* 1996;137:5109–5118.
33. Karaplis AC, Luz A, Glowacki J, et al. Lethal skeletal dysplasia from targeted disruption of the parathyroid hormone-related peptide gene. *Genes Dev* 1994;8:277–289.
34. Vortkamp A, Lee K, Lanske B, Segre GV, Kronenberg HM, Tabin CJ Regulation of rate of cartilage differentiation by Indian hedgehog and PTH-related protein. *Science* 1996;273:613–622.
35. Lanske B, Karaplis AC, Luz A, et al. PTH/PTHrP receptor in early development and Indian hedgehog-regulated bone growth. *Science* 1996;273:663–666.
36. Weir EC, Philbrick WM, Amling M, Neff LA, Baron R, Broadus AE. Targeted overexpression of parathyroid hormone-related peptide in chondrocytes causes skeletal dysplasia and delayed endochondral bone formation. *Proc Natl Acad Sci USA* 1996;93:10240–10245.
37. Usdin TB. Evidence for a parathyroid hormone-2 receptor selective ligand in the hypothalamus. *Endocrinology* 1997;138:831–834.
38. Usdin TB, Gruber C, Bonner TI. Identification and functional expression of a receptor selectively recognizing parathyroid hormone, the PTH2 receptor. *J Biol Chem* 1995;270:15455–15458.
39. Suda T, Udagawa N, Takahashi N. Cells of bone: osteoclast generation. In: Bilezikian JP, Raisz LG, Rodan GA, eds. *Principles of bone biology.* New York: Academic Press, 1996:87–102.
40. Talmage RV, Elliott JR. Removal of calcium from bone as influenced by the parathyroids. *Endocrinology* 1958;62:717–722.
41. Mundy GR, Roodman GD. Osteoclast ontogeny and function. In: Meunier PW, ed. *Bone and mineral research.* Vol 5. Amsterdam: Elsevier, 1987:209–280.

42. Finkelstein JS. Pharmacological mechanisms of therapeutics: parathyroid hormone. In: Bilezikian JP, Raisz LG, Rodan GA, eds. *Principles of bone biology.* New York: Academic Press, 1996:993–1005.

43. Mears DC. Effects of parathyroid hormone and thyrocalcitonin on the membrane potential of osteoclasts. *Endocrinology* 1971;88:1021–1028.

44. Ferrier J, Ward A, Kanehisa J, Heersche JN. Electrophysiological responses of osteoclasts to hormones. *J Cell Physiol* 1986;128:23–26.

45. Teti A, Rizzoli R, Zallone AZ. Parathyroid hormone binding to cultured avian osteoclasts. *Biochem Biophys Res Commun* 1991;174:1217–1222.

46. Hakeda Y, Hiura K, Sato T, et al. Existence of parathyroid hormone binding sites on murine hemopoietic blast cells. *Biochem Biophys Res Commun* 1989;163:1481–1486.

47. Rouleau MF, Mitchell L, Goltzman D. In vivo distribution of parathyroid hormone receptors in bone: evidence that a predominant osseous target cell is not the mature osteoblast. *Endocrinology* 1988;123:187–191.

48. Silve CM, Hradek GT, Jones AL, Arnaud CD. Parathyroid hormone receptor in intact embryonic chicken bone: characterization and cellular localization. *J Cell Biol* 1982;94:379–386.

49. Liu BY, Guo J, Lanske B, Divieti P, Kronenberg HM, Bringhurst FR. Conditionally immortalized murine bone marrow stromal cells mediate parathyroid hormone-dependent osteoclastogenesis in vitro. *Endocrinology* 1998;139:1952–1964.

50. Yasuda H, Shima N, Nakagawa N, et al. Osteoclast differentiation factor is a ligand for osteoprotegerin/osteoclastogenesis-inhibitory factor and is identical to TRANCE/RANKL. *Proc Natl Acad Sci USA* 1998;95:3597–3602.

51. Löwik CWGM, van der Pluijm G, Bloys H, et al. Parathyroid hormone (PTH) and PTH-like protein (PLP) stimulate interleukin-6 production by osteogenic cells: a possible role of interleukin-6 in osteoclastogenesis. *Biochem Biophys Res Commun* 1989;162:1546–1552.

52. Felix R, Fleisch H, Elford PR. Bone-resorbing cytokines enhance release of macrophage colony-stimulating activity by the osteoblastic cell MC3T3-E1. *Calcif Tissue Int* 1989;44:356–60.

53. Lacey DL, Timms E, Tan HL, et al. Osteoprotegerin ligand is a cytokine that regulates osteoclast differentiation and activation. *Cell* 1998;93:165–176.

54. Yamamoto M, Murakami T, Nishikawa M, et al. Hypocalcemic effect of osteoclastogenesis inhibitory factor/osteoprotegerin in the thyroparathyroidectomized rat. *Endocrinology* 1998;139:4012–4015.

55. Simonet SW, Lacey DL, Dunstan CR, et al. Osteoprotegerin: a novel secreted protein involved in the regulation of bone density. *Cell* 1997;89:309–319.

56. Tsuda E, Goto M, Mochizuki S, et al. Isolation of a novel cytokine from human fibroblasts that specifically inhibits osteoclastogenesis. *Biochem Biophys Res Commun* 1997;234:137–142.

57. Bucay N, Sarosi I, Dunstan DR, et al. Osteoprotegerin-deficient mice develop early onset osteoporosis and arterial calcification. *Genes Dev* 1998;12:1260–1268.

58. Bringhurst FR. Calcium and phosphate distribution, turnover, and metabolic actions. In: DeGroot LJ, ed. *Endocrinology,* 2nd ed. Vol 2. Philadelphia: WB Saunders, 1989:805–843.

59. Cheng L, Sacktor B. Sodium gradient-dependent phosphate transport in renal brush border vesicles. *J Biol Chem* 1981;256:1556–1564.

60. Pfister MF, Ruf I, Stange G, et al. Parathyroid hormone leads to the lysosomal degradation of the renal type II Na/P_i cotransporter. *Proc Natl Acad Sci USA* 1998;95:1909–1914.

61. Malmström K, Murer H. Parathyroid hormone regulates phosphate transport in OK cells via an irreversible inactivation of a membrane protein. *FEBS Lett* 1997;216:257–260.

62. Beck L, Karaplis AC, Amizuka N, Hewson AS, Ozawa H, Tenenhouse HS. Targeted inactivation of Ntp2 in mice leads to severe renal phosphate wasting, hypercalciuria, and skeletal abnormalities. *Proc Natl Acad Sci USA* 1998;95:5372–5377.

63. Drezner MK. Phosphorus homeostasis and related disorders. In: Bilezikian JP, Raisz LG, Rodan GA, eds. *Principles in bone biology.* New York: Academic Press, 1996:263–276.

64. Suki WN. Calcium transport in the nephron. *Am J Physiol* 1979;237:F1–F6.

65. Torikai S, Wang M-S, Klein KL, Kurokawa K. Adenylate cyclase and cell cyclic AMP of rat cortical thick ascending limb of Henle. *Kidney Int* 1981;20:649–654.

66. Morel F, Imbert-Teboul M, Charbardes D. Distribution of hormone-dependent adenylate cyclase in the nephron and its physiological significance. *Annu Rev Physiol* 1981;43:569–581.

67. Garabedian M, Holick MF, Deluca HF, Boyle IT. Control of 25-hydroxycholecalciferol metabolism by parathyroid glands. *Proc Natl Acad Sci USA* 1972;69:1673–1676.

68. Fraser DR, Kodicek E. Regulation of 25-hydroxycholecalciferol-1-hydroxylase activity in kidney by parathyroid hormone. *Nature* 1973;241:163–166.

69. Fox J, Mathew MB. Heterogeneous response to PTH in aging rats: evidence for skeletal PTH resistance. *Am J Physiol* 1991;260:E933–E937.

70. Norman AW, Roth J, Orci L. The vitamin D endocrine system: steroid metabolisms, hormone receptors and biological response. *Endocr Rev* 1982;3:331–366.

71. Shigematsu T, Horiuchi N, Ogura Y. Human parathyroid hormone inhibits renal 24-hydroxylase activity of 25-hydroxyvitamin D_3 by a mechanism involving adenosine 3′,5′-monophosphate in rats. *Endocrinology* 1986;118:1583–1589.

72. Brenza HL, Kimmel-Jehan C, Jehan F, et al. Parathyroid hormone activation of the 25-hydroxyvitamin D_3-1α-hydroxylase gene promoter. *Proc Natl Acad Sci USA* 1998;95:1387–1391.

73. Levine MA, Aurbach GD. Pseudohypoparathyroidism. In: DeGroot LJ, ed. *Endocrinology.* Philadelphia: Saunders, 1989:1065–1079.

74. Schipani E, Weinstein LS, Bergwitz C, et al. Pseudohypoparathyroidism type Ib is not caused by mutations in the coding exons of the human parathyroid hormone (PTH)/PTH-related peptide receptor gene. *J Clin Endocrinol Metab* 1995;80:1611–1621.

75. Bettoun JD, Minagawa M, Kwan MY, et al. Cloning and characterization of the promoter regions of the human parathyroid hormone (PTH)/PTH-related peptide receptor gene: analysis of deoxyribonucleic acid from normal subjects and patients with pseudohypoparathyroidism type Ib. *J Clin Endocrinol Metab* 1997;82:1031–1040.

76. Jüppner H, Schipani E, Bastepe M, et al. The gene responsible for pseudohypoparathyroidism type Ib is paternally imprinted and maps in four unrelated kindreds to chromosome 20q13.3. *Proc Natl Acad Sci USA* 1998;95:11798–11803.

77. Schipani E, Langman CB, Parfitt AM, et al. Constitutively activated receptors for parathyroid hormone and parathyroid hormone-related peptide in Jansen's metaphyseal chondrodysplasia. *N Engl J Med* 1996;335:708–714.

78. Jobert AS, Zhang P, Couvineau A, et al. Absence of functional receptors parathyroid hormone and parathyroid hormone-related peptide in Blomstrand chondrodysplasia. *J Clin Invest* 1998;102:34–40.

79. Zhang P, Jobert AS, Couvineau A, Silve C. A homozygous inactivating mutation in the parathyroid hormone/parathyroid hormone-related peptide receptor causing Blomstrand chondrodysplasia. *J Clin Endocrinol Metab* 1998;83:3373–3376.

80. Karaplis AC, Bin He MT, Nguyen A, Young ID, Semeraro D, Ozawa H, Amizuka N. Inactivating mutation in the human parathyroid hormone receptor type I gene in Blomstrand chondrodysplasia. *Endocrinology* 1998;139:5255–5258.

14. Parathyroid Hormone-Related Protein

Gordon J. Strewler, M.D. and *Robert A. Nissenson, Ph.D.

*Department of Medicine, Harvard Medical School, Boston, Massachusetts and Boston Healthcare System, West Roxbury Campus Veterans Affairs Medical Center, West Roxbury, Massachusetts; and *Department of Medicine and Physiology, University of California, San Francisco, and Endocrine Research Unit, Veterans Affairs Medical Center, San Francisco, California*

The parathyroid hormone-related protein (PTHrP) is a second member of the parathyroid hormone (PTH) family. Originally discovered as the cause of hypercalcemia in malignancy (1), PTHrP has proven to act in many tissues to regulate both development and function, and its recognition has expanded our concept of the role of the PTH/PTHrP family beyond the horizons of calcium homeostasis, to include developmental and regulatory functions in a variety of tissues (2–4).

The characteristics of the clinical syndrome of humoral hypercalcemia are discussed in Chapter 34. As in primary hyperparathyroidism, hypercalcemia in malignancy is characterized by a decreased renal threshold for phosphate, leading to hypophosphatemia, and by increased urinary excretion of cyclic adenosine monophosphate (cAMP) (5). Yet PTH is suppressed in malignancy-associated hypercalcemia. The finding that PTH was suppressed in a syndrome that so resembled primary hyperparathyroidism biochemically suggested that a distinct molecule secreted by tumors could mimic PTH, and this led to the development of bioassay techniques to search for a PTH-like factor in tumors that produced hypercalcemia. These assays guided the isolation and ultimate identification of what proved to be a PTH-related protein (also called PTH-like protein). As predicted, the tumor-derived protein proved to be an able mimic of PTH, for reasons that became clear when its structure could be determined.

Human PTHrP is encoded by a single-copy gene located on chromosome 12 (3). The human PTHrP gene, with three promoters, nine exons, and complex patterns of alternative exon splicing, is much more complicated than the PTH gene. Yet it is clear from the protein structure and from similarities in gene organization that both arose from a common ancestral gene. The amino acid sequence of PTHrP is homologous with the sequence of PTH only at the amino terminus, where eight of the first 13 amino acids in PTH and PTHrP are identical (Fig. 1). This homologous domain, limited as it is, involves a crucial region of the molecule that is known to be required for activation of the shared PTH/PTHrP receptor, and thus explains the ability of PTHrP to mimic PTH as an inducer of bone resorption, renal phosphate wasting, and hypercalcemia in malignancy. Beyond this region, the sequences of PTH and PTHrP have little in common. Even in the primary receptor-binding domain (amino acids 18 to 34), PTH and PTHrP do not have recognizable primary sequence similarities, although the binding domain has a common α-helical secondary structure in both peptides. Compared with the 84-amino-acid peptide PTH, PTHrP is considerably longer, with three isoforms of 139, 141, and 173 amino acids, whose sequences are identical through amino acid 139 (3). These isoforms arise from alternative RNA splicing. Although the protein isoforms are expressed differentially in individual tissues and tumors, their relative importance in normal physiology and humoral hypercalcemia are unknown.

The isoforms of PTHrP are cleaved by prohormone convertases within cells that secrete them to produce a variety of secreted peptides (Fig. 2). These include an amino-terminal fragment that possesses the ability to bind to the classic PTH/PTHrP receptor and a midregion fragment that has biologic actions distinct from those of amino-terminal PTHrP [e.g., stimulation of placental calcium transport (see later)]. Carboxyl-terminal fragments also are predicted to be secretory fragments, and they can be detected in the blood. Carboxyl-terminal PTHrP peptides that induce calcium transients in hippocampal neurons (6) also appear to be capable of inhibiting bone resorption in some systems (7,8), and one peptide, PTHrP(107 to 139), has been named "osteostatin." Thus PTHrP is a polyhormone, the precursor of multiple biologically active peptides. In this regard, PTHrP resembles proopiomelanocortin, the pituitary precursor of adrenocorticotropic hormone (ACTH), melanocyte-stimulating hormone (MSH), β-lipotropin, and the endorphins and enkephalins.

Parathyroid hormone-related protein and PTH bind with equivalent affinities to a common receptor, the PTH/PTHrP receptor (9,10), and consequently they have very similar ranges of biologic activities. Both produce hypercalcemia, hypophosphatemia as a consequence of reduced renal reabsorption of phosphate, and accelerated production of 1,25-dihydroxyvitamin D by the kidney (2,9). However, each of the hormones also has its own receptors: in the case of PTH, the PTH-2 receptor does not recognize PTHrP. In the case of PTHrP, receptors in brain (11) and skin (12) recognize the amino-terminal domain of PTHrP exclusively. There must be additional PTHrP receptors to mediate the effects of midregion and carboxyl-terminal PTHrP peptides, but these have yet to be identified.

There is little doubt that PTHrP is the major cause of hypercalcemia in malignancy (1). Infusion of PTHrP can reproduce most aspects of the clinical syndrome of hypercal-

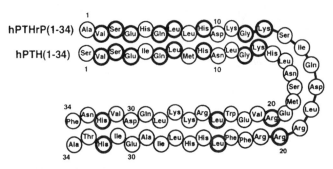

FIG. 1. Amino-terminal amino acid sequence of human parathyroid-hormone-related protein (hPTHrP) is compared with that of hPTH.

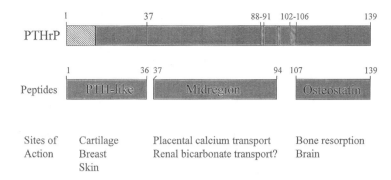

FIG. 2. Top: Structural features of parathyroid-hormone-related protein (PTHrP). The PTH-homologous domain PTHrP(1–13) is delineated by *slashed lines*, and potential cleavage sites are shown as *lines* or *cross-hatched regions*. **Middle:** Peptides known or postulated to be derived from PTHrP. **Bottom:** Proven or postulated sites of action of individual PTHrP peptides are shown beneath each peptide.

cemia, serum levels of PTHrP are increased in hypercalcemia (13) (see Chapter 34), and neutralizing antibodies to PTHrP can reverse hypercalcemia induced in animals by human tumor cells (14). This indicates that secretion of PTHrP is not merely associated with hypercalcemia but is necessary for its development. The specific tumors that characteristically produce humoral hypercalcemia by secreting PTHrP include squamous, renal, and breast carcinoma. Parathyroid hormone-related protein also plays a causative role in the hypercalcemia associated with islet cell tumors, pheochromocytoma, and the adult T-cell leukemia syndrome, where PTHrP is produced by malignant T lymphocytes infected with the etiologic agent of this disorder, the human T-cell lymphotrophic virus (15). It recently was suggested that PTHrP also has a role in some cases of multiple myeloma (16) and in sarcoidosis (17).

The normal circulating level of PTHrP is considerably lower than the level of PTH, and it is doubtful that PTHrP has a major role in the day-to-day maintenance of calcium homeostasis. It is clear, however, that PTHrP has vital functions in development and in normal physiology, primarily local ones at the cell or tissue level. Parathyroid hormone-related protein is widely present in fetal tissues, including cartilage, many epithelial surfaces, skeletal and heart muscle, distal renal tubules, hair follicles, brain, and placenta (18,19).

It was recently possible to disrupt both copies of the PTHrP gene in the mouse by targeted mutations introduced by homologous recombination (20). Although mice heterozygous for the loss of PTHrP have a subtle phenotype (21), in the homozygous state, loss of the PTHrP gene is an embryonic lethal mutation. Homozygotes survive until near the time of parturition but have multiple anomalies in the development of cartilage and bone. Their limbs are short and their rib cages are small, because of defective proliferation of chondrocytes during endochondral bone formation, as well as premature maturation and apoptosis of chondrocytes (20,22). In the regulation of endochondral bone formation, PTHrP is under the control of the secreted morphogen Indian hedgehog, one of a family of developmental patterning genes, the vertebrate orthologs of the *Drosophila* segmentation gene *Hedgehog* (23).

The PTHrP gene is widely expressed in developing and adult tissues, and it has a number of physiological functions. Genetic models to elucidate these functions are now available, as it has been possible to rescue PTHrP knockout mice from lethality by expressing either PTHrP or a constitutively active receptor in cartilage (24,25), allowing other phenotypes to be expressed. To date, these models have disclosed important roles of PTHrP in mammary gland, which is virtually absent in rescued PTHrP knockout mice, the teeth, which fail to erupt, and the skin and hair. In each case, PTHrP is a signaling molecule in epithelial–mesenchymal interactions, in which PTHrP is secreted by epithelial cells and signals for a mesenchymal response. (See Table 1.)

Secretion of PTHrP from the ingrowing epithelial sprouts in developing breast tissue permits branching morphogenesis

TABLE 1. *Sites of expression and proposed actions of PTHrP*

Sites of expression	Proposed actions
Mesenchymal tissues	
Cartilage	Promotes proliferation of chondrocytes; inhibits terminal differentiation and apoptosis of chondrocytes
Bone	Inhibits bone resorption
Smooth muscle	Released in response to stretch; relaxes smooth muscle
Vascular Myometrium Urinary bladder	
Cardiac muscle	Positive chronotropic stimulus; indirect positive inotropic stimulus
Skeletal muscle	Unknown
Epithelial tissues	
Mammary	Induces branching morphogenesis; secreted into milk; possible roles in lactation
Epidermis	Unknown
Hair follicle	Inhibits anagen
Intestine	Unknown
Tooth enamel	Induces osteoclastic resorption of overlying bone
Endocrine tissues	
Parathyroid	Stimulates placental calcium transport
Pancreatic islets	Stimulates insulin secretion and somatic growth
Pituitary	Unknown
Placenta	Unknown
Central nervous system	Released from cerebellar granular neurons in response to L-type calcium channels; receptors in cerebellum, hippocampus, hypothalamus

of mammary glands by activating receptors in the underlying mesenchyme (24). Presumably this interaction induces a mesenchymal signal that is sent back to the epithelium of the ducts to induce their proliferation. PTHrP appears to have additional roles to play in lactating mammary tissue. There, expression of PTHrP is under the control of prolactin (26), and PTHrP is secreted into milk at concentrations 10,000-fold higher than its serum concentration (27). It is not clear whether these findings reflect a role for PTHrP in lactation itself, in the neonate who ingests large quantities of PTHrP in milk, or in both.

The failure of tooth eruption in rescued PTHrP knockout mice can be attributed to another epithelial–mesenchymal interaction. The formation of the teeth appears normal, but PTHrP is absent from the enamel epithelium, which caps the tooth rudiment as it pushes its way through the overlying alveolar bone to erupt. Restoration of PTHrP expression to enamel epithelium restores tooth eruption (28). This implies that PTHrP secreted by the epithelial layer is targeted to receptors in the overlying bone, where it activates resorption of alveolar bone by osteoclasts to allow passage of the tooth. The signaling circuit in alveolar bone is distinctive, because there is no general defect in osteoclast function in transgenic mice to produce an osteopetrotic phenotype.

PTHrP is expressed in epidermal keratinocytes (the parental cells for squamous carcinomas in which secretion of PTHrP is the cause of hypercalcemia) and in the inner root sheath of the hair follicle. The PTH/PTHrP receptor is present in the underlying dermis. Treatment with a PTHrP antagonist enhances entry of hair follicles into anagen, the active phase of hair growth (29). Skin is excessively keratinized and the hair coat is shaggy in rescued knockout mice (personal communication, A. E. Broadus); conversely, alopecia occurs when PTHrP is overexpressed in the skin (30). This suggests that PTHrP secreted by epithelial cells may interact with mesenchymal receptors to regulate the differentiation of epidermis and the hair follicle, another example of epithelial–mesenchymal interactions in which PTHrP serves as the messenger.

It has long been known that to supply calcium to the mineralizing skeleton of the fetus, calcium is transported across the placenta by a placental pump, maintaining a serum calcium level that is higher in the fetus than in the mother. This maternal–fetal gradient is abolished in PTHrP knockout mice (31), indicating that PTHrP is the principal regulator of placental calcium transport. Placental transport of calcium in the sheep is sharply reduced after parathyroidectomy (32), suggesting that the source of PTHrP is, at least in part, the fetal parathyroid glands. The transport of calcium can be restored by infusion of midregional fragments or PTHrP, but not by amino-terminal PTHrP or by PTH (33,34). Thus for the regulation of systemic calcium economy, the fetus uses a midregion peptide from PTHrP, perhaps secreted from the parathyroid gland, in much the same way that PTH is used in the postnatal state.

PTHrP is secreted by a variety of smooth-muscle beds (35), where it is released in response to stretch (36,37), and it acts as a smooth-muscle dilator by binding to the PTH/PTHrP receptor (38). This sets up the circuitry for a short-loop feedback system in which PTHrP would respond to stretch by relaxing smooth muscle locally. This circuitry could be operative in uterine smooth muscle at the time of parturition (37), in the urinary bladder (36), and in arterial hypertension (39). In the heart, PTHrP is released by atrial and ventricular myocytes (40) and has a positive chronotropic effect, as well as a positive inotropic effect that probably results from coronary vasodilation (41,42). PTHrP also is released from stromal cells of the spleen and other organs in response to endotoxic shock (43), and neutralization of PTHrP effects with antibodies prolongs survival after administration of lethal doses of endotoxin (44). In the arterial wall, PTHrP is expressed in proliferating vascular smooth-muscle cells in culture and after balloon angioplasty *in vivo* (45). The level of PTHrP is increased in atherosclerotic coronary arteries (46). Exposure of rat vascular smooth-muscle cells to PTHrP has an antimitotic effect, suggesting that locally released PTHrP would act to throttle the response to a proliferative stimulus (47). In contrast, when transfected into A10 rat vascular smooth-muscle cells, PTHrP markedly induces proliferation (48). The proliferative response does not occur with transfection of mutant forms of PTHrP from which polybasic amino acid sequences between residues 88 and 106 have been deleted. These sequences have been shown to function as a nuclear-localization sequence in other cells (49), and wild-type PTHrP, but not the deletion mutants, is targeted to the nucleus of A10 cells. It thus appears possible that in addition to binding to cell-surface receptors, PTHrP can have direct nuclear actions, termed *intracrine* actions. Because secreted fragments of PTHrP and its intracrine actions appear to have opposing effects on proliferation, PTHrP could interplay in a complex fashion with other proliferative factors in determining the response of the vascular wall to injury or atherosclerosis.

REFERENCES

1. Wysolmerski JJ, Broadus AE. Hypercalcemia of malignancy: the central role of parathyroid hormone-related protein. *Annu Rev Med* 1994;45:189–200.
2. Halloran BP, Nissenson RA. *Parathyroid hormone-related protein: normal physiology and its role in cancer.* Boca Raton: CRC Press, 1992.
3. Broadus A, Stewart A. Parathyroid hormone-related protein: structure, processing, and physiological actions. In: Bilezikian J, Levine M, Marcus R, eds. *The parathyroids.* New York: Raven Press, 1994:259–339.
4. Wysolmerski JJ, Stewart AF. The physiology of parathyroid hormone-related protein: an emerging role as a developmental factor. *Annu Rev Physiol* 1998;60:431–460.
5. Stewart AF, Horst R, Deftos LJ, Cadman EC, Lang R, Broadus AE. Biochemical evaluation of patients with cancer-associated hypercalcemia. *N Engl J Med* 1980;303:1377–1383.
6. Fukayama S, Tashjian AH Jr, Davis JN, Chisholm JC. Signaling by N- and C-terminal sequences of parathyroid hormone-related protein in hippocampal neurons. *Proc Natl Acad Sci USA* 1995;92:10182–10186.
7. Fenton AJ, Kemp BE, Kent GN, et al. A carboxyl-terminal peptide from the parathyroid hormone-related protein inhibits bone resorption by osteoclasts. *Endocrinology* 1991;129:1762–1768.
8. Cornish J, Callon KE, Nicholson GC, Reid IR. Parathyroid hormone-related protein(107-139) inhibits bone resorption in vivo. *Endocrinology* 1997;138:1299–1304.
9. Orloff JJ, Wu TL, Stewart AF. Parathyroid hormone-like proteins: biochemical responses and receptor interactions. *Endocr Rev* 1989;10:476–495.
10. Orloff JJ, Reddy D, de Papp AE, Yang KH, Soifer NE, Stewart AF. Parathyroid hormone-related protein as a prohormone: posttranslational processing and receptor interactions. *Endocr Rev* 1994;15:40–60.
11. Yamamoto S, Morimoto I, Yanagihara N, et al. Parathyroid hormone-related peptide-(1-34) [PTHrP-(1-34)] induces vasopressin release from

the rat supraoptic nucleus in vitro through a novel receptor distinct from a type I or type II PTH/PTHrP receptor. *Endocrinology* 1997; 138:2066–2072.

12. Orloff JJ, Ganz MB, Ribaudo AE, Burtis WJ, Reiss M, Milstone LMS. Analysis of PTHrP binding and signal transduction mechanisms in benign and malignant squamous cells. *Am J Physiol* 1992;262:E599–E607.

13. Burtis WJ, Brady TG, Orloff JJ, et al. Immunochemical characterization of circulating parathyroid hormone-related protein in patients with humoral hypercalcemia of cancer. *N Engl J Med* 1990;322:1106–1112.

14. Kukreja SC, Shevrin DH, Wimbiscus SA, et al. Antibodies to parathyroid hormone-related protein lower serum calcium in athymic mouse models. *J Clin Invest* 1988;82:1798–1802.

15. Ikeda K, Ohno H, Hane M, et al. Development of a sensitive two-site immunoradiometric assay for parathyroid hormone-related peptide: evidence for elevated levels in plasma from patients with adult T-cell leukemia/lymphoma and B-cell lymphoma. *J Clin Endocrinol Metab* 1994;79:1322–1327.

16. Firkin F, Seymour JF, Watson AM, Grill V, Martin TJ. Parathyroid hormone-related protein in hypercalcaemia associated with haematological malignancy. *Br J Haematol* 1996;94:486–492.

17. Zeimer HJ, Greenaway TM, Slavin J, et al. Parathyroid hormone-related protein in sarcoidosis. *Am J Pathol* 1998;152:1721.

18. Moseley JM, Hayman JA, Danks JA, et al. Immunohistochemical detection of parathyroid hormone-related protein in human fetal epithelia. *J Clin Endocrinol Metab* 1991;73:478–484.

19. Ferguson JE II, Gorman JV, Bruns DE, et al. Abundant expression of parathyroid hormone-related protein in human amnion and its association with labor. *Proc Natl Acad Sci USA* 1992;89:8384–8388.

20. Karaplis AC, Luz A, Glowacki J, et al. Lethal skeletal dysplasia from targeted disruption of the parathyroid hormone-related peptide gene. *Genes Dev* 1994;8:277–289.

21. Amizuka N, Karaplis AC, Henderson JE, et al. Haploinsufficiency of parathyroid hormone-related peptide (PTHrP) results in abnormal postnatal bone development. *Dev Biol* 1996;175:166–176.

22. Amling M, Neff L, Tanaka S, et al. BCL2 lies downstream of parathyroid hormone-related peptide in a signaling pathway that regulates chondrocyte maturation during skeletal development. *J Cell Biol* 1997;136:205–213.

23. Vortkamp A, Lee K, Lanske B, Segre GV, Kronenberg HM, Tabin CJ. Regulation of rate of cartilage differentiation by Indian hedgehog and PTH-related protein [Comments]. *Science* 1996;273:613–622.

24. Wysolmerski JJ, Philbrick WM, Dunbar ME, et al. Rescue of the parathyroid hormone-related protein knockout mouse demonstrates that parathyroid hormone-related protein is essential for mammary gland development. *Development* 1998;125:1285–1294.

25. Schipani E, Lanske B, Hunzelman J, et al. Targeted expression of constitutively active receptors for parathyroid hormone and parathyroid hormone-related peptide delays endochondral bone formation and rescues mice that lack parathyroid hormone-related peptide. *Proc Natl Acad Sci USA* 1997;94:13689–13694.

26. Thiede MA, Rodan GA. Expression of a calcium-mobilizing parathyroid hormone-like peptide in lactating mammary tissue. *Science* 1998;242:278–280.

27. Budayr AA, Halloran BP, King JC, Diep D, Nissenson RA, Strewler GJ. High levels of a parathyroid hormone-like protein in milk. *Proc Natl Acad Sci USA* 1989;86:7183–7185.

28. Philbrick WM, Dreyer BE, Nakchbandi IA, Karaplis AC. Parathyroid hormone-related protein is required for tooth eruption. *Proc Natl Acad Sci USA* 1998;95:11846–11851.

29. Holick MF, Ray S, Chen TC, Tian X, Persons KS. A parathyroid hormone antagonist stimulates epidermal proliferation and hair growth in mice. *Proc Natl Acad Sci USA* 1994;91:8014–8016.

30. Wysolmerski JJ, Mccaugherncarucci JF, Daifotis AG, Broadus AE, Philbrick WM. Overexpression of parathyroid hormone-related protein or parathyroid hormone in transgenic mice impairs branching morphogenesis during mammary gland development. *Development* 1995; 121:3539–3547.

31. Kovacs CS, Lanske B, Hunzelman JL, Guo J, Karaplis AC, Kronenberg HM. Parathyroid hormone-related peptide (PTHrP) regulates fetal-placental calcium transport through a receptor distinct from the PTH/PTHrP receptor. *Proc Natl Acad Sci USA* 1996;93:15233–15238.

32. Care AD, Caple IW, Abbas SK, Pickard DW. The effect of fetal thyroparathyroidectomy on the transport of calcium across the ovine placenta to the fetus. *Placenta* 1986;7:417–424.

33. Abbas SK, Pickard DW, Rodda CP, et al. Stimulation of ovine placental calcium transport by purified natural and recombinant parathyroid hormone-related protein (PTHrP) preparations. *Q J Exp Physiol* 1989; 74:549–552.

34. Care AD, Abbas SK, Pickard DW, et al. Stimulation of ovine placental transport of calcium and magnesium by midmolecule fragments of human parathyroid hormone-related protein. *Exp Physiol* 1990; 75: 605–608.

35. Massfelder T, Helwig JJ, Stewart AF. Parathyroid hormone-related protein as a cardiovascular regulatory peptide. *Endocrinology* 1996; 137:3151–3153.

36. Yamamoto M, Harm SC, Grasser WA, Thiede MA. Parathyroid hormone-related protein in the rat urinary bladder: a smooth muscle relaxant produced locally in response to mechanical stretch. *Proc Natl Acad Sci USA* 1992;89:5326–5330.

37. Thiede MA, Daifotis AG, Weir EC, et al. Intrauterine occupancy controls expression of the parathyroid hormone-related peptide gene in preterm rat myometrium. *Proc Natl Acad Sci USA* 1990;87:6969–6973.

38. Nickols GA, Nana AD, Nickols MA, DiPette DJ, Asimakis GK. Hypotension and cardiac stimulation due to the parathyroid hormone-related protein, humoral hypercalcemia of malignancy factor. *Endocrinology* 1989;125:834–841.

39. Takahashi K, Inoue D, Ando K, Matsumoto T, Ikeda K, Fujita T. Parathyroid hormone-related peptide as a locally produced vasorelaxant regulation of its mRNA by hypertension in rats. *Biochem Biophys Res Commun* 1995;208:447–455.

40. Deftos LJ, Burton DW, Brandt DW. Parathyroid hormone-like protein is a secretory product of atrial myocytes. *J Clin Invest* 1993;92: 727–735.

41. Ogino K, Burkhoff D, Bilezikian JP. The hemodynamic basis for the cardiac effects of parathyroid hormone (PTH) and PTH-related protein. *Endocrinology* 1995;136:3024–3030.

42. Hara M, Liu YM, Zhen LC, et al. Positive chronotropic actions of parathyroid hormone and parathyroid hormone-related peptide are associated with increases in the current, IF, and the slope of the pacemaker potential. *Circulation* 1997;96:3704–3709.

43. Funk JL, Krul EJ, Moser AH, et al. Endotoxin increases parathyroid hormone-related protein mRNA levels in mouse spleen: mediation by tumor necrosis factor. *J Clin Invest* 1993;92:2546–2552.

44. Funk JL, Moser AH, Strewler GJ, Feingold KR, Grunfeld C. Parathyroid hormone-related protein is induced during lethal endotoxemia and contributes to endotoxin-induced mortality in rodents. *Mol Med* 1996;2:204–210.

45. Ozeki S, Ohtsuru A, Seto S, et al. Evidence that implicates the parathyroid hormone-related peptide in vascular stenosis increased gene expression in the intima of injured rat carotid arteries and human restenotic coronary lesions. *Arterioscler Thromb Vasc Biol* 1996;16:565–575.

46. Nakayama T, Ohtsuru A, Enomoto H, et al. Coronary atherosclerotic smooth muscle cells overexpress human parathyroid hormone-related peptides. *Biochem Biophys Res Commun* 1994;200:1028–1035.

47. Pirola CJ, Wang HM, Kamyar A, et al. Angiotensin II regulates parathyroid hormone-related protein expression in cultured rat aortic smooth muscle cells through transcriptional and posttranscriptional mechanisms. *J Biol Chem* 1993;268:1987–1994.

48. Massfelder T, Dann P, Wu TL, Vasavada R, Helwig JJ, Stewart AF. Opposing mitogenic and antimitogenic actions of parathyroid hormone-related protein in vascular smooth muscle cells: a critical role for nuclear targeting. *Proc Natl Acad Sci USA* 1997;94:13630–13635.

49. Henderson JE, Amizuka N, Warshawsky H, et al. Nucleolar localization of parathyroid hormone-related peptide enhances survival of chondrocytes under conditions that promote apoptotic cell death. *Mol Cell Biol* 1995;15:4064–4075.

15. Vitamin D: Photobiology, Metabolism, Mechanism of Action, and Clinical Applications

Michael F. Holick, Ph.D., M.D.

Department of Medicine and Section of Endocrinology, Nutrition, and Diabetes, Boston University Medical Center, Boston, Massachusetts

Vitamin D is a secosteroid that is made in the skin by the action of sunlight (1). Vitamin D is biologically inert and must undergo two successive hydroxylations in the liver and kidney to become the biologically active 1,25-dihydroxyvitamin D [1,25 $(OH)_2$ D] (1–3). The main biologic effect of 1,25 $(OH)_2$ D is to maintain the serum calcium level within the normal range. This is accomplished by increasing the efficiency of intestinal absorption of dietary calcium and by recruiting stem cells in the bone to become mature osteoclasts, which in turn mobilize calcium stores from the bone into the circulation. The renal production of 1,25 $(OH)_2$ D is tightly regulated by serum calcium levels through the action of parathyroid hormone (PTH) and phosphorus. A wide variety of inborn and acquired disorders in the metabolism of vitamin D can lead to both hypo- and hypercalcemic conditions. Recently it was appreciated that 1,25 $(OH)_2$ D not only regulates calcium metabolism but also is capable of inhibiting the proliferation and inducing terminal differentiation of a variety of cells not associated with calcium metabolism (1). This unique property of 1,25 $(OH)_2$ D was effectively used to develop a new generation of active vitamin D compounds for the treatment of the hyperproliferative skin disease, psoriasis.

PHOTOBIOLOGY OF VITAMIN D_3

The skin is the organ responsible for the production of vitamin D_3. During exposure to sunlight, 7-dehydrocholesterol (7-DHC, provitamin D_3), the immediate precursor of cholesterol, absorbs solar radiation with energies between 290 and 315 nm [ultraviolet B (UVB)], which, in turn, causes the transformation of 7-DHC to previtamin D_3 (Fig. 1) (4). Once formed, previtamin D_3 undergoes a thermally induced isomerization over a period of a few hours and is transformed into vitamin D_3. Vitamin D_3 is translocated from the skin into the circulation, where it is bound to the vitamin D–binding protein (4).

There are no documented cases of vitamin intoxication resulting from excessive exposure to sunlight. The likely reason for this is that once previtamin D_3 is formed, it absorbs solar UVB radiation and is transformed into biologically inert photoproducts, lumisterol and tachysterol. Furthermore, vitamin D_3 that is made in the skin is exquisitely sensitive to sunlight and is photoisomerized to suprasterol 1, suprasterol 2, and 5,6-*trans*-vitamin D_3 (4).

A variety of factors can alter the cutaneous production of vitamin D_3. Melanin is an excellent natural sunscreen and competes with 7-DHC for UVB photons. Therefore, increased skin melanin pigmentation decreases the photosynthesis of vitamin D_3 (1). People with darker skin color require longer exposure to sunlight to make the same amount of vitamin D_3 as those with lighter skin color (4). Aging signifi-

cantly diminishes the concentration of unesterified 7-DHC in the epidermis. This results in a marked reduction in the production of vitamin D_3. Compared with a young adult, a person older than 70 years produces <30% of the amount of vitamin D_3 when exposed to the same amount of simulated sunlight (Fig. 2) (5). Latitude, time of day, and season of the year can dramatically affect the production of vitamin D_3 in the skin. At a latitude of 42°N (Boston), sunlight is incapable of producing vitamin D_3 in the skin between the months of November and February. At 52°N (Edmonton, Canada), this period is extended to include the months of

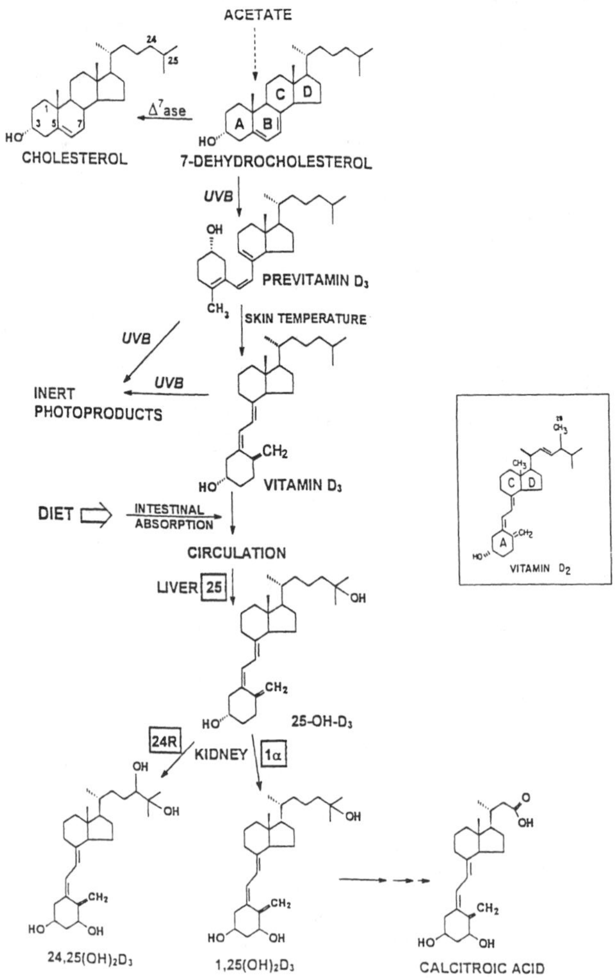

FIG. 1. The photochemical, thermal, and metabolic pathways for vitamin D_3. Boxed letters and numbers denote specific enzymes: D7ase, 7-dehydrocholesterol reductase; 25, vitamin D-25-hydroxylase; 1α, 25 (OH) D-1α-hydroxylase; 24R, 25 (OH) D-24R-hydroxylase. **Inset:** the structure of vitamin D_2.

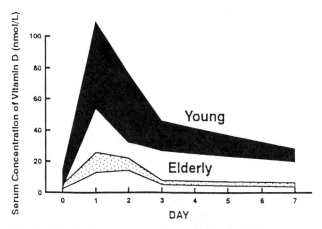

FIG. 2. Circulating concentrations of vitamin D in response to a whole-body exposure to one minimal erythemal dose in healthy young and elderly subjects. (Adapted from Holick MF, Matsuoka LY, Wortsman J. Age, vitamin D, and solar ultraviolet radiation. *Lancet* 1989;4:1104–1105.)

October through March (4). Casual exposure to sunlight provides most of our vitamin D requirement. For children and young adults, the cutaneous production of vitamin D_3 during the spring, summer, and fall is adequate to produce enough that can be stored in the fat for use during the winter months. However, because the elderly may not make enough vitamin D_3 and therefore would have insufficient stores for winter use, the inability of the sun to produce vitamin D_3 in northern and southern latitudes during the winter may require them to take a vitamin D supplement to prevent vitamin D deficiency. Exposure to sunlight at lower latitudes, such as Los Angeles, (24°N), Puerto Rico (18°N), and Buenos Aires (34°S), results in the cutaneous production of vitamin D_3 during the entire year (4). During the summer months in Boston, exposure to sunlight from the hours of 700 to 1700 Eastern Daylight Savings Time (EDT) contains sufficient UVB radiation to produce vitamin D_3 in the skin. In the spring and fall months, vitamin D_3 production commences at ~900 and ceases after 1500 EDT. The topical use of a sunscreen with a sun-protection factor of 8 will substantially reduce, by >95%, the cutaneous production of vitamin D_3 (4). Prolonged use of sunscreens can result in vitamin D insufficiency (4). Although sunscreen use is extremely valuable for the prevention of skin cancer and the damaging effects of excessive exposure to the sun, the elderly who depend on sunlight for their vitamin D_3 should consider exposure to suberythemal amounts of sunlight before topically applying a sunscreen. Thus they can take advantage of the beneficial effect of sunlight while preventing the damaging effects of prolonged excessive exposure to sunlight.

FOOD SOURCES OF VITAMIN D AND THE RDA

Vitamin D (either vitamin D_2 or vitamin D_3) is rare in foods. The major natural sources of vitamin D are fatty fish, such as salmon and mackerel, and fatty fish oils, including cod liver oil. Vitamin D also can be obtained from foods

fortified with vitamin D, including some cereals, bread products, and milk. Other dairy products, including ice cream, yogurt, and cheese, are not fortified with vitamin D. A recent survey of the vitamin D content in milk throughout the United States and Canada, however, revealed that approximately 80% of the samples did not contain between 400 (10 μg) and 600 IU/qt (6). Almost 50% of the milk samples did not contain within 50% of the amount of vitamin D stated on the label, and approximately 15% of skim milk samples contained no detectable vitamin D. Multivitamin preparations containing vitamin D were found to contain between 400 and 600 IU of vitamin D, and pharmaceutical preparations labeled as 50,000 IU of vitamin D_2 contained the stated amount $\pm10\%$. The Institute of Medicine in 1997 recommended adequate intake (AI) for vitamin D for infants (birth to 6 months), children older than 6 months, and adults up to the age of 50 years is 200 IU (5 μg)/day. For adults 51 to 70 years and 71 years and older, the new recommended AIs are 400 IU (10 μg)/day and 600 IU (15 μg)/day, respectively. For pregnant and lactating women of all ages, the AI is 200 IU. In the absence of sunlight, the AI for vitamin D for all age groups should be increased by 200 IU (4,7,8). The tolerable upper intake was recommended to be 1000 IU for 0 to 12 months and 2000 IU for ages older than 1 year.

METABOLISM OF VITAMIN D

Vitamin D_2, which comes from yeasts and plants, and vitamin D_3, which is found in the fatty fish and cod liver oil and is made in the skin, have the same biologic potency in humans. The only difference between vitamin D_2 and vitamin D_3 is that vitamin D_2 contains a double bond between C_{22} and C_{23}, and a methyl group on C_{24} (Fig. 1) (1). Once either vitamin D_2 or vitamin D_3 enters the circulation, it is bound to the vitamin D–binding protein and transported to the liver, where the cytochrome P_{450}–vitamin D–25-hydroxylase introduces an OH on carbon 25 to produce 25-hydroxyvitamin D [25 (OH) D; Fig. 1] (1–4). 25 (OH) D enters the circulation and is the major circulating form of vitamin D. Because the hepatic vitamin D–25-hydroxylase is not tightly regulated, an increase in the cutaneous production of vitamin D_3 or ingestion of vitamin D will result in an increase in circulating levels of 25 (OH) D (1,3). Therefore its measurement is used to determine whether a patient is vitamin D deficient, vitamin D sufficient, or vitamin D intoxicated (1). 25 (OH) D is biologically inert. It is transported to the kidney, where the cytochrome P_{450}-monooxygenase, 25 (OH) D–1α-hydroxylase, metabolizes 25 (OH) D to 1,25-dihydroxyvitamin D [1,25 (OH)$_2$ D; Fig. 3] (1–3). Although the kidney is the major source of the circulating 1,25 (OH)$_2$ D, there is strong evidence that a wide variety of cells, including monocytes and skin cells, express 25 (OH) D 1α-hydroxylase, have the ability to produce 1,25 (OH)$_2$ D (1,9). In addition, during pregnancy, the placenta produces 1,25 (OH)$_2$ D (1,10). However, because anephric patients have very low or undetectable levels of 1,25 (OH)$_2$ D in their blood, the extrarenal sites of 1,25 (OH)$_2$ D production do not appear to play a role in calcium homeostasis. The local production of 1,25 (OH)$_2$ D in tissues not associated with calcium homeostasis may be for the purpose of

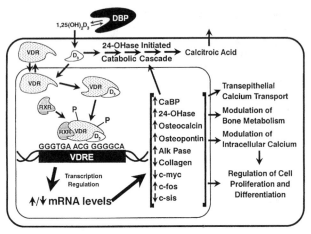

FIG. 3. Proposed mechanism of action of 1,25 (OH)₂ D₃ in target cells, resulting in a variety of biologic responses. The free form of 1,25 (OH)₂ D₃ (D3) enters the target cell and interacts with its nuclear vitamin D receptor (VDR), which is phosphorylated (P). The 1,25 (OH)₂ D₃–VDR complex combines with the retinoic acid X receptor (RXR) to form a hetero-dimer, which, in turn, interacts with the vitamin D–responsive element (VDRE), causing an enhancement or inhibition of transcription of vitamin D–responsive genes such as the 25 (OH) D-24-hydroxylase (24-OHase).

regulating cell growth (1,2,9,11). When serum ionized calcium declines, there is an increase in the production and secretion of PTH, which has a variety of biologic functions on calcium metabolism (see Chapters 8, 9, and 11). It also regulates calcium homeostasis by enhancing the renal conversion of 25 (OH) D to 1,25 (OH)₂ D (Fig. 1) (1–3). It does this indirectly through its renal wasting of phosphorus, resulting in decreased intracellular and blood levels of phosphorus. 1,25 (OH)₂ D strongly regulates its own renal synthesis directly by its negative feedback regulation on the 25 (OH) D 1α-ase and indirectly by its inhibition of the expression of the PTH gene. Hypophosphatemia and hyperphosphatemia are associated with increased and decreased circulating concentrations of 1,25 (OH)₂ D, respectively (12). A variety of other hormones associated with growth and development of the skeleton or calcium regulation, including growth hormone and prolactin, indirectly increase the renal production of 1,25 (OH)₂ D (1). Aged osteoporotic patients may lose their ability to upregulate the renal production of 1,25 (OH)₂ D by PTH (13,14). This may help explain the age-related decrease in the efficiency of intestinal calcium absorption (13,14). 1,25 (OH)₂ D is metabolized in its target tissues (the intestine and bone) as well as in the liver and kidney (1–3). It undergoes several hydroxylations in the sidechain, resulting in the cleavage of the sidechain between carbons 23 and 24, resulting in the biologically inert, water-soluble acid, calcitroic acid (Fig. 1) (1,2). Both 25 (OH) D and 1,25 (OH)₂ D undergo a 24-hydroxylation to form 24,25-dihydroxyvitamin D [24,25 (OH)₂ D] and 1,24,25 trihydroxyvitamin D, respectively. These metabolites are considered to be biologically inert and are the first step in the biodegradation. Although >40 different metabolites of vitamin D have been identified, only 1,25 (OH)₂ D is believed to be important for most if not all of the biologic actions of

vitamin D on calcium and bone metabolism (1,3). There continue to be intriguing data to suggest that 24,25 (OH)₂ D may have some role in bone formation and on the fracture-healing process (15).

MOLECULAR BIOLOGY OF VITAMIN D

Once vitamin D is dihydroxylated, it becomes more hydrophilic. However, this hormone is still very lipid soluble, and therefore it acts like a steroid hormone. The mechanism of action of this hormone is similar to that of estrogen and other steroids. All target tissues for vitamin D contain a nuclear vitamin D receptor (VDR) for 1,25 (OH)₂ D. This vitamin D receptor has a 1000-fold higher affinity for 1,25 (OH)₂ D, compared with 25 (OH) D and other dihydroxylated metabolites of vitamin D (1,3). Analogous to other steroid hormones, the free 1,25 (OH)₂ D in the circulation enters its target cell, where it is recognized by its nuclear receptor (Fig. 3). The exact sequence by which 1,25 (OH)₂ D interacts with its receptor and causes activation of transcription of specific genes whose products are involved in the stimulation of biologic responses to vitamin D has not been completely clarified (Fig. 3). However, it is known that the VDR must complex with a retinoic acid X receptor (RXR) to form a heterodimeric complex with 1,25 (OH)₂ D₃ (15). Once formed, this heterodimer complex interacts with a specific vitamin D–responsive element within the DNA. The DNA-binding motif for VDR, which is present in the N-terminus part of the molecule containing the zinc fingers (Fig. 4), interacts with the vitamin D–responsive element (VDRE), which is composed of two tandemly repeated hexanucleotide sequences separated by three base pairs (Fig. 3). This interaction leads to the transcription of the gene and the synthesis of new messenger RNAs (mRNAs) for a variety of proteins (1) (Fig. 3). The best-characterized proteins identified from osteoblasts are osteocalcin, osteopontin, and alkaline phos-

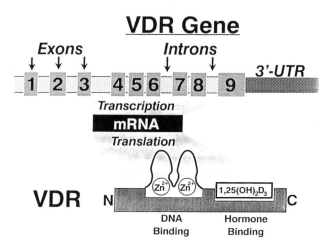

FIG. 4. Structure of the vitamin D–receptor (VDR) gene showing the nine exons and intervening introns and the 3'-untranslated region (3'-UTR). The nine exons are transcribed into the VDR messenger RNA, which, in turn, is translated into the VDR that contains a DNA- and a hormone-binding domain.

phatase, and, from the intestine, calcium-binding protein (CaBP) (1,3,16,17). The VDR gene has nine exons that give rise to the VDR, which contains a DNA-binding domain in the N-terminal region and a hormone-binding domain in the C-terminal region (Fig. 4). Specific exon mutations have been identified that cause resistance to 1,25 (OH)₂ D, causing vitamin D–dependent rickets type II (18). There are also mutations in the exons and introns that can lead to polymorphisms of the VDR gene that do not cause any alteration in the amino acid composition of the VDR. These polymorphisms are thought to be important in the transcription of the VDR gene or stabilization of the resultant VDR mRNA or both (19). There is some evidence that these polymorphisms may lead to a differential responsiveness to 1,25 (OH)₂ D₃ in the intestine and bone, thereby playing a role in peak bone mass and the development of osteoporosis (19). Although several studies supported the concept that homozygotes for bb, TT VDR genotypes have a higher bone mineral density at various sites, other studies have not found the association (20).

BIOLOGIC FUNCTION OF VITAMIN D IN THE INTESTINE

The major biologic function of vitamin D is to maintain calcium homeostasis by increasing the efficiency of the small intestine to absorb dietary calcium (1–3). Specific nuclear receptors for 1,25 (OH)₂ D (VDR) are found in nuclei throughout the small intestine, with the highest concentration in the duodenum. 1,25 (OH)₂ D directly affects the entry of calcium through the plasma membrane into the intestinal absorptive cell, enhances the movement of calcium through the cytoplasm, and transfers the calcium across the basilateral membrane into the circulation (1–3,16,17). Although the exact mechanism by which 1,25 (OH)₂ D alters the flux of calcium across the intestinal absorptive cell is not known, 1,25 (OH)₂ D increases the production and activity of several proteins in the small intestine, including the CaBP, alkaline phosphatase, low-affinity Ca adenosine triphosphatase (ATPase), brush-border actin, calmodulin, and brush-border proteins of 80 to 90 kDa (1–3,16,17). CaBP is specifically induced by 1,25 (OH)₂ D and is thought to be one of the major proteins responsible for the alteration in the flux of calcium across the gastrointestinal mucosa. When 1,25 (OH)₂ D is given as a single intravenous dose to vitamin D–deficient animals, it causes a biphasic response. A rapid response occurs within 2 hours and peaks by 6 hours, and another begins after 12 hours and peaks at 24 hours, implying that several mechanisms may be involved in intestinal calcium absorption (1,2,16,17). 1,25 (OH)₂ D₃ also increases the efficiency of the small intestine to absorb dietary phosphorus. Although both calcium and phosphorus absorption occur along the entire length of the small intestine, most of the phosphorus-transport activity is located in the jejunum and ileum, whereas calcium absorption occurs principally in the duodenum (1,2).

PHYSIOLOGIC ACTIONS OF 1,25 (OH)₂ D ON BONE

The major biologic function of vitamin D on bone is to enhance the mobilization of calcium stores at a time when dietary calcium is inadequate to maintain blood calcium in the normal range. 1,25 (OH)₂ D accomplishes this by inducing monocytic stem cells in the bone marrow to differentiate into osteoclasts (1). Once the osteoclasts have matured, they lose their ability to recognize 1,25 (OH)₂ D (21). Osteoclastic activity appears to be regulated indirectly by 1,25 (OH)₂ D₃ through its action on osteoblasts, which produce a variety of osteoclast-sensitive cytokines and hormones. Mature osteoblasts in the bone possess nuclear receptors for 1,25 (OH)₂ D. 1,25 (OH)₂ D increases the expression of alkaline phosphatase, osteopontin, and osteocalcin, as well as a variety of cytokines in these cells (1). Although vitamin D has long been recognized as important for bone mineralization, there is little direct evidence that 1,25 (OH)₂ D actively participates in this process (1,2). Instead, 1,25 (OH)₂ D promotes the mineralization of osteoid laid down by osteoblasts, by maintaining the extracellular calcium and phosphorus concentrations within the normal range, which results in the deposition of calcium hydroxyapatite into the bone matrix (1,2).

BIOLOGIC FUNCTION OF 1,25 (OH)₂ D ON THE KIDNEY

The kidney, which produces 1,25 (OH)₂ D, is responsible for maintaining circulating concentrations of 1,25 (OH)₂ D for calcium homeostasis. The renal tubular cells have a VDR. It remains controversial whether 1,25 (OH)₂ D alters tubular reabsorption or excretion of calcium and phosphorus. It is well documented, however, that 1,25 (OH)₂ D, through its receptor, induces the metabolic cascade for catabolizing the hormone to the water-soluble inactive calcitroic acid (Fig. 1). 1,25 (OH)₂ D, through its receptor, also strongly negatively regulates by feedback the production of 1,25 (OH)₂ D.

BIOLOGIC FUNCTION OF 1,25 (OH)₂ D₃ IN NONCALCEMIC TISSUES

A wide variety of tissues and cells possess nuclear receptors for 1,25 (OH)₂ D (1–3,9,11). Tumor cells that possess a VDR, when exposed to 1,25 (OH)₂ D, decrease their proliferative activity and also may terminally differentiate (22). For example, cells from the promyelocytic leukemic cell line HL-60, when exposed to physiologic amounts of 1,25 (OH)₂ D₃, are induced to become biochemically functioning macrophages (1,23). Of great interest is that, whereas resting T and B lymphocytes do not possess VDR, when the cells are activated, they express a VDR and become responsive to 1,25 (OH)₂ D (24). Activated T lymphocytes respond to 1,25 (OH)₂ D₃ by decreasing the production of interleukin-2. 1,25 (OH)₂ D₃ also was reported to inhibit DNA synthesis and immunoglobulin production in stimulated B lymphocytes (1). Peripheral mononuclear cells have a VDR, and, when exposed to 1,25 (OH)₂ D in vitro, they are induced to become macrophages. Epidermal skin cells also possess a VDR (1,4,9,11). 1,25 (OH)₂ D₃ inhibits the proliferation of cultured human keratinocytes and induces them to differentiate terminally (1,4,9). The clinical use of 1,25 (OH)₂ D₃ for treating hyperproliferative diseases such as breast cancer and leukemia does not yet appear to be promising because of recurrence of disease and complications resulting from hypercalcemic activity of the vitamin D compounds (11,25). Several noncalcemic 1,25 (OH)$_2$ D analogues are being investigated as a new therapeutic approach for treating several cancers including breast, prostate, and colon cancer. The potent antiproliferative activity of 1,25 (OH)$_2$ D$_3$ and its analogue calcipotriene (Dovonex), with its attendant prodifferentiating properties, has been effectively used for the treatment of the nonmalignant hyperproliferative skin disorder psoriasis (4,26,27).

REGULATION OF PARATHYROID HORMONE SECRETION BY 1,25 (OH)$_2$ D$_3$

Parathyroid hormone is the principal regulator for the renal production of 1,25 (OH)$_2$ D (1,2). 1,25 (OH)$_2$ D, in turn, increases serum calcium levels through its action on the intestine and bone, which results in the decrease in synthesis and production of PTH. In addition to its action of increasing serum ionized calcium concentrations, 1,25 (OH)$_2$ D$_3$ is recognized by the VDR that is present in chief cells in the parathyroid glands. 1,25 (OH)$_2$ D$_3$ decreases the expression of the PTH gene, thereby decreasing the production and secretion of PTH (28). Patients with long-standing secondary and tertiary hyperparathyroidism can develop nests of PTH-secreting cells that have little or no VDR, and, therefore, they are probably not responsive to the PTH-reducing effect of 1,25 (OH)$_2$ D (29). Therefore the treatment of patients with moderate and severe renal failure with 1,25 (OH)$_2$ D$_3$ not only maintains calcium homeostasis but also helps decrease the risk of secondary hyperparathyroidism (30).

CLINICAL APPLICATIONS

Hypocalcemic Disorders

A variety of hypocalcemic disorders are directly associated with acquired and inherited disorders in the acquisition of vitamin D and its metabolism to 1,25 (OH)$_2$ D (1,2,31). Vitamin D deficiency can be caused by a decreased synthesis of vitamin D$_3$ in the skin, resulting from (a) excessive sunscreen use, (b) clothing of all sun-exposed areas, (c) aging, (d) changes in season of the year, and (e) increased latitude. Intestinal malabsorption of vitamin D associated with fat-malabsorption syndromes, including Crohn's disease, sprue, Whipple's disease, and hepatic dysfunction, is recognizable by low or undetectable concentrations of circulating 25 (OH) D. Dilantin and phenobarbital can alter the kinetics for the metabolism of vitamin D to 25 (OH) D, requiring that patients using the drugs receive 2 to 5 times the RDA for vitamin D to correct this abnormality (1,31). Because the liver has such a large capacity to produce 25 (OH) D, usually >90% of the liver has to be dysfunctional before it is incapable of making an adequate quantity of 25 (OH) D. Often the fat malabsorption associated with the liver failure is the cause for vitamin D deficiency (1,31,32). Patients with nephrotic syndrome, who excrete >4 gm of protein per 24 hours, can have lower 25 (OH) D because of the coexcretion of the vitamin D–binding protein with its 25 (OH) D (1,31,33).

Acquired disorders in the metabolism of 25 (OH) D to 1,25 (OH)$_2$ D can cause hypocalcemia. Patients with chronic renal failure with a glomerular filtration rate of <30% of normal have decreased reserve capacity to produce 1,25 (OH)$_2$ D (1,3,31). Hyperphosphatemia and hypoparathyroidism will result in the decreased production of 1,25 (OH)$_2$ D (1,31). Oncogenic osteomalacia, a rare acquired disorder, is associated with hypocalcemia, hypophosphatemia, and low levels of 1,25 (OH)$_2$ D (31). Two rare inherited hypocalcemic disorders are caused by either a deficiency in the renal production of 1,25 (OH)$_2$ D (vitamin D–dependent rickets type I) or a defect in or deficiency of the VDR (vitamin D–dependent rickets type II, or 1,25 (OH)$_2$ D-resistant syndrome) (3,31,34). Although patients with X-linked hypophosphatemic rickets have low-normal or normal 1,25 (OH)$_2$ D levels, they are considered to have a defect in the renal production of 1,25 (OH)$_2$ D because these levels are inappropriately low for the degree of hyposphosphatemia (31).

Hypercalcemic Disorders

Excessive ingestion of vitamin D (usually >5000 to 10,000 IU/day) for many months can cause vitamin D intoxication that is recognized by markedly increased levels of 25 (OH) D (usually >125 ng/ml), hypercalcemia, and hyperphosphatemia (1,31). Ingestion of excessive quantities of 25 (OH) D$_3$, 1α (OH) D$_3$, 1,25 (OH)$_2$ D$_3$, dihydrotachysterol, or exuberant use of topical calcipotriene (Dovonex) for psoriasis can cause vitamin D intoxication (4,31). Because activated macrophages convert in an unregulated fashion 25 (OH) D to 1,25 (OH)$_2$ D, chronic granulomatous diseases such as sarcoidosis and tuberculosis are often associated with increased serum levels of 1,25 (OH)$_2$ D, which results in hypercalciuria and hypercalcemia (1,31,35). Rarely, lymphoma associated with hypercalcemia is caused by increased production of 1,25 (OH)$_2$ D by lymphomatous tissue (1). Primary hyperparathyroidism and hypophosphatemia also are associated with increased renal production of 1,25 (OH)$_2$ D (1,12,31).

CONSEQUENCES AND TREATMENT OF VITAMIN D DEFICIENCY

Vitamin D plays a critically important role in the mineralization of the skeleton at all ages. As the body depletes its stores of vitamin D because of lack of exposure to sunlight or a deficiency of vitamin D in the diet, the efficiency of intestinal calcium absorption decreases from approximately 30% to no more than 15%. This results in a decrease in the ionized calcium concentration in the blood, which signals the calcium sensor in the parathyroid glands, resulting in an increase in the synthesis and secretion of PTH. PTH not only tries to conserve calcium by increasing renal tubular reabsorption of calcium, but it also plays an active role in mobilizing stem cells to become active calcium-resorbing osteoclasts. PTH also increases tubular excretion of phosphorus, causing hypophosphatemia. The net effect of vitamin D insufficiency and vitamin D deficiency is a normal serum calcium, increased PTH and alkaline phosphatase, and a low or low-normal fasting serum phosphorus. The hallmark of vitamin D insufficiency and deficiency is low-normal (between 10 and 20 ng/ml) and low or undetectable (>10 ng/ml) 25 (OH) D, respectively, in the blood. The secondary hyperparathyroidism and low plasma calcium phosphorus product are thought to be responsible for the increase in unmineralized osteoid, which is the hallmark of rickets/osteomalacia. In addition, the secondary hyperparathyroidism causes increased osteoclastic activity, resulting in calcium wasting from the bone, which in turn exacerbates osteoporosis in older adults.

Vitamin D insufficiency and vitamin D deficiency are now recognized as significant causes of metabolic bone disease in older adults. It has been estimated that upward of 57% of inpatients and 40% of outpatients (ages 49 to 83 years in Boston) were vitamin D deficient (37). In New England during the winter, when sunlight is incapable of producing sufficient quantities of vitamin D in the skin, a marked loss of bone mineral density of the hip and spine can be detected, which can be related to a decrease in circulating levels of 25 (OH) D and secondary hyperparathyroidism. During the summer, serum 25 (OH) D levels increase, PTH levels decrease, and the bone density partially or completely recovers (8,38).

A multivitamin that contains 400 IU of vitamin D is an excellent source of the vitamin and will help maintain circulating concentrations of 25 (OH) D. However, in the absence of sunlight, a multivitamin may not be adequate to maintain a normal vitamin D status. For patients who are vitamin D deficient, treatment once a week with 50,000 IU of vitamin D_2 for 8 weeks increased serum 25 (OH) D levels by >100% from <15 ng/ml to 35 ng/ml and decreased PTH levels by 35% (Fig. 5). This treatment, along with a multivitamin that contains 400 IU of vitamin D, will maintain 25 (OH) D levels in the normal range for 2 to 4 months.

Casual exposure to sunlight provides most of our vitamin D requirement. The skin has a large capacity to produce vitamin D_3. For a young adult, a whole-body exposure to a minimal erythemal dose of simulated sunlight is equivalent to taking a single oral dose of between 10,000 and 75,000 IU of vitamin D (4). Therefore, adults older than 50 years will benefit from exposure of hands, face, and arms to suberythemal doses of sunlight. For example, in Boston, 5 to 15 minutes a day (depending on the skin's sensitivity to sunlight) in the spring, summer, and fall is usually adequate, as is sitting in sunlight on a verandah for 15 to 30 minutes in New Zealand (39).

CONCLUSIONS

When evaluating patients for hypo- and hypercalcemic conditions, it is appropriate to consider the patients' vitamin D status, as well as whether they suffer from either an acquired or inherited disorder in the acquisition or metabolism (or both) of vitamin D. Because the assay for vitamin D is not available to clinicians, the best compound to assay to determine vitamin D status is 25 (OH) D. Only when there is a suspicion that there is an acquired or inherited disorder in the metabolism of 25 (OH) D is it reasonable to measure circulating 1,25 (OH)$_2$ D concentrations. The measurement of other vitamin D metabolites, of which there

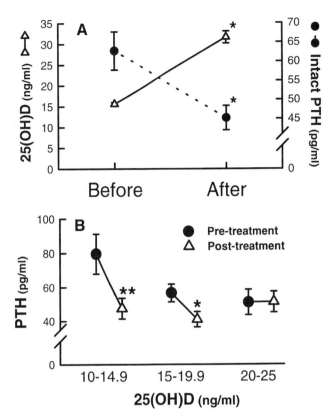

FIG. 5. Top: Serum levels of 25 (OH) D and intact parathyroid hormone (PTH) before and after receiving 50,000 IU of vitamin D_2 once a week for 8 weeks. **Bottom:** Patients (ages 49 to 83 years) with serum 25 (OH) D > 10 ng/ml (considered to be the lowest limit of the normal range) and <25 ng/ml received 50,000 IU of vitamin D_2 for 8 weeks. The PTH levels were measured before and immediately after therapy. The data clearly show significant declines in PTH when the serum 25 (OH) D levels were between 11 and 19 ng/ml, suggesting that the patients were deficient in vitamin D until the 25 (OH) D reached 20 ng/ml. (From Malabanan A, Veronikis IE, Holick MF. Redefining vitamin D deficiency. *Lancet* 1998;351:805–806, with permission.)

are a variety in the circulation, has not proved to be of any significant value. It was suggested that there may be a correlation of the development of metabolic bone disease with polymorphism for the VDR gene (19,20). Although these data are intriguing, the information is, at this time, of limited clinical value; it may someday provide an insight into a person's potential maximal bone density. The noncalcemic actions of 1,25 (OH)$_2$ D_3 have great promise for clinical applications in the future. Already activated vitamin D compounds such as 1,25 (OH)$_2$ D_3, 1,24 (OH)$_2$ D_3, and calcipotriene herald a new pharmacologic approach for treating psoriasis. 1,25 (OH)$_2$ D_3 and its analogues are actively being tested for treating autoimmune disorders such as diabetes type I and some cancers (11).

ACKNOWLEDGMENT

This work was supported in part by National Institutes of Health grants AR 36963, DK 43690, M01RR 00533, and AG 04390.

REFERENCES

1. Holick MF. Vitamin D: photobiology, metabolism, and clinical applications. In: DeGroot L, Besser H, Burger HG, et al., eds. *Endocrinology,* 3rd ed. Philadelphia: WB Saunders, 1995:990–1013.
2. DeLuca H. The vitamin D story: a collaborative effort of basic science and clinical medicine. *Fed Proc Am Soc Exp Biol* 1988;2:224–236.
3. Reichel H, Koeffler HP, Norman AW. The role of the vitamin D endocrine system in health and disease. *N Engl J Med* 1989; 320:981–991.
4. Holick MF. Vitamin D: new horizons for the 21st century. *Am J Clin Nutr* 1994;60:619–630.
5. Holick MF, Matsuoka LY, Wortsman J. Age, vitamin D, and solar ultraviolet radiation. *Lancet* 1989;4:1104–1105.
6. Holick MF, Shao Q, Liu WW, Chen TC. The vitamin D content of fortified milk and infant formula. *N Engl J Med* 1992;326:1178–1181.
7. Chapuy MC, Arlot M, Duboeuf F, et al. Vitamin D_3 and calcium to prevent hip fracture in elderly women. *N Engl J Med* 1992;327:1637–1642.
8. Dawson-Hughes B, Dallal GE, Krall EA, Harris S, Sokoll LJ, Falconer G. Effect of vitamin D supplementation on wintertime and overall bone loss in healthy postmenopausal women. *Ann Intern Med* 1991; 115:505–512.
9. Pillai S, Bikle DD, Elias PM. 1,25-Dihydroxyvitamin D production and receptor binding in human keratinocytes varies with differentiation. *J Biol Chem* 1987;263:5390–5395.
10. Gray TK, Lester GE, Lorenc RS. Evidence for extrarenal 1-hydroxylation of 25-hydroxyvitamin D_3 in pregnancy. *Science* 1979;204:1311–1313.
11. Holick MF. Noncalcemic actions of 1,25-dihydroxyvitamin D_3 and clinical applications. *Bone* 1995;17:107S–111S.
12. Portale AA, Booth BE, Halloran BP, Morris RC Jr. Effect of dietary phosphorus on circulating concentrations of 1,25-dihydroxyvitamin D and immunoreactive parathyroid hormone in children with moderate renal insufficiency. *J Clin Invest* 1984;73:1580–1589.
13. Slovik DM, Adams JS, Neer RM, Holick MF, Potts JT. Deficient production of 1,25-dihydroxyvitamin D in elderly osteoporotic patients. *N Engl J Med* 1981;305:372–374.
14. Riggs BL, Hamstra A, DeLuca HF. Assessment of 25-hydroxyvitamin D-1α-hydroxylase reserve in postmenopausal osteoporosis by administration of parathyroid extract. *J Clin Endocrinol Metab* 1981;53:833–835.
15. Kato A, Seo EG, Einhorn TA, Bishop JE, Norma AW. Studies on 24R,25-dihydroxyvitamin D_3: evidence for a nonnuclear membrane receptor in chick tibial fracture-healing callus. *Bone* 1998;23:141–146.
16. Ozono K, Sone T, Pike JW. Perspectives: the genomic mechanism of action of 1,25-dihydroxyvitamin D_3. *J Bone Miner Res* 1991;6:1021–1027.
17. Wasserman RH, Fullmer CS, Shimura F. Calcium absorption and the molecular effects of vitamin D_3. In: Kumar R, ed. *Vitamin D: basic and clinical aspects.* Boston: Nijhoff, 1984:233–257.
18. Yagi H, Ozono K, Miyake H, Nagashima K, Kuroume T, Pike JW. A new point mutation in the deoxyribonucleic acid-binding domain of the vitamin D receptor in a kindred with hereditary 1,25-dihydroxyvitamin D-resistant rickets. *J Clin Endocrinol Metab* 1992;76:509–512.
19. Morrison NA, Qi JC, Tokita A, et al. Prediction of bone density from vitamin D receptor alleles. *Nature* 1994;367:284–287.
20. Hustmyer FG, Peacock M, Hui S, Johnston CC, Christian J. Bone

21. Merke J, Klaus G, Hugel U, et al. No 1,25-dihydroxyvitamin D_3 receptors on osteoclasts of calcium-deficient chicken despite demonstrable receptors on circulating monocytes. *J Clin Invest* 1986;77:312–314.
22. Miyaura C, Abe E, Suda T, Kuroki T. Alternative differentiation of human promyelocytic leukemia cells (HL-60) induced selectively by retinoic acid and 1,25-dihydroxyvitamin D_3. *Cancer Res* 1985;45:4244–4248.
23. Tanaka H, Abe E, Miyaura C, et al. 1,25-Dihydroxycholeciferol and human myeloid leukemia cell line (HL-60): the presence of cytosol receptor and induction of differentiation. *Biochem J* 1982;204:713–719.
24. Provvedine DM, Tsoukaas CD, Deftos LJ, Manolagas SC. 1,25-Dihydroxyvitamin D_3 receptors in human leukocytes. *Science* 1983;221:118.
25. Koeffler HP, Hirjik J, Iti L, and the Southern California Leukemia Group. 1,25-Dihydroxyvitamin D_3: in vivo and in vitro effects on human preleukemic and leukemic cells. *Cancer Treat Rep* 1985; 69:1399–1407.
26. Smith EL, Pincus SH, Donovan L, Holick MF. A novel approach for the evaluation and treatment of psoriasis. *J Am Acad Dermatol* 1988;19:516–528.
27. Kragballe K. Treatment of psoriasis by the topical application of the novel vitamin D_3 analogue MC 903. *Arch Dermatol* 1989;125:1647–1652.
28. Naveh-Many T, Silver J. Regulation of parathyroid hormone gene expression by hypocalcemia, hypercalcemia, and vitamin D in the rat. *J Clin Invest* 1990;86:1313–1319.
29. Fukuda N, Tanaka H, Tominaga R, Fukagawa M, Kurokawa K, Seino Y. Decreased 1,25-dihydroxyvitamin D_3 receptor density is associated with a more severe form of parathyroid hyperplasia in chronic uremic patients. *J Clin Invest* 1993;92:1436–1443.
30. Delmez JA, Tindira C, Grooms P, Dusso A, Windus DW, Slatopolsky E. Parathyroid hormone suppression by intravenous 1,25-dihydroxyvitamin D: a role for increased sensitivity to calcium. *J Clin Invest* 1989;83:1349–1355.
31. Holick MF, Krane S, Potts JR Jr. Calcium, phosphorus, and bone metabolism: calcium-regulating hormones. In: Isselbacher KJ, Braunwald E, Wilson JD, et al., eds. *Harrison's principles of internal medicine.* 13th ed. New York: McGraw-Hill, 1994:2137–2151.
32. Bengoa JM, Sitrin MD, Meredith S, et al. Intestinal calcium absorption and vitamin D status in chronic cholestatic liver disease. *Hepatology* 1984;4:261–265.
33. Pietrek J, Kokot F. Serum 25-hydroxyvitamin D in patients with chronic renal disease. *Eur J Clin Invest* 1977;7:283–287.
34. Demay MB. Hereditary defects in vitamin D metabolism and vitamin D receptor defects. In: Degroot LJ, ed. Cahil GF Jr, Martini L, Nelson DH, consulting eds. *Endocrinology.* Vol 2, 13th ed. Philadelphia: Saunders, 1995:1173–1178.
35. Adams JS, Gacad MA, Anders A, Endres DB, Sharma OP. Biochemical indicators of disordered vitamin D and calcium homeostasis in sarcoidosis. *Sarcoidosis* 1986;3:1–6.
36. Thomas MK, Lloyd-Jones DM, Thadhani RI, et al. Hypovitaminosis D in medical inpatients. *N Engl J Med* 1998;338:777–783.
37. Malabanan A, Veronikis IE, Holick MF. Redefining vitamin D deficiency. *Lancet* 1998;351:805–806.
38. Rosen CJ, Morrison A, Zhou H, Storm D, et al. Elderly women in northern New England exhibit seasonal changes in bone mineral density and calciotropic hormones. *Bone Miner* 1994;25:83–92.
39. Reid IR, Gallagher DJA, Bosworth J. Prophylaxis against vitamin D deficiency in the elderly by regular sunlight exposure. *Age Ageing* 1985;15:35–40.

mineral density in relation to polymorphism at the vitamin D receptor gene locus. *J Clin Invest* 1994;94:2130–2134.

16. Calcitonin

Leonard J. Deftos, M.D., J.D., *Bernard A. Roos, M.D., and †Edward L. Oates, Ph.D.

*Department of Medicine and Endocrine Research Laboratory, University of California, San Diego, and Veterans Affairs San Diego Healthcare System, San Diego, California; *Divisions of Endocrinology and Gerontology and Geriatric Medicine, University of Miami School of Medicine; and *†Geriatric Research, Education, and Clinical Center, Veterans Affairs Medical Center, Miami, Florida*

Calcitonin (CT) is a 32-amino-acid peptide that is secreted primarily by thyroidal C cells in mammals and by the ultimobranchial gland in submammals. Its main biologic effect is to inhibit osteoclastic bone resorption. This property led to its use for disorders characterized by increased bone resorption. Calcitonin is approved by the Food and Drug Administration (FDA). Parenteral and nasal formulations of the peptide are used for the treatment of Paget's disease, osteoporosis, and the hypercalcemia of malignancy. The secretion of CT is regulated acutely by blood calcium and chronically by gender and perhaps age. CT is metabolized by the kidney and the liver. It is also a tumor marker for medullary thyroid carcinoma and the signal tumor of multiple endocrine neoplasia (MEN) type 2 (1,2).

BIOCHEMISTRY

Structures of CT have been determined in more than a dozen species (2) (Fig. 1). Common features include a 17-amino-terminal disulfide bridge, a glycine at residue 28, and a carboxy-terminal proline amide residue. Five of the nine amino-terminal residues are identical in all CT species. The greatest divergence resides in the interior 27 amino acids. Basic amino acid substitutions enhance potency. Thus the nonmammalian CTs have the most potency, even in mammalian systems. Unlike that for parathyroid hormone (PTH), a biologically active fragment of CT has not been discovered. However, an amphipathic backbone seems to enhance potency.

MOLECULAR BIOLOGY

The CT gene consists of six exons separated by introns (3,4) (Fig. 2). Two distinct mature messenger RNAs (mRNAs) are generated from differential splicing of the exon regions in the initial gene transcript. One translates as a 141-residue CT precursor and the other as a 128-residue precursor for calcitonin gene–related peptide (CGRP). Calcitonin is the major posttranslationally processed peptide in C cells, whereas CGRP, a 37-amino-acid peptide, is the major processed peptide in neurons. The main biologic effect of CGRP is vasodilation, but it also functions as a neurotransmitter and does react with the CT receptor. The relevance of CGRP to skeletal metabolism is unknown, but it may be produced locally in skeletal tissue and exert a local regulatory effect. An alternative splicing pathway for the CT gene produces a carboxy-terminal C-pro CT with eight different terminal amino acids (5). The CT gene predicts the presence of other processed peptides, and there is more than one copy of this gene (1–3,5).

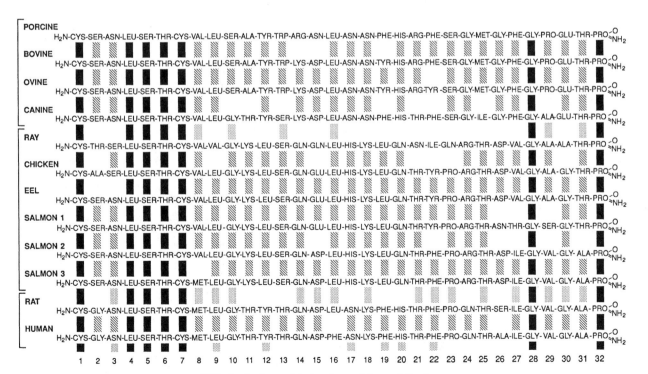

FIG. 1. Amino acid structure of the calcitonins.

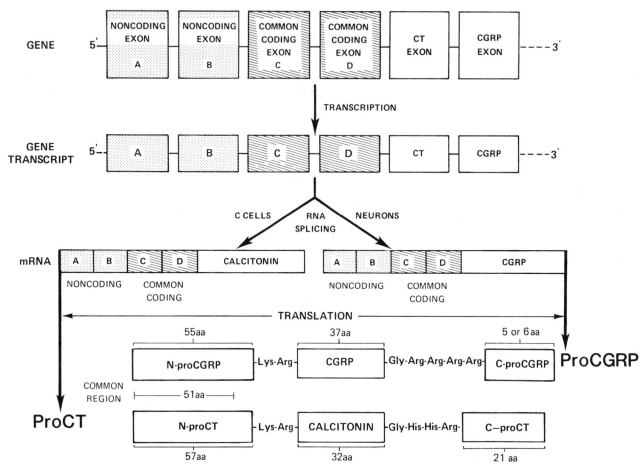

FIG. 2. Model for calcitonin gene expression.

BIOSYNTHESIS

Thyroidal C cells are the primary source of CT in mammals, and the ultimobranchial gland is the primary source in submammals (1–3). C cells are neural crest derivatives, and they also produce CGRP, the second CT gene product. Other tissue sources of CT have been described, notably the pituitary cells and widely distributed neuroendocrine cells (2,6). Although CT may have paracrine effects at these sites, the nonthyroidal sources of CT are not likely to contribute to its peripheral concentration. However, malignant transformation can occur in both ectopic and eutopic cells that produce CT, and the peptide then becomes a tumor marker. The best example of the latter is medullary thyroid carcinoma and of the former, small-cell lung cancer. Many of the tumors associated with ectopic CT production probably derive this potential from their common neural crest origin with thyroidal C cells (1).

BIOLOGIC EFFECTS

The main biologic effect of CT is to inhibit osteoclastic bone resorption (2). Within minutes of its administration, CT causes the osteoclast to shrink and to decrease its bone-resorbing activity. This dramatic and complex event is mediated by the CT receptor, which is robustly expressed by osteoclasts (7). When bone turnover is sufficiently high, CT will produce hypocalcemia and hypophosphatemia. Calcitonin also was reported to inhibit osteocytes and stimulate osteoblasts, but these effects are controversial. Analgesia is a commonly reported effect of CT treatment. Calciuria, phosphaturia, and gastrointestinal effects on calcium flux have been reported for CT, but they occur at concentrations of the hormone that are supraphysiologic (1). It should be noted, however, that the concentration of the peptide at its several sites of biosynthesis may be sufficiently high to explain some extraskeletal effects of CT by a paracrine mechanism. Thus CT may exert physiologic effects on the pituitary and central nervous system. Furthermore, the demonstration of CT and CT receptors at intracranial sites may qualify CT as a neurotransmitter. Other effects of CT have been reported. It has been observed to act as an antiinflammatory agent, to promote fracture and wound healing, to be uricosuric, to be antihypertensive, and to impair glucose tolerance. Calcitonin may regulate and be regulated by other calcitropic hormones, and there is some evidence to suggest that it exerts an autoregulatory effect. The importance of these effects is yet to be determined (4).

CT as a Drug

The main biologic action of CT, its inhibition of osteoclastic bone resorption, has resulted in its successful use in disease states characterized by increased bone resorption and the consequent hypercalcemia. Calcitonin is FDA approved for Paget's disease, in which osteoclastic bone resorption is dramatically increased, and in osteoporosis, in which the increase of bone resorption may be more subtle, and in the treatment of hypercalcemia of malignancy. A nasal preparation of CT is receiving increasing clinical application (4).

SECRETION

Calcium

Ambient calcium concentration is the most important regulator of CT secretion (1). When blood calcium increases acutely, there is a proportional increase in CT secretion, and an acute decrease in blood calcium produces a corresponding decrease in plasma CT. However, the effects of chronic hypercalcemia and chronic hypocalcemia are not fully defined, and conflicting results have been reported. It seems likely that the C cells can respond to sustained hypercalcemia by increasing CT secretion, but if the hypercalcemia is severe or prolonged or both, the C cells probably exhaust their secretory reserve (8). The inhibitory effect on CT secretion by hypocalcemia is difficult to demonstrate. Chronic hypocalcemia seems to decrease the secretory challenge to C cells, and they increase their stores of CT; these stores can be released on appropriate stimulation (9).

Metabolism

The metabolism of CT is a complex process that involves many organ systems. Evidence has been reported for degradation of the hormone by kidney, liver, bone, and even the thyroid gland (1,2). Like many other peptide hormones, CT disappears from plasma in a multiexponential manner that includes an early half-life measured in minutes. In most studies, the kidney seems to be the most important organ of clearance for CT. Inactivation of the hormone seems more important than renal excretion, because relatively little CT can be detected in urine (1–3).

Gastrointestinal Factors

Gastrointestinal peptides, especially those of the gastrin–cholecystokinin family, are potent CT secretagogues when administered parenterally in supraphysiologic concentrations (10). This observation has led to the postulate that there is an entero-C-cell regulatory pathway for CT secretion. However, only meals that contain sufficient calcium to increase the blood calcium have been demonstrated to increase CT secretion in humans (11). Thus the secretory relation between the gastrointestinal tract and C cells in humans is of unknown physiologic significance.

Other Factors

Although a variety of neuroendocrine and ionic factors have been demonstrated to regulate CT secretion under experimental conditions (1), it is unlikely that these agents participate in the physiologic regulation of CT secretion (1–3).

Provocative Testing for CT-Producing Tumors

The stimulatory effect of calcium and gastrin-related peptides, especially pentagastrin, on CT secretion has led to the use of these agents as provocative tests for the secretion of CT (2). These procedures are widely used in patients suspected of having medullary thyroid carcinoma (MTC), especially when the basal concentration of the hormone is not diagnostically elevated. Medullary thyroid carcinoma is a neoplastic disorder of thyroidal C cells that can occur in a familial pattern as part of MEN type 2, for which genetic tests are now available. Most tumors respond with increased CT secretion to the administration of either calcium or pentagastrin or their combination, but either agent can sometimes give misleading results. Therefore, in clinically compelling situations, both agents should be considered for diagnostic testing.

Gender and Age

Most investigators find that women have lower CT levels than men (11). The mechanism of this difference is unclear but may be accounted for in part by a stimulating effect of gonadal steroids on CT secretion. The effect of age on CT secretion is more controversial: newborns seem to have a higher serum level of the hormone, and in adults, a progressive decline with age was reported by several laboratories. However, stable adult levels also were observed. It is likely that the different assay procedures used in different studies account for the conflicting results. Thus the serum concentration of some forms of CT may decline with age, whereas others do not. The physiologic significance of the various circulating forms of CT measured by different assay procedures has not been defined. Nonmonomeric, as well as monomeric, forms of circulating CT species are biologically active, and some procedures may not accurately reflect biologically active CT in blood.

THE CALCITONIN RECEPTOR AND RECEPTOR MODULATION

Ligand and Receptor Structural Features

CT mediates its biologic effects through the CT receptor (CTR) (1,7). CTRs have been cloned from the pig, human, rat, mouse, and rabbit, but a nonmammalian CTR has yet to be cloned. CTRs are most robustly expressed in osteoclasts but also are expressed in several other sites, including the central nervous system. The mammalian CTRs share common structural and functional motifs, signal through several pathways, and can exist in several isoforms with insert sequences or deletions or both in their intracellular and extracellular domains. These isoforms arise from alternative splicing of receptor mRNA transcribed from a single gene. Some of the isoforms of the CTR seem to have differential ligand specificity.

Studies with mutations and chimeras suggested the following model for CT–CTR interaction: the ligand is sandwiched between the receptor's amino terminus and transmembrane loops, with high affinity being conferred by the helicity of the internal, nonconserved basic sequences of the CT. Signal transduction through several pathways results from the interaction of the amino terminus of CT with the transmembrane domain of the receptor. Thus the ligand specificity of the CTR is determined by the membrane-embedded portion of the receptors, whereas the amino-terminal, extracellular domain of the receptors affects binding affinity for the respective agonist (7).

SCT apparently conforms best to these structural requirements for binding and signaling of mammalian CTRs, perhaps explaining its greater potency in humans and mammals and its sustained receptor binding and activation of cyclic adenosine monophosphate (cAMP) (2,7). An isoform of the CTR that is expressed in rat brain seems to preferentially recognize SCT, and binding sites for SCT are present at several sites in the central nervous system (CNS). It is thus speculated that an SCT-like ligand is produced by mammals. There is some evidence for this in both humans and murine. Finally, it is also notable that another nonmammalian CT, chicken CT (CCT), also seems more potent in humans than human CT and that a CCT-like ligand may be expressed in humans.

Ligand Families

Long known to be related to CGRP1 and 2 (Fig. 2), CT recently was recognized to be related in sequence to two other bioactive peptides, adrenomedullin and amylin (Fig. 3). Except for CT and CGRP1, each of these peptides derives from a separate gene and exerts characteristic actions at a distinct array of targets (12). Although all of these peptides share the feature of being neuromodulators, they also appear to have unique hormone actions. The effects of CT were described earlier. CGRP1 and CGRP2 are potent vasodilators and immunomodulators, with actions in the CNS and at many other targets. Adrenomedullin also is a potent vasodilator with some CNS actions. The actions of amylin are

related to carbohydrate metabolism, to gastric emptying, and to CNS function.

Receptor Modulation

Despite their distinct bioactivities, this family of peptides shows some cross-reactivity at each other's receptors, even though they generally bear only partial homology. These receptors are members of the family of the heptahelical, G protein–coupled receptors (GPCRs) that can be structurally subclassified into subtypes A and B, with the CT receptor belonging to subtype B and certain CGRP and adrenomedullin receptors to A or B. The interaction of ligands among these receptors is influenced by newly discovered receptor-modulating proteins (13–15). This modulation expands the repertoire of biologic actions that can be mediated by receptors and their ligands. One modulator, termed CGRP-receptor component protein (CGRP-RCP), consists of a hydrophilic protein that is highly conserved across species and found in virtually all tissues (13,15). It was discovered by its ability to modulate a CGRP-unresponsive receptor to a responsive state (13). The second group of receptor modulators is a family of proteins termed receptor-activity-modifying proteins (RAMPs) and comprises three members, RAMPs1 to 3 (14). The RAMPs are membrane proteins with one transmembrane domain. RAMPs interact with a distinct calcitonin receptor–like receptor (CRLR) that has >50% homology with the CT receptor (GPCR, subtype B) and transports it to the cell-membrane surface. RAMP1 transport of CRLR results in a terminally glycosylated receptor that recognizes CGRP, whereas RAMP2 and 3 expression produces a core glycosylated receptor that recognizes adrenomedullin. Figure 4 is a schematic representation of the GPCRs comparing subtypes A and B.

Receptor modulation is another molecular mechanism of genetic economy whereby specific ligands can acquire functions beyond those allowed by a simple lock-and-key model of receptor specificity.

Role of Calcitonin in Mineral Metabolism

The exact physiologic role of CT in calcium homeostasis and skeletal metabolism has not been established in humans, and many questions remain unanswered about the significance of this hormone in humans. Does CT secretion decline with age? Do gonadal steroids regulate the secretion of CT?

```
HUM A-TYPE CALC         CGNLSTCMLGTYTQDFNKFHTFPQTAIGVGAP-amide
A-HUMAN CGRP            AC DTATCVTHRLAGLLSRSGGVVKNNFVPTNVGS KAF-amide
B-HUMAN CGRP            AC NTATCVTHRLAGLLSRSGGMVKSNFVPTNVGS KAF-amide
Human ADM    YRQSMNNFQGLRSFGC RFGTCTVQKLAHQIYQFTDKDKDNVAPRSKISPQGY-amide
HUMAN AMYLIN            KC NTATCATQRLANFLVHSSNNFGAILSSTNVGS NTY-amide
Consensus               C *taTC t+rla  l +s   k n ptnvgS +  -amide
```

FIG. 3. The calcitonin family of peptides. The alignment of the human peptides shows that the generally hydrophobic hormones are highly homologous in sequence, with a conserved C-C 6-7 amino acid loop at or close to the N terminus. Bioactivity is confined to this portion of the hormones, whereas regions more carboxyl bind their specific receptors.

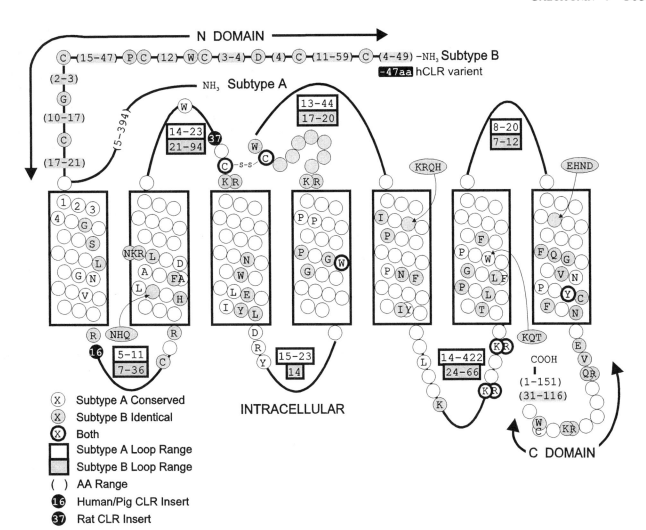

FIG. 4. Schematic representation of subtypes A and B of the G protein–coupled receptor (GPCR) family. The calcitonin family of peptides (Fig. 2) acts by binding to a specific type of seven transmembrane spanning GPCRs called the calcitonin–secretin group or subtype B. With the possible exception of related receptors for CGRP and adrenomedullin (RDC1 and G10D, respectively, which are in subtype A), this group of receptors (comprising >20 members) differs greatly from the much larger subtype A group, as shown in the comparison of conserved amino acids for the two receptor subtypes. Differences include an N-terminal region that is longer than most subtype A receptors and more conserved (notably the positions of six Cys residues). Subtype B receptors have greater overall sequence conservation than subtype A GPCRs.

Do the lower levels of serum CT in women contribute to the pathogenesis of age-related loss of bone mass and osteoporosis? Do extrathyroidal sources of CT participate in the regulation of skeletal metabolism? Are there primary and secondary abnormalities of CT secretion in diseases of skeletal and calcium homeostasis? The conclusive answers to these questions await clinical studies with an assay procedure that directly measures the biologic activity of CT in blood. Furthermore, accurate local measurements of CT and its effects may be necessary to elucidate the emerging role of CT as a paracrine and autocrine agent.

REFERENCES

1. Deftos LJ, JJ Nolan. Syndromes involving multiple endocrine glands. In: Greenspan FS, Strewler GJ, eds. *Basic and clinical endocrinology.* 5th ed. Norwalk, CT: Lange Medical Books, Appleton & Lange, 1997: 753–769.
2. Deftos LJ. Calcitonin. In: Favus MJ, ed. *Primer on the metabolic bone diseases and disorders of mineral metabolism.* 3rd ed. New York: Lippincott-Raven, 1996:82–87.
3. Deftos LJ. Multiple endocrine neoplasia. In: *Clinical essentials of calcium and skeletal disorders.* 1st ed. Professional communications, 1998:137–151.
4. Carstens JH, Feinblatt JD. Future horizons for calcitonin. *J Bone Miner Res* 1991;49:2–6.
5. Minvielle S, Giscard-Dartevelle S, Cohen R, et al. A novel calcitonin carboxyl-terminal peptide produced in medullary thyroid carcinoma by alternative RNA processing of the calcitonin/calcitonin gene-related peptide gene. *J Biol Chem* 1991;266:24627–24631.
6. Deftos LJ. Pituitary cells secrete calcitonin in the reverse hemolytic plaque assay. *Biochem Biophys Res Commun* 1987;146:1350–1356.
7. Deftos LJ. There's something fishy and perhaps fowl about the mammalian calcitonin receptor and its ligand [Editorial]. *Endocrinology* 1997; 138:519–520.
8. Parthemore JG, Deftos LJ. Secretion of calcitonin in primary hyperparathyroidism. *J Clin Endocrinol Metab* 1979;49:223–226.

9. Deftos LJ, Powell D, Parthemore JG, Potts JT Jr. Secretion of calcitonin in hypocalcemic states in man. *J Clin Invest* 1973;52:3109–3114.
10. Austin LA, Health H III. Calcitonin: physiology and pathophysiology. *N Engl J Med* 1981;304:269–278.
11. Deftos LJ, Weisman MH, Williams GH, et al. Influence of age and sex on plasma calcitonin in human beings. *N Engl J Med* 1980;302:1351–1353.
12. Muff R, Born W, Fischer JA. Calcitonin, calcitonin gene related peptide, adrenomedullin and amylin: homologous peptides, separate receptors and overlapping biological actions. *Eur J Endocrinol* 1995; 133:17–20.
13. Luebke AE, Dahl GP, Roos BA, Dickerson IM. Identification of a protein that confers calcitonin gene-related peptide responsiveness to oocytes by using a cystic fibrosis transmembrane conductance regulator assay. *Proc Natl Acad Sci USA* 1996;93:3455–3460.
14. McLatchie LM, Fraser NJ, Main MJ, et al. RAMPs regulate the transport and ligand specificity of the calcitonin-receptor-like receptor. *Nature* 1998;393:333–338.
15. Balkan W, Oates EL, Howard GA, Roos BA. Testes exhibit elevated expression of calcitonin gene-related peptide receptor component protein. *Endocrinology* 1999;140:1459–1469.

17. Gonadal Steroids and Receptors

Katrina M. Waters, Ph.D. and *Thomas C. Spelsberg, Ph.D.

*Endocrine, Reproductive, and Developmental Toxicology, Chemical Industry Institute of Toxicology, Research Triangle Park, North Carolina; and *Department of Biochemistry and Molecular Biology, Mayo Graduate and Medical Schools, Mayo Clinic, Rochester, Minnesota*

INTRODUCTION

Since steroid hormones were discovered in the early 1900s, studies of their molecular actions have extended from the whole body, to the target organs, to specific functions within those target tissues, to the specific cells, and finally to specific genes and their protein products. It is well accepted that sex steroids play an important role in bone cell metabolism, including the regulation of osteoblast and osteoclast activities and reinforcing the coupling between these cells by paracrine factors. The overall function of the gonadal steroids in bone is to maintain a steady state in bone metabolism to prevent the loss of bone mass in humans. Type I osteoporosis is believed to be an acceleration of the rapid phase of bone loss during the first 5 to 10 years after menopause. Estrogen-replacement therapy reinstates the homeostasis between the osteoblasts and osteoclasts and prevents bone loss, thereby supporting the role of estrogen deficiency in osteoporosis. This chapter presents a brief overview of the structure and function of gonadal steroid hormones, their receptors, and the mechanisms by which they regulate cell function.

STEROID HORMONES

There are three categories of steroid hormones: glucocorticoids, mineralocorticoids, and the gonadal steroids (estrogens, androgens, and progesterone). Sex steroids are synthe-sized in response to signals from the brain. Input from the central nervous system initiates the stimulus from the hypothalamus to the pituitary gland, which releases hormones that target the reproductive organs. These hormones, luteinizing hormone and follicle-stimulating hormone, stimulate the synthesis of progesterone and estrogens in the female ovaries and testosterone in the male testes. Comprehensive reviews of these processes are available (1–3). Traditionally, sex steroids were thought to regulate activity only in reproductive organs, but the discovery of steroid hormone receptors throughout the body has implicated functionality in many other tissues.

Biosynthesis of Steroid Hormones

The synthesis of steroid hormones from cholesterol involves pathways with ten or more enzymes (Fig. 1A). The level of steroid hormones in the bloodstream is primarily controlled by its rate of synthesis, because little steroid is stored. The increase of these hormones in the serum takes from hours to days, so cellular responses are delayed but last longer than the effects mediated by peptide hormones.

In ovulating women and during pregnancy, progesterone is secreted by the ovaries. Progesterone not only exhibits biologic activity but, as shown in Fig. 1A, also serves as a precursor for all other steroid hormones.

Estrone and estradiol are formed from androstenedione and testosterone, respectively (Fig. 1A). This reaction is

---

FIG. 1. A: Pathways of steroid hormone biosynthesis from cholesterol. The initiation of steroid hormone synthesis involves the hydrolysis of cholesterol esters and the uptake of cholesterol into mitochondria of cells in the target organ. Dehydrogenation of pregnenolone produces progesterone, which serves as a precursor molecule for the generation of all other gonadal steroid hormones. (Adapted from Khosla S, Spelsberg TC, Riggs BL. Sex steroid effects on bone metabolism. In: Seibel M, Robins S, Bilezikian J, eds. *Dynamics of bone and cartilage metabolism.* San Diego: Academic Press (in press), with permission.) **B:** Chemical structures of common steroid analogues.

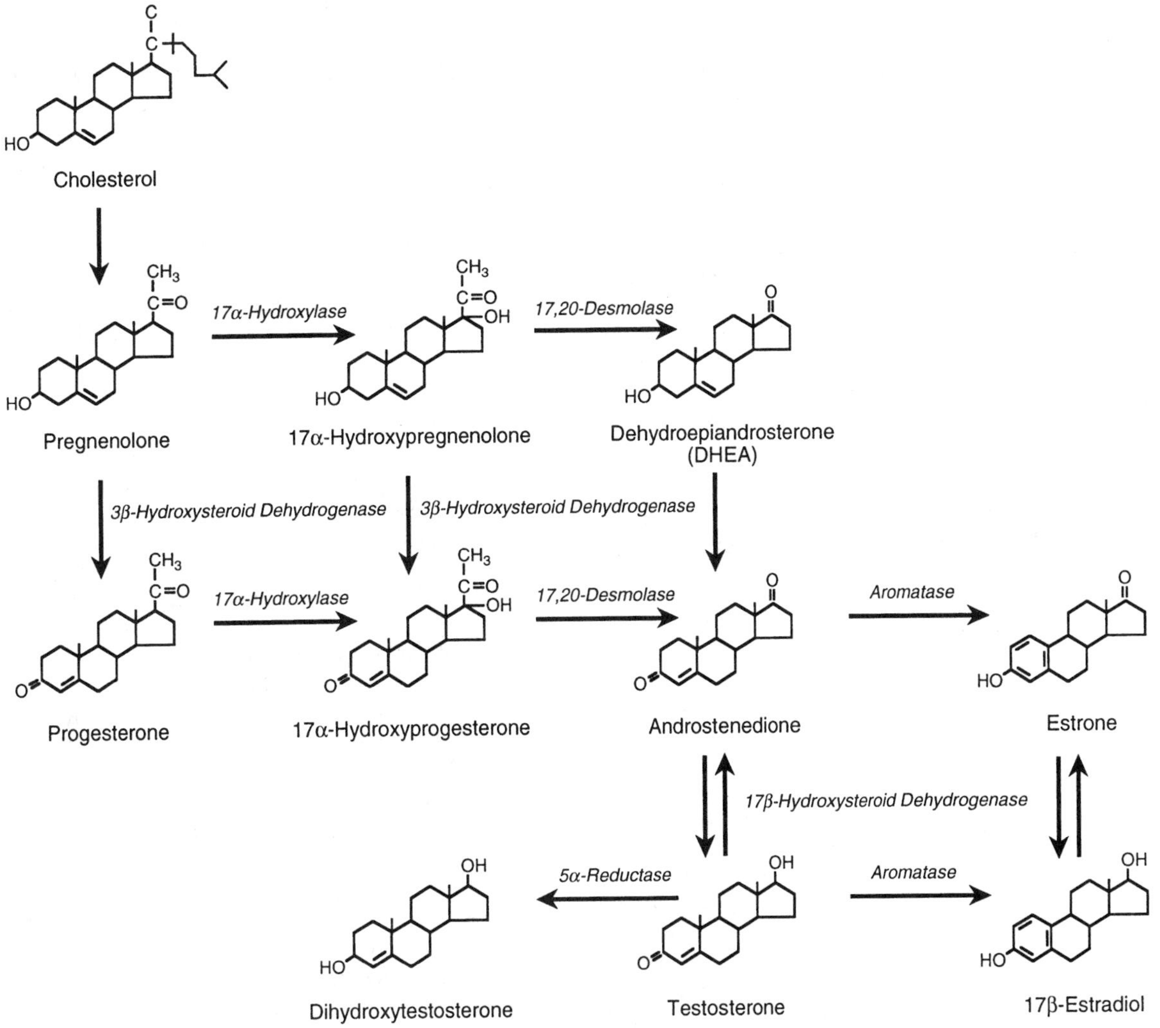

Cholesterol

Pregnenolone

17α-Hydroxypregnenolone

Dehydroepiandrosterone (DHEA)

17α-Hydroxylase

17,20-Desmolase

3β-Hydroxysteroid Dehydrogenase

3β-Hydroxysteroid Dehydrogenase

Progesterone

17α-Hydroxyprogesterone

Androstenedione

Estrone

17α-Hydroxylase

17,20-Desmolase

Aromatase

17β-Hydroxysteroid Dehydrogenase

5α-Reductase

Aromatase

Dihydroxytestosterone

Testosterone

17β-Estradiol

A

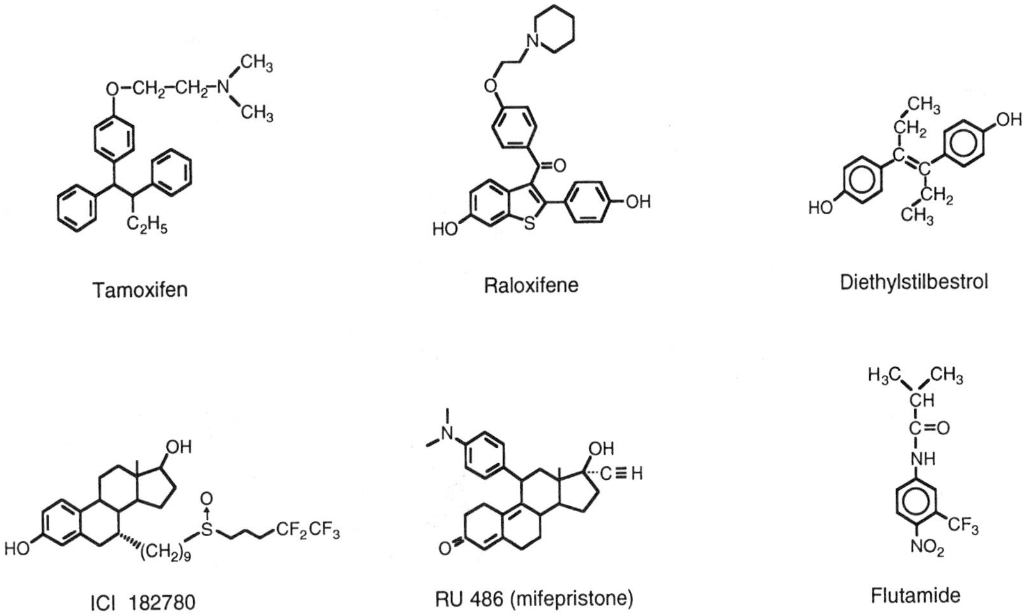

Tamoxifen

Raloxifene

Diethylstilbestrol

ICl 182780

RU 486 (mifepristone)

Flutamide

B

mediated by the enzyme aromatase, a cytochrome P-450 enzyme present in the ovary, as well as the testis, adipocytes, and bone cells. Estradiol and estrone are in reversible equilibrium caused by hepatic and intestinal 17β-hydroxysteroid dehydrogenases. The major circulating estrogen in postmenopausal women is estrone, which, in turn, follows two main pathways of metabolism to 16α-hydroxyestrone and 2-hydroxyestrone. The balance in the ratio of these hydroxylated estrones has been implicated as playing a role in several disease states, including breast cancer, osteoporosis, systemic lupus erythematosus, and liver cirrhosis.

The steroidogenic pathway is essentially the same in the testes as in the ovaries, with the exception that testosterone is the major secretory product, although small amounts of estradiol also are secreted. Testosterone is converted to more active metabolites in target tissues, including the gonads, brain, and bone. This modification is accomplished by two enzymes: 5α-reductase and aromatase. As depicted in Fig. 1A, the 5α-reductase irreversibly converts testosterone to dihydroxytestosterone, which then cannot be aromatized to estrogens. Conversely, aromatase irreversibly converts testosterone into estrogenic molecules.

Transport through the Bloodstream

The major sex steroids in circulation are androgens and estrogens (estradiol and estrone). Because their chemical structure makes them fat soluble, most are bound to specific carrier proteins for transportation through the bloodstream to hormone receptors, which reside in the cells of target tissues. Only 1% to 3% of the total circulating sex steroids are free in solution. Both the free steroid and the albumin-bound fraction (35% to 55%) can enter target tissues, thereby representing the "bioavailable" steroid pool. The remaining fraction, bound to sex hormone-binding globulin, is unable to enter the cells. The sex steroids enter all cells by simple diffusion through the cell membrane and then, in target cells, bind to specific receptor molecules in the nucleus to regulate gene transcription.

Selective Estrogen-Receptor Modulators

Steroid analogues have been developed to elicit tissue-specific rather than systemic effects, avoiding common side effects of steroid-replacement therapy. One particular class of these compounds is called selective estrogen-receptor modulators (SERMs) because they bind to estrogen receptors as a ligand but can act as an agonist, antagonist, or even have no apparent effect, depending on the cell/tissue type (Fig. 1B). For example, the SERM tamoxifen is an antagonist in reproductive tissues with little effect on bone, and raloxifene is an agonist in bone with little effect in reproductive tissues. Diethylstilbestrol is not a steroid but mimics estrogen action in reproductive and bone tissues. The synthetic steroid ICI 182,780 is a pure antiestrogen, with no estrogenic activity in any tissue investigated to date. Similarly, both RU 486 and flutamide are synthetic antagonists of progesterone and testosterone, respectively. Further studies with SERM analogues will provide new alternatives to steroid-replacement therapy (4).

STEROID HORMONE RECEPTORS

Steroid hormones generate and transmit an intracellular signal by binding proteins called receptors. There are three steps in the general mechanism of action for steroid receptors: (a) binding of the steroid ligand to the receptor in the nucleus, (b) translocation of the steroid–receptor complex to a specific site on the DNA, and (c) the regulation of gene transcription.

Specific receptors exist for each of the steroid hormones because of their unique structure that allows them to differentiate between the diverse species of steroid and nonsteroid molecules. Steroid-receptor proteins have multiple "domains," each of which has specific functions, as shown in Fig. 2. All steroid-receptor species share significant homology in terms of their sequence and their four domains. There are currently two sites in domains I and IV identified as having transcriptional activation functions (TAFs). These domains are responsible for activation of gene transcription, once the steroid–receptor complex interacts with the regulatory regions of genes. In addition, a sequence of basic amino acids near the second zinc finger in domain III represents a nuclear localization sequence, which directs the receptor to the nucleus. Additional nuclear-localization signals have been identified in the hormone-binding domain, and many of these have been shown to be hormone dependent (5,6).

Heat-Shock Proteins

In their inactive state (i.e., steroid unbound), steroid receptors exist as part of a large complex in association with other nonsteroid-binding proteins within cells not exposed to the steroid, as depicted in Fig. 3. One of these nonsteroid-binding proteins, a 90-kDa heat-shock protein (hsp90), is associated with most inactive steroid hormone receptors studied thus far (7). Although the role of these associated proteins in steroid-receptor function is not fully understood, it is believed that they play a role in some aspect of receptor transport, stability, or transformation or a combination of these.

Receptor Activation

Each receptor reversibly binds its respective steroid with high affinity, but few steroid ligands exhibit absolute specificity (e.g., most ligands bind to more than one receptor, especially at high concentrations). This lack of specificity is not unexpected in view of the significant homology among the ligand-binding domains of these receptors. The primary effect of ligand binding to domain IV is to "activate" the receptor molecule by inducing a conformational change in the whole protein, so that it can interact with DNA. This conformational change in the receptor on ligand binding seems to be conserved across steroid family members.

CONTROL OF GENE EXPRESSION

The mechanism by which steroid-hormone receptors exert their effect is fundamentally different from that for receptors

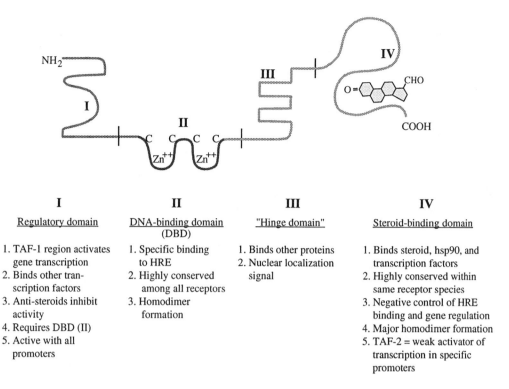

I	II	III	IV
Regulatory domain	DNA-binding domain (DBD)	"Hinge domain"	Steroid-binding domain
1. TAF-1 region activates gene transcription	1. Specific binding to HRE	1. Binds other proteins	1. Binds steroid, hsp90, and transcription factors
2. Binds other transcription factors	2. Highly conserved among all receptors	2. Nuclear localization signal	2. Highly conserved within same receptor species
3. Anti-steroids inhibit activity	3. Homodimer formation		3. Negative control of HRE binding and gene regulation
4. Requires DBD (II)			4. Major homodimer formation
5. Active with all promoters			5. TAF-2 = weak activator of transcription in specific promoters

A

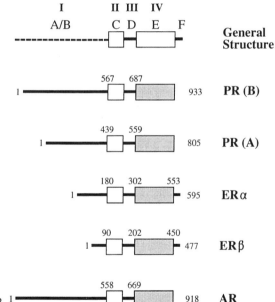

B

FIG. 2. A: Structure and functional domains of steroid-hormone receptors. Proceeding in the N-terminal to C-terminal direction, the receptors contain a variable domain *(I* or *A/B),* thought to be involved in cell type–specific regulation of gene transcription; a DNA-binding domain *(II* or *C)* of 66 to 68 amino acids, which shows a high degree of homology among members of the steroid receptor family; a "hinge" domain *(III* or *D);* a steroid-binding domain *(IV* or *E),* showing some homology; and variable regions *(V* or *F)* with little homology that somehow contribute to optimal function of the receptor. **B:** Structural homology among sex steroid receptor family members. The sex steroid receptors range in size from 595 amino acids for the estrogen receptor to 933 amino acids for the progesterone receptor. Human progesterone receptors exist in two isoforms, *A* and *B,* generated by the same gene through differential promoters. The estrogen receptor also exists in two forms *(ERα* and *ERβ);* however, they arise from different genes, each with unique domains that allow tissue- and ligand-specific functions. (Adapted from Oursler MJ, Kassem M, Turner R, Riggs BL, Spelsberg TC. Regulation of bone cell function by gonadal steroids. In: Marcus R, Feldman D, Kelsey J, eds. *Osteoporosis.* San Diego: Academic Press, 1996:237–260, with permission.) TAF, transcriptional activation function; DBD, DNA-binding domain; HRE, hormone response element.

of other types of hormones. Once bound by their specific ligand, cell-surface (membrane) receptors initiate signal-transduction cascades that eventually alter the activities of selected transcription factors. In contrast, the activated sex steroid receptors become capable of interacting either with a specific response DNA sequence, called a hormone response element (HRE), or with specific transcription factors, as shown in Fig. 3. Either process enhances or suppresses the expression (transcription) of specific genes by the binding of the steroid–receptor complex to one of several types of sites on the regulatory "promoter" region neighboring each gene.

The Receptor Binding to DNA

The DNA-binding domain of the receptor contains two "zinc fingers," looped structures involving chelated metal ions that are responsible for the binding to the HREs of target genes. A characteristic hexanucleotide inverted palindromic repeat allows the receptor to bind the DNA as a dimer. The orientation, sequence, and space between the hexanucleotide repeats are unique for each steroid hormone. Again, the similarity among the steroid-receptor superfamily results in cross-reactivity between ligands, receptors, and DNA sequences (8,9).

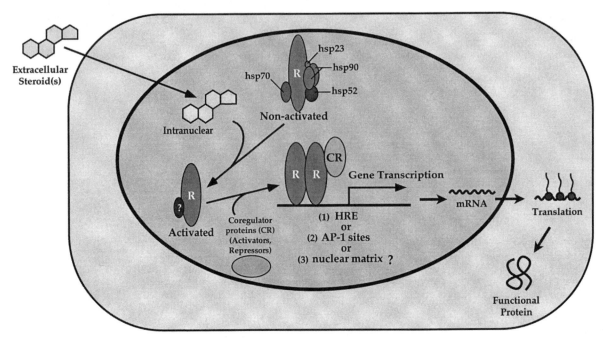

FIG. 3. Activation of steroid hormone receptors by ligand binding. The inactive receptor protein is complexed to several heat-shock proteins (hsp). On binding of the steroid hormone, a conformational change in the receptor allows transcriptional regulation by binding to HREs on DNA. In many cases, hsp90 may function as a protein "chaperone," which regulates and directs the assembly of receptor/coregulator protein complexes. It has been suggested that these hsp proteins are required for signal transduction or that they may function in the general maintenance of the cell.

Coregulators/Coactivators/Corepressors

Over the last few years, numerous cofactor proteins, or coregulators, were found to associate with receptors, and are thought to mediate the action of receptors. The designation of a protein as a coactivator, or corepressor, is based on a steroid-dependent gene response in the presence of the coregulator, or sometimes the demonstration of altered transactivation with binding of the coregulator protein. A common theme for all of these cofactors is that their association with receptors is almost always modulated by ligand binding, suggesting that the interaction may be directly with the ligand-binding domain of the receptor (10).

Steroid receptors also were shown to interact with the c-*jun*/c-*fos* transcription factors at the AP-1 DNA element, often regulating genes in opposite patterns from the HRE site (8–10).

There is strong evidence that the nuclear chromatin and especially the nuclear matrix structure play important roles in the nuclear binding of steroid receptors and regulation of gene transcription (8,11).

Chronology of Steroid Hormone Action

The chronologic order in which genes are regulated by steroids is important to both the physiologic and mechanistic responses to steroid treatments, as depicted in Fig. 4. In animals, the diffusion of steroids into cells and the nuclear binding of the steroid–receptor complex occurs within minutes after injection. This is followed by "early" gene transcription and translation of regulatory proteins, which activate "late" gene expression within 2 to 10 hours by the cascade model of steroid action (12,13). The late genes code for other proteins, including enzymes and cytokines, that trigger cell proliferation and in turn act as paracrine factors to regulate neighboring cells. The major physiologic effects of steroids in cells are usually observed 24 to 48 hours after steroid treatment.

NONGENOMIC EFFECTS

There is a growing body of evidence that steroids can alter cell metabolism by nongenomic effects (i.e., without interaction with DNA). These effects have been characterized by rapid responses ranging from seconds to minutes, involving steroid interaction with membrane receptors or steroid-receptor activation in the absence of ligand. Nongenomic estrogen effects signal through the activation of cell-surface receptors, leading to alterations in cyclic adenosine monophosphate (cAMP) levels, calcium influx, and direct channel gating. Covalent modification of the steroid receptor, such as a change in phosphorylation state, also is thought to be responsible for activation by nonsteroid effectors (14,15).

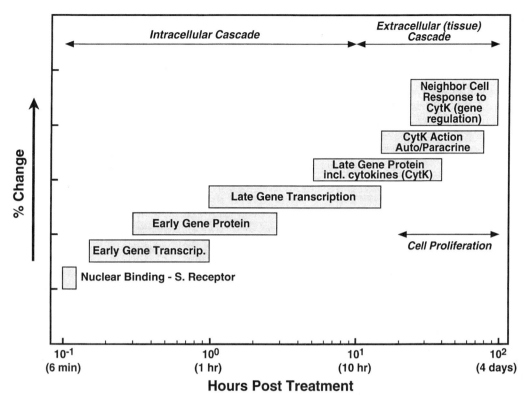

FIG. 4. Chronology of events in steroid action on target cells. After the steroid–receptor complex formation (1 to 4 minutes) is the binding of this complex to the specific "acceptor" sites on the promoter of the gene (2 to 5 minutes). The resulting regulation of gene transcription occurs within minutes for "early" genes but not until several hours for "late" genes. The late genes, in turn, code for enzymes and cytokines within 10 hours, which act as paracrine/autocrine factors to regulate neighboring cells for 12 to 24 hours and beyond. (Adapted from Robinson JA, Spelsberg TC. Mode of action at the cellular level with specific reference to bone cells. In: Lindsay R, Dempster DW, Jordan VC, eds. *Estrogens and antiestrogens: basic and clinical aspects.* Philadelphia: Lippincott-Raven, 1997:43–62.)

PHYSIOLOGY OF STEROID EFFECTS ON BONE

The two major types of cells in bone that are responsible for the maintenance of normal bone density are osteoblasts (OBs) and osteoclasts (OCLs). Normal bone-remodeling processes involve bone resorption by OCLs and bone formation by OBs, which are tightly coupled to prevent a net loss of bone mass. Many factors that influence bone resorption can either act directly on the OCLs or indirectly through the OBs. Some of these factors are local regulators, including interleukins, tumor necrosis factor, prostaglandins, and transforming growth factor-β (TGF-β), or systemic factors, including parathyroid hormone, vitamin D_3, calcitonin, glucocorticoid, and the sex steroid hormones.

Estrogens

Estrogen has been shown to play an important role in maintaining bone mass. The major effect of estrogen is on reducing bone resorption indirectly by inhibiting osteoclastogenesis and directly by inhibiting OCL function. In postmenopausal women, there is an increase in bone-remodeling activity in which resorption is no longer coupled to equal bone formation, resulting in a net loss of bone. Estrogen deficiency is recognized as the most important factor in the pathogenesis of postmenopausal bone loss, because estrogen-replacement therapy has been shown to be effective in preventing and treating osteoporosis. The identification of estrogen receptors in human OBs and OCLs implicated estrogen as a direct effector on bone, as opposed to previous theories that other calcitropic hormones were the primary mediators of the skeletal effects of estrogen deficiency (13,16,17).

Progesterone

At menopause, there is a decrease in circulating levels of progesterone as well as estrogens, which implicates progesterone in postmenopausal bone loss. However, in contrast to the abundance of work on the effects of estrogens on bone metabolism, there is little evidence of direct effects of progesterone on bone (18). Clinical studies suggest that the effects of progesterone treatment on postmenopausal women are similar to those of estrogen, but combined estrogen and progesterone treatment has effects that differ from those of treatment with either steroid alone. Because of the adverse side effects of estrogen-alone therapy, alternative therapies, such as the combined estrogen and progesterone treatments, are worth pursuing. Although estrogen is usually required to induce their synthesis, progesterone receptors have been identified in human OB cells, so progesterone could exert direct effects on bone through its own receptor. Another possible mechanism for progesterone action is through interaction with glucocorticoid receptor. Progesterone displaces glucocorticoids from their receptors without activating the receptor, effectively blocking glucocorticoid responses.

Androgens

Like estrogens, androgens influence bone development and metabolism with dramatic clinical manifestations. Decreased androgen levels have been linked to lower bone density in men, and there is a strong correlation between hypogonadism in elderly men and hip fracture and spinal osteoporosis. Clinical studies also demonstrated that treatment of osteoporosis with androgens is effective in increasing bone density in both men and women. Human bone cells have androgen-receptor concentrations similar to those of estrogen receptors and 5α-reductase and aromatase activity, for the conversion of testosterone to dihydroxytestosterone and estrogen, respectively. Androgens decrease bone resorption by acting directly on human OCL cells. In addition, androgens also regulate the production of a number of bone-resorbing factors by mature OBs or by marrow stromal cells, which contain OB progenitor cells. As with progesterone, further studies are needed to determine the complete role of androgens in bone metabolism (19).

SUMMARY

The steroid receptors are nuclear transcription factors whose structure is altered by steroid ligand binding, such that the transcription-activating domains of the receptor molecule are free to regulate gene transcription. The binding of steroid analogues to these receptors can alter the receptor structure, thereby modulating which protein factors are bound to the receptor and which TAF region is active. The types and relative amounts of steroid receptors in a cell determine the response as much as the circulating hormone levels [e.g., estrogen receptor-α (ERα) and ERβ in different ratios can modulate a particular cell type response to a steroid and have identified new target cells for estrogens]. The interaction of steroids with nonsteroid receptors and activation of steroid receptors in the absence of ligand can cause alternative biologic/physiologic responses. These molecular discoveries are explaining the physiologic actions of steroid hormones and their selected steroid-receptor modulators.

ACKNOWLEDGMENTS

Special thanks to Drs. David Toft, M. Subramaniam, B. Lawrence Riggs, Sundeep Khosla, Eric Wieben, and William Karnes for their helpful suggestions and review of this manuscript.

REFERENCES

1. Becker KL, ed. *Principles and practice of endocrinology and metabolism.* Philadelphia: JB Lippincott, 1990.
2. Wilson JD, Foster DW, eds. *Williams textbook of endocrinology*, 8th ed. Philadelphia: WB Saunders, 1992.
3. Milgrom E. Steroid hormones. In: Baulieu EE, Kelly PA, eds. *Hormones: from molecules to disease.* New York: Chapman & Hall, 1990:387–437.
4. Lindsay R, Dempster DW, Jordan VC, eds. *Estrogens and antiestrogens: basic and clinical aspects.* Philadelphia: Lippincott-Raven, 1997.
5. Ing NH, O'Malley BW. The steroid hormone receptor superfamily: molecular mechanisms of action. In: Weintraub BD, ed. *Molecular endocrinology: basic concepts and clinical correlations.* New York: Raven Press, 1995:195–215.
6. Vegeto E, Wagner BL, Imhof MO, McDonnell DP. The molecular pharmacology of ovarian steroid receptors. *Vitam Horm* 1996;52: 99–128.
7. Pratt WB, Toft DO. Steroid receptor interactions with heat shock protein and immunophilin chaperones. *Endocr Rev* 1997;18:306–360.
8. Freeman LP, ed. *Molecular biology of steroid and nuclear hormone receptors.* Boston: Birkhauser, 1998.
9. Parker MG, ed. *Nuclear hormone receptors: molecular mechanisms, cellular functions, clinical abnormalities.* London: Academic Press, 1991.
10. Shibata H, Spencer TE, Onate SA, et al. Role of co-activators and co-repressors in the mechanism of steroid/thyroid receptor action. *Recent Prog Horm Res* 1997;52:141–165.
11. Barrett TJ, Spelsberg TC. Nuclear matrix and steroid hormone action. In: Litwack G, ed. *Vitamins and hormones*, Vol 55. San Diego: Academic Press, 1999:127–163.
12. Landers JP, Spelsberg TC. Updates and new models for steroid hormone action. *Ann NY Acad Sci* 1991;637:26–55.
13. Robinson JA, Spelsberg TC. Mode of action at the cellular level with specific reference to bone cells. In: Lindsay R, Dempster DW, Jordan VC, eds. *Estrogens and antiestrogens: basic and clinical aspects.* Philadelphia: Lippincott-Raven, 1997:43–62.
14. Moss RL, Gu Q, Wong M. Estrogen: nontranscriptional signaling pathways. *Recent Prog Horm Res* 1997;52:33–69.
15. Weigel NL. Steroid hormone receptors and their regulation by phosphorylation. *Biochem J* 1996;319:657–667.
16. Oursler MJ, Kassem M, Turner R, Riggs BL, Spelsberg TC. Regulation of bone cell function by gonadal steroids. In: Marcus R, Feldman D, Kelsey J, eds. *Osteoporosis.* San Diego: Academic Press, 1996:237–260.
17. Khosla S, Spelsberg TC, Riggs BL. Sex steroid effects on bone metabolism. In: Seibel M, Robins S, Bilezikian J, eds. *Dynamics of bone and cartilage metabolism.* San Diego: Academic Press (in press).
18. Prior JC. Progesterone as a bone-trophic hormone. *Endocr Rev* 1990;11:386–398.
19. Vanderschueren D, Bouillon R. Androgens and bone. *Calcif Tissue Int* 1995;56:341–346.

SECTION IV

Clinical Evaluation of Bone and Mineral Disorders

18. History and Physical Examination

Peter M. Sklarin, M.D., *Dolores M. Shoback, M.D., and †Craig B. Langman, M.D.

*Menlo Medical Clinic, Menlo Park, California; and *Departments of Medicine and Endocrine, Veterans Affairs Medical Center, and Department of Medicine, University of California, San Francisco, California; and †Department of Pediatrics, Northwestern University Medical School, and Department of Nephrology and Mineral Metabolism, Children's Memorial Hospital, Chicago, Illinois*

With the availability of treatments that can prevent, control, or cure most metabolic bone diseases, early recognition is essential. An experienced clinician can accurately diagnose many bone disorders by history and physical examination alone. Many of these diseases have a subtle and insidious onset and are not often recognized until they have reached a severe stage. The clinician's challenge, therefore, is not only early diagnosis of existing disease, but also the identification of patients at risk. A careful history and thorough physical examination are the physician's most powerful tools in choosing whom to screen with diagnostic tests and deciding which patients will benefit most from preventive intervention or therapy (for review see references 1 and 2).

MEDICAL HISTORY

For the adult, an initial assessment should include the patient's age, gender, race, menopausal status, and a complete medical, pharmacologic, nutritional, and family history. For the child, a careful maternal gestational history with an emphasis on perinatal or neonatal mortality, birth history, feeding history, and level of usual activity is warranted. In some situations, the chief complaint leads directly to the diagnosis: for example, a hip fracture from osteoporosis, bowing deformity of the legs from rickets, numbness and tingling around the mouth and in the tips of the fingers in a patient with hypocalcemia, or polyuria with hypercalcemia. Other factors may provide strong evidence that an unspecified bone disease is present and prompt the physician to explore further. For example, severe back or bone pain, history of fracture with minimal trauma, prolonged immobilization, loss of height in elderly people, and sunlight deprivation all raise the index of suspicion for the presence of skeletal disease. In children, additional features of growth retardation or short stature, bone pain, muscle weakness, skeletal deformities, extraskeletal calcifications, and waddling gait are suggestive of the presence of metabolic bone disease.

The duration of symptoms also is important: are they lifelong or new? Does the diet contain adequate calcium, phosphorus, and vitamin D? If the diet is insufficient, is there adequate sunlight exposure? Does the patient engage in regular weight-bearing exercise? Does an adult or child with osteopenia engage in activities at play or work that involve a high risk of trauma? A drug history is of vital importance, because many medicines, including over-the-counter preparations, can adversely affect the skeleton. Glucocorticoids, whether inhaled, taken orally, or administered systemically, thyroid hormone, anticonvulsants, and heparin may cause or worsen osteoporosis. Current use of long-acting benzodiazepines and high caffeine intake may increase the risk of osteoporotic hip fracture. Excessive alcohol intake is associated with hypomagnesemia, nutritional deficiencies of calcium, vitamin D, and protein, reduced sunlight exposure, and tendency to fall. Alcohol ingestion also may directly impair osteoblast function. Antacids containing aluminum may lead to aluminum-induced bone disease, typically in the setting of renal insufficiency. Cancer chemotherapy, even years previously, may affect bone. Long-term lithium therapy is associated with hypercalcemia and parathyroid hormone (PTH) hypersecretion (1). Prolonged use of sodium fluoride or the bisphosphonate etidronate can result in osteomalacia. Hypervitaminosis A is associated with excessive bone resorption and bone pain, and vitamin D excess can result in hypercalcemia. Gonadotropin-releasing hormone agonists induce an estrogen-deficient state when given in a continuous manner and may result in reduced bone mass. Diuretics can confound test interpretation by increasing or decreasing urine calcium or by increasing serum alkaline phosphatase activity (2).

The patient should be asked about any history of endocrine, renal, or gastrointestinal disease. Hyper- and hypoparathyroidism, hyperthyroidism, Cushing's syndrome, and sex hormone deficiency all may affect bone remodeling. Gastrectomy or gastric stapling, intestinal-malabsorption syndromes, chronic obstructive biliary disease, and pancreatic insufficiency all can result in osteopenia. Children with cystic fibrosis or chronic cholestatic liver disease are prone to osteopenia.

Data from the Study of Osteoporotic Fractures (SOF), a multicenter cohort of 9709 white women aged 65 years or older, identified historical factors that help to predict hip fracture in older women (3). This study suggests that the risk of hip fracture is higher among women who have had previous fractures of any type after age 50 years, women who rate their own health as fair or poor, and women who spend ≤4 hours a day on their feet. Among the SOF cohort, investigators found that the more weight a woman had gained since age 25 years, the lower her risk of hip fracture. However, if a woman weighed less than she had at age 25 years, this doubled her risk of hip fracture. Women who were tall at age 25 years also had a greater risk.

Because many of the metabolic bone disorders are heritable, a careful family history is important for purposes of screening and educating those at risk, or for recommending genetic counseling. In the SOF cohort, women with a maternal history of hip fracture had a twofold increased risk of hip fracture, independent of bone mass, height, and weight (3). In certain conditions, the diagnosis is firmly established when other family members are tested. For example, in X-linked hypophosphatemic rickets (also called vitamin D–resistant rickets; see Chapter 64), the presence of isolated hypophosphatemia in a heterozygous woman confirms the presence of the trait and its hereditary pattern.

PHYSICAL EXAMINATION

Height and weight should be measured in all patients, and head circumference in children younger than 3 years. A Tanner sexual-maturity rating should be given to all children and adolescents. The clinician should look specifically for any bony deformities or masses, leg-length inequality, vertebral tenderness, a surgical scar on the neck (suggesting previous thyroid or parathyroid surgery), and abnormal gait. Often a single physical finding leads to a specific diagnosis. Blue or gray sclerae suggest osteogenesis imperfecta. These patients also may have deafness, ligamentous laxity with joint hypermobility, diaphoresis, dental defects, and they may bruise easily. Café au lait spots are present in the McCune–Albright syndrome, soft-tissue or mesenchymal tumors in oncogenic rickets/osteomalacia, and premature loss of deciduous teeth in hypophosphatasia. Alopecia, ranging from sparse hair to total alopecia without eyelashes, occurs in two thirds of kindreds with vitamin D–dependent rickets type II.

In rickets, a constellation of physical findings provides the diagnosis. The patient may have short stature, bony tenderness, softened skull (craniotabes), parietal flattening, and frontal bossing. There is often palpable enlargement of the costochondral junctions (the "rachitic rosary"), thickening of the wrists and ankles, flared wrists from metaphyseal widening, Harrison's groove (a horizontal depression along the lower border of the chest, corresponding to the costal insertions of the diaphragm), bowing deformity of the long bones from weight bearing, and waddling gait. The patient also may have reduced muscle strength and tone, lax ligaments, an indentation of the sternum in response to the force exerted by the diaphragm and intercostal muscles, delayed eruption of permanent teeth, and enamel defects. Rickets affects the most rapidly growing bone. Because the skull is growing rapidly at birth, craniotabes is found in congenital rickets. A rachitic rosary is prominent during the first year of life, when the rib cage grows rapidly. Late rickets, which occurs at the time of the adolescent growth spurt, results in a knock-knee deformity. In infants and young children, listlessness and irritability are common. In infants, floppiness and hypotonia are characteristic. Associated syndromic features in children should be evaluated as well during the examination, including ocular and otic abnormalities.

Hypocalcemia is characterized by neuromuscular irritability. This may include varying degrees of tetany, which usually begins with numbness and tingling around the mouth and in the tips of fingers, followed by muscle spasms in the extremities and face. There may be thumb adduction, metacarpophalangeal joint flexion, and interphalangeal joint extension. Latent tetany can be demonstrated by eliciting Chvostek's sign or Trousseau's sign. Chvostek's sign is spasm of facial muscles elicited by tapping the facial nerve in the region of the parotid gland, just anterior to the ear lobe, below the zygomatic arch, or between the zygomatic arch and the corner of the mouth. The response ranges from a twitching of the lip at the corner of the mouth to a twitching of all of the facial muscles on the stimulated side. Slightly positive reactions may occur in up to 10% to 15% of normal adults; it is commonly present in neonates without evidence of pathology. To elicit Trousseau's sign, a sphygmomanometer is inflated on the arm to 20 mm above the systolic blood pressure for 2 to 5 minutes. A positive response consists of carpal spasm with relaxation occurring 5 to 10 seconds after the cuff is deflated. Relaxation should not be immediate. Both Chvostek's and Trousseau's signs can be absent, however, even in severe hypocalcemia.

In patients with idiopathic hypoparathyroidism, the physician should look for signs of the polyglandular failure syndromes: chronic mucocutaneous candidiasis, Addison's disease, alopecia, vitiligo, premature ovarian failure, diabetes mellitus, autoimmune thyroid disease, and pernicious anemia. Pseudohypoparathyroidism presents a constellation of signs, including those of long-standing hypocalcemia and hyperphosphatemia. Symptoms of tetany are common and include carpopedal spasm, tetanic convulsions, paresthesias, muscle cramps, and stridor. There may be soft-tissue calcifications, and posterior subcapsular cataracts develop frequently. Albright's hereditary osteodystrophy refers to a constellation of findings seen in pseudohypoparathyroidism or pseudo-pseudohypoparathyroidism. It includes round facies, short stature, obesity, shortening of the digits (brachydactyly), subcutaneous ossification, and dental hypoplasia. Many patients are mentally retarded. A characteristic shortening of the fourth and fifth digits can be recognized as dimpling over the knuckles of a clenched fist (Archibald's sign).

Most patients with primary hyperparathyroidism usually have no abnormal physical findings. Enlarged parathyroid glands are usually palpable only when parathyroid carcinoma is present, and band keratopathy (calcium–phosphate deposition in the medial and lateral limbic margins of the cornea) is seen rarely and usually only by slit-lamp examination. Extreme elevations of serum calcium may produce an altered sensorium, hypertension, and nonspecific abdominal pain.

Patients with renal osteodystrophy often have characteristic physical findings. Spontaneous tendon rupture may occur in patients with advanced renal failure, almost always in association with marked secondary hyperparathyroidism. Bone deformities are common, especially in patients with severe aluminum toxicity. A funnel-chest abnormality may be produced by rib deformities and kyphoscoliosis. Pseudoclubbing may result from enlargement of the distal tufts of the fingers as a result of osteitis fibrosa. Bowing of long bones, genu valgum, and ulnar deviation of the wrist may be seen in children before epiphyseal closure has occurred, and slipped epiphyses may occur in the periadolescent period.

Patients with Paget's disease usually have no signs of the disease. Over many years, however, progressive cranial involvement can produce increased head size, whereas bowing and enlargement of the long bones may occur with disease of the femur and tibia. Slowly progressive hearing loss, vertigo, tinnitus, or a combination of these can occur in up to 25% of patients with skull involvement. Commonly, there is redness with increased skin temperature over an affected bone. Defects in Bruch's membrane of the retina, termed angioid streaks, may be observed in about 10% of patients. Deformity of the facial bones (leontiasis ossea) may be seen in Paget's disease but is more common in fibrous dysplasia.

Patients with established osteoporosis often exhibit dorsal kyphosis or a gibbus (dowager's hump) and loss of height. They may have a protuberant abdomen (that the patient may confuse with obesity), ribs within the pelvic rim that may be bruised, paravertebral muscle spasm, and thin skin (McConkey's sign). The clinician should look for signs of secondary causes of osteoporosis (e.g., hypogonadism, Cushing's syndrome). In the SOF, four physical findings indicated an increased risk of hip fracture: the inability to rise from a chair without using one's arms, a resting pulse rate of >80 beats/min, poor depth perception, and poorer low-frequency contrast sensitivity (3). By combining these clinical findings with a careful history and bone-density measurement, it may be possible to make a good assessment of hip-fracture risk.

With the availability of sophisticated diagnostic techniques to assess bone density and remodeling, the clinician is faced with new and difficult decisions about test interpretation and resource allocation. A complete history and physical examination continue to be the clinician's most important guides, often providing crucial clues to the origin of skeletal disorders in children and adults.

REFERENCES

1. Bilezikian JP, Marcus R, Levine MA, eds. *The parathyroids, basic and clinical concepts.* New York: Raven Press, 1994:457–470, 721–746, 781–800.
2. DeGroot LJ, Besser M, Burger HG, eds. *Endocrinology.* Philadelphia: WB Saunders, 1995:1136–1150, 1204–1227, 1259–1273.
3. Cummings SR, Nevitt MC, Browner WS, et al. Risk factors for hip fracture in white women: study of Osteoporotic Fractures Research Group. *N Engl J Med* 1995:322:767–773.

19. Blood Calcium, Phosphorus, and Magnesium

Anthony A. Portale, M.D.

Departments of Pediatrics and Medicine, University of California, San Francisco, California

SERUM CALCIUM CONCENTRATION

Calcium in serum exists in three fractions: protein-bound calcium (40%), which is not filtered by the renal glomerulus, and ionized calcium (48%) and complexed calcium (12%), which are filtered by the renal glomerulus (1). Complexed calcium is that bound to various anions, such as phosphate, citrate, and bicarbonate. For clinical purposes, the total concentration of calcium in serum is the most commonly evaluated index of calcium status, although the blood ionized calcium concentration provides a more precise estimate of an individual's calcium status, particularly in critically ill patients.

Total Calcium Concentration

Albumin accounts for 90% of the protein binding of calcium in serum; globulins account for the remainder. Calcium binds to anionic carboxylate groups on the albumin molecule, and in normal serum, fewer than 20% of the binding sites are occupied. Conditions that change the serum concentration of albumin will affect the measurement of total calcium concentration, and under such circumstances, the total calcium concentration may not then accurately reflect the calcium status of the patient. For example, in patients with nephrotic syndrome or hepatic cirrhosis, in whom serum albumin concentration is reduced, the total calcium concentration will decrease, whereas the ionized calcium concentration may remain normal. Several algorithms or nomograms have been developed to correct the total calcium concentration for abnormal values of total protein or albumin or to estimate the "free" calcium concentration (2). Such algorithms, however, do not provide precise estimates of the free calcium concentration and incorrectly predicted the calcium status in 20% to 30% of subjects, as judged from actual measurement of ionized calcium concentration (2). For routine clinical interpretation of serum calcium levels, the simplest formula for "correction" of the total serum calcium concentration for changes in albumin concentration is the following (3): For each 1 g/dL decrease in serum albumin concentration <4.0 g/dL, add 0.8 mg/dL to the measured total calcium concentration; conversely, for each 1 g/dL increase in serum albumin concentration >4.0 g/dL, subtract 0.8 mg/dL from the measured total calcium concentration. Given that the measurement of blood ionized calcium concentration is now widely available in clinical laboratories, the use of estimated values for "free" calcium should be abandoned.

The total calcium concentration in serum exhibits a circadian rhythm characterized by a single nadir and peak, with amplitude (nadir to peak) of approximately 0.5 mg/dL (Table 1) (4,5). This rhythm is thought to reflect hemodynamic changes in serum albumin concentration that result from changes in body posture (6). Prolonged upright posture or venostasis can cause hemoconcentration and thus potentially misleading increases of about 0.5 mg/dL in serum calcium concentration. There is little difference between values taken in fasting and nonfasting states.

Normal values for serum total calcium concentration vary somewhat among clinical laboratories, and in general range from 9.0 to 10.6 mg/dL. In men, the calcium concentration decreases with advancing age from a mean of about 9.6 mg/dL at age 20 years to about 9.2 mg/dL at age 80 years, and the decrease can be accounted for by decrease in serum

TABLE 1. *Characteristics of the circadian rhythms in blood mineral concentration in humans*

	Concentration (mg/dL)		Amplitude (mg/dL)	Phase (h)	
	Fasting	24-h mean	(Nadir to peak)	Nadir	Peak
Total serum calcium	9.6	9.4	0.5	0300	1300
Blood ionized calcium	4.67	4.52	0.3	1900	1000
Serum phosphorus	3.6	4.0	1.2	1100	0200

From Markowitz M, Rotkin L, Rosen JF. Circadian rhythms of blood minerals in humans. *Science* 1981;213:672–674 and Portale AA, Halloran BP, Morris RC JR. Dietary intake of phosphorus modulates the circadian rhythm in serum concentration of phosphorus: implications for the renal production of 1,25-dihydroxyvitamin D. *J Clin Invest* 1987;80:1147–1154.

albumin concentration (7). In women, no change is observed with age. In children, the serum calcium concentration is higher than that in adult subjects, being highest at age 6 to 24 months, the mean about 10.2 mg/dL, decreasing to about 9.8 mg/dL at 6 to 8 years, and decreasing further to adult values at 16 to 20 years (8,9) (Table 2).

For routine determination of total serum calcium concentration, most clinical laboratories use automated spectrophotometric techniques, such as the *o*-cresolphthalein complexone method; the reference method is atomic absorption spectrophotometry (10). Calcium concentrations expressed in mg/dL can be converted to mmol/L (m*M*) by dividing by 4, and to mEq/L by dividing by 2. The atomic weight of calcium is 40.08, and its valence is 2.

Ionized Calcium

Ionized calcium is the fraction of plasma calcium that is important for physiologic processes, such as muscle contraction, blood coagulation, nerve conduction, hormone secretion (parathyroid hormone and 1,25-dihydroxyvitamin D) and action, ion transport, and bone mineralization. In the past, measurement of blood ionized calcium concentration was technically difficult and not widely available in clinical settings. Now readily and accurately measured in most hospital laboratories (11), this measurement is most useful in critically ill patients, particularly those in whom serum protein levels are decreased, acid–base disturbances are present, or to whom large amounts of citrated blood products are

TABLE 2. *Representative normal values for concentrations of blood ionized calcium, serum total calcium, phosphorus, and magnesium*

	Age (yr)	Blood ionized calcium		Serum total calcium (mg/dL)	Phosphorus (mg/dL)	Magnesium (mg/dL)
		(mg/dL)	(m*M*)			
Infants	0–0.25	4.9–5.6	(1.22–1.40)	8.8–11.3	4.8–7.4	1.6–2.5
	1–5	4.9–5.3	(1.22–1.32)	9.4–10.8	4.5–6.2	1.6–2.5
Children	6–12	4.6–5.3	(1.15–1.32)	9.4–10.3	3.6–5.8	1.7–2.3
Men	20	4.5–5.2	(1.12–1.30)	9.1–10.2	2.5–4.5	1.7–2.6
	50	4.5–5.2	(1.12–1.30)	8.9–10.0	2.3–4.1	1.7–2.6
	70	4.5–5.2	(1.12–1.30)	8.8–9.9	2.2–4.0	1.7–2.6
Women	20	4.5–5.2	(1.12–1.30)	8.8–10.0	2.5–4.5	1.7–2.6
	50	4.5–5.2	(1.12–1.30)	8.8–10.0	2.7–4.4	1.7–2.6
	70	4.5–5.2	(1.12–1.30)	8.8–10.0	2.9–4.8	1.7–2.6

Values are approximate, and normal ranges must be determined for each laboratory. Data are from Keating FRJ, Jones JD, Elveback LR, Randall RV. The relation of age and sex to distribution of values in healthy adults of serum, calcium inorganic phosphorus, magnesium, alkaline phosphatase, total proteins, albumin, and blood urea. *J Lab Clin Med* 1961;73:825–834, Arnaud SB, Goldsmith RS, Stickler GB, McCall JT, Arnaud CD. Serum parathyroid hormone and blood minerals: interrelationships in normal children. *Pediatr Res* 1973;7:485–493, Burritt MF, Slockbower JM, Forsman RW, Offord KP, Bergstralh EJ, Smithson WA. Pediatric reference intervals for 19 biologic variables in healthy children. *Mayo Clin Proc* 1990;65:329–336, Bowers GN, Brassard C, Sena S. Measurement of ionized calcium in serum with ion-selective electrodes: a mature technology that can meet the daily service needs. *Clin Chem* 1986;32:1437–1447, Loughead JL, Mimouni F, Tsang RC. Serum ionized calcium concentrations in normal neonates. *Am J Dis Child* 1988;142:516–518, Nelson N, Finnstrom O, Larsson L. Neonatal reference values for ionized calcium, phosphate and magnesium: selection of reference population by optimality criteria. *Scand J Clin Lab Invest* 1987;47:111–117, Specker BL, Lichenstein P, Mimouni F, Gormley C, Tsang RC. Calcium-regulating hormones and minerals from birth to 18 months of age: a cross-sectional study: II. effects of sex, race, age, season, and diet on serum minerals, parathyroid hormone, and calcitonin. *Pediatrics* 1986;77:891–896, Brodehl J, Gellissen K, Weber HP. Postnatal development of tubular phosphate reabsorption. *Clin Nephrol* 1982;17:163–171, Greenberg BG, Winters RW, Graham JB. The normal range of serum inorganic phosphorus and its utility as discriminant in the diagnosis of congenital hypophosphatemia. *J Clin Endocrinol* 1960;20:364–379, and Meites S, ed. *Pediatric clinical chemistry.* Washington: The American Association for Clinical Chemistry, 1989.

given, such as with cardiac surgery or liver transplantation.

The range of values of ionized calcium for normal individuals must be established for each laboratory and will vary depending on which technique is used and whether the measurement is made in serum, plasma, or heparinized whole blood. Measured with currently available, ion-selective electrodes, serum ionized calcium concentrations in healthy adult men and women range from approximately 4.5 to 5.2 mg/dL (1.12 to 1.30 mmol/L), without significant sex differences (10,11). In healthy infants, ionized calcium levels decrease from about 5.8 mg/dL (1.45 mmol/L) at birth to a nadir of 4.9 mg/dL (1.22 mmol/L) at 24 hours of life (12), and increase slightly during the first week of life to 5.4 mg/dL (1.35 mmol/L) (13). Values in young children are slightly higher (by about 0.1 mg/dL) than those in adults until after puberty (10,14).

Calcium binding to albumin is strongly pH dependent between pH 7 and 8; an acute increase or decrease in pH of 0.1 pH units will increase or decrease, respectively, the protein-bound fraction of calcium by about 0.12 mg/dL. Thus in hypocalcemic patients with metabolic acidosis, rapid correction of acidemia with sodium bicarbonate can precipitate tetany, because of increased binding of calcium to albumin and thereby a decrease in ionized calcium concentration. Blood ionized calcium concentrations exhibit a low-amplitude circadian rhythm characterized by a peak at 1000 hours and a nadir at 1800 to 2000 hours, with amplitude (nadir to peak) of 0.3 mg/dL (4). Thus specimens for analysis drawn after the morning give slightly lower values. Specimens must be obtained anaerobically to avoid spurious results due to ex vivo changes in pH. Measurements made in heparinized whole blood tend to be slightly lower than those in serum because of binding of calcium by heparin. Calcium binding to heparin can be minimized by using calcium-titrated heparin (Radiometer Corporation, Copenhagen, Denmark) at a concentration of ≤50 IU/mL, or sodium or lithium heparin at a concentration of ≤15 U/mL (15); under these circumstances, values from serum, plasma, or whole blood are similar. For hospitalized patients, it is recommended that specimens be obtained in the morning fasting state to avoid possible effects of posture, diurnal variation, and food ingestion.

SERUM PHOSPHORUS CONCENTRATION

Phosphorus exists in plasma in two forms: an organic form principally consisting of phospholipids, and an inorganic form (16). Of the total plasma phosphorus of approximately 14 mg/dL, about 8 mg/dL is in the organic form and about 4 mg/dL in the inorganic form. In clinical settings, only the inorganic orthophosphate form is routinely measured. About 15% to 20% of total plasma inorganic phosphorus is protein bound; the remainder, which is filtered by the renal glomerulus, exists principally either as the undissociated or "free" phosphate ions, HPO_4^{2-} and $H_2PO_4^-$, which are present in serum in a ratio of 4 : 1 at pH 7.4, or as phosphate complexed with sodium, calcium, or magnesium.

The terms *phosphorus concentration* and *phosphate concentration* are often used interchangeably, and for clinical purposes, the choice matters little. Phosphorus in the form of the phosphate ion circulates in blood, is filtered by the glomerulus, and is transported across plasma membranes. However, the content of phosphate in plasma, urine, tissue, or foodstuffs is measured and expressed in terms of the amount of elemental phosphorus contained in the specimen: hence use of the term phosphorus concentration.

In healthy subjects ingesting typical diets, the serum phosphorus concentration exhibits a circadian rhythm, characterized by a decrease to a nadir just before noon, an increase to a plateau in late afternoon, and a small further increase to a peak shortly after midnight (Table 1) (4,17). The amplitude (nadir to peak) is approximately 1.2 mg/dL, or 30% of the 24-hour mean level. Increases or decreases in dietary intake of phosphorus induce substantial increases or decreases, respectively, in serum phosphorus levels during late morning, afternoon, and evening, but less or no change in morning-fasting phosphorus levels (17). To minimize the effect of dietary phosphorus on the serum phosphorus concentration, specimens for analysis should be obtained in the morning-fasting state. Specimens obtained in the afternoon are more likely to be affected by diet and may be more useful in monitoring the effect of changes in dietary phosphorus on serum levels of phosphorus, as in patients with renal insufficiency receiving phosphorus-binding agents to suppress secondary hyperparathyroidism. With administration of the phosphorus-binding agent aluminum hydroxide, the decrease in morning-fasting phosphorus levels underestimated the severity of hypophosphatemia observed throughout much of the day (17,18).

Factors other than time of day and diet can affect the serum phosphorus concentration. Presumably because of movement of phosphorus into the cell, the serum phosphorus concentration can be decreased acutely by intravenous infusion of glucose or insulin, ingestion of carbohydrate-rich meals, acute respiratory alkalosis, or infusion or endogenous release of epinephrine. The decrease in phosphorus concentration induced by acute respiratory alkalosis can be as great as 2.0 mg/dL (19). Serum phosphorus concentration can be increased acutely by metabolic acidosis or by intravenous infusion of calcium, the latter presumably due to efflux of inorganic phosphate from red blood cells (20).

There are substantial effects of age on the fasting serum concentration of phosphorus. Serum phosphorus levels are high in infants, ranging from 4.8 to 7.4 mg/dL (mean, 6.2 mg/dL) in the first 3 months of life and decreasing to 4.5 to 5.8 mg/dL (mean, 5.0 mg/dL) at age 1 to 2 years (21). In midchildhood, values range from 3.5 to 5.5 mg/dL (mean, 4.4 mg/dL) and decrease to adult values by late adolescence (8,9,22). In adult men, serum phosphorus levels decrease with age from about 3.5 mg/dL at age 20 years to 3.0 mg/dL at age 70 years (7,22). In women, the values are similar to those of men until after the menopause, when they increase slightly from about 3.4 mg/dL at age 50 to 3.7 mg/dL at age 70 years. Representative normal ranges for serum phosphorus concentration are depicted in Table 2.

The normal range for serum phosphorus concentration is laboratory specific. Phosphorus concentration is most commonly determined by using automated spectrophotometric techniques based on the reaction of phosphate ions with molybdate (10). Phosphorus concentrations should be determined in serum or plasma that has been separated promptly from red blood cells. Prolonged standing or hemolysis of the specimen can lead to a spurious increase in phosphorus concentration. Concentrations of phosphorus expressed as mg/dL can be converted to mmol/L by dividing by 3.1. The atomic weight of phosphorus is 30.98. Because plasma phosphate is a mixture of monovalent and divalent ions, the composite valence of phosphorus in serum (or intravenous solutions) at pH 7.4 is 1.8. At this pH, 1 mmol phosphorus is equal to 1.8 mEq.

SERUM MAGNESIUM CONCENTRATION

As with calcium, magnesium exists in serum in three distinct forms, protein-bound magnesium (30%), which is not filtered by the renal glomerulus, and ionized (55%) and complexed (15%) magnesium, which are (16). Magnesium is bound principally to albumin in a pH-dependent manner similar to that of calcium. Ionized magnesium is the fraction that is important for physiologic processes, including neuromuscular transmission and cardiovascular tone. Measurement of ionized magnesium concentration by using ion-selective electrodes has recently become available in some laboratories; however, its clinical usefulness in evaluating body magnesium status remains to be determined (23–25). For most clinical purposes, the total concentration of magnesium in serum is determined. Most laboratories use automated spectrophotometric techniques; the reference method is atomic absorption spectrophotometry (10).

The serum total magnesium concentration is closely maintained within the narrow range of 1.7 to 2.6 mg/dL. There are no significant differences in magnesium concentration between men and women, nor with respect to age, and values in children are similar to those in adults (Table 2). The circadian variation in magnesium concentration is of low amplitude and not clinically significant. Prolonged standing or hemolysis of the specimen can lead to a spurious increases in serum magnesium concentration. The whole-blood ionized magnesium concentration in healthy volunteers ranges from 0.44 to 0.59 mmol/L, the mean about 0.52 mmol/L. Concentrations expressed as mg/dL can be converted to mmol/L by dividing by 2.4, and to mEq/L by dividing by 1.2. The atomic weight of magnesium is 24.31.

REFERENCES

1. Moore EW. Ionized calcium in normal serum, ultrafiltrates, and whole blood determined by ion-exchange electrodes. *J Clin Invest* 1970; 49:318–334.
2. Ladenson JH, Lewis JW, Boyd JC. Failure of total calcium corrected for protein, albumin, and pH to correctly assess free calcium status. *J Clin Endocrinol Metab* 1978;46:986–993.
3. Serum calcium. *Lancet* 1978;11:858–859.
4. Markowitz M, Rotkin L, Rosen JF. Circadian rhythms of blood minerals in humans. *Science* 1981;213:672–674.
5. Halloran BP, Portale AA, Castro M, Morris RCJ, Goldsmith RS. Serum concentration of 1,25-dihydroxyvitamin D in the human: diurnal variation. *J Clin Endocrinol Metab* 1985;60:1104–1110.
6. Jubiz W, Canterbury JM, Reiss E, Tyler FH. Circadian rhythm in serum parathyroid hormone concentration in human subjects: correlation with serum calcium, phosphate, albumin, and growth hormone levels. *J Clin Invest* 1972;51:2040–2046.
7. Keating FRJ, Jones JD, Elveback LR, Randall RV. The relation of age and sex to distribution of values in healthy adults of serum, calcium inorganic phosphorus, magnesium, alkaline phosphatase, total proteins, albumin, and blood urea. *J Lab Clin Med* 1961;73:825–834.
8. Arnaud SB, Goldsmith RS, Stickler GB, MCcall JT, Arnaud CD. Serum parathyroid hormone and blood minerals: interrelationships in normal children. *Pediatr Res* 1973;7:485–493.
9. Burritt MF, Slockbower JM, Forsman RW, Offord KP, Bergstralh EJ, Smithson WA. Pediatric reference intervals for 19 biologic variables in healthy children. *Mayo Clin Proc* 1990;65:329–336.
10. Pesce AJ, Kaplan LA, eds. *Methods in clinical chemistry*. St. Louis: CV Mosby, 1987.
11. Bowers GN, Brassard C, Sena S. Measurement of ionized calcium in serum with ion-selective electrodes: a mature technology that can meet the daily service needs. *Clin Chem* 1986;32:1437–1447.
12. Loughead JL, Mimouni F, Tsang RC. Serum ionized calcium concentrations in normal neonates. *Am J Dis Child* 1988;142:516–518.
13. Nelson N, Finnstrom O, Larsson L. Neonatal reference values for ionized calcium, phosphate and magnesium: selection of reference population by optimality criteria. *Scand J Clin Lab Invest* 1987; 47:111–117.
14. Specker BL, Lichenstein P, Mimouni F, Gormley C, Tsang RC. Calcium-regulating hormones and minerals from birth to 18 months of age: a cross-sectional study: II. effects of sex, race, age, season, and diet on serum minerals, parathyroid hormone, and calcitonin. *Pediatrics* 1986;77:891–896.
15. Boink ABTJ, Buckley BM, Christiansen TF, et al. IFCC recommendation: recommendation on sampling, transport and storage for the determination of the concentration of ionized calcium in whole blood, plasma and serum. *Clin Chim Acta* 1991;202:S13–S22.
16. Marshall RW. Plasma fractions. In: Nordin BEC, ed. *Calcium, phosphate and magnesium metabolism*. London: Churchill Livingston, 1976:162–185.
17. Portale AA, Halloran BP, Morris RC JR. Dietary intake of phosphorus modulates the circadian rhythm in serum concentration of phosphorus: implications for the renal production of 1,25-dihydroxyvitamin D. *J Clin Invest* 1987;80:1147–1154.
18. Cam JM, Luck VA, Eastwood JB, De Wardener HE. The effect of aluminium hydroxide orally on calcium, phosphorus and aluminium metabolism in normal subjects. *Clin Sci Mol Med* 1976;51:407–414.
19. Mostellar ME, Tuttle EP. Effects of alkalosis on plasma concentration and urinary excretion of inorganic phosphate in man. *J Clin Invest* 1964;43:138–149.
20. Peraino RA, Suki WN. Influence of calcium on renal handling of phosphate. In: Massry SG, Fleisch H, eds. *Renal handling of phosphate*. New York: Plenum, 1980:287–306.
21. Brodehl J, Gellissen K, Weber HP. Postnatal development of tubular phosphate reabsorption. *Clin Nephrol* 1982;17:163–171.
22. Greenberg BG, Winters RW, Graham JB. The normal range of serum inorganic phosphorus and its utility as discriminant in the diagnosis of congenital hypophosphatemia. *J Clin Endocrinol* 1960;20:364–379.
23. Saha H, Harmoinen A, Pietila K, Morsky P, Pasternack A. Measurement of serum ionized versus total levels of magnesium and calcium in hemodialysis patients. *Clin Nephrol* 1996;46:326–331.
24. Cook LA, Mimouni FB. Whole blood ionized magnesium in the healthy neonate. *J Am Coll Nutr* 1997;16:181–183.
25. Steinberger HA, Hanson CW. Outcome-based justification for implementing new point-of-care tests: there is no difference between magnesium replacement based on ionized magnesium and total magnesium as a predictor of development of arrhythmias in the postoperative cardiac surgical patient. *Clin Lab Manag Rev* 1998;12:87–90.
26. Meites S, ed. *Pediatric clinical chemistry*. Washington: The American Association for Clinical Chemistry, 1989.

20. Assay Methods: Parathyroid Hormone, Parathyroid Hormone-Related Protein, and Calcitonin

Eberhard Blind, M.D. and *Robert F. Gagel, M.D.

*Department of Medicine, Endocrinology, University of Würzburg, Würzburg, Germany; and *Department of Internal Medicine Specialties, Section of Endocrine Neoplasia and Hormonal Disorders, University of Texas M.D. Anderson Cancer Center, Houston, Texas*

PARATHYROID HORMONE

Improvements in parathyroid hormone (PTH) measurement methods over the last 20 years have simplified the diagnosis of parathyroid disease. Current assay technology makes it possible to approach the evaluation of an increased or decreased serum calcium concentration with the expectation that parathyroid function can be determined accurately in most patients.

Background: PTH Synthesis, Secretion, and Catabolism

Parathyroid hormone is synthesized as a precursor hormone, which undergoes cleavage during intracellular processing to the major secretory form, an 84-amino-acid straight-chain polypeptide (1). Several features of PTH physiology make measurement of PTH challenging. The first is the low level of circulating hormone; the normal range for the intact PTH (iPTH) molecule is 10 to 65 ng/L (1 to 6 pmol/L) (2), and it is rapidly cleared by liver and kidney (3,4) with a half-life of 2 to 4 minutes. The second is the extensive proteolytic cleavage of PTH during intracellular processing and after secretion by the liver. These cleavage products have different half-lives, resulting in molar concentrations of these fragments that may vary by as much as 5- to 20-fold. The biologically active form of the hormone, PTH 1 to 27 (amino acids 1 to 27; amino fragment) has the shortest half-life and is therefore present at the lowest concentration (Fig. 1). The larger mid- and carboxy-terminal fragments (Fig. 1) have longer half-lives and may interfere with the immunologic measurement of the intact hormone.

Measurement Methods

Two techniques for the measurement of PTH are currently in widespread use: the traditional radioimmunoassay (RIA) and two-site immunologic assays, by using either radioisotopic (IRMA), colorimetric, or chemiluminescence detection methods.

The RIA uses an antibody directed against PTH. A radiolabeled fragment of PTH will bind to the antibody and can be displaced from the antibody by the addition of unlabeled PTH. The assay is performed by adding a constant amount of antibody and radiolabeled PTH to a series of tubes with increasing amounts of unlabeled PTH. The amount of PTH in an unknown sample can be determined by comparing the binding of radiolabeled PTH in the unknown with that in the series of tubes with known amounts of PTH. PTH RIAs for the amino terminal (PTH 1 to 34), midregion (PTH 44 to 68 or PTH), or carboxy terminal (PTH 69 to 84) have been developed. The amino-terminal assays detect the biologically active portion of the molecule, but have had limited usefulness because this PTH fragment has a very short half-life and circulates at very low concentrations, making it unsuitable for normal clinical use. The midregion-specific assays (PTH 44 to 68) provide the greatest sensitivity: the

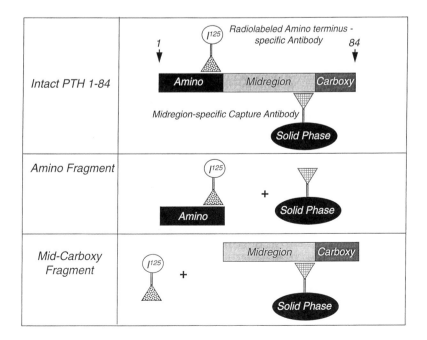

FIG. 1. Two-site immunoradiometric assay for parathyroid hormone (PTH). The capture antibody is bound to a solid phase (plastic bead or test-tube wall) and is used to extract PTH from the serum sample. In this example, the capture antibody is midregion specific and captures the three types of PTH peptides. Intact PTH is completely captured, but an excess of unoccupied capture antibody remains. The bound intact PTH is the only captured species that will bind the 125I-labeled signal antibody (amino-terminal specific in this example). Any amino-terminal PTH fragments that are present also will bind the 125I-labeled antibody, but they will be washed away when the solid phase is rinsed before counting. The number of counts bound to the solid phase after washing increases in direct proportion to the amount of intact PTH in the sample.

antibodies directed against this fragment are of high affinity, and this fragment is normally present in higher concentrations because of its longer half-life. Carboxy-terminal antibodies, although directed against a fragment with long half-life, generally have lower affinity and are therefore less useful for clinical purposes.

Although the midregion PTH RIA provided the first clinically useful measurement technique for PTH, this technique has been supplanted by development of two-site immunologic assays that measure the concentration of intact PTH (5). This type of assay uses two different anti-PTH antibodies (or antibody pools), each recognizing epitopes in a separate region of the intact PTH molecule (top, Fig. 1). One antibody is bound to a solid phase to extract (capture) PTH from the serum sample. The second antibody is labeled (radioisotope, colorimetric, or chemiluminescence) and is used as a "probe" to detect captured molecules that bear both epitopes. Because antibodies are large molecules, multiple sites on each antibody can be labeled, further enhancing the sensitivity of the assay. Hormone fragments that do not bind both antibodies will not be detected (middle and lower panels of Fig. 1). Current assay techniques use capture antibodies directed against epitopes in the 44 to 84 region and a probe antibody directed against epitopes in the 1 to 33 region (top, Fig. 1).

Influence of Renal Function on PTH Assay Results

Fragments of PTH are cleared largely by glomerular filtration. In particular, midregion and carboxy-terminal fragments accumulate in the serum at glomerular filtration rates <40 mL/min and will be detected by RIAs specific for these fragments. This can lead to a false-positive elevation of PTH and an incorrect diagnosis. Midregion PTH values also increase with aging, largely a result of the declining glomerular filtration rate, although secondary hyperparathyroidism caused by inadequate calcium and vitamin D intake in older patients is common.

Intact PTH is cleared in the kidney by peritubular uptake, a process that is better preserved during progressive renal failure than is glomerular filtration (3). Hepatic clearance of intact PTH also continues in renal insufficiency. For these reasons, intact PTH levels are less likely to be falsely elevated when there is a decreased glomerular filtration rate. Renal failure does, however, prolong the half-life of bioactive PTH by a factor of roughly 2, and it has been shown that, in the first few minutes after parathyroidectomy, intact PTH values may decrease less rapidly in those with renal insufficiency.

Specific Uses of PTH Assays

Differential Diagnosis of Hypercalcemia

Parathyroid hormone assays can help differentiate primary hyperparathyroidism from other (nonparathyroid-mediated) forms of hypercalcemia, such as malignancy, sarcoidosis, and thyrotoxicosis. Ninety percent to 95% of patients with primary hyperparathyroidism have elevated values in either intact or midregion PTH assays (6), with a slightly higher

percentage of elevated values found in midregion compared with intact PTH assays.

Intact PTH values are suppressed below the normal range in 70% to 80% of patients with nonparathyroid hypercalcemia and are in the lower half of the normal range in the remainder (7). The suppression of intact PTH in most patients makes it possible to separate patients with nonparathyroid hypercalcemia from those with mild hyperparathyroidism, who will have high normal or slightly abnormal PTH values. The occasional patient with an elevated PTH value in the context of nonparathyroid hypercalcemia may have either concomitant hyperparathyroidism or decreased renal function.

Differential Diagnosis of Hypocalcemia

Measurement of PTH with either intact or midregion assays may help establish the cause of hypocalcemia. The PTH value should be undetectable in total hypoparathyroidism, but it may lie within the normal range if there is only a partial loss or inhibition of parathyroid function (partial hypoparathyroidism or magnesium deficiency, for example). In hypomagnesemic hypocalcemia, PTH values will increase within minutes after parenteral magnesium administration, a change that can be used to confirm the diagnosis of hypomagnesemia-induced parathyroid dysfunction. The PTH value will be increased in pseudohypoparathyroidism.

Measurement of PTH can detect mild degrees of secondary hyperparathyroidism and is useful in situations that predispose to a deficiency of vitamin D or its action (intestinal malabsorption, dietary or environmental vitamin deficiency, resistance to vitamin D action). PTH values also can be used to monitor the adequacy of treatment of secondary hyperparathyroidism. In mild degrees of secondary hyperparathyroidism, without overt hypocalcemia, the PTH value should return to normal with a few days of adequate treatment. If the deficiency of vitamin D action is chronic or severe enough to have caused symptomatic hypocalcemia, however, the PTH values may be markedly elevated (a reflection of parathyroid hyperplasia) and may take several weeks to return to normal after normocalcemia is restored.

Evaluation of Renal Osteodystrophy

One of the goals of managing patients with renal failure is to minimize the rate of parathyroid growth. Measurement of intact PTH provides the clearest indication of parathyroid hyperfunction, because clearance of intact PTH is affected only slightly in renal failure. Values >300 pg/mL often are associated with hyperparathyroid bone disease, although intact PTH values have been shown to decrease rapidly as serum calcium increases during hemodialysis, and there may be considerable variation on this basis.

Midregion PTH measurements are affected to a greater extent by reduced glomerular filtration. One midregion assay was shown to give 4- to 40-fold elevated values in renal patients first entering dialysis and without clinical evidence of bone disease, whereas hemodialysis patients with radiographic and clinical evidence of significant hyperparathyroid bone disease showed values from 60- to 600-fold above normal (6).

Use in Other Metabolic Bone Diseases

The incidence of hyperparathyroidism may be >10% in Paget's disease of bone, and there is evidence for greater activation of Paget's disease in hyperparathyroidism. Screening of pagetic patients with hypercalcemia or those with bone pain for hyperparathyroidism may be appropriate.

Measurement of PTH also may be useful in the assessment of normocalcemic hypophosphatemia. In the hereditary form of hypophosphatemic rickets/osteomalacia, serum PTH values are usually normal unless treatment with neutral phosphate has been instituted. Parathyroid hyperfunction, however, may be found in other forms of hypophosphatemia. Patients with mild vitamin D deficiency may have hypophosphatemia and a normal or minimally reduced serum calcium value, yet show a significant increase in PTH. Patients with the syndrome of oncogenic osteomalacia and hypophosphatemia may have a low serum 1,25-dihydroxyvitamin D_3 values and elevated PTH values.

PARATHYROID HORMONE-RELATED PROTEIN

In 1987, parathyroid hormone-related protein (PTHrP) was identified as the cause of the humoral form of malignancy-associated hypercalcemia. Unlike the PTH gene, PTHrP is expressed in many tissues, and it is thought to act mostly as an autocrine or paracrine local regulator of tissue-specific functions (8).

PTHrP becomes detectable in plasma in states of hypersecretion, of which the most important is the hypercalcemia of malignancy syndrome. It also may have a systemic role during lactation. PTHrP has limited homology with PTH (8 of the first 13 amino acids are identical) and exerts its effects on calcium metabolism by activating the classic PTH/PTHrP receptor of bone and kidney.

PTHrP Fragments in Circulation

PTHrP peptides with lengths of 139, 141, and 173 amino acids are encoded by alternatively processed forms of PTHrP messenger RNA (mRNA). The synthesized proteins may undergo further intracellular or extracellular processing, resulting in several shorter circulating forms of PTHrP. These include an amino-terminal fragment (amino acids 1 to 36), a midregion peptide starting with alanine in position 38 of 50 to 70 amino acids length, and a carboxyl-terminal peptide (9). The amino-terminal PTHrP fragments have PTH-like effects, whereas midregion PTHrP fragments (amino acids 67 to 86) are probably involved in transplacental calcium transport; and some carboxyl-terminal fragments (amino acids 107 to 111) are thought to be osteoclast inhibitors.

PTHrP Immunoassays

Measuring PTHrP plasma levels may be useful (a) in the differential diagnosis of hypercalcemia in the presence of a known or suspected tumor, (b) as a tumor marker in patients with tumors known to be associated with hypercalcemia of malignancy undergoing treatment, and (c) possibly as a prognostic factor for the development of bone metastases, especially in breast cancer.

Methods of Measurement

PTHrP can be determined by using competitive immunoassays [RIAs, enzyme-linked immunosorbent assays (ELISAs)] using antibodies directed against the amino-terminal (amino acids 1 to 34) or the midregion (amino acids 44 to 68 or 53 to 84) fragment, or by using two-site immunometric assays (commercially available) with antibodies against the amino-terminal fragments 1 to 74 or 1 to 86 (similar in design to some PTH assays; see Fig. 1). There is no cross-reactivity with PTH because most assays use antisera directed against nonhomologous portions of the molecule. Because these assays measure different PTHrP fragments, values obtained by different assays cannot be compared easily. The most sensitive assays have a detection level of 0.2 pmol/L; immunoreactive PTHrP is detected in <50% of healthy individuals (10,11). At room temperature, the half-life of PTHrP is approximately 4 hours (12) and is more rapidly degraded in whole blood than in plasma, leading to the recommendation that plasma be separated from blood cells immediately after collection in a tube containing heparin or EDTA (10,13).

Carboxyl-terminal and, to a smaller degree, midregion fragments of PTHrP are cleared by the kidney, and, therefore, a rise in plasma PTHrP is anticipated in renal insufficiency. A specific peptide containing the carboxyl-terminal PTHrP sequence 109 to 136 has been found to be elevated in patients with malignancy-associated hypercalcemia or renal insufficiency (14).

Uses of PTHrP Measurements

PTHrP in Malignancy-Associated Hypercalcemia

Typically, 60% to 80% of all patients with malignancy-associated hypercalcemia have increased amino-terminal PTHrP values (Fig. 2) (15). Similarly, up to 80% of patients have increased values in a midregion PTHrP assay (16). PTHrP values with midregion assays are approximately 10 times higher than those found with amino-terminal assays. More than 80% of patients with malignancy-associated hypercalcemia measured by using a two-site immunometric assay (which requires the amino-terminal and midregion section PTHrP 1 to 74 or 1 to 86) have elevated PTHrP values in plasma (11,14), with a mean concentration of 20 pmol/L and normal values of <5.1 pmol/L in one assay (Fig. 2).

PTHrP in Patients with Solid Tumors

Patients with malignancy-associated hypercalcemia and no evidence of bone metastases almost always have increased PTHrP concentrations (humorally mediated hypercalcemia), as do most hypercalcemic patients with a squamous cell carcinoma (14). The tumors most often associated with increased PTHrP concentrations are cancers of the lung, breast, kidney, bladder, and esophagus.

Patients with breast cancer and hypercalcemia frequently have increased PTHrP values, even when there is extensive bone metastasis (17), blurring the distinction between humorally mediated and locally osteolytic malignancy-associ-

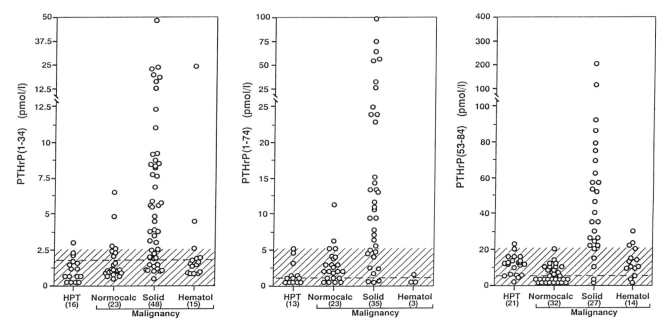

FIG. 2. Plasma concentrations of parathyroid hormone-related protein (PTHrP) in patients with hyperparathyroidism (HPT), normocalcemic patients with malignancy (normocalc), patients with hypercalcemia of malignancy due to a solid tumor (solid), or a hematologic malignancy (hematol). Measurements were performed with a radioimmunoassay for amino-terminal PTHrP(1–34) [**left panel** (15)], an immunoradiometric assay (IRMA) for PTHrP(1–74) [**middle panel** (14)], and a radioimmunoassay (RIA) for midregion PTHrP(53–84) [**right panel** (16)]. The *hatched area* represents the normal ranges; the *dotted line*, the limits of detection. The numbers in parentheses below each group indicate the number of patients. In the PTHrP(1–74) assay group (middle), five patients classified in the "solid" group had local osteolytic hypercalcemia, and two had lymphoma. Reproduced in corrected form from Blind E, Nissenson RA, Strewler GJ. Parathyroid hormone-related protein. In: Becker K, ed. *Principles and practice of endocrinology and metabolism.* Philadelphia: Lippincott, 1995:467–474, with permission.)

ated hypercalcemia. PTHrP is found by immunohistochemical techniques in breast carcinoma bone metastases much more frequently than in extraosseous metastases.

An increased plasma PTHrP is rarely identified in normocalcemic tumor patients, possibly related to lack of assay sensitivity. When these patients become hypercalcemic, however, PTHrP levels become elevated (14,17).

PTHrP in Malignant Hematologic Disease

PTHrP plays only a minor role in the causation of hypercalcemia associated with hematologic malignancy. An exception is adulthood T-cell leukemia/lymphoma syndrome in which human T-cell leukemia/lymphoma virus (HTLV-1) infection-induced hypercalcemia is caused by PTHrP in >50% of the patients. Elevated levels of PTHrP have been found in rare hypercalcemic patients with multiple myeloma, and there is evidence of local production of PTHrP by myeloma cells in some patients.

PTHrP in Primary Hyperparathyroidism and in Differentiating Causes of Hypercalcemia

Plasma PTHrP concentrations are normal in hyperparathyroidism and other nonmalignant causes of hypercalcemia.

It should be clearly stated, however, that an intact PTH measurement is a more powerful discriminator between PTHrP- and PTH-mediated hypercalcemia. Serum intact PTH levels are normally elevated in primary hyperparathyroidism and suppressed in PTHrP-mediated hypercalcemia (see preceding section).

CALCITONIN

The primary RNA transcript of a single gene, CALC I, is alternatively processed to produce an mRNA encoding either calcitonin or calcitonin gene–related peptide. Calcitonin is synthesized as a prohormone and the 32-amino-acid calcitonin monomer is released from the prohormone by amino- and carboxy-terminal proteolytic cleavage (Fig. 3). Calcitonin is produced predominantly in the thyroidal C-cell, although other neuroendocrine cell types produce small amounts, and neoplastic transformation of a variety of cell types is associated with calcitonin production. Secretion of calcitonin from the C-cell is regulated by the extracellular calcium concentration through a calcium-sensing receptor-mediated mechanism.

Measurement Methods

It is now possible to measure normal circulating concentrations of calcitonin by using one of several methods. The

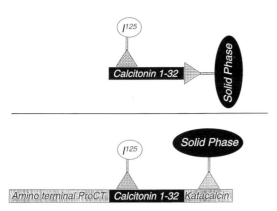

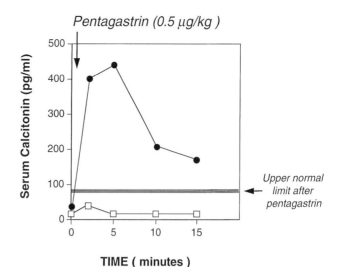

FIG. 4. Pentagastrin test for diagnosis of medullary carcinoma of the thyroid. Pentagastrin was injected intravenously, and serum calcitonin was measured by a standard calcitonin radioimmunoassay at the indicated times (see Appendix). The response of calcitonin to pentagastrin is compared in a normal subject (*open squares*) and a patient with medullary thyroid carcinoma (*closed circles*). The upper limit of normal after pentagastrin stimulation is indicated.

FIG. 3. Two-site immunoradiometric assay for calcitonin **(A)** or procalcitonin **(B)**. Calcitonin is extracted by antibody bound to a solid phase. This antibody recognizes an antigenic site that is present only after cleavage of the carboxyl-flanking peptide of the procalcitonin molecule (katacalcin), so procalcitonin is not extracted. The bound calcitonin is then quantitated with a second antibody labeled with [125]I. The assay for procalcitonin uses an extracting antibody against katacalcin and a labeled antibody against calcitonin.

first is a standard RIA using polyclonal antisera (18,19). Sensitive assays can detect normal circulating concentrations of calcitonin (2 to 10 pg/mL). A second method for calcitonin measurement is the two-site IRMA, chemiluminescent, or colorimetric (ELISA) assay (20), which use affinity-purified polyclonal antibodies directed against two epitopes within the calcitonin monomer to provide a specific and sensitive (2 to 10 pg/mL) assay for calcitonin monomer (Fig. 3). A two-site IRMA with specificity only for procalcitonin has also been developed (20). Its antisera are directed against an epitope in the sequence for calcitonin monomer and a second in the flanking region of calcitonin (katacalcin or carboxy-terminal-adjacent peptide; Fig. 3). Both standard and two-site calcitonin assays are available commercially.

Specific Uses of Calcitonin Assays

Measurement of serum calcitonin is useful in several clinical situations. It is the primary diagnostic tool for diagnosis of medullary thyroid carcinoma (19,21) and may be useful for diagnosis of other tumors in which ectopic production of calcitonin is observed (22). The best diagnostic accuracy is provided by use of a provocative-stimulation technique such as the pentagastrin test (19,21) (Fig. 4), the combined calcium–pentagastrin test, or the short calcium infusion (see Appendix) (19). Interpretation of calcitonin values from these tests is usually straightforward, and most commercial laboratories have well-established normal ranges for basal and provocative-stimulation tests. There are, however, diagnostic pitfalls. In 1% to 5% of tests, measurement of calcitonin with a standard RIA will give an elevated basal serum calcitonin with no additional increase after the provocative stimulation (Fig. 4) (23). This type of result has several possible causes. First, the elevated serum calcitonin may represent a nonspecific RIA result. Such false-positive test results are usually assay specific, and reassay of the samples with an RIA by using a different antiserum or measurement

by using a two-site assay will usually yield a normal result. A second possibility is that the elevated value represents a higher-molecular-weight form of calcitonin, ectopically produced by a tumor other than a medullary thyroid carcinoma (22). It is possible to separate monomeric calcitonin from procalcitonin by use of two-site assays specific for each.

The identification of mutations of the RET protooncogene causative for hereditary medullary thyroid carcinoma (multiple endocrine neoplasia type 2) and the ready availability of mutational analysis has replaced pentagastrin or calcium–pentagastrin testing for routine detection of individuals at risk for hereditary medullary thyroid carcinoma (24). Pentagastrin or combined calcium–pentagastrin testing is of use after total thyroidectomy for medullary thyroid carcinoma to confirm complete removal of all calcitonin-producing C-cells and should be performed periodically in such patients. Serum calcitonin may also be elevated in sepsis (25) and in Williams syndrome.

ACKNOWLEDGMENTS

We thank Lawrence E. Mallette, M.D., Ph.D., for providing an earlier version of a portion of this chapter and for sharing his insight regarding parathyroid hormone measurement.

REFERENCES

1. Keutmann HT, Sauer MM, Hendy GN, O'Riordan JLH, Potts JT Jr. Complete amino acid sequence of human parathyroid hormone. *Biochemistry* 1978;17:5723–5729.
2. Nussbaum SR, Zahradnik RJ, Lavigne JR, et al. Highly sensitive two-site immunoradiometric assay of parathyrin, and its clinical utility in evaluating patients with hypercalcemia. *Clin Chem* 1988;33:1364–1367.

3. Martin KJ, Hruska KA, Lewis J, Anderson C, Slatopolsky E. The renal handling of parathyroid hormone: role of peritubular uptake and glomerular filtration. *J Clin Invest* 1977;60:808–814.

4. Segre GV, Perkins AS, Witters LA, Potts JT Jr. Metabolism of parathyroid hormone by isolated rat Kupffer cells and hepatocytes. *J Clin Invest* 1981;67:449–457.

5. Blind E, Schmidt-Gayk H, Scharla S, et al. Two-site assay of intact parathyroid hormone in the investigation of primary hyperparathyroidism and other disorders of calcium metabolism compared with a midregion assay. *J Clin Endocrinol Metab* 1988;67:353–360.

6. Mallette LE, Tuma SN, Berger RE, Kirkland J. Radioimmunoassay for the middle region of human parathyroid hormone using an homologous antiserum with a carboxy-terminal fragment of bovine PTH as radioligand. *J Clin Endocrinol Metab* 1982;54:1017–1024.

7. Mallette LE, Beck P, VandePol C. Malignancy hypercalcemia: evaluation of parathyroid function and response to treatment. *Am J Med Sci* 1991;302:205–210.

8. Blind E, Nissenson RA, Strewler GJ. Parathyroid hormone-related protein. In: Becker K, ed. *Principles and practice of endocrinology and metabolism.* Philadelphia: Lippincott, 1995:467–474.

9. Orloff JJ, Reddy D, de Papp A, Yang K, Soifer NE, Stewart A. Parathyroid hormone-related protein as a prohormone: posttranslational processing and receptor interactions. *Endocr Rev* 1994;15:40–60.

10. Pandian MR, Morgan CH, Carlton E, Segre GV. Modified immunoradiometric assay of parathyroid hormone-related protein: clinical application in the differential diagnosis of hypercalcemia. *Clin Chem* 1992; 38:282–288.

11. Ratcliffe WA, Norbury S, Heath DA, Ratcliffe JG. Development and validation of an immunoradiometric assay of parathyrin-related protein in unextracted plasma. *Clin Chem* 1991;37:678–685.

12. Wu T, Taylor R, Kao P. Parathyroid-hormone-related peptide immunochemiluminometric assay. *Ann Clin Lab Sci* 1997;27:384–389.

13. Ratcliffe JG. Ectopic hormones—biochemical aspects. *Scott Med J* 1980;25:146–150.

14. Burtis WJ, Brady TG, Orloff JJ, et al. Immunochemical characterization of circulating parathyroid hormone-related protein in patients with humoral hypercalcemia of cancer. *N Engl J Med* 1990;322:1106–1112.

15. Budayr AA, Nissenson RA, Klein RF, et al. Increased serum levels of a parathyroid hormone-like protein in malignancy-associated hypercalcemia. *Ann Intern Med* 1989;111:807–812.

16. Blind E, Raue F, Götzmann J, Schmidt-Gayk H, Kohl B, Ziegler R. Circulating levels of midregional parathyroid hormone-related protein in hypercalcaemia of malignancy. *Clin Endocrinol (Oxf)* 1992;37: 290–297.

17. Bundred NJ, Ratcliffe WA, Walker RA, Coley S, Morrison JM, Ratcliffe JG. Parathyroid hormone related protein and hypercalcemia in breast cancer. *Br Med J* 1991;303:1506–1509.

18. Gagel RF, OBriain DS, Voelkel EF, et al. Pituitary immunoreactive calcitonin-like material: lack of evidence for cross-reactivity with pro-opiomelanocortin. *Metabolism* 1983;32:686–696.

19. Parthemore JG, Bronzert D, Roberts G, Deftos LJ. A short calcium infusion in the diagnosis of medullary thyroid carcinoma. *J Clin Endocrinol Metab* 1974;39:108–111.

20. Seth R, Motte P, Kehely A, et al. A sensitive and specific two-site enzyme-immunoassay for human calcitonin using monoclonal antibodies. *J Endocrinol* 1988;119:351–357.

21. Gagel RF, Tashjian AH, Jr, Cummings T, et al. The clinical outcome of prospective screening for multiple endocrine neoplasia type 2a: an 18-year experience. *N Engl J Med* 1988;318:478–484.

22. Samaan NA, Castillo S, Schultz PN, Khalil-K G, Johnston DA. Serum calcitonin after pentagastrin stimulation in patients with bronchogenic and breast cancer compared to that in patients with medullary thyroid carcinoma. *J Clin Endocrinol Metab* 1980;51:237–241.

23. Body JJ, Heath HI. Nonspecific increases in plasma immunoreactive calcitonin in healthy individuals: discrimination from medullary thyroid carcinoma by a new extraction technique. *Clin Chem* 1984;30:511–514.

24. Eng C, Clayton D, Schuffenecker I, et al. The relationship between specific RET proto-oncogene mutations and disease phenotype in multiple endocrine neoplasia type 2: international RET mutation consortium analysis. *JAMA* 1996;276:1575–1579.

25. Snider RH Jr, Nylen ES, Becker KL. Procalcitonin and its component peptides in systemic inflammation: immunochemical characterization. *J Invest Med* 1997;45:552–560.

21. Vitamin D Metabolites

Bruce W. Hollis, Ph.D., *Thomas L. Clemens, Ph.D., and †John S. Adams, M.D.

*Departments of Pediatrics, Biochemistry, and Molecular Biology, Medical University of South Carolina, Charleston, South Carolina; and *Departments of Medicine and Molecular and Cellular Physiology, University of Cincinnati College of Medicine, Cincinnati, Ohio; and †Department of Medicine, University of California, Los Angeles School of Medicine, and Division of Endocrinology and Metabolism, Cedars-Sinai Medical Center, Los Angeles, California*

Many improvements have been introduced within the last few years with respect to the methods of assessing circulating antirachitic vitamin D sterols. The current assays are all stand-alone types as opposed to multiple-metabolite assays described in years past (1–3); the stand-alone format was chosen because in a clinical situation, a battery of vitamin D metabolite values is seldom required. Further, the assays for 25-hydroxyvitamin D [25 (OH) D] and 1,25-dihydroxyvitamin D [1,25 (OH)$_2$ D] have been optimized as single metabolite procedures (4,5). From a clinical standpoint (see section Clinical Utility of Assays), only measurements of circulating 25 (OH) D and 1,25 (OH)$_2$ D supply useful information, so this chapter deals only with their quantitation. Further information describing the assay of other vitamin D compounds can be found in a more detailed publication (6).

ANALYTIC METHODS

Measurement of 25-Hydroxyvitamin D

Historical Perspective

One of the major factors responsible for the explosion of knowledge related to vitamin D metabolism was the introduction of a valid competitive protein-binding assay for 25 (OH) D in the early 1970s (7,8). Assays for 25 (OH) D involving direct UV-quantitation after high-performance-liquid chromatography appeared soon thereafter (9,10). These assays were all quite cumbersome and involved the use of tritiated tracers, which mandate the use of liquid scintillation counting. The first valid radioimmunoassay (RIA) for assessing circulating 25 (OH) D was introduced

TABLE 1. *Currently available bone biochemical markers*

A. Formation
   Serum
      Bone-specific alkaline phosphatase (BSAP)
      Osteocalcin (OC)
      Carboxy-terminal propeptide of type I collagen (PICP)
      Amino-terminal propeptide of type I collagen (PINP)
B. Resorption
   Urine
      Hydroxyproline
      Free and total pyridinolines (Pyd)
      Free and total deoxypyridinolines (Dpd)
      N-telopeptide of collagen cross-links (NTx)
      C-telopeptide of collagen cross-links (CTx)
   Serum
      Cross-linked C-telopeptide of type I collagen
        (ICTP)
      Tartrate-resistant acid phosphatase (TRAP)

ization of bones and teeth (1). The precise role of BSAP in the mineralization process, however, remains unclear. It may increase local concentrations of inorganic phosphate, destroy local inhibitors of mineral crystal growth, transport phosphate, or act as a calcium-binding protein or Ca^{2+}-adenosine triphosphatase (ATPase).

Circulating alkaline phosphatase (AP) activity is derived from several tissues, including intestine, spleen, kidney, placenta (in pregnancy), liver, and bone, or from various tumors. Thus measurement of total AP activity does not provide specific information on bone formation. However, because the two most common sources of elevated AP levels are liver and bone, a number of techniques, including heat denaturation, chemical inhibition of selective activity, gel electrophoresis, and precipitation by wheat germ lectin have been used to distinguish the liver from bone isoforms of the enzyme. Recent assays, however, have used tissue specific monoclonal antibodies to measure the bone isoform, which has on the order of 10% to 20% cross-reactivity with the liver isoform.

Osteocalcin (OC) is another noncollagenous protein secreted by osteoblasts and is widely accepted as a marker for osteoblastic activity and hence, bone formation. However, it should be kept in mind that OC is incorporated into the matrix and is released into the circulation from the matrix during bone resorption, so the serum level at any one time has a component of both bone formation and resorption. Therefore OC is more properly a marker of bone turnover rather than a specific marker of bone formation. It is a small protein of 49 amino acids and, in most species, contains three residues (at 17, 21, and 24) of γ-carboxyglutamic acid (Gla). The function of OC has not been identified, although its deposition in the bone matrix increases with hydroxyapatite deposition during skeletal growth. *In vitro* studies suggest that OC may function to limit the process of mineralization (2) and *in vivo* studies using OC ''knockout mice'' have found that these mice actually have increases in bone mass (3).

In the circulation, OC is present as the intact molecule and as a fragment or fragments of the intact molecule. It is

unclear whether fragmentation of the intact molecule occurs in the blood or whether this occurs during bone resorption, or both. Whereas older immunoassays that measured various OC fragments often gave widely discordant results even in the same individuals, newer assays measuring the major circulating forms of OC, which are either the intact molecule or a large N-terminal fragment spanning residues 1 to 43 (4), have shown much greater reliability as bone-turnover markers.

As noted earlier, the major synthetic product of osteoblasts is type I collagen, so in principle, indices of type I collagen synthesis would appear to be ideal bone-formation markers. Several such assays have been developed in recent years, directed against either the carboxy- or amino-extension peptides of the procollagen molecule. These extension peptides (carboxy-terminal propeptide of type I collagen, PICP, and amino-terminal propeptide of type I procollagen, PINP) guide assembly of the collagen triple helix and are cleaved from the newly formed molecule in a stoichiometric relation with collagen biosynthesis. However, because type I collagen is not unique to bone, these peptides are also produced by other tissues that synthesize type I collagen, including skin.

Several immunoassays for PICP and PINP have been developed (5,6). Clinically, however, neither of these appears to be as useful as either BSAP or OC in terms of distinguishing normal from disease states. This may, in part, be the result of the inability of current assays to distinguish between bone and soft-tissue contributions to the circulating levels of these peptides.

In contrast to the bone-formation markers, of which the noncollagenous proteins produced by osteoblasts appear to be the most useful markers, the collagen-degradation products, rather than specific osteoclast proteins, are most useful as markers of bone resorption. As the skeleton is resorbed, the collagen-breakdown products are released into the circulation and ultimately cleared by the kidney.

The recent development of rapid and relatively inexpensive immunoassays for various collagen-breakdown products represents perhaps the major advance in this area and one that is likely to greatly increase the clinical utility of the bone-resorption markers. Collagen molecules in the bone matrix are staggered to form fibrils that are joined by covalent cross-links (Fig. 1). These cross-links consist of hydroxylysyl-pyridinolines (pyridinoline, Pyd) and lysyl-pyridinolines (deoxypyridinoline, Dpd). Pyd is present in the skeleton more abundantly than Dpd, but Dpd has greater specificity because Pyd is present to some extent in type II collagen of cartilage and other connective tissues. The Pyd and Dpd cross-links occur at two intermolecular sites in the collagen molecule: at or near residue 930, where two aminotelopeptides are linked to a helical site (N-telopeptide of collagen cross-links, NTx), and at residue 87, where two carboxytelopeptides are linked to a helical site (C-telopeptide of collagen cross-links, CTx; Fig. 1).

When osteoclasts resorb bone, they release a variety of collagen-degradation products into the circulation that are metabolized further by the liver and the kidney. Thus urine contains both free Pyd and Dpd (approximately 40%) and peptide-bound Pyd and Dpd (approximately 60%). The initial assays for Pyd and Dpd measured both free and after acid hydrolysis of urine, total Pyd and Dpd by fluorimetry

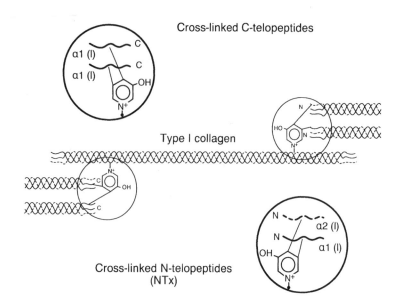

Cross-linked C-telopeptides

Type I collagen

Cross-linked N-telopeptides
(NTx)

FIG. 1. Cross-linked N- and C-telopeptides of type I collagen (Adapted from Calvo MS, Eyre DR, Gundberg CM. Molecular basis and clinical applications of biological markers of bone turnover. *Endocr Rev* 1996;17:333–368, with permission.)

after high-performance liquid chromatography (HPLC) (7). Although this likely remains the gold standard for measuring Pyd and Dpd in urine, it is relatively time consuming and expensive, and there are now a number of immunoassays that can measure free Pyd and Dpd in urine (8).

In addition to the free Pyd and Dpd assays, immunoassays also are available to measure the amino- and carboxy-terminal telopeptides released during bone resorption (NTx and CTx, respectively) (9,10). There are, therefore, a number of rapid and relatively inexpensive methods for assessing urinary bone-resorption markers, each with certain advantages and limitations (discussed later). Moreover, assays also are being developed to measure Dpd, NTx, and CTx in the circulation, which would obviate the need for urine collections. However, these serum markers have not as yet been adequately evaluated and are thus not available for clinical use.

In addition to these assays, there has been another assay available for measuring serum cross-linked C-telopeptide of type I collagen (ICTP), which recognized an antigen in serum, but not in urine. Although this assay has been available for several years, it has been relatively disappointing as a bone-resorption marker (11), and the peptides being recognized in serum have not been fully characterized.

Finally, the only osteoclast-specific product that has been evaluated to any extent as a bone-resorption marker is tartrate-resistant acid phosphatase (TRAP). Acid phosphatase is a lysosomal enzyme that is present in a number of tissues, including bone, prostate, platelets, erythrocytes, and the spleen. Osteoclasts contain a TRAP that is released into the circulation. However, plasma TRAP is not entirely specific for the osteoclast, and the enzyme is relatively unstable in frozen samples. Because of these limitations, TRAP has not been used to any significant extent in the clinical assessment of patients, although the development of immunoassays using monoclonal antibodies specifically directed against the bone isoenzyme of TRAP may improve its clinical utility.

GENERAL CONSIDERATIONS IN THE USE OF BONE BIOCHEMICAL MARKERS

Before discussing the specific clinical settings in which bone biochemical markers might be useful, it is helpful to review certain general issues regarding the use of these markers. First, because all of the currently available bone-resorption markers are based on urinary measurements, they are generally reported after normalizing to creatinine excretion. This has certain limitations, including variability in the creatinine measurement, which contributes to the overall variability in the measurement of the urinary markers (see later), as well as potential artifactual changes in the urinary markers based on alterations in muscle mass. Thus a more appropriate correction might be to express the urinary markers in terms of deciliters or liters of glomerular filtrate, although this is relatively cumbersome in the clinical setting. Nonetheless, this potential for artifact should be kept in mind when interpreting the urinary-excretion markers.

A second issue is that many of the bone-turnover markers have circadian rhythms, so the timing of sampling is of some importance. Thus both serum OC and PICP levels peak in the early morning hours (between 4 a.m. and 8 a.m.), and have nadirs in the middle to late afternoon (12,13). BSAP, which has a long half-life in serum (1 to 2 days), however, does not show much circadian variability. All of the urinary bone-resorption markers also have significant circadian patterns, with peak levels occurring between 4 a.m. and 8 a.m. (14) (Fig. 2). For the urine markers, therefore, it is best to obtain a 24-hour urine collection, or, if that is inconvenient for the patient, a second morning void sample can be used.

A third consideration is that most of the bone-turnover markers tend to be positively associated with age (15), except for a significant decline from adolescence to about age 25 years, as the phase of skeletal consolidation is completed (12). This issue must be kept in mind when normative data for each of the markers are established. Moreover, unlike the

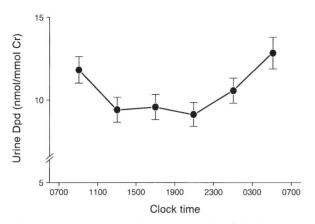

FIG. 2. Urinary Dpd excretion as a function of time in a group of elderly women (mean ± SD, 71 ± 2 years). (Adapted from McKane WR, Khosla S, Egan KS, Robins SP, Burritt MF, Riggs BL. Role of calcium intake in modulating age-related increases in parathyroid function and bone resorption. *J Clin Endocrinol Metab* 1996;81:1699–1703, with permission.)

current World Health Organization definitions for osteopenia and osteoporosis (see Chapter 25), there are currently no accepted criteria for defining high bone turnover. Thus the clinician obtaining the bone-turnover marker should be aware as to whether the reference range for that particular marker is based on young-adult individuals (i.e., age 20 or 25 to 40 years) or on age-matched individuals.

A fourth issue is the potential for differential changes in the various bone-formation or bone-resorption markers in different disease states or in response to different therapies. Thus BSAP tends to show much larger increases in Paget's disease than does OC; conversely, glucocorticoid therapy is associated with larger decrements in OC levels as opposed to BSAP levels (16). Similarly, the urinary excretion of free and peptide-bound fractions of Pyd appears to be differently affected by bisphosphonate and estrogen therapy. Bisphosphonate treatment has been reported to induce a specific decrease of cross-linked peptides without any change in the excretion of free cross-links, whereas estrogen therapy decreases the urinary excretion of both forms of Pyd and Dpd (10).

Finally, one has to be aware of the potential variability (technical and biologic) of the various bone-turnover markers. BMD can be measured by dual-energy x-ray absorptiometry with an accuracy of >95% and a precision error for repeated measurements of between 0.5% and 2.5%. The technology needs to be this good because the rate of change in BMD is slow, and in many circumstances, the annual rate of change is less than the precision error of the measurement. In contrast, the biochemical markers of bone remodeling are subject to intra- and interassay variability (technical variability) as well as individual patient biologic variability. As noted earlier, for the urine-based markers, this variability is compounded by the normalization to creatinine excretion, because there is considerable day-to-day variation of creatinine excretion in individual patients. In general, the long-term variability of the urine-based markers is on the order of 20% to 30% (17,18), and the serum-based markers of

formation on the order of 10% to 15% (19). This issue is considered further later, because it is critical to keep this in mind when these markers are used in the clinical setting.

POTENTIAL CLINICAL USES OF BONE BIOCHEMICAL MARKERS

The Prediction of Bone Mass

Bone biochemical markers assess balance between resorption and formation, and although bone-turnover markers are generally inversely correlated with BMD (20), these correlations are not strong enough to have any value in terms of predicting bone mass for a given individual. Thus these markers cannot and should not be used to diagnose osteoporosis or to predict bone mass; direct measurement of BMD is extremely effective at accomplishing that.

The Prediction of Fracture Risk

This represents perhaps the most intriguing use of bone biochemical markers because, in principle, assessment of bone turnover may provide additional information on fracture risk beyond that provided by BMD. Several studies suggested that bone turnover may be an independent predictor of fracture risk (20–22). Thus, in a prospective cohort study of elderly (older than 75 years) French women, urinary CTx and free Dpd excretion above the upper limit of the premenopausal range (i.e., mean + 2 SD) was associated with an increased risk of hip fracture (Fig. 3), even after adjusting for femoral-neck BMD (22). In recent population-based studies in women, bone-resorption markers were negatively correlated with BMD of the hip, spine, and forearm,

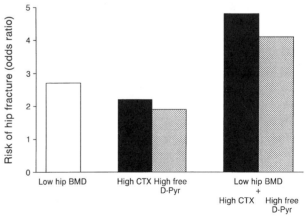

FIG. 3. Combination of the assessment of bone mineral density (BMD) and bone-resorption rate to predict hip fracture risk in a cohort of elderly (mean age, 82.5 years) French women. Low BMD was defined by a value <2.5 SD of the young-adult mean, and high bone resorption by urinary CTx or free Dpd values >2.0 SD of the young-adult mean. (Adapted from Garnero P, Hausherr E, Chapuy MC, et al. Markers of bone resorption predict hip fracture in elderly women: the EPIDOS Prospective Study. *J Bone Miner Res* 1996;11:1531–1538, with permission.)

and women with osteoporosis were more likely to have high bone turnover (20). Moreover, a history of osteoporotic fractures of the hip, spine, or distal forearm was associated with reduced hip BMD and with elevated levels of biochemical markers of bone resorption (20). The mechanisms by which increased bone turnover adversely affects fracture risk include exacerbation of rates of bone loss (23) (see later), microarchitectural deterioration of the skeleton due to perforation of trabeculae and loss of structural elements of bone (24), or a reduction in bone strength due to an enlarged remodeling space (21,25). Thus bone turnover, as assessed by biochemical markers, appears to have a significant impact on the risk of fracture, independent of BMD. However, until more prospective data are available, particularly in younger women than those studied in the French cohort (22), the routine use of bone biochemical markers to complement BMD measurements for prediction of fracture risk cannot be recommended at this time.

The Prediction of Bone Loss

Estrogen deficiency at the menopause increases the rate of bone remodeling, which results in high bone-turnover loss. This is reflected by a significant increase in the mean value of markers of resorption and formation from before to after menopause. Moreover, the individual variability in the bone-turnover markers also increases after the menopause, reflecting a variable skeletal response among different individuals to estrogen deficiency. This also is reflected in the variable rates of bone loss observed among women after the menopause. Several studies have indicated that, at least for groups of individuals, bone biochemical markers can be used to predict the rate of bone loss. Hansen et al. (23) measured the bone mineral content of the forearm at baseline and 12 years later and attempted to predict the observed rate of bone loss by using a biochemical model that included fat mass, serum AP activity, fasting urinary calcium-to-creatinine ratio, and fasting urinary hydroxyproline-to-creatinine ratio. By using these relative crude bone-turnover markers, they were able to predict the observed bone mass 12 years later with a high degree of accuracy (Fig. 4). These and other data (26) suggest that bone-turnover markers, either individually or in combination, may be able to predict rates of bone loss, thus complementing the static measurement of BMD. However, although this appears to be the case for groups of individuals, whether bone-turnover markers can predict the rate of bone loss in a given individual, particularly given the day-to-day variability in some of the markers, remains to be established.

Selection of Patients for Antiresorptive Therapy

Several studies indicated that individuals with the highest levels of bone turnover appear to have the best response to antiresorptive therapy (i.e., with estrogen, calcitonin, or bisphosphonates). In a prospective 2-year study of hormone-replacement therapy (HRT), Chesnut et al. (27) found that subjects in the highest quartiles for baseline urinary NTx excretion demonstrated the greatest gain in BMD in response to HRT (Fig. 5). However, because all of the currently

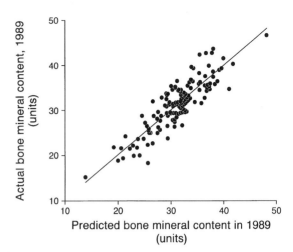

FIG. 4. Predicted versus actual bone mineral content of the forearm in a group of early postmenopausal women studied 12 years apart. Bone mineral content was predicted by using a combination of bone biochemical markers. (Adapted from Hansen MA, Overgaard K, Riis BJ, Christiansen C. Role of peak bone mass and bone loss in postmenopausal osteoporosis: 12 year study. *Br Med J* 1991;303:1548–1549, with permission.)

approved drugs for the prevention or treatment or both of osteoporosis are antiresorptive drugs, it is not clear how useful the ability to predict a gain in BMD in response to therapy would be at present. Nonetheless, this ability will likely become more important as new classes of therapies, such as formation-stimulation agents, become available.

Monitoring Effectiveness of Therapy

This is perhaps the best established clinical use of bone biochemical markers. Considerable data now indicate that

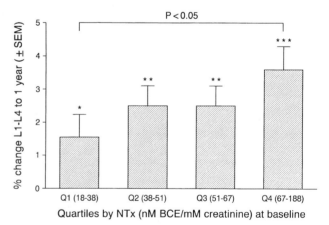

FIG. 5. Response to hormone-replacement therapy at the spine by quartiles of baseline NTx excretion in a group of early postmenopausal women (*p* values vs. baseline bone mineral density: **p* < 0.05; ***p* < 0.001; and ****p* < 0.0001). (Adapted from Chesnut CHI, Bell NH, Clark GS, et al. Hormone replacement therapy in postmenopausal women: urinary N-telopeptide of type I collagen monitors therapeutic effect and predicts response of bone mineral density. *Am J Med* 1997;102:29–37, with permission.)

TABLE 1. *Examples of clinical utilization of DXA in pediatric patients*

Disorder	Findings
Leukemia	Decreased lumbar bone mineral density (BMD) during therapy. Thought to be related primarily to glucocorticoid therapy
(JRA) Juvenile rheumatoid arthritis	Decreased BMD at multiple cortical sites. Related to clinical severity of JRA
JRA	Decreased whole-body BMD. Related to clinical severity of JRA
Turner syndrome	Normal bone mineralization when corrected for weight and pubertal status
Congenital adrenal hyperplasia	Normal bone mineralization on replacement steroids. Not a risk factor for adult osteoporosis
Idiopathic hypercalciuria	Osteopenia in 30%. May be accompanied by low urine citrate and/or high urine uric acid. Negative correlation of BMD and serum calcitriol
Cerebal palsy	Progressive osteopenia with increasing age. Fracture risk more related to spica casting and previous fracture than BMD
Osteogenesis imperfecta	Study showing beneficial effect of bisphosphonate (pamidronate) in two of three patients[a]
JRA (review)	Appendicular skeleton predominantly affected and appendicular measurements best reflect overall bone mineral status
Inflammatory bowel disease	Osteopenia common in IBD. May be related to corticosteroid use, disease activity, or biochemical markers of bone metabolism
Spinal cord injury	Proximal femur demineralization. Different sites in proximal femur correlated with different clinical parameters

[a] From Glorieux FH, Bishop NJ, Plotkin H, Chabot G, Lanoue G, Travers R. Cyclic administration of pamidronate in children with severe osteogenesis imperfecta. *N Engl J Med* 1998;339:986–987.

tween radial and lumbar BMD as measured by DXA is simply due to their individual correlations with age, height, and weight (12). The *Z* scores (standard deviations from the mean) for radial and lumbar DXA examinations had no meaningful correlation. Thus the conclusions regarding the normality or degree of abnormality of bone mineralization for one site were not related to those at another site. In particular, significant demineralization was demonstrated by radial DXA in many patients whose lumbar DXA measurements were within normal limits (12). This may be related to different factors that influence mineralization of cortical bone, as measured in the radius, and of trabecular bone, as measured in the lumbar spine. Evaluation of the effects of different disease states on cortical and trabecular bone will be important. In another pediatric study that compared *Z* scores for the lumbar spine and proximal femur, two sites that contain largely trabecular bone, there was much better correlation (*r* = 0.73). However, even with this seemingly good correlation, the *Z* scores were often disparate, and in many cases different conclusions would be reached for the lumbar spine and proximal femur when a *Z* score of −2 or lower was used to define abnormal (13). The advent of DXA made possible evaluation of the lumbar spine, and because pediatric standards are best established for this site, it is often the only site that is measured. However, measurement of lumbar BMD alone fails to provide the information on cortical bone status that had been measured previously by SPA. Therefore DXA of the lumber spine should be combined with measurement of the radial diaphysis by either

DXA or other methods for overall assessment of bone mineralization in children.

Quantitative Computed Tomography

Quantitative computed tomography is a method whereby computed tomography (CT) scanning is used to measure bone mineral, and this has been performed by using both single-energy and dual-energy techniques. The attenuation numbers for specific regions of interest from the CT scan are compared with those for a phantom with several known concentrations of hydroxyapatite, which is scanned simultaneously. With QCT, the region of interest for bone mineral measurement is a well-defined volume, permitting examination of the trabecular bone within the vertebral bodies without including cortical bone. Furthermore, QCT defines the volume that is being measured rather than its two-dimensional projection, and thus QCT measures bone mineral as a true volume density (g/cm^3), which is less influenced by bone size. By analyzing the difference between regions of interest for the entire vertebra and the trabecular component, one also can determine vertebral cortical bone. By using these techniques, normal values for children have been established, and the factors that influence growth of the cortical and trabecular components of vertebrae in children have been studied (14,15). Cortical BMD increases throughout childhood and correlates well with height, weight, and muscle volume (15), which is similar to the linear growth of

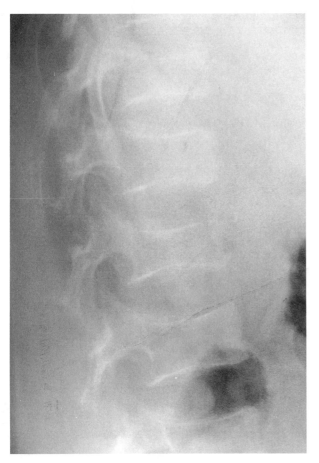

FIG. 2. Multiple compression fractures from osteoporosis in a boy with Crohn's disease. The vertebral bodies are flatter than normal, with indentations on the end plates. Compare with the vertebrae in Fig. 5, which show normal vertebral shape but are abnormally sclerotic.

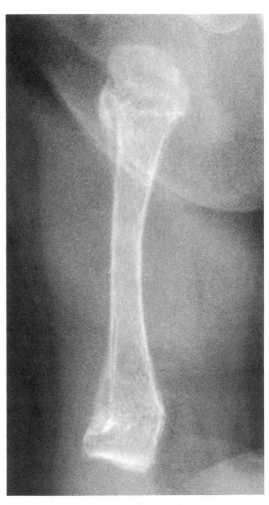

FIG. 3. Multiple femoral fractures in a premature neonate with bronchopulmonary dysplasia. There is callus around the upper femoral fracture. The lower fracture is angulated, with some callus on the lateral side. This is evidence of healing. The poorly mineralized bones in this infant fractured with no known trauma, but from normal handling in the nursery.

diaphyseal cortical bone as demonstrated by SPA (16). Trabecular BMD is relatively constant, however, in preadolescent children and then increases significantly with puberty (14,15). QCT has proven useful is several clinical investigations in children. The osteosclerosis of osteopetrosis has been shown to be due to increased amounts of cortical bone with normal density of the femoral diaphysis, whereas trabecular bone density in the lumbar spine is increased (17). In primary hyperparathyroidism, cortical BMD is decreased, whereas trabecular BMD is increased, suggesting that parathyroid hormone (PTH) may cause a redistribution of bone mineral from cortical to trabecular bone (18). QCT also has been used to investigate the genetic factors that underlie bone mineral development (19). In this study, two of the polymorphisms for the vitamin D–receptor gene were associated with higher vertebral BMD and slightly higher femoral BMD with no difference in cross-sectional area of these sites. Although the ability of QCT to isolate specific regions within the vertebrae is useful, particularly in a research setting, there are several disadvantages, including the cost of the equipment and thus the cost of the examination, the need to compete with other examinations for scanner time,

and the larger radiation dose. The skin-entrance dose has been estimated to be 2 to 15 mSv, and the effective dose equivalent is approximately 50 μSv. QCT also does not have the ability to evaluate regional and whole-body composition, which can be studied by DXA.

QUALITATIVE EVALUATION OF RADIOGRAPHS FOR BONE LOSS

Overall Density

Subjective evaluation of radiographic density is a very inaccurate and inconsistent method for evaluation of bone loss (20). In the spine, >50% of bone can be lost without any evidence on the radiograph because it is mostly cortical bone that is seen on plain radiographs, and much loss of cancellous bone can occur before it is visualized. The apparent density is very dependent on the radiographic technique used; the higher the kilovoltage, the more "washed out" the bone appears. Similarly, not using a high-ratio grid can make the bones look more osteopenic.

Appearance of the Cortex Compared with the Center of Bone

Although both cortical and trabecular bone are usually deficient in patients with osteopenia, there is often relative preservation of the thinned cortex, which stands out sharply against the very lucent trabecular region. This sign is sometimes useful in evaluation of the vertebrae (21), producing a "picture-frame vertebra" with the well-defined vertebral margins surrounding the lucent trabecular center. Similarly, relative cortical preservation in the epiphyses characterizes Wimberger's ring of scurvy, which is simply a manifestation of severe osteopenia. Sometimes focal areas of cortical lucency may be associated with endosteal scalloping (21). Although these findings are useful when present, they are technique dependent.

Appearance of Trabecular Pattern

A coarse trabecular pattern may be useful in evaluating the presence and type of osteopenia; however, it can also be quite inaccurate. Trabecular orientation is related to stress, and with osteopenia, there is relative preservation of those trabeculae that are aligned in the direction of maximal stress. In the spine, the vertically oriented trabeculae are preserved, and thus prominent vertical striations are usually a sign of osteoporosis. Similarly, in the hip, coarse trabeculation may be an indication of osteopenia; in adults, the degree of osteopenia can be graded by the number of trabecular patterns present (22). There is some difference in appearance between the coarse trabecular patterns in osteoporosis and hyperparathyroidism, but usually this is not a reliable differential sign.

Presence of Compression Fractures of the Spine or Fractures of Other Bones

The appearance of anterior wedging or concave end-plate deformities in the spine, seen best in the lateral projections, is a good sign of bone loss (21) (Fig. 2). In children, vertebral compression fractures may occur without any history of trauma in diseases associated with severe bone loss, such as osteogenesis imperfecta, rickets, juvenile rheumatoid arthritis, Crohn's disease, or corticosteroid therapy. Vertebral compressions may be the presenting sign of leukemia or neuroblastoma. Other disorders producing wedged vertebrae include Langerhans' cell histiocytosis, juvenile osteoporosis, Gaucher's disease, and Scheuermann's disease. A square impression on the end plate is seen characteristically in sickle cell disease.

Bone loss can be associated with a variety of fractures of the long bones and of the spine. In hyperparathyroidism, fractures through the growth plates and metaphyses are not uncommon. In osteogenesis imperfecta or in osteoporosis

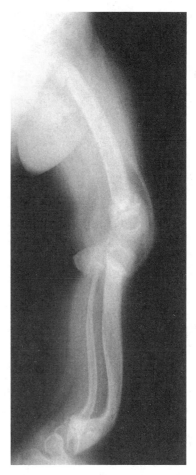

FIG. 4. Bowing of the lower extremity bones in a child with treated rickets. The legs may bend in any direction, depending on the stresses involved.

associated with neuromuscular abnormalities, particularly myelodysplasia, fracture healing with overabundant callus can be seen. In premature neonates receiving total parenteral nutrition, most fractures occur without a history of trauma (Fig. 3).

Presence of Bowing of the Bones in Children

A number of conditions with osteopenia in children will result in bowing of the long bones, particularly rickets (Fig. 4), osteogenesis imperfecta, and fibrous dysplasia. In some cases, there may be associated small cortical breaks on the convex surface. In children with rickets, the bowing is a manifestation of osteomalacia. After treatment for rickets, the bones tend to straighten with growth over time.

Presence of Subperiosteal Resorption and Other Signs of Hyperparathyroidism

Subperiosteal resorption is a pathognomonic manifestation of hyperparathyroidism (23,24). These resorptions are best seen on hand radiographs obtained with either industrial

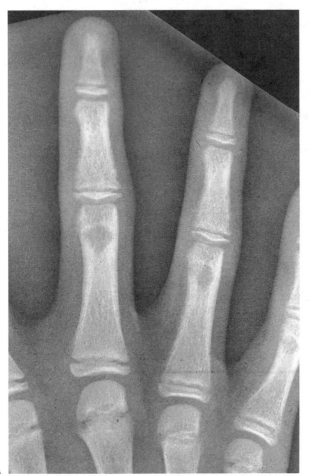

A

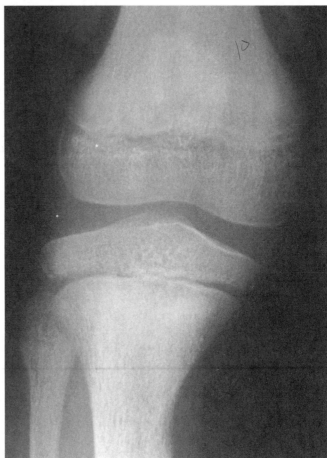

C

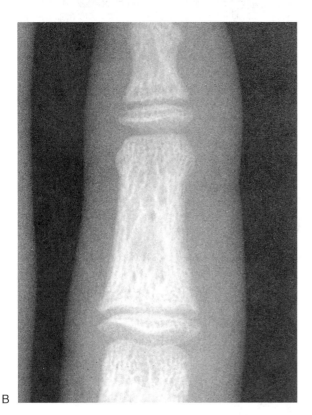

B

FIG. 5. Hyperparathyroidism. **A:** Moderately severe findings. Subperiosteal resorption is present, more prominent along the radial than the ulnar aspects of the middle phalanges, and there also are erosions of the terminal tufts. Lucent defects in the distal portions of the proximal phalanges are brown tumors of hyperparathyroidism. **B:** Child with more subtle findings of hyperparathyroidism. Subperiosteal erosion is more marked on the radial side of the finger. **C:** Erosion of the medial aspect of the proximal tibia in hyperparathyroidism due to renal osteodystrophy.

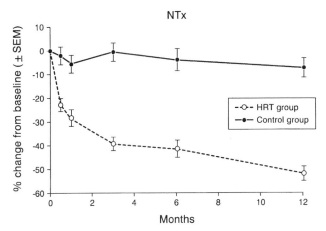

FIG. 6. Percentage change from baseline NTx excretion in early postmenopausal women treated with hormone-replacement therapy or in control women. (Adapted from Chesnut CHI, Bell NH, Clark GS, et al. Hormone replacement therapy in postmenopausal women: urinary N-telopeptide of type I collagen monitors therapeutic effect and predicts response of bone mineral density. *Am J Med* 1997;102:29–37, with permission.)

after initiation of antiresorptive therapy, there is a significant reduction in markers of bone resorption within 4 to 6 weeks (11,28) and in markers of bone formation in 2 to 3 months (11). Thus bone-turnover markers can be used to determine when therapy is ineffective. Antiresorptive agents should produce a reduction in the markers of resorption of between 20% and 80%, depending on the agent and the markers. Despite the potential technical and biologic variability of the markers, changes of this magnitude should be clinically meaningful. For most treatments, the nadir will be reached between 2 to 3 months after initiation and will remain constant as long as the patient is receiving therapy (Fig. 6) (27). Failure to show the expected reduction in resorption markers could indicate noncompliance with therapy or the possible need to change the dose or type of therapy. This use of bone biochemical markers offers a marked advantage over using BMD to assess the effectiveness of therapy, because the interval between serial measurements of BMD must be at least 12 (and possibly 24) months before significant changes in BMD can be documented or, more important, the lack of change in BMD can be established with any certainty.

SUMMARY AND CONCLUSIONS

The availability of biochemical markers of bone formation and resorption that can be measured rapidly and relatively inexpensively is a significant advance in the evaluation and treatment of patients at risk for or with osteoporosis. The markers provide a dynamic assessment of the skeleton that can potentially complement the static measurement of BMD. As with any new technology, however, one needs to understand their limitations and use them in the appropriate clinical setting. The use of these markers is likely to continue to increase with further clinical experience and technical

refinements in the assays. This, in turn, has the potential for resulting in better selection of patients for therapy, tailoring specific therapies to different patients, and better monitoring of the effectiveness of therapy.

REFERENCES

1. Whyte MP. Hypophosphatasia and the role of alkaline phosphatase in skeletal mineralization. *Endocr Rev* 1994;15:439–461.
2. Zhou H, Choong P, McCarthy R, Chou S, Martin T, Ng K. In situ hybridization to show sequential expression of osteoblast gene markers during bone formation in vivo. *J Bone Miner Res* 1994;9:1489–1500.
3. Ducy P, Desbois C, Boyce B, et al. Increased bone formation in osteocalcin-deficient mice. *Nature* 1996;382:448–452.
4. Deftos LJ, Wolfert RL, Hill CS, Burton DW. Two-site assays of bone Gla protein (osteocalcin) demonstrate immunochemical heterogeneity of the intact molecule. *Clin Chem* 1992;38:2318–2321.
5. Melkko J, Niemi S, Risteli L, Risteli J. Radioimmunoassay of the carboxyterminal propeptide of human type I procollagen. *Clin Chem* 1990;36:1328–1332.
6. Melkko J, Kauppila S, Niemi S, et al. Immunoassay for intact amino-terminal propeptide of human type I procollagen. *Clin Chem* 19956; 42:947–954.
7. Black D, Duncan A, Robins SP. Quantitative analysis of the pyridinium crosslinks of collagen in urine using ion-paired reversed-phase high-performance liquid chromatography. *Anal Biochem* 1988;169:197–203.
8. Robins SP, Woitge H, Hesley R, Ju J, Seyedin S, Seibel M. Direct enzyme-linked immunoassay for urinary deoxypyridinoline as a specific marker for measuring bone resorption. *J Bone Miner Res* 1994; 9:1643–1649.
9. Hanson DA, Weis MAE, Bollen A, Maslan SL, Singer FR, Eyre DR. A specific immunoassay for monitoring human bone resorption: quantitation of type I collagen cross-linked N-telopeptides in urine. *J Bone Miner Res* 1992;7:1251–1258.
10. Garnero P, Gineyts E, Arbault P, Christiansen C, Delmas PD. Different effects of bisphosphonate and estrogen therapy on free and peptide-bound bone cross-links excretion. *J Bone Miner Res* 1995;10:641–649.
11. Garnero P, Shih WJ, Gineyts E, Karpf DB, Delmas PD. Comparison of new biochemical markers of bone turnover in late postmenopausal osteoporotic women in response to alendronate treatment. *J Clin Endocrinol Metab* 1994;79:1693–1700.
12. Eastell R, Simmons PS, Colwell A, et al. Nyctohemeral changes in bone turnover assessed by serum bone Gla-protein concentration and urinary deoxypyridinoline excretion: effects of growth and ageing. *Clin Sci* 1992;83:375–382.
13. Hassager C, Risteli J, Risteli L, Jensen SB, Christiansen C. Diurnal variation in serum markers of type I collagen synthesis and degradation in healthy premenopausal women. *J Bone Miner Res* 1992;7:1307–1311.
14. McKane WR, Khosla S, Egan KS, Robins SP, Burritt MF, Riggs BL. Role of calcium intake in modulating age-related increases in parathyroid function and bone resorption [Comments]. *J Clin Endocrinol Metab* 1996;81:1699–1703.
15. Khosla S, Melton LJI, Atkinson EJ, Klee GG, O'Fallon WM, Riggs BL. Relationship of serum sex steroid levels with bone mineral density in aging women and men: a key role for bioavailable estrogen. *J Clin Endocrinol Metab* 1998;83:2266–2274.
16. Duda RJ Jr, O'Brien JF, Katzmann JA, Peterson JM, Mann KG, Riggs BL. Concurrent assays of circulating bone Gla-protein and bone alkaline phosphatase: effects of sex, age, and metabolic bone disease. *J Clin Endocrinol Metab* 1988;66:951–957.
17. Kleerekoper M, Wilson PS, Simpson P. Within subject variability of biochemical markers of bone remodeling in normal older women. *J Bone Miner Res* 1994;9(Suppl 1):S394.
18. Gertz BJ, Shao P, Hanson DA, Quan H, Harris ST, Genant HK. Monitoring bone resorption in early postmenopausal women by an immunoassay for cross-linked collagen peptides in urine. *J Bone Miner Res* 1994;9:135–140.

19. Panteghini M, Pagani F. Biological variation in bone-derived biochemical markers in serum. *Scan J Clin Lab Invest* 1995;55:609–616.

20. Melton LJI, Khosla S, Atkinson EJ, O'Fallon WM, Riggs BL. Relationship of bone turnover to bone density and fractures. *J Bone Miner Res* 1997;12:1083–1091.

21. Riggs BL, Melton LJ III, O'Fallon WM. Drug therapy for vertebral fractures in osteoporosis: evidence that decreases in bone turnover and increases in bone mass both determine antifracture efficacy [Review]. *Bone* 1996;18:197S–201S.

22. Garnero P, Hausherr E, Chapuy MC, et al. Markers of bone resorption predict hip fracture in elderly women: the EPIDOS Prospective Study. *J Bone Miner Res* 1996;11:1531–1538.

23. Hansen MA, Overgaard K, Riis BJ, Christiansen C. Role of peak bone mass and bone loss in postmenopausal osteoporosis: 12 year study. *Br Med J* 1991;303:1548–1549.

24. Parfitt AM. Age-related structural changes in trabecular and cortical bone: cellular mechanisms and biomechanical consequences. *Calcif Tissue Int* 1984;36:S123–S128.

25. Einhorn TA. Bone strength: the bottom line. *Calcif Tissue Int* 1992; 51:333–339.

26. Uebelhart D, Schlemmer A, Johansen JS, Gineyts E, Delmas PD. Effect of menopause and hormone replacement therapy on the urinary excretion of pyridinium cross-links. *J Clin Endocrinol Metab* 1991; 72:367–373.

27. Chesnut CHI, Bell NH, Clark GS, et al. Hormone replacement therapy in postmenopausal women: urinary N-telopeptide of type I collagen monitors therapeutic effect and predicts response of bone mineral density. *Am J Med* 1997;102:29–37.

28. Prestwood KM, Pilbeam CC, Burleson JA, et al. The short term effects of conjugated estrogen on bone turnover in older women. *J Clin Endocrinol Metab* 1994;79:366–371.

23. Radiologic Evaluation of Bone Mineral in Children

Richard M. Shore, M.D. and Andrew K. Poznanski, M.D.

Department of Radiology, Northwestern University Medical School, and Children's Memorial Hospital, Chicago, Illinois

Bone mineral evaluation in childhood is performed for different reasons than that in adults, and the approaches used for this evaluation are consequently different. A major use of bone mineral evaluation in children is in the diagnosis and management of renal osteodystrophy and rickets. It also is useful in many other chronic conditions associated with bone loss, such as inflammatory bowel disease and juvenile rheumatoid arthritis. Bone-mass evaluation also is of value in diverse congenital disorders, such as osteogenesis imperfecta and osteopetrosis. In premature infants, severe bone loss can occur, and radiologic evaluation may be useful in determining its causes.

Bone mineral evaluation in childhood includes both quantitative and qualitative assessments. Because subjective assessment of bone density from skeletal radiographs is a poor indicator of bone mineral status, several techniques are more useful in determining the amount of bone mineral present. These methods are essential in following up bone mineralization longitudinally to evaluate the effects of therapy. Furthermore, children with mild bone mineral disorders often have skeletal radiographs that are within normal limits, and an abnormality can be recognized only with the quantitative techniques. Although these children are often asymptomatic, recognition of subtle mineral abnormalities is important because the disease process may lead to significantly reduced bone mineral mass at the completion of growth and thus predispose to symptomatic osteoporosis during adulthood. Quantitative evaluation alone is nonspecific, however, and should be used in conjunction with qualitative assessment of skeletal radiographs, as well as with other clinical and laboratory data, to determine the mechanism and etiology of bone loss. Rickets, other vitamin deficiencies or poisonings, osteoporosis, hyperparathyroidism, and osteogenesis imperfecta may have typical radiographic appearances. Qualitative findings indicate that bone mineral deficiency is present, and these are important to recognize because they may be the first clinical indication of a bone mineral abnormality.

QUANTITATIVE MEASUREMENTS OF BONE LOSS IN CHILDREN

The techniques that are available for measuring bone mineral in children are similar to those used in adults, although their selection is influenced by the availability of normal values. Quantitative methods that have pediatric applications include radiogrammetry (measurement of cortical dimensions) and multiple methods of quantifying photon absorption by bone, including dual x-ray absorptiometry (DXA) and quantitative computed tomography (QCT).

Radiogrammetry

Measurements of cortical dimensions are usually performed on hand films, although the humerus also is useful in neonates. The second metacarpal is the bone that is most frequently used, and standards have been established for different populations (1). In the United States, the most commonly used standards are those of Garn et al. (2), with the cortical measurements performed at the midshaft of the second metacarpal. A high-detail film screen combination should be used, and the measurements are best made by using a magnifying comparator scaled to measure one tenth of a millimeter. The outside and inside diameters of the cortex are measured. Based on these measurements, cortical thickness, cortical area, and percentage cortical area can all be calculated. One difficulty is that the inside diameter may be poorly defined; this occurs primarily in conditions with rapid bone loss, producing a permeative pattern with a ragged margin.

Cortical bone standards also have been developed for the humerus for neonates of varying gestational ages (3). These humeral measurements are obtained at the midshaft just above the level of the nutrient canal, which is profiled on the frontal view and seen *en face* on the lateral view. As for the second metacarpal, humeral cortical thickness is calculated from measurements of the outside and inside diameters. Premature infants can be monitored longitudinally from birth to determine whether cortical bone mineral is growing along the normal growth curve, as would have occurred *in utero,* or whether significant bone loss has occurred (Fig. 1). In severely ill premature infants, a rapid bone loss occurs mainly by endosteal resorption. This may predispose the infant to fractures, after even ordinary handling.

Virtama and Helela (4) also developed cortical standards for a number of sites in other long bones in a Finnish population. Their values for the second metacarpal are reasonably close to the standards of Garn et al. (2).

Advantages

Radiogrammetry is the simplest, least expensive technique of measuring bone mineral. It is particularly useful in children because good age- and sex-specific standards have been developed for several population groups in the United States, including whites, African Americans, and Mexican Americans (1). In addition to calculation of cortical thickness, these measurements can be used to evaluate whether the bone loss is due to endosteal resorption or lack of periosteal surface apposition. In most causes of pediatric osteoporosis, other than renal osteodystrophy, the usual mechanism of bone loss is increased resorption along the endosteal surface, resulting in a larger medullary space (5). There is also a lack of growth on the outer surface in osteogenesis imperfecta, as well as in chronically ill children with poor nutrition, juvenile rheumatoid arthritis, or Crohn's disease (1,2,5). Because little or no bone is lost from the outer surface, other than with subperiosteal resorption in hyperparathyroidism, a diminished outside diameter is indicative of lack of growth. From the hand radiograph, one can determine the presence or absence of subperiosteal resorption, which is indicative of hyperparathyroidism, or intracortical resorption, which is seen with either hyperparathyroidism or other causes of rapid bone loss. These findings indicate that additional evaluation is needed to determine the mechanism and cause of bone loss. Another advantage of the hand radiograph in children is that skeletal age can be determined, allowing bone mineralization to be compared with either chronologic age or skeletal age-matched control values (5). The latter may be more realistic, particularly for disorders in which there is marked retardation of skeletal maturation or in delayed puberty.

Disadvantages

Radiogrammetry does not measure cancellous bone and does not recognize bone loss within the cortex. The inability to measure cancellous bone mass may seem to be less a problem in children than in adults because osteoporotic fractures of the hip seldom occur in children. Trabecular bone accumulation during childhood is important, however, because it determines how much bone can be lost subsequently during adulthood before symptomatic osteoporosis develops. Intracortical bone loss is not recognized by measurement of cortical thickness, and thus if subperiosteal resorption or increased intracortical striations are seen on the hand radiograph, cortical measurements should not be used. This is seen most often in children with renal osteodystrophy, and in these cases, single-photon absorptiometry (SPA) or DXA is more accurate. Because radiogrammetry has lower precision than SPA or DXA, it is less sensitive than those techniques for recognizing changes over serial examinations.

Dual X-Ray Absorptiometry

Dual x-ray absorptiometry (DXA) was developed to measure bone mineral at multiple sites. By analyzing photon absorption at two different energies, one can calculate the amount of bone mineral, soft tissue, and fat without the need to have constant body-part thickness. This allows determination of whole-body composition as well as the bone mineral content of multiple skeletal sites. The most frequently studied site is the lumbar spine. Additional regions often studied include the proximal femur, the radius, and whole body measurements of both bone mineral and body composition (lean body mass, fat, and mineral).

The major advantage of DXA is its ability to measure skeletal density at sites other than the extremities, especially the lumbar spine and proximal femur. Lumbar examinations typically include the first four lumbar vertebrae, usually studied in the frontal projection. Because DXA is a projectional rather than a cross-sectional method, it includes both the cortical and trabecular components of the vertebra. Normal standards for the lateral view are not as well established as those for the frontal view in adults, and they are not available in children. Studies of normal lumbar bone mineral growth as measured by DXA (frontal view) showed that bone mineral density (BMD) increases throughout childhood, with the greatest rate of increase during puberty (6–8). Similarly, weight and pubertal development were found to be the best clinical predictors of lumbar bone mineral during childhood and adolescence (7). In another study, the major independent determinants of lumbar and whole body BMD were found to be pubertal development in female and weight in male subjects (9).

Although measurement of the lumbar spine by DXA is relatively new, there is a growing amount of clinical experience with using the lumbar spine to monitor children with bone mineral disorders. Table 1 summarizes some of the clinical studies that evaluated the lumbar spine by either dual photoabsorptiometry (DPA) or DXA.

For adequate evaluation of overall bone mineral status, both cortical and trabecular sites should be examined. Several studies in adults showed a poor correlation between those sites that contain mostly cortical bone and those that contain more trabecular bone, such as the spine and hip (10,11). Similarly, in children, most of the correlation be-

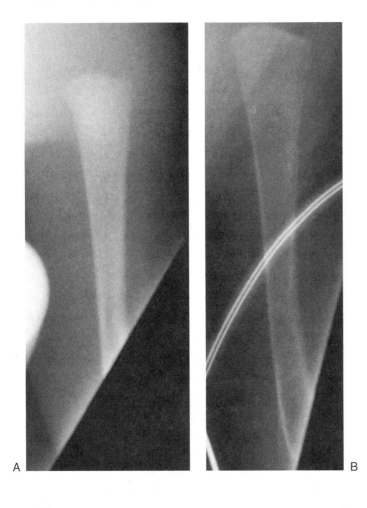

A
B

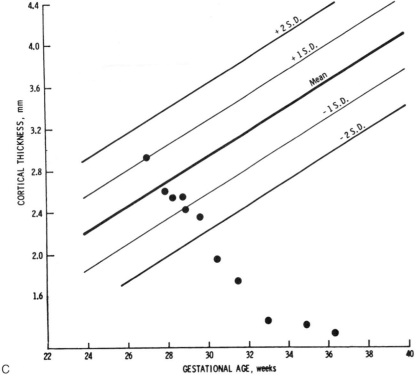

C

FIG. 1. Humerus of a premature infant at birth **(A)** and 6 weeks later **(B)**. Note the marked thinning of the cortex postnatally. Most of the loss occurred by endosteal resorption. The outer diameter has shown little change, but the medullary diameter is considerably wider. Longitudinal humeral cortical-thickness measurements for this patient are shown against the *in utero* growth curve for humeral cortical thickness at birth. **(C)**. At birth, the cortical thickness was 1 SD above the mean, but it decreased rapidly thereafter. At 10 weeks after birth, equivalent to just older than 36 weeks' gestational age, the bone mineral was very low, much lower than that of even a 22-week gestational age infant. (From Poznanski AK, Kuhns LR, Guire KE. New standards of cortical mass in the humerus of neonates: a means of evaluating bone loss in the premature infant. *Radiology* 1980;134:639–644.)

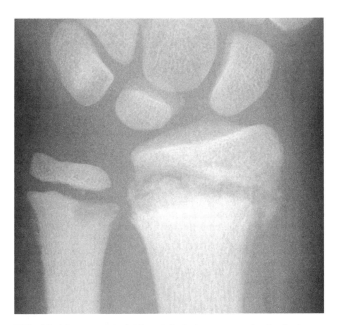

FIG. 11. Trauma mimicking rickets in a young football player who continued to play with a sore wrist for a few weeks. Widening and irregularity of the growth plates is due to un-healed growth-plate fractures of the radius and ulna, which had not been allowed to heal because of motion between the fragments. After casting, healing was complete.

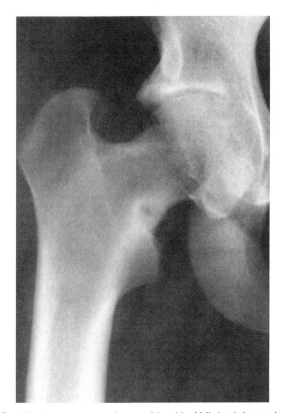

FIG. 12. Looser zone in a girl with X-linked hypophos-phatemic rickets and painful hips. The linear lucency in the medial portion of the femoral neck with sclerosis around it is a typical Looser zone (also called pseudofracture) and is indicative of osteomalacia.

standards for most age groups. When SPA is used in children, a radiograph of the hand and forearm also should be obtained. This permits the evaluation of qualitative signs of bone mineral abnormalities, skeletal maturation, and focal bone abnormalities that would invalidate the bone mineral study. DXA has become more widely available, and because of its versatility, it is a more useful clinical tool that is replacing SPA. DXA examinations should include the lumbar spine and the forearm because evaluation of the lumbar spine alone often fails to recognize cortical demineralization, which can be demonstrated by DXA or SPA studies of the radial diaph-ysis (12). Pending the development of normal values for DXA of the radius in children, DXA measurements can be converted to SPA-equivalent values and used with existing SPA standards (see 12 for conversion). Although QCT is a useful research tool, in most settings, it is not practical for standard clinical monitoring of children with bone mineral disorders.

For determining the presence of rickets, radiography of the knees is the best single view because this is the site of most rapid growth. However, an anteroposterior view of the ankle or wrist also may be used. To detect the pseudofrac-tures of osteomalacia, the best views are the hips or shoul-ders. Radiography of painful areas should be obtained be-cause pseudofractures can occur in other areas.

For evaluating bone mineral status in premature neonates, measurement of cortical thickness of the humerus is probably the simplest and best method. This is often readily obtained from available chest radiographs, so that additional films need not be taken. Because most of the bone loss appears to be the result of endosteal resorption, this measure is an accurate means for evaluating appendicular bone loss. SPA has been used in infants; however, it is difficult to perform, and normal values for infants also are not as well established. DXA may be a potentially useful tool in neonates, but few data are currently available.

REFERENCES

1. Poznanski AK. *The hand in radiologic diagnosis.* Philadelphia: WB Saunders, 1974.
2. Garn SM, Poznanski AK, Nagy JM. Bone measurement in the differen-tial diagnosis of osteopenia and osteoporosis. *Radiology* 1971;100:509–518.
3. Poznanski AK, Kuhns LR, Guire KE. New standards of cortical mass in the humerus of neonates: a means of evaluating bone loss in the premature infant. *Radiology* 1980;134:639–644.
4. Virtama P, Helela T, eds. *Radiographic measurements of cortical bone.* Stockholm: Turku Auraprint Oy, 1969.
5. Poznanski AK. Radiologic evaluation of growth. In: Davidson M, ed. *Growth retardation among children and adolescents with inflammatory bowel disease: report of workshop conducted in Reston, Virginia, March 6–8, 1981.* New York: National Foundation for Ileitis and Colitis, 1983:53–81.
6. Glastre C, Braillon P, David L. Measurement of bone mineral content of the lumbar spine by dual energy X-ray absorptiometry in normal children: correlations with growth parameters. *J Clin Endocrinol Metab* 1990;70:1330–1333.
7. Southard RN, Morris JD, Mahan JD, et al. Bone mass in healthy children: measurement with quantitative DXA. *Radiology* 1991;179:735–738.
8. Kröger H, Kotaniemi A, Kröger L, Alhava E. Development of bone mass and bone density of the spine and femoral neck: a prospective study of 65 children and adolescents. *Bone Miner* 1993;23:171–182.

9. Boot AM, de Ridder MA, Krenning EP, de Muinck Keizer-Schrama SM. Bone mineral density in children and adolescents: relation to puberty, calcium intake, and physical activity. *J Clin Endocrinol Metab* 1997;82:57–62.

10. Mazess RB, Pepper WW, Chesney RW, Lange TA, Lindgren U, Smith E Jr. Does bone measurement on the radius indicate skeletal status? *J Nucl Med* 1984;25:281–288.

11. Seldin DW, Esser PD, Alderson PO. Comparison of bone density measurements from different skeletal sites. *J Nucl Med* 1988;29:158–173.

12. Shore RM, Langman CB, Donovan JM, Conway JJ, Poznanski AK. Bone mineral disorders in children: evaluation with dual X-ray absorptiometry. *Radiology* 1995;196:535–540.

13. Henderson RC. The correlation between dual-energy X-ray absorptiometry measures of bone density in the proximal femur and lumbar spine of children. *Skeletal Radiol* 1997;26:544–547.

14. Gilsanz V, Gibbens DT, Roe TF, et al. Vertebral bone density in children: effect of puberty. *Radiology* 1988;166:847–850.

15. Mora S, Goodman WG, Loro ML, Roe TF, Sayre J, Gilsanz V. Age-related changes in cortical and cancellous vertebral bone density in girls: assessment with quantitative CT. *AJR Am J Roentgenol* 1994;162:405–409.

16. Mazess RB, Cameron JR. Growth of bone in school children: comparison of radiographic morphometry and photon absorptiometry. *Growth* 1972;36:77–92.

17. Kovanlikaya A, Loro ML, Gilsanz V. Pathogenesis of osteosclerosis in autosomal dominant osteopetrosis. *AJR Am J Roentgenol* 1997;168:929–932.

18. Boechat MI, Westra SJ, Van Dop C, Kaufman F, Gilsanz V, Roe TF. Decreased cortical bone and increased cancellous bone in two children with primary hyperparathyroidism. *Metabolism* 1996;45:76–81.

19. Sainz J, Van Tornout JM, Loro ML, Sayre J, Roe TF, Gilsanz V. Vitamin D-receptor gene polymorphisms and bone density in prepubertal American girls of Mexican descent. *N Engl J Med* 1997;337:77–82.

20. Epstein DM, Dalinka MK, Kaplan FS, Arochick JM, Marinelli DL, Kundel HL. Observer variation in the detection of osteopenia. *Skeletal Radiol* 1986;15:347–349.

21. Schneider R. Radiologic methods of evaluating generalized osteopenia. *Orthop Clin North Am* 1984;15:631–651.

22. Singh M, Nagrath AR, Maini PS. Changes in trabecular pattern of the upper end of the femur as an index of osteoporosis. *J Bone Joint Surg Am* 1970;52:457–467.

23. Meema HE, Oreopoulos DG. The mode of progression of subperiosteal resorption in the hyperparathyroidism of chronic renal failure. *Skeletal Radiol* 1983;10:157–160.

24. Debnam JW, Bates ML, Kopelman RC, Teitelbaum SL. Radiological pathological correlations in uremic bone disease. *Radiology* 1977;125:653–658.

25. Weiss A. Incidence of subperiosteal resorption in hyperparathyroidism studied by fine detail bone radiography. *Clin Radiol* 1974;25:273–276.

26. Parfitt AM. Clinical and radiographic manifestations of renal osteodystrophy. In: Davis DS, ed. *Calcium metabolism in renal failure and nephrolithiasis.* New York: John Wiley, 1977:145–195.

27. Meema HE, Oreopoulos DG, DeVeber GA. Arterial calcifications in severe chronic renal disease and their relationship to dialysis treatment, renal transplant, and parathyroidectomy. *Radiology* 1976;121:315–321.

28. Mehls O, Ritz E, Krempien B, et al. Slipped epiphyses in renal osteodystrophy. *Arch Dis Child* 1975;50:545–554.

29. Meema HE, Meema S. Comparison of microradioscopic and morphometric findings in the hand bones with densitometric findings in the proximal radius in thyrotoxicosis and in renal osteodystrophy. *Invest Radiol* 1972;7:88–96.

30. Meema HE, Oreopoulos DG, Meema S. A roentgenologic study of cortical bone resorption in chronic renal failure. *Radiology* 1978;126:67–74.

31. Frame B, Poznanski AK. Conditions that may be confused with rickets. In: DeLuca HJ, ed. *Pediatric diseases related to calcium.* Holland/New York: Elsevier, 1980:269–289.

24. Scintigraphy in Metabolic Bone Disease

Ignac Fogelman, B.Sc., M.D., F.R.C.P. and Gary J. R. Cook, M.B.B.S., M.Sc., M.R.C.P., F.R.C.R.

Department of Radiological Sciences, Guy's, King's College and St. Thomas' Hospital Medical School, and Department of Nuclear Medicine, Guy's Hospital, London, England

Bone scintigraphy was first described by Fleming et al. (1) in 1961 by using strontium 85 as the radiopharmaceutical. Since then both gamma cameras and radiopharmaceuticals have undergone progressive development. Gamma cameras are now able to perform high-resolution imaging routinely in short scan times either as whole-body acquisitions or as a number of localized views of the skeleton. More recently, tomographic imaging has become widely available, and its use has become routine in clinical nuclear medicine, leading to improved sensitivity for lesion detection.

The most commonly used radiopharmaceuticals for bone imaging are labeled with technetium 99m (^{99m}Tc), a radionuclide available to all nuclear medicine departments and with physical properties that make it ideal for acquiring high-resolution data on many physiologic and pathologic processes. Diphosphonate compounds such as methylene diphosphonate (MDP), labeled with ^{99m}Tc, are the most commonly used radiopharmaceuticals for bone scintigraphy. These compounds have the basic structure illustrated in Fig. 1.

The exact mechanism of localization of these compounds in bone is not fully understood, but it is probable that they attach to bone surfaces and are chemisorbed to hydroxyapatite crystals. In a normal skeleton, approximately 30% of an injected dose of ^{99m}Tc-MDP remains in the skeleton, with the majority of uptake being within the first hour. Remaining tracer is cleared from extracellular fluid and blood by renal excretion, and imaging is usually performed at 3 to 4 hours, before there has been significant physical decay of ^{99m}Tc and when the ratio between bone activity and background activity is maximal. The degree of accumulation in bone is

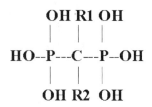

FIG. 1. Structure of diphosphonates where R1 and R2 may differ in different radiopharmaceuticals.

dependent on local blood flow but is influenced more strongly by the degree of osteoblastic activity and hence bone formation. Most pathologic processes that involve bone result in increased local bone turnover, with both osteoblast and osteoclast activity being increased. A bone scan is therefore a functional map of bone turnover, which may be either focal or generalized throughout the skeleton.

Conventionally bone scans are acquired and displayed as planar images, but in recent years, the use of tomography (SPECT, single photon emission computed tomography) in nuclear medicine has become widely available and is increasingly used, particularly in the investigation of back pain. Although spatial resolution is not improved by tomography, there is heightened contrast between abnormalities and adjacent normal structures, increasing the sensitivity of lesion detection. In addition, tomography provides data in three dimensions, so anatomic localization of abnormalities is improved, allowing more specific diagnoses.

In clinical practice, the bone scan is most widely used in malignancy to assess skeletal metastases. In recent years there has been an increase in the applications and use in benign bone diseases including the metabolic bone disorders.

OSTEOPOROSIS

In clinical management of the metabolic bone diseases, the isotope bone scan is most useful in osteoporotic patients, in whom it has a valuable role in evaluation and management. The bone scan has no role in the diagnosis of uncomplicated osteoporosis but is most often used in established osteoporosis to diagnose vertebral fracture. The characteristic appearance of this type of fracture is of intense, linearly increased tracer uptake at the affected site. It should be noted that whereas the bone scan may be positive immediately after fracture, it can take 2 weeks for the scan to become abnormal (2), and thereafter there is a gradual reduction in tracer uptake, with the scan normalizing between 3 and 18 months after the incident, the average being between 9 and 12 months (3) (Fig. 2). Because of this, the bone scan also is extremely useful in assessing the age of fractures. If a patient complains of back pain with multiple vertebral fractures on radiographs, and the bone scan is normal, then this essentially excludes recent fracture as a cause of symptoms, and other causes of pain should then be considered. Currently a vertebral fracture is defined on the basis of morphometry (4), but morphometric abnormalities are not specific to fracture and, for example, may be due to congenital vertebral anomalies. The bone scan may therefore have a role in deciding whether a morphometric abnormality is related to a fracture, provided that it is acquired within several months of the start of symptoms. Ryan and Fogelman (5), by comparing vertebral fractures identified with scintigraphy with morphometric radiographic changes, concluded that only in vertebrae with morphometric deformities >3 standard deviations below the normal mean can fractures be confidently diagnosed. To date this approach has not been used in clinical practice, however.

Because of its great sensitivity, the bone scan also is useful in identifying unsuspected osteoporotic fractures at

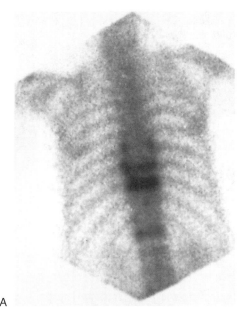

A

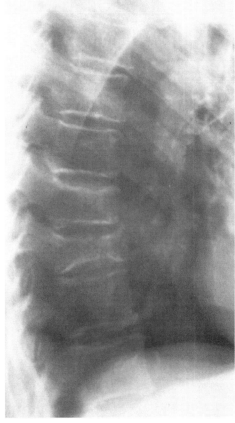

B

FIG. 2. A: ^{99m}Tc-methylene diphosphonate (MDP) bone scan showing typical linear uptake of vertebral fractures. The different intensity suggests they occurred at different times. The fractures are confirmed on the corresponding lateral radiograph **(B)**.

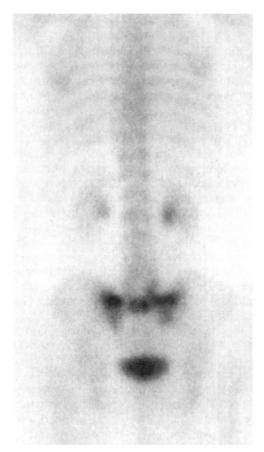

FIG. 3. ^{99m}Tc-methylene diphosphonate (MDP) bone scan performed in a woman with known osteoporosis and buttock pain showing typical features of a sacral insufficiency fracture, which was not detected radiologically.

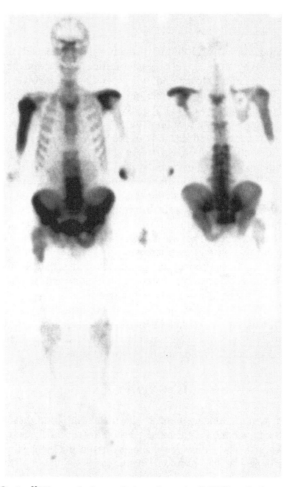

FIG. 5. ^{99m}Tc-methylene diphosphonate (MDP) anterior and posterior whole-body bone scan demonstrating intense activity within a number of bones, with features typical of Paget's disease.

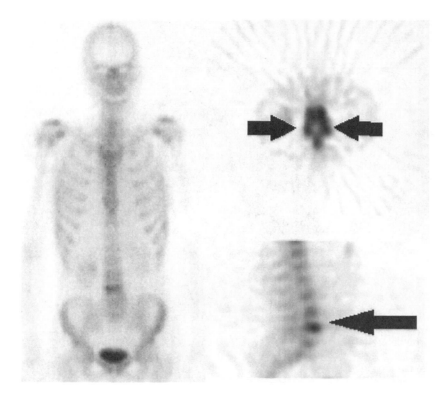

FIG. 4. ^{99m}Tc-methylene diphosphonate (MDP) planar *(left)* and single photon emission computed tomography (SPECT) transaxial *(top)* and sagittal *(bottom)* images. Linear uptake typical of vertebral fracture is seen at L4 on the planar and sagittal images *(large arrow),* but transaxial slices also show increased activity in the facet joints bilaterally *(arrows).*

DIAGNOSIS OF OSTEOPOROSIS BY USING BONE DENSITOMETRY: THE WORLD HEALTH ORGANIZATION CRITERIA

For bone densitometry to be used for the purpose of identifying asymptomatic individuals at risk for fracture, a paradigm shift in the definition of osteoporosis had to occur. Osteoporosis had to be defined on the basis of a level of bone mineral density (BMD) or bone mineral content (BMC) rather than by the presence of a fracture. This process was begun in 1991 by the Consensus Development Conference on Osteoporosis and completed in 1994 by a highly regarded committee of the World Health Organization (WHO) (2). The major justification for changing the diagnostic criteria for osteoporosis from one of prevalent fragility fracture to one of BMD or BMC is the data establishing the higher risk for the second fracture once the first fracture has occurred. This risk is far greater than the increased risk of a first fracture in elderly individuals who have low bone mass[1] alone (4). The logical corollary of these data is the need to identify individuals with low bone mass before the occurrence of the first fracture.

The WHO criteria for the diagnosis of normalcy, osteopenia, and osteoporosis (Table 1) are based on comparisons with peak adult bone mass (PABM). The cutoff of ≥ -2.5 standard deviations (SD) below PABM for the diagnosis of osteoporosis was derived from a population of postmenopausal white women. This cutoff results in a diagnosis of osteoporosis in 30% of postmenopausal white women on an epidemiologic basis, 50% of whom will already have had a fragility fracture. It is important to distinguish the use of bone-density measurements for diagnosis from the use for the prediction of fracture risk. There is a gradient of fracture risk with declining levels of bone mass or density (5). Recognizing this, the WHO created a second diagnostic category of osteopenia (low bone mass) to alert the clinician that individuals with lesser degrees of reduction in bone mass merit attention, particularly if they are postmenopausal or have secondary conditions associated with bone loss. Postmenopausal women not receiving hormone replacement therapy (HRT) will predictably lose bone, as will most women and men receiving medications or diagnosed with medical conditions associated with bone loss. As the emphasis on skeletal health shifts from treatment to prevention, a diagnosis of osteopenia takes on increasing importance. Individuals with osteopenia may experience fragility fractures, particularly when other factors that increase fracture risk above the risk implied by the bone density are present (6). Such factors include, but are not limited to, increased rates of bone turnover, advancing age, and increased likelihood of falling. It is not surprising, therefore, that some of these patients with lesser reductions in BMD and other risk factors may have fragility fractures.

As in all diagnostic criteria, there are strengths and limita-

TABLE 1. *World Health Organization Criteria for the Diagnosis of Osteoporosis based on bone mass or density*

Category	Criteria
Normal	Bone mineral density (BMD) or bone mineral content (BMC) ≤ 1 standard deviations (SD) below average peak young adult
Osteopenia	BMD or BMC >1 SD but <2.5 SD below average peak young adult
Osteoporosis	BMD or BMC ≥ 2.5 SD below average peak young adult
Severe osteoporosis	BMD or BMC ≥ 2.5 SD below average peak young adult and fragility fracture

tions in the WHO criteria for the diagnosis of osteoporosis (Table 2). The WHO criteria provide the practitioner with a straightforward and objective number for the diagnosis of osteoporosis, akin to the classic level of blood pressure of 140/90 mm Hg for the diagnosis of hypertension. Practitioners are now provided with objective criteria that trigger the cognitive process of assessment leading to intervention. In addition, the WHO criteria stress the importance of making a diagnosis of low bone mass (osteopenia) or osteoporosis *before* the first fracture occurs. On the other hand, the cutoff of -2.5 for the diagnosis of osteoporosis has been misinterpreted as an intervention cutoff as well. In addition, with these somewhat arbitrary cutoff levels for diagnosis, a

TABLE 2. *Strengths and limitations of World Health Organization Criteria for the Diagnosis of Osteoporosis based on bone mineral density or bone mineral content*

Strengths	Limitations
Provides a straightforward number for busy practitioners to use for diagnosis	Misused by third-party payors to deny reimbursement
Emphasizes the need to diagnose osteoporosis before first fracture	Based only on data derived from postmenopausal white women
Provides uniform terminology previously lacking in the field	Dependent on accuracy of peak adult bone mass and standard deviations in manufacturers' reference databases
Creates analogous definition of disease based on presence of risk factors for an outcome but not requiring the outcome itself, such as seen with hypertension and hypercholesterolemia	Misinterpreted as intervention thresholds rather than as diagnostic thresholds
	Implies a threshold of bone mass or density rather than gradient for fracture risk
	Classifies sufficiently low bone mass as osteoporosis regardless of pathophysiology

---

[1] In this chapter the terms *bone mass* and *bone mineral density* are used interchangeably and synonymously. It is recognized that bone mass has different connotations for the histomorphologist, and bone mineral density is predominantly an areal-density expression in grams per square centimeter rather than a volumetric-density expression in grams per cubic centimeter.

threshold for fracture is suggested rather than emphasizing the true gradient of fracture risk with declining levels of bone density that actually exists.

Although the limitations appear to outnumber the strengths of the WHO criteria in Table 2, this belies the beneficial impact that the WHO criteria have had on both densitometry and the prevention and management of osteoporosis. The WHO criteria have facilitated the widespread use of bone mass measurement for the identification of individuals at risk for fracture by providing objective criteria with which to interpret densitometry data.

One of the limitations of the WHO criteria is the lack of applicability to women of other races and to men in general. The WHO criteria were based on fracture prevalence in postmenopausal white women. Similar data for men and women of other racial groups is much less well established. Two initial studies suggested that fracture rates in white men per standard deviation reduction in BMD parallel those seen in white women (7,8). It may therefore be reasonable to apply WHO criteria to white men as well. As prospective fracture data are obtained for other races, the applicability of the WHO criteria can be judged. WHO criteria were not intended to be applied to premenopausal women of any race.

Bone mineral density data for the total hip and femoral neck from the National Health and Examination Survey III (NHANES III), acquired in women and men of different races, helped to define the prevalence of osteoporosis at the hip between men and women of different races, based on the BMD levels of the WHO criteria (9). The incorporation of these common reference data into the databases of the three major manufacturers of central dual-energy x-ray (DXA) equipment has eliminated the potential for machine-specific diagnoses of osteoporosis or osteopenia at the hip (10). As mentioned previously, however, the relation between the WHO diagnostic categories and hip fracture risk is unknown, except in elderly white women. Nevertheless, regardless of gender or race, low bone mass, which can be objectively measured by the clinician, is the most important contributor to fragility fracture risk.

A continuing issue is the nonuniform reference databases for skeletal sites other than the hip. A basic principle of statistics is that each sample derived from any given population will yield a different mean and potentially different SD. The mean PABM and the SD from that mean form the basis of the calculation of the T score.[2] As a consequence, an individual may be classified quite differently if different sample populations are used to create the reference database with which the patient is compared (11). This presents substantial clinical difficulties and potential credibility and reimbursement issues. These issues could be resolved by the creation of a standardized reference database for each skeletal site and technique, which could be adopted by all the major manufacturers. This uniform database would then become the "gold standard" with which future databases could be compared. At present, there is no such standard. As

a consequence, different manufacturers' devices, including ultrasound devices, may yield different T scores and possibly different diagnoses when used to measure the same skeletal site or different skeletal sites in the same individual. The lack of a standardized reference database notwithstanding, the various devices themselves can be used to measure BMC per unit volume of bone with extraordinary accuracy and precision (12).

The WHO chose to define osteoporosis based on comparisons of the patient's BMD/BMC with the average BMD/BMC of the young adult by using the T score rather than comparing the patient with age-matched peers. Although bone mass declines with advancing age (13), it is illogical to assume that such bone loss is beneficial or inevitable. If only those individuals who lose more bone than predicted for their age were termed "diseased," many individuals with increased risk of fracture would go unrecognized and untreated. Such individuals would be inappropriately termed "normal." If the prevalence of osteoporosis were defined by using age-matched BMD data, the prevalence of osteoporosis would not increase with age. This is an illogical approach, because declining bone mass increases the risk for fracture, and the prevalence of fracture does increase with age. The use of aged-matched z scores would result in underdiagnosis of osteoporosis (2). This would damage the credibility of bone densitometry by incorrectly reporting "no osteoporosis" or "normal for age" in elderly patients with fragile skeletons and even prevalent fractures. Even if 80% of white women older than 80 years have osteoporosis by using the WHO criteria and by measuring multiple skeletal sites, this is not overdiagnosis, because 50% of these will have a fragility fracture if left untreated (14). Use of young normal BMD as the diagnostic level for subsequent BMD comparisons recognizes the true magnitude of the osteoporotic problem. Therefore osteoporosis was defined as being characterized by low bone mass, resulting in skeletal fragility and susceptibility to fracture, by the 1991 Consensus Conference. The WHO amplified this definition in 1994 with the creation of diagnostic categories based on BMC/BMD expressed as the number of standard deviations below peak bone mass or the T score.

Aged-matched data are appropriate for comparisons in the growing child or adolescent. Once PABM is achieved, the desirable clinical goal is to maintain the bone density at that level, not to prevent losses in excess of those predicted with age. It has often been stated that aged-matched z scores poorer than −2 in the postmenopausal population may indicate the presence of a secondary metabolic process causing bone loss (i.e., something other than aging or estrogen deficiency). Although this is intuitively correct, this suggestion remains an untested hypothesis.

The WHO criteria have been inappropriately applied to healthy, estrogen-replete premenopausal women. This may cause undue fear about fracture risk and the initiation of inappropriate or excessive treatments. The majority of longitudinal data suggest that healthy, estrogen-replete premenopausal women do not lose bone mass (15). Healthy premenopausal women with low bone mass may not have any greater current fracture risk than their age-matched peers with a normal BMD. The scant fracture data available in young people are cross-sectional, include small numbers, or have wide confidence intervals. Healthy young individuals may be

---

[2] T score = (PABM in g/cm^2 − Measured BMD in g/cm^2) ÷ SD of the PABM in g/cm^2. A minus sign is placed in front of the value if the measured BMD lies below the PABM; a plus sign is placed in front of the value if the measured BMD lies above the PABM.

TABLE 3. *Characteristics of central bone densitometry techniques*

Technique	Regions of interest	Precision (%CV)	Units reported
DXA	PA spine	~1	BMD as g/cm^2
	Lateral spine	1.5–3.0	BMC as g
	Proximal femur	1.4–2.3	
	Total body	0.5–1.0	
QCT	Spine	1.0–3.0	BMD as mg/cm^3

BMC, bone mineral content; BMD, bone mineral density; %CV, percentage coefficient of variation; DXA, dual-energy x-ray absorptiomtry; QCT, quantitative computed tomography.

inappropriately restricted in their activities or have reduced quality of life by the inappropriate application of the WHO criteria to a population to whom it was not intended to be applied. Peak adult bone mass follows a normal distribution. The discovery of the low bone mass in otherwise healthy premenopausal women during an initial bone density study does not necessarily mean that bone loss has occurred. This may simply represent a genetically determined low PABM. Such individuals deserve an assessment to exclude secondary causes of potential bone loss, conservative prevention advice, and a repeated bone mass measurement in 2 years to assure stability of the bone mass and prompt protection of their skeleton at the menopause.

No data suggest that additional pharmacologic intervention with bisphosphonates, calcitonin, or estrogen analogues has any value in the premenopausal, estrogen-replete woman. As with all epidemiology-based criteria, the WHO criteria for the diagnosis of osteoporosis based on bone density must be properly applied to be useful.

WHY DO WE PERFORM BONE MASS MEASUREMENTS?

There are three clinical applications of bone mass measurements. Each has a distinct value in clinical decision making. These three applications are (a) diagnosis of osteopenia or osteoporosis, (b) fracture risk prediction, and (c) serial monitoring of BMD to measure response to intervention(s) or diseases/medications that affect bone.

The clinician has at his or her disposal various devices that can measure BMD. Both for practical and reimbursement issues, these devices are generally characterized as those that measure predominantly the central (spine and hip) or peripheral skeleton (wrist, heel, finger; Tables 3 and 4). For each of the three applications of bone-density measurements listed earlier, the central and peripheral devices have both advantages and disadvantages (16,17). All of today's x-ray–based densitometers are accurate and precise. Radiation exposure, whether expressed as the skin dose or effective dose, is correctly characterized as low or negligible. The greatest advantage of the central devices is their versatility. Software applications for these machines make possible the study of virtually every skeletal site. Body composition analysis and skeletal morphometry also are possible with the central devices. The disadvantages of central devices are capital cost and lack of portability, although it should be noted that small table models can be rolled from room to room. These smaller tables, however, tend to be designed to measure only the anteroposterior (AP) spine and proximal femur, sacrificing some versatility for portability. The greatest advantages of peripheral devices are lower capital cost and portability. They lack versatility, however, being designed to measure only one or perhaps two skeletal sites.

The Diagnosis of Osteopenia and Osteoporosis

The diagnosis of osteopenia (*T* score of >-1.0 but <-2.5) is clinically important, independent of any fracture

TABLE 4. *Characteristics of peripheral bone densitometry techniques*

Technique	Regions of interest	Precision (%CV)[a]	Units reported
pDXA	Forearm	1.0–1.7	BMD as g/cm^2 or BMC as g
	Calcaneus	1.0–1.5	
	Phalanges	~1.0	
SXA	Calcaneus	1.3	BMD as g/cm^2
RA	Phalanges	~1.0	
pQCT	Forearm	~1.0	BMD as mg/cm^3
QUS	Calcaneus	0.3–5.4	BUA in db/MHz
	Tibia	0.3	SOS in m/s
			BMD in g/cm^2
			SI, QUI

[a] Precision will vary by the parameter reported and site of measurement. %CV, percentage coefficient of variation; pDXA, peripheral dual-energy x-ray absorptiometry; BMD, bone mineral density; BMC, bone mineral content; SXA, single-energy x-ray absorptiometry; RA, radiographic absorptiometry; pQCT, peripheral quantitative computed tomography; QUS, quantitative ultrasound; BUA, broadband ultrasound attenuation; SOS, speed of sound; SI (stiffness index) and QUI (quantitative ultrasound index) are calculated from BUA and SOS.

risk implications. This diagnostic category represents the range of bone density for which prevention strategies for early postmenopausal bone loss are designed. The recognition of low bone mass in early postmenopausal women facilitates the acceptance of HRT in those who are undecided whether to use it (18). It will most likely be the same for the other Food and Drug Administration (FDA)-approved interventions for the prevention of early postmenopausal bone loss such as bisphosphonates and selective estrogen-receptor modulators (SERMs). These agents are recommended for the prevention of bone loss in postmenopausal women who are unwilling or unable to use HRT.

The utility of central or peripheral sites in detecting osteopenia is dependent on the age of the patient and the particular skeletal site measured. BMD is not the same throughout the skeleton, that is, it is discordant, and this discordance is greater in the early postmenopausal population than in individuals age 65 years and older (19). In older individuals, the greater concordance in BMD at various skeletal sites reduces the likelihood of missing a diagnosis of osteopenia or osteoporosis when measuring only one skeletal site such as the wrist, heel, finger, or hip. The exception in the elderly is a single measurement of the AP spine by DXA, where osteophytes or facet sclerosis of the posterior elements may increase the AP spine BMD values (20). In individuals age 65 years and older then, with the exception of the AP spine, central measurements and peripheral measurements have equivalent value for diagnosing osteopenia or osteoporosis. The lack of prospective fracture data for lateral spine DXA measurements has been a major obstacle to its utilization for this purpose by clinicians. The very strong correlation between BMD of the lumbar spine measured in the lateral projection by DXA and BMD of the spine measured by quantitative computed tomography (QCT), which has adequate fracture predictive value, would strongly suggest that in the elderly, low lateral-spine DXA values should predict increased fracture risk (21).

Although central and peripheral BMD sites appear to have equal diagnostic utility in elderly women, the same may not be true for younger, perimenopausal women because of discordance in BMD among the sites. Discordance in BMD values is greater in the perimenopausal population. There are at least three potential explanations for this discordance:

1. Differences in development of PABM at various sites (22);
2. Differences in rates of bone loss between cancellous bone and cortical bone in the early postmenopausal years; and
3. Differences in the accuracy of measuring BMC by various technologies.

Published studies have not clarified how many early postmenopausal women have normal BMD at one site and osteopenia at another. These differences may not be insignificant. Many early postmenopausal women may need additional BMD testing if a single skeletal site measurement is normal (Table 5). This is particularly true if the woman has additional risk factors for low BMD or if a diagnosis of osteopenia would make a difference in deciding whether to initiate pharmacologic preventive interventions. It is difficult from the standpoint of economics and geographic accessibility to argue that all postmenopausal women with a normal peripheral BMD result need additional BMD testing.

TABLE 5. *Patients with a normal peripheral bone mineral density who may need additional bone-mass testing*

- Patients concerned about osteoporosis, not receiving ERT (estrogen-replacement therapy) but who would accept ERT, bisphosphonates, or selective estrogen-receptor modulators if bone mineral density is found to be low
- Patients at high risk for hip fracture such as those with maternal history of hip fracture, height >5'7", weight <127 lb, or history of smoking
- Patients taking medications associated with bone loss such as glucocorticoids, antiseizure medications, chronic heparin therapy, etc.
- Patients with secondary conditions associated with low bone mass or bone loss such as hyperparathyroidism, malabsorption, hemigastrectomy, hyperthyroidism, etc.
- Patients found to have elevated collagen cross-links >1 SD above upper limit of premenopausal range
- Patients with a history of fragility fracture(s)

Adapted with permission from Miller PD, Bonnick SL, Johnstons CC, et al. The challenges of peripheral bone density testing: which patients need additional central density skeletal measurements? *J Clin Den* 1998;1:211–217.

Therefore guidelines are needed in this circumstance to minimize the potential for misdiagnosis.

There are other patient populations in which a diagnosis of osteopenia may lead to intervention. The prevention of glucocorticoid-induced bone loss is recommended in patients with T scores >-1.0 (23). It also may be appropriate to intervene pharmacologically in other secondary forms of bone loss (i.e., hyperthyroidism, hyperparathyroidism, posttransplantation) on the basis of a finding of osteopenia.

The Prediction of Fracture Risk

There is little debate that low bone mass is the most important predictor of fragility fracture. Approximately 80% of the variance in bone strength and resistance to fracture in animal models is explained by the BMC per unit volume of bone. Other risk factors are predictive of fracture, but the risk is either not so objectively quantifiable as bone mass or it is not modifiable (24). Examples of such risk factors are height >5 ft 7 in, body weight <127 lb, smoking, and maternal history of hip fracture, all of which are strong predictors of hip fracture. BMD, however, is an objective, quantitative measurement that offers clinical value akin to showing a patient's blood pressure or cholesterol measurement on a printed sheet. Bone loss can be halted. Gains in bone density can be achieved. The observation that increased height or maternal history of hip fracture increases fracture risk leads to no intervention that will modify those specific risk factors.

The relation between fracture risk and bone density is best described as a gradient rather than a threshold. Nevertheless, in addition to using the category of osteopenia as a diagnostic cut-off for early postmenopausal intervention decisions, the category can be used as an indicator of current fragility fracture risk in elderly women. A 1.0 SD reduction in BMD is associated with an increased fracture risk and is greater at the same level of BMD as age increases (25). Because bone loss is an otherwise asymptomatic process, identifying lesser reductions in bone mass in early postmenopausal patients with densitometry becomes important. Without intervention to halt bone loss, fracture risk increases as BMD decreases and age increases. Some patients will fracture with a BMD that is only minimally reduced (osteopenia) because of the effects of other factors that increase bone fragility. In some of these patients, the rate of bone turnover, or the nature of a fall, may lead to fracture with only minimal reductions in BMD (6,26,27).

Fracture prediction can be expressed as current fracture risk or lifetime fracture risk. Current fracture risk is the risk potential 3 to 5 years after the bone mass has been measured. Current fracture risk can be expressed as relative risk, absolute risk or incidence, or annual risk. Relative risk, the ratio of two absolute risks, is increased 1.5 to 3.0 times for each SD reduction in BMD (4,28). All of the fracture-risk data in the elderly suggest that fracture prediction is nearly equal regardless of the skeletal site measured or the technique (central or peripheral) used (28,29). This observation is probably related to the high concordance of bone mass at different sites in the elderly population. Thus low BMD measured at one site is more likely to represent a global reduction in BMD. The only exception is in predicting hip-fracture risk, in which the predictive value per SD reduction in BMD appears to be greater at the proximal femoral sites than at other sites (28). This observation does not, however, diminish the strong predictive value that peripheral bone mass measurements have for hip fracture. Data on current fracture risk have been obtained only in older white women. This is primarily because younger women fracture infrequently and are not therefore included in studies designed to determine current fracture risk.

Current fracture risk data should not be applied to younger perimenopausal women or premenopausal healthy women with low PABM. Even though some few cross-sectional data exist to suggest that low BMD in adolescents or premenopausal women is associated with higher current fracture risk, the numbers of patients studied is small or the confidence intervals so wide that conclusions should be drawn cautiously (30,31). Clearly, advancing age older than 60 years is an independent predictor for fracture. In discussing the fracture risk of a 50-year-old woman, it is correct to state that her current fracture risk at any given level of low BMD is substantially lower than that of a 70-year-old with an identical BMD (25). The 50-year-old woman with a low BMD may have a greater lifetime fracture risk than her comparable 50-year-old counterpart with a normal BMD, but no direct data exist to allow the physician to support this conclusion. Most postmenopausal women lose bone mass after the menopause without intervention. Their bone mass is expected to be much lower as they age, which will be associated with an increased current fracture risk. However, all lifetime fracture predictive models are hypothetical, statistical models not yet validated by longitudinal data (32,33). Clinically, however, it is useful to discuss the implications of a low bone mass at the menopause relative to lifetime fracture-risk projections, because it may facilitate the acceptance of HRT or other pharmacologic prevention interventions when indicated. Certainly if the 50-year-old

woman with low bone mass is postmenopausal, she should be strongly advised to investigate all options to maintain her BMD, but projecting beyond what current data will support may lead to substantial alterations in normal life activities that should be avoided.

Serial Assessments of Bone Mass

Bone densitometry can be used for the serial monitoring of BMD of the natural progression of disease processes or the response of bone to pharmacologic interventions. Here there is a clear advantage to central skeletal site testing. In monitoring the response of bone to estrogens, SERMs, bisphosphonates, or calcitonin, the axial skeleton consistently demonstrates the greatest magnitude of change in the shortest time (34,35). The regions of interest in the proximal femur tend to show smaller changes in response to pharmacologic intervention than those in the spine, whereas little or no change is seen at the wrist, finger, or heel. Why these peripheral skeletal sites have a limited response to pharmacologic intervention is unclear. It is not due to the measurement error (precision error) of the peripheral bone mass techniques, which is excellent, usually <1.0%. Several hypotheses have been proposed to explain this observation, such as differences in the bone marrow environment of the peripheral skeleton versus the central skeleton, differences in surface area of bone, and differences in blood flow between the two bone compartments. No matter which hypothesis is correct, the spine and hip are more responsive skeletal sites.

There are some data, although limited, to suggest that forearm sites may be useful in showing a response to estrogen-replacement therapy (ERT) in individual patients (36) and that calcaneal ultrasound may show changes after pharmacologic interventions as well. These data need confirmation by additional studies.

The forearm appears to be the best site to monitor the effects of excess parathyroid hormone activity (37). It also may be a valuable skeletal region to monitor in deciding the timing of parathyroidectomy.

The magnitude of the change between serial BMD measurements can be expressed as either the percentage change (% change) between two measurements or the absolute change (in g/cm^2) between two measurements. Expressing change in either form is acceptable, provided that the precision of the measurement is available from the testing facility. DXA manufacturers may correctly claim, for example, that their devices are capable of a precision error of ≤1% at the AP spine. This in fact may be 3% to 4% in the elderly population with BMD values that are low (38). This is because the precision error, when expressed as the percentage coefficient of variation (%CV) at each skeletal site, increases as the BMD declines (Fig. 1). In addition, variability may be introduced by the technologist during positioning or analysis that will increase the precision error even in individuals with normal BMDs. This variability must be quantified by each densitometry facility if any significance is to be attached to interpretation of serial BMD changes. The change in BMD between two measurements must be at least 2.77 times the precision error for 95% statistical confidence that any real change has occurred. For example, if the precision error

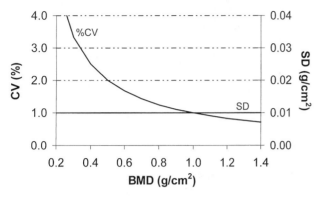

FIG. 1. Precision expressed as %CV or SD across a range of bone mineral density (BMD). Precision, when expressed as the %CV, increases dramatically at lower levels of BMD. When expressed as the SD in g/cm², however, precision remains relatively constant across a wide range of BMD. Graph reproduced courtesy of Dr. K. G. Faulkner, Oregon Osteoporosis Center. %CV, percentage coefficient of variation; SD, standard deviation.

were expressed as a %CV of 1.5%, then a 4.16%[3] change between two BMD measurements would be significant at the 95% confidence level. However, if the precision error were 3%, then almost a 9%[4] change is needed to be 95% confident that a true change in BMD has occurred. Misleading conclusions may be drawn based on the failure to recognize nonsignificant serial changes with attending inappropriate alterations in treatments if precision errors are not known.

Using absolute change in BMD expressed in g/cm² rather than percentage change has a smaller margin of error in expressing interval BMD change, because precision expressed as the SD of BMD is rather constant over wide ranges of BMD (Fig. 1). Any change in BMD >0.04 g/cm² at the AP spine or 0.05 g/cm² at the femoral neck will generally be significant at the 95% confidence level. Absolute change is calculated by subtracting the second BMD measurement from the baseline measurement. In the medical literature, serial change has generally been expressed as percentage change. Both ways of expressing interval BMD change are valid, but it is imperative that clinical facilities document their precision error. BMD testing for serial monitoring is generally performed no more often than every 12 to 24 months, depending on the disease process or therapeutic intervention being monitored and the precision error of the site being measured. In patients who have a documented response in bone density to pharmacologic intervention, which may be defined as either a gain or no loss in BMD, annual BMD measurements are not necessary. In patients with a documented response to ERT, BMD measurements every 3 to 5 years are reasonable in the anticipation of improving the recognized poor long-term compliance to

HRT. Even in elderly women who have previously been documented as estrogen responders, a 3- to 5-year BMD testing interval may be used to document continuing skeletal preservation, because age-related factors may induce BMD loss even with continued estrogen use (39).

It is very difficult to compare serial changes in BMD when measurements are performed on different manufacturers' machines. It is often difficult to compare values obtained on different machines from the same manufacturer. It would be ideal if patients had serial measurements performed on the same machine by the same technician. This is unrealistic, as patients move from city to city or from one payer's plan to another within the same city. Given the proprietary design of these devices and differences in calibration, the absolute BMD values in an individual patient will not be the same. Even when the machines are from the same manufacturer, slight differences in calibration or differences in technique during data acquisition will introduce sources of error. The creation of the standardized BMD (sBMD) by the International Bone Densitometry Standards Committee has made better comparisons possible for data obtained on different manufacturers' machines. Utilizing the calculated sBMD of the spine and total hip for serial comparison reduces but does not eliminate the variance in the measurements. As a general clinical rule, even when using the sBMD, an additional 1% precision error should be added in calculating the percentage change between measurements performed on machines from different manufacturers.

IMPLICATIONS OF YOUNG-NORMAL REFERENCE DATABASES: FROM CHILDHOOD TO THE ACHIEVEMENT OF PABM

Bone mineral content increases during linear growth in children and adolescents and appears to plateau around age 20 years. Many clinical situations often require the measurement of BMC/BMD in growing children. Such situations include children with multiple fractures, children receiving medications such as long-term glucocorticoids for asthma or posttransplantation or antiseizure medications and some forms of chemotherapy, and adolescents with eating disorders. All of these situations may be associated with impaired BMC accretion and increased skeletal fragility. In addition, multiple fractures in children with BMC/BMD consistent with their chronologic and Tanner-stage peers may raise the suspicion of child abuse.

To attach any significance to BMC or BMD in growing children, prospective data that are race and gender-specific from birth to 20 years must be available. Whereas a substantial amount of cross-sectional normative data exist, very little prospective, longitudinal normative data exist, which also adjusts for body mass index, body fat, and height or bone age (40). As more prospective normative data are acquired, it will need to be incorporated into manufacturers' software. Until such time as data from longitudinal studies are incorporated, any given child's BMC/BMD can be compared only with the existing manufacturer's database. The association between bone age, assessed predominantly by wrist or hand radiographs and pubertal age, chronologic age, and BMC/BMD is very high. Therefore bone age does not need to be

---

[3] Magnitude of change necessary for 95% confidence ≥1.5% × 2.77 or 4.16%.

[4] Magnitude of change necessary for 95% confidence ≥3% × 2.77 or 8.31%.

assessed if there is no large gap between chronologic age and pubertal age (41).

CONCLUSIONS

Bone densitometry has revolutionized the clinical approach to the disease osteoporosis much as the sphygmomanometer revolutionized the field of hypertension and the prediction of the risk of stroke. Densitometry provides a measurement of BMD that is directly related to fracture. If densitometry is used responsibly and competently, patient care will be enhanced. The measurement of BMD enables physicians and their patients to make informed decisions regarding preventive and therapeutic strategies. It also allows physicians to monitor the efficacy of these interventions.

REFERENCES

1. Miller PD, Bonnick SL, Rosen CJ. Clinical utility of bone mass measurements in adults: consensus of an international panel. *Semin Arthritis Rheum* 1996;25:361–372.
2. The WHO Study Group. *Assessment of fracture risk and its application to screening for postmenopausal osteoporosis.* Geneva: World Health Organization, 1994.
3. Pouilles JM, Ribot C, Tremollieres F, Bonneu M, Brun S. Risk factors of vertebral osteoporosis: results of a study of 2279 women referred to a menopause clinic. *Rev Rhum Mal Osteo-Artic* 1991;58:169–177.
4. Ross PD, Davis JW, Epstein RS, Wasnich RD. Pre-existing fractures and bone mass predict vertebral fracture incidence in women. *Ann Intern Med* 1991;114:919–923.
5. Huang C, Ross PD, Wasnich RD. Short-term and long-term fracture prediction by bone mass measurements: a prospective study. *J Bone Miner Res* 1998;13:107–113.
6. Riis BJ, Hansen MA, Jensen AM, Overgaard K, Christiansen C. Low bone mass and fast rate of bone loss at menopause: equal risk factors for future fracture: a 15-year follow-up study. *Bone* 1996;19:9–12.
7. Lunt M, Felsenberg D, Reeve J, et al. Bone density variation and its effect on risk of vertebral deformity in men and women studied in thirteen European centers: the EVOS study. *J Bone Miner Res* 1997;12:1883–1894.
8. Mussolino ME, Looker AC, Madans JH, Langlois JA, Orwoll ES. Risk factors for hip fracture in white men: the NHANES I epidemiological follow-up study. *J Bone Miner Res* 1998;13:918–925.
9. Looker AC, Wahner HW, Dunn WL, et al. Proximal femur bone mineral levels of US adults. *Osteoporos Int* 1995;5:389–409.
10. Faulkner KG, Roberts LA, McClung MR. Discrepancies in normative data between Lunar and Hologic DXA system. *Osteoporos Int* 1996;6:432–436.
11. Ahmed AIH, Blake GM, Rymer JM, Fogelman I. Screening for osteopenia and osteoporosis: do the accepted normal ranges lead to overdiagnosis? *Osteoporos Int* 1997;7:432–438.
12. Genant HK, Engelke K, Furst T, et al. Noninvasive assessment of bone mineral and structure: state of the art. *J Bone Miner Res* 1996;11:707–730.
13. Arlot ME, Sornay-Rendu E, Garnero P, Vey-Marty B, Delmas PD. Apparent pre- and postmenopausal bone loss evaluated by DXA at different skeletal sites in women: the OLEFY cohort. *J Bone Miner Res* 1997;12:683–690.
14. Cummings SR, Black DM, Rubin SM. Lifetime risks of hip, Colles' or vertebral fracture and coronary heart disease among white postmenopausal women. *Arch Intern Med* 1989;149:2556–2448.
15. Riis BJ. Premenopausal bone loss: fact or artifact? *Osteoporos Int* 1994;S1:S35–S37.
16. Miller PD, McClung M. Prediction of fracture risk I: bone density. *Am J Med Sci* 1996;312:257–259.
17. Baran DT, Faulkner KG, Genant HK, Miller PD, Pacifici R. Diagnosis and management of osteoporosis: guidelines for the utilization of bone densitometry. *Calcif Tissue Int* 1997;61:433–440.
18. Rubin SM, Cummings SR. Results of bone densitometry affect women's decisions about taking measures to prevent fractures. *Ann Intern Med* 1992;116:990–995.
19. Pouilles JM, Tremollieres F, Ribot C. Spine and femur densitometry at the menopause: are both sites necessary in the assessment of the risk of osteoporosis? *Calcif Tissue Int* 1993;52:344–347.
20. Greenspan SL, Maitland-Ramsey L, Myers E. Classification of osteoporosis in the elderly is dependent on site-specific analysis. *Calcif Tissue Int* 1995;58:409–414.
21. Finkelstein JS, Cleary RL, Butler JP, et al. A comparison of lateral versus anterior-posterior spine dual energy x-ray absorptiometry for the diagnosis of osteopenia. *J Clin Endocrinol Metab* 1994;78:724–730.
22. Bonnick SL, Nichols DL, Sanborn CF, et al. Dissimilar spine and femoral z-scores in premenopausal women. *Calcif Tissue Int* 1997;61:263–265.
23. Reid I. Glucocorticoid-induced osteoporosis: assessment and treatment. *J Clin Densitometry* 1998;1:55–65.
24. Cummings SR, Nevitt MC, Browner WS, et al. Risk factors for hip fracture in white women. *N Engl J Med* 1995;332:767–773.
25. Hui SL, Slemenda CW, Johnston CC Jr. Age and bone mass as predictors of fracture in a prospective study. *J Clin Invest* 1988;81:1804–1809.
26. Garnero P, Hausherr E, Chapuy M-C, et al. Markers of bone resorption predict hip fracture in elderly women: the EPIDOS prospective study. *J Bone Miner Res* 1996;11:1531–1537.
27. Greenspan SL, Myers ER, Maitland LA, Resnick NM, Hayes WC. Fall severity and bone mineral density as risk factors for hip fracture in ambulatory elderly. *JAMA* 1994;271:128–133.
28. Cummings SR, Black DM, Nevitt MC, et al. Bone density at various sites for prediction of hip fracture. *Lancet* 1993;341:72–75.
29. Yates AJ, Ross PD, Lydick E, Epstein RS. Radiographic absorptiometry in the diagnosis of osteoporosis. *Am J Med* 1995;98(S2A):41S–47S.
30. Duppe H, Gardsell P, Nilsson B, Johnell O. A single bone density measurement can predict fractures over 25 years. *Calcif Tissue Int* 1997;60:171–174.
31. Goulding A, Cannan R, Williams SM, Gold EJ, Taylor RW, Lewis-Barned NJ. Bone mineral density in girls with forearm fractures. *J Bone Miner Res* 1998;13:143–148.
32. Kanis JA. Diagnosis of osteoporosis. *Osteoporos Int* 1997;7(S3):S108–S116.
33. Huang C, Ross PD, Wasnich RD. Short-term and long-term fracture prediction by bone mass measurements: a prospective study. *J Bone Miner Res* 1998;13:107–113.
34. Lufkin EG, Wahner HW, O'Fallon WM, et al. Treatment of postmenopausal osteoporosis with transdermal estrogen. *Ann Intern Med* 1992;117:1–9.
35. Watts NB, Harris ST, Genant HK, et al. Intermittent cyclic etidronate treatment of postmenopausal osteoporosis. *N Engl J Med* 1990;323:73–79.
36. Christiansen C, Lindsay R. Estrogens, bone loss and preservation. *Osteoporos Int* 1990;1:7–12.
37. Silverberg SJ, Shane E, de la Cruz L, et al. Skeletal disease in primary hyperparathyroidism. *J Bone Miner Res* 1989;4:283–291.
38. Faulkner KG, McClung MR. Quality control of DXA instruments in multicenter trials. *Osteoporos Int* 1995;5:218–227.
39. Cauley JA, Seeley DG, Ensrud K, Ettinger B, Black D, Cummings SR. Estrogen replacement therapy and fracture in older women. *Ann Intern Med* 1995;122:9–16.
40. Theintz G, Buchs B, Rizzoli R, et al. Longitudinal monitoring of bone mass accumulation in healthy adolescents: evidence for a marked reduction after 16 years of age at the levels of lumbar spine and femoral neck in female subjects. *J Clin Endocrinol Metab* 1992;75:1060–1065.
41. Glastre C, Braillon P, David L, Cochat P, Meunier PJ, Delmas PD. Measurement of bone mineral content of the lumbar spine by dual energy x-ray absorptiometry in normal children: correlations with growth parameters. *J Clin Endocrinol Metab* 1990;70:1330–1333.

26. Radiology of Osteoporosis

Michael D. Jergas, M.D. and *Harry K. Genant, M.D.

*Department of Radiology, Ruhr-University Bochum, and St. Josef-Hospital, Bochum, Germany; and *Osteoporosis and Arthritis Research Group, University of California, San Francisco, California*

The term osteoporosis is widely used clinically to mean generalized loss of bone, or osteopenia, accompanied by relatively atraumatic fractures of the spine, wrist, hips, or ribs. Because of uncertainties of specific radiologic interpretation, the term osteopenia (''poverty of bone'') has been used as a generic designation for radiographic signs of decreased bone density. Radiographic findings suggestive of osteopenia and osteoporosis are frequently encountered in daily medical practice and can result from a wide spectrum of diseases, ranging from highly prevalent causes such as postmenopausal and involutional osteoporosis to very rare endocrinologic and hereditary or acquired disorders (Table 1). Histologically, the result in each of these disorders is a deficient amount of osseous tissue, although different pathogenic mechanisms may be involved. The value of conventional radiographs for detecting and quantifying osteopenia

and osteoporosis has raised scientific interest for many years. With the advent of highly accurate and precise quantitative techniques such as single and dual photon absorptiometry (SPA, DPA), single and dual x-ray absorptiometry (SXA, DXA), and quantitative computed tomography (QCT), the status of conventional radiography for the diagnosis and follow-up of osteoporosis has changed (1). Nevertheless, conventional radiography is widely available, and it remains useful for the detection of specific alterations in certain instances (e.g., subperiosteal resorption in hyperparathyroidism). Alone and in conjunction with modern imaging techniques such as bone scintigraphy and magnetic resonance imaging, conventional radiography is still widely used for the detection of complications of osteopenia, such as fractures, for the differential diagnosis of osteopenia, or for follow-up examinations in specific clinical settings (progression of soft-tissue calcifications or signs of secondary hyperparathyroidism and osteomalacia in renal osteodystrophy).

TABLE 1. *Disorders associated with radiographic osteoporosis (osteopenia).*

Primary osteoporosis
    Involutional osteoporosis (postmenopausal and senile)
    Juvenile osteoporosis
Secondary osteoporosis
  Endocrine
    Adrenal cortex (Cushing's disease)
    Gonadal disorders (hypogonadism)
    Pituitary (hypopituitarism)
    Pancreas (diabetes)
    Thyroid (hyperthyroidism)
    Parathyroid (hyperparathyroidism)
  Marrow replacement and expansion
    Myeloma
    Leukemia
    Metastatic disease
    Gaucher's disease
    Anemias (sickle cell disease, thalassemia)
  Drugs and substances
    Corticosteroids
    Heparin
    Anticonvulsants
    Immunosuppressants
    Alcohol (in combination with malnutrition)
  Chronic disease
    Chronic renal disease
    Hepatic insufficiency
    Gastrointestinal malabsorption
    Chronic inflammatory polyarthropathies
    Chronic immobilization
  Deficiency states
    Vitamin D
    Vitamin C (scurvy)
    Calcium
    Malnutrition
  Inborn errors of metabolism
    Osteogenesis imperfecta
    Homocystinuria

PRINCIPAL RADIOGRAPHIC FINDINGS IN OSTEOPENIA AND OSTEOPOROSIS

In osteoporosis, the amount of calcium per unit mineralized bone volume remains constant at about 35% (2,3). Therefore, a decrease in the mineralized bone volume results in a decrease of the total bone calcium and a decreased absorption of the x-ray beam. This phenomenon is then referred to as increased radiolucency. As bone mass is lost, changes in the bone structure occur. Bone is composed of two compartments: cortical bone and trabecular bone. The structural changes seen in cortical bone represent bone resorption at different sites (e.g., the inner and outer surfaces of the cortex, or within the cortex in the Haversian and Volkmann channels). These three sites (endosteal, intracortical, and periosteal) may react differently to distinct metabolic stimuli.

Cortical bone remodeling typically occurs in the endosteal ''envelope,'' and the interpretation of subtle changes in this layer may be difficult. With increasing age, there is a widening of the marrow canal due to an imbalance of endosteal bone formation and resorption that leads to a ''trabeculization'' of the inner surface of the cortex (Fig. 1). Endosteal scalloping due to resorption of the inner bone surface can be seen in high-bone-turnover states such as reflex sympathetic dystrophy.

Intracortical bone resorption may cause longitudinal striation or tunneling. These changes are seen in various high-turnover metabolic diseases affecting the bone such as hyperparathyroidism, osteomalacia, renal osteodystrophy, and acute osteoporoses from disuse or the reflex sympathetic dystrophy syndrome, but also postmenopausal osteoporosis (Figs. 2 and 3). Intracortical tunneling is a hallmark of rapid bone turnover. It is usually not apparent in disease states with relatively low bone turnover such as senile osteoporosis.

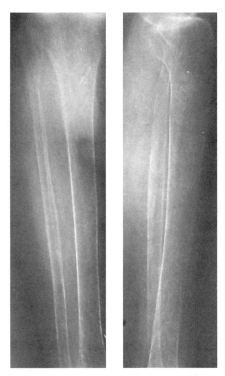

FIG. 1. Advanced involutional osteoporosis producing marked thinning of the cortices of the tibia and fibula because of chronic endosteal resorption and widening of the medullary space.

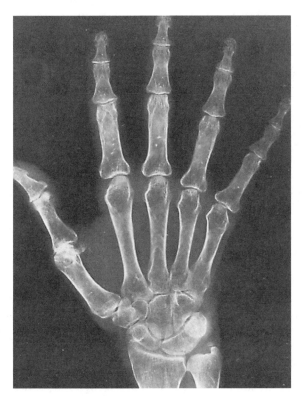

FIG. 2. Advanced involutional osteoporosis with generalized cortical thinning and uniform trabecular resorption as depicted on this hand radiograph.

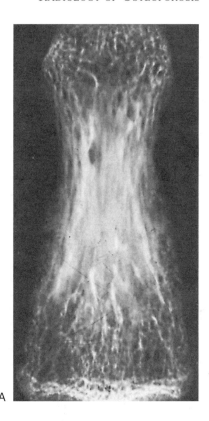

A

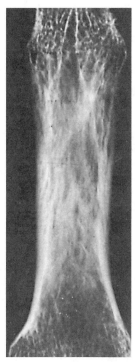

B

FIG. 3. High-resolution radiographs of the phalanges. **A:** This middle phalanx shows marked subperiosteal and intracortical bone resorption in primary hyperparathyroidism. **B:** Proximal phalanx showing endosteal scalloping and intracortical striation, indicating aggressive bone resorption in a recently (2 years before this radiograph) oophorectomized woman.

Accelerated endosteal and intracortical resorption, with intracortical tunneling and indistinct border of the inner cortical surface, is best depicted with high-resolution radiographic techniques (Fig. 3).

Subperiosteal bone resorption is associated with an irregular definition of the outer bone surface. This finding is pronounced in diseases with a high bone turnover, principally primary and secondary hyperparathyroidism (see also later in this chapter). However, rarely it may also be present in other diseases.

The trabecular bone responds faster to metabolic changes than does cortical bone (4). Trabecular bone changes are most prominent in the axial skeleton and in the ends of the long and tubular bones of the appendicular skeleton (juxtaarticular; e.g., proximal femur, distal radius). These are sites with a relatively great proportion of trabecular bone. Loss of trabecular bone (in cases of low rates of loss) occurs in a predictable pattern. Non–weight-bearing trabeculae are resorbed first. This leads to a relative prominence of the weight-bearing trabeculae. The remaining trabeculae may even become thicker, which may result in a distinct radiographic trabecular pattern. For example, early changes of osteopenia in the lumbar spine include a rarefaction of the horizontal trabeculae accompanied by a relative accentuation of the vertical trabeculae. This may lead to an appearance of vertical striation (Fig. 4).

The anatomic distribution of osteopenia or osteoporosis depends on the underlying cause. Osteopenia can be generalized, affecting the whole skeleton, or regional, affecting only a part of the skeleton, usually in the appendicular skeleton. Typical examples of generalized osteopenias are involutional and postmenopausal osteoporosis and osteoporosis caused by endocrine disorders such as hyperparathyroidism, hyperthyroidism, osteomalacia, and hypogonadism. Regional forms of osteoporosis result from factors affecting only parts of the appendicular skeleton such as disuse, reflex sympathetic syndrome, and transient osteoporosis of large joints.

The detection of osteopenia by conventional radiography is inaccurate because it is influenced by many technical factors such as radiographic exposure factors, film development, soft-tissue thickness of the patient, and so on. It has been estimated that as much as 20% to 40% of bone mass must be lost before a decrease in bone density can be seen in lateral radiographs of the thoracic and lumbar spine (5).

DISEASES CHARACTERIZED BY GENERALIZED OSTEOPENIA

Involutional Osteoporosis

Involutional osteoporosis is the most common generalized skeletal disease. It has been classified as a type I or postmenopausal osteoporosis and a type II or senile osteoporosis (6,7). Gallagher (8) added a third type, secondary osteoporosis (Table 2). Even though the importance of estrogen deficiency for postmenopausal osteoporosis has been established, the distinction between the first two types of osteoporosis is not generally accepted. Postmenopausal osteoporosis is believed to represent that process occurring in a subset of postmenopausal women, typically between ages 50 and 65 years. There is accelerated trabecular bone resorption related to estrogen deficiency, and the fracture pattern in this group of women primarily involves the spine and the wrist. In senile osteoporosis, there is a proportionate loss of cortical and trabecular bone. Characteristic fractures of senile osteoporosis include fractures of the hip, the proximal humerus, the tibia, and the pelvis in elderly women and men. Major factors in the etiology of senile osteoporosis include the age-related decrease in bone formation, diminished adrenal function, reduced intestinal calcium absorption, and secondary hyperparathyroidism. Distinctions between postmenopausal and senile osteoporosis may sometimes be arbitrary, and the assignment of fracture sites to the different types of osteoporosis is uncertain.

Osteopenia and Osteoporosis of the Axial Skeleton

A major radiographic manifestation of osteopenia of the axial skeleton is increased radiolucency of the vertebrae, which may assume the radiographic density of the intervertebral disk space. Further findings include vertical striation of the vertebrae due to reinforcement of vertical trabeculae in the osteopenic vertebra, framed appearance of the vertebrae (*picture framing* or *empty box*) due to an accentuation of the cortical outline, and increased biconcavity of the vertebral endplates (Figs. 4–6). The biconcavity of the vertebrae results from protrusion of the intervertebral disk into the weakened vertebral body.

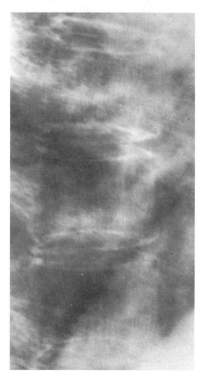

FIG. 4. Moderate postmenopausal osteoporosis of the thoracic spine with overall loss of bone density. The cortices are thinned, and the vertebral bodies have a striated appearance because of loss of secondary trabeculae and reinforcement of sharply defined primary trabeculae.

TABLE 2. *Classification of osteoporosis*

Type	I Postmenopausal	II Senile	III Secondary
Age (yr)	55–70	75–90	Any age
Years past menopause	5–15	25–40	—
Sex ratio (female/male)	20:1	2:1	1:1
Fracture site	Spine	Hip, spine, pelvis, humerus	Spine, hip, peripheral skeleton
Bone loss			
Trabecular	+++	++	+++
Cortical	+	++	+++
Contributing factor			
Menopause	+++	++	++
Age	+	+++	++

From Albright F. Osteoporosis. *Ann Intern Med* 1947;27:861–882, Riggs BL, Melton LJ. Evidence for two distinct syndromes of involutional osteoporosis. *Am J Med* 1983;75:899–901, and Gallagher JC. The pathogenesis of osteoporosis. *Bone Miner* 1990;9:215–227.

Vertebral Fractures and Their Diagnosis

Vertebral fractures are the hallmarks of osteoporosis, and even though one may argue that osteopenia *per se* may not be diagnosed reliably from spinal radiographs, spinal radiography continues to be a substantial aid in diagnosing and following up vertebral fractures. Changes in the gross morphology of the vertebral body have a wide range of appearances from increased concavity of the end plates to a complete destruction of the vertebral anatomy in vertebral crush fractures (Fig. 6). In clinical practice, conventional radiographs of the thoracolumbar region in lateral projection are analyzed qualitatively by radiologists or experienced clinicians to identify vertebral deformities or fractures. The most frequent fractures in early postmenopausal women, vertebral fractures have become the most important end points in epidemiologic studies and clinical drug trials. In these settings, conventional radiography is usually the only method applied to assess vertebral fractures. Several quantitative morphometric methods that rely entirely on measurements of vertebral heights for vertebral fracture diagnosis have been proposed to reduce the subjectivity that is inherent in a radiologist's reading (9,10).

Osteopenia and Osteoporosis at Other Skeletal Sites

The axial skeleton is not the only site where characteristic changes of osteopenia and osteoporosis can be depicted radiographically. Changes in the trabecular and cortical bone also can be seen in the appendicular skeleton. It is first apparent at the ends of long and tubular bones due to the predominance of cancellous bone in these regions. Endosteal resorption has a prominent role, particularly in senile osteoporosis. The result of this chronic process is widening of the medullary canal and thinning of the cortices (Figs. 1 and 2). In late stages of senile osteoporosis, the cortices are paper-thin, and the endosteal surfaces are smooth. In rapidly evolving postmenopausal osteoporosis, accelerated endosteal and intracortical bone resorption may be seen and can be directly assessed by high-resolution radiographic techniques. Methods to quantitate the changes at the peripheral skeleton have been proposed and also applied clinically.

Radiogrammetry is the simple measurement of cortical thickness potentially applied in virtually every long bone (Fig. 7). It is easy to perform with a caliper or with a graduated magnifying glass. Simple cortical measurements may be represented in several ways. For example, one method involves summing the thickness of both cortices as an index of bone mass; another method uses the combined cortical thickness divided by the total bone width as a measure of density. These methods have proven to be reproducible within 5% to 10%, depending on the specific site that is measured (11,12). Radiogrammetry is applied most often to the metacarpal bones. One major limitation leading to the potential insensitivity of radiogrammetry is related to the

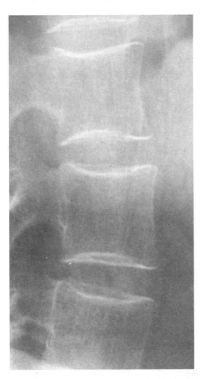

FIG. 5. As trabecular bone is lost, there is a relative accentuation of the cortex, resulting in the appearance of "picture framing."

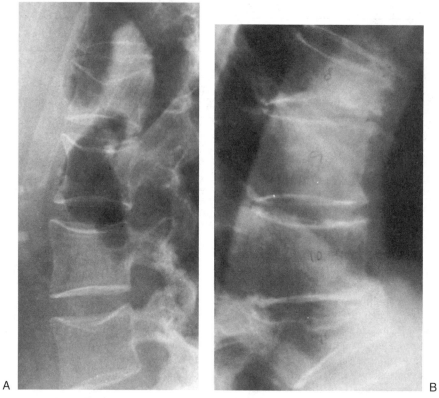

FIG. 6. A: Moderate osteoporotic fractures with end-plate deformities of the vertebrae and biconcave vertebrae in the lumbar spine in involutional osteoporosis. **B:** Advanced osteoporosis and vertebral fractures in the thoracic spine. Wedging and compression fractures have occurred.

failure to measure intracortical resorption or porosity and irregular endosteal scalloping or erosion. Because intracortical resorption and trabecular bone resorption are indicators of high-bone-turnover states, the fact that they are not measured by this technique is significant. Despite its shortcomings when applied to individual patients, radiogrammetry remains an important research tool to study changes in cortical bone (13,14).

Other Causes of Generalized Osteoporosis

Aside from senile and postmenopausal states leading to a generalized osteoporosis, various other conditions may be accompanied by generalized osteoporosis. Although most of the previously mentioned radiographic characteristics are shared by a variety of conditions, there may be some apparent differences in the appearance of osteoporosis as compared with involutional osteoporosis.

Endocrine Disorders Associated with Osteoporosis

Increased serum concentrations of the parathyroid hormone in hyperparathyroidism may result from autonomous hypersecretion by a parathyroid adenoma or diffuse hyperplasia of the parathyroid glands (primary hyperparathyroidism). A long-sustained hypocalcemic stimulus may result in

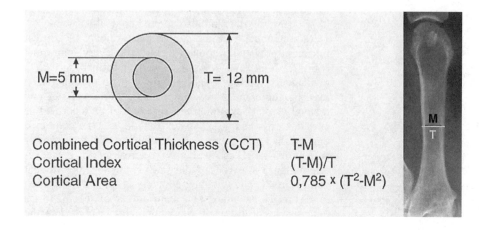

Combined Cortical Thickness (CCT)	T-M
Cortical Index	(T-M)/T
Cortical Area	$0,785 \times (T^2-M^2)$

FIG. 7. Schematic representation of a cross section of a tubular bone showing several parameters that may be determined by using radiogrammetry *(right)*. The left figure illustrates the measurement performed at a metacarpal bone.

hyperplasia of all parathyroid glands and secondary hyperparathyroidism. The cause of hypocalcemia usually is chronic renal failure or rarely malabsorption states. Patients with long-standing hyperparathyroidism may develop autonomous function and hypercalcemia (tertiary hyperparathyroidism). Whereas it is the increase in serum parathyroid hormone and calcium that establishes the diagnosis, radiographs document the severity and the course of the disease. Hyperparathyroidism leads to both increased bone resorption and bone formation. In fact, the skeletal changes and their radiographic appearance induced by hyperparathyroidism are quite complex (15). Bone resorption can affect all bone surfaces including subperiosteal, intracortical, endosteal, subchondral, subepiphyseal, subligamentous and subtendinous, and trabecular bone resorption.

Subperiosteal bone resorption is the most characteristic radiographic feature of hyperparathyroidism (16). It is especially prominent in the hand, wrist, and foot but may also be seen at other sites (Fig. 8). Radiographically, the outer margin of the bone becomes indistinct. Scalloping and spiculations of the cortex may occur in later stages. A distinctive type of acroosteolysis also may be observed (17). Intracortical resorption results in longitudinally oriented linear striations within the cortex, and endosteal bone resorption leads to scalloping of the inner cortex, cortical thinning, and widening of the medullary canal (18).

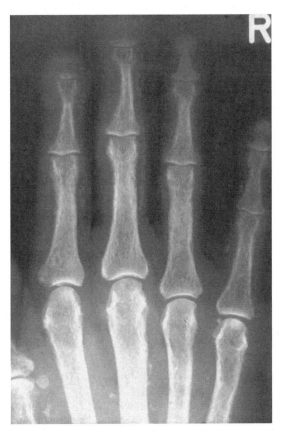

FIG. 8. Radiograph of the hand in secondary hyperparathyroidism showing subperiosteal resorption with scalloping and spiculations of the outer cortex, endosteal tunneling, acroosteolysis, and soft-tissue calcifications.

Subchondral bone resorption is another common manifestation of hyperparathyroidism that most frequently affects the joints of the axial skeleton (19). For example, it may mimic widening of the sacroiliac joint space, leading to "pseudo-widening" of the joint. The osseous surface may collapse and thus may simulate subchondral lesions of inflammatory disease. Osteopenia occurs frequently in hyperparathyroidism and may be observed throughout the skeleton (20).

Other radiographic signs of hyperparathyroidism include focal bone lesions ("brown tumors"), cartilage calcification, and also bone sclerosis (21). Increased amounts of trabecular bone leading to bone sclerosis may occur, especially in patients with renal osteodystrophy and secondary hyperparathyroidism (22,23). Increased bone density may occur preferably in the axial skeleton, sometimes leading to deposition of bone in subchondral areas of the vertebral body, resulting in an appearance of radiodense bands across the superior and inferior border and normal or decreased density of the center (rugger-jersey spine).

Whereas osteoporosis is defined by a reduction of regularly mineralized osteoid, findings in osteomalacia include an abnormally high amount of nonmineralized osteoid and a reduction in mineralized bone volume. Thus radiographic abnormalities in osteomalacia include osteopenia (reduction of mineralized bone), coarsened, indistinct trabeculae, and unsharp delineation of cortical bone (excessive apposition of nonmineralized osteoid), deformities, insufficiency fractures, and true fractures (bone softening and weakening). The deformations include bowing and bending of the long bones and biconcave deformities of the vertebrae. Pseudofractures, or Looser's zones (focal accumulations of osteoid in compact bone at right angles to the long axis), are diagnostic of osteomalacia and often occur bilaterally and symmetrically (24). More than 50 different diseases may cause osteomalacia, of which chronic renal insufficiency, hemodialysis, and renal transplantation are the most common (Fig. 9) (25). The destruction of renal parenchyma impairs the metabolism of calcium, phosphorus, and vitamin D, which is essential for the normal development of bone mineral. A decrease of this vitamin and reduced responsiveness in chronic renal insufficiency results in osteomalacia and rickets. The additional secondary hyperparathyroidism leads to a superimposition of radiographic changes from both osteomalacia and secondary hyperparathyroidism (26). This radiographic appearance is termed renal osteodystrophy. A common finding in secondary hyperparathyroidism associated with renal osteodystrophy is the osteosclerosis resulting in typical appearance of the vertebral bodies, as seen in the rugger-jersey spine (Fig. 10) (25). Several other radiographic abnormalities may be frequently seen in renal osteodystrophy including amyloid deposits, destructive spondyloarthropathy, inflammatory changes, and avascular necrosis, soft-tissue calcification, and arteriosclerosis (27).

Hyperthyroidism is a high-turnover disease, and it is associated with an increase in both bone resorption and bone formation. Because bone resorption exceeds bone formation, rapid bone loss may occur and result in generalized osteoporosis (28). This effect is especially pronounced in patients with thyrotoxicosis or with a history of thyrotoxicosis (29). Thyroid-stimulating hormone (TSH)-suppressive doses of

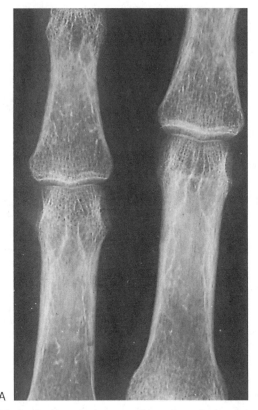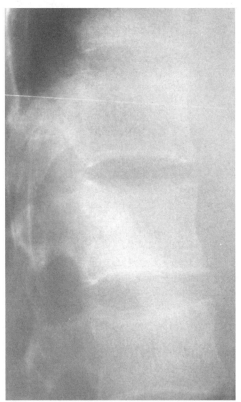

A

B

FIG. 9. Osteomalacia secondary to intestinal malabsorption. The high-resolution radiograph of the hand **(A)** demonstrates osteopenia accompanied by intracortical tunneling due to secondary hyperparathyroidism. The lateral radiograph of the spine **(B)** demonstrates osteopenia with indistinct cortical and trabecular outlines. Biconcave deformities of the vertebral bodies are also present.

thyroid hormone have been reported to decrease or to have no effect on bone density (30). Radiologic findings of hyperthyroidism-induced osteoporosis are those that are commonly seen in involutional or senile osteoporosis, including generalized osteopenia and cortical thinning and tunneling (31). The fractures associated with this condition affect the spine, the hip, and the distal radius (32).

Medication-Induced Osteoporosis

Hypercortisolism is probably the most common cause of medication-induced generalized osteoporosis, whereas the endogenous form of hypercortisolism, Cushing's disease, is relatively rare (33–36). Decreased bone formation and increased bone resorption have been observed in hypercortisolism. This has been attributed to inhibition of osteoblast formation, either direct stimulation of osteoclast activity or increased secretion of parathyroid hormone. The typical radiographic appearance of steroid-induced osteoporosis comprises generalized osteoporosis, at predominantly trabecular sites, with decreased bone density and fractures of the axial but also of the appendicular skeleton. A characteristic finding in steroid-induced osteoporosis is the marginal condensation of the vertebral bodies resulting from exuberant callus formation. Osteonecrosis is another complication of hypercortisolism, most frequently involving the femoral

head, and to a lesser extent, the humeral head and the femoral condyles (37,38).

Generalized osteoporosis has been observed in patients receiving high-dose heparin therapy (39,40). The radiologic features of heparin-induced osteoporosis include generalized osteopenia and vertebral compression fractures (41). The pathologic mechanism of heparin-induced osteoporosis is not completely clear, and the changes may be reversible with cessation of therapy (42).

Other Causes of Generalized Osteoporosis

Other causes of generalized osteoporosis include malnutrition, chronic alcoholism (if associated with malnutrition), smoking and caffeine intake, Marfan syndrome, and rather uncommonly, pregnancy (43–47). Marrow abnormalities associated with osteoporosis are anemias (sickle cell anemia, thalassemia), plasma cell myeloma, leukemia, Gaucher's disease, and glycogen storage disease (48,49). This list is certainly far from complete, but it represents some of the major causes of osteoporosis. Additional imaging techniques such as computed tomography, magnetic resonance tomography, and bone scintigraphy as well as clinical information may be helpful in differential diagnosis of the various conditions associated with osteoporosis (50,51).

Some conditions of the juvenile skeleton result in general-

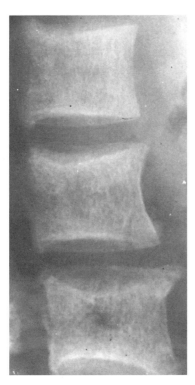

FIG. 10. Lateral radiograph of the lumbar spine in renal osteodystrophy demonstrates mottled subchondral bands of sclerosis, the "rugger jersey" spine.

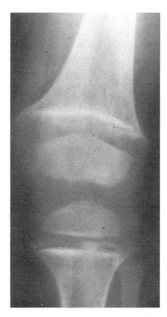

FIG. 11. Radiograph of the knee in a child with rickets demonstrating diffuse osteopenia. The growth plates have widened and protrude into the weakened metaphyseal region, causing cupping and widening of the metaphyses. Note also the irregular, indistinct borders of the femoral epiphysis.

ized osteoporosis. Rickets is characterized by inadequate mineralization of the bone matrix, and some of its radiographic appearance may resemble that of osteomalacia (52). Widening of the growth plates, cupping of the metaphysis, and decreased density and irregularities of the metaphyseal margins may be present (Fig. 11) (53). Epiphyseal ossification centers may show delayed ossification and unsharp borders (54). Overgrowth of the hyaline cartilage may lead to prominence of costochondral junctions of the ribs (rachitic rosary). The child's age at the onset of the disease determines the pattern of bone deformity, with bowing of the long bone being more pronounced in infancy and early childhood, and vertebral deformities and scoliosis in older children. Further deformities that may be observed in rickets include pseudofractures, basilar invagination, and triradiate configuration of the pelvis (55).

Idiopathic juvenile osteoporosis is a self-limited disease of childhood with recovery occurring as puberty progresses (56). A typical feature of this condition is the increased vulnerability of the metaphyses, often resulting in metaphyseal injuries of the knees and ankles. Idiopathic juvenile osteoporosis must be distinguished from osteogenesis imperfecta, another disease often seen with radiographic signs of generalized osteoporosis. The pathogenesis of osteogenesis imperfecta is quantitative or qualitative abnormalities of type I collagen. Osteogenesis imperfecta is divided into four major types, and the degree of osteoporosis in osteogenesis imperfecta depends strongly on the particular type (57). The clinical features of each type usually correspond to the type of mutation. The abnormal maturation of collagen seen in this disorder results in a primary defect in bone matrix.

Combined with a defective mineralization, this results in overall loss of bone density involving both the axial and peripheral skeleton. Patients with type III disease have a significantly decreased bone density, seen with generalized osteopenia, thinned cortices, fractures of long bones and ribs, exuberant callus formation, and bone deformation (58). The degree of osteopenia is highly variable, however, and at the mildest end of the spectrum, some patients do not have any radiographic signs of osteopenia.

REGIONAL OSTEOPOROSIS

Osteoporosis may also be confined to only a segment of the body. This type of osteoporosis is called regional osteoporosis, and it is commonly caused by some disorder of the appendicular skeleton. Osteoporosis due to immobilization or disuse characteristically occurs in the immobilized regions of patients with fractures, motor paralysis due to central nervous system disease or trauma, and bone and joint inflammation (59). Chronic and acute disease may vary somewhat in their radiographic appearance, showing diffuse osteopenia, linear radiolucent bands, speckled radiolucent areas, and cortical bone resorption.

Reflex sympathetic dystrophy, sometimes also termed Sudeck's atrophy or algodystrophy, has the radiographic appearance of a high-turnover process. It most often occurs in patients with trauma, such as Colles' fracture, but also in patient with any neurally related musculoskeletal, neurologic, or vascular condition such as hemiplegia or myocardial infarction (60–62). This condition probably related to overactivity of the sympathetic nervous system with increased blood flow and increased intravenous oxygen saturation in the affected extremity. Its radiographic appearance includes soft-tissue swelling as well as regional osteoporosis, with band-like, patchy, or periarticular osteoporosis, subperiosteal bone resorption, intracortical tunneling, endosteal bone resorption with initial excavation and scalloping of the endosteal surface and subsequent remodeling and widening of the medullary canal, and subchondral and juxtaarticular erosions (63). Especially in the early stages of reflex sympathetic dystrophy, bone scintigraphy may be helpful to establish the diagnosis (64).

Transient regional osteoporosis includes conditions that have in common the development of self-limited pain and radiographic osteopenia affecting one or several joints, most commonly the hip. Transient osteoporosis typically occurs in middle-aged men and in women in the third trimester of pregnancy (65). At the onset of clinical symptoms, there may be normal radiographic findings, and within several weeks, patients develop variable osteopenia of the hip, sometimes involving the acetabulum. Some patients later develop similar changes in the opposite hip or in other joints, in which case, the term regional migratory osteoporosis may be used (66). No specific therapy is required, because all patients recover. The cause of transient regional osteoporosis is not known, and it appears that it may be related to reflex sympathetic dystrophy. In some patients with clinically similar or identical manifestations, magnetic resonance imaging shows transient regional bone marrow edema (67). Because not all patients with identical clinical symptoms and transient bone marrow edema develop regional osteoporosis, the sensitivity as to the detection of regional osteoporosis must be questioned, as well as the interrelation between transient regional osteoporosis and transient bone marrow edema. A relation between transient bone marrow edema and ischemic necrosis of bone has been suggested. There is a need to define criteria allowing differentiation of transient bone marrow edema and the edema pattern associated with osteonecrosis (68).

REFERENCES

1. Genant HK, Engelke K, Fuerst T, et al. Noninvasive assessment of bone mineral and structure: state of the art. *J Bone Miner Res* 1996; 11:707–730.
2. Albright F, Smith PH, Richardson AM. Postmenopausal osteoporosis: its clinical features. *JAMA* 1941;116:2465–2474.
3. LeGeros RZ. Biological and synthetic apatites. In: Brown PW, Constantz B, eds. *Hydroxyapatite and related materials.* Boca Raton: CRC Press, 1994:3–28.
4. Frost HM. Dynamics of bone remodeling. In: Frost HM, ed. *Bone biodynamics.* Boston: Little Brown, 1964:315–334.
5. Lachmann E, Whelan M. The roentgen diagnosis of osteoporosis and its limitations. *Radiology* 1936;26:165–177.
6. Albright F. Osteoporosis. *Ann Intern Med* 1947;27:861–882.
7. Riggs BL, Melton LJ. Evidence for two distinct syndromes of involutional osteoporosis. *Am J Med* 1983;75:899–901.
8. Gallagher JC. The pathogenesis of osteoporosis. *Bone Miner* 1990;9: 215–227.
9. Black D, Palermo L, Nevitt MC, et al. Comparison of methods for defining prevalent vertebral deformities: the study of osteoporotic fractures. *J Bone Miner Res* 1995;10(6):890–902.
10. Genant HK, Jergas M, Palermo L, et al. Comparison of semiquantitative visual and quantitative morphometric assessment of prevalent and incident vertebral fractures in osteoporosis. *J Bone Miner Res* 1996;11: 984–996.
11. Rico H, Hernandez ER. Bone radiogrametry: caliper versus magnifying glass. *Calcif Tissue Int* 1989;45:285–287.
12. Kalla AA, Meyers OL, Parkyn ND, Kotze TJvW. Osteoporosis screening-radiogrammetry revisited. *Br J Rheumatol* 1989;28:511–517.
13. Gallagher JC, Kable WT, Goldgar D. Effect of progestin therapy on cortical and trabecular bone: comparison with estrogen. *Am J Med* 1991;90:171–178.
14. Danielsen CC, Mosekilde L, Svenstrup B. Cortical bone mass, composition, and mechanical properties in female rats in relation to age, long-term ovariectomy, and estrogen substitution. *Calcif Tissue Int* 1993; 52:26–33.
15. Genant HK, Vander Horst J, Lanzl LH, Mall JC, Doi K. Skeletal demineralization in primary hyperparathyroidism. In: Mazess RB, ed. *Proceedings of international conference on bone mineral measurement.* Washington, DC: National Institute of Arthritis, Metabolism and Digestive Diseases, 1974:177.
16. Camp JD, Ochsner HC. The osseous changes in hyperparathyroidism associated with parathyroid tumor: a roentgenologic study. *Radiology* 1931;17:63.
17. Resnick D, Niwayama G. Parathyroid disorders and renal osteodystrophy. In: Resnick D, ed. *Diagnosis of bone and joint disorders,* 3rd ed. Philadelphia: W.B. Saunders Company, 1995:2012–2075.
18. Meema HE, Meema S. Microradioscopic and morphometric findings in the hand bones with densitometric findings in the procimal radius in thyrotoxicosis and in renal osteodystrophy. *Invest Radiol* 1972;7:88.
19. Resnick D, Niwayama G. Subchondral resorption of bone in renal osteodystrophy. *Radiology* 1976;118:315.
20. Richardson ML, Pozzi-Mucelli RS, Kanter AS, Kolb FO, Ettinger B, Genant HK. Bone mineral changes in primary hyperparathyroidism: *Skeletal Radiol* 1986;15:85–95.
21. Steinbach HL, Gordan GS, Eisenberg E, Carne JT, Silverman S, Goldman L. Primary hyperoarthyroidism: a correlation of roentgen, clinical and pathologic features. *Am J Roentgenol Radium Ther Nucl Med* 1961;86:239–243.
22. Crawford T, Dent CE, Lucas P. Osteosclerosis associated with chronic renal failure. *Lancet* 1954;2:981.
23. Davis JG. Osseous radiographic findings of chronic renal insufficiency. *Radiology* 1953;60:406.
24. Steinbach HL, Noetzli M. Roentgen appearance of the skeleton in osteomalacia and rickets. *Am J Radiol* 1964;91:955.
25. Pitt MJ. Rickets and osteomalacia are still around. *Radiol Clin North Am* 1991;29:97–118.
26. Sundaram M. Renal osteodystrophy. *Skeletal Radiol* 1989;18:415–426.
27. Murphey MD, Sartoris DJ, Quale JL, Pathria MN, Martin NL. Musculoskeletal manifestations of chronic renal insufficiency. *Radiographics* 1993:13:357–379.
28. Eriksen EF. Normal and pathological remodeling of human trabecular bone: three dimensional reconstruction of the remodeling sequence in normals and in metabolic bone disease. *Endocr Rev* 1986;7:379–408.
29. Toh SH, Claunch BC, Brown PH. Effect of hyperthyroidism and its treatment on bone mineral content. *Arch Intern Med* 1985;145: 883–886.
30. Krølner B, Jørgensen JV, Nielsen SP. Spinal bone mineral content in myxoedema and thyrotoxicosis: effects of thyroid hormone(s) and antithyroid treatment. *Clin Endocrinol* 1983;18:439–446.
31. Chew FS. Radiologic manifestations in the musculoskeletal system of miscellaneous endocrine disorders. *Radiol Clin North Am* 1991; 29:135–147.
32. Solomon BL, Wartofsky L, Burman KD. Prevalence of fractures in postmenopausal women with thyroid disease. *Thyroid* 1993;3:17–23.
33. Laan RF, Buijs WC, van Erning LJ, et al. Differential effects of glucocorticoids on cortical appendicular and cortical vertebral bone mineral content. *Calcif Tissue Int* 1993;52:5–9.
34. Brandli DW, Golde G, Greenwald M, Silverman SL. Glucocorticoid-induced osteoporosis: a cross-sectional study. *Steroids* 1991;56: 518–523.
35. Saito JK, Davis JW, Wasnich RD, Ross PD. Users of low-dose glucocorticoids have increased bone loss rates: a longitudinal study. *Calcif Tissue Int* 1995;57:115–119.
36. Adachi JD, Bensen WG, Hodsman AB. Corticosteroid-induced osteoporosis. *Semin Arthr Rheum* 1993;22:375–384.
37. Heimann WG, Freiberger RH. Avascular necrosis of the femoral and humeral heads after high-dosage corticosteroid therapy. *N Engl J Med* 1969;263:672–674.

38. Hurel SJ, Kendall-Taylor P. Avascular necrosis secondary to postoperative steroid therapy. *Br J Neurosurg* 1997;11:356–358.
39. Griffith GC, Nichols G, Ashey JD, Flannagan B. Heparin osteoporosis. *JAMA* 1965;193:85–88.
40. Rupp WM, McCarthy HB, Rohde TD, Blackshear PJ, Goldenberg FJ, Buchwald H. Risk of osteoporosis in patients treated with long-term intravenous heparin therapy. *Curr Surg* 1982;39:419–422.
41. Sackler JP, Liu L. Heparin-induced osteoporosis. *Br J Radiol* 1973;46:548–550.
42. Walenga JM, Bick RL. Heparin-induced thrombocytopenia, paradoxical thromboembolism, and other side-effects of heparin therapy. *Med Clin North Am* 1998;82:635–658.
43. Seeman E, Szmukler GI, Formica C, Tsalamandris C, Mestrovic R. Osteoporosis in anorexia nervosa: the influence of peak bone density, bone loss, oral contraceptive use, and exercise. *J Bone Miner Res* 1992;7:1467–1474.
44. Kohlmeyer L, Gasner C, Marcus R. Bone mineral status of women with Marfan syndrome. *Am J Med* 1993;95:568–572.
45. Smith R, Stevenson JC, Winearls CG, Woods CG, Wordsworth BP, Osteoporosis of pregnancy. *Lancet* 1985;1178–1180.
46. Hopper JL, Seeman E. The bone density of twins discordant for tobacco use. *N Engl J Med* 1994;330:387–392.
47. Diez A, Puig J, Serrano S, Marinoso M-L, Bosch J, Marrugat J. Alcohol-induced bone disease in the absence of severe chronic liver damage. *J Bone Miner Res* 1994;9:825–831.
48. Resnick D. Hemoglobinopathies and other anemias. In: Resnick D, ed. *Diagnosis of bone and joint disorders,* 3rd ed. Philadelphia: W.B. Saunders Company, 1995:2107–2146.
49. Resnick D. Plasma cell dyscrasias and dysgammaglobulinemias. In: Resnick D, ed. *Diagnosis of bone and joint disorders,* 3rd ed. Philadelphia: W.B. Saunders Company, 1995:2147–2189.
50. Hosten N, Neumann K, Zwicker C, et al. Diffuse Demineralisation der Lendenwirbelsaule: Magnetresonanztomographische Untersuchungen bei Osteoporose und Plasmozytom. *Röfo Fortschr Geb Röntgenstr Neuen Bildgeb Verfahr* 1993;159:264–268.
51. Lecouvet F, Van de Berg B, Maldague B, et al. Vertebral compression fractures in multiple myeloma: part I: distribution and appearance at MR imaging. *Radiology* 1997;204:195–199.
52. Molpus WM, Pritchard RS, Walker CW, Fitzrandolph RL. The radiographic spectrum of renal osteodystrophy. *Am Fam Physician* 1991;43:151–158.
53. Pitt MJ. Rickets and osteomalacia. In: Resnick D, ed. *Diagnosis of bone and joint disorders,* 3rd ed. Philadelphia: W.B. Saunders Company, 1995:1885–1922.
54. Steinbach HL, Kolb FO, Gilfillan R. A mechanism of the production of pseudofractures in osteomalacia (Milkman's syndrome). *Radiology* 1954;62:388.
55. Rosenberg AE. The pathology of metabolic bone disease. *Radiol Clin North Am* 1991;29:19–35.
56. Smith R. Idiopathic juvenile osteoporosis: experience of twenty-one patients. *Br J Rheumatol* 1995;34:68–77.
57. Minch CM, Kruse RW. Osteogenesis imperfecta: a review of basic science and diagnosis. *Orthopedics* 1998;21:558–567.
58. Hanscom DA, Winter RB, Lutter L, Lonstein JE, Bloom BA, Bradford DS. Osteogenesis imperfecta: radiographic classification, natural history, and treatment of spinal deformities. *J Bone Joint Surg Am* 1992;74:598–616.
59. Kiratli BJ. Immobilization osteopenia. In: Marcus R, Feldman D, Kelsey J, eds. *Osteoporosis.* San Diego: Academic Press, 1996:833–853.
60. Mitchell SW. *Gunshot wounds and other injuries.* Philadelphia: J.B. Lippincott; 1872.
61. Sudeck P. Über die akute (reflectorische) Knochenatrophie nach entzündungen und Verletzungen an den Extremitäten und ihre klinischen Erscheinungen. *RöFo* 1901;5:277.
62. Gellman H, Keenan MA, Stone L, Hardy SE, Waters RL, Stewart C. Reflex sympathetic dystrophy in brain-injured patients. *Pain* 1992;51(3):307–311.
63. Resnick D, Niwayama G. Osteoporosis. In: Resnick D, ed. *Diagnosis of bone and joint disorders,* 3rd ed. Philadelphia: W.B. Saunders Company, 1995:1783–1853.
64. Todorovic Tirnanic M, Obradovic V, Han R, et al. Diagnostic approach to reflex sympathetic dystrophy after fracture: radiography or bone scintigraphy? *Eur J Nucl Med* 1995;22:1187–1193.
65. Rosen RA. Transitory demineralization of the femoral head. *Radiology* 1970;94:509–512.
66. Gupta RC, Popovtzer MM, Huffer WE, Smyth CJ. Regional migratory osteoporosis. *Arthritis Rheum* 1973;21:363–368.
67. Hayes CW, Conway WF, Daniel WW. MR imaging of bone marrow edema pattern: transient osteoporosis, transient bone marrow edema syndrome, or osteonecrosis. *Radiographics* 1993;13(5):1001–1011.
68. Froberg PK, Braunstein EM, Buckwalter KA. Osteonecrosis, transient osteoporosis, and transient bone marrow edema: current concepts. *Radiol Clin North Am* 1996;34:273–291.

27. Bone Biopsy and Histomorphometry in Clinical Practice

Robert R. Recker, M.D., F.A.C.P., F.A.C.E.

Department of Medicine, Creighton University School of Medicine, Section of Endocrinology, Creighton University Medical Center, St. Joseph Hospital, Osteoporosis Research Center, and Omaha Veterans Affairs Hospital, Omaha, Nebraska

Bone modeling is the coordinated system of bone cell function that shapes and sculpts the skeleton. It is very active during growth and development and, in humans, is largely extinguished at the time adulthood is reached. Bone remodeling is the coordinated system of bone cell function that removes and replaces bone tissue with no net change in bone mass (1). Modeling results in bone gain, and remodeling results in no change or loss in bone. Metabolic bone diseases are manifest as derangements of one or both of these systems. In humans, the bone-remodeling system is directly examined *in vivo* by histomorphometric analysis of microscopic sections of trabecular bone from transilial bone biopsies. Fluorochromes must be given as tissue-time markers before biopsy, and the specimens must be processed without removal of mineral. Because the remodeling system is most prominent in adult metabolic bone disease, it is the focus of discussion here.

THE BONE-REMODELING SYSTEM

The bone remodeling system was characterized in numerous publications in the recent past (2). A brief summary is presented here. Remodeling occurs on trabecular and haversian bone surfaces. The first step is activation of osteoclast precursors to form osteoclasts, which then begin to excavate a cavity. After removal of about 0.05 mm³ of bone tissue, the site remains quiescent for a short time. Then activation of osteoblast precursors occurs at the site, and the excavation is refilled. In normal adults there is no net change in the amount of bone after the work is finished. The average length of time required to complete the remodeling cycle is approximately 6 months (3), about 4 weeks for resorption and the rest for formation. This process serves several functions. It serves to remove aged, microdamaged bone tissue and replace it with new mechanically competent bone tissue. It serves to rearrange bone architecture to meet changing mechanical needs. Weakening of the skeleton by bone loss, abnormal accumulation of microdamage, or errors in geometry can come about only through defects in this system. Derangements in bone cell function, such as vitamin D deficiency, are manifest through this system. Figures 1 through 3 contain representative photomicrographs from human transilial biopsies. An extensive atlas is available (4).

Active bone remodeling units, termed basic multicellular units, or BMUs, are populations having a birthrate and life span. Frost (5) pointed out that population dynamics (census = birthrate × life span) can be applied to the remodeling events that occur continuously in the skeleton (5). These dynamics can be examined by the use of histomorphometry of nondecalcified sections of trabecular bone from biopsies taken after appropriate labeling with tissue-time markers.

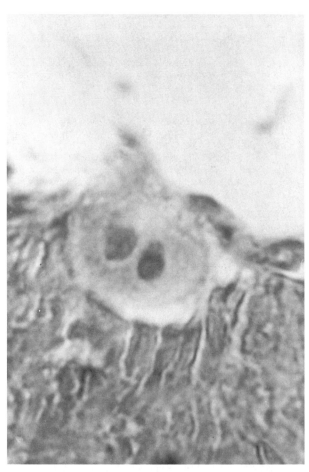

FIG. 2. Example of a normal bone-resorbing surface. Multinucleated osteoclasts are located in a Howship's lacuna.

THE BIOPSY PROCEDURE

The transilial approach is preferred to the vertical one by most workers because there is less discomfort to the patient and because most of the normal reference data from living subjects come from transilial biopsies (3). The preferred site is approximately 2 cm posterior to the anterior superior spine immediately inferior to the crest. While the patient is supine and the hip slightly elevated on a folded sheet, the biopsy site is located by grasping the ala of the ilium immediately posterior to the anterior superior spine between the thumb and forefinger. The thumb then falls into the spot where the skin incision should be made and the trephine should be inserted.

After mild sedation with intravenous midazolam (<5 mg), the area for infiltration of local anesthetic is marked with a felt-tipped pen. The surgeon performs a complete scrub (dons a cap, mask, gown, and gloves) and prepares and drapes the operative site. He or she removes the core of bone through a 1.5-cm incision and closes the skin wound with two to four 5-0 monofilament sutures. The patient returns to usual activities after 2 hours of quiet rest with instructions to keep the dressing dry and to avoid heavy physical activity for a few days. After 7 days, the suture is removed.

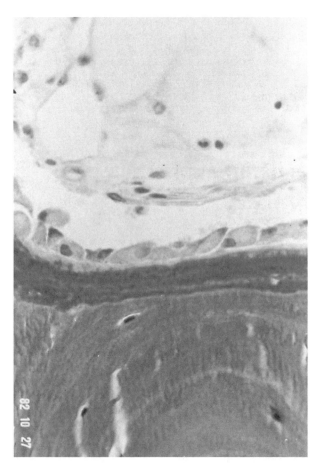

FIG. 1. Example of a normal bone-forming surface. Unmineralized osteoid is covered with plump osteoblasts.

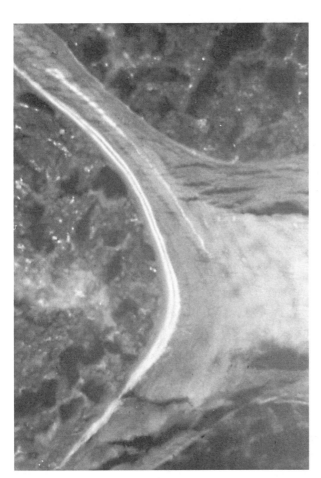

FIG. 3. Mineralizing surface containing two tetracycline labels given on a 3-14-3:5 schedule. One label is tetracycline hydrochloride, and the other is demeclocycline.

It is most important for the surgeon to use very gentle pressure to advance the trephine through the ilium. This requires patience because the tendency is to hurry through the biopsy site, pressing ever harder as the trephine advances. Excessive pressure on the trephine will crush most osteopenic specimens and will create excessive artifact in others.

In a survey of 9,131 biopsies (6,7), complications included 22 with hematomas, 17 with pain for >7 days, 11 with transient neuropathy, 6 with wound infection, 2 with fracture, and 1 with osteomyelitis, for a total incidence of complications of 0.7%. There were no deaths and no permanent disabilities. The procedure itself should be nearly pain free.

THE BIOPSY INSTRUMENT

The trephine should have an inner diameter of at least 7.5 mm, the dimension of the Bordier needle as modified by Meunier (Lepine a Lyon, Instruments de Chirurge, Lyon, France) or the Rochester needle (Accurate Tool & Machining Co. Inc., Rochester, MN). The needle should *always* be very sharp. Sharpen (and recondition if necessary) after every three to five procedures.

TETRACYCLINE LABELING

The ideal tissue-time bone fluorochrome label for use in humans is one of the tetracycline antibiotics. Demeclocycline fluoresces with an orange color, and all of the others fluoresce with a light lemon color. Most observers possess enough color acuity to distinguish between demeclocycline and the others. This difference in the color of fluorescence can be exploited to distinguish between pairs of labels given at different points in time. I use tetracycline hydrochloride, 250 mg, 4 times daily, or demeclocycline, 150 mg, 4 times daily. Tetracycline must be taken on an empty stomach. No dairy products or calcium supplements should be taken for 1 hour before or after the tetracycline.

There are practical limits for optimal timing of the labels. The minimum schedule is 2 days of label, 10 days free, 2 days of label, and then 5 days before biopsy (2-10-2:5). The maximum schedule is 3-14-3:5. I routinely use 3-14-3:5. A thorough analysis of the optimal labeling schedule has been published (8). Longer labeling schedules will result in few surfaces taking the double label because of the "label-escape" phenomenon, and shorter schedules will result in labels spaced too closely together for accurate interlabel width measurements.

HANDLING THE SPECIMENS

The biopsy core specimen should be placed in 70% ethanol immediately after removal. It can be stored for very long times in this solution without deterioration, but to ensure proper fixation, it should not be removed in less than 48 hours. The specimen is then dehydrated, defatted, embedded, and sectioned by using one of the published methods (9). Methyl methacrylate is the preferred embedding agent in my laboratory, but several hard plastics are available and seem to work well. Five-micrometer sections are cut for light microscopy and 10-micrometer sections for fluorescence microscopy. A number of stains are used, as previously described (9), and unstained sections are used with epifluorescence to analyze the fluorochrome labels.

A microscope with integrating eyepiece reticule or with camera lucida and drawing tablet can be used to obtain the histomorphometric data. Histomorphometry laboratories with high-volume workloads generally use one of the interactive image-analysis systems such as Bioquant-True Color Windows™ (BIOQUANT-R&M Biometrics, Inc., Nashville, TN). The basic microscope measurements are trabecular bone volume (TV/BV), bone surface (BS), eroded surface (ES/BS), osteoid surface (OS/BS), mineralized surface (MS/BS), wall thickness (W.Th), osteoid thickness (O.Th), and mineral apposition rate (MAR). Numerous important variables are calculated from these primary data (10) (Table 1).

INDICATIONS FOR BONE BIOPSY

The most important purpose in choosing a diagnostic procedure in clinical medicine is to establish a diagnosis, a necessary prerequisite for making a treatment decision. Another is to establish information on prognosis. Further, the risk, discomfort, and expense of a diagnostic procedure

TABLE 1. *Histomorphometry variables with operational definitions (human transilial bone biopsy)*

Abbreviation	Units	Name
BFR/BS	mm^2/mm/yr	Bone-formation rate (surface referent)
BFR/BV	mm^3/mm/yr	Bone-formation rate (bone volume referent)
BFR/TV	mm^3/mm/yr	Bone-formation rate (total volume referent)
BV/TV	%	Bone volume
Cn.Wi	mm	Cancellous width
C.Wi	mm	Core width
Ct.Wi1	mm	Cortical width (thicker cortex)
Ct.Wi2	mm	Cortical width (thinner cortex)
ES/BS	%	Eroded surface
FP	yr	Formation period
MS/BS	%	Mineralizing surface (as double-label surface)
MS/BS″	%	Mineralizing surface (as double-label plus one-half single-label surface)
MAR	μm/day	Mineral apposition rate
MS/OS	%	Mineralizing surface
Mlt/Os	day	Mineralization lag time/osteoid surface referent
Mlt	day	Mineralization lag time
Oft	day	Off time
Oft/FP	%	Off time (formation-period referent)
Oc.S/BS	%	Osteoclast surface
OAR	μm/day	Osteoid apposition rate
OS/BS	%	Osteoid surface
O.Th	μm	Osteoid thickness
OV/TV	%	Osteoid volume
OV/BV	%	Osteoid volume
RmP	yr	Remodeling period
RP	yr	Resorption period
TbT.Ar	mm^2	Trabecular tissue area (area analyzed including marrow and bone)
Tb.Pm	mm	Trabecular perimeter (surface analyzed)
Tb.Th	μm	Trabecular thickness
Tb.N	mm^{-1}	Trabecular number
Tb.Sp	μm	Trabecular separation
W.Th	μm	Wall thickness

should be appropriate to the importance of the information. Given these caveats, the number of clinical indications for transilial bone biopsy is small (Table 2). A clinician can manage most metabolic bone diseases without the aid of a bone biopsy. The following list contains some situations in which bone biopsy after fluorochrome labeling is useful. One impediment to widespread use of the biopsy is that availability of processing is limited. Most pathology laboratories cannot handle nondecalcified bone specimens or perform histomorphometry.

Vitamin D–Resistant Rickets

There are many variants of this disorder. Descriptions of the identifying characteristics of each is contained in Chapters 63 and 64. Several recent reviews are available (11).

These patients are first seen with disordered growth and development. In patients with a spontaneous mutation, when a family history is not present, bone biopsy may be necessary to make the diagnosis, although even under these circumstances, most clinicians can recognize the diagnosis from clinical and laboratory information, not including a bone biopsy. Perhaps the most important use of transilial biopsy with fluorochrome labeling is to judge the success of treatment and to evaluate the effect of changes in treatment in patients from families with a known diagnosis and in patients with nonfamilial varieties. The evaluation of new treatments requires the use of the biopsy.

Renal Osteodystrophy

This provides the most important diagnostic use of the transilial bone biopsy, because treatment decisions may depend on the results of the biopsy. The most dramatic example is the evaluation of bone pain and fractures in patients receiving prolonged dialysis who have hypercalcemia. If the biopsy shows predominantly osteitis fibrosa with brisk bone turnover, then partial parathyroidectomy may be indicated. On the other hand, if the biopsy shows little turnover (little or no fluorochrome label), with or without extensive aluminum deposits, then parathyroidectomy is contraindicated, and treatment with a chelating agent may be indicated. Current dialysis practice has reduced the number of cases with extensive aluminum deposits, although the biopsy can also help

TABLE 2. *Indications for transilial bone biopsy*

Vitamin D resistant rickets (various forms)
Renal osteodystrophy
Nutritional rickets and osteomalacia
Anticonvulsant osteomalacia

determine the extent of vitamin D deprivation and indicate the adequacy of vitamin D treatment.

Nutritional Rickets and Osteomalacia

This is very uncommon in the developed world, and thus the call for biopsy to evaluate it is relatively rare. Nevertheless, the problem may be present in occult form among the elderly that reside in nursing homes, retirement centers, or in their own homes and thus do not get sufficient sunlight exposure. There has been uncertainty about the biochemical definition of nutritional vitamin D deficiency. The bone biopsy may be more sensitive than measurement of serum vitamin D to make the diagnosis (see Chapter 61). In my experience, careful histomorphometric analysis and comparison with a valid database from age- and sex-matched normal subjects is surprisingly sensitive when the measurements of osteoid seam width, osteoid surface, and appositional rate are combined to calculate mineralization lag time (10). It is important to emphasize that simple measurement of osteoid seam width alone is not sufficient to determine whether osteomalacia or "hypovitaminosis D osteopathy" is present.

Anticonvulsant Osteomalacia

Long-term anticonvulsant therapy, particularly in elderly patients, may cause musculoskeletal pain and vertebral and hip fractures (see Chapters 55 and 67). In addition to osteopenia, patients may have a mineralization defect that produces prolonged mineralization lag time and accumulation of unmineralized osteoid. Transilial bone biopsy may be the only method of discovering this lesion, which may require changing the anticonvulsant therapy or adding treatment with one of the vitamin D preparations.

Transilial Biopsy as a Research Tool

The most important use of the transilial bone biopsy coupled with fluorochrome labeling is in the study of metabolic bone disease and assessing the mechanism of action, safety, and efficacy of new pharmaceutical agents. For example, recent clinical trials of bisphosphonates included subsets of patients who underwent biopsy for evaluation of bone-remodeling rates and for assessment of mineralization (14). Two important safety questions answered by the biopsy data were whether the agent stopped remodeling completely (it did not) and whether it created a defect in the mineralization of osteoid (it did not). Further, the biopsies indicated that the mechanism of the bisphosphonate in causing increased bone density was largely the reduction of the remodeling space. There is need to include transilial biopsy after fluorochrome labeling in any trials of new bone-active agents, at least at the beginning of study, and the pharmaceutical industry has responded by including transilial biopsies in the protocols. Further, in preclinical animal studies, serial biopsy sampling at multiple skeletal sites, by using different colored fluorochrome labels (calcein or xylenol orange) has become a standard means of predicting the safety, efficacy, and mechanism of action of new pharmaceutical agents.

AVAILABILITY OF BONE HISTOMORPHOMETRY

Laboratory facilities that process transilial bone are scarce. However, the surgical procedure of obtaining the specimen is not difficult, and specimens can be mailed to one of the centers now performing bone histomorphometry. Physicians who contemplate performing the biopsy should contact a biopsy-processing center ahead of time to obtain explicit instructions on the patient's history, the fluorochrome labeling schedule, performance of the biopsy, fixing solution, mailing, and so on. Most centers require 4 weeks or more to report the results from a specimen.

POSTMENOPAUSAL OSTEOPOROSIS

The role of transilial bone biopsy in postmenopausal osteoporosis should be mentioned. In clinical practice, biopsy is rarely needed. However, in clinical osteoporosis research, transilial biopsy coupled with fluorochrome labeling is quite useful. For example, in treatment trials, it is desirable to have baseline biopsies to rule out confounding diagnoses and to compare with biopsies during treatment. With paired biopsies, we can learn whether remodeling characteristics at the beginning of treatment affect the outcome of treatment. We can obtain some understanding of the mechanism of a treatment response before waiting the length of time required to detect a positive bone-mass effect or an antifracture effect. In some trials bone biopsy is mandatory to determine safety of a test drug suspected of suppressing remodeling or of producing abnormal bone tissue.

Every new treatment tested for osteoporosis should be accompanied with bone biopsy in the early stages of development in at least a subset of study subjects until safety and efficacy are assured. Some treatments can be predicted to fail, based on the biopsy findings during treatment. An example would be continuous treatment with an agent that stops activation of remodeling or impairs bone formation significantly or both in those remodeling sites undergoing formation at the time the agent was introduced. Such an agent might harm the mechanical strength of the skeleton in the long term rather than improve it. This problem can be detected earlier with biopsy than with other technology.

The incidence and prevalence of postmenopausal osteoporosis is very high in modern societies (15–21). Thus it is clearly unrealistic and not necessary for every patient with postmenopausal osteoporosis to undergo transilial bone biopsy with tetracycline labeling, because confounding diagnoses are usually ruled out by noninvasive clinical methods.

REFERENCES

1. Frost HM. *Intermediary organization of the skeleton.* Boca Raton, FL: CRC Press, 1986.
2. Parfitt AM. Osteonal and hemi-osteonal remodeling: the spatial and temporal framework for signal traffic in adult human bone. *J Cell Biochem* 1994;55:273–286.
3. Recker RR, Kimmel DB, Parfitt AM, Davies KM, Keshawarz N, Hinders S. Static and tetracycline-based bone histomorphometric data from 34 normal postmenopausal females. *J Bone Miner Res* 1988;3:133–144.
4. Malluche HH, Faugere MC, Malluche HH, Faugere MC, eds. *Atlas of mineralized bone histology.* New York: Karger, 1986.

5. Frost HM. Tetracycline-based histological analysis of bone remodeling. *Calcif Tissue Res* 1969;3:211–237.
6. Duncan H, Rao DS, Parfitt AM. Complications of bone biopsy. *Metab Bone Dis Relat Res* 1980;2:475.
7. Rao DS. Practical approach to biopsy. In: Recker RR, ed. *Bone histomorphometry: techniques and interpretation.* Boca Raton, FL: CRC Press, 1983:3–11.
8. Frost HM. Bone histomorphometry: correction of the labeling ''escape error.'' In: Recker RR, ed. *Bone histomorphometry: techniques and interpretation.* Boca Raton, FL: CRC Press, 1983: 133–142.
9. Baron R, Vignery A, Neff L, Silvergate A, Santa Maria A. *Processing of undecalcified bone specimens for bone histomorphometry.* Boca Raton, FL: CRC Press, 1983:13–36.
10. Parfitt AM, Drezner MK, Glorieux FH, et al. Bone histomorphometry: standardization of nomenclature, symbols, and units. *J Bone Miner Res* 1987;2:595–610.
11. Econs MJ, Drezner MK. Bone disease resulting from inherited disorders of renal tubule transport and vitamin D metabolism. In: Coe FL, Favus MJ, eds. *Disorders of bone and mineral metabolism.* 1st ed. New York: Raven Press, 1992:935–950.
12. Rao SD, Villanueva A, Mathews M, et al. *Histologic evolution of vitamin-D depletion in patients with intestinal malabsorption or dietary deficiency.* Amsterdam: Excerpta Medica, 1983:224–226.
13. Kragstrup JMFML. Reduced wall thickness of completed remodeling sites in iliac trabecular bone following anticonvulsant therapy. *Metab Bone Dis Rel Res* 1982;4:181–185.
14. Chavassieux PM, Arlot ME, Reda C, Wei L, Yates AJ, Meunier PJ. Histomorphometric assessment of the long-term effects of alendronate on bone quality and remodeling in patients with osteoporosis. *J Clin Invest* 1997;100:1475–1480.
15. Riggs BL, Melton L III. Involutional osteoporosis. *N Engl J Med* 1986;314:1676–1686.
16. Black DM, Cummings SR, Melton LJ. Appendicular bone mineral and a woman's lifetime risk of hip fracture. *J Bone Miner Res* 1992;7: 639–646.
17. Cummings SR, Black DM, Rubin SM. Lifetime risks of hip, Colles', or vertebral fracture and coronary heart disease among white postmenopausal women. *Arch Intern Med* 1989;149:2445–2448.
18. Cooper C, Atkinson EJ, O'Fallon WM, Melton LJ. Incidence of clinically diagnosed vertebral fractures: a population-based study in Rochester, Minnesota, 1985-1989. *J Bone Miner Res* 1992;7:221–227.
19. Melton LJ III. The prevalence of osteoporosis. *J Bone Miner Res* 1997;12:1769–1771.
20. Melton LJ III, Chrischilles EA, Cooper C, Lane AW, Riggs BL. Perspective: how many women have osteoporosis? *J Bone Miner Res* 1992;7:1005–1010.
21. Melton LJ III, Thamer M, Ray NF, et al. Fractures attributable to osteoporosis: report from the National Osteoporosis Foundation. *J Bone Miner Res* 1997;12:16–23.

28. Molecular Diagnosis of Bone and Mineral Disorders

Robert F. Gagel, M.D. and *Gilbert J. Cote, Ph.D.

*Department of Internal Medicine Specialties and *Section of Endocrine Neoplasia and Hormonal Disorders, University of Texas M. D. Anderson Cancer Center, Houston, Texas*

Discoveries during the past 5 to 10 years have greatly expanded our understanding of how genetic abnormalities cause bone and mineral disorders. Examples of such discoveries include the identification of mutations of type I collagen genes in osteogenesis imperfecta, vitamin D and estrogen-receptor polymorphisms associated with osteoporosis, genes responsible for certain types of hereditary hypercalcemia, and mutations found in a wide variety of dysplasias, providing a greater understanding of the signaling pathways involved in the formation and patterning of developing bones.

Diagnostic use of this type of information is very quickly making its way into clinical practice. For example, within 3 years of the description of point mutations in the *RET* protooncogene in multiple endocrine neoplasia type II (MEN II), genetic testing for these mutations replaced the pentagastrin-stimulation test, the previous ''gold standard'' for diagnosing this condition (see Chapter 16). In addition, mutational analysis of the calcium receptor can be an important component in the differential diagnosis of hypercalcemia, especially in cases in which the diagnosis of hyperparathyroidism is equivocal (see Chapters 31 and 32). This rapid acquisition of new information and its application to disease management underscore the importance for clinicians in the bone and mineral field to acquire a fundamental knowledge of testing strategies and to understand the power and limitations of current approaches to genetic testing.

The single most important resource for up-to-date information related to specific genetic syndromes is provided by Online Mendelian Inheritance in Man (OMIM), available to all physicians without charge on the World Wide Web (details provided in Table 1). This concise but complete reference is an excellent starting point for genetic information relating to bone and mineral disorders and provides an intuitive, searchable textual database that is updated on a regular basis. What follows is a description of the principles behind the most commonly used molecular genetic techniques and approaches.

POLYMERASE CHAIN REACTION

A basic understanding of the principles underlying polymerase chain reaction (PCR) is vital to molecular genetic diagnosis. The DNA used in diagnostic studies is most commonly extracted from peripheral white blood cells and occasionally from other tissues. It is important, if possible, to obtain blood from an affected family member as well as the patient at risk. Occasionally, a DNA copy of messenger RNA (mRNA) from a specific tissue can be made by a

TABLE 1. *Summary of molecular defects in bone and mineral disorders*

Genetic disorder	Affected gene
Achondrogenesis	Collagen-2-A1 or diastrophic dysplasia sulfate transporter
Achondroplasia	Fibroblast growth factor receptor-3
Acromesomelic dysplasia	Cartilage-derived morphogenetic protein-1
Albright osteodystrophy	G-Protein, α subunit
Apert syndrome	Fibroblast growth factor receptor-2
Atelosteogenesis	Diastrophic dysplasia sulfate transporter
Autosomal dominant hypocalcemia	Calcium-sensing receptor
Bartter syndrome	Na-K-Cl cotransporter-2
Brachydactly	Cartilage-derived morphogenetic protein-1
Campomelic dysplasia	SRY box-related-9 (SOX9)
Chondrodysplasia punctata	Arylsulfatase E
Chrondrosarcoma	Exostosis-1
Cleidocranial dysplasia syndrome	Core-binding factor, α subunit 1
Crouzon syndrome	Fibroblast growth factor receptor-2
Diastrophic dysplasia	Diastrophic dysplasia sulfate transporter
Epiphyseal dysplasia	Cartilage oligomeric matrix protein-1
Familial hypocalciuric hypercalcemia	Calcium-sensing receptor
Familial hypoparathyroidism	Calcium-sensing receptor or parathyroid hormone
Greig cephalopolysyndactyly syndrome	GLI-Kruppel member
Hereditary multiple exostoses	Exostosis-1 or -2
Hydrochrondroplasia	Fibroblast growth factor receptor-3
Hypophosphataemic rickets, X-linked	PHEX endopeptidase
Hypophosphatasia	Alkaline phosphatase
Jackson–Weiss syndrome	Fibroblast growth factor receptor-2
Kniest dyplasia	Collagen-2-A1
Langer mesomelic dysplasia	Short stature homeo box
Leprechaunism	Insulin receptor
Leri–Weill synchondrosteosis	Short stature homeo box
Marfan syndrome	Fibrillin-1
Marshall syndrome	Collagen-11-A1
McCune–Albright syndrome	G-Protein, α subunit
Metaphyseal chondrodysplasia	Collagen-10-A1 or parathyroid hormone receptor
Multiple endocrine neoplasia, type 1	MEN1
Multiple endocrine neoplasia, type 2	RET protooncogene
Nephrolithiasis, X-linked, Dent disease	Renal-specific chloride channel
Neonatal hyperparathyroidism	Calcium-sensing receptor
Osteopetrosis with renal tubular acidosis	Carbonic anhydrase II
Osteogenesis imperfecta	Collagen-1-A1, Collagen-2-A1
Otospondylomegaepiphyseal dysplasia	Collagen-11-A1
Pallister–Hall syndrome	GLI-Kruppel member
Pfeiffer syndrome	Fibroblast growth factor receptor-1 or -2
Pituitary dwarfism	Growth hormone, growth hormone receptor
Postaxial polydactyly, type A1	GLI-Kruppel member
Pseudoachondroplasia	Cartilage oligomeric matrix protein-1
Pycnodysostosis	Cathepsin-K
Rhizomelic chondrodysplasia punctata	Peroxin-7
Simpson–Golabi–Behmel overgrowth syndrome	Glypican-3
Spondyloepiphyseal dysplasia	Collagen-2-A1
Spondyloepimetaphyseal dysplasia	Collagen-2-A1
Stickler syndrome	Collagen-2-A1, collagen-11-A1
Thanatophoric dysplasia	Fibroblast growth factor receptor-3
Trichodentoosseous syndrome	Distal-less homeo box
Vitamin D–resistant rickets, type IIA	Vitamin D receptor
Waardenburg syndrome	PAX3 or microphthalmia-associated transcription factor
Wagner syndrome	Collagen-2A1
Williams syndrome	Elastin
Zellweger syndrome	Peroxin-1, -2, -5, -6, or -12

Information identifying the disorders and their respective affected genes was obtained by key-word search of the Online Mendelian Inheritance in Man, OMIM™. Center for Medical Genetics, Johns Hopkins University (Baltimore, MD) and National Center for Biotechnology Information, National Library of Medicine (Bethesda, MD), 1997. World Wide Web URL: http://www.ncbi.nlm.nih.gov/omim/

technique called reverse transcription. The genomic DNA or the copy of the mRNA is used as a template for PCR, a method for amplification of a selected portion of a specific DNA sequence (1).

The specific portion of the gene of interest to be copied is targeted by using small single-stranded DNA fragments that are complementary to and flank the DNA sequence of interest (oligonucleotide primers). The addition of nucleotides and a thermostabile DNA polymerase, an enzyme that synthesizes new DNA, followed by heating and cooling through 20 to 30 cycles, results in the formation of millions of copies of the targeted DNA (Fig. 1). Copies will be made of both parental alleles of the target DNA sequence (one derived from each parent). The sensitivity of the PCR reaction is so great that appropriate controls must be included in each amplification to exclude the possibility of DNA

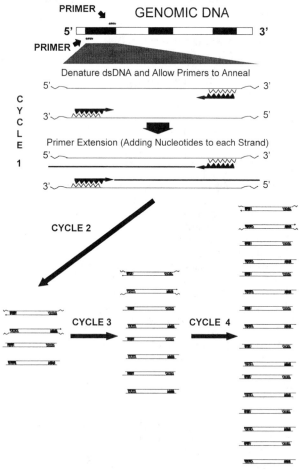

FIG. 1. Polymerase chain reaction. DNA from the patient to be tested is denatured by heating. Oligonucleotides, which complement a small sequence flanking the targeted piece of DNA, are added to the mixture. The oligonucleotides hybridize to the target DNA and serve as a template for extension of the DNA strand by a thermostabile polymerase. The DNA is again denatured by heating, followed by a new cycle of DNA synthesis (cycle 2). In subsequent cycles, there is a logarithmic increase in the number of copies of the targeted DNA. After 20 to 30 cycles, most of the DNA copies are of a single size.

contamination. The amplified DNA serves as the starting material for all subsequent mutational analysis techniques.

GENERAL SCREENING TECHNIQUES TO DETECT MUTATIONS

There are many different strategies for identification of specific mutations. This summary focuses on the six commonly used techniques and discusses the advantages and disadvantages of each (Fig. 2). Major factors for deciding which techniques to use include the size of the DNA sequence to be examined and the spectrum of mutations that cause the disease. For example, mutations affecting the collagen type I α-1 gene in osteogenesis imperfecta (see Chapter 57) may affect any of the >50 exons in the gene, and a broad screening approach (such as single-strand conformational polymorphism, dideoxy fingerprinting, or denaturing gradient gel electrophoresis, discussed later) may provide the best approach to identifying a mutation. Identification of a potential sequence abnormality would lead to the use of a more focused approach (such as DNA sequencing, restriction endonuclease analysis, or allele-specific hybridization).

The majority of the techniques for DNA analysis use gel electrophoresis. A sample containing the DNA molecules to be examined is applied to a gel (a thin layer of acrylamide or agarose), and an electrical current is applied to move the molecules along the long axis through the gel. Small differences in charge, size, or conformational state of an individual molecule can affect the mobility of the molecule (Fig. 2), making it possible to separate two pieces of DNA with as little as a single nucleotide difference. The descriptions are intended to provide an introduction to these methods; more detailed discussion and protocols can be found elsewhere (2,3).

Single-Strand Conformational Polymorphism

Single-strand conformational polymorphism (SSCP) relies on the theory that a denatured DNA molecule (one in which the two complementary strands of DNA that form the double helix are separated) forms a unique single-stranded three-dimensional structure (2–4). The major determinants of this structure are the specific DNA sequence and internal base pairing. A single nucleotide change may result in a conformation that differs from that of the normal sequence. In many genetic disorders, an affected individual will inherit one normal and one mutated copy of a gene, which can be detected by differences in DNA mobility on nondenaturing polyacrylamide gels (Fig. 2). This technique is particularly suited for analysis of large stretches of DNA sequence when the specific mutation is not known, such as the mutations described for osteogenesis imperfecta. DNA sequence analysis of the entire gene would be prohibitively expensive and time consuming. A disadvantage of SSCP is that it does not identify the specific mutation and generally cannot distinguish between mutations and nucleotide polymorphisms (a change in the DNA that does not alter the coding sequence of a protein). This technique cannot detect a mutation in which two copies of the mutated DNA (one from each parent) are inherited unless an external control

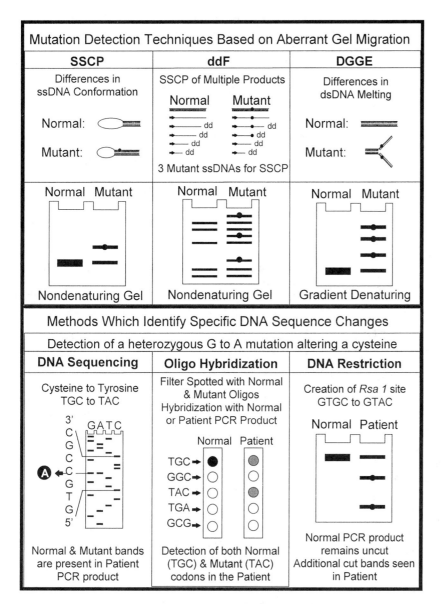

FIG. 2. Six different techniques for detecting a single nucleotide mutation. This figure schematically shows the results of six common methods used to detect a mutations. The upper panels illustrate the methods of single-strand conformational polymorphism analysis (SSCP), dideoxy fingerprinting (ddF), and denaturing gradient gel electrophoresis (DGGE), which detect mutations by differential migration of the normal and mutant DNA fragments in a gel. Within each panel, the fundamental mechanism or principle for each technique is diagrammed. A specific point mutation is denoted by a solid circle. In the lower part of each panel, gel electrophoretic profiles of products derived from a normal and mutant DNA fragment analyzed by the respective technique is shown, with mutant bands designated by a solid circle. SSCP separates single-stranded DNA molecules in a nondenaturing gel. The point mutation alters the mobility of the mutant band. Dideoxynucleotide fingerprinting creates a ladder of mutant SSCP products in which fragments containing normal sequence are separated from mutant bands by using nondenaturing conditions. The sequencing ladder is provided by the inclusion of dideoxynucleotides in the reaction mixture to terminate the chain at different points. Normal and bands containing mutant sequence migrate differently in the nondenaturing gel, creating a ladder-like effect. DGGE identifies four bands: normal homoduplex, mutant homoduplex, and two additional bands that represent two variants of normal–mutant heteroduplexes. In the lower panels, three additional methods are shown that identify specific DNA mutations. The example shown is a heterozygous G-to-A mutation that converts cysteine (TGC) to tyrosine (TAC). Direct DNA sequencing of the PCR product *(lower left)* shows the presence of two bands at the mutated codon (G and A, respectively), indicating that one allele (PCR product) contains the normal sequence, and the other, the mutated sequence. The lower central panel shows allele-specific oligonucleotide hybridization, which uses oligonucleotides with specific mutant sequences and detects the mutation by interaction of mutant sequence with its complementary oligonucleotide. In the example shown, four possible mutations (GGC, TAC, TGA, GCG) of a single cysteine codon (TGC) are examined by dotting of oligonucleotides containing these mutations onto a filter. Hybridization of a PCR product from a normal shows labeling only of the TGC dot, whereas the PCR product with normal and mutant sequence (heterozygous mutation) hybridizes to both TGC and TAC. The G-to-A substitution creates an *Rsa* I restriction site. Addition of this endonuclease to the reaction mixture that contains the normal PCR product identifies only a single electrophoretic band *(lower right)*. Addition of the same enzyme to a PCR product that contains one mutated allele results in the appearance of two new bands *(solid circles)* as well as the band derived from the normal allele.

from another patient is included in the analysis. More focused techniques, discussed later, are used to determine the nature of the DNA abnormality.

Dideoxy Fingerprinting

Dideoxy fingerprinting (ddF) is a method that combines SSCP with a step reminiscent of dideoxy DNA sequencing

(discussed later), in an effort to improve on the ability to detect single base mutations in PCR-amplified segments (5) (Fig. 2). After PCR, a DNA sequencing reaction with the Sanger chain-termination procedure is performed by using an end-labeled internal primer and a mixture containing a single dideoxynucleotide [e.g., dideoxyguanosine triphosphate (ddGTP)]. This results in the production of several DNA products, which vary in length depending on where the polymerase terminated. The radiolabeled products are denatured, renatured by using SSCP-type conditions, and analyzed by nondenaturing gel electrophoresis (Fig. 2). The resulting pattern resembles that seen in a single lane (e.g, G) of a sequencing gel, with one important difference. DNA fragments that contain a mutation will migrate differently from the normal fragment. The presence of multiple bands that contain the mutant sequence will create a series of bands, making it easier to detect the mutation and determine its general location (Fig. 2). However, like SSCP, other techniques are needed to determine the nature of the DNA abnormality. This technique was used successfully to screen a large number of genes in the mapping and identification of multiple endocrine neoplasia type 1 (MEN I) as the causative gene for MEN type I (6).

Denaturing Gradient Gel Electrophoresis

Like SSCP and ddF, denaturing gradient gel electrophoresis (DGGE) identifies mutations based on differences in DNA migration patterns (2,3,7). In this method, double-stranded DNA produced by PCR is applied to a gradient gel containing urea and formamide, which results in gradient-dependent denaturation (separation of the double helix into single strands) as gel electrophoresis proceeds. Separation of the DNA strands is responsible for altering the DNA mobility. DNA denaturation is sequence dependent. Therefore a single nucleotide change will frequently generate a specific denaturation pattern. This effect is enhanced by the addition of "GC-clamps" or stretches of GCs to a single end of the PCR product to stimulate unidirectional DNA denaturation. This is a more complex technique, requiring a period of development for optimal results. The technique is, however, more sensitive than SSCP, more easily detects single base differences, and may be so specific that a characteristic electrophoretic pattern may be produced by a single base mutation. In most cases, however, the suspected mutation should be confirmed by a more specific technique.

SPECIFIC TECHNIQUES FOR DETECTION OF DNA SEQUENCE ABNORMALITIES

Direct DNA Sequencing

Direct DNA sequencing of PCR products is the most sensitive and specific method for detection of specific mutations (2,8). This technique is impractical to apply on a widespread basis, however, unless the region to be analyzed has been narrowed to several hundred to 1000 nucleotides. Direct DNA sequencing of a PCR product derived from genomic DNA permits analysis of both alleles or copies of the gene and the identification of new or unreported mutations. The disadvantages include its complexity and the difficulty of analyzing more than 200 nucleotides in a single sequencing reaction. In a disease such as MEN type II, in which more than 90% of known mutations are clustered in a small region of the *RET* protooncogene, this approach offers the ability to detect most mutations in a single sequencing run (8,9).

One strategy used is to focus initially on the most common

mutations and to extend sequencing to include other regions of the gene only in those individuals for whom the initial analysis does not identify a mutation.

Allele-Specific Hybridization

Short DNA sequences will hybridize (create a double-stranded piece of DNA by nucleotide pairing) most readily to a sequence with perfect complementarity (i.e., A's will hybridize best to T's, and G's to C's). In a disease caused by a single or finite number of nucleotide changes within a gene, it is possible to exploit complementarity to develop a detection system for a specific mutation (2,9).

There are several variations of this technique, but in its simplest form, oligonucleotides containing all possible disease-causing sequence changes are synthesized, dotted, and immobilized on a nylon membrane (Fig. 2). The complementary fragment of DNA from the patient is amplified by PCR and radiolabeled, and DNA/DNA hybridization is performed by using conditions in which only a perfectly matched DNA sequence will hybridize. Only those DNA molecules from the patient that contain the mutant sequence will hybridize to the synthetic oligonucleotide. This method is rapid, technically easy to perform, and permits rapid analysis of large numbers of samples. The major drawback is its inability to detect mutations beyond those included in the dotted oligonucleotides, making it almost certain that a new or previously unidentified mutation will not be detected. This technique is best used for rapid screening of a family whose specific mutation is already known.

Restriction Endonuclease Analysis

This provides a simple and effective method for detecting the presence or absence of mutations at a single site and is useful when a mutation creates or destroys a restriction site. For example, a single nucleotide change in the sequence GTGC to GTAC would create a new restriction site for the endonuclease *Rsa* I. A PCR amplification product from a patient who inherited this mutation from a single parent would contain one normal DNA sequence and one containing the single nucleotide mutation. Addition of the restriction enzyme *Rsa* I to a PCR product from this patient would result in cleavage of the allele containing the mutant sequence into two fragments, whereas the allele containing the normal sequence would remain uncleaved. Separation of these fragments by gel electrophoresis (Fig. 2) would show one uncut fragment representing the normal sequence and two smaller fragments representing the cleaved mutant allele. Mutations that destroy an existing restriction site provide an additional analytic challenge because it is necessary to document that the enzyme is active before concluding that the failure to cleave the DNA fragment into two pieces is caused by a mutation. To establish the activity of the enzyme, a positive control (a piece of DNA that contains the normal restriction site) is included with each analysis. This technique is used most effectively when a single DNA sequence change causes all examples of the disease or in a family whose specific mutation is known.

SOURCES OF ERROR IN GENETIC TESTING

It is important that clinicians be aware of the frequency and nature of genetic testing errors (9). Sample mix-up, especially in family screening in which many family members share a common last name, may occur in up to 5% of analyses. These errors may occur at the time of blood drawing or during subsequent analysis or recording. A second potential source of error is contamination by DNA from individuals who harbor a disease-causing mutation. The funneling of large numbers of samples to a few laboratories for analysis of a single disease further increases the chance of contamination. The extreme sensitivity of PCR analysis makes it possible that a positive result could occur as a result of airborne contamination of a reaction tube. A third source of error is the failure to amplify both alleles, thereby resulting in the possibility of a false-negative result because only the normal allele is included in the analysis. The most common explanation for amplification failure is a random polymorphism (DNA sequence change) acting to reduce oligonucleotide primer hybridization during the PCR reaction.

If genetic testing is to be used as the sole determinant for decision making in disease management, it is important for the clinician to be aware of the possibility of errors and to take steps to minimize their impact on patient care. One simple approach that will eliminate the majority of these errors is to repeat each analysis, whether positive or negative, in a different laboratory on an independently obtained sample. This approach will identify most sample mix-up, DNA contamination, and technical errors. Sending the sample to a separate laboratory that uses a different primer set for PCR amplification also will reduce the likelihood of a single allele amplification error.

INTEGRATION OF GENETIC INFORMATION INTO CLINICAL MANAGEMENT

Genetic testing has several important clinical uses. Identification of a specific disease-causing mutation may clarify and simplify patient management. For example, the identification of a mutation of the calcium receptor causative of familial hypercalcemic hypocalciuria (see Chapter 32) in an individual with an atypical clinical presentation may prevent unnecessary parathyroid surgery. In other situations, such as MEN type II (see Chapter 31), the identification of a specific mutation may lead to a specific action (thyroidectomy) in a child (9).

In other situations, the benefits of genetic screening may be more ambiguous. The identification of a mutation in an individual with a severe and fatal form of osteogenesis imperfecta may not alter therapy for the patient; however, detection of the mutation may make prenatal genetic screening possible. Identification and categorization of these muta-

tions also are important because gene-therapy strategies, especially for single gene defects, are evolving rapidly. Table 1 provides a current summary of gene defects that cause bone and mineral diseases in humans.

An evolving area of genetic research implicates subtle DNA differences in the pathogenesis of disease (10). For example, genetic studies examining polymorphism identified several candidate genes that may be involved in osteoporosis, including the vitamin D receptor (11), the estrogen receptor (12), and the collagen type I α1 gene (13). Although the role of these polymorphisms is currently controversial, there are examples in other systems that clearly point to population-based genetic differences that may influence disease expression. The techniques for identification of these polymorphisms can use any of the methods described in Fig. 2, but typically look for differences in the size of a PCR product on a denaturing gel. Further characterization and clarification of the roles that these genetic polymorphisms play in disease genesis may permit us to identify high-risk populations for application of preventive strategies.

REFERENCES

1. Saiki RK, Gelfand DH, Stoffel S, et al. Primer-directed enzymatic amplification of DNA with a thermostable DNA polymerase. *Science* 1988;239:487–491.
2. Cotton RGH. Current methods of mutation detection. *Mutat Res* 1993;285:125–144.
3. Birren B, Green ED, Klapholz S, Meyers RM, Roskams J. *Genome analysis, Vol 2, detecting genes: a laboratory manual.* New York: Cold Spring Harbor Laboratory Press, 1998.
4. Ainsworth PJ, Surh LC, Coulter-Mackie MB. Diagnostic single-strand conformational polymorphism (SSCP): A simplified non-radioisotopic method as applied to a Tay-Sachs B1 variant. *Nucleic Acids Res* 1991;19:405–406.
5. Sarkar G, Yoon H-S, Sommer SS. Dideoxy fingerprinting (ddF): a rapid and efficient screen for the presence of mutations. *Genomics* 1992;13:441–443.
6. Chandrasekharappa SC, Guru SC, Manickam P, et al. Positional cloning of the gene for multiple endocrine neoplasia-type I. *Science* 1997; 276:404–407.
7. Fodde R, Losekoot M. Mutation detection by denaturing gradient gel electrophoresis (DGGE). *Hum Mutat* 1994;3:83–94.
8. Khorana S, Gagel RF, Cote GJ. Direct sequencing of PCR products in agarose gel slices. *Nucleic Acids Res* 22:3425–3426.
9. Cote GJ, Wohllk N, Evans D, Goepfert H, Gagel RF. *RET* proto-oncogene mutations in multiple endocrine neoplasia type II and medullary thyroid carcinoma. *Baillieres Clin Endocrinol Metab* 1995;9: 609–630.
10. Ralston SH. The genetics of osteoporosis. *Q J Med* 1997;90:247–251.
11. Morrison NA, Qi JC, Tokita A, et al. Prediction of bone density from vitamin D receptor alleles. *Nature* 1994;367:284–287.
12. Sano M, Inoue S, Hosoi T, et al. Association of estrogen receptor dinucleotide repeat polymorphism with osteoporosis. *Biochem Biophys Res Commun* 1995;217:378–383.
13. Uitterlinden AG, Burger H, Huang Q, et al. Relation of alleles of the collagen type I alpha1 gene to bone density and the risk of osteoporotic fractures in postmenopausal women. *N Engl J Med* 1998;338:1016–1021.

SECTION V

Disorders of Serum Minerals

29. Hypercalcemia: Pathogenesis, Clinical Manifestations, Differential Diagnosis, and Management

Elizabeth Shane, M.D.

Department of Medicine, Columbia University College of Physicians and Surgeons,
and New York Presbyterian Hospital, New York, New York

The clinical presentation of hypercalcemia varies from a mild, asymptomatic, biochemical abnormality detected during routine screening to a life-threatening medical emergency. In this chapter, pathogenesis, clinical manifestations, differential diagnosis, and management of hypercalcemia are discussed.

PATHOGENESIS

The concentration of calcium in the extracellular fluid is critical for many physiologic processes. Under normal circumstances, the range is remarkably constant, between 8.5 and 10.5 mg/dL (2.1 to 2.5 mm). The exact normal range varies slightly, depending on the laboratory. Approximately half the total serum calcium is bound to plasma proteins, primarily albumin. A small component of the total calcium is complexed to anions such as citrate or sulfate. The remaining half circulates as the free calcium ion. It is only this ionized portion of the total serum calcium that is physiologically important, regulating neuromuscular contractility, the process of coagulation, and a variety of other cellular activities.

In a variety of chronic illnesses, a substantial reduction in the serum albumin concentration may reduce the total serum calcium concentration, whereas ionized calcium concentrations remain normal. A simple correction for hypoalbuminemia may be made by adding 0.8 mg/dL to the total serum calcium concentration for every 1.0 g/dL by which the serum albumin concentration is <4.0 g/dL. Thus a patient with a total serum calcium of 10.5 mg/dL and a serum albumin level of 2.0 g/dL has a corrected total serum calcium of 12.1 mg/dL. Conversely, falsely elevated serum calcium levels may be observed, usually the result of an elevation of the serum albumin due to dehydration or hemoconcentration during venipuncture. A similar maneuver can be performed to correct the serum calcium in this situation, except that the correction factor must be subtracted from the serum calcium level.

In contrast to changes in the serum albumin concentration, which affect the total but not the ionized calcium level, alterations in pH affect the ionized but not the total calcium concentration. Acidosis increases the ionized calcium by decreasing the binding of calcium ions to albumin, whereas alkalosis decreases the ionized calcium by enhancing binding of calcium ions to albumin. Measurement of total serum calcium, particularly if corrected for the serum albumin, is usually adequate for most situations. However, in complex cases (changes in both albumin and pH), a direct measurement of the ionized calcium should be performed.

Under normal circumstances, the plasma calcium concentration reflects a balance between the flux of calcium into the extracellular fluid from the gastrointestinal (GI) tract, the skeleton, and the kidney, and the flux of calcium out

of the extracellular fluid into the skeleton and the urine. Hypercalcemia develops when the rate of calcium entry into the blood compartment is greater than its rate of removal. This occurs most commonly when accelerated osteoclastic bone resorption or excessive GI calcium absorption delivers quantities of calcium into the blood that exceed the capacities of the kidney to eliminate it and of the skeleton to reclaim it. Less commonly, normal rates of calcium entry into the extracellular fluid may result in hypercalcemia if the process of renal excretion or that of bone mineralization is impaired.

Accelerated bone resorption by osteoclasts, multinucleated bone-resorbing cells, is the primary pathogenetic mechanism in most instances of hypercalcemia (1). Osteoclasts may be stimulated to resorb bone by parathyroid hormone (PTH), PTH-related protein (PTHrP), and 1,25-dihydroxy-vitamin D [1,25 (OH)$_2$ D], all of which have been shown to cause hypercalcemia (2,3). A number of cytokines (interleukin-1α, interleukin-1β, interleukin-6, tumor necrosis factor, lymphotoxin, and transforming growth factor-α) also stimulate osteoclastic bone resorption either alone or in concert with PTHrP (4). Some cytokines have been linked to the development of hypercalcemia in human malignancy (4). Excessive GI absorption of calcium is a much less common cause of hypercalcemia, although it may play a role in hypercalcemic states characterized by excess vitamin D, such as lymphoma or vitamin D intoxication. Whether the primary cause of the hypercalcemia is accelerated bone resorption or excessive GI tract absorption of calcium, the kidney is the primary defender against an increase in the serum calcium. Thus hypercalcemia is usually preceded by hypercalciuria, and it is only when the capacity of the kidney to excrete calcium has been exceeded that the patient becomes hypercalcemic (5).

Several other factors may contribute to the pathogenesis of hypercalcemia. In addition to stimulating osteoclast-mediated bone resorption, both PTH and PTHrP increase reabsorption of calcium from the distal tubule, thus interfering with the ability of the kidneys to clear the filtered calcium load. Hypercalcemia interferes with the action of antidiuretic hormone on the distal tubule, causing a form of nephrogenic diabetes insipidus that results in polyuria. The thirst mechanism may not be fully operative because of the nausea and vomiting that frequently accompany hypercalcemia; thus urinary fluid losses may not be replaced, and dehydration may ensue. The resulting reduction in the extracellular fluid volume and associated reduction in the glomerular filtration rate exacerbate the hypercalcemia. Finally, immobilization also may contribute to hypercalcemia by virtue of associated increases in bone resorption.

CLINICAL MANIFESTATIONS

The clinical presentation of the hypercalcemic patient (6) may involve several organ systems. The signs and symptoms

183

tend to be similar regardless of the etiology of the hypercalcemia. Because an optimal extracellular calcium concentration is necessary for normal neurologic function, symptoms of neurologic dysfunction often predominate in hypercalcemic states. The patient (or family members) may notice subtle changes in the ability to concentrate or an increased sleep requirement. With increasing severity of the hypercalcemia, symptoms may gradually progress to depression, confusion, and even coma. Muscle weakness is common.

Gastrointestinal symptoms are often prominent, with constipation, anorexia, nausea, and vomiting present in varying degrees. Pancreatitis and peptic ulcer disease are unusual but have been reported. They may be somewhat more common if the hypercalcemia is due to primary hyperparathyroidism than to other causes of hypercalcemia.

Polyuria, resulting from the impaired concentrating ability of the distal nephron, is common, particularly during the early phases. Polydipsia also is usually present. The combination of polyuria and diminished fluid intake due to GI symptoms may lead to severe dehydration. Nephrolithiasis occurs in patients with primary hyperparathyroidism (15% to 20% in recent series), but along with nephrocalcinosis, it also may develop in patients with hypercalcemia due to other causes, particularly when the hypercalcemia is chronic.

Hypercalcemia increases the rate of cardiac repolarization. Thus shortening of the QT interval is observed commonly on the electrocardiogram. Bradycardia and first-degree atrioventricular block, as well as other arrhythmias, may occur. Caution should be exercised when treating the hypercalcemic patient with digitalis, because increased sensitivity to this drug has been observed.

In general, the presence or absence of symptoms correlates with the degree of elevation of the serum calcium and with the rapidity of its increase. Most patients do not begin to show clinical features of hypercalcemia until the total calcium concentration exceeds 12 mg/dL, and patients are almost invariably symptomatic at levels >14 mg/dL. However, there is much individual variation in this regard. Certain patients will be quite symptomatic with moderate hypercalcemia of 12.0 to 14.0 mg/dL, whereas others may show no overt symptoms at a similar level. The latter situation occurs most often in chronic hypercalcemia. In other circumstances, the absence of symptoms in the severely hypercalcemic patient should prompt one to measure the ionized calcium level to be certain that hypercalcemia is not the result of excessive binding of calcium to plasma proteins (Chapter 37).

DIFFERENTIAL DIAGNOSIS

Detection of an elevated serum calcium level requires that the etiology be established. The many causes of hypercalcemia are listed in Table 1, and most are covered separately in subsequent chapters. However, certain general principles that apply to the differential diagnosis of hypercalcemia are covered here.

Malignancy and primary hyperparathyroidism are by far the most common causes of hypercalcemia, accounting for >90% of hypercalcemic patients (6). Differentiating between these two diagnoses is generally not difficult on clini-

TABLE 1. *Differential diagnosis of hypercalcemia*

Most common
  Primary hyperparathyroidism
  Malignant disease
    Parathyroid hormone–related protein (carcinoma of lung, esophagus, head and neck, renal cell, ovary, and bladder)
    Ectopic production of 1,25-dihydroxyvitamin D (lymphoma)
    Lytic bone metastases (multiple myeloma and breast carcinoma)
    Other factor(s) produced locally or ectopically
Uncommon
  Endocrine disorders
    Thyrotoxicosis
  Granulomatous diseases
    Sarcoidosis
  Drug induced
    Vitamin D
    Thiazide diuretics
    Lithium
    Estrogens and antiestrogens
    Androgens (breast cancer therapy)
    Aminophylline
    Vitamin A
    Aluminum intoxication (in chronic renal failure)
  Miscellaneous
    Immobilization
    Renal failure (acute and chronic)
    Total parenteral nutrition
Rare
  Endocrine disorders
    Pheochromocytoma
    Vasoactive intestinal polypeptide–producing tumor
    Familial hypocalciuric hypercalcemia
  Granulomatous diseases
    Tuberculosis
    Histoplasmosis
    Cocidioidomycosis
    Leprosy
  Miscellaneous
    Milk-alkali syndrome
    Hypophosphatasia

cal grounds alone. The vast majority of patients with primary hyperparathyroidism have relatively mild hypercalcemia, within 1.0 mg/dL above the upper limits of normal and usually <12.0 mg/dL. They are often asymptomatic. Review of medical records may reveal that the hypercalcemia has been present for months to years. When symptoms of hypercalcemia are present, they tend to be chronic, such as nephrolithiasis. In contrast, patients with hypercalcemia of malignancy are usually ill and are more likely to manifest the classic signs and symptoms of an elevated serum calcium. In general, the malignancy itself is readily apparent and presents little diagnostic challenge to the physician. Less commonly, occult malignancy may be seen with hypercalcemia, or the patient with primary hyperparathyroidism may have moderate to severe elevation of the serum calcium that is associated with symptoms or with the acute onset of severe hypercalcemia (parathyroid crisis). Such cases pose a greater diagnostic problem.

The availability of reliable assays for intact PTH based on double-antibody techniques (two-site, immunoradiometric, or immunochemiluminescent assays) has been of great diagnostic value in the evaluation of the hypercalcemic patient. The majority of patients with primary hyperparathyroidism have intact PTH levels that are frankly elevated. Patients with hypercalcemia of malignancy virtually always demonstrate suppressed or undetectable levels of intact PTH. It is distinctly unusual for a patient with malignancy (excepting parathyroid cancer) to show elevated levels of PTH. When this occurs, two possibilities exist: the patient may have concomitant primary hyperparathyroidism, or the malignancy itself may be secreting PTH, an uncommon event.

In most patients with malignancy-associated hypercalcemia, the hypercalcemia is a result of secretion of PTHrP by the tumor (2). Commercial assays for PTHrP are now available; when elevated, they can prove helpful in the diagnosis of hypercalcemia of malignancy. However, a negative result does not exclude malignancy, particularly because certain tumors cause hypercalcemia by mechanisms independent of PTHrP, such as secretion of other bone-resorbing cytokines, or extrarenal conversion of 25-hydroxyvitamin D to $1,25 (OH)_2$ D. Local bone-resorbing effects of tumors such as breast cancer also may be involved.

Hypercalcemia from causes other than malignancy or primary hyperparathyroidism also may occur. A thorough history and physical examination are invaluable in arriving at the correct diagnosis. Each of the etiologies listed in Table 1 is covered in one of the other chapters in this section.

MANAGEMENT

The decision to institute therapy for the hypercalcemic patient depends on the level of the serum calcium and the presence or absence of clinical manifestations of an elevated serum calcium. In general, patients with mild hypercalcemia (<12.0 mg/dL) do not have symptoms of hypercalcemia and do not derive significant clinical benefit from normalization of their serum calcium. Thus immediate intervention is not usually necessary. In contrast, when the serum calcium is >14.0 mg/dL, therapy should be initiated regardless of whether the patient has signs or symptoms of hypercalcemia. Moderate elevation of the serum calcium (12.0 to 14.0 mg/dL) should be treated aggressively if the patient demonstrates clinical signs or symptoms consistent with hypercalcemia. However, if such a patient is asymptomatic, a more conservative approach may be appropriate. It also is important to consider the underlying cause of the hypercalcemia when deciding whether therapy is necessary and the type of therapy to institute. For example, a patient with acute primary hyperparathyroidism, a completely curable condition, would warrant more aggressive treatment than a patient with diffuse metastatic cancer and a poor prognosis. Another difficult situation arises in the patient whose serum calcium is about 12.0 mg/dL, not within the range one would usually treat aggressively, yet who has an altered mental status or other symptoms that could conceivably be ascribed to a hypercalcemic state. In such situations, it is important to consider other potential causes for the symptoms before instituting therapy.

TABLE 2. *Management of hypercalcemia*

General
  Hydration
  Saline diuresis
  Loop diuretics
  Dialysis
  Mobilization
Specific
  Bisphosphonates
    Pamidronate
    Etidronate
    Clodronate
  Plicamycin (mithramycin)
  Calcitonin
  Gallium nitrate
Therapy of underlying causes

The management of hypercalcemia is outlined in Table 2. When the serum calcium exceeds 12.0 mg/dL, and signs and symptoms are present, a series of general measures should be instituted. Most of these therapeutic maneuvers tend to lower serum calcium by increasing urinary calcium excretion (7,8). Dehydration, resulting from the pathophysiologic events induced by the hypercalcemia (anorexia, nausea, vomiting, defective urinary concentrating mechanism, and polyuria) is very common. Hydration with normal saline, to correct the extracellular fluid deficit, is central to the early management of hypercalcemia from any cause. Restoration of the volume deficit can usually be achieved by the continuous infusion of 3 to 4 L of 0.9% sodium chloride over a 24- to 48-hour period. This maneuver generally lowers the serum calcium by 1.0 to 3.0 mg/dL. Hydration with saline enhances urinary calcium excretion by increasing glomerular filtration of calcium and decreasing both proximal and distal tubular reabsorption of sodium and calcium. However, saline hydration alone does not usually establish normocalcemia unless the calcium concentration is only modestly elevated. Moreover, this form of therapy must be used with caution in elderly patients or in others with compromised cardiovascular or renal function.

Under certain circumstances, a loop diuretic, such as furosemide or ethacrynic acid, may be added to saline hydration in the therapy of hypercalcemia. Loop diuretics act on the thick ascending loop of Henle to inhibit both sodium and calcium reabsorption. Thus the use of such agents enhances urinary calcium losses, increases the likelihood of normalization of the serum calcium level, and mitigates the dangers of hypernatremia and volume overload that may accompany the use of intravenous saline. Only after extracellular fluid volume has been replenished should small doses of furosemide (10 to 20 mg) be administered as necessary to control clinical manifestations of volume excess. Overzealous use of loop diuretics before intravascular volume has been restored can worsen hypercalcemia by exacerbating volume depletion. Hypokalemia and other electrolyte abnormalities can ensue. Intensive therapy with large doses of furosemide (80 to 100 mg every 1 to 2 hours) and replacement of fluid and electrolytes based on measured urinary losses is rarely indicated. It must be emphasized that thiazide diuretics are contraindicated in this setting because they decrease renal calcium excretion and may worsen hypercalcemia.

Dialysis, another general measure, is usually reserved for the severely hypercalcemic patient. Peritoneal dialysis or hemodialysis with a low or zero calcium dialysate will lower serum calcium rapidly in those patients who are refractory to other measures or who have renal insufficiency. Finally, the patient should be mobilized as soon as clinically feasible to minimize the negative calcium balance that accompanies immobilization.

Specific approaches to the hypercalcemic patient are based on the underlying pathophysiology. Excessive mobilization of calcium from the skeleton resulting from an accelerated rate of bone resorption is the most important factor in the pathogenesis of hypercalcemia in the majority of patients. Numerous pharmacologic agents specifically block osteoclast-mediated bone resorption and effectively lower serum calcium in most hypercalcemic patients (Table 2).

Inorganic pyrophosphates are naturally occurring inhibitors of bone resorption. Bisphosphonates are analogues of pyrophosphate that are resistant to phosphatases. These drugs are bone-seeking compounds that bind to hydroxyapatite and prevent its dissolution. Osteoclast function is impaired after exposure to bisphosphonates, and these drugs have had increasing use in disorders characterized by excessive bone resorption. GI absorption of bisphosphonates is very poor, and therefore intravenous administration is usually necessary when they are used to treat hypercalcemia. Bisphosphonates should be administered in large volumes (>500 mL) over 4 hours to prevent nephrotoxicity due to precipitation of calcium bisphosphonate. Three bisphosphonates, pamidronate, etidronate, and alendronate are currently approved for use in the United States. Another effective bisphosphonate, clodronate, is available in Europe and the United Kingdom but is unavailable in the United States. Other more potent bisphosphonates are under investigation.

Pamidronate is the most potent bisphosphonate available for the treatment of hypercalcemia. Although a variety of regimens have been reported, the recommended dose is 60 to 90 mg intravenously as a single infusion. Pamidronate may cause transient fever (20% of patients) and myalgias during the day after the infusion. Preemptive treatment with acetaminophen ameliorates these side effects in the majority of patients. Occasionally, transient leukopenia may develop. Mild, usually asymptomatic, hypocalcemia (10%) and hypophosphatemia (10% to 30%) may occur in some patients, particularly with higher doses (90 mg). The 90-mg dose also has been associated with infusion reactions. Both pamidronate and clodronate have been reported to reduce the progression of skeletal metastases and prevent the onset of hypercalcemia in patients with breast cancer, and monthly pamidronate infusions reduce the skeletal complications of multiple myeloma. The duration of the hypocalcemic effect of pamidronate is variable, ranging from several days to several weeks.

Etidronate, a first-generation bisphosphonate, can be administered by intravenous infusion for therapy of hypercalcemia (9–11). However, a single 4-hour infusion of pamidronate (60 mg) is associated with a more rapid duration of action, a larger decline in serum calcium, and a longer duration of action than a 3-day course of etidronate. Therefore,

pamidronate has largely replaced etidronate in the therapy of hypercalcemia.

Plicamycin, previously called mithramycin, is a cytotoxic antibiotic that blocks RNA synthesis in osteoclasts and therefore inhibits bone resorption. When administered intravenously in a dose of 15 to 25 μg/kg over a period of 4 to 6 hours, plicamycin effectively lowers elevated calcium levels in most patients. The serum calcium usually begins to decline within 12 hours of administration and generally reaches its nadir within 48 to 72 hours. Often a single dose may be sufficient to achieve normocalcemia. However, if necessary, the dose may be repeated several times at 24- to 48-hour intervals. The duration of the normocalcemia depends on the intensity of underlying bone resorption and may vary from days to weeks. Administration is commonly associated with nausea, which may be minimized by slow infusion rates. Plicamycin has considerable toxicity (bone marrow, renal, hepatic); it may be associated with transient elevation of transaminases, serum creatinine, or both, with proteinuria, and with thrombocytopenia, particularly when repeated administrations (more than three or four) are required. These toxicities make this drug of limited usefulness in chronic hypercalcemia. Bisphosphonates are replacing plicamycin as a less toxic first-line therapy in the severely hypercalcemic patient. However, when serum calcium requires rapid correction, plicamycin remains a reasonable choice.

Calcitonin is a polypeptide hormone that is secreted by the parafollicular C-cells of the thyroid gland. Salmon calcitonin is the most potent and frequently used form of the drug. Calcitonin inhibits osteoclastic bone resorption, increases urinary calcium excretion, and is a very safe drug. Moreover, calcitonin has the most rapid onset of action of the available calcium-lowering drugs, causing the serum calcium to fall within 2 to 6 hours of administration. The usual dose ranges from 4 to 8 IU/kg, administered by intramuscular or subcutaneous injection every 6 to 8 hours. Unfortunately, the hypocalcemic effect of calcitonin is transient, not as pronounced as either plicamycin or the bisphosphonates, and rarely normalizes the serum calcium. The serum calcium concentration usually declines by a mean of 2 mg/dL and may begin to rise again within 24 hours, despite continued therapy. Calcitonin given in combination with bisphosphonates or plicamycin appears to achieve a more rapid and greater decrease in the serum calcium than when either drug is administered by itself. Used in this way, calcitonin has a role at the outset of therapy in instances of severe hypercalcemia, when it is desirable to lower the serum calcium more rapidly than can be accomplished with either plicamycin or a bisphosphonate alone (7).

Gallium nitrate, originally studied as a therapeutic agent for cancer, also is approved by the Food and Drug Administration for the therapy of hypercalcemia. Although its precise mechanism of action is uncertain, it appears to adsorb to hydroxyapatite crystals (1) and may inhibit bone resorption by reducing crystal solubility. A direct inhibitory effect on the osteoclast also was observed (12). When administered as a continuous 5-day infusion at a dose of 200 mg/m^2/day, it was reported to normalize the serum calcium in a majority of patients. The rate of fall of the serum calcium was rather slow, in that a normal level was not reached until the end of the 5-day infusion, and the nadir was not achieved until

3 days later. Gallium nitrate causes elevation of the serum creatinine that may be potentiated by volume depletion and concomitant administration of other nephrotoxic drugs. Its use is contraindicated in renal insufficiency (i.e., serum creatinine >2.5 mg/dL) and when other nephrotoxic agents are being used. It also may be associated with reduction in the serum phosphate and hemoglobin concentrations. For these reasons, it is not the ideal agent for therapy of hypercalcemia and is not in common use.

Glucocorticoid therapy has been used for many years to treat hypercalcemia, particularly when due to hematologic malignancies such as lymphoma and multiple myeloma. Glucocorticoids also are effective in situations such as vitamin D toxicity or granulomatous diseases in which the hypercalcemia is mediated by the actions of $1,25\ (OH)_2\ D$. Glucocorticoids are seldom effective in patients with solid tumors or primary hyperparathyroidism. The usual dose is 200 to 300 mg of intravenous hydrocortisone, or its equivalent, daily for 3 to 5 days.

Intravenous phosphate was used in the past to lower serum calcium in hypercalcemic patients. However, intravenous phosphate is accompanied by a substantial risk of precipitation of calcium–phosphate complexes, leading to severe organ damage and even death. This form of therapy should rarely be necessary today and is not recommended.

Therapy for the underlying cause of the hypercalcemia should not be neglected, because specific therapy may be the most effective approach to the problem. However, patients with widespread metastatic disease, in whom no further specific antitumor chemotherapy is to be given, may be approached with the realization that reduction of the serum calcium per se will achieve little in the long run. In these circumstances, sometimes the best approach is to resist specific measures to reduce the serum calcium and to make the patient as comfortable as possible.

REFERENCES

1. Attie MF. Treatment of hypercalcemia. *Endocrinol Metab Clin North Am* 1989;18:807–828.
2. Halloran BP, Nissenson BA, eds. *Parathyroid hormone-related protein: normal physiology and its role in cancer.* Boca Raton, FL: CRC Press, 1992.
3. Adams JS, Fernandez M, Gacad MA, et al. Vitamin-D metabolite-mediated hypercalcemia and hypercalciuria in patients with AIDS and non-AIDS associated lymphoma. *Blood* 1989;73:235–239.
4. Mundy GR. Role of cytokines, parathyroid hormone and growth factors in malignancy. In: Bilezikian JP, Raisz LG, Rodan GA, eds. *Principles of bone biology.* New York: Academic Press, 1996:827–836.
5. Harinck HIJ, Bijvoet OLM, Plantingh AST, et al. Role of bone and kidney in tumor-induced hypercalcemia and its treatment with bisphosphonate and sodium chloride. *Am J Med* 1987;82:1133–1142.
6. Bilezikian JP, Singer FR. Acute management of hypercalcemia due to parathyroid hormone and parathyroid hormone-related protein. In: Bilezikian JP, Marcus R, Levine MA, eds. *The parathyroids.* New York: Raven Press, 1994:359–372.
7. Bilezikian JP. Management of acute hypercalcemia. *N Engl J Med* 1992;326:1196–1203.
8. Grill V, Murray RML, Ho PWM, et al. Circulating PTH and PTHrP levels before and after treatment of tumor induced hypercalcemia with pamidronate disodium. *J Clin Endocrinol Metab* 1990;74:1468–1470.
9. Nussbaum SR. Pathophysiology and management of severe hypercalcemia. *Endocrinol Metab Clin North Am* 1993;22:343–362.
10. Jacobs TP, Gordon AC, Silverberg SJ, et al. Neoplastic hypercalcemia: physiologic response to intravenous etidronate disodium. *Am J Med* 1987;82(suppl 2a):42–50.
11. Flores JF, Singer FR, Rude RK. Twenty-four hour infusion of etidronate for hypercalcemia of malignancy. *Miner Electrolyte Metab* 1991;17:390–395.
12. Hall TJ, Chambers TJ. Gallium inhibits bone resorption by a direct action on osteoclasts. *Bone Miner* 1990;8:211–216.

30. Primary Hyperparathyroidism

John P. Bilezikian, M.D.

Departments of Medicine and Pharmacology, and Division of Endocrinology, College of Physicians and Surgeons, and Department of Medicine, Columbia Presbyterian Medical Center, New York, New York

Primary hyperparathyroidism is one of the two most common causes of hypercalcemia and thus ranks high as a key diagnostic possibility in anyone with an elevated serum calcium concentration. It is a relatively common endocrine disease with an incidence as high as 1 in 500 to 1 in 1000 (1). The high visibility of primary hyperparathyroidism in the population today marks a dramatic change from several generations ago when it was considered to be a rare disorder. The fourfold to fivefold increase in incidence since the early 1970s is due primarily to the widespread use of the autoanalyzer, gratuitously providing serum calcium determinations when the test is usually ordered for another reason (2). A recent decline in the incidence in primary hyperparathyroidism was reported by Wermers et al (3). It is not clear whether that experience reflects a particular demographic characteristic of Rochester, Minnesota, or whether it portends a more general decline in incidence, a possible outcome if automated screening tests are to be restricted in the United States. Primary hyperparathyroidism occurs at all ages but is most frequent in the sixth decade of life. Women are affected more often than men by a ratio of 3 : 1. The majority of individuals are postmenopausal women. When it is found in children, an unusual event, it is likely to be a component of one of several endocrinopathies with a genetic basis, such as multiple endocrine neoplasia, type I or II (Chapter 31).

Primary hyperparathyroidism is a hypercalcemic state due to excessive secretion of parathyroid hormone (PTH) from one or more parathyroid glands. The disease is caused by a benign, solitary adenoma 80% of the time. A parathyroid adenoma is a collection of chief cells surrounded by a rim of normal tissue at the outer perimeter of the gland. In the patient with a parathyroid adenoma, the remaining three parathyroid glands are normal. Less commonly, primary hyperparathyroidism is due to a pathologic process characterized by hyperplasia of all four parathyroid glands. Four-gland parathyroid hyperplasia is seen in 15% to 20% of patients with primary hyperparathyroidism. Four-gland disease may occur sporadically, but also in association with multiple endocrine neoplasia, types I or II (Chapter 31). A very rare presentation of primary hyperparathyroidism is parathyroid carcinoma, occurring in fewer than 0.5% of patients with hyperparathyroidism (4). Pathologic examination of the malignant tissue might show mitoses, vascular invasion, and fibrous trabeculae but is often not definitive. Unless local invasion or distant metastases are present, the diagnosis of parathyroid cancer can be exceedingly difficult to make.

The pathophysiology of primary hyperparathyroidism relates to the loss of normal feedback control of PTH by extracellular calcium. With virtually all other hypercalcemic conditions, the parathyroid gland is suppressed, and PTH levels are low. Why the parathyroid cell loses its normal sensitivity to calcium is unknown, but in adenomas, this appears to be the major mechanism. In primary hyperparathyroidism due to hyperplasia of the parathyroid glands, the "set point" for calcium is not changed for a given parathyroid cell, but the increased number of cells per se gives rise to the hypercalcemia.

The underlying cause of primary hyperparathyroidism is not known. External neck irradiation in childhood, recognized in some patients, is unlikely to be causative in the majority of patients. The clonal origin of most parathyroid adenomas suggests a defect at the level of the gene controlling growth of the parathyroid cell or in the expression of PTH. Patients with primary hyperparathyroidism have been discovered in whom the protooncogene PRAD 1 (or cyclin D1) is rearranged to a site in close proximity to specific enhancer elements of the PTH gene (5). This realignment places a growth promoter under the control of a regulatory element that normally controls PTH synthesis exclusively. Thus when the synthesis of PTH is stimulated, tissue growth also is stimulated. Although this genetic mechanism is attractive, such rearrangements have been documented in only a small number of parathyroid adenomas. On the other hand, increased levels of PRAD 1 protein have been seen in up to 20% of parathyroid adenomas (6). Another molecular explanation for clonal expansion of a parathyroid cell into an adenoma is inactivation of a tumor-suppressor gene. The tumor-suppressor gene identified in association with multiple endocrine neoplasia, type I (7,8) has been demonstrated to be abnormal in up to 17% of patients with parathyroid adenomas (9). Another candidate tumor-suppressor gene is located in chromosomal region 1p (10). The possibility that the calcium-sensing receptor gene could be abnormal in primary hyperparathyroidism has not received much experimental support (11,12).

SIGNS AND SYMPTOMS

Primary hyperparathyroidism is associated classically with skeletal and renal complications. At skeletal sites, excess PTH can lead to a condition called *osteitis fibrosa cystica*. Subperiosteal resorption of the distal phalanges, tapering of the distal clavicles, a "salt and pepper" appear-ance of the skull, bone cysts, and brown tumors of the long bones are all overt manifestations of hyperparathyroid bone disease. The skeletal features are readily seen by conventional radiographs if they are present. Along with the major increase in incidence of primary hyperparathyroidism, however, overt hyperparathyroid bone disease has become most unusual. It is now seen in well under 5% of patients with primary hyperparathyroidism (13).

Similar to the skeleton, the kidney also is involved in primary hyperparathyroidism much less commonly than before. The incidence of kidney stones has declined from approximately 33% in the 1960s to 20% now. Nephrolithiasis, nevertheless, is still the most common complication of the hyperparathyroid process (14). Other renal features of primary hyperparathyroidism include diffuse deposition of calcium–phosphate complexes in the parenchyma (nephrocalcinosis). Hypercalciuria [>250 mg (women) or >300 mg (men) daily calcium excretion] is seen in up to 30% of patients. Primary hyperparathyroidism may be associated with a reduction in creatinine clearance, in the absence of any other cause.

The classic neuromuscular syndrome of primary hyperparathyroidism, which is associated with a definable myopathy, has virtually disappeared (15). In its place, however, is a less well-defined syndrome characterized by easy fatigability, a sense of weakness, and a feeling that the aging process is advancing faster than it should. This is sometimes accompanied by an intellectual weariness and a sense that cognitive faculties are less sharp. In some studies, psychometric evaluation has appeared to reveal a distinct psychiatric profile (16). Whether these nonspecific features of primary hyperparathyroidism are truly part and parcel of the disease process, reversible on successful parathyroid surgery, is an issue that has not yet been settled by definitive studies (17).

Gastrointestinal manifestations of primary hyperparathyroidism have classically included peptic ulcer disease and pancreatitis. Peptic ulcer disease is not likely to be linked in a pathophysiologic way to primary hyperparathyroidism unless type I multiple endocrine neoplasia is present. Pancreatitis is virtually never seen any more as a complication of primary hyperparathyroidism because the hypercalcemia tends to be so mild. Like peptic ulcer disease, the association between primary hyperparathyroidism and hypertension is tenuous. Although there may be an increased incidence of hypertension in primary hyperparathyroidism, it is rarely corrected or improved after successful surgery. Reports from series typified by more active primary hyperparathyroidism described coronary and left ventricular calcifications, septal and ventricular hypertrophy, and valvular calcifications (18). Such involvement is not routinely seen in asymptomatic primary hyperparathyroidism. Still other potential organ systems that in the past were affected by the hyperparathyroid state are now relegated to being archival curiosities. These include gout and pseudogout, anemia, band keratopathy, and loose teeth.

CLINICAL FORMS OF PRIMARY HYPERPARATHYROIDISM

In its most common clinical form, asymptomatic hypercalcemia, serum calcium levels are not usually higher than 1 mg/dL above the upper limits of normal. These patients do not have specific complaints and do not show evidence of any target-organ complications. Rarely a patient will demonstrate serum calcium levels in the life-threatening range, so-called acute primary hyperparathyroidism or parathyroid crisis. These patients are invariably symptomatic of hypercalcemia (19). Although this is an unusual presentation of primary hyperparathyroidism, it should always be considered in any patient who presents with acute hypercalcemia of unclear etiology.

Unusual clinical presentations of primary hyperparathyroidism include the multiple endocrine neoplasias, types I and II, familial primary hyperparathyroidism not associated with any other endocrine disorder, familial cystic parathyroid adenomatosis, and neonatal primary hyperparathyroidism (Chapter 31).

EVALUATION AND DIAGNOSIS OF PRIMARY HYPERPARATHYROIDISM

The history and the physical examination rarely give any clear indications of primary hyperparathyroidism but are helpful because of the paucity of specific manifestations of the disease. The diagnosis of primary hyperparathyroidism is established by laboratory tests. Hypercalcemia is virtually always present. Occasionally a patient with known mild hypercalcemia will have a normal serum calcium concentration. However, it is distinctly unusual for a patient with primary hyperparathyroidism regularly to show serum calcium levels within the normal range. The serum phosphorus tends to be in the lower range of normal. In approximately one third of patients, it is frankly low. The serum alkaline phosphatase activity may be elevated. More specific markers of bone formation (bone-specific alkaline phosphatase, osteocalcin) and bone resorption (urinary pyridinoline, deoxypyridinoline, N-telopeptide of collagen) can be above normal even in the absence of overt bone disease. Elevations in circulating levels of bone-resorbing cytokines, such as interleukin-6 and tumor necrosis factor (TNF), also can be detected (20). These indices of active metabolic dynamics in the skeleton are likely to reflect the extent to which the hyperparathyroid process is influencing bone turnover. The actions of PTH to alter acid–base handling in the kidney will lead in some patients to a small increase in the serum chloride concentration and a concomitant decrease in the serum bicarbonate concentration. Urinary calcium excretion is elevated in approximately 25% of patients. The circulating 1,25-dihydroxyvitamin D [1,25 $(OH)_2$ D] concentration is elevated in some patients with primary hyperparathyroidism, although it is of little diagnostic value because 1,25 $(OH)_2$ D levels are increased in other hypercalcemic states such as sarcoidosis, other granulomatous diseases, and some lymphomas (21). The 25-hydroxyvitamin D concentration tends to be in the lower range of normal.

Measurement of the circulating PTH concentration is the most definitive way to make the diagnosis of primary hyperparathyroidism. In the presence of hypercalcemia, an elevated level of PTH virtually establishes the diagnosis. In 85% to 90% of patients with primary hyperparathyroidism, the PTH level will be elevated. Moreover, it is distinctly

unusual for other causes of hypercalcemia to be associated with elevated concentrations of PTH. Thus the assay for PTH helps also to rule out other causes of hypercalcemia. The immunoradiometric (IRMA) and immunochemiluminometric (ICMA) assays for PTH that measure the intact molecule have replaced older radioimmunoassays as the "gold standard" (22). The utility of the PTH measurement in the differential diagnosis of hypercalcemia is due to the fact that the most common other cause of hypercalcemia, hypercalcemia of malignancy, is associated with suppressed levels of hormone. This is true even for the syndrome of humoral hypercalcemia of malignancy (Chapter 34) in which parathyroid hormone-related protein (PTHrP) is the major causative factor. There is no cross-reactivity with PTHrP in the IRMA and ICMA assays for PTH. The only hypercalcemic disorders in which the PTH concentration might be elevated are those related to lithium or thiazide diuretic use (Chapter 37). It is relatively easy to exclude either of these two possibilities by the history. If it is conceivable that the patient has drug-related hypercalcemia, the only secure way to make the diagnosis of primary hyperparathyroidism is to discontinue the medication and to confirm persistent hypercalcemia and elevated PTH levels 2 to 3 months later.

Specific radiologic manifestations of primary hyperparathyroidism are not seen in the vast majority of patients. On the other hand, bone mineral densitometry has great sensitivity to detect early changes in bone mass (Chapter 25) and thus is used as an integral aspect of the evaluation. Patients with primary hyperparathyroidism tend to show a pattern of bone involvement that preferentially affects the cortical as opposed to the cancellous skeleton (23). The typical pattern is a reduction in bone density of the distal third of the forearm (a site enriched in cortical bone) and relative preservation of the lumbar spine (a site enriched in cancellous bone). The hip region shows values intermediate between the distal radius and the lumbar spine because its composition is a more equal mixture of cortical and cancellous elements. Bone-mass measurements in primary hyperparathyroidism are used to help make recommendations for parathyroid surgery or for conservative medical observation (see later).

TREATMENT OF PRIMARY HYPERPARATHYROIDISM

Surgery

Primary hyperparathyroidism is cured when the abnormal parathyroid tissue is removed. The decision to recommend surgery is tempered by the realization that the majority of patients with primary hyperparathyroidism are asymptomatic. Moreover, we lack predictive indices that indicate who among the asymptomatic are at risk for complications of this disease (24). In the absence of such data, the following guidelines, originally recommended by the Consensus Development Conference on the Management of Asymptomatic Primary Hyperparathyroidism (25), are used:

1. Serum calcium >1 mg/dL above the upper limit of normal;

2. Any complication of primary hyperparathyroidism (e.g., overt bone disease, nephrolithiasis);
3. An episode of acute primary hyperparathyroidism with life-threatening hypercalcemia;
4. Marked hypercalciuria (>400 mg daily excretion);
5. Reduction in bone mass at the distal radius, as determined by bone densitometry >2 standard deviations below age and sex-matched control subjects; or
6. Age younger than 50 years.

Approximately 50% of patients with primary hyperparathyroidism will meet at least one of these criteria and thereby become candidates for surgery. Among candidates for surgery, approximately two thirds will be asymptomatic but will have met criteria because of the serum or urinary calcium level or low bone mass.

These guidelines for surgery, however, may not exclusively influence decisions for or against surgery. Such decisions are influenced by both the physician and the patient. Some physicians will recommend surgery for *all* patients with primary hyperparathyroidism, regardless of these guidelines. Other physicians will not recommend surgery unless overt complications of primary hyperparathyroidism are present. The patient enters into this therapeutic dialogue as well. Some patients cannot tolerate the idea of living with a curable disease and will seek surgery in the absence of any of the aforementioned guidelines. Other patients with coexisting medical problems may not wish to face the risks of surgery even though surgical indications are present.

Parathyroid surgery requires exceptional expertise and experience. The glands are notoriously variable in location, requiring knowledge by the surgeon of typical ectopic sites such as intrathyroidal, retroesophageal, the lateral neck, and the mediastinum. The surgeon also must be aware of the proper operation to perform. In the case of the adenoma, the other glands are ascertained to be normal but not removed. In the case of multiglandular disease, the approach is to remove all tissue except a remnant that is left *in situ* or autotransplanted in the nondominant forearm. Most parathyroid surgery is still performed under general anesthesia. In some centers, the operation is being performed increasingly under local anesthesia.

Normal parathyroid glands regain their sensitivity to calcium within the first few days after surgery (26). It is unusual for the patient to experience a brief postoperative period of symptomatic hypocalcemia. Thus it is usually not necessary to treat the postoperative patient aggressively with calcium. If overt skeletal disease is present, however, there may be a prolonged postoperative period of symptomatic hypocalcemia due to rapid deposition of calcium and phosphate into bones ("hungry bone syndrome"). These patients require parenteral calcium to control symptomatic hypocalcemia. In patients who have had previous neck surgery or who undergo subtotal parathyroidectomy (for multiglandular disease), permanent hypoparathyroidism may ensue. Another long-term complication of parathyroid surgery is damage to the recurrent laryngeal nerve, which can lead to hoarseness and reduced voice volume.

A number of localization tests are available to define the site of abnormal parathyroid tissue preoperatively. Among the noninvasive tests, ultrasonography, computed tomography, magnetic resonance imaging, and scintigraphy with technetium-99m sestamibi are available (27,28). Over the past 5 years, the sestamibi scan has become established as the best and the most convenient to perform (29,30). It can be done as a two-phase test with a 2-hour image compared with an earlier time point. This approach takes advantage of a property of sestamibi: it is "washed out" rapidly by thyroid tissue but persists in abnormal parathyroid tissue. Another approach is to use subtraction imaging with iodine 123 or [^{99m}Tc]pertechnetate. The thyroid image, but not the parathyroid image, is visualized by the ^{123}iodine or the [^{99m}Tc]pertechnetate. Sestamibi scanning also can be performed with computed tomographic techniques (SPECT), thus giving a three-dimensional image and greater anatomic resolution (31). In patients who have had prior neck surgery, preoperative localization can be extremely helpful, even to the expert parathyroid surgeon. There is an appreciable incidence of false-positive studies with all noninvasive localization procedures, so that confirmation with two approaches gives better confidence of accurate localization.

Invasive localization tests with arteriography and selective venous sampling for PTH in the draining thyroid veins are options when noninvasive studies have been unsuccessful (27). Marked elevation of PTH in blood samples obtained from neck veins selectively draining abnormal parathyroid tissue can provide very useful information. When combined with arteriographic demonstration of the tumor, complete identification is established. Unfortunately, arteriography and selective venous catheterization are time-consuming, expensive, and difficult procedures. Their success is dependent on the skill of the angiographer. When the need for these tests arises in a patient, referral is usually made to one of the few sites in the United States that do these studies on a regular basis.

Recent attempts to streamline the approach to the difficult patient about to undergo repeated parathyroid surgery have used a sophisticated mixture of surgical and imaging expertise along with intraoperative measurements of PTH (32,33). This approach uses administration of ^{99m}Tc sestamibi, 2 to 3 hours before surgery, detection of the area of increased uptake by a hand-held gamma counter in the operative field, removal of the identified tissue, and immediate intraoperative confirmation of the expected dramatic fall in PTH levels by "quick" ICMA assay for PTH (34). In extremely difficult cases, this approach, which requires more broad-based expertise than is found in most medical centers, may have merit.

Whereas all agree that preoperative localization tests in patients who have had prior neck surgery are clearly indicated, it is not as clear that those who have not had prior neck surgery should undergo these tests. In view of the general success of the sestamibi scan in locating parathyroid adenomas, some have been tempted to recommend it uniformly to all patients, whether or not they have had prior neck surgery. This argument is strengthened by the fact that the expert parathyroid surgeon is not always available. However, arguments against using preoperative localization with sestamibi imaging in all patients are many. First, no studies have yet shown that operative time is reduced or even that the success rate of parathyroid surgery is greater with imaging among those who have not had prior neck surgery (30,35). The expert parathyroid surgeon still has a better success rate than sestamibi imaging (30). Moreover, medical centers that lack such surgical expertise also may lack expertise in imaging technology. In addition, the sestamibi test tends to be much less helpful when more than one gland is abnormal. An asymmetrically large parathyroid gland in a patient with four-gland hyperplasia could lead to the erroneous impression of a single overactive gland (30). The dictum that all parathyroid glands must be identified at the time of surgery, irrespective of the results of imaging, is still advisable.

In patients who undergo successful parathyroid surgery, the hyperparathyroid state is completely cured. Serum biochemistries normalize and the PTH level returns to normal. In addition, bone mass improves substantially, as documented by bone densitometry (36). It is particularly noteworthy that the lumbar spine, a site where PTH appears to protect against age-related and postmenopausal bone loss, is a site of rapid gains in bone mass.

Medical Management

If patients with primary hyperparathyroidism are not to undergo parathyroid surgery, a set of general medical guidelines is recommended (25). Adequate hydration and ambulation are always encouraged. Thiazide diuretics are to be avoided because they may lead to worsening hypercalcemia. Dietary intake of calcium should be moderate. There is no good evidence that patients with primary hyperparathyroidism show significant fluctuations of their serum calcium as a function of dietary calcium intake. High calcium intakes should be avoided, however, especially in patients whose $1,25 (OH)_2 D$ level is elevated (37). Low-calcium diets also should be avoided because they could theoretically lead to further stimulation of PTH secretion.

We still lack an effective and safe therapeutic agent for the medical management of primary hyperparathyroidism. Oral phosphate will lower the serum calcium in patients with primary hyperparathyroidism by approximately 0.5 to 1 mg/dL. Phosphate appears to act by three mechanisms: interference with absorption of dietary calcium, inhibition of bone resorption, and inhibition of renal production of $1,25 (OH)_2 D$. Phosphate, however, is not used widely as a therapy for primary hyperparathyroidism because of concerns related to ectopic calcification in soft tissues as a result of increasing the calcium–phosphate product. Moreover, oral phosphate leads to an undesirable, further elevation of PTH levels.

In postmenopausal women, estrogen therapy has been considered (38). The rationale for estrogen use in primary hyperparathyroidism is based on the known antagonism by estrogen of PTH-mediated bone resorption. Even though the serum calcium concentration does tend to decline after estrogen administration, PTH levels and the serum phosphorus concentration do not change.

Bisphosphonates also have been considered as a possible medical approach to primary hyperparathyroidism. Two of the original bisphosphonates, etidronate and dichloromethylene bisphosphonate, have been studied. Although etidronate is not effective (39), dichloromethylene bisphosphonate was shown in early studies to reduce the serum calcium in primary hyperparathyroidism (40). The drug, however, does not appear to lead to sustained reductions in the serum calcium concentration (41). It remains to be seen whether alendronate, a potent bisphosphonate that is efficacious in Paget's disease and in osteoporosis, will be shown to be effective in primary hyperparathyroidism.

Finally, a more targeted approach to the medical therapy of primary hyperparathyroidism is to interfere specifically with the production of PTH. A new class of agents, termed calcimimetics, alter the function of the extracellular calcium-sensing receptor (42) and could conceivably reduce PTH levels in primary hyperparathyroidism. In a recent pilot study, a calcimimetic agent was shown to reduce PTH and serum calcium levels in 20 postmenopausal women with asymptomatic primary hyperparathyroidism (43). The results of this study prove the validity of this approach in concept. Larger clinical trials are ongoing to establish further the clinical potential of the calcimimetics in primary hyperparathyroidism.

Patients who are not surgical candidates for parathyroidectomy appear to do well when they are managed conservatively (44,45). In general, they do not show substantial changes in serum or urinary indices or in bone density. Long-term epidemiologic data also indicate that these patients do well with respect to morbid and fatal events (46). Their long-term survival is not adversely affected. Routine medical follow-up usually includes visits twice yearly with serum calcium determinations. Yearly urinary calcium excretion and bone densitometry also are recommended.

REFERENCES

1. Silverberg SJ, Fitzpatrick LA, Bilezikian JP. Hyperparathyroidism In: Becker KL, ed. *Principles and practice of endocrinology and metabolism*. 2nd ed. Philadelphia: JB Lippincott, 1995:512–519.
2. Heath H III, Hodgson SF, Kennedy MA. Primary hyperparathyroidism: incidence, morbidity, and potential economic impact in a community. *N Engl J Med* 1980;302:189.
3. Wermers RA, Khosla S, Atkinson EJ, Hodgson SF, O'Fallon WM, Melton LJ III. The rise and fall of primary hyperparathyroidism: a population-based study in Rochester, Minnesota 1965–1992. *Ann Intern Med* 1997;126:433–440.
4. Wynne AG, Van Heerden J, Carney JA, Fitzpatrick LA. Parathyroid carcinoma: clinical and pathological features in 43 patients. *Medicine* 1992;71:197–205.
5. Arnold A. Molecular genetics of parathyroid gland neoplasia. *J Clin Endocrinol Metab* 1993;77:1108–1112.
6. Hsi ED. Zukerberg LR, Yang W-I, Arnold A. Cyclin D1/PRAD 1 expression in parathyroid adenomas: an immunohistological study. *J Clin Endocrinol Metab* 1996;81:1736–1739.
7. Chandrasekharappa SC, Guru SC, Manickam P et al. Positional cloning of the gene for multiple endocrine neoplasia type I. *Science* 1997; 276:404–407.
8. European consortium on MEN1 gene. *Hum Mol Genet* 1997;6:1177–1183.
9. Heppner C, Kester MB, Agarwal SK, et al. Somatic mutation of the MEN I gene in parathyroid tumors. *Nat Genet* 1997;16:375–378.
10. Cryns VL, Yi SM, Tahara H, Gaz RD, Arnold A. Frequent loss of chromosome arm 1p DNA in parathyroid adenomas. *Genes Chromosomes Cancer* 1995;13:9–17.

11. Hosokawa Y, Pollak MR, Brown EM, Arnold A. The extracellular calcium-sensing receptor gene in human parathyroid tumors. *J Clin Endocrinol Metab* 1995;80:3107–3110.

12. Thakker RV. Molecular genetics of parathyroid disease. *Curr Opin Endocrinol Diabetes* 1996;3:521–528.

13. Bilezikian JP, Silverberg SJ, Gartenberg F, et al. Clinical presentation of primary hyperparathyroidism. In: Bilezikian JP, Marcus R, Levine MA, eds. *The parathyroids*. New York: Raven Press, 1994: 457–470.

14. Silverberg SJ, Shane E, Jacobs TP, et al. Nephrolithiasis and bone involvement in primary hyperparathyroidism. *Am J Med* 1990;89: 327–334.

15. Turken SA, Cafferty M, Silverberg SJ, et al. Neuromuscular involvement in mild, asymptomatic primary hyperparathyroidism. *Am J Med* 1989;87:553–557.

16. Solomon BL, Schaaf M, Smallridge RC. Psychologic symptoms before and after parathyroid surgery. *Am J Med* 1994;96:101–106.

17. Kleerekoper M, Bilezikian JP. Parathyroidectomy for non-traditional features of primary hyperparathyroidism. *Am J Med* 1994;96:99–100.

18. Stefenelli T, Abela C, Frank H, eds. Cardiac abnormalities in patients with primary hyperparathyroidism: implications for follow-up. *J Clin Endocrinol Metab* 1997;82:106–112.

19. Fitzpatrick LA. Acute primary hyperparathyroidism. In: Bilezikian JP, Marcus R, Levine MA, eds. *The parathyroids*. New York: Raven Press, 1994:583–589.

20. Grey A, Mitnick M, Shapses S, Ellison A, Gundberg C, Insogna K. Circulating levels of interleukin-6 and tumor necrosis factor-alpha are elevated in primary hyperparathyroidism and correlate with markers of bone resorption. *J Clin Endocrinol Metab* 1996;81:3450–3454.

21. Thys-Jacobs S, Chan FKW, Koberle LMC, Bilezikian JP. Hypercalcemia due to vitamin D toxicity. In: Feldman D, ed. *Vitamin D*. San Diego: Academic Press, 1997:883–901.

22. Nussbaum SR, Potts JT Jr. Advances in immunoassays for parathyroid hormone. In: Bilezikian JP, Marcus R, Levine MA, eds. *The parathyroids*. New York: Raven Press, 1994:157–169.

23. Silverberg SJ, Shane E, de la Cruz L, et al. Skeletal disease in primary hyperparathyroidism. *J Bone Miner Res* 1989;4:283–291.

24. Kleerekoper M. Clinical course of primary hyperparathyroidism. In: Bilezikian JP, Marcus R, Levine MA, eds. *The parathyroids*. New York: Raven Press, 1994:471–484.

25. Consensus Development Conference Panel. Diagnosis and management of asymptomatic primary hyperparathyroidism: Consensus Development Conference Statement. *Ann Intern Med* 1991;114:593–597.

26. Brasier AR, Wang C, Nussbaum SR. Recovery of parathyroid hormone secretion after parathyroid adenomectomy. *J Clin Endocrinol Metab* 1988;61:495–500.

27. Doppman JL. Preoperative localization of parathyroid tissue in primary hyperparathyroidism. In: Bilezikian JP, Marcus R, Levine MA, eds. *The parathyroids*. New York: Raven Press, 1994:553–566.

28. Turton DB, Miller DL. Recent advances in parathyroid imaging. *Trends Endocrinol Metab* 1996;7:163–168.

29. Johnston LB, Carrol MJ, Britton KE, et al. The accuracy of parathyroid gland localization in primary hyperparathyroidism using sestamibi radionuclide imaging. *J Clin Endocrinol Metab* 1996;81:346–352.

30. McIntyre RC, Ridgway EC. Sestamibi: opening a new era of parathyroid surgical procedures. *Endocrine Pract* 1998;4:241–244.

31. Chen CC, Holder LE, Scovill WA, Tehan AM, Gann DS. Comparison of parathyroid imaging with technetium-99m-pertechnetate/sestamibi subtraction, double-phase technetium-99m-sestamibi and technetium-99m-SPECT. *J Nucl Med* 1997;38:637–640.

32. Norman J, Chheda H. Minimally invasive parathyroidectomy facilitated by intraoperative nuclear mapping. *Surgery* 1997;122:998–1003.

33. Feng S, Moore FD Jr. Parathyroid reoperative with use of technetium 99m sestamibi radiolocalization and an intraoperative gamma counter. *Endocrine Pract* 1996;2:382–384.

34. Boggs JE, Irvin GI, Molinari AS, Deriso GT. Intraoperative parathyroid hormone monitoring as an adjunct to parathyroidectomy. *Surgery* 1996;120:954–958.

35. Roe SM, Burns RP, Graham LD, Brock WB, Russell WL. Cost-effectiveness of preoperative localization studies in primary hyperparathyroid disease. *Ann Surg* 1994;219:582–586.

36. Silverberg SJ, Gartenberg F, et al. Increased bone density after parathyroidectomy in primary hyperparathyroidism. *J Clin Endocrinol Metab* 1995;80:729–734.

37. Locker FG, Silverberg SJ, Bilezikian JP. Optimal dietary calcium intake in primary hyperparathyroidism. *Am J Med* 1997;102:543–550.

38. Stock JL, Marcus R. Medical management of primary hyperparathyroidism. In: Bilezikian JP, Marcus R, Levine ML, eds. *The parathyroids*. New York: Raven Press, 1994:519–530.

39. Kaplan RA, Geho WB, Poindexter C, Haussler M, Dietz GW, Pak CYC. Metabolic effects of diphosphonate in primary hyperparathyroidism. *J Clin Pharmacol* 1977;17:410–419.

40. Shane E, Baquiran DC, Bilezikian JP. Effects of dichloromethylene diphosphonate on serum and urine calcium in primary hyperparathyroidism. *Ann Intern Med* 1981;95:23.

41. Adami S, Mian M, Bertoldo F, et al. Regulation of calcium-parathyroid hormone feedback in primary hyperparathyroidism: effects of bisphosphonate treatment. *Clin Endocrinol* 1990;33:391–397.

42. Nemeth EF. Calcium receptors as novel drug targets. In: Bilezikian JP, Raisz LG, Rodan GA, eds. *Principles of bone biology*. San Diego: Academic Press, 1996:1019–1036.

43. Silverberg SJ, Bone HG III, Marriott TB, et al. Short-term inhibition of parathyroid hormone secretion by a calcium receptor agonist in primary hyperparathyroidism. *N Engl J Med* 1997;337:1506–1510.

44. Rao DS, Wilson RJ, Kleerekoper M, Parfitt AM. Lack of biochemical progression or continuation of accelerated bone loss in mild asymptomatic primary hyperparathyroidism: evidence for a biphasic disease course. *J Clin Endocrinol Metab* 1988;67:1294–1298.

45. Silverberg SJ, Gartenberg F, Jacobs TP, et al. Longitudinal measurements of bone density and biochemical indices in untreated primary hyperparathyroidism. *J Clin Endocrinol Metab* 1995;80:723–728.

46. Wermers RA, Khosla S, Atkinson EJ, et al. Survival after the diagnosis of hyperparathyroidism. *Am J Med* 1998;104:115–122.

31. Familial Hyperparathyroid Syndromes

Maurine R. Hobbs, Ph.D. and *Hunter Heath III, M.D.

*Department of Internal Medicine, Division of Endocrinology, University of Utah, Salt Lake City, Utah; and *Endocrine Medical Affairs, U.S. Medical Division, Eli Lilly and Company, and Department of Internal Medicine, The Wishard Hospital, Iupui Medical Center, Indianapolis, Indiana*

As described in Chapter 30, most cases of primary hyperparathyroidism (HPT) result from sporadic, benign parathyroid tumors (adenomas). However, up to 10% of cases may occur as hereditary forms of isolated HPT or HPT associated with other genetically determined abnormalities. Recent genetic linkage and mutational analyses confirmed the hereditary nature of these syndromes and, in some cases, led to identification of specific genetic mutations responsible for parathyroid neoplasia or hyperfunction. The most common variety of hereditary HPT occurs in the syndrome of multiple endocrine neoplasia type I (MEN I) (1), whereas the relative frequencies of the other disorders are poorly documented.

MULTIPLE ENDOCRINE NEOPLASIA TYPE I (WERMER SYNDROME)

The familial occurrence of parathyroid, anterior pituitary, and pancreatic tumors—today called MEN I (1)—was recognized as a distinct syndrome by Wermer in 1954 (Table 1). MEN I is transmitted in an autosomal dominant mode of inheritance with a high degree of penetrance. The most common feature of MEN I is HPT, which is almost always present. The clinical and biochemical presentation of HPT in MEN I resembles that of nonfamilial or sporadic HPT, except that MEN I occurs in both sexes equally, whereas sporadic HPT is more frequent in women. In general, patients with MEN I are younger at the time of diagnosis than are patients with sporadic HPT. In fact, childhood and neonatal cases have been reported.

The only definitive therapy for HPT in MEN I, as in sporadic cases, is surgical. The indications for surgery also are generally the same. Given the younger average age of MEN I patients, however, surgical intervention is generally undertaken fairly early.

The surgical approach to patients with HPT as part of the MEN I syndrome is dictated by the underlying pathology of the parathyroid glands. Although solitary adenomas have been noted, HPT in MEN I is usually a multiglandular disorder, with hyperplasia of all four parathyroids. The importance of recognizing hyperplasia in MEN I is that resection of a single gland or even fewer than three glands frequently leads to persistent or recurrent hypercalcemia. About 70% of patients with HPT and MEN I have remission of hypercalcemia after removal of three or more glands, whereas only about a third respond to resection of $2\frac{1}{2}$ glands or fewer.

Most centers now perform a subtotal parathyroidectomy in hypercalcemic patients with MEN I, resecting $3\frac{1}{2}$ glands and leaving about 50 mg of viable tissue. To avoid persistent hypercalcemia or permanent postoperative hypoparathyroidism, some surgeons perform total parathyroidectomy with autotransplantation of the abnormal parathyroid tissue into forearm muscles, reasoning that recurrent HPT will not require a second neck exploration. However, graft-dependent persistent or recurrent hypercalcemia may occur and be difficult to manage. Regardless of the approach, close follow-up and expert management of this frustrating condition is mandatory.

Patients with MEN I also frequently develop pancreatic and pituitary neoplasms. The pancreatic lesions are usually islet cell tumors, two thirds secreting excess gastrin, leading to Zollinger-Ellison syndrome, and about one third hypersecreting insulin, leading to fasting hypoglycemia. In a minority, a variety of other substances are secreted, including vasoactive intestinal peptide, prostaglandins, glucagon, pancreatic polypeptide, adrenocorticotropic hormone (ACTH), and serotonin.

The pituitary tumors in MEN I, thought initially to be largely nonfunctional, are now increasingly recognized as prolactinomas. These tumors also may secrete growth hormone, leading to acromegaly, or ACTH, resulting in Cushing's disease.

Up to one third of MEN I patients have enlargement of the adrenal glands. The histopathology includes diffuse and nodular cortical hypertrophy, cortical hyperplasia, adenomas, and rarely, adrenocortical carcinoma. The cause(s) of the adrenal cortical hyperplasia are unknown.

The recently identified MEN I gene, Menin (2), maps to chromosome 11q13. Mutations identified in MEN I families have been found in all ten exons of the gene, with approximately 10% of mutations characterized as *de novo* mutations (3). Thus siblings of a proband may not be at risk of developing the disease, whereas offspring of MEN I patients have a 50% risk of inheriting the mutant copy of the gene. MEN

TABLE 1. *Characteristics of familial hyperparathyroid syndromes*

Feature	MEN I	MEN IIA	HPT-JT	Familial HPT	FBHH
Hyperparathyroidism	>95%	Histologically, ≤50%; ~10% hyper-calcemic	>95%	100%	100%
Parathyroid carcinoma	Reported	Rare	6/15 families	Reported	—
Pancreatic tumors	30%–80%	—	—	—	—
Pituitary adenomas	15%–50%	—	—	—	—
Adrenocortical hyperplasia	<33%	—	—	—	—
Medullary CA thyroid	—	100%	—	—	—
Pheochromocytoma or adrenal medullary hyperplasia	—	Up to 50%	—	—	—
Lichen amyloidosis	—	Reported	—	—	—
Fibroosseous jaw tumors	—	—	10/15 families	—	—
Wilms' tumor, hamartomas, or renal cysts	—	—	7/15 families	—	—
Inheritance	AD	AD	AD	AD, AR (1 kindred)	AD
Genetic locus	11q13	10q11.2	1q21-q31	Not mapped	3q13.3-q21, 19p, and 19q
Gene mutated	Menin	*RET* proto-oncogene	Unknown	Unknown	Ca^{2+} receptor (FBHH$_{3q}$), others unknown

MEN, multiple endocrine neoplasia; HPT-JT, hyperparathyroidism–jaw tumor syndrome; FBHH, familial benign hypocalciuric hypercalcemia; CA, carcinoma; AD, autosomal dominant inheritance; AR, autosomal recessive inheritance.

I–associated lesions may manifest as late as age 35 years in persons at genetic risk. Even extensive biochemical testing, including serum calcium, glucose, gastrin, and serum prolactin assays, may not identify all affected persons before overt symptoms develop (4). It is nonetheless important to screen first-degree relatives of affected individuals; serum calcium measurement alone will identify many cases. Genetic sequencing is cumbersome, but it can be used for informed genetic counseling in some cases.

MULTIPLE ENDOCRINE NEOPLASIA TYPE IIA (SIPPLE SYNDROME)

Multiple endocrine neoplasia type IIA (MEN IIA) syndrome is characterized by medullary thyroid carcinoma (MTC), bilateral pheochromocytomas, and parathyroid hyperplasia (Table 1) (5). Originally described by Sipple in 1961, this syndrome is inherited as an autosomal dominant trait.

The dominant feature of the MEN IIA syndrome is MTC, a calcitonin-secreting neoplasm derived from the thyroid C-cells, which occasionally leads to death from metastatic disease. Until recently, early detection of MTC was achieved primarily by the measurement of plasma calcitonin after infusion of calcium or pentagastrin. Once hypercalcitoninemia was detected in persons at risk, early total thyroidectomy generally was performed. However, molecular genetic diagnosis is rapidly supplanting diagnosis by calcitonin assay (6).

The other major feature of MEN IIA is pheochromocytoma, present in up to 50% of patients, which may precede or follow detection of thyroid cancer. In contrast to sporadic pheochromocytoma, the tumor in MEN IIA is virtually always bilateral and often requires total adrenalectomy. Unrecognized pheochromocytoma can be lethal during surgical procedures, so this lesion should be diagnosed and treated before neck exploration. Indeed, patients with MEN IIA are far more likely to die of unrecognized pheochromocytoma than of MTC.

Hyperparathyroidism is less common and milder in MEN IIA than in MEN I, but here also, it is a result of diffuse parathyroid hyperplasia. However, the hyperplastic glands may be quite heterogeneous in size, leading to an erroneous diagnosis of adenomatous HPT. The surgical management is similar to that for HPT in MEN I.

Pruritic, pigmented cutaneous lesions localized to the upper back, and generally containing amyloid (''lichen amyloidosis''), have occurred in some MEN IIA families (7). The lesions are thought to be a form of dorsal neuropathy that could be an early clinical marker for MEN IIA.

The MEN IIA gene was localized by linkage analysis to the centromeric region of chromosome 10, and then identified as the *RET* protooncogene (8). MEN IIA results from a limited number of mutations in the *RET* protooncogene, and molecular genetic tests are now available commercially to permit presymptomatic diagnosis of MEN IIA in individuals (6). Persons at risk who are found to have a *RET* mutation may undergo appropriate testing and surgery electively, before complications have arisen (e.g., metastatic MTC or renal damage from HPT). Affected persons may ultimately have total thyroidectomy, bilateral adrenalectomy, and subtotal parathyroidectomy.

THE HYPERPARATHYROIDISM–JAW TUMOR SYNDROME

The hyperparathyroidism–jaw tumor syndrome (HPT-JT) syndrome, first reported in 1958 by Jackson et al. (9,10), was recently localized to chromosome 1q21-q31 (Table 1). Affected families show autosomal dominant inheritance of a highly penetrant disorder encompassing early-onset parathyroid tumors that may recur and fibroosseous jaw tumors (10). Parathyroid carcinoma and various renal tumors occur at lesser frequencies (40% and 46% of families, respectively) (10).

Patients having HPT-JT may become severely hypercalcemic in childhood and up to the late teenage years. In contrast to the parathyroid hyperplasia found in other forms of inherited HPT, however, they usually have a solitary enlarged parathyroid gland (adenoma), sometimes cystic, and they become normocalcemic on removal of the lesions. The severe HPT has resulted in crippling skeletal disease and death in several individuals.

The bone lesions of HPT-JT occur exclusively in the maxilla and mandible, appearing as punched-out ''cystic'' lesions on radiographs, and running a course independent of the HPT. Although often small and asymptomatic, the lesions may be large, destructive, persistent, or recurrent. The jaw tumors consist of trabeculae of woven bone set in a cytologically bland fibrocellular stroma; the original abnormal cell type is unknown. They differ strikingly from classic hyperparathyroid ''brown tumors,'' which may occur anywhere in the skeleton, in their lack of osteoclasts. HPT-JT bone tumors occur mostly in adolescence or young adulthood. The renal lesions in these families have been reported as Wilms' tumors, hamartomas, and polycystic kidney disease. In HPT-JT families, it is important for the clinician to seek these various manifestations on a regular basis.

FAMILIAL ISOLATED PRIMARY HYPERPARATHYROIDISM

The existence of familial HPT as a disorder distinct from the MEN I, MEN IIA, and HPT-JT syndromes has been a subject of debate. Several kindreds with familial hypercalcemia and no other endocrine abnormalities have subsequently been reclassified as having MEN I, familial benign hypocalciuric hypercalcemia (FBHH; Chapter 32), or HPT-JT (11). Isolated HPT in some families has been mapped by genetic linkage analysis to 11q13 (the MEN I locus) (12), or 1q21-q31 (the HPT-JT locus) (11). Thus, isolated HPT may sometimes represent an allelic variant of MEN I or HPT-JT. One kindred was described with apparent autosomal recessive inheritance of HPT and recurrent large parathyroid adenomas (13). Space does not permit detailed presentation here, but there appear to be many other variants of isolated familial HPT, some with adenomatous and some with hyperplastic parathyroid disease, and some in association with other disorders. We suspect that there are many genetically distinct forms of isolated familial HPT.

THE FAMILIAL BENIGN HYPOCALCIURIC HYPERCALCEMIAS

FBHH comprises at least three distinct genetic variants, the most common of which is $FBHH_{3q}$ (mutations of the cell-surface calcium receptor) (14). A chromosome 19p variant ($FBHH_{19p}$) has been reported, as well as one family in which the genetic locus is on 19q ($FBHH_{19q}$) (Table 1). These functional (nonneoplastic) disorders of the parathyroids are described in more detail in Chapter 32.

SUMMARY AND CONCLUSIONS

Hereditary forms of HPT are increasingly recognized, and their genetic bases are becoming clearer; molecular genetic diagnosis is possible for some of them. Physicians should be aware of the characteristics of familial HPT syndromes and seek clues to these diseases in newly diagnosed HPT patients. The implications of finding hereditary HPT are many, including the need for family screening, the necessity for special approaches to the parathyroid surgery, and the existence of serious concomitant diseases such as thyroid cancer, pheochromocytoma, or Wilms' tumor.

REFERENCES

1. Metz DC, Jensen RT, Bale AE, et al. Multiple endocrine neoplasia type I. In: Bilezikian JP, Marcus R, Levine MA, eds. *The parathyroids: basic and clinical concepts.* New York: Raven Press, 1994:591–646.
2. Chandrasekharappa SC, Guru SC, Manickam P, et al. Positional cloning of the gene for multiple endocrine neoplasia-type 1. *Science* 1997;276:404–407.
3. Bassett JHD, Forbes SA, Pannett AAJ, et al. Characterization of mutations in patients with multiple endocrine neoplasia type 1. *Am J Hum Genet* 1998;62:232–244.
4. Friedman E, Larsson C, Amorosi A, et al. Multiple endocrine neoplasia type I: pathology, pathophysiology, molecular genetics, and differential diagnosis. In: Bilezikian JP, Marcus R, Levine MA, eds. *The parathyroids: basic and clinical concepts.* New York: Raven Press, 1994: 591–646.
5. Gagel RF. Multiple endocrine neoplasia type II. In: Bilezikian JP, Marcus R, Levine MA, eds. *The parathyroids: basic and clinical concepts.* New York: Raven Press, 1994:591–646.
6. Ledger GA, Khosla S, Lindor NM, Thibodeau SN, Gharib H. Genetic testing in the diagnosis and management of multiple endocrine neoplasia type II. *Ann Intern Med* 1995;122:118–124.
7. Gagel RF, Levy ML, Donovan DT, Alford BR, Wheeler T, Tschen JA. Multiple endocrine neoplasia type 2a associated with cutaneous lichen amyloidosis. *Ann Intern Med* 1989;111:802–806.
8. Mulligan LM, Kwok JB, Healey CS, et al. Germ-line mutations of the RET proto-oncogene in multiple endocrine neoplasia type 2A. *Nature* 1993;363:458–460.
9. Jackson CE, Norum RA, Boyd SB, et al. Hereditary hyperparathyroidism and multiple ossifying jaw fibromas: a clinically and genetically distinct syndrome. *Surgery* 1990;108:1006–1012; discussion 1012–1013.
10. Szabo J, Heath B, Hill VM, et al. Hereditary hyperparathyroidism-jaw tumor syndrome: the endocrine tumor gene HRPT2 maps to chromosome 1q21-q31. *Am J Hum Genet* 1995;56:944–950.
11. Teh BT, Farnebo F, Twigg S, et al. Familial isolated hyperparathyroidism maps to the hyperparathyroidism-jaw tumor locus in 1q21-q32 in a subset of families. *J Clin Endocrinol Metabol* 1998;83:2114–2120.
12. Kassem M, Zhang X, Brask S, Eriksen EF, Mosekilde L, Kruse TA. Familial isolated primary hyperparathyroidism. *Clin Endocrinol (Oxf)* 1994;41:415–420.
13. Law WM Jr, Hodgson SF, Heath H III. Autosomal recessive inheritance of familial hyperparathyroidism. *N Engl J Med* 1983;309: 650–653.
14. Heath H III, Odelberg S, Jackson CE, et al. Clustered inactivating mutations and benign polymorphisms of the calcium receptor gene in familial benign hypocalciuric hypercalcemia suggest receptor functional domains. *J Clin Endocrinol Metab* 1996;81:1312–1317.

32. Familial Hypocalciuric Hypercalcemia

Stephen J. Marx, M.D.

Genetics and Endocrinology Section, National Institute of Diabetes and Digestive and Kidney Diseases, National Institutes of Health, Bethesda, Maryland

Familial hypocalciuric hypercalcemia (FHH) [also termed familial benign hypercalcemia (FBH)] is an autosomal dominant trait characterized by moderate hypercalcemia and relative hypocalciuria (i.e., urine calcium that is low considering the simultaneous hypercalcemia) with high penetrance for both of these features throughout life (1,2).

CLINICAL FEATURES

Symptoms and Signs

Patients with FHH are usually asymptomatic. Occasionally they note easy fatigue, weakness, thought disturbances, or polydipsia. Although these symptoms also are common in typical primary hyperparathyroidism, they are less common and less severe in FHH. There seems to be an increased incidence of relapsing pancreatitis (1,3), and this can occasionally be severe and life threatening. There may be an increased incidence of gallstones, diabetes mellitus, and myocardial infarction (1,2). The rate of nephrolithiasis or of peptic ulcer disease is the same as in a normal population.

Radiographs and Indices of Bone Function

Radiographs are usually normal. Nephrocalcinosis has the same incidence as in a normal population. There is an increased incidence of chondrocalcinosis (usually clinically silent) and premature vascular calcification (1). Bone turnover measured by indices of bone formation (serum bone gla-protein or serum alkaline phosphatase or both) or by indices of bone resorption (ratio of urine hydroxyproline to creatinine) is mildly increased (4). Mean bone mass is normal, and there is not increased susceptibility to fracture (2,4).

Serum Electrolytes

Serum calcium in gene carriers is elevated throughout life. Typically, the degree of elevation decreases modestly from infancy to old age (1). The degree of elevation is similar to that in typical primary hyperparathyroidism. Both free and bound calcium are increased, with a normal ratio of free to bound calcium (5). Serum magnesium is typically in the high range of normal or modestly elevated, and serum phosphate is modestly depressed.

Renal Function Indices

Creatinine clearance is generally normal. Urinary excretion of calcium is normal, with affected and unaffected family members showing a similar distribution of values. The normal urinary calcium in the face of hypercalcemia reflects increased renal tubular resorption of calcium (i.e., relative hypocalciuria). The renal tubular resorption of magnesium also is modestly increased. Because calcium excretion depends heavily on glomerular filtration rate, total calcium excretion is not a useful index to distinguish FHH from typical primary hyperparathyroidism. The ratio of calcium clearance to creatinine clearance,

$$
\begin{aligned}
\mathrm{ClCa/ClCr} &= [\mathrm{Ca_u} \times \mathrm{V/Ca_s}]/\mathrm{Cr_u} \times \mathrm{V/Cr_s} \\
&= [\mathrm{Ca_u} \times \mathrm{Cr_s}]/[\mathrm{Cr_u} \times \mathrm{Ca_s}]
\end{aligned} \tag{1}
$$

(where Cl is renal clearance, Ca is total calcium, Cr is creatinine, u is urine, V is volume, and s is serum) corrects for most of the variation from glomerular filtration. The clearance ratio in FHH is one third of that in typical primary hyperparathyroidism, and a cutoff value at 0.01 (note that the clearance ratio has no units) is helpful for this distinction in a patient with hypercalcemia.

Parathyroid Function Indices

Biochemical testing of parathyroid function, including serum PTH and 1,25-dihydroxyvitamin D [1,25 (OH)$_2$ D] is usually normal, with modest elevations in 5% to 10% of cases (6,7). The normal parathyroid function indices in the presence of lifelong hypercalcemia are inappropriate and indicative of a specific role for the parathyroids in maintenance of hypercalcemia. There is often mild parathyroid gland hyperplasia (evident only by careful measurement of gland size) (8,9).

Response to Parathyroidectomy

Subtotal parathyroidectomy results in only very transient lowering of serum calcium, with restoration of hypercalcemia within a week (2). Familial hypocalciuric hypercalcemia has been a common cause of unsuccessful parathyroidec-

tomy, accounting for 10% of unsuccessful operations in several large series during the 1970s, before wider recognition of the implications of this diagnosis (10). Total parathyroidectomy in FHH leads to decreased production of 1,25 (OH)$_2$ D, hypocalcemia, and features of chronic hypoparathyroidism. In several FHH cases, deliberate total parathyroidectomy has been attempted without induction of hypocalcemia; presumably, small amounts of residual parathyroid tissue were sufficient to sustain hypercalcemia.

GENETICS OF FAMILIAL HYPOCALCIURIC HYPERCALCEMIA AND RELATION TO NEONATAL SEVERE PRIMARY HYPERPARATHYROIDISM

There is virtually 100% penetrance for hypercalcemia at all ages among heterozygotes for the FHH gene (1). The hypercalcemia has been documented in the first week of life (11). The degree of hypercalcemia shows clustering within kindreds, with several kindreds showing very modest hypercalcemia, and several showing rather severe hypercalcemia (12.5 to 14 mg/dL) in all affected members (1,12). Genetic linkage analyses in eight families indicated that a gene for FHH is on the long arm of chromosome 3 (13,14). In one large kindred, the FHH trait was linked to the short arm of chromosome 19 (14). In another it was linked to the long arm of chromosome 19 (14a).

The prevalence of FHH has not been established, but it is probably similar to that for familial multiple endocrine neoplasia type I; each of these diseases may account for about 2% of cases with asymptomatic hypercalcemia.

Neonatal severe primary hyperparathyroidism is an unusual state of life-threatening, severe hypercalcemia with massive hyperplasia of all parathyroid glands. Most of these neonates had FHH in one or both parents (12,15). Some cases clearly reflected a double dose of FHH genes (16). Other cases may result from an FHH heterozygote having gestated in a normocalcemic (i.e., FHH-negative) mother, which caused superimposed intrauterine secondary hyperparathyroidism (15,17,18). The maternal contribution to neonatal hyperparathyroidism in this latter setting may be self-limited.

PATHOPHYSIOLOGY

Biochemical testing has established that the parathyroid gland functions abnormally in FHH (see preceding sections). A surgically decreased gland mass can maintain the same calcium level by increasing hormone secretion rate per cell. Parathyroid function shows features expected from a selective and mild increase in glandular "setpoint" for calcium suppression of PTH secretion. Setpoint was measured in parathyroid cells from a neonate presumed to have a double dose of FHH genes (19); these cells showed a setpoint higher than ever seen in any parathyroid adenoma. Depending on definition, FHH can therefore be labeled as a form of primary hyperparathyroidism. We prefer to consider it an atypical form of primary hyperparathyroidism in distinct contrast to the more typical form associated with hypercalciuria, nephrolithiasis, markedly increased gland mass, clear elevations of plasma PTH, and generally excellent response to subtotal parathyroidectomy.

In addition to the disturbance presumed to be intrinsic to the parathyroids in FHH, there also is a disturbance intrinsic to the kidneys. The tubular reabsorption of calcium, normally regulated by parathyroid hormone, remains strikingly increased even after total parathyroidectomy in FHH (20).

Most cases are probably caused by inactivating mutations in the calcium-ion–sensing receptor (CaSR) gene (Chapter 13) (21). The encoded product is predicted to be a seven transmembrane cell-surface receptor (like adrenergic and many other receptors) that interacts with extracellular calcium ion, translating it into an intracellular signal through coupling to a cytoplasmic guanyl nucleotide-binding protein. The unusual FHH kindreds not linked to the locus at chromosome 3q, such as those linked to 19p or 19q, represent mutation in other genes of unknown function.

MANAGEMENT

Intervention in the Typical Case of Familial Hypocalciuric Hypercalcemia

Because of the generally benign course and the lack of response to subtotal parathyroidectomy, virtually all patients should be advised against parathyroidectomy. Attempts to regulate serum calcium with medications (diuretics, estrogens, and phosphates) have not changed serum calcium. Familial hypocalciuric hypercalcemia is compatible with survival into the ninth decade, and it is uncertain whether there is any decrease in average life expectancy.

Indications for Parathyroidectomy

In rare situations, such as (a) neonatal severe primary hyperparathyroidism resulting from a double dose of FHH gene, (b) an adult with relapsing pancreatitis, and (c) a child or an adult with serum calcium persistently above 14 mg/dL, parathyroidectomy may be necessary. Attempted total parathyroidectomy is recommended in these unusual situations. Several patients have had parathyroidectomy with fresh parathyroid autografts; most have developed graft-dependent recurrent hypercalcemia.

Sporadic Hypocalciuric Hypercalcemia

Without a positive family history, the decision about management of sporadic hypocalciuric hypercalcemia is difficult. Because there is a wide range of urine calcium values in patients with FHH and with typical primary hyperparathyroidism, an occasional patient with parathyroid adenoma will show a very low calcium-to-creatinine clearance ratio. Moreover, occasionally a patient with FHH may show a high ratio. Coexistent FHH and idiopathic hypercalciuria was clearly documented in at least one case (1). Sporadic hypocalciuric hypercalcemia should generally be managed as typical FHH. In time, the underlying diagnosis may become evident; low morbidity in such patients should be anticipated for the same reasons that morbidity is low in

FHH. Detection of a calcium-ion–sensing receptor mutation can be helpful. Failure to find one does not exclude FHH, as there may be mutation outside the open reading frame or in other FHH genes.

Pregnancy

Pregnancy in an FHH carrier or in the spouse of an FHH carrier requires special understanding, because of possible antagonism between fetal and maternal calcium regulation. The affected offspring of a mother with FHH should show asymptomatic hypercalcemia. The unaffected offspring of a mother with FHH may show symptomatic hypocalcemia from fetal parathyroid suppression as a result of maternal hypercalcemia. The affected offspring of an unaffected mother may show rather severe neonatal hypercalcemia because of intrauterine secondary hyperparathyroidism; this will usually evolve into asymptomatic hypercalcemia without parathyroidectomy.

Family Screening

Because of the high penetrance for expression of hypercalcemia in FHH carriers, accurate genetic assignments can usually be made from one determination of total calcium (or preferably ionized or albumin-adjusted calcium). Family screening is particularly valuable to avoid unnecessary parathyroidectomy in those patients in whom hypercalcemia is initially recognized during blood testing for routine care. Genetic linkage testing and CaSR mutation analysis also have important roles.

CONCLUSIONS

Familial hypocalciuric hypercalcemia is a rather common cause of asymptomatic hypercalcemia, particularly when the hypercalcemia presents at early ages. The diagnosis requires evaluation of to urinary calcium. In the past, FHH was a common cause of unsuccessful parathyroidectomy. Although mild symptoms similar to those in typical primary hyperparathyroidism are quite common, virtually all patients should be followed without any intervention.

REFERENCES

1. Marx SJ, Attie MF, Levine MA, Spiegel AM, Downs RW Jr, Lasker RD. The hypocalciuric or benign variant of familial hypercalcemia: clinical and biochemical features in fifteen kindreds. *Medicine* 1981;60:397–412.
2. Law WM Jr, Heath H III. Familial benign hypercalcemia (hypocalciuric hypercalcemia): clinical and pathogenetic studies in 21 families. *Ann Intern Med* 1985;102:511–519.
3. Davies M, Klimiuk PS, Adams PH, Lumb GA, Anderson DC. Familial hypocalciuric hypercalcemia and acute pancreatitis. *Br Med J* 1981;282:1029–1031.
4. Kristiansen JH, Rødbro P, Christiansen C, Johansen J, Jensen JT. Familial hypocalciuric hypercalcemia III: bone mineral metabolism. *Clin Endocrinol* 1987;26:713–716.
5. Marx SJ, Spiegel AM, Brown EM, et al. Divalent cation metabolism: familial hypocalciuric hypercalcemia versus typical primary hyperparathyroidism. *Am J Med* 1978;65:235–242.
6. Firek AF, Kao PC, Heath H III. Plasma intact parathyroid hormone

(PTH) and PTH-related peptide in familial benign hypercalcemia: greater responsiveness to endogenous PTH than in primary hyperparathyroidism. *J Clin Endocrinol Metab* 1991;72:541–546.

7. Kristiansen JH, Rødbro P, Christiansen C, Brochner MJ, Carl J. Familial hypocalciuric hypercalcemia II: intestinal calcium absorption and vitamin D metabolism. *Clin Endocrinol* 1985;23:511–515.

8. Thorgeirsson U, Costa J, Marx SJ. The parathyroid glands in familial hypocalciuric hypercalcemia. *Hum Pathol* 1981;12:229–237.

9. Law WM Jr, Carney JA, Heath H III. Parathyroid glands in familial benign hypercalcemia (familial hypocalciuric hypercalcemia). *Am J Med* 1984;76:1021–1026.

10. Marx SJ, Stock JL, Attie MF, et al. Familial hypocalciuric hypercalcemia: recognition among patients referred after unsuccessful parathyroid exploration. *Ann Intern Med* 1980;92:351–356.

11. Orwoll E, Silbert J, McClung M. Asymptomatic neonatal familial hypercalcemia. *Pediatrics* 1982;69:109–111.

12. Marx SJ, Fraser D, Rapoport A. Familial hypocalciuric hypercalcemia: mild expression of the gene in heterozygotes and severe expression in homozygotes. *Am J Med* 1985;78:15–22.

13. Chou Y-HW, Brown EM, Levi T, et al. The gene responsible for familial hypocalciuric hypercalcemia maps to chromosome 3q in four unrelated families. *Nat Genet* 1992;1:295–300.

14. Heath H III, Jackson CE, Otterud B, Leppart MF. Familial benign hypercalcemia (FBH) phenotype results from mutations at two distant loci on chromosomes 3q and 19p. *Clin Res* 1993;41:270A.

14a. Lloyd SE, Pannett AA, Dixon PH, Whyte MP, Thakker RV. Localization of familial benign hypercalcemia, Oklahoma variant (FBHOk), to chromosome 19q13. *Am J Hum Genet* 1999;64:189–195.

15. Marx SJ, Attie MF, Spiegel AM, Levine MA, Lasker RD, Fox M. An association between neonatal severe primary hyperparathyroidism and familial hypocalciuric hypercalcemia in three kindreds. *N Engl J Med* 1982;306:257–264.

16. Pollak MR, Chou YH-W, Marx SJ, et al. Familial hypocalciuric hypercalcemia and neonatal severe hyperparathyroidism: effects of mutant gene dosage on phenotype. *J Clin Invest* 1994;93:1108–1112.

17. Eftekhari F, Yousefzadeh DK. Primary infantile hyperparathyroidism: clinical, laboratory, and radiographic features in 21 cases. *Skeletal Radiol* 1982;8:201–208.

18. Page LA, Haddow JE. Self-limited neonatal hyperparathyroidism in familial hypocalciuric hypercalcemia. *J Pediatr* 1987;111:261–264.

19. Marx SJ, Lasker RD, Brown EM, et al. Secretory dysfunction in parathyroid cells from a neonate with severe primary hyperparathyroidism. *J Clin Endocrinol Metab* 1986;62:445–449.

20. Attie MF, Gill JR Jr, Stock JL, et al. Urinary calcium excretion in familial hypocalciuric hypercalcemia: persistence of relative hypocalciuria after induction of hypoparathyroidism. *J Clin Invest* 1983;72:667–676.

21. Brown EM, Pollak M, Seidman CE, et al. Calcium-ion-sensing cell-surface receptors. *N Engl J Med* 1995;333:234–240.

33. Tertiary Hyperparathyroidism and Refractory Secondary Hyperparathyroidism

Olafur S. Indridason, M.D., M.H.Sc. and L. Darryl Quarles, M.D.

Department of Medicine, Division of Nephrology, Duke University Medical Center, Durham, North Carolina

Physiologic parathyroid hormone (PTH) actions on bone result in mobilization of calcium and phosphorus. In the kidney, PTH enhances the reabsorption of calcium in the distal renal tubule, decreases the reabsorption of phosphorus, and increases the production of 1,25-dihydroxyvitamin D_3 [1,25 $(OH)_2$ D_3] in the proximal tubule (see Chapters 11 and 13). In turn, calcium, phosphorus, and 1,25 $(OH)_2$ D_3 exert direct and indirect effects on the parathyroid gland. Calcium regulates parathyroid gland function through activation of the parathyroid cell-surface G protein-coupled calcium receptor (CaR) (1), resulting in decreased production and secretion of PTH, through an increase in intracellular calcium acting as a second messenger. Changes in serum calcium levels also modulate cellular PTH synthesis at the level of pre-pro-PTH transcription and may directly regulate parathyroid cell proliferation as well (2). 1,25 $(OH)_2$ D_3 enhances calcium and phosphorus uptake by the intestine and augments the osseous effects of PTH. In contrast to calcium, 1,25 $(OH)_2$ D_3 has no acute effects on PTH secretion but displays potent suppressive effects on PTH gene transcription and cell growth that are mediated by the vitamin D receptor (VDR), a classic nuclear steroid receptor. The role of phosphorus is less well established. In addition to decreased 1,25 $(OH)_2$ D_3 production in response to hyperphosphatemia, recent studies also suggest a direct effect of phosphorus on parathyroid gland function (3,4). Finally, autocrine and paracrine regulators of PTH secretion, including PTH itself, chromogranin A, chromogranin A-related peptides, and endothelin-1 may be important.

PATHOGENESIS OF TERTIARY/REFRACTORY SECONDARY HYPERPARATHYROIDISM

Secondary hyperparathyroidism (2°HPT) is an acquired disorder representing parathyroid hyperfunction in response to perturbations in the feedback systems described earlier. It is most commonly encountered in end-stage renal disease (ESRD) but also is seen in other vitamin D-deficiency and vitamin-D-resistant states. Prolonged abnormalities in mineral metabolism may eventually result in the evolution of 2°HPT to a state of apparent autonomous PTH secretion, resulting in elevated levels of serum calcium, resembling 1°HPT. Traditionally, the term *tertiary hyperparathyroidism* (3°HPT) is used to describe such patients. Refractory 2°HPT defines another group of patients with severe 2°HPT without spontaneous hypercalcemia, who display nonsuppressible PTH secretion after correcting the inciting metabolic abnormalities [hypocalcemia, hyperphosphatemia, and calcitriol deficiency (see following sections)]. In both 3°HPT and refractory 2°HPT, the parathyroid gland has reached a hyperfunctioning state that no longer responds appropriately to physiologic regulation.

Several changes in the parathyroid gland at the tissue, cellular, and molecular levels potentially explain the inability to restore PTH secretion to normal in some patients with 2°HPT. The most important factors appear to be an increased number of parathyroid cells, possible alterations in the calcium-sensing mechanism, and abnormalities of VDR function. Additionally, hyperphosphatemia and end-organ resistance to PTH actions may contribute to persistent HPT in spite of calcium and vitamin D treatment.

Role of Increased Gland Size

A great deal of evidence supports the notion that parathyroid hyperplasia is important in the pathogenesis of refractory hyperfunction. Both human and animal studies showed that there is a nonsuppressible component of PTH secretion in hypercalcemic states (5). Implantation of excessive amounts of normal parathyroid tissue into nonuremic rats produces hypercalcemia, suggesting that an increase in the number of cells secreting nonsuppressible amounts of PTH can overcome the homeostatic mechanisms that normally control steady-state serum PTH levels. Clinical studies also illustrate that refractoriness to therapy correlates with the degree of parathyroid gland enlargement. Additionally, in a series describing the histologic features of 128 parathyroid glands taken from patients with chronic renal insufficiency, the parathyroid glands of subjects with 3°HPT were usually larger than those from patients with 2°HPT. The average weight of a single gland from patients with 3°HPT was 25 times the weight of a normal parathyroid gland. A significant correlation between parathyroid gland size and the resistance to calcium-mediated PTH suppression is observed in hemodialysis patients with moderate to severe 2°HPT (6) and is similar to the relation that exists between adenoma mass and calcium-mediated PTH suppression in 1°HPT (Fig. 1). Moreover, PTH-secreting cells have a long life span with a limited ability to involute (undergo apoptosis), resulting in persistently increased cell numbers (7). In animal studies of 2°HPT, calcitriol can prevent but not reverse glandular hyperplasia (8). Most human studies have also shown that calcitriol therapy does not cause involution of the enlarged parathyroid gland. However, when such involution occurs, it has been associated with successful therapy of 2°HPT (9). Thus gland size or other factors associated with increased parathyroid mass [e.g., nodular dysplasia (*vide infra*)] may play an important role in the development of refractory 2°HPT/3°HPT.

Phenotypic Alterations of the Parathyroid Gland in Tertiary Hyperparathyroidism

Several studies on excised human parathyroid glands have shown changes indicative of monoclonal cellular expansion in refractory 2°HPT and 3°HPT. These changes include demonstration of allelic loss of chromosome 11, the location of the MEN-I gene, which is associated with primary parathyroid hyperplasia (10). Further data have come from immunohistochemical and X-chromosome inactivation analysis studies showing monoclonal proliferation of a single parathyroid cell, identical to that seen in 1°HPT (11). This monoclonal expansion may be confined to nodular areas of the parathyroid glands; in contrast, diffuse hyperplasia stems from polyclonal cell growth. Thus a nodular histologic pattern in the parathyroid glands may be a marker of cellular transformation, which in turn is associated with deranged regulation of PTH secretion. In this regard, nodules are more common in the glands of hypercalcemic patients with 3°HPT than in

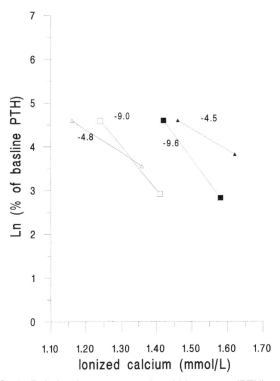

FIG. 1. Relation between parathyroid hormone (PTH) suppression and serum ionized calcium concentration. PTH levels were expressed as the natural logarithm of the percentage of baseline serum PTH concentration. Numbers indicate the slopes of the respective lines. Each line represents the mean of the individual subject curves. The slope in familial benign hypocalciuric hypercalcemia (FBHH) subjects (*solid squares*) was similar to that of normal subjects (*open squares*); (−9.6 and −9.0, respectively). In contrast, 1° hyperparathyroidism (HPT) (*solid triangles*) and 2°HPT (*open triangles*) had slopes (−4.5 and −4.8, respectively) that were significantly different from those of normal subjects. The rightward shift of the lines for FBHH and 1°HPT compared with the normal group is consistent with impaired calcium sensing (that is, setpoint changes), whereas the steepness of the slope correlated with gland size in 1°HPT and 2°HPT. (Reprinted from Indridason OS, Heath H, Khosla S, Yohay DA, Quarles LD. Non-suppressible parathyroid hormone secretion is related to gland size in uremic secondary hyperparathyroidism. *Kidney Int* 1996;50:1663–1671, with permission.)

2°HPT. The histology of such nodular areas bears a strong resemblance to that of primary parathyroid adenomas. Furthermore, the density of vitamin D receptors is low in such nodular areas. Similarly, decreased expression of the CaR has been demonstrated at both messenger RNA (mRNA) and protein level in parathyroid nodules (12). *In vitro* studies have also demonstrated altered regulation of PTH secretion in nodular hyperplastic tissue as compared with diffuse hyperplastic tissue, indicating a degree of insensitivity to calcium that resembles regulatory characteristics of primary adenomas. Finally, autotransplantation of nodular hyperplastic glands may predispose to recurrent HPT after parathyroidectomy. Thus prolonged physiologic stimuli that result in polyclonal parathyroid hyperplasia may eventually progress to adenomatous transformation, possibly with the monoclonal cells displaying a more autonomous phenotype.

Role of Abnormal Calcium Sensing (Altered Setpoint)

To what extent altered calcium sensing plays a role in the pathology of secondary hyperparathyroidism is not certain and clinical studies examining setpoint changes have yielded variable results. Recently new insight into potential calcium-sensing abnormalities has been gained by comparing 2°HPT with other pathologic conditions of the parathyroid glands [i.e., familial benign hypocalciuric hypercalcemia (FBHH) and 1°HPT]. FBHH, a disorder in which there is an allelic loss of functional CaR gene (Chapter 32) is characterized by a pure right shift of the relation between extracellular calcium and PTH during hypercalcemic PTH suppression [i.e., increased setpoint but normal response to changes in ionized calcium (normal suppression)]. 1°HPT (Chapter 30) also is characterized by an elevated setpoint; however, there also is an abnormal response to changes in extracellular calcium (decreased calcium-mediated PTH suppression), which is related to adenoma size. In comparison, normocalcemic patients with moderate to severe 2°HPT demonstrated decreased suppression, which was related to gland size, but no setpoint shift, indicating normal calcium sensing (12) (Fig. 1). On the other hand, preliminary results from similar studies in hypercalcemic patients with 3°HPT prior to parathyroidectomy indicate elevated setpoint in addition to reduced suppression, giving a picture resembling 1°HPT.

The molecular mechanisms underlying impaired calcium sensing in 1°HPT and 3°HPT are not completely understood as yet. There have been no documented somatic mutations of CaR in either parathyroid adenomas or uremic 2°HPT. Indeed, cloned CaR cDNA from a primary parathyroid adenoma lacked any coding-region mutation and was shown to have functional properties similar to that of normal parathyroid CaR cDNA when expressed in *Xenopus* oocytes (13). *In situ* hybridization and immunohistochemical studies demonstrated that both CaR mRNA and protein expression are decreased in 1°HPT and 2°HPT, particularly within nodular areas (12). However, in a study with quantitative reverse transcriptase polymerase chain reaction (PCR) technique found no decrease in CaR mRNA (14). Furthermore, no differences in the parathyroid gland CaR mRNA levels have been observed in animal models of 2°HPT.

Regardless, setpoint alterations and abnormalities in CaR, when present in patients with 2°HPT may be limited to glands with adenomatous transformation. However, the possibilities that posttranscriptional processing, downstream signaling pathways, changes in CaR promoter activity, or other mechanisms could be responsible for abnormal CaR function need further studies in these patients.

Role of Abnormal Vitamin D Metabolism

Persistent abnormalities in vitamin D homeostasis likely contribute to the development of refractory 2°HPT and 3°HPT. Vitamin D affects both PTH biosynthesis and parathyroid cellular proliferation. 1,25 $(OH)_2$ D_3 deficiency is sufficient to stimulate parathyroid gland hyperplasia in nor-

mocalcemic dogs, and administration of calcitriol can prevent parathyroid gland hyperplasia in animal models of 2°HPT (8,15). Vitamin D also has a marked inhibitory effect on cellular proliferation in culture. Furthermore, vitamin D, but not calcium, down-regulates expression of protooncogenes associated with cellular proliferation in parathyroid tissue and other cell models. The importance of this antiproliferative effect in the progression to 3°HPT is not clear, however. Nevertheless, vitamin D has profound effects on PTH production. Vitamin-D-deficient rats are unable to modulate PTH mRNA levels in response to alterations of ambient calcium (16), and calcitriol has been shown to decrease PTH mRNA levels in parathyroid cells in animal and *in vitro* studies. In addition to calcitriol deficiency, there is marked down-regulation of the VDR number in uremic parathyroid glands, a finding that is particularly prominent in nodular areas in severe forms of parathyroid hyperplasia. Whereas the VDR can be up-regulated by calcitriol treatment, uremia may both diminish the ability of calcitriol to induce the expression of VDR (17) and impair the VDR–DNA interactions (18). Finally, the expression of chromogranin A mRNA, which has been implicated in autocrine/paracrine PTH regulation, is increased by calcitriol treatment of normal rats and is low in uremic rats with low vitamin D levels.

Role of Phosphorus

There is increasing evidence to suggest that phosphorus has a direct effect on parathyroid gland function and proliferation. In isolated parathyroid glands, extracellular phosphorus increases PTH secretion independent of ambient calcium concentration (19). In animal studies, hypophosphatemia reduces PTH mRNA and parathyroid cell proliferation independent of calcium and calcitriol, whereas high serum phosphorus accelerates parathyroid hyperplasia (3,4). Furthermore, rat studies linked hyperphosphatemia to reductions in calcium-mediated PTH suppression. More important, in dialysis patients treated with calcitriol, resistance to therapy has been directly related to high serum phosphorus concentration (9). Hyperphosphatemia may thus play a key role in both parathyroid proliferation and resistance to calcium and calcitriol actions on the parathyroid gland through mechanisms that remain to be identified.

Although the exact molecular mechanisms of refractory 2°HPT/3°HPT remain to be defined, a combination of hypertrophy, hyperplasia, and dysregulated control of PTH secretion and production combine to produce a state in which PTH production remains excessive in spite of adequate replacement of calcium and calcitriol and control of serum phosphorus.

CLINICAL CONDITIONS ASSOCIATED WITH TERTIARY/REFRACTORY SECONDARY HYPERPARATHYROIDISM

Refractory 2°HPT has been observed in many chronic disorders of mineral metabolism, including those that are associated with ESRD, nutritional vitamin D deficiency, high-dose phosphate treatment of chronic hypophosphatemic disorders, various VDR/dependent states, and certain hepatobiliary diseases.

End-stage Renal Disease

The uremic state presents multiple stimuli to the parathyroid gland leading to 2°HPT. These include hypocalcemia, hyperphosphatemia, 1,25 $(OH)_2$ D_3 deficiency, down-regulation of the VDR, and possibly altered calcium sensing (or setpoint). The presence of 2°HPT is probably best defined in ESRD by a circulating level of intact PTH above 150 to 200 pg/mL, the values associated with histologic evidence of increased bone remodeling (20). These reference values are roughly threefold greater than that of circulating PTH levels in normal individuals (65 pg/mL). The upper limit of PTH is likely higher in uremia because of the end-organ resistance to PTH. Uremic 2°HPT is a heterogeneous disorder characterized by variable suppressible PTH levels that are likely related to the degree of parathyroid gland hyperplasia and acquired alterations in PTH regulation (see earlier). In mild to moderate 2°HPT, most patients normalize serum PTH levels in response to correction of hyperphosphatemia, hypocalcemia, and calcitriol deficiency. Responsive subjects probably have minimal parathyroid gland enlargement and appear to display normal sensitivity to calcium-mediated PTH suppression. The major abnormality identified by dynamic testing is an increased capacity to secrete PTH in response to hypocalcemic stimuli. Today only a few patients with ESRD develop 3°HPT (roughly 5% in most series; 21). Its development is related to the duration of ESRD requiring dialysis. Refractory 2°HPT occurs in 12% to 55% of chronic maintenance hemodialysis patients (22). This range is consistent with the reported 30% of hemodialysis patients treated with vitamin D analogs that display progression of 2°HPT (21). In general, patients with 3°HPT or refractory 2°HPT have intact PTH levels exceeding 1500 pg/mL, although there is no absolute circulating PTH threshold for establishing this diagnosis. Renal transplantation may unmask 3°HPT/refractory 2°HPT in patients with preexisting severe 2°HPT of long duration. Indeed, hypercalcemia has been reported to occur in as many as one third of successfully transplanted subjects. The restoration of 1,25 $(OH)_2$ D_3 production by the renal allograft and amelioration of end-organ resistance to PTH may increase the susceptibility to hypercalcemia during the slow involution of hypersecreting parathyroid glands. Autopsy specimens taken from renal transplant patients without clinically evident 2°HPT confirm that parathyroid gland hyperplasia does not rapidly resolve, even with the nearly normal metabolic milieu resulting from transplantation. In addition, the degree of elevation of PTH following hypocalcemic stimulation correlates with the residual parathyroid gland volume in renal transplant subjects (23).

Vitamin-D-Resistant/Dependent States

Large doses of oral phosphorus used to treat children with X-linked hypophosphatemic rickets can result in chronic stimulation of PTH secretion via lowering of the serum ionized calcium. A subset of these patients appear to develop 3°HPT associated with diffuse parathyroid gland hyperpla-sia. Occasionally, parathyroid adenomas are observed. It is not clear whether these adenomas represent concurrence of 1°HPT or monoclonal expansion derived from diffuse hyperplasia. In any event, subtotal parathyroidectomy and, more recently, total parathyroidectomy with autotransplantation have been effectively used to decrease functional parathyroid mass in these children.

Vitamin-D-Deficient States

Chronic vitamin D deficiency has been shown to result in refractory 2°HPT. Detailed studies of a cohort of vitamin-D-deficient Asian vegetarians revealed inability to suppress PTH levels completely, even after a full year of therapy with calcium and calcitriol. The duration of parathyroid stimulation may be essential to development of a nonsuppressible state, because treatment of vitamin-D-deficient children with calcium and vitamin D typically results in rapid normalization of elevated PTH levels. In addition, unlike that in ESRD and treatment of hypophosphatemic disorders, the 2°HPT of chronic dietary vitamin D deficiency is usually mild to moderate.

Hepatobiliary Disorders

A similar cause of PTH hypersecretion has been postulated in patients with primary biliary cirrhosis, a disease state characterized by low 25 (OH) D_3 and 1,25 $(OH)_2$ D_3 levels (secondary to inability of the liver to convert vitamin D effectively to 25 (OH) D_3 via vitamin D 25-hydroxylase). A group of patients with primary biliary cirrhosis who had been adequately supplemented with calcium and 1,25 $(OH)_2$ D_3 were found to have an average PTH level significantly higher than normal controls. Thirty percent of the patients had a PTH level above the normal range. Again, severe hypercalcemia was absent, and other clinical manifestations of 2°HPT were not severe enough to warrant parathyroidectomy in this group of patients.

THERAPY

Controversy exists over the role of 1,25 $(OH)_2$ D_3 in the management of refractory 2°HPT disorders. Although by definition these disorders are resistant to medical therapy, earlier studies suggested that high-dose intravenous calcitriol administration might effectively accomplish a "medical" parathyroidectomy. These initial results, however, have not been substantiated by controlled studies (22). Although there may be some advantage to pulse administration of 1,25 $(OH)_2$ D_3 by either the intravenous or the oral route, more recent studies suggest that pharmacologic calcitriol therapy, regardless of route of administration, is poorly tolerated (50% of subjects developed hypercalcemia and 75% developed hyperphosphatemia) and often ineffective in suppressing elevated PTH levels in chronic maintenance hemodialysis patients (22). A search for parathyroid gland-specific vitamin D analogues with minimal effect on intestinal calcium and phosphate transport has not yet been successful. Several promising compounds, including 1α-hydroxyvitamin D_2, 19-*nor*-1,25-dihydroxyvitamin D_2, and 22-oxacalcitriol have been identified, but limited human experience suggests that these analogues may still lead to hypercalcemia and hyperphosphatemia (24). The novel class of calcimimetic compounds also has shown promise in animal models of 2°HPT and results from a recent short-term study of one such calcium-receptor agonist in 1°HPT (25) suggest it may be beneficial in 3°HPT as well. However, it is not clear whether these new compounds offer any benefit over calcitriol, as direct comparisons have not been performed. Moreover, they have not been examined in the setting of refractory 2°HPT or 3°HPT, in which abnormalities in VDR or calcium sensing or both may limit their usefulness.

Cure of refractory 2°HPT/3°HPT requires surgical intervention designed to "debulk" the parathyroid gland. Surgical treatment is indicated in symptomatic patients with nonsuppressible serum PTH levels. Symptoms may include those related to hypercalcemia, hyperparathyroid bone disease, nephrocalcinosis, and nephrolithiasis. In ESRD patients, intractable pruritus, bone pain, severe hyperphosphatemia, calciphylaxis, and soft-tissue calcification may be additional indications. In renal transplant patients with persistent 2°HPT, serum calcium levels >12.5 mg/dL after 1 year and progressive and unexplained renal insufficiency in the setting of hypercalcemia are usual indications for parathyroidectomy. Patients with persistently elevated circulating PTH concentrations, but without hypercalcemia or symptoms, after intensive medical therapy are often managed expectantly, like patients with asymptomatic 1°HPT. There are, however, no controlled studies that evaluate conservative management of asymptomatic refractory 2°HPT compared with parathyroidectomy.

Early approaches used subtotal parathyroidectomy that reduced parathyroid mass by approximately seven eighths. With this procedure, some patients remained hyperparathyroid, requiring a second neck exploration for further tissue removal. Another alternative is total parathyroidectomy and autografting of parathyroid tissue fragments into the muscle of the forearm. The advantages of this procedure are lower failure rates and ability to reduce further parathyroid mass without another neck exploration. The disadvantages are the occasional induction of hypoparathyroidism and, rarely, continued 3°HPT resulting from adenomatous growth of fragments reimplanted in the arm. Perhaps the ability to determine clonality in hyperplastic parathyroid tissue will someday enable a surgeon to avoid autotransplantation of potentially autonomous parathyroid tissue. The exception to the use of parathyroid autografting may be the renal transplant patient with 2°HPT. In prospective renal transplant patients, to minimize the risk of hypoparathyroidism, some clinicians prefer subtotal parathyroidectomy.

REFERENCES

1. Brown EM, Gamba G, Riccardi D, et al. Cloning and characterization of an extracellular Ca(2+)-sensing receptor from bovine parathyroid. *Nature* 1993;366:575–580.
2. Naveh-Many T, Rahamimov R, Livni N, Silver J. Parathyroid cell proliferation in normal and chronic renal failure rats: the effects of calcium, phosphate, and vitamin D. *J Clin Invest* 1995;96:1786–1793.
3. Denda M, Finch J, Slatopolsky E. Phosphorus accelerates the development of parathyroid hyperplasia and secondary hyperparathyroidism in rats with renal failure. *Am J Kidney Dis* 1996;28:596–602.
4. Kilav R, Silver J, Naveh-Many T. Parathyroid hormone gene expression in hypophosphatemic rats. *J Clin Invest* 1995;96:327–333.
5. Mayer GP, Habener JF, Potts JT Jr. Parathyroid hormone secretion in vivo: demonstration of a calcium-independent nonsuppressible component of secretion. *J Clin Invest* 1976;57:678–683.
6. Indridason OS, Heath H, Khosla S, Yohay DA, Quarles LD. Nonsuppressible parathyroid hormone secretion is related to gland size in uremic secondary hyperparathyroidism. *Kidney Int* 1996;50:1663–1671.
7. Parfitt AM. Hypercalcemic hyperparathyroidism following renal transplantation: differential diagnosis, management, and implications for cell population control in the parathyroid gland. *Miner Electrolyte Metab* 1982;8:92–112.
8. Szabo A, Merke J, Beier E, Mall G, Ritz E. 1,25(OH)$_2$ vitamin D_3 inhibits parathyroid cell proliferation in experimental uremia. *Kidney Int* 1989;35:1049–1056.
9. Quarles LD, Yohay DA, Carroll BA, et al. Prospective trial of pulse oral versus intravenous calcitriol treatment of hyperparathyroidism in ESRD. *Kidney Int* 1994;45:1710–1721.
10. Friedman E, Sakaguchi K, Bale AE, et al. Clonality of parathyroid tumors in familial multiple endocrine neoplasia type 1. *N Engl J Med* 1989;321:213–218.
11. Arnold A, Brown MF, Urena P, et al. Monoclonality of parathyroid tumors in chronic renal failure and in primary parathyroid hyperplasia. *J Clin Invest* 1995;95:2047–2053.
12. Gogusev J, Duchambon P, Hory B, et al. Depressed expression of calcium receptor in parathyroid gland tissue of patients with hyperparathyroidism. *Kidney Int* 1997;51:328–336.
13. Garrett JE, Capuano IV, Hammerland LG, et al. Molecular cloning and functional expression of human parathyroid calcium receptor cDNAs. *J Biol Chem* 1995;270:12919–12925.
14. Garner SC, Hinson TK, McCarty KS, Leight M, Leight GSJ, Quarles LD. Quantitative analysis of the calcium-sensing receptor messenger RNA in parathyroid adenomas. *Surgery* 1997;122:1166–1175.
15. Hendy GN, Stotland MA, Grunbaum D, Fraher LJ, Loveridge N, Goltzman D. Characteristics of secondary hyperparathyroidism in vitamin D-deficient dogs. *Am J Physiol* 1989;256:E765–E772.
16. Naveh-Many T, Silver J. Regulation of parathyroid hormone gene expression by hypocalcemia, hypercalcemia, and vitamin D in the rat. *J Clin Invest* 1990;86:1313–1319.
17. Hsu CH, Patel SR, Vanholder R. Mechanism of decreased intestinal calcitriol receptor concentration in renal failure. *Am J Physiol* 1993;264:F662–F669.
18. Patel SR, Ke HQ, Vanholder R, Koenig RJ, Hsu CH. Inhibition of calcitriol receptor binding to vitamin D response elements by uremic toxins. *J Clin Invest* 1995;96:50–59.
19. Slatopolsky E, Finch J, Denda M, et al. Phosphorus restriction prevents parathyroid gland growth: high phosphorus directly stimulates PTH secretion in vitro. *J Clin Invest* 1996;97:2534–2540.
20. Quarles LD, Lobaugh B, Murphy G. Intact parathyroid hormone overestimates the presence and severity of parathyroid-mediated osseous abnormalities in uremia. *J Clin Endocrinol Metab* 1992;75:145–150.
21. Mizumoto D, Watanabe Y, Fukuzawa Y, Yuzawa Y, Yamazaki C. Identification of risk factors on secondary hyperparathyroidism undergoing long-term haemodialysis with vitamin D_3. *Nephrol Dial Transplant* 1994;9:1751–1758.
22. Indridason OS, Quarles LD. Oral versus intravenous calcitriol: is the route of administration really important? *Curr Opin Nephrol Hypertens* 1995;4:307–312.
23. McCarron DA, Muther RS, Lenfesty B, Bennett WM. Parathyroid function in persistent hyperparathyroidism: relationship to gland size. *Kidney Int* 1982;22:662–670.
24. Frazao JM, Chesney RW, Coburn JW. Intermittent oral 1-alpha-hydroxyvitamin D_2 is effective and safe for the suppression of secondary hyperparathyroidism in hemodialysis patients. *Nephrol Dial Transplant* 1998;13:68–72.
25. Silverberg SJ, Bone HG, Marriott TB, et al. Short-term inhibition of parathyroid hormone secretion by a calcium receptor agonist in patients with primary hyperparathyroidism. *N Engl J Med* 1997;337:1506–1510.

34. Humoral Hypercalcemia of Malignancy

Michelle M. Roberts, M.D. and *Andrew F. Stewart, M.D.

*Department of Medicine, University of Pittsburgh School of Medicine and *Division of Endocrinology,
University of Pittsburgh Medical Center, Pittsburgh, Pennsylvania*

The term humoral hypercalcemia of malignancy (HHM) describes, in broad terms, a clinical syndrome characterized by hypercalcemia caused by the secretion by a cancer of a circulating calcemic factor. The tumor typically has limited or no skeletal involvement. The term describes a classic endocrine system, with the secretory gland being the tumor and the target organs being the skeleton and the kidney. The term can be used in a general sense to describe the production by tumors of any humoral calcemic factor. For example, hypercalcemia resulting from the production of 1,25-dihydroxyvitamin D [1,25 $(OH)_2$ D] in patients with lymphoma and hypercalcemia resulting from ectopic secretion of parathyroid hormone by an ovarian carcinoma would both fulfill the literal criteria for being humoral forms of hypercalcemia. These examples are discussed further at the conclusion of this chapter. As currently used, however, the term HHM describes a very specific clinical syndrome that results from the production of parathyroid hormone-related protein (PTHrP) (see Chapters 14 and 20). The large majority of patients with humorally mediated hypercalcemia have HHM. Several recent detailed reviews of the syndrome are listed at the end of this section.

The syndrome was first described in 1941, in a patient with a renal carcinoma and a solitary skeletal metastasis. Subsequent studies in the 1950s and 1960s documented the humoral nature of the syndrome by demonstrating that (a) typical patients had little or no skeletal tumor involvement, and (b) the hypercalcemia and other biochemical abnormalities were reversed when the tumor was resected or treated. Evidence provided in the 1960s and 1970s suggested that the responsible factor was either prostaglandin E_2, a vitamin-D-like sterol, or parathyroid hormone (PTH). It is now clear that none of these is responsible.

From a clinical standpoint, patients with HHM have advanced disease with tumors that are usually obvious clinically and therefore carry a poor prognosis. As a rule, by the time hypercalcemia occurs in a patient with cancer, survival can be measured in weeks to a few months. Exceptions to this rule include small, well-differentiated endocrine tumors such a pheochromocytomas or islet cell tumors. In contrast to patients with hypercalcemia due to skeletal involvement with cancer (see Chapter 35), who typically have breast cancer, multiple myeloma, or lymphomas, patients with HHM most often have squamous carcinomas (involving lung, esophagus, cervix, vulva, skin, or head and neck). Other tumor types commonly associated with HHM are renal, bladder, and ovarian carcinomas. Breast carcinomas may cause typical HHM, or they may lead to hypercalcemia through skeletal metastatic involvement. Finally, the subset of hypercalcemic patients with lymphomas due to human T-cell leukemia virus I appear to have classic biochemical HHM. Patients with HHM account for up to 80% of patients with malignancy-associated hypercalcemia. Certain common tumors (e.g., colon, prostate, thyroid, oat cell, and gastric carcinomas) rarely cause hypercalcemia of any type.

Biochemically and histologically, patients with HHM share certain features with patients with primary hyperparathyroidism (HPT) and differ in other respects (Table 1; Figs. 1–4). Both groups of patients have a humoral syndrome, both are hypercalcemic, and both are hypophosphatemic and display reductions in the renal tubular phosphorus threshold. Both groups display increased nephrogenous or urinary cyclic adenosine monophosphate (AMP) excretion, indicating an interaction of the respective humoral mediator with proximal tubular PTH receptors. Both groups display increases in osteoclastic bone resorption when bone is examined histologically (Fig. 2).

In contrast, patients with HHM differ from those with HPT in several important respects (Fig. 1; Table 1). PTH is a potent stimulus for distal tubular calcium reabsorption, and patients with HPT therefore display only modest hypercalciuria. In contrast, most patients with HHM demonstrate marked increases in calcium excretion, perhaps reflecting a weaker effect of PTHrP on distal tubular calcium reabsorption. PTH also is a potent stimulus for the renal production of 1,25 $(OH)_2$ D. Patients with HPT therefore often demonstrate increases in circulating 1,25 $(OH)_2$ D and a resultant increase in calcium absorption by the intestine. In contrast, patients with HHM display reductions in serum 1,25 $(OH)_2$ D values and in intestinal calcium absorption. The physiology underlying this observation is uncertain, because N-terminal PTHrPs *in vitro* and *in vivo* stimulate renal 1α-hydroxylase, the enzyme that synthesizes 1,25 $(OH)_2$ D. Osteoblastic bone formation is increased and coupled to the increased bone resorption rate in patients with HPT (Fig. 2). In patients with HHM, osteoblastic bone formation, however, is reduced and is therefore dissociated or uncoupled from the increased osteoclastic bone resorption (Fig. 2). The reasons for this uncoupling also are unclear, because synthetic N-terminal PTHrPs *in vitro* and *in vivo* in animals stimulate osteoblastic activity. Of course, immunoreactive PTH concentrations in

TABLE 1. *Similarities and differences between patients with primary hyperparathyroidism (HPT) and HHM*

	HPT	HHM
Humorally mediated hypercalcemia	+	+
Hypophosphatemia	+	+
Phosphaturia	+	+
Nephrogenous cAMP elevation	+	+
Increased osteoclastic bone resorption	+	+
Increased renal calcium reabsorption	+	±
Increased plasma 1,25$(OH)_2$D	+	−
Increased osteoblastic bone formation	+	−
Increased circulating immunoreactive PTH	+	−
Increased circulating immunoreactive PTHrP	−	+
Hypercalcemia due primarily to effects on kidney and GI tract	+	−
Hypercalcemia due primarily to bone resorption	−	+

203

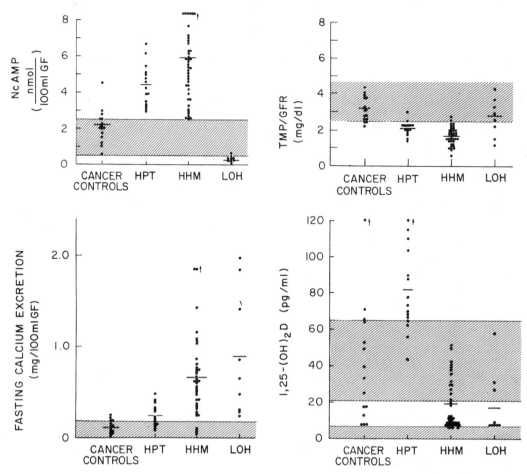

FIG. 1. Nephrogenous cyclic adenosine monophosphate excretion (NcAMP), renal tubular maximum for phosphorus (TmP/GFR), fasting calcium excretion, and plasma 1,25-dihydroxyvitamin D values in normocalcemic patients with cancer (cancer controls) and in patients with primary hyperparathyroidism (HPT), with humoral hypercalcemia of malignancy (HHM), and with hypercalcemia due to bone metastases or local osteolytic hypercalcemia (LOH). (Adapted from Stewart AF, Horst R, Deftos LJ, Cadman EC, Lang R, Broadus AE. Biochemical evaluation of patients with cancer-associated hypercalcemia: evidence for humoral and non-humoral groups. *N Engl J Med* 1980;303:1377–1383, with permission.)

plasma are elevated in patients with HPT, but they are normal or suppressed, depending primarily on the assay used, in patients with HHM (Fig. 3). Conversely, immunoreactive PTHrP values are elevated in HHM, but they are normal in patients with HPT (Fig. 4). Preliminary studies suggested that the immunoreactive PTHrP concentration may be useful in monitoring responses to surgery, chemotherapy, or radiotherapy in patients in whom levels are elevated prior to therapy.

Hypercalcemia in patients with HHM has both skeletal and renal components. The skeletal component, as noted earlier, reflects increased osteoclast activity and uncoupling of osteoblasts from osteoclasts. The renal component reflects variable increases in distal tubular calcium reabsorption. Equally or more important, patients with HHM are usually volume depleted, partly as a result of their hypercalcemia, with resultant inability to concentrate the urine, and partly as a result of poor oral fluid intake. The volume depletion leads to a reduction in the filtered load of calcium and a reduction in the fractional excretion of calcium.

Therapy of HHM is discussed in more detail in Chapter 29; it should include measures aimed at (a) reducing the tumor burden, (b) reducing osteoclastic bone resorption, and (c) augmenting renal calcium clearance. Measures aimed at reducing tumor burden (surgery, radiotherapy, and chemotherapy) lead to a reduction in the circulating concentration of PTHrP. Measures aimed at inhibiting osteoclastic bone resorption (use of bisphosphonates, mithramycin, or calcitonin) may reverse hypercalcemia but have no effect on circulating PTHrP concentrations.

UNUSUAL FORMS OF HUMORAL HYPERCALCEMIA

The two broad categories of malignancy-associated hypercalcemia, described in this chapter (HHM) and in Chapter 35 (hypercalcemia due to hematologic malignancies and

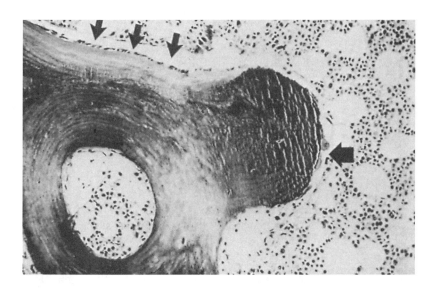

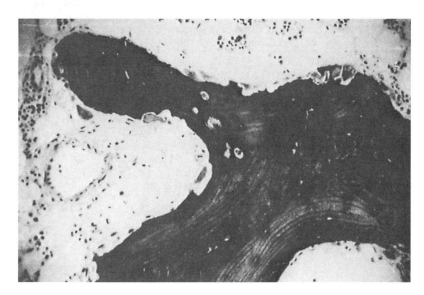

FIG. 2. Comparison of bone histology in a patient with hyperparathyroidism (HPT; **top**) and humoral hypercalcemia of malignancy (HHM; **bottom**). In both groups, osteoclastic activity is accelerated, although it is higher in HHM than in HPT. In HPT, osteoblastic activity and osteoid are increased, but both are markedly decreased in HHM. This uncoupling of formation from resorption in HHM plays the major role in causing hypercalcemia.

solid tumors associated with extensive skeletal involvement), compose the vast majority of patients with cancer and hypercalcemia. It should, however, be clear that other mechanisms, although uncommon, may be encountered. For example, patients who clearly display humorally mediated hypercalcemic syndromes (i.e., hypercalcemia that is reversed by tumor resection) have been reported who do not fit into the HHM biochemical categorization described. The humoral mediator in these patients is unknown. Rare patients with renal carcinomas have been described who appear to have *bona fide* tumor secretion of prostaglandin E_2 as a cause.

Finally, it is important to emphasize that patients with cancer may develop hypercalcemia as a result of other coexisting conditions, such as primary HPT, tuberculosis, sarcoidosis, immobilization, and use of calcium-containing hyperalimentation solutions. These causes should be actively sought and corrected.

In addition to these poorly characterized syndromes, two types of malignancy-associated hypercalcemia, although rare, have been well characterized and are interesting mechanistically. These are discussed later.

1,25-Dihydroxyvitamin-D-Secreting Lymphomas

Breslau et al. and Rosenthal et al. in 1984 described six patients with malignant lymphomas in whom circulating concentrations of 1,25 $(OH)_2$ D were found to be elevated, in some cases strikingly so. Seymour et al. presented a review and update of this syndrome in 1994. The elevation of plasma 1,25 $(OH)_2$ D is in contrast to findings in other types of malignancy-associated hypercalcemia (Fig. 1). No evidence for a role for either PTH or PTHrP has been found. Resection or therapy of the lymphomas reversed the hypercalcemia and reversed the elevations of 1,25 $(OH)_2$ D in plasma. No unifying histologic theme was present among the lymphomas. Rather, lymphomas of several differ-

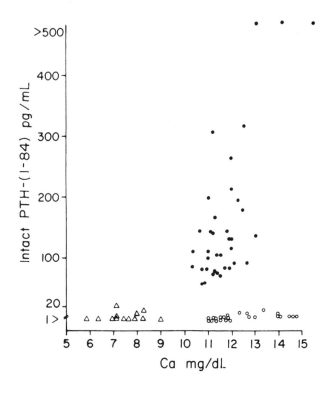

FIG. 3. Immunoreactive parathyroid hormone (PTH) concentration of PTH by using a two-site immunoradiometric assay for PTH(1–84) in patients with primary hyperparathyroidism *(solid circles),* in patients with hypoparathyroidism *(open triangles),* and in patients with hypercalcemia of malignancy *(open circles).* (From Nussbaum S, Zahradnik RJ, Lavigne JR, et al. Highly sensitive two-site immunoradiometric assay of parathyrin and its clinical utility in evaluating patients with hypercalcemia. *Clin Chem* 1987;33:1364–1367, with permission.)

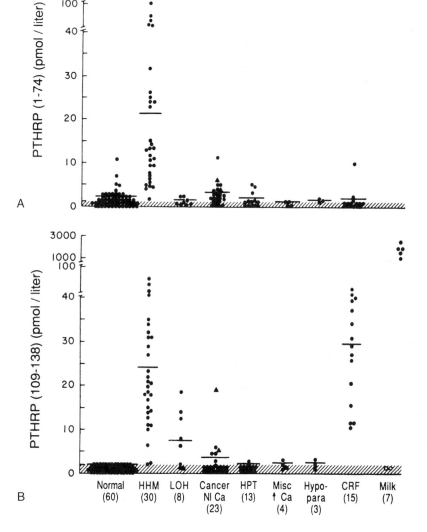

FIG. 4. Immunoreactive parathyroid hormone-related protein (PTHrP) values in patients with humoral hypercalcemia of malignancy (HHM) and in various control groups. iPTHrP values shown were obtained by using a two-site immunoradiometric assay (IRMA) directed against PTHrP(1–74). See Chapter 20 for a complete discussion. (From Burtis WJ, Brady TG, Orloff JJ, et al. Immunochemical characterization of circulating PTH-related protein in patients with humoral hypercalcemia of malignancy. *N Engl J Med* 1980;322:1106–1112, with permission.)

ent subcategories are included in this group. The elevations and hypercalcemia are corrected with glucocorticoid therapy. This syndrome appears to be the malignant counterpart of sarcoidosis (Chapter 36), with malignant lymphocytes, macrophages, or both converting diet- and sun-derived 25 (OH) D to 1,25 (OH)$_2$ D.

Ectopic Hyperparathyroidism

From the 1940s through the 1970s, what is now called HHM was widely attributed to ectopic secretion of parathyroid hormone by malignant tumors. Terms such as "ectopic hyperparathyroidism" and "pseudohyperparathyroidism" were in common use. In the 1980s, as described earlier, it was recognized that the vast majority of cases of HHM were caused by PTHrP, and it was questioned whether "ectopic secretion" of PTH even existed. In the 1990s, this question was clearly answered. At the time of this writing, seven cases of what can be described as authentic "ectopic hyperparathyroidism" have been reported. These tumors included two small-cell carcinomas (one of the lung and one of the ovary), a squamous carcinoma of the lung, an adenocarcinoma of the ovary, a thymoma, an undifferentiated neuroendocrine tumor, and a papillary carcinoma of the thyroid. Immunoreactive PTH was found to be elevated in state-of-the-art PTH two-site assays and declined with the hypercalcemia after tumor resection. In most cases, PTH was present immunohistochemically; the tumors secreted PTH, but not PTHrP, into their culture medium *in vitro*; the tumors contained PTH, but not PTHrP, messenger RNA. In one case, PTH overexpression by an ovarian tumor resulted from a rearrangement of the PTH gene, which placed it under the control of an ovarian promoter. These findings make it clear that authentic ectopic secretion of PTH, although exceedingly rare, can occur. This entity should be considered in the diagnosis of patients with hypercalcemia and increased concentrations of PTH.

SUGGESTED READINGS

Humoral Hypercalcemia of Malignancy

1. Bonjour J-P, Phillipe J, Guelpa G, et al. Bone and renal components of hypercalcemia in malignancy and responses to a single infusion of clodronate. *Bone* 1988;9:123–130.
2. Budayr AA, Zysset E, Jenzer A, et al. Effects of treatment of malignancy-associated hypercalcemia on serum parathyroid hormone-related protein. *J Bone Miner Res* 1994;9:521–526.
3. Everhart-Caye M, Inzucchi SE, Guinness-Henry J, Mitnick MA, Stewart AF. Parathyroid hormone-related protein(1–36) is equipotent with parathyroid hormone(1–34) in humans. *J Clin Endocrinol Metab* 1995;81:199–208.
4. Godsall JW, Burtis WJ, Insogna KL, Broadus AE, Stewart AF. Nephrogenous cyclic AMP, adenylate cyclase-stimulating activity, and the humoral hypercalcemia of malignancy. In: Greep RO, ed. *Recent progress in hormone research*. Boca Raton, FL: Academic Press, 1986:705–750.
5. Grill V, Ho P, Body JJ, et al. Parathyroid hormone-related protein: elevated levels in both humoral hypercalcemia of malignancy and hypercalcemia complicating metastatic breast cancer. *J Clin Endocrinol Metab* 1991;73:1309–1315.
6. Grill V, Murray RML, Ho PWM, et al. Circulating PTH and PTHrP levels before and after treatment of tumor induced hypercalcemia with pamidronate disodium (APD). *J Clin Endocrinol Metab* 1992;74:468–470.
7. Ikeda K, Ohno H, Hane M, et al. Development of a sensitive two-site immunoradiometric assay for parathyroid hormone-related peptide: evidence for elevated levels in plasma from patients with adult T-cell leukemia/lymphoma and B-cell lymphoma. *J Clin Endocrinol Metab* 1994;79:1322–1327.
8. Isales C, Carcangiu ML, Stewart AF. Hypercalcemia in breast cancer: a reassessment of the mechanism. *Am J Med* 1987;82:1143–1147.
9. Motokura T, Fukumoto S, Matsumoto T, et al. Parathyroid hormone-related protein in adult T-cell leukemia-lymphoma. *Ann Intern Med* 1989;111:484–488.
10. Nagai Y, Yamato H, Akaogi K, et al. Role of interleukin 6 in uncoupling of bone in vivo in a human squamous carcinoma co-producing PTHrP and interleukin 6. *J Bone Miner Res* 1998;13:664–672.
11. Nakayama K, Fukumoto S, Takeda S, et al. Differences in bone and vitamin D metabolism between primary hyperparathyroidism and malignancy-associated hypercalcemia. *J Clin Endocrinol Metab* 1996;81:607–611.
12. Ralston SH, Gallacher SJ, Patel U, Campbell J, Boyle IT. Cancer-associated hypercalcemia: morbidity and mortality: clinical experience in 126 treated patients. *Ann Intern Med* 1990;112:499–504.
13. Skrabanek P, McPartlin J, Powell D. Tumor hypercalcemia and ectopic hyperparathyroidism. *Medicine (Baltimore)* 1980;59:262–282.
14. Stewart AF, Insogna KL, Broadus AE. Malignancy-associated hypercalcemia. In: DeGroot L, ed. *Endocrinology*. 3rd ed. Philadelphia: WB Saunders, 1995:1061–1074.
15. Stewart AF, Vignery A, Silverglate A, et al. Quantitative bone histomorphometry in humoral hypercalcemia of malignancy. *J Clin Endocrinol Metab* 1982;55:219–227.
16. Yamato H, Nagai Y, Inoue D, et al. In vivo evidence for progressive activation of parathyroid hormone-related peptide gene transcription with tumor growth and stimulation of osteoblastic bone formation at an early stage of humoral hypercalcemia of malignancy. *J Bone Miner Res* 1995;10:36–44.

1,25-Dihydroxyvitamin D and Lymphoma

17. Breslau NA, McGuire JL, Zerwekh JE, Frenkel ED, Pak CYC. Hypercalcemia associated with increased serum calcitriol levels in three patients with lymphoma. *Ann Intern Med* 1984;100:1–7.
18. Rosenthal NR, Insogna KL, Godsall JW, Smalldone L, Waldron JA, Stewart AF. Elevations in circulating 1,25(OH)$_2$D in three patients with lymphoma-associated hypercalcemia. *J Clin Endocrinol Metab* 1985;60:29–33.
19. Seymour JF, Gagel RF, Hagemeister FB, Dimopoulos MA, Cabanillas F. Calcitriol production in hypercalcemia and normocalcemia patients with non-Hodgkin lymphoma. *Ann Intern Med* 1994;121:633–640.

Ectopic Parathyroid Hormone Secretion

20. Nussbaum SR, Gaz RD, Arnold A. Hypercalcemia and ectopic secretion of parathyroid hormone by an ovarian carcinoma with rearrangement of the gene for PTH. *N Engl J Med* 1990;323:1324–1328.
21. Iguchi H, Miyagi C, Tomita K, et al. Hypercalcemia caused by ectopic production of parathyroid hormone in a patient with papillary adenocarcinoma of the thyroid gland. *J Clin Endocrinol Metab* 1998;83:2653–2657.

35. Hypercalcemia in Hematologic Malignancies and in Solid Tumors Associated with Extensive Localized Bone Destruction

Gregory R. Mundy, M.D., Toshiyuki Yoneda, Ph.D., D.D.S., and Theresa A. Guise, M.D.

Department of Medicine, Division of Endocrinology and Metabolism, The University of Texas
Health Science Center, San Antonio, Texas

HYPERCALCEMIA AND BONE DESTRUCTION IN MYELOMA

Almost all patients with myeloma have extensive bone destruction. Bone destruction may occur either as discrete local lesions or diffuse involvement throughout the axial skeleton. This increased bone resorption is responsible for a number of disabling features including susceptibility to pathologic fracture, intractable bone pain, and in some patients, hypercalcemia. Approximately 80% of patients with myeloma present with the chief complaint of bone pain. Hypercalcemia occurs in between 20% and 40% of patients at some time during the course of the disease.

The bone destruction that occurs in myeloma is due to an increase in the activity of osteoclasts. Myeloma cells in the marrow cavity produce cytokines that activate adjacent endosteal osteoclasts to resorb bone. This was first recognized by observations on cultured human myeloma cells, which were found to release local factors that stimulate osteoclast activity (1,2). Over the years, the identity of the cytokines responsible for stimulating osteoclasts has been sought but still remains elusive. Established cultures of human myeloma cells produce lymphotoxin (3), and a major portion of bone-resorbing activity produced by these cells in vitro can be accounted for by lymphotoxin. Lymphotoxin is produced normally by activated T lymphocytes. It is a member of the same family of immune cell products as tumor necrosis factor (TNF) and interleukin-1, both of which are produced by cells in the monocyte–macrophage lineage. Lymphotoxin has overlapping biologic properties with those of TNF and binds to the same receptor. TNF is thought to be one of the major mediators of the systemic effects of endotoxic shock. In bone, these cytokines stimulate osteoclast precursors to replicate but also stimulate the differentiation of committed osteoclast precursors into mature cells. In addition to these actions, they act on mature multinucleated cells to cause them to form resorption lacunae (4,5). Lymphotoxin is not the only cytokine implicated in myeloma, however. Other studies show that interleukin-1, interleukin-6, and parathyroid hormone-related protein (PTHrP) also may be involved in the bone destruction in some cases (6–8). Studies showing interleukin-1 production have used freshly isolated collections of myeloma cells (which also contain normal bone marrow mononuclear cells). Myeloma cells are known frequently to produce interleukin-6, but interleukin-6 is not by itself a powerful bone-resorbing factor. PTHrP has been shown to be expressed in myeloma cells in some patients and to be increased in the plasma of some hypercalcemic patients (8). The difficulties in interpreting some of these results is knowing whether the *in vitro* behavior of the myeloma cells is the same as their behavior *in vivo*. As a consequence, we cannot at this time be sure of the cytokine(s) responsible for bone destruction in myeloma.

Although essentially all patients with myeloma develop extensive bone destruction, less than 40% become hypercalcemic. Moreover, there is not a close correlation between the extent of bone destruction and the development of hypercalcemia (9). The explanation is that increased bone resorption is most likely to lead to hypercalcemia in those patients with impaired glomerular filtration. Impairment of glomerular filtration decreases the kidney's capacity to excrete calcium and to clear it from the circulation. Impairment of glomerular filtration is common in patients with myeloma (10) for a number of reasons. Probably the most important is the development of Bence Jones nephropathy, otherwise called "myeloma kidney." In this circumstance, free light chain fragments of immunoglobulin molecules (Bence Jones proteins) are filtered by the glomerulus but impair both glomerular and tubular function. Patients with myeloma also may develop azotemia because of recurrent infections, uric acid nephropathy, and amyloidosis.

Because the mechanisms responsible for hypercalcemia are different in patients with myeloma from patients with other types of malignancy, there are subtle differences in laboratory tests at the time of diagnosis. Because renal function is impaired, many patients with myeloma have increased serum phosphorus rather than a decreased serum phosphorus, which is common with other types of malignancy. In addition, serum alkaline phosphatase, a marker of osteoblast activity, is usually not increased in patients with myeloma because there is little active new bone formation. For similar reasons, bone scans also may be negative. The reason for the decrease in osteoblast activity in patients with myeloma is not known.

Treatment of myeloma patients with hypercalcemia may be difficult because of the impairment in glomerular filtration. Nephrotoxic agents should be avoided if possible. For example, plicamycin (also called mithramycin) is not an ideal therapeutic agent for hypercalcemia in myeloma because it is directly nephrotoxic and is dependent on the kidneys for its elimination. As a consequence, its use will often be associated with toxicity. Parenteral pamidronate (a bisphosphonate) and gallium nitrate are both extremely effective in this situation, although there is more experience with pamidronate. Pamidronate can be expected to reverse hypercalcemia in essentially all patients with myeloma. However, caution should be used with these agents in patients with severely impaired renal function. Hypercalcemia in many patients with myeloma responds well to treatment of the primary disease with alkylating agents and corticosteroids (11). Corticosteroids themselves are more frequently useful in the treatment of hypercalcemia in myeloma than they are in other malignancies. The combination of calcitonin and corticosteroids is usually effective in myeloma and may be useful particularly in those cases in which glomerular filtration is impaired or other antihypercalcemic drugs are contraindicated, because neither agent is nephrotoxic. It is generally not advisable to treat an osteopenic patient with corticosteroids, although in myeloma, the prognosis for the patient is usually so poor once hypercalcemia has developed that the objectives of therapy are usually to keep the patient symptom free from hypercalcemia in the remaining months left to live, and corticosteroids may be very effective in this regard.

For a number of years, clinicians have attempted to devise therapeutic approaches in myeloma that would relieve those disabling symptoms due to skeletal destruction and bone fragility. This was first attempted with the use of fluoride and later calcium and fluoride, although this combination was ineffective and, in fact, potentially detrimental because of the associated side effects. More recently, several groups showed that the newer generation bisphosphonates will relieve bone pain and produce a rapid, sustained, and significant decrease in the urinary excretion of calcium and hydroxyproline, indicating decreased bone turnover (12,13). This was shown first with pamidronate (12) and then with clodronate (13). Pamidronate was recently approved by the Food and Drug Administration (FDA) for this use in myeloma patients without hypercalcemia. A large study by Berenson et al. (14) showed that in several hundred patients with myeloma, there was a satisfactory response in bone pain, reduced need for radiation therapy, and prevention of fractures. The skeleton-related events associated with myeloma were reduced by approximately 50%. This study confirmed other large studies in Europe and is consistent with the results of the VIth MRC myeloma trial, in which clodronate was the bisphosphonate used (15). Outstanding residual questions include which is the best bisphosphonate for this purpose, what is the ideal dose, for how long should it be administered, should it be given to patients early in the course of the disease, and most important, do these drugs have a beneficial effect on survival. Active research in this area is likely soon to lead to the introduction of other suitable and nontoxic agents of this class that will be useful as oral forms of therapy to relieve the symptoms caused by bone destruction and its complications in patients with myeloma.

It is controversial whether bisphosphonates have any direct effects on myeloma cells, which influence tumor burden. Although there have been suggestions that there may be some improvement in survival for patients with advanced disease treated with the bisphosphonates (14), this has not been confirmed. In animal models of myeloma bone disease, bisphosphonates had no effect on tumor burden. In spite of this, there is *in vitro* and *in vivo* evidence that bisphosphonates may affect rates of apoptosis in myeloma cells, suggesting that it is possible they could have beneficial effects on survival by decreasing tumor burden (16). New generations of bisphosphonates are being developed by a number of pharmaceutical companies, and their use is certain to become even more widespread during the next 5 years. As this happens, knowledge also may increase on the extent of the benefits to patients with these advanced malignancies and the role of bisphosphonates as an adjuvant therapy in patients with osteolytic bone disease.

There are other important issues in the management of myeloma bone disease. This crippling form of bone disease is associated with the most severe and intractable bone pain, as well as frequent fractures after trivial injury. When the bone pain is localized to specific areas such as in the vertebral spine or the ribs, a course of local radiation therapy may be very effective. Analgesics should be used liberally for the severe pain. Patients require frequent counseling because of the bone pain, deformity, and loss of height associated with progressive myeloma bone disease and will in general manage their symptoms best when they understand the nature of the bone disease and those activities that are hazardous. Similar principles that guide the lifestyles of patients with osteoporosis also apply to myeloma bone disease. For example, patients should avoid those situations that put them at risk for fractures, such as climbing ladders, slipping on ice, or tripping on loose bathroom rugs.

HYPERCALCEMIA ASSOCIATED WITH LYMPHOMAS

Occasional patients with various lymphomas develop hypercalcemia (17). This can occur in Hodgkin's disease, in B-cell lymphomas, in T-cell lymphomas, and in Burkitt's lymphoma. In T-cell lymphomas, it is frequently associated with the human T-cell lymphotrophic virus-type I (HTLV-I). This is a recently described oncogenic type C retrovirus that is related to the acquired immunodeficiency syndrome virus, infects certain T cells, and results in a lymphoproliferative T-cell disorder (18). The cause of hypercalcemia and bone destruction in these lymphomas has been well characterized. In most cases, it is probably due to a bone-resorbing factor produced by the neoplastic lymphoid cells. In Japan, where hypercalcemia associated with human T-cell lymphoma virus (HTLV)-lymphoproliferative disorders is common, serum 1,25-dihydroxyvitamin D [1,25 $(OH)_2$ D] is not increased, but production of the PTHrP by neoplastic cells was clearly demonstrated (19). In a few patients, hypercalcemia may be due, at least in part, to increased 1,25 $(OH)_2$ D production by the lymphoid cells. Several patients with different types of lymphoma and hypercalcemia have been found to have increased serum 1,25 $(OH)_2$ D concentrations (20). When measured, this has been associated with increased absorption of calcium from the intestine. Lymphoid cells transformed by inoculation with HTLV-I virus develop the capacity to synthesize 1,25 $(OH)_2$ D (21). However, there has been controversy about the relative frequency of increased serum 1,25 $(OH)_2$ D in patients with hypercalcemia associated with lymphoproliferative disorders. One group in California reported that half of their patients have increased serum 1,25 $(OH)_2$ D concentrations (22).

Hypercalcemia also occurs occasionally in other hematologic malignancies such as chronic lymphocytic leukemia, acute leukemia, and chronic myelogenous leukemia, particularly during acute blast transformation. However, the association of hypercalcemia with these disorders is unusual enough that these patients should be carefully evaluated for another cause of hypercalcemia. In most patients, if another cause is present, this other cause will be primary hyperparathyroidism.

HYPERCALCEMIA IN SOLID TUMORS ASSOCIATED WITH EXTENSIVE LOCALIZED BONE DESTRUCTION

Solid tumors frequently spread to involve the skeleton, and when they do so, the bone lesions are usually destructive (osteolytic) (23). Approximately one third to one half of all tumors spread to bone. Bone is the third most common site of metastasis of solid tumors after the liver and the lung. However, there is a distinct pattern of tumor cell metastasis to bone. Common tumors such as lung, breast, and prostate cancer frequently metastasize to bone, and bone metastases are present in nearly all patients with advanced breast or prostate cancer. Therefore bone metastasis is a very important clinical problem.

There are two distinct types of tumor metastases, osteoblastic metastases and osteolytic metastases. Osteolytic metastases are much more common and more significant as a clinical problem. Lytic metastases are usually destructive and are much more likely to be associated with pathologic fracture and hypercalcemia.

Osteolytic bone metastasis is one of the most feared complications of malignancy. The consequences for the patient include intractable bone pain at the site of the metastasis, pathologic fracture after trivial injury, nerve compression syndromes due to obstruction of foramina (the most serious example is spinal cord compression), and hypercalcemia, when bone destruction is advanced. Once tumor cells are housed in the skeleton, curative therapy is no longer possible in most patients, and only palliative therapy is available.

Tumor cells metastasize most frequently to the axial skeleton, and particularly the vertebrae, pelvis, proximal ends of the long bones, and skull. It is clear that there are important properties of both the tumor cell (the seed) and the skeleton (the soil) that determine the likelihood that any particular tumor will metastasize to bone. These properties are only now being identified, with the goal that understanding what they are and how they affect tumor growth should lead to more effective treatments for metastatic cancer.

Because hypercalcemia of breast cancer is associated with extensive bone metastasis in the majority of patients, under-standing the mechanism for tumor cell migration to bone and subsequent bone destruction also should clarify the mechanisms by which breast cancer cells cause hypercalcemia. Tumor cells spread to bone after being shed from the primary tumor. Release from the primary site is probably associated with the production of proteolytic enzymes by the cancer cells, which causes the cells to detach one from another. Once tumor cells enter the circulation, they traverse vascular organs including the red bone marrow. Within the bone marrow cavity, they migrate through wide-channeled sinusoids to the endosteal bone surface.

The migration of tumor cells from the bloodstream to the endosteal surfaces of bone involves a number of distinct steps (24) (Fig. 1). These steps include (a) attachment to the basement membrane, probably via the basement membrane glycoprotein laminin and laminin receptors on the tumor cell surface; (b) production of proteolytic enzymes (including matrix metalloproteinases) by tumor cells, which disrupt the basement membrane and allow tumor cells access to the organ stroma; (c) directed migration of tumor cells via chemotactic processes through the basement membrane; and (d) production of mediators that activate osteoclasts at the bone surface. These processes are now being unraveled by both *in vitro* and *in vivo* techniques. Some facts have become apparent. For example, it was recently shown that (a) laminin receptors on tumor cells are important for metastasis to form, and antagonists of laminin may block the metastatic process to bone (25); (b) metastatic tumor cells in the bone microenvironment show properties different from the same tumor cells at the primary site (for example, they may produce PTHrP in bone but not at the primary site); (c) it is likely that the bone-derived factors stored in bone and released locally when bone is resorbed may alter function of tumor cells in the bone microenvironment; (d) tumor cells can be stimulated to migrate unidirectionally in response to the products of resorbing bone cultures (26), as well as to fragments of type-1 collagen (27), which is the most abundant protein in the bone matrix (possibly breast cancer cells are attracted by these mechanisms to sites of relatively active bone turnover, where they form a nidus that eventually becomes an osteolytic deposit); and (e) inhibitors of osteoclas-

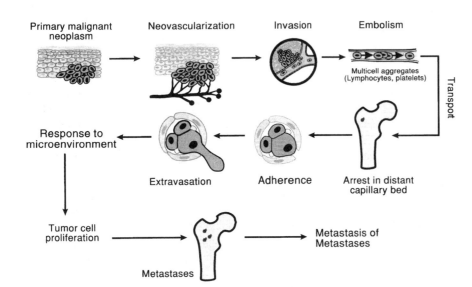

FIG. 1. Multiple steps involved in tumor migration from primary site in breast to bone. Each of these steps involves specific interactions between tumor cells and host cells and represents a potential target for drugs that may inhibit the process.

tic bone resorption can not only inhibit skeletal complications of cancer, but also impair tumor growth at the metastatic site (28).

Recently it has become apparent that the tumor peptide PTHrP has special importance in breast cancer that metastasizes to bone. PTHrP is produced in excessive amounts, particularly in patients with metastatic breast cancer, but produced relatively specifically in the bone microenvironment (29,30). This production of PTHrP in the bone microenvironment is due to bone-derived transforming growth factor β (TGF$_\beta$), which is released in active form as a consequence of bone resorption. Thus the sequence of events is that bone destruction caused by the presence of the tumor leads to the production of active TGF$_\beta$, which in turn interacts with the tumor cells to enhance the production of PTHrP. A vicious cycle is set up in which tumor cell production of PTHrP leads to production by bone of more TGF$_\beta$, which in turn leads to more PTHrP. This vicious cycle can be interrupted either by neutralizing PTHrP effects or by making tumor cells less susceptible to TGF$_\beta$.

It is likely that this TGF$_\beta$/PTHrP relation is not the only growth factor/osteotropic agent interaction that is important in the bone marrow microenvironment. For example, insulin-like growth factor and the fibroblast growth factor family also may be important in stimulating proliferation of tumor cells at the metastatic site.

TREATMENT OF OSTEOLYTIC BONE DISEASE

Because bone metastasis is such an important complication of the most common tumors that affect humans, lung cancer and breast cancer, understanding the cellular events involved and devising therapeutic strategies to prevent new metastasis and inhibit continued growth of established metastases is a very important therapeutic goal for cancer management.

There has been a tremendous upsurge of interest in the role of the bisphosphonates in the management of patients with osteolytic bone disease during the last 5 years. It has been known that these compounds are effective in disorders associated with increased osteoclastic bone resorption for over 25 years. However, their role in patients with malignant disease but without hypercalcemia was not widely accepted in the United States until the last several years, during which time they have been approved by the FDA for treatment in osteolytic bone disease due to myeloma (1995) and in osteolytic bone disease due to breast cancer (1996). They are now widely used in patients with myeloma and even extensively used in patients with advanced breast cancer. They decrease the skeleton-related events associated with malignancies by approximately one half (14,31). Data on experimental models of breast cancer metastasis to bone indicate that in addition to decreasing osteolytic lesions, they also decrease tumor burden in bone (28). There are not as yet such comparable data in humans, although there are some preliminary data that bisphosphonates may reduce tumor burden in bone and possibly other sites when used as adjuvant therapy with other agents (32). This is also seen in the animal models of breast cancer metastasis. However, when it is used alone and without other therapy, the tumor burden in soft-tissue sites may actually increase (33).

The principles of treatment of hypercalcemic patients with metastatic bone disease and hypercalcemia are the same as those for other patients with hypercalcemia of malignancy (34).

REFERENCES

1. Mundy GR, Raisz LG, Cooper RA, Schechter GP, Salmon SE. Evidence for the secretion of an osteoclast stimulating factor in myeloma. *N Engl J Med* 1974;291:1041–1046.
2. Mundy GR, Bertolini DB. Bone destruction and hypercalcemia in plasma cell myeloma. *Semin Oncol* 1986;13:291–299.
3. Garrett IR, Durie BGM, Nedwin GE, et al. Production of the bone resorbing cytokine lymphotoxin by cultured human myeloma cells. *N Engl J Med* 1987;317:526–532.
4. Thomson BM, Saklatvala J, Chambers TJ. Osteoblasts mediate interleukin-1 stimulation of bone resorption by rat osteoclasts. *J Exp Med* 1986;164:104–112.
5. Thomson BM, Mundy GR, Chambers TJ. Tumor necrosis factors alpha and beta induce osteoblastic cells to stimulate osteoclastic bone resorption. *J Immunol* 1987;138:775–779.
6. Bataille R, Jourdan M, Zhang Xue-Guang, Klein B. Serum levels of interleukin-6, a potent myeloma cell growth factor, as a reflection of disease severity in plasma cell dyscrasias. *J Clin Invest* 1989;84:2008–2011.
7. Cozzolino F, Torcia M, Aldinucci D, et al. Production of interleukin-1 by bone marrow myeloma cells. *Blood* 1989;74:387–390.
8. Firkin F, Seymour JF, Watson AM, Grill V, Martin TJ. Parathyroid hormone-related protein in hypercalcemia associated with haematological malignancy. *Br J Haematol* 1996;94:486–492.
9. Durie BGM, Salmon SE, Mundy GR. Relation of osteoclast activating factor production to the extent of bone disease in multiple myeloma. *Br J Haematol* 1981;47:21–30.
10. Harinck HIJ, Bijvoet OLM, Plantingh AST. Role of bone and kidney in tumor-induced hypercalcemia and its treatment with bisphosphonate and sodium chloride. *Am J Med* 1987;82:1113–1142.
11. Binstock ML, Mundy GR. Effects of calcitonin and glucocorticoids in combination with hypercalcemia of malignancy. *Ann Intern Med* 1980;93:269–272.
12. Van Breukelen FJM, Bijvoet OLM, Van Oosterom AT. Inhibition of osteolytic bone lesions by (3-amino-1-hydroxypropylidene)-1,1-bisphosphonate (A.P.D.). *Lancet* 1979;1:803–805.
13. Siris ES, Sherman WH, Baquiran DC, Schlatterer JP, Osserman EF, Canfield RE. Effects of dichloromethylene diphosphonate on skeletal mobilization of calcium in multiple myeloma. *N Engl J Med* 1980;302:310–315.
14. Berenson JR, Lichtenstein A, Porter L, et al. Efficacy of pamidronate in reducing skeletal events in patients with advanced multiple myeloma. *N Engl J Med* 1996;334:488–493.
15. McCloskey EV, MacLennan IC, Drayson MT, Chapman C, Dunn J, Kanis JA. A randomized trial of the effect of clodronate on skeletal morbidity in multiple myeloma. *Br J Haematol* 1998;100:317–325.
16. Shipman CM, Rogers MJ, Apperley JF, Russell RGG, Croucher PI. Bisphosphonates induce apoptosis in human myeloma cell lines: a novel anti-tumour activity. *Br J Haematol* 1997;98:665–672.
17. Canellos GP. Hypercalcemia in malignant lymphoma and leukemia. *Ann N Y Acad Sci* 1974;230:240–246.
18. Bunn PA, Schechter GP, Jaffe E, et al. Clinical course of retrovirus-associated adult T-cell lymphoma in the United States. *N Engl J Med* 1983;309:247–264.
19. Motokura T, Fukumoto S, Matsumoto T, et al. Parathyroid hormone related protein in adult T-cell leukemia-lymphoma. *Ann Intern Med* 1989;111:484–488.
20. Breslau NA, McGuire JL, Zerwekh JE, Frenkel EP, Pak CYC. Hypercalcemia associated with increased serum calcitriol levels in three patients with lymphoma. *Ann Intern Med* 1984;100:107.
21. Fetchick DA, Bertolini DR, Sarin PS, Weintraub ST, Mundy GR, Dunn JD. Production of 1,25 dihydroxyvitamin D by human T-cell lymphotrophic virus-I transformed lymphocytes. *J Clin Invest* 1986;78:592–596.
22. Adams JS, Fernandez M, Gacad MA, et al. Vitamin D metabolite-

mediated hypercalcemia and hypercalciuria in patients with AIDS- and non-AIDS-associated lymphoma. *Blood* 1989;73:235–239.

23. Mundy GR, Martin TJ. Pathophysiology of skeletal complications of cancer. In: Mundy GR, Martin TJ, eds. *Physiology and pharmacology of bone: handbook of experimental pharmacology*. Springer, 1993:641–671.

24. Liotta LA. Tumor invasion: role of the extracellular matrix. *Cancer Res* 1986;46:1–7.

25. Nakai M, Mundy GR, Williams PJ, Boyce B, Yoneda T. A synthetic antagonist to laminin inhibits the formation of osteolytic metastases by human melanoma cells in nude mice. *Cancer Res* 1992;52:5395–5399.

26. Orr W, Varani J, Gondek MD, Ward PA, Mundy GR. Chemotactic responses of tumor cells to products of resorbing bone. *Science* 1972;203:176–179.

27. Mundy GR, DeMartino S, Rowe DW. Collagen and collagen fragments are chemotactic for tumor cells. *J Clin Invest* 1981;68:1102–1105.

28. Sasaki A, Boyce BF, Story B, et al. The bisphosphonate risedronate reduces metastatic human breast cancer burden in bone in nude mice. *Cancer Res* 1995;55:3551–3557.

29. Powell GJ, Southby J, Danks JA, et al. Localization of parathyroid hormone-related protein in breast cancer metastases: increased incidence in bone compared with other sites. *Cancer Res* 1991;51:3059–3061.

30. Guise TA, Yin JJ, Taylor SD, et al. Evidence for a causal role of parathyroid hormone-related protein in the pathogenesis of human breast cancer-mediated osteolysis. *J Clin Invest* 1996;98:1544–1549.

31. Hortobagyi GN, Theriault RL, Porter L, et al. Efficacy of pamidronate in reducing skeletal complications in patients with breast cancer and lytic bone metastases. *N Engl J Med* 1996;335:1785–1791.

32. Diel LJ, Solgmayer EF, Goerner R. Adjuvant treatment of breast cancer patients with the bisphosphonate clodronate reduces incidence and number of bone and non-bone metastases. *Proc Am Soc Clin Oncol* 1997;16:461.

33. Michigami T, Dallas SL, Mundy GR, Yoneda T. Interactions of myeloma cells with bone marrow stromal cells via $\alpha_4\beta_1$ integrin-VCAM-1 is required for the development of osteolysis. *J Bone Miner Res* 1997;12(suppl):104.

34. Mundy GR, Martin TJ. The hypercalcemia of malignancy: pathogenesis and treatment. *Metabolism* 1982;31:1247–1277.

36. Hypercalcemia Due to Granuloma-Forming Disorders

John S. Adams, M.D.

Department of Medicine, University of California, Los Angeles School of Medicine, and Division of Endocrinology and Metabolism, Burns and Allen Research Institute, Cedars-Sinai Medical Center, Los Angeles, California

PATHOGENESIS

The association of dysregulated calcium homeostasis and granuloma-forming disease was established in 1939 by the work of Harrell and Fisher (1). With the advent of automated serum chemistry testing, more recent studies indicate that mild to severe hypercalcemia is detected in 10% of patients with sarcoidosis, and up to 50% of patients will become hypercalciuric at some time during the course of their disease (2). Vitamin D was implicated in the pathogenesis of abnormal calcium metabolism after it was appreciated that patients with sarcoidosis who had hypercalcemia or hypercalciuria (or both) absorbed high amounts of dietary calcium, and that normocalcemic patients were prone to hypercalcemia after receiving small amounts of vitamin D or ultraviolet light (3). It has been proposed that bone resorption is also an important contributor to the pathogenesis of hypercalciuria and hypercalcemia (4), based on the observations that a diet low in calcium seldom induces a normocalcemic state in sarcoidosis patients with moderate to severe hypercalcemia, and that urinary calcium excretion often exceeds dietary calcium intake. Recent studies (5) demonstrated that generalized, accelerated trabecular bone loss occurs in patients with sarcoidosis before institution of steroid therapy. Rizzato et al. (5) showed that (a) bone mass was significantly decreased in patients with active sarcoidosis, (b) bone loss was most marked in patients with hypercalcemia and/or hypercalciuria, and (c) bone loss was most prominent in postmenopausal women with long-standing disease.

For many years, these and similar clinical observations suggested that hypercalcemia and/or hypercalciuria in patients with sarcoidosis resulted from a heightened sensitivity to the biologic effects of vitamin D. However, the discovery that a high proportion of these patients had elevated circulating concentrations of 1,25-dihydroxyvitamin D [1,25 (OH)$_2$ D] indicated that the endogenous overproduction of an active vitamin D metabolite was the etiology of disordered calcium regulation in this disease. More recently, high serum 1,25 (OH)$_2$ D concentrations were reported in hypercalcemic pa-

TABLE 1. *Human disease associated with 1,25-dihydroxy-vitamin-D–mediated hypercalcemia/hypercalciuria*

Granuloma-forming diseases	
Noninfectious	
Sarcoidosis	Adams et al. (6)
Silicone-induced granulomatosis	Kozeny et al. (7)
Paraffin-induced granulomatosis	Albitar et al. (8)
Berylliosis	Stoeckle (9)
Wegener's	Edelson (10)
Eosinophilic granuloma	Jurney (11)
Infantile fat necrosis	Cook (12)
Infectious	
Tuberculosis	Gkonos (13)
Candidiasis	Kantarijian (14)
Leprosy	Hoffman (15)
Histoplasmosis	Walker (16)
Coccidiodmycosis	Parker (17)
Cat-scratch disease	Bosch (18)
Malignant lymphoproliferative disease	
B-cell lymphoma	Adams et al. (19)
Hodgkin's disease	Seymor and Gagel (20)
Lymphomatoid granulomatosis	Schienman et al. (21)

tients with other granuloma-forming diseases and in patients harboring lymphoproliferative neoplasms (Table 1); in all of these disorders, there is a presumed extrarenal source for the hormone.

Four major lines of clinical evidence suggest that the endogenous extrarenal synthesis of 1,25 (OH)₂ D in some hypercalcemic/hypercalciuric patients with granulomatous disease and lymphoma is not subject to normal, physiologic regulatory influences (22–24). First, hypercalcemic patients possess a frankly high or inappropriately elevated serum 1,25 (OH)₂ D concentration, although their serum immunoreactive parathyroid hormone levels are suppressed and serum phosphorus concentrations are relatively elevated. If 1,25 (OH)₂ D synthesis were under the trophic control of parathyroid hormone and phosphorus, then 1,25 (OH)₂ D concentrations should be low. Second, unlike in normal individuals, whose serum 1,25 (OH)₂ D concentrations are not influenced by small to moderate increments of circulating 25-hydroxyvitamin D [25 (OH) D] concentrations, the serum 1,25 (OH)₂ D concentration in patients with active sarcoidosis is exquisitely sensitive to an increase in the availability of substrate. Third, serum calcium and 1,25 (OH)₂ D concentrations are positively correlated to indices of disease activity; patients with sarcoidosis who have widespread disease and high serum angiotensin-converting enzyme activity are more likely to be hypercalciuric or frankly hypercalcemic. And fourth, the rate of endogenous 1,25 (OH)₂ D production, which is significantly increased in patients with sarcoidosis, is unusually sensitive to inhibition by factors (e.g., glucocorticoids) that do not influence the renal 1-hydroxylase.

CELLULAR SOURCE OF ACTIVE VITAMIN D METABOLITES

The experiments of Barbour et al. (25) proved the source of 1,25 (OH)₂ D to be extrarenal in sarcoidosis. These investigators described an anephric patient with sarcoidosis, hypercalcemia, and a high serum 1,25 (OH)₂ D concentration. The elevated 1,25 (OH)₂ D concentration in patients with sarcoidosis is now known to result from increased production of 1,25 (OH)₂ D by the macrophage (6), a prominent constituent of the sarcoid granuloma. Synthesis of 1,25 (OH)₂ D₃ in lymphoma is likely the result of overproduction of hormone by the tumor cell.

Although similar to the authentic renal 25 (OH) D-1-hydroxylase in terms of kinetics and substrate specificity (26), factors that exert a regulatory influence on the synthetic reaction in the kidney vary considerably from those that influence the sarcoid macrophage. The sarcoid macrophage 1-hydroxylation reaction is immune to the stimulatory effects of parathyroid hormone, but it is very sensitive to stimulation by interferon-γ (IFN-γ) (26), a lymphokine produced by activated lymphocytes, and to stimulation by modulators of this lymphokine's postreceptor signal-transduction pathway, including nitric oxide (27). The macrophage hydroxylation reaction is very sensitive to inhibition by glucocorticoid (26), chloroquine, and related analogues (28), and the cytochrome P-450 inhibitor ketoconazole (29), but it is refractory to inhibition by 1,25 (OH)₂ D (26). The renal enzyme, on the other hand, is relatively insensitive to inhibi-

tion by glucocorticoids and is downregulated by 1,25 (OH)₂ D. These differences in regulated expression of the hydroxylation reaction in the kidney and macrophage may not result from expression of two different genes but from differential regulation of the vitamin D-1-hydroxylase gene in the two cell types (30). The 1-hydroxylase gene in the kidney (31) is regulated at the level of transcription. In contrast, it is likely that the macrophage 1-hydroxylase gene is constitutively expressed with hormone production controlled by the flow of substrate (32) and electrons (28) to the cytochrome P-450.

IMMUNOACTIVITY OF 1,25-DIHYDROXYVITAMIN D

1,25-Dihydroxyvitamin D is known to exert a potent immunoinhibitory effect on activated human lymphocytes *in vitro*. These actions include inhibition of lymphocyte proliferation, lymphokine production, and immunoglobulin synthesis (33). It was suggested (34) that 1,25 (OH)₂ D produced by the macrophage in granulomatous diseases exerts a paracrine immunoinhibitory effect on neighboring, activated lymphocytes that express receptors for the hormone, and that this acts to slow an otherwise "overzealous" immune response that may be detrimental to the host. Despite the theoretic attractiveness of this model, few data support a role for 1,25 (OH)₂ D as a paracrine immunoinhibitor *in vivo* (35).

TREATMENT OF HYPERCALCEMIA/ HYPERCALCIURIA

The most important factor in the successful management of disordered vitamin D metabolism of sarcoidosis is recognition of patients at risk. Those at risk include patients with (a) indices of active, widespread disease (i.e., elevated serum angiotensin-converting enzyme levels, diffuse infiltrative pulmonary disease); (b) preexistent hypercalciuria; (c) a previous history of hypercalcemia or hypercalciuria; (d) a diet enriched in vitamin D and calcium; and (e) a recent history of sunlight exposure or treatment with vitamin D. All patients with active sarcoidosis should be screened for hypercalciuria. In a timed, fasting urine collection, a fractional urinary calcium excretion rate exceeding 0.16 mg calcium per 100 mL glomerular filtrate is considered hypercalciuria. If the fractional urinary calcium excretion rate is elevated, serum 25 (OH) D and 1,25 (OH)₂ D concentrations should be determined as a disease marker and to judge the efficacy of therapy. Because hypercalciuria frequently precedes the development of overt hypercalcemia, the occurrence of either is an indication for therapy.

Glucocorticoids (40 to 60 mg prednisone or equivalent, daily) are the mainstay of therapy of disordered calcium homeostasis resulting from the endogenous overproduction of active vitamin D metabolites. Institution of glucocorticoid therapy results in a prompt decrease in the circulating 1,25 (OH)₂ D concentration (within 3 days), presumably by inhibition of the macrophage hydroxylation reaction. Normalization of the serum or urine calcium usually occurs within a matter of days (23). Failure to normalize the serum calcium after 10 days of therapy suggests the coexistence of another hypercalcemic process (e.g., hyperparathyroidism or humoral hypercalcemia of malignancy). Obviously the dietary intake of calcium and vitamin D should be limited in such patients, as should sunlight (UV light) exposure. After a hypercalcemic episode, urinary calcium excretion rates should be monitored intermittently to detect recurrence. Glucocorticoids also appear to be effective in the management of vitamin D–mediated hypercalcemia or hypercalciuria in other granuloma-forming diseases and lymphoma. Chloroquine (28,35) or hydroxychloroquine (36) and ketoconazole (29) are also capable of reducing the serum $1,25 (OH)_2$ D and calcium concentration in patients with sarcoidosis, but chloroquine and its analogues are not effective in lymphoma patients (36); this differential responsiveness likely results from the failure of chloroquine to act in lymphoma cells as it does in macrophages. Because of the limited experience with these drugs as antihypercalcemic agents, they should be limited to patients in whom steroid therapy is unsuccessful or contraindicated. The theoretic advantage of these agents over glucocorticoids is that correction of the serum $1,25 (OH)_2$ D concentration should result in rapid recovery of at least some of the bone mineral density lost to the disease (37). The utility of the newer bisphosphonates in blocking bone resorption in hypercalcemic/hypercalciuric patients with sarcoidosis is still unknown.

REFERENCES

1. Harrell GT, Fisher S. Blood chemical changes in Boeck's sarcoid with particular reference to protein, calcium and phosphatase values. *J Clin Invest* 1939;18:687–693.
2. Studdy PR, Bird R, Neville E, James DG. Biochemical findings in sarcoidosis. *J Clin Pathol* 1980;33:528–533.
3. Bell NH, Gill JR Jr, Bartter FC. On the abnormal calcium absorption in sarcoidosis: evidence for increased sensitivity to vitamin D. *Am J Med* 1964;36:500–513.
4. Fallon MD, Perry HM III, Teitelbaum SL. Skeletal sarcoidosis with osteopenia. *Metab Bone Dis Res* 1981;3:171–174.
5. Rizzato G, Montemurro L, Fraioli P. Bone mineral content in sarcoidosis. *Semin Resp Med* 1992;13:411–423.
6. Adams JS, Singer FR, Gacad MA, et al. Isolation and structural identification of 1,25-dihydroxyvitamin D3 produced by cultured alveolar macrophages in sarcoidosis. *J Clin Endocrinol Metab* 1985;60:960–966.
7. Kozeny GA, Barbato AL, Bansal VK, Vertuno LL, Hano JE. Hypercalcemia associated with silicone-induced granulomas. *N Engl J Med* 1984;311:1103–1105.
8. Albitar S, Genin R, Fen-Chong M, et al. Multisystem granulomatous injuries 28 years after paraffin injections. *Nephrol Dial Transplant* 1997;12:1974–1976.
9. Stoeckle JD, Hardy HL, Weber AL. Chronic beryllium disease: long-term follow-up of sixty cases and selective review of the literature. *AM J Med* 1969;46:545–561.
10. Edelson GW, Talpos GB, Bone HG III. Hypercalcemia associated with Wegener's granulomatosis and hyperparathyroidism: etiology and management. *Am J Nephrol* 1993;13:275–277.
11. Jurney TH. Hypercalcemia in a patient with eosinophilic granuloma. *AM J Med* 1984;76:527–528.
12. Cook JS, Stone MS, Hansen JR. Hypercalcemia in association with subcutaneous fat necrosis of the newborn: studies of calcium regulating hormones. *Pediatrics* 1992;90:93–96.
13. Gkonos PJ, London R, Hendler ED. Hypercalcemia and elevated 1,25-dihydroxyvitamin D levels in a patient with end stage renal disease and active tuberculosis. *N Engl J Med* 1984;311:1683–1685.
14. Kantarijian HM, Saad MF, Estey EH, Sellin RV, Samaan NA. Hypercalcemia in disseminated candidiasis. *Am J Med* 1983;74:721–724.
15. Hoffman VH, Korzeniowski OM. Leprosy, hypercalcemia, and elevated serum calcitriol levels. *Ann Intern Med* 1986;105:890–891.
16. Walker JV, Baran D, Yakub YN, Freeman RB. Histoplasmosis with hypercalcemia, renal failure, and papillary necrosis: confusion with sarcoidosis. *JAMA* 1977;237:1350–1352.
17. Parker MS, Dokoh S, Woolfenden JM, Buchsbaum HW. Hypercalcemia in coccidioidomycosis. *Am J Med* 1984;76:341–343.
18. Bosch X. Hypercalcemia due to endogenous overproduction of active vitamin D in identical twins with cat-scratch disease. *JAMA* 1998;279:532–534.
19. Adams JS, Fernandez M, Gacad MA, et al. Vitamin D metabolite mediated hypercalcemia and hypercalciuria patients with AIDS and non-AIDS-associated lymphoma. *Blood* 1989;73:235–239.
20. Seymour JF, Gagel RF. Calcitriol: the major humoral mediator of hypercalcemia in Hodgkin's disease and non-Hodgkin's lymphomas. *Blood* 1993;82:1383–1394.
21. Schienman SJ, Kelberman MW, Tatum AH, Zamkoff KW. Hypercalcemia with excess serum 1,25-dihydroxyvitamin D in lymphomatoid granulomatosis/angiocentric lymphoma. *Am J Med Sci* 1991; 301:178–181.
22. Sandler LM, Wineals CG, Fraher LJ, Clemens TL, Smith R, O'Riordan JLH. Studies of the hypercalcaemia of sarcoidosis: effects of steroids and exogenous vitamin D3 on the circulating concentration of 1,25-dihydroxyvitamin D3. *Q J Med* 1984;53:165–180.
23. Meyrier A, Valeyre D, Bouillon R, Paillard F, Battesti JP, Georges R. Resorptive versus absorptive hypercalciuria: correlations with 25-hydroxyvitamin D3 and 1,25-dihydroxyvitamin D3 and parameters of disease activity. *Q J Med* 1985;54:269–281.
24. Insogna KL, Dreyer BE, Mitnick M, Ellison AF, Broadus AE. Enhanced production rate of 1,25-dihydroxyvitamin D in sarcoidosis. *J Clin Endocrinol Metab* 1988;66:72–75.
25. Barbour GL, Coburn JW, Slatopolsky E, Norman AW, Horst RL. Hypercalcemia in an anephric patient with sarcoidosis: evidence for extrarenal generation of 1,25-dihydroxyvitamin D. *N Engl J Med* 1981;305:440–443.
26. Adams JS, Gacad MA. Characterization of 1 hydroxylation of vitamin D3 sterols by cultured alveolar macrophages from patients with sarcoidosis. *J Exp Med* 1985;161:755–765.
27. Adams JS, Ren SY, Arbelle JE, Clemens TL, Shany S. A role for nitric oxide in the regulated expression of the 25 hydroxyvitamin D-1-hydroxylation reaction in the chick myelomonocytic cell line HD-11. *Endocrinology* 1994;134:499–502.
28. Adams JS, Diz MM, Sharma OP. Effective reduction in the serum 1,25-dihydroxyvitamin D and calcium concentration in sarcoidosis-associated hypercalcemia with short-course chloroquine therapy. *Ann Intern Med* 1989;111:437–438.
29. Adams JS, Sharma OP, Diz MM, Endres DB. Ketoconazole decreases the serum 1,25-dihydroxyvitamin D and calcium concentration in sarcoidosis-associated hypercalcemia. *J Clin Endocrinol Metab* 1990; 70:1090–1095.
30. St-Arnaud R, Messerlian S, Moir JM, Omdahl JL, Glorieux FH. The 25-hydroxyvitamin D 1-alpha-hydroxylase gene maps to the pseudovitamin D-deficiency rickets (PDDR) diseases locus. *J Bone Min Res* 1997;12:1552–1559.
31. Gacad MA, Chen H, Arbelle JE, LeBon T, Adams JS. Functional characterization and purification of an intracellular vitamin D-binding protein in vitamin D-resistant New World primate cells. *J Biol Chem* 1997;272:8433–8440.
32. Rigby WFC. The immunobiology of vitamin D. *Immunol Today* 1988;9:54–58.
33. Adams JS. Hypercalcemia and hypercalciuria. *Semin Respir Med* 1992;13:402–410.
34. Barnes PF, Modlin RL, Bickle DD, Adams JS. Transpleural gradient of 1,25-dihydroxyvitamin D in tuberculous pleuritis. *J Clin Invest* 1989;83:1527–1532.
35. O'Leary TJ, Jones G, Yip A, et al. The effects of chloroquine on serum 1,25-dihydroxyvitamin D and calcium metabolism in sarcoidosis. *N Engl J Med* 1986;315:727–730.
36. Adams JS, Kantorovich V. Inability of short-term, low-dose hydroxychloroquine to resolve vitamin D-mediated hypercalcemia in patients with B-cell lymphoma. *J Clin Endocrinol Metab* 1999;84:799–801.
37. Adams JS, Lee G. Recovery of bone mineral density with resolution of exogenous vitamin D intoxication. *Ann Intern Med* 1997;127:203–206.

37. Miscellaneous Causes of Hypercalcemia

Andrew F. Stewart, M.D.

Department of Medicine, University of Pittsburgh School of Medicine and Division of Endocrinology,
University of Pittsburgh Medical Center, Pittsburgh, Pennsylvania

Hypercalcemia resulting from parathyroid disorders, from cancer, and from granulomatous disorders compose the majority of cases of hypercalcemia. These are discussed in the preceding chapters. In this chapter, attention is focused on less common causes of hypercalcemia. At the beginning of each of the ensuing sections is a reference to an article or articles that contain recent, more detailed reviews of the area under discussion.

PROTEIN-BINDING ABNORMALITIES

Hypocalcemia due to hypoalbuminemia is widely recognized (1–3). That hypercalcemia may result as a consequence of hyperproteinemia is less widely appreciated. This occurs in two settings. First, patients with dehydration and volume contraction may display hyperalbuminemia. Because albumin is the primary binding protein for calcium in blood, hyperalbuminemia leads to an elevation in the total, but not the ionized, serum calcium. Because the ionized serum calcium concentration is normal, symptoms and signs of hypercalcemia are not present. A number of formulae have been developed to predict or correct the serum calcium for reductions or elevations in serum calcium. In general, these are only moderately reliable. The firm diagnosis of a calcium–protein interaction rests on the direct measurement of ionized serum calcium concentration.

A second and far less common scenario was described in patients with multiple myeloma or Waldenstrom's macroglobulinemia who have an abnormal immunoglobulin that specifically binds calcium ions. The globulin fraction, the total protein, and total serum calcium concentrations are elevated, but the ionized serum calcium is normal. Another variant of this syndrome occurs when elevated immunoglobulins interfere with total calcium determination by autoanalyzer methods. In this case, the total calcium determined by autoanalyzer is elevated, but the total calcium determined by atomic absorption and the ionized serum calcium is normal. In both of these artefactual hypercalcemia syndromes, symptoms and signs of hypercalcemia do not occur. Because elevations in ionized serum calcium can occur in multiple myeloma, hypercalcemia resulting from the immunoglobulin abnormality may be unrecognized and inappropriately treated. In multiple myeloma, physicians may be alerted to this type of artefactual hypercalcemia by the presence of moderate to severe hypercalcemia in the absence of symptoms, with normal QT intervals on electrocardiogram, and with normal rates of urinary calcium excretion.

ENDOCRINE CAUSES OF HYPERCALCEMIA OTHER THAN HYPERPARATHYROIDISM

Thyrotoxicosis

Mild hypercalcemia (serum calcium values of 10.5 to 11.5 mg/dL) frequently accompanies thyrotoxicosis (4–9).

Although coexisting hyperparathyroidism has proved to be the cause of hypercalcemia in some of these patients, it is clear that thyrotoxicosis alone can lead to hypercalcemia, a scenario that has been reported to occur in up to 50% of hyperthyroid patients. Renal calcium reabsorption and circulating 1,25-dihydroxyvitamin D [1,25 (OH)₂ D] values are reduced in such patients, reflecting suppression of parathyroid function. Bone turnover and resorption are increased. Thus hypercalcemia is believed to result from thyroxine- and triiodothyronine-induced bone resorption, a phenomenon that, over the long term, would appear to account at least in part for the osteopenia associated with thyrotoxicosis. Hypercalcemia may respond to therapy with β-adrenergic antagonists. Establishment of a diagnosis of hyperthyroidism as the cause of hypercalcemia requires that hypercalcemia be reversed with therapy of the thyrotoxicosis.

Pheochromocytoma

Hypercalcemia, at times severe, has been reported to occur in patients with pheochromocytoma (10,11). In most instances, hypercalcemia results from coexistent primary hyperparathyroidism due to parathyroid hyperplasia and constitutes a manifestation of the multiple endocrine neoplasia syndrome type IIa (see Chapter 31). Occasionally, however, hypercalcemia reverses after adrenalectomy for the pheochromocytoma. This observation suggests that the hypercalcemia resulted from the secretion by the pheochromocytoma of a circulating factor that stimulates bone resorption or that induces hyperparathyroidism. Some evidence, albeit weak, suggests that catecholamines may play these roles. More recently, however, pheochromocytomas were demonstrated to produce parathyroid hormone-related protein (PTHrP; see Chapters 14 and 34). Pheochromocytomas should be suspected and excluded prior to parathyroidectomy in all hypertensive patients with hyperparathyroidism.

Hypoadrenalism

Hypercalcemia has been reported to occur in patients with adrenal insufficiency, typically during Addisonian crisis (12–14). It also has been encountered in patients with secondary (pituitary) hypoadrenalism. The majority of reports are in the older literature, and the pathophysiology has not been thoroughly evaluated. Hypercalcemia may simply reflect hemoconcentration and volume contraction, with elevation in the serum albumin. In more recent studies, it was shown that, at least in some patients, ionized calcium is elevated, and parathyroid hormone (PTH), PTHrP and 1,25 (OH)₂ vitamin D are suppressed. Hypercalcemia responds to volume expansion and glucocorticoids. This diagnosis should be considered in the acquired immunodeficiency syndrome (AIDS) era in patients who are susceptible to *Mycobacterium avium-intracellulare* and other infectious forms of adrenal insufficiency.

Islet Cell Tumors of the Pancreas

Islet cell tumors may secrete PTHrP (see Chapters 14 and 34) or may occur with parathyroid gland hyperplasia as a feature of the multiple endocrine neoplasia type I syndrome (Chapter 31) (15–18). However, 90% of patients with islet cell tumors that secrete vasoactive intestinal polypeptide (VIP) develop hypercalcemia. These "VIP-omas" are manifested clinically by the WDHA syndrome: severe watery diarrhea ("pancreatic cholera"), hypokalemia, and achlorhydria. The mechanism responsible for hypercalcemia is unknown.

IMMOBILIZATION

Weightlessness (as occurs in space flight) and complete, prolonged bed rest due to orthopedic casting or traction, to spinal cord injury, or to other neurologic disorders regularly leads to accelerated bone resorption and hypercalcemia in individuals whose underlying rate of bone turnover is high (19–22). These individuals include children, adolescents, and young adults, patients with primary hyperparathyroidism, secondary hyperparathyroidism (as occurs in renal failure), patients with Paget's disease of bone (see Chapter 77), and patients with early, mild, or "subclinical" instances of malignancy-associated hypercalcemia. Hypercalcemia develops within days to weeks of the onset of bed rest, and is associated with (a) uncoupling of bone cell activity (i.e., increases in osteoclastic bone resorption and decreases in osteoblastic bone formation); (b) hypercalciuria leading to both upper and lower urinary tract nephrolithiasis; and (c) if the condition is allowed to continue, osteopenia. The osteoclastic bone resorption, hypercalciuria, and hypercalcemia promptly reverse with the resumption of normal weight-bearing, but passive range-of-motion exercises are ineffective. Circulating PTH and 1,25 (OH)$_2$ D levels are reduced, as is urinary cyclic adenosine monophosphate (cAMP) excretion. Preliminary evidence suggests that treatment with bisphosphonates may reverse or diminish immobilization-induced hypercalcemia and osteopenia. The cellular mechanisms responsible for immobilization-induced bone resorption remain speculative.

THE MILK-ALKALI SYNDROME

Hypercalcemia resulting from overingestion of calcium was first described in the 1930s, generally in the context of ulcer treatment with large quantities of milk together with sodium bicarbonate (23,24). The presentation of the syndrome has changed over the years in the sense that today, the offending agent is almost always calcium carbonate, in the form of over-the-counter antacids or osteoporosis supplements/preventives. However, consumption of large quantities of milk or other dairy products such as yogurt still may be a part of the presentation. In one recent hospital survey, this syndrome was responsible for 7% of inpatient admissions for hypercalcemia.

The classic features of the syndrome include moderate to severe hypercalcemia, alkalosis, and renal failure. Pathogenetically, some have argued that alkalosis (from the antacid or from vomiting) is a critical etiologic component of the syndrome, leading to enhanced calcium absorption from the gut as well as enhanced renal calcium reabsorption. Others might argue that the critical issue is simply calcium overingestion. The threshold for calcium ingestion (i.e., the minimal quantity of calcium that must be ingested for hypercalcemia to occur may be as low as 2000 to 3000 mg/day), but most reported patients have ingested quantities in the 5000 to 15,000 mg/day range. Therapy consists of making the diagnosis (a common problem because calcium supplements are often not considered to be medications by either the patient or the physician); discontinuing the offending source of calcium and/or antacid; rehydration; and diuresis. In severe cases, particularly if renal failure precludes large-volume diuresis, acute hemodialysis against a low-calcium dialysate has been very effective. The restoration of full renal function is likely in cases of brief duration but may not occur in more chronic cases.

TOTAL PARENTERAL NUTRITION

Hypercalcemia may occur in patients receiving total parenteral nutrition (25–27). In the early phases of therapy (days to weeks), hypercalcemia may result from excessive addition of calcium or vitamin D to the hyperalimentation fluid. This can be documented by correcting hypercalcemia after reformulation of the hyperalimentation solution by the pharmacy. Over the longer term (months to years), hypercalcemia associated with an osteomalacic osteodystrophy has been reported to occur in patients receiving hyperalimentation with little or no calcium in the hyperalimentation fluid. This disorder has been ascribed to the inadvertent addition of aluminum to the hyperalimentation solution in amino acid hydrolysates, with resultant aluminum intoxication. With the removal of aluminum from hyperalimentation solutions in recent years, this chronic syndrome appears to have disappeared.

HYPERCALCEMIA RESULTING FROM MEDICATIONS

Vitamin D and Related Compounds

Hypercalcemia is regularly encountered in patients receiving vitamin D or its analogues [25-hydroxyvitamin D; 1,25 (OH)$_2$ D; and dihydrotachysterol] (28–31). Recently an "outbreak" of hypercalcemia due to vitamin D intoxication was described that resulted from the accidental oversupplementation by a commercial dairy of cow's milk with vitamin D. The recommended daily allowance for vitamin D is 400 to 800 U/day. The amount of vitamin D required to produce hypercalcemia is in excess of 50,000 U/week. Thus hypercalcemia occurs not from over-the-counter multivitamin overdose but from prescribed vitamin D doses, usually used in the treatment of osteoporosis, hypoparathyroidism, malabsorption, or renal osteodystrophy. The vitamin D analogues described earlier also are prescription drugs and frequently cause hypercalcemia when used in excessive doses. The hypercalcemia that occurs in this setting has gastrointestinal, renal, and skeletal components and responds to withdrawal of the vitamin D compound, volume expansion, and calciuresis. Occasionally glucocorticoid treatment is required. The biologic half-life of vitamin D is very long (weeks to months), whereas that of its metabolites is relatively short (hours to days).

Vitamin A and Related Compounds

Vitamin A in large doses (greater than 50,000 IU/day) may cause hypercalcemia (32–35). Vitamin A–induced hypercalcemia was once a medical curiosity limited to occasional intentional drug overdoses and to Arctic explorers forced to consume sled-dog and polar bear liver. More recently, however, the widespread use of vitamin A analogues such as cis-retinoic acid and all-trans-retinoic acid for the treatment of acne and other dermatologic disorders, as well as for the treatment of neuroblastoma, hematologic, and other malignancies, has been associated with the occasional occurrence of hypercalcemia. PTH, PTHrP, and plasma 1,25 $(OH)_2$ D are suppressed. The hypercalcemia appears to result from osteoclast-mediated bone resorption.

Estrogens and Antiestrogens

Estrogens and antiestrogens cause hypercalcemia in approximately 30% of patients when used to treat breast cancer metastatic to the skeleton (36,37). The physiologic basis of this "estrogen" or "antiestrogen flare" is unknown. It has been associated with subsequent tumor regression when the offending drug can be continued. The hypercalcemia appears to be skeletal in origin, responsive to hydration and glucocorticoids, and self-limiting.

Lithium

Lithium carbonate in doses of 900 to 1500 mg/day has been reported to cause hypercalcemia in approximately 5% of patients receiving the drug (38). There is an upward resetting of the parathyroid gland setpoint for calcium sensing. That is, the hypercalcemia is the result of lithium-induced failure of suppression of PTH secretion by calcium. The precise parathyroid cellular defect remains to be defined but appears to be distal to the cell-surface calcium receptor. Evidence suggests an additional, anticalciuric renal action of lithium. Except in patients with previously unrecognized coincidental primary hyperparathyroidism, the hypercalcemia will resolve if lithium therapy is discontinued.

Thiazide Diuretics

Thiazide diuretics regularly cause hypercalcemia (39). The hypercalcemia appears to be largely renal in origin because thiazide diuretics enhance calcium reabsorption in the distal tubule. On the other hand, it was reported that thiazide diuretics may cause hypercalcemia in anephric patients, suggesting that extrarenal effects of thiazides may be important. Hypercalcemia reverses rapidly with discontinuation of the offending drug. The thiazide effect on the kidney is used in the treatment of hypoparathyroidism and nephrolithiasis due to renal calcium wasting.

Aminophylline

Aminophylline and its derivatives have been reported to cause hypercalcemia (40). This has usually been in an asthmatic patient receiving a loading dose of theophylline that raised serum theophylline levels above the therapeutic range. Serum calcium values become normal when patients are placed on maintenance therapy and serum theophylline levels fall into the therapeutic range. Theophylline-induced hypercalcemia is typically mild. Its mechanism is not known.

Growth Hormone Therapy

Growth hormone has been used in surgical intensive care settings and in patients with AIDS to prevent or reverse the catabolic consequences of severe illness (41,42). In these settings, the use of growth hormone has been associated with the development of moderate degrees of hypercalcemia (serum calcium concentrations of 11.5 to 13.5 mg/dL). PTH and 1,25 $(OH)_2$ D are suppressed. The underlying mechanisms are unknown.

8-Chloro-cyclic AMP

8-Chloro-cAMP is an antineoplastic protein kinase A modulator (43). Phase I trials indicated that moderate hypercalcemia routinely occurs when the drug is administered to humans and that the hypercalcemia results, at least in part, from activation of renal 1,25 $(OH)_2$ D synthesis.

Foscarnet

Foscarnet is an antiviral agent used in the treatment of patients with AIDS (44). It has been associated both with hypocalcemia (see Chapter 43) and hypercalcemia. The mechanism responsible is unknown.

NONGRANULOMATOUS INFLAMMATORY DISEASES

As reviewed in Chapter 36, granulomatous disorders such as sarcoidosis and tuberculosis can lead to hypercalcemia (45–48). Recently a number of other inflammatory disorders not associated with granuloma formation were reported to cause hypercalcemia. These conditions include systemic lupus erythematosus, juvenile rheumatoid arthritis, unexplained elevated systemic interleukin-6 concentrations, and recent hepatitis B vaccination. In general, the mechanisms for hypercalcemia induction are less than perfectly understood: this clearly represents an area for additional investigation.

AIDS

The AIDS syndrome has been associated with hypercalcemia through a number of mechanisms, several of which are listed in the preceding sections (42,44,49). Given the complexity and frequency of the AIDS syndrome, it is given a separate heading here. Causes of hypercalcemia listed earlier, particularly linked to the AIDS syndrome, include foscarnet use, hypoadrenalism due to infection (viral/parasite/mycobacterial), secondary neoplasms such as lymphomas with resultant malignancy-associated hypercalcemia, and growth hormone therapy for wasting syndromes. One additional syndrome that has been described is direct skeletal resorption due to human immunodeficiency virus (HIV), HTLV-III, or cytomegalovirus (CMV) infection of the skeleton.

CHRONIC AND ACUTE RENAL FAILURE

Hypercalcemia may occur in both acute and chronic renal failure (50,51). In the former, hypercalcemia was reported to occur in the recovery phase of acute tubular necrosis due to rhabdomyolysis. It was postulated that the severe hyperphosphatemia that accompanies the early phases of acute renal failure in this syndrome exceeds the calcium–phosphate solubility product and leads to the deposition of calcium phosphate salts in soft tissues, as well as to hypocalcemia-mediated secondary hyperparathyroidism. As renal function recovers, the combination of excessive circulating PTH concentrations and of reentry of calcium salts into the circulation from soft tissues leads to hypercalcemia.

In chronic renal failure, particularly in patients receiving hemodialysis, hypercalcemia is common and may result from vitamin D intoxication, calcium antacid overingestion, immobilization, aluminum intoxication, or combinations of these. These are discussed in more detail in Chapter 69.

GAUCHER'S DISEASE

A single case describing hypercalcemia in an adult with Gaucher's disease with an acute pneumonia recently was reported (52). In this patient, the serum calcium had been normal prior to the development of pneumonia, and the mechanisms underlying the hypercalcemia could not be fully defined.

MANGANESE INTOXICATION

Manganese intoxication has been reported to produce severe hypercalcemia in workers exposed to toxic concentrations of manganese in contaminated industrial settings or in wells (53,54). The mechanisms responsible for hypercalcemia are unknown.

ADVANCED CHRONIC LIVER DISEASE

Patients with end-stage chronic liver disease awaiting liver transplantation have been reported to display hypercalcemia (55). Again, the mechanisms underlying the hypercalcemia are unknown but are likely multifactorial.

PRIMARY OXALOSIS

Adults with primary oxalosis have been reported to develop severe hypercalcemia (56,57). These cases are difficult to sort out in mechanistic terms, because the affected patients have frequently undergone kidney and liver transplantation and are immunosuppressed. Circulating calcitropic hormones are suppressed. It has been hypothesized that oxalate-induced granulomas form in the marrow space and lead to bone resorption, findings that are apparent both histologically and radiologically.

REFERENCES

1. Ladenson JH, Lewis JH, McDonald JM, Slatopolsky E, Boyd JC. Relationship of free and total calcium in hypercalcemic conditions. *J Clin Endocrinol Metab* 1978;48:393–397.
2. Merlini G, Fitzpatrick LA, Siris ES, et al. A human myeloma immunoglobulin G binding four moles of calcium associated with asymptomatic hypercalcemia. *J Clin Immunol* 1984;4:185–196.
3. Rhys J, Oleesky D, Issa D, et al. Pseudohypercalcemia in two patients with IgM paraproteinemia. *Ann Clin Biochem* 1997;34:694–696.
4. Peerenboom H, Keck E, Kruskemper GL, Strohmeyer G. The defect in intestinal calcium transport in hyperthyroidism and its response to therapy. *J Clin Endocrinol Metab* 1984;59:936–940.
5. Burman KD, Monchick JM, Earll JM, Wartofski L. Ionized and total serum calcium and parathyroid hormone in hyperthyroidism. *Ann Intern Med* 1976;84:668–671.
6. Ross DS, Nussbaum SR. Reciprocal changes in parathyroid hormone and thyroid function after radioiodine treatment of hyperthyroidism. *J Clin Endocrinol Metab* 1989;68:1216–1219.
7. Britto JM, Fenton AJ, Holloway WR, Nicholson GC. Osteoblasts mediate thyroid hormone stimulation of osteoclastic bone resorption. *Endocrinology* 1994;123:169–176.
8. Rosen HN, Moses AC, Gundberg C, et al. Therapy with parenteral pamidronate prevents thyroid hormone-induced bone turnover in humans. *J Clin Endocrinol Metab* 1993;77:664–669.
9. Rude RK, Oldham SB, Singer FR, Nicoloff JT. Treatment of thyrotoxic hypercalcemia with propranolol. *N Engl J Med* 1976;294:431–433.
10. Stewart AF, Hoecker J, Segre GV, Mallette LE, Amatruda T, Vignery A. Hypercalcemia in pheochromocytoma: evidence for a novel mechanism. *Ann Intern Med* 1985;102:776–779.
11. Mune T, Katakami H, Kato Y, Yasuda K, Matsukura S, Miura K. Production and secretion of parathyroid hormone-related protein in pheochromocytoma: participation of an α-adrenergic mechanism. *J Clin Endocrinol Metab* 1993;76:757–762.
12. Muls E, Bouillon R, Boelaert J, et al. Etiology of hypercalcemia in a patient with Addison's disease. *Calcif Tissue Int* 1982;34:523–526.
13. Vasikaran SD, Tallis GA, Braund WJ. Secondary hypoadrenalism presenting with hypercalcaemia. *Clin Endocrinol* 1994;41:261–265.
14. Diamond T, Thornley S. Addisonian crisis and hypercalcaemia. *Aust N Z J Med* 1994;24:316.
15. Mao C, Carter P, Schaefer P, et al. Malignant islet cell tumor associated with hypercalcemia. *Surgery* 1994;117:37–40.
16. Ratcliffe WA, Bowden SJ, Dunne FP, et al. Expression and processing of parathyroid hormone-related protein in a pancreatic endocrine cell tumour associated with hypercalcaemia. *Clin Endocrinol* 1994; 40:679–686.
17. Asa SL, Henderson J, Goltzman D, Drucker DJ. Parathyroid hormone-like peptide in normal and neoplastic human endocrine tissues. *J Clin Endocrinol Metab* 1990;71:1112–1118.
18. Verner JV, Morrison AB. Endocrine pancreatic islet disease with diarrhea. *Arch Intern Med* 1974;133:492–500.
19. Stewart AF, Adler M, Byers CM, Segre GV, Broadus AE. Calcium homeostasis in immobilization: an example of resorptive hypercalciuria. *N Engl J Med* 1982;306:1136–1140.
20. Bergstrom WH. Hypercalciuria and hypercalcemia complicating immobilization. *Am J Dis Child* 1978;132:553–554.
21. Chappard D, Minaire P, Privat C, et al. Effects of tiludronate on bone loss in paraplegic patients. *J Bone Miner Res* 1995;10:112–118.
22. Roberts D, Lee W, Cuneo RC, et al. Longitudinal study of bone turnover after acute spinal cord injury. *J Clin Endocrinol Metab* 1998; 83:415–422.
23. Beall DP, Scofield RH. Milk-alkali syndrome associated with calcium carbonate consumption. *Medicine* 1995;74:89–96.

24. Orwoll ES. The milk-alkali syndrome: current concepts. *Ann Intern Med* 1982;97:242–248.

25. Ott SM, Maloney NA, Klein GL, et al. Aluminum is associated with low bone formation in patients receiving chronic parenteral nutrition. *Ann Intern Med* 1983;96:910–914.

26. Klein GL, Horst RL, Norman AW, Ament ME, Slatopolsky E, Coburn JW. Reduced serum levels of 1a, 25-dihydroxyvitamin D during long-term total parenteral nutrition. *Ann Intern Med* 1981;94:638–643.

27. Shike M, Sturtridge WC, Tam CS, et al. A possible role of vitamin D in the genesis of parenteral-nutrition-induced metabolic bone disease. *Ann Intern Med* 1981;95:560–568.

28. Haussler MR, McCain TA. Basic and clinical concepts related to vitamin D metabolism and action. *N Engl J Med* 1977;297:974–1041.

29. Holick MF, Shao Q, Liu WW, Chen TC. The vitamin D content of fortified milk and infant formula. *N Engl J Med* 1992;326:1178–1181.

30. Jacobus CH, Holick MF, Shao Q, et al. Hypervitaminosis D associated with drinking milk. *N Engl J Med* 1992;326:1173–1177.

31. Pettifor JM, Bikle DD, Cavalerso M, Zachen D, Kamdar MC, Ross FP. Serum levels of free 1,25-dihydroxyvitamin D in vitamin D toxicity. *Ann Intern Med* 1995;122:511–513.

32. Valente JD, Elias AN, Weinstein GD. Hypercalcemia associated with oral isotretinoin in the treatment of severe acne. *JAMA* 1983;250:1899.

33. Suzumiya J, Asahara F, Katakami H, et al. Hypercalcaemia caused by all-trans retinoic acid treatment of acute promyelocytic leukaemia: case report. *Eur J Haematol* 1994;53:126–127.

34. Bourke JF, Berth-Jones J, Hutchinson PE. Hypercalcemia with topical calcipotriol. *Br Med J* 1993;306:1334–1335.

35. Villablanca J, Khan AA, Avramis VI, et al. Phase I trial of 13-*cis*-retinoic acid in children with neuroblastoma following bone marrow transplantation. *J Clin Oncol* 1995;13:894–901.

36. Legha SS, Powell K, Buzdar AU, Blumen-Schein GR. Tamoxifen-induced hypercalcemia in breast cancer. *Cancer* 1981;47:2803.

37. Valentin-Opran A, Eilon G, Saez S, Mundy GR. Estrogens and antiestrogens stimulate release of bone-resorbing activity in cultured human breast cancer cells. *J Clin Invest* 1985;75:726.

38. Haden ST, Stoll AL, McCormick S, Scott J, Fuleihan GE. Alterations in parathyroid dynamics in lithium-treated subjects. *J Clin Endocrinol Metab* 1979;82:2844–2848.

39. Porter RH, Cox BG, Heaney D, Hostetter TH, Stinebaugh BJ, Suki WN. Treatment of hypoparathyroid patients with chlorthalidone. *N Engl J Med* 1978;298:577.

40. McPherson ML, Prince SR, Atamer E, Maxwell DB, Ross-Clunis H, Estep H. Theophylline-induced hypercalcemia. *Ann Intern Med* 1986;105:52–54.

41. Knox JB, Demling RH, Wilmore DW, Sarraf P, Santos AA. Hypercalcemia associated with the use of human growth hormone in an adult surgical intensive care unit. *Arch Surg* 1995;130:442–445.

42. Sakoulas G, Tritos NA, Lally M, Wanke C, Hartzband P. Hypercalcemia in an AIDS patient treated with growth hormone. *AIDS* 1997;11:1353–1356.

43. Saunders M, Salisbuy AJ, O'Byrne KJ, et al. A novel cyclic adenosine monophosphate analog induces hypercalcemia via production of 1,25-dihydroxyvitamin D in patients with solid tumors. *J Clin Endocrinol Metab* 1997;83:4044–4048.

44. Gayet S, Ville E, Durand JM, et al. Foscarnet-induced hypercalcemia in AIDS. *AIDS* 1997;11:1068–1070.

45. Schurman SJ, Bergstrom WH, Root AW, Souid AK, Hannah WP. Interleukin 1 beta-mediated calcitropic activity in serum of children with juvenile rheumatoid arthritis. *J Rheumatol* 1998;25:161–165.

46. Cathebras P, Odile C, Lafage-Proust M-H, et al. Arthritis, hypercalcemia and lytic bone lesions after hepatitis B vaccination. *J Rheumatol* 1996;23:558–560.

47. Deftos LJ, Burton DW, Baird SM, Terkeltaub RA. Hypercalcemia and systemic lupus erythematosus. *Arthritis Rheum* 1996;39:2066–2069.

48. Greenwald RA, Stein B, Miller F. Rapid skeletal turnover and hypercalcemia associated with markedly elevated interleukin 6 levels in a young black man. *Bone* 1998;22:285–288.

49. Zaloga GP, Chernow B, Eil C. Hypercalcemia and disseminated cytomegalovirus infection in the acquired immunodeficiency syndrome. *Ann Intern Med* 1985;102:331–333.

50. Llach F, Felsenfeld AJ, Haussler MR. The pathophysiology of altered calcium metabolism in rhabdomyolysis-induced acute renal failure. *N Engl J Med* 1981;305:117–123.

51. Lane JT, Boudrea RJ, Kinlaw WB. Disappearance of muscular calcium deposits during resolution of prolonged rhabdomyolysis-induced hypercalcemia. *Am J Med* 1990;89:523–525.

52. Byrne CD, Bermann L, Cox TM. Pathologic bone fractures preceded by sustained hypercalcemia in Gaucher disease. *J Inherit Metab Dis* 1997;20:709–710.

53. Chandra SV, Seth PK, Mankeshwar JK. Manganese poisoning: clinical and biochemical observations. *Environ Res* 1974;7:374–380.

54. Chandra SV, Shukla GS, Srivastava RS. An exploratory study of manganese exposure to welders. *Clin Toxicol* 1981;18:407–416.

55. Gerhardt A, Greenberg A, Reilly JJ, Van Thiel DH. Hypercalcema complication of advanced chronic liver disease. *Arch Intern Med* 1987;147:274–277.

56. Yamaguchi K, Grant J, Noble-Jamieson G, Jamieson N, Barnes ND, Compston JE. Hypercalcemia in primary oxalosis: role of increased bone resorption and effects of treatment with pamidronate. *Bone* 1995;16:61–67.

57. Toussaint C, DePauw C, Tielmans C, Abramowicz D. Hypercalcemia complicating systemic oxalosis in primary hyperoxaluria type 1. *Nephrol Dial Transplant* 1995;10(suppl 8):17–21.

38. Hypercalcemic Syndromes in Infants and Children

Craig B. Langman, M.D.

Department of Pediatrics, Northwestern University Medical School, and Nephrology and Mineral Metabolism Department, Children's Memorial Hospital, Chicago, Illinois

Blood ionized calcium levels in normal infants and young children are similar to those of adults, with a mean $\pm$ 2 SD = 1.21 $\pm$ 0.13 mM. In neonates, the normal blood ionized calcium level is dependent on postnatal age (1). In the first 72 hours after birth, there is a significant decrease in the blood ionized calcium level in term newborns, from 1.4 to 1.2 mM; the decrease is exaggerated in preterm neonates.

Chronic hypercalcemia in young infants and children may not be associated with the usual signs and symptoms described in Chapter 29. Rather, the predominant manifestation of hypercalcemia is "failure to thrive," in which linear growth is arrested and there is lack of appropriate weight gain. Additional features of chronic hypercalcemia in children include nonspecific symptoms of irritability, gastrointestinal reflux, abdominal pain, and anorexia. Acute hypercalcemia is very uncommon in infants and children; when it occurs, its manifestations are similar to those of older children and adults, with potential alterations in the nervous system, the conduction system of the heart, and kidney functions

WILLIAMS SYNDROME

Williams et al. (2) described a syndrome in infants with supravalvular aortic stenosis and peculiar ("elfin-like") facies; hypercalcemia during the first year of life also was noted (3). However, the severe elevations in serum calcium initially described failed to appear with equal frequency in subsequent series of such infants. Other series of children with the cardiac lesion failed to demonstrate the associated facial dysmorphism. It is thought that there exists a spectrum of infants with some or all of these abnormalities, and a scoring system has been described to assign suspected infants as lying within or outside of the syndrome classification (4).

Two thirds of infants with Williams syndrome are small for their gestational age, and many are born past their expected date of birth. The facial abnormalities consist of structural asymmetry, temporal depression, flat malae with full cheeks, microcephaly, epicanthal folds, lacy or stellate irises, a short nose, long philtrum, arched upper lip with full lower lip, and small, maloccluded teeth. The vocal tone is often hoarse. Neurologic manifestations include hypotonia, hyperreflexia, and mild-to-moderate motor retardation. The personality of affected children has been described as "cocktail party," in that they are unusually friendly to strangers. Other vascular abnormalities have been described in addition to supravalvular aortic stenosis, including other congenital heart defects and many peripheral organ arterial stenoses (renal, mesenteric, and celiac). Hypertension may be present in infancy in a minority of children but increases in incidence after the first decade of life.

Hypercalcemia, if initially present, rarely persists to the end of the first year of life and generally disappears spontaneously. Despite the rarity of chronic hypercalcemia, persistent hypercalciuria is not uncommon. Additionally, many of the signs and symptoms of hypercalcemia mentioned previously and in the introduction to this section have been noted in these infants. The long-term prognosis for patients with Williams syndrome seems to depend on features other than the level of blood calcium, such as the level of mental retardation and the clinical significance of the cardiovascular abnormalities. Approximately 25% of patients may have radioulnar synostosis, which may impede normal developmental milestones of fine-motor activities of the upper extremities if not recognized (5).

A search for the gene(s) responsible for Williams syndrome localized the cardiac component, supravalvular aortic stenosis, to the long arm of chromosome 7 (6). It appears that translocations of the elastin gene may be responsible for isolated or familial supravalvular aortic stenosis (7,8), whereas a heterozygous microdeletion of chr 7q11.23, which encompasses the elastin gene (9), produces Williams syndrome. Rarely it may involve a defect of chromosome 11 [del(11)(q13.5q14.2)], or of chromosome 22 [r(22)(p11—>q13)] (10).

Despite the potential localization of the disorder to a deletion of the elastin locus on chromosome 7, the pathogenesis of the disorder remains unknown, although many studies focused on disordered control of vitamin D metabolism. Previous studies of affected children demonstrated increased circulating levels of 25-hydroxyvitamin D after vitamin D administration (11), increased levels of calcitriol (1,25-dihydroxyvitamin D [1,25 $(OH)_2$ D]) during periods of hypercalcemia (12) but not during normocalcemia (13,14), or diminished levels of calcitonin during calcium infusions (15). Although excess administration of vitamin D to pregnant rabbits may produce an experimental picture not dissimilar to that in humans with Williams syndrome, the overwhelming majority of children with Williams syndrome are not the result of maternal vitamin D intoxication.

IDIOPATHIC INFANTILE HYPERCALCEMIA

In the early 1950s in England, Lightwood (16) reported a series of infants with severe hypercalcemia. Epidemiologic investigations revealed that the majority of affected infants were born to mothers ingesting foods heavily fortified with vitamin D. The incidence of the disease declined dramatically with reduction of vitamin D supplementation. Other cases have been described without previous exposure to excessive maternal vitamin D intake, and the incidence of idiopathic infantile hypercalcemia (IIH) has remained fixed over the past 20 years. Affected infants have polyuria, increased thirst, and the general manifestations of hypercalcemia previously noted. Severely affected neonates may have cardiac lesions similar to those seen in Williams syndrome and may even manifest the dysmorphic features of those infants and children. The distinction between the two syndromes remains problematic (17). Other clinical manifestations include chronic arterial hypertension, strabismus, inguinal hernias, musculoskeletal abnormalities (disordered posture and mild kyphosis), and bony abnormalities (radioulnar synostosis and dislocated patella). Hyperacusis is present in the majority of affected children with IIH, but not Williams syndrome, and it is persistent.

As in Williams syndrome, disordered vitamin D metabolism with increased vitamin D sensitivity with respect to gastrointestinal transport of calcium has been posited as the cause of this disorder (18), although the data are conflicting. We recently identified seven consecutive children with IIH in whom the presence of an elevated level of N-terminal parathyroid hormone-related protein (PTHrP) was demonstrated at the time of hypercalcemia (19). Further, in five of those children who achieved normocalcemia, the levels of PTHrP normalized or were unmeasurably low, and in one child with persistent hypercalcemia, the level of PTHrP remained elevated. No other nonmalignant disorder of childhood that we have examined, including two children with hypercalcemia from Williams syndrome, has had elevated levels of PTHrP, although a recent report of an infantile fibrosarcoma and hypercalcemia demonstrated PTHrP production from the soft-tissue tumor (20). In contrast to the hypercalcemia of Williams syndrome, the level of blood calcium in IIH remains elevated for a prolonged period in the most severely affected children. Therapy includes the use of glucocorticoids to reduce gastrointestinal absorption of calcium, as well as the avoidance of vitamin D and excess dietary calcium.

FAMILIAL HYPOCALCIURIC HYPERCALCEMIA

This disorder also is called familial benign hypercalcemia and has been recognized since 1972 (21) as a cause of elevated total and serum ionized calcium. The onset of the change in calcium is commonly before age 10 years and was described in newborns (22) (see Chapter 32 for a fuller discussion).

NEONATAL PRIMARY HYPERPARATHYROIDISM

Primary hyperparathyroidism (Chapter 30) is uncommon in neonates and children (23), with less than 100 cases reported. Additionally, only 20% of cases occur in children younger than 10 years. Hypercalcemia in the first decade of life may more likely be caused by the other disorders discussed in this chapter. The presenting clinical manifestations are weakness, anorexia, and irritability, which are seen in a multitude of pediatric disorders. The association with other endocrine disorders occurs with decreased frequency in young children with primary hyperparathyroidism. Histologic examination of the parathyroid glands demonstrates that 20% to 40% of affected children may have hyperplasia rather than the more typical adenoma in older individuals.

However, the neonate may demonstrate one unusual form of hyperparathyroidism. Neonatal severe primary hyperparathyroidism is now known to result from inheritance of two mutant alleles associated with the calcium-sensing receptor gene on chromosome 3 (24). Extreme elevations of serum calcium (total calcium, $\geq$20 mg/dL; blood ionized calcium levels, $\geq$3 mM) is a hallmark of the disorder, and emergency total surgical parathyroidectomy is required for life-saving reasons. An attempt to salvage one of the parathyroid glands and perform autotransplantation is suggested for such infants. A recent report emphasizes that certain heterozygous inactivating mutations in the extracellular calcium-receptor gene may still produce neonatal hypercalcemia (25), leading to the conclusion that even the heterozygous state has important clinical implications for the neonate.

JANSEN SYNDROME

Jansen syndrome (26–28) presents in neonates with hypercalcemia and skeletal radiographs that resemble a rachitic condition. It is a form of metaphyseal dysplasia, and after infancy, the radiographic condition evolves into a more typical picture, with resultant mottled calcifications in the distal end of the long bones. These areas represent patches of partially calcified cartilage protruding into the diaphyseal portion of bone. The skull and spine may be affected also. The hypercalcemia appears to be lifelong.

Biochemical findings in patients with Jansen syndrome are consistent with primary hyperparathyroidism (see Chapter 30), but there are no measurable levels of PTH or PTHrP. The disorder results from a defect in the gene for the PTH/PTH-like protein receptor. One of three different amino acid substitutions produces a mutant receptor that is capable of autoactivation in the absence of ligand. This produces unopposed PTH/PTH-like protein actions in such patients, and thereby explains the absence of circulating levels of either hormone. Such patients appear to be at risk for the development of the complications of hyperparathyroidism in the adult years. However, other patients have been given the diagnosis of Jansen syndrome without either hypercalcemia or the finding of a mutation in the gene for the PTH/PTHrP receptor.

MISCELLANEOUS DISORDERS

Subcutaneous Fat Necrosis

Michael et al. (29) reported the association of significant birth trauma with fat necrosis in two small-for-gestational-age infants who subsequently developed severe hypercalcemia (serum calcium >15 mg/dL) and violaceous discolorations in pressure sites. Histologic examination of the affected pressure sites in such patients demonstrated both an inflammatory, mononuclear cell infiltrate and crystals that contain calcium. We also noted hypercalcemia in several children with subcutaneous fat necrosis associated with major trauma or disseminated varicella. The mechanism of the hypercalcemia is unknown, but it may be related to mildly elevated levels of 1,25 (OH)$_2$ D (30) or excess prostaglandin E production (31). The prognosis for infants and children with subcutaneous fat necrosis depends on the duration of the hypercalcemia. Reductions in serum calcium have been noted with the use of exogenous corticosteroids, saline, and furosemide diuresis, and the avoidance of excess dietary calcium and vitamin D. Recurrence of hypercalcemia has not been seen.

Hypophosphatasia

This disorder is discussed in detail in Chapter 66 and is mentioned here only for completeness. Severe infantile hypophosphatasia is associated with markedly elevated serum calcium levels and a reduction in circulating alkaline phosphatase, increase in urinary phosphoethanolamine, and elevated serum pyridoxal-5-phosphate concentrations. The use of calcitonin in a neonate with hypercalcemia was reported as beneficial to long-term outcome (32).

Sarcoidosis and Other Granulomatous Disorders of Childhood

Thirty percent to 50% of children with the autoimmune disorder sarcoidosis (33) (see Chapter 36) manifest hypercalcemia, and an additional 20% to 30% demonstrate hypercalciuria with normocalcemia. Many of the presenting manifestations of children with sarcoidosis may be related to the presence of hypercalcemia. A recent report of hypercalcemia in twin children with cat-scratch disease (34), a granulomatous disorder resulting from infection with *Bartonella henselae*, demonstrates that the granuloma may represent a source of 1,25 (OH)$_2$ D production that leads to the hypercalcemia. Successful therapy of these disorders reduces the circulating levels of that hormone to normal.

Limb Fracture

Isolated weight-bearing limb fracture (35) (see Chapter 37) that requires immobilization for even several days may be associated with elevated blood ionized calcium levels and hypercalciuria in young children and adolescents. Although prolonged immobilization itself commonly produces hypercalcemia and hypercalciuria, the occurrence after short-term bed rest in children probably reflects their more rapid skeletal turnover.

Vitamin D (or Vitamin D Metabolite)

Hypervitaminosis D (vitamin D intoxication) produces symptomatic hypercalcemia. In childhood, vitamin D intoxication has been seen after excessively prolonged feeding of premature infants with a vitamin D–fortified formula (36), after ingestion of improperly fortified dairy milk (37,38), and in children receiving therapeutic vitamin D or vitamin D metabolites (39).

An outbreak of hypercalcemia in eight patients was reported from the incorrect dosing of dairy milk with vitamin D (37), and in addition, a defect was found in the concentrate used to fortify the milk (containing cholecalciferol rather than the expected ergocalciferol). These same investigators extended their measurements of the vitamin D content to both commercial dairy milks and fortified infant formulas, and they found that only 29% of the milks and formulas contained a vitamin D content within 20% of the stated amount (38). These studies suggest that improved monitoring of the fortification process is mandatory and may explain the rare finding of clinical vitamin D deficiency in children drinking fortified milk.

Children with renal osteodystrophy are commonly treated with 1,25-dihydroxyvitamin D$_3$ [1,25 (OH)$_2$ D$_3$] and develop hypercalcemia once every 12 to 15 treatment months (see Chapter 69), whereas the use of 25-hydroxyvitamin D$_3$ is associated with a lower incidence of hypercalcemia. Children with frank hypocalcemic disorders treated with 1,25 (OH)$_2$ D$_3$ develop hypercalcemia at one third the frequency of children with renal osteodystrophy treated with any vitamin D metabolite (39). Treatment with the parent vitamin D compound is associated with the production of hypercalcemia similar to the rate produced with calcitriol. However, the hypercalcemia associated with vitamin D is prolonged four- to sixfold in comparison with hypercalcemia with metabolite therapy because of retention in body fat stores.

Prostaglandin E

Bartter syndrome may result from one of several mutations in the genes for various sodium-linked chloride transporters (40). A neonatal form may produce a marked increase in prostaglandin E production and lead to hypercalcemia, in part, from excessive bone resorption (41). Such a disturbance in bone also may contribute to the hypercalcemia seen in neonates who receive prostaglandin E infusions for congenital cardiovascular diseases that mandate patency of the fetal ductus arteriosus.

Congenital Lactase Deficiency

A recent report emphasized that seven of 10 infants with congenital lactase deficiency manifested hypercalcemia within the first 3 months of life, and was associated with renal medullary nephrocalcinosis (42). A lactose-free diet was associated with return of elevated serum calcium levels to normal. The mechanism of the hypercalcemia remains unclear but may reflect the known effects of lactose to promote direct calcium absorption through the intestine.

REFERENCES

1. Specker BL, Lichtenstein P, Mimouni F, Gormley C, Tsang RC. Calcium-regulating hormones and minerals from birth to 18 months of age: a cross-sectional study. II. Effects of sex, race, age, season, and diet on serum minerals, parathyroid hormone and calcitonin. *Pediatrics* 1986;77:891–896.
2. Williams JCP, Barratt-Boyes BG, Lowe JB. Supravalvular aortic stenosis. *Circulation* 1961;24:1311–1316.
3. Black JA, Bonham Carter RE. Association between aortic stenosis and facies of severe infantile hypercalcemia. *Lancet* 1963;2:745–748.
4. Preus M. The Williams syndrome: objective definition and diagnosis. *Clin Genet* 1984;25:422–428.
5. Charvat KA, Hornstein L, Oestreich AE. Radio-ulnarsynostosis in Williams syndrome: a frequently associated anomaly. *Pediatr Radiol* 1991;21:508–510.
6. Ewart AK, Morris CA, Ensing GJ, et al. A human vascular disorder, supravalvular aortic stenosis, maps to chromosome 7. *Proc Natl Acad Sci USA* 1993;90:3226–3230.
7. Curran ME, Atkinson DL, Ewart AK, Morris CA, Keppert MF, Keating MT. The elastin gene is disrupted by a translocation associated with supravalvular aortic stenosis. *Cell* 1993;73:159–168.
8. Ewart AK, Jin W, Atkinson D, Morris CA, Keating MT. Supravalvular aortic stenosis associated with a deletion disrupting the elastin gene. *J Clin Invest* 1994;93:1071–1077.
9. Perez Jurado LA, Peoples R, Kaplan P, Hamel BC, Francke U. Molecular definition of the chromosome 7 deletion in Williams syndrome and parent-of-origin effects on growth. *Am J Hum Genet* 1996;59:781–792.
10. Joyce CA, Zorich B, Pike SJ, Barber JC, Dennis NR. Williams-Beuren syndrome: phenotypic variability and deletions of chromosomes 7, 11, and 22 in a series of 52 patients. *J Med Genet* 1996;33:986–992.
11. Taylor AB, Stern PH, Bell NH. Abnormal regulation of circulating 25OHD in the Williams syndrome. *N Engl J Med* 1982;306:972–975.
12. Garabedian M, Jacqz E, Guillozo H, et al. Increased plasma 1,25(OH)$_2$D$_3$ concentrations in infants with hypercalcemia and an elfin facies. *N Engl J Med* 1985;312:948–952.
13. Martin NDT, Snodgrass GJAI, Makin HLJ, Cohen RD. [Letter]. *N Engl J Med* 1986;313:888–889.
14. Chesney RW, DeLuca HF, Gertner JM, Genel M. [Letter]. *N Engl J Med* 1986;313:889–890.
15. Culler FL, Jones KL, Deftos LJ. Impaired calcitonin secretion in patients with Williams syndrome. *J Pediatr* 1985;107:720–723.
16. Lightwood RL. Idiopathic hypercalcemia with failure to thrive. *Arch Dis Child* 1952;27:302–303.
17. Martin NDT, Snodgrass GJAI, Cohen RD. Idiopathic infantile hypercalcemia: a continuing enigma. *Arch Dis Child* 1984;59:605–613.
18. Aarskog D, Asknes L, Markstead T. Vitamin D metabolism in idiopathic infantile hypercalcemia. *Am J Dis Child* 1981;135:1021–1025.

19. Langman CB, Budayr AA, Sailer DE, Strewler GJ. Nonmalignant expression of parathyroid hormone-related protein is responsible for idiopathic infantile hypercalcemia. *J Bone Miner Res* 1992;7:593S.

20. Micigami T, Yamato H, Mushiake S, et al. Hypercalcemia associated with infantile fibrosarcoma producing parathyroid hormone-related protein. *J Clin Endocrinol Metab* 1996;81:1090–1095.

21. Foley TP Jr, Harrison HC, Arnaud CD, Harrison HE. Familial benign hypercalcemia. *J Pediatr* 1972;81:1060–1067.

22. Marx SJ, Attie MF, Spiegel AM, Levine MA, Lasker RD, Fox M. An association between neonatal severe primary hyperparathyroidism and familial hypocalciuric hypercalcemia. *N Engl J Med* 1982; 306:257–264.

23. Bernulf J, Hall K, Sjogren I, Werner I. Primary hyperparathyroidism in children. *Acta Pediatr Scand* 1970;59:249–258.

24. Pollak MR, Chou YH, Marx SJ, et al. Familial hypocalciuric hypercalcemia and neonatal severe hyperparathyroidism: effects of mutant gene dosage on phenotype. *J Clin Invest* 1994;93(3):1108–1112.

25. Cole DE, Janicic N, Salisbury SR, Hendy GN. Neonatal severe hyperparathyroidism, secondary hyperparathyroidism, and familial hypocalciuric hypercalcemia: multiple different phenotypes associated with an inactivating Alu insertion mutation of the calcium-sensing receptor gene. *Am J Med Genet* 1997;71:202–210.

26. Frame B, Poznanski AK. Conditions that may be confused with rickets. In: Deluca HF, Anast CN, eds. *Pediatric diseases related to calcium.* New York: Elsevier, 1980:269–289.

27. Schipiani E, Kruse K, Jüppner H. A constitutively active mutant PTH-PTHrp receptor in Jansen-type metaphyseal chondrodysplasia. *Science* 1995;268:98–100.

28. Schipani E, Langman CB, Parfitt AM, et al. Two different constitutively active PTH/PTHrP receptor mutations cause Jansen-type metaphyseal chondrodysplasia. *N Engl J Med* 1996;335:708–714.

29. Michael AF, Hong R, West CD. Hypercalcemia in infancy. *Am J Dis Child* 1962;104:235–244.

30. Sharata H, Postellon DC, Hashimoto K. Subcutaneous fat necrosis, hypercalcemia and prostaglandin E. *Pediatr Dermatol* 1995;12:43–47.

31. Kruse K, Irle U, Uhlig R. Elevated 1,25-dihydroxyvitamin D serum concentrations in infants with subcutaneous fat necrosis. *J Pediatr* 1993;122:460–463.

32. Barcia JP, Strife CF, Langman CB. Infantile hypophosphatasia: treatment options to control acute hypercalcemia and chronic bone demineralization. *J Pediatr* 1997;130:825–828.

33. Jasper PL, Denny FW. Sarcoidosis in children. *J Pediatr* 1968; 73:499–512.

34. Bosch X. Hypercalcemia due to endogenous overproduction of active vitamin D in identical twins with cat-scratch disease. *JAMA* 1998;279:532–534.

35. Rosen JF, Wolin DA, Finberg L. Immobilization hypercalcemia after single limb fractures in children and adolescents. *Am J Dis Child* 1978;132:560–564.

36. Nako Y, Fukushima N, Tomomasa T, Nagashima K, Kuroume T. Hypervitaminosis D after prolonged feeding with a premature formula. *Pediatrics* 1993;92:862–864.

37. Jacobus CH, Holick MF, Shao Q, et al. Hypervitaminosis D associated with drinking milk. *N Engl J Med* 1992;326:1173–1177.

38. Holick MF, Shao Q, Liu WW, Chen TC. The vitamin D content of fortified milk and infant formula. *N Engl J Med* 1992;326:1178–1181.

39. Chan JCM, Young RB, Alon U, Manunes P. Hypercalcemia in children with disorders of calcium and phosphate metabolism during long-term treatment with 1,25(OH)₂D₃. *Pediatrics* 1983;72:225–233.

40. Karolyi L, Koch MC, Grzeschik KH, Seyberth HW. The molecular genetic approach to Bartter's syndrome. *J Mol Med* 1998;76:317–325.

41. Welch TR. The hyperprostaglandin E syndrome: a hypercalciuric variant of Bartter syndrome. *J Bone Miner Res* 1997;12:1753–1754.

42. Saarela T, Simila S, Koivisto M. Hypercalcemia and nephrocalcinosis in patients with congenital lactase deficiency. *J Pediatr* 1995; 127:920–923.

39. Hypocalcemia: Pathogenesis, Differential Diagnosis, and Management

Elizabeth Shane, M.D.

Department of Medicine, Columbia University College of Physicians and Surgeons, and New York Presbyterian Hospital, New York, New York

Hypocalcemia is encountered commonly in medical practice. Like hypercalcemia, hypocalcemia varies in its clinical presentation from an asymptomatic biochemical abnormality to a severe life-threatening condition. The many causes of hypocalcemia are listed in Tables 1 and 2, and also are considered separately in subsequent chapters. General principles that apply to the differential diagnosis and management of hypocalcemia are covered in this chapter.

PATHOGENESIS AND DIFFERENTIAL DIAGNOSIS

The concentration of calcium in the extracellular fluid is critical for many physiologic processes. Under normal circumstances, the range is kept remarkably constant, between 8.5 and 10.5 mg/dL (2.1 to 2.5 mM). The exact normal ranges vary slightly depending on the laboratory. Approximately half the total serum calcium is bound to plasma proteins, primarily albumin. A small component is complexed to anions such as citrate or sulfate. The remaining half circulates as free calcium ion. It is only this ionized portion of the total serum calcium that is physiologically important, regulating neuromuscular contractility, the activity of many enzymes, the process of coagulation, and a variety of other cellular activities.

In many chronic illnesses, substantial reductions may occur in the serum albumin concentration that may lower total serum calcium concentration while the ionized calcium concentration remains normal. A simple correction for hypoalbuminemia can be made by adding 0.8 mg/dL to the total serum calcium for every 1.0 g/dL by which the serum albumin is lower than 4.0 g/dL. Thus a patient with a serum calcium of 7.8 mg/dL and a serum albumin of 2.0 mg/dL has a corrected total serum calcium of 9.4 mg/dL. In contrast to changes in the serum albumin, which affect the total but not the ionized calcium level, alterations in pH affect the ionized calcium concentration without altering the total calcium level. Acidosis increases the ionized calcium by decreasing the binding of calcium ions to albumin, whereas alkalosis decreases the ionized calcium by enhancing bind-

TABLE 1. *Hypoparathyroid states resulting in hypocalcemia*

Autoimmune
  Isolated
  End-organ deficiency syndrome
Congenital
  DiGeorge syndrome
  Calcium sensor mutation
Postsurgical
Severe magnesium deficiency
Neck irradiation
Infiltrative
  Hemochromatosis
  Sarcoidosis
  Thalassemia
  Wilson's disease
  Amyloidosis
  Metastatic carcinoma
Neonatal hypocalcemia
Hungry-bone syndrome (postparathyroidectomy)

TABLE 2. *Nonhypoparathyroid states resulting in hypocalcemia*

Vitamin D deficiency
  Lack of sunlight exposure
  Dietary lack
  Malabsorption
  Upper gastrointestinal tract surgery
  Liver disease
  Renal disease
  Anticonvulsants
  Vitamin-D–dependent rickets, type I (1α-hydroxylase deficiency)
Parathyroid hormone resistance
  Pseudohypoparathyroidism
  Severe magnesium deficiency
Vitamin D resistance
  Vitamin-D–resistant rickets
  Vitamin-D–dependent rickets, type II (resistance to 1,25-dihydroxyvitamin D)
  Familial vitamin D resistance
Drugs
  Hypocalcemic agents
    Bisphosphonates
    Plicamycin
    Calcitonin
    Gallium nitrate
    Phosphate
  Anticancer agents
    Asparaginase
    Cisplatinum
    Cytosine arabinoside
    Doxorubicin
    WR 2721
  Other
    Ketaconazole
    Pentamidine
    Foscarnet
Miscellaneous
  Acute pancreatitis
  Massive tumor lysis
  Osteoblastic metastases
  Phosphate infusion
  Multiple citrated blood transfusions
  Toxic shock syndrome
  Acute rhabdomyolysis
  Acute severe illness

ing of calcium ions to albumin. Measurement of total serum calcium is usually adequate for most clinical situations, but in complex cases, direct measurement of the ionized calcium should be performed.

The parathyroid glands are extremely sensitive to small changes in the serum ionized calcium level. Parathyroid hormone, through its acute effects on bone resorption and renal calcium reabsorption in the distal tubule, is responsible for the minute-to-minute regulation of the serum calcium level. Adjustments in intestinal calcium absorption via parathyroid hormone–stimulated renal 1,25-dihydroxyvitamin D [1,25 $(OH)_2$ D] production require 24 to 48 hours to become maximal, and therefore they come into play only when the hypocalcemic stimulus is of a more chronic nature. Hypocalcemia occurs when there is a failure of, or incomplete compensation by, the parathyroid hormone–controlled homeostatic mechanisms that defend against a hypocalcemic stimulus (see Chapter 12). The most common causes of hypocalcemia include hypoparathyroidism, deficiency or abnormal metabolism of vitamin D, hypomagnesemia, and acute or chronic renal failure. In general, hypocalcemic states may be classified according to whether they are associated with inappropriately low levels of parathyroid hormone (hypoparathyroid states) (Table 1) or whether parathyroid hormone levels are increased, indicating normal parathyroid gland responsiveness to the low serum calcium (secondary hyperparathyroid states) (Table 2).

Idiopathic hypoparathyroidism is manifested by hypocalcemia and coexistent low or absent parathyroid hormone levels. It most often occurs as part of an autoimmune syndrome associated with deficient function of one or more endocrine glands (adrenals, thyroid, and ovaries), pernicious anemia, alopecia, vitiligo, and mucocutaneous candidiasis. This disorder may be sporadic or familial. When familial, its inheritance appears to be autosomal recessive. Familial hypoparathyroidism may also occur as an isolated defect, the mode of inheritance varying in each kindred. Rarely congenital aplasia of the parathyroid glands may occur, usually in conjunction with defective development of the thymus (DiGeorge syndrome).

Postsurgical hypoparathyroidism, transient or permanent, may develop after neck surgery for thyroid disease as a result of inadvertent removal of or trauma to the parathyroid glands or their vascular supply. The widespread use of radioactive iodine to treat thyrotoxicosis has decreased the frequency of this occurrence. Neck exploration for primary hyperparathyroidism is now the most frequent situation in which postsurgical hypoparathyroidism occurs. Severe and prolonged hypocalcemia frequently develops after parathyroid surgery for osteitis fibrosis due to chronic renal insufficiency. In this situation, the relative hypoparathyroidism induced by the surgical procedure is complicated by deposition of available calcium into the healing bony lesions (hungry-bone syndrome). Severe magnesium deficiency (see Chapter 44) is a rather common cause of hypocalcemia. The normal serum magnesium level is 1.8 to 3.0 mg/dL (0.8 to

1.2 mmol/L). In general, the serum magnesium is less than 1.0 mg/dL (0.4 mmol/L) when hypocalcemia is due to hypomagnesemia. At least two pathogenetic mechanisms have been implicated. Impaired secretion of parathyroid hormone resulting in absolute or relative hypoparathyroidism is present in the vast majority of patients with hypocalcemia secondary to hypomagnesemia. Increased resistance to the action of parathyroid hormone at bone and kidney also was demonstrated in some patients with severe hypomagnesemia. A number of less common causes of hypoparathyroidism resulting from parathyroid hormone deficiency are listed in Table 1.

Hypocalcemia also may complicate a large number of primary disorders (Table 2) in patients who have intrinsically normal parathyroid glands. In these conditions, the fall in serum calcium caused by the underlying disease process results in a compensatory increase in parathyroid hormone secretion. This state of ''secondary hyperparathyroidism'' has the effect of raising the serum calcium, frequently into the low-normal range, by enhancing bone resorption, renal tubular calcium reabsorption, and where possible, gastrointestinal (GI) calcium absorption. The most common causes of hypocalcemia with normal parathyroid function (nonhypoparathyroid hypocalcemia) are related to deficiencies in vitamin D and/or its active metabolites (see Chapters 61, 62, 63) that accompany a large number of GI or renal diseases. The syndromes of parathyroid hormone resistance (pseudohypoparathyroidism) and vitamin D resistance, also accompanied by secondary hyperparathyroidism, are reviewed in Chapters 41 and 64, respectively. Other causes of hypocalcemia include acute pancreatitis (Chapter 43), osteoblastic metastases, multiple transfusions of citrated blood, and acute rhabdomyolysis. In each of these situations, when the secondary hyperparathyroidism is insufficient to compensate for the hypocalcemic stimulus, hypocalcemia ensues.

CLINICAL FEATURES OF HYPOCALCEMIA

The signs and symptoms of acute hypocalcemia (Table 3) primarily result from enhanced neuromuscular irritability. Sensations of numbness and tingling involving the fingertips, toes, and circumoral region are early symptoms. Increased neuromuscular irritability may be demonstrated at the bedside by eliciting Chvostek's sign or Trousseau's sign. Chvostek's sign is twitching of the circumoral muscles in response to gently tapping the facial nerve just anterior to the ear. It

TABLE 3. *Clinical features of hypocalcemia*

Neuromuscular irritability
Paresthesias
Chvostek's sign
Trousseau's sign
Laryngospasm
Bronchospasm
Tetany
Seizures
Prolonged QT interval on ECG

should be noted that approximately 10% of normal individuals will demonstrate a slight twitch in response to this maneuver. Trousseau's sign is carpal spasm elicited by inflation of a blood pressure cuff to 20 mm Hg above the patient's systolic blood pressure for 3 minutes. The classic response (flexion of the wrist and metacarpophalangeal joints, extension of the interphalangeal joints, and adduction of the digits) reflects the heightened irritability of the nerves resulting from ischemia in the region of the cuff. A positive Trousseau's sign is rare in the absence of significant hypocalcemia.

Muscle cramps are often experienced by hypocalcemic patients. They most commonly involve the lower back, legs, and feet. In severe or acute hypocalcemia, the muscle cramps may progress to spontaneous carpopedal spasm (tetany). Laryngospasm or bronchospasm also may develop. Seizures of all types (syncopal episodes, petit mal, grand mal, and focal) may occur whether the hypocalcemia is acute or chronic. Other central nervous system manifestations include irritability, impaired intellectual capacity, and personality disturbances. Severe hypocalcemia may be accompanied by prolongation of the QT interval on the electrocardiogram, and rarely, congestive heart failure; both cardiac manifestations are reversible with correction of the hypocalcemia. Although the presence of symptoms primarily reflects the degree of the hypocalcemia, a rapid rate of fall of the serum calcium and/or the concomitant presence of alkalosis, which enhances binding of ionized calcium to albumin, also may be associated with more severe signs and symptoms.

Patients with chronic hypocalcemia due to idiopathic hypoparathyroidism or pseudohypoparathyroidism also may have calcification of the basal ganglia and extrapyramidal neurologic symptoms. Subcapsular cataracts and abnormal dentition also are common in such patients (see Chapters 40, 41).

MANAGEMENT OF ACUTE HYPOCALCEMIA

Management of acute hypocalcemia is considered in this chapter. Therapy of chronic hypocalcemia is discussed in Chapters 40, 41, 63, and 64.

The decision to treat the hypocalcemic patient depends on the severity of the hypocalcemia, the rapidity with which it developed, and the presence or absence of clinical signs and symptoms. At one end of the spectrum, an asymptomatic patient with mild hypocalcemia (7.5 to 8.5 mg/dL, or 1.9 to 2.1 mmol/L) may warrant cautious observation and require only oral calcium supplements (500 to 1000 mg elemental calcium every 6 hours). In contrast, a patient with tetany, a sign of severe hypocalcemia, must be treated aggressively with intravenous calcium administration. Serum calcium levels of less than 7.5 mg/dL (1.9 mmol/L), or any level in a patient with symptoms, require parenteral calcium therapy.

The mainstay of therapy for acute symptomatic hypocalcemia is intravenous administration of calcium salts. Calcium should be administered with caution in digitalized patients, because sensitivity to the adverse effects of digitalis, particularly arrhythmias, is increased by hypercalcemia. Calcium gluconate (90 mg elemental calcium/10-mL ampule) is preferred to calcium chloride (272 mg elemental calcium/10-mL ampule) because it is less irritating to the veins. Initially, 1 to 2 ampules of calcium gluconate diluted in 50 to 100 mL of 5% dextrose (180 mg of elemental calcium) should be infused over a period of 5 to 10 minutes. This procedure should be repeated as necessary to control symptomatic hypocalcemia. Persistent or less severe hypocalcemia may be managed by administration of more dilute calcium solutions over longer periods. In general, 15 mg/kg of elemental calcium infused over a period of 4 to 6 hours will raise the serum calcium by 2 to 3 mg/dL (0.5 to 0.75 mmol/L). One practical approach is to initiate therapy with 10 ampules of calcium gluconate in 1 L of 5% dextrose infused at a rate of 50 mL/h (45 mg of elemental calcium/h); the rate of the infusion then may be titrated to maintain the serum calcium in the low-normal range. When volume is a concern, the concentration of the solution may be increased. However, solutions of greater than 200 mg/100 mL of elemental calcium (more than 2 ampules of calcium gluconate/100 mL) should be avoided because of the propensity for irritation of veins and, in the event of extravasation, soft tissues. If hypocalcemia is likely to persist, therapy should be initiated early with oral calcium supplements (1 to 2 g elemental calcium) and 1,25 (OH)$_2$ D (0.5 to 1.0 mg) daily.

The hypomagnesemic patient who is also hypocalcemic will require treatment of the hypomagnesemia before the hypocalcemia will resolve (Chapter 44). Moreover, in the acutely hypocalcemic patient in whom magnesium deficiency is clinically likely, it is appropriate to add magnesium to the treatment regimen while awaiting laboratory confirmation of hypomagnesemia.

SUGGESTED READINGS

1. Shane EJ, Bilezikian JP. Disorders of calcium, phosphate and magnesium metabolism. In: Askanazi J, Starker PM, Weissman C, eds. *Fluid and electrolyte management in critical care.* London: Butterworth, 1986:337–353.
2. Guise TA, Mundy GR. Evaluation of hypocalcemia in children and adults. *J Clin Endocrinol Metab* 1995;80:1473–1478.
3. Tohme JF, Bilezikian JP. Hypocalcemic emergencies. *Endocrinol Metab Clin North Am* 1993;22:363–375.

40. Hypoparathyroidism

David Goltzman, M.D. and *David E. C. Cole, M.D., Ph.D., F.R.C.P.C.

*Department of Medicine, McGill University and Royal Victoria Hospital, Montreal, Quebec, Canada; and *Departments of Laboratory Medicine and Pathobiology, University of Toronto, and Genetic Repository, The Toronto Hospital, Toronto, Ontario, Canada*

Hypoparathyroidism is a clinical disorder that manifests when the parathyroid hormone (PTH) produced by the parathyroid gland is insufficient to maintain extracellular fluid (ECF) calcium in the normal range, or when adequate circulating concentrations of PTH are unable to function optimally in target tissues to maintain normal ECF calcium levels. The causes of hypoparathyroidism (Table 1) can be classified broadly as (a) failure of parathyroid gland development, (b) destruction of the parathyroid glands, (c) reduced parathyroid gland function due to altered regulation, and (d) impaired PTH action. The common aspect of these conditions is the presence of reduced, biologically active PTH. This results in characteristic clinical and laboratory features, which may be influenced, however, by the specific pathogenetic mechanism.

CLINICAL MANIFESTATIONS

The acute clinical signs and symptoms of hypoparathyroidism of any etiology include evidence of latent or overt increased neuromuscular irritability due to hypocalcemia (Chapter 39). The acute symptoms may occur more readily during times of increased demand on the calcium homeostatic system (pregnancy and lactation, the menstrual cycle, and states of alkalosis). Chronically, patients may manifest muscle cramps, pseudopapilledema, extrapyramidal signs, mental retardation, and personality disturbances, as well as cataracts, dry rough skin, coarse brittle hair, alopecia, and abnormal dentition. The dental abnormalities may include defects due to enamel hypoplasia, defects in dentin, shortened premolar roots, thickened lamina dura, delayed tooth eruption, and increased frequency of dental caries. Occasionally patients may be edentulous. Finally, some patients may be diagnosed only after a low serum calcium is detected on routine blood screening.

LABORATORY ABNORMALITIES

The biochemical hallmarks of hypoparathyroidism are hypocalcemia and hyperphosphatemia in the presence of normal renal function. Serum calcium concentrations are often 6 to 7 mg/dL (1.50 to 1.75 mM) and serum phosphorus levels, 6 to 9 mg/dL (1.93 to 2.90 mM). In most instances, an ionized calcium concentration of less than 4 mEq/L (1.0 mM) also is observed. Serum concentrations of immunoreactive PTH are low or undetectable except in cases of PTH resistance, in which they are elevated or high normal (Chapter 41 and Appendix). Serum concentrations of 1,25-dihydroxyvitamin D are usually low or low normal, but alkaline phosphatase activity is unchanged. The 24-hour urinary excretion of calcium is reduced, although the fractional excretion of calcium is increased, because the filtered load is

TABLE 1. *Pathogenetic classification of hypoparathyroidism*

A. Failure of parathyroid gland development
  Isolated hypoparathyroidism
    X-linked (307700)[a]
    Autosomal recessive (241400)
  DiGeorge sequence (188400 and 601362)
    Barakat/Hypoparathyrodism, nerve deafness, and renal dysplasia (146255 and 256340)
    Hypoparathyroidism with short stature, mental retardation, and seizures (241410)
    Kenny–Caffey syndrome (127000 and 244460)
    Mitochondrial neuromyopathies
      Kearns–Sayre syndrome (530000)
      Pearson syndrome (557000)
      tRNA-Leu mutations (590050)
    Long-chain hydroxyacyl-CoA dehydrogenase deficiency (600890)
B. Destruction of the parathyroid glands
  Surgical
  Polyglandular autoimmune disease (APECED[c]) (240300)
  Radiation
  Metal overload (iron, copper)
  Granulomatous infiltration
  Neoplastic invasion
C. Reduced parathyroid gland function due to altered regulation
  Primary
    Autosomal dominant (146200)
      Calcium-sensing receptor mutation (145980)[b]
      Parathyroid hormone (PTH) mutation (168450.0001)
    Autosomal recessive
      PTH mutation (168450.0002)
  Secondary
    Maternal hyperparathyroidism
    Hypomagnesemia
D. Impaired parathyroid hormone action
  Hypomagnesemia
  Pseudohypoparathyroidism

[a] Numbers refer to standardized entries in the McKusick catalog, "Online Mendelian Inheritance in Man." It can be accessed through the internet address http://www3.ncbi.nlm.nih.gov/Omim/ or by browsing the web by using the search term OMIM.

[b] May also be sporadic if the mutation is *de novo*.

[c] APECED, Autoimmune polyglandular candidiasis ectodermal dystrophy syndrome.

lower still, because of the hypocalcemia induced by lower intestinal calcium absorption and diminished bone resorption. Nephrogenous cyclic adenosine monophosphate (AMP) excretion is low, and renal tubular reabsorption of phosphorus is elevated. Urinary cyclic AMP and phosphorus excretion both increase markedly after administration of exogenous bioactive PTH (Ellsworth–Howard test; see Chapter 41) except in PTH-resistant states.

Calcification of the basal ganglia or more widespread intracranial structures may be detected on routine radiographs or by enhanced imaging [computed tomography (CT) scan or magnetic resonance imaging (MRI)], and electroencephalographic changes may be present. These are occasionally the only clinical evidence of disease. Detection of limited parathyroid gland reserve may require an ethylenediaminetetraacetate (EDTA)-infusion study, which should be conducted only under close supervision.

CAUSES OF HYPOPARATHYROIDISM

Failure of the Parathyroid Glands to Develop

Congenital agenesis or hypoplasia of the parathyroid glands can produce hypoparathyroidism that manifests in the newborn period. This may occur as isolated hypoparathyroidism (autosomal recessive or X-linked; the precise molecular genetic defects are unknown). It also is seen in infants who have thymic aplasia with immunodeficiency and congenital conotruncal cardiac anomalies. Genetic studies indicate that a wide range of etiologies, both genetic and environmental (Table 2), may underlie the developmental abnormalities of the third and fourth branchial pouches that lead to this group of disorders. Syndromologists have termed this condition the DiGeorge sequence to emphasize its etiologic heterogeneity and focus attention on other clinical findings that may suggest a primary cause (Table 2). Hypoparathyroidism is a potential problem in any syndrome that includes the DiGeorge sequence. If the DiGeorge sequence of anomalies (now considered to include distinctive facial features, cleft lip/palate, and a wider variety of congenital heart disease) is not clearly part of another syndrome, it is likely the result of a microdeletion on the long arm of chromosome 22. Detection of the microdeletion of chromosomal band 22q11.21-q11.23 by using Fluorescence In Situ Hybridization (FISH) is diagnostic. A negative result does not completely exclude the possibility of a 22q abnormality. A small group of DiGeorge patients have been shown to carry deletions on the short arm of chromosome 10, but

TABLE 2. *Conditions with DiGeorge sequence*

Chromosomal
  dup(1q)
  del(5p)
  dup(8q)
  del(10p)—(601362)[a]
  del(22q)—(188400 and 192430)[a]
Monogenic
  Isolated autosomal dominant
  Isolated autosomal recessive
  Velocardiofacial syndrome or "CATCH 22"
  Zellweger syndrome
Teratogenic
  Diabetic embryopathy
  Fetal alcohol syndrome
  Retinoid embryopathy
Associational
  Arhinencephalia/DiGeorge
  CHARGE/DiGeorge[b]
  Cardiofacial/DiGeorge

[a] Small interstitial deletions at these loci may be detected by FISH or related cytogenetic techniques.

[b] CHARGE association: **C**oloboma of the iris, **H**eart disease, Choanal **a**tresia, **R**etarded growth and development, **G**enital anomalies, **E**ar anomalies.

detailed molecular studies suggest there may be no shortest-region-of-overlap (SRO), and more than one contiguous locus on 10p for parathyroid development has been proposed. Karyotypic abnormalities on other chromosomes also were reported (Table 2), and the possibility that still other genetic loci will be identified as essential for parathyroid development should be kept in mind.

Individuals with the velocardiofacial (or Schprintzen) syndrome also have microdeletions of 22q, and it is now believed that the two conditions overlap. The term "CATCH 22" has been applied to this cluster of disorders, as a mnemonic for the characteristic features (**C**ardiac anomalies, **A**bnormal facies, **T**hymic aplasia, **C**left palate, **H**ypocalcemia with **22**q deletion). All patients with otherwise unexplained persistent hypoparathyroidism in infancy should be karyotyped ($\pm$ FISH for 22q11 or 10p microdeletions) and evaluated for other occult anomalies, including subclinical cardiac disease, renal dysplasia, and occasionally gastrointestinal maldevelopment. Although many cases of DiGeorge sequence are the result of *de novo* deletions, autosomal dominant inheritance is not uncommon. Demonstration of decreased parathyroid reserve in an otherwise healthy parent may require provocative testing, but evidence of dominant inheritance may depend on other features (conotruncal cardiac anomalies, renal dysplasia, decreased cell-mediated immunity, etc.).

As a rule, microdeletions are associated with a variable phenotype, even within a family. Less well-defined syndromes with hypoparathyroidism (Table 1), such as the Barakat or HDR (**H**ypoparathyroidism, Nerve **D**eafness and **Re**nal Dysplasia) syndrome, may be extremes of the identified chromosomal microdeletion phenotypes, rather than entities of a different genetic etiology. In one patient with HDR syndrome, a 10p deletion was identified. In patients with congenital hypoparathyroidism, short stature, and mental retardation syndrome, similarities to the DiGeorge sequence have been noted, but genetic mapping suggests a locus on chromosome 1q42-43. The Kenny–Caffey syndrome, another congenital anomaly, is associated with absent parathyroid tissue, growth retardation, and medullary stenosis of tubular bones. Analysis of the PTH gene in this syndrome revealed no defect. Both dominant and recessive modes of inheritance have been observed.

Hypoparathyroidism also is a variable component of the neuromyopathies caused by mitochondrial gene defects. Among the clinical conditions are the Kearns–Sayre syndrome (ophthalmoplegia, retinal degeneration, and cardiac-conduction defects), the Pearson marrow pancreas syndrome (lactic acidosis, neutropenia, sideroblastic anemia, and pancreatic exocrine dysfunction), and mitochondrial encephalomyopathy. The molecular defects range from large deletions of the mitochrondrial genomes in an extensive range of tissues (Pearson syndrome) to single base-pair mutations in one of the transfer RNA genes found only in a restricted range of cell types (mitochondrial encephalomyopathy). Another unusual myopathy associated with an inborn error of fatty acid oxidation (**L**ong-**C**hain **H**ydroxy**A**cyl**C**oA **D**ehydrogenase deficiency or LCHAD) also may be accompanied by hypoparathyroidism. This condition manifests as nonketotic hypoglycemia, cardiomyopathy, hepatic dysfunction, and developmental delay and is associated with maternal fatty liver of pregnancy.

Destruction of the Parathyroid Glands

The most common cause of hypoparathyroidism is surgical excision of or damage to the parathyroid glands as a result of total thyroidectomy for thyroid cancer, radical neck dissection for other cancers, or repeated operations for primary hyperparathyroidism. Transient and reversible hypocalcemia following parathyroid surgery may be due to (a) edema or hemorrhage into the parathyroids, (b) hungry-bone syndrome due to severe hyperparathyroidism, or (c) postoperative hypomagnesemia. Prolonged hypocalcemia, which may develop immediately or weeks to years after neck surgery, suggests permanent hypoparathyroidism. The incidence of this condition after neck exploration for primary hyperparathyroidism is usually less than 5%. In patients with a higher risk of developing permanent hypoparathyroidism, such as those with primary parathyroid hyperplasia or with repeated neck explorations required to identify an adenoma, parathyroid tissue may be autotransplanted into the brachioradialis or sternocleidomastoid muscle at the time of parathyroidectomy or cryopreserved for subsequent transplantation, as necessary.

Rarely hypoparathyroidism was described in a small number of patients who received extensive radiation to the neck and mediastinum. It also was reported in metal overload diseases such as hemochromatosis (iron), thalassemia (iron), and Wilson's disease (copper), and in neoplastic or granulomatous infiltration of the parathyroid glands.

Hypoparathyroidism also may occur as a presumed autoimmune disorder either alone or in association with other endocrine deficiency states. Antibodies directed against parathyroid tissue can be detected in 33% of patients with isolated disease and 41% of patients with hypoparathyroidism and other endocrine deficiencies. The genetic etiology of the autosomal recessive polyglandular disorder, APECED (**A**utoimmune **P**olyglandular **E**ndocrinopathy **C**andidiasis **E**ctodermal **D**ystrophy syndrome), has been traced to mutations of the autoimmune regulator (AIRE) gene on chromosome 21q22.3, which encodes a unique protein with characteristics of a transcription factor. This condition also has been called "hypoparathyroidism, Addison's disease, moniliasis" (HAM), polyglandular autoimmune syndrome (PGA), and autoimmune polyglandular syndrome (APS). The most common associated manifestations are mucocutaneous candidiasis (65% to 75%) and Addison's disease (55% to 60%). Adrenal insufficiency occurs in only 10% of all patients with hypoparathyroidism, and moniliasis, in only 15%, so that their presence together should suggest polyglandular deficiency. Hypoparathyroidism, either as an isolated autoimmune disorder or as part of APECED, may present between age 6 months and 20 years (average age, 7 to 8 years). Because hypoparathyroidism presents 1 to 4 years after candidiasis or Addison's disease manifests, few individuals with isolated autoimmune adrenal insufficiency later develop hypoparathyroidism. Candidiasis may affect the skin, nails, and mucous membranes of the mouth and vagina and is often intractable. Addison's disease can mask the presence of hypoparathyroidism or may manifest only in improvement of the hypoparathyroidism with a reduced requirement for calcium and vitamin D. The etiology of this association is not understood. By diminishing gastrointestinal absorption of calcium and increasing renal calcium excretion, glucocorticoid therapy for the adrenal insufficiency may exacerbate the hypocalcemia and could prove lethal if introduced before the hypoparathyroidism is recognized.

In addition to Addison's disease and moniliasis, hypoparathyroidism in APECED may be associated with insulin-dependent diabetes mellitus, primary hypogonadism, autoimmune thyroiditis, keratoconjunctivitis, pernicious anemia, chronic active hepatitis, steatorrhea (malabsorption resembling celiac disease), alopecia (totalis or areata), and vitiligo. Pernicious anemia and diabetes mellitus usually develop after hypoparathyroidism.

Reduced Parathyroid Gland Function Due to Altered Regulation

Altered regulation of parathyroid gland function may be primary or secondary. Secondary causes include maternal hyperparathyroidism and hypomagnesemia. The infant of a mother with primary hyperparathyroidism generally develops hypocalcemia within the first 3 weeks of life, but it may occur up to a year after birth (Chapter 42). Although therapy may be required acutely, the disorder is usually self-limited. Hypomagnesemia due to defective intestinal absorption or renal tubular reabsorption of magnesium may impair secretion of PTH, and in this way, contribute to hypoparathyroidism (Chapter 44). Magnesium replacement will correct the hypoparathyroidism.

Primary alterations of parathyroid gland regulation now have a firm genetic basis. To date, three rare genetic defects have been defined.

The largest group involves the calcium-sensing receptor (CASR or CaR). Discovery of this plasma membrane G-protein linked receptor and cloning of the CASR gene found on chromosome 3q13.3-q21 led to new insights into the regulation of PTH secretion. CASR mutations that result in constitutive activated protein (that is, a receptor with a decreased setpoint for extracellular calcium concentrations) cause a functional hypoparathyroid state with hypocalcemia and hypercalciuria. In cases in which the mutations are transmitted through several generations, the picture is one of familial autosomal dominant hypoparathyroidism. In other cases, sporadic disease has been shown to arise from *de novo* activating mutations of the gene. The consequence of the activated parathyroid gland CASR is chronic suppression of PTH secretion, whereas the activated CASR receptor in kidney induces hypercalciuria, which exacerbates the hypocalcemia. In many instances, however, the degree of hypocalcemia and hypercalciuria may be mild and therefore well tolerated. For subjects without symptoms, the greatest threat can be excessive intervention with vitamin D. On the other hand, individuals who are aware of the condition are more likely to identify the early, nonspecific signs and symptoms of hypocalcemia and thereby avert the sudden, unexpected onset of more serious manifestations, such as tetany and seizures.

Isolated hypoparathyroidism also has been found with a single base substitution in exon 2 of the *PTH* gene. This mutation in the signal sequence of PTH apparently impedes conversion of pre-pro-PTH to pro-PTH, thereby reducing normal production of the mature hormone. In another family with autosomal recessive isolated hypoparathyroidism, the

entire exon 2 of the *PTH* gene was deleted. This exon contains the initiation codon and a portion of the signal sequence required for peptide translocation at the endoplasmic reticulum in the process of generating a mature secretory peptide.

Impaired PTH Action

Although in theory, a bioinactive form of PTH could be synthesized and secreted by the parathyroid gland, this has not been documented. An early report suggesting this as a mechanism underlying hypoparathyroidism was not supported in a follow-up study. More commonly, ineffective PTH action appears to be due to peripheral resistance to the effects of PTH. Such resistance may occur secondary to hypomagnesemia (Chapter 44) or as a primary disorder (pseudohypoparathyroidism, Chapter 41).

THERAPY

The major goal of therapy in all hypoparathyroid states is to restore serum calcium and phosphorus as close to normal as possible. The main pharmacologic agents available are supplemental calcium and vitamin D preparations. Phosphate binders and thiazide diuretics may be useful ancillary agents. The major impediment to restoration of normocalcemia is the development of hypercalciuria, with a resulting predilection for renal stone formation. With the loss of the renal calcium-retaining effect of PTH, the enhanced calcium absorption of the gut induced by vitamin D therapy results in an increased filtered load of calcium, which is readily cleared through the kidney. Consequently, urinary calcium excretion frequently increases in response to vitamin D supplementation well before serum calcium is normalized. It is often necessary or even desirable to aim for a low normal serum calcium concentration to prevent chronic hypercalciuria. If urine calcium concentrations are high and the serum calcium is still less than 8 mg/dL (2 mM), addition of a thiazide diuretic may reduce urinary calcium and raise serum calcium into the normal range. If serum calcium is normalized and the serum phosphorus remains greater than 6 mg/dL (1.93 mM), a nonabsorbable antacid may be added to reduce the hyperphosphatemia and prevent metastatic calcification. Dairy products, which are high in phosphate, should be avoided, and calcium administered in the form of supplements. Generally, at least 1 g/day of elemental calcium is required.

A variety of vitamin D preparations may be used including (a) vitamin D_3 or D_2, 25,000 to 100,000 U (1.25 to 5 mg) per day; (b) dihydrotachysterol, 0.2 to 1.2 mg per day; (c) 1-α-hydroxyvitamin D_3, 0.5 to 2.0 μg/day; or (d) calcitriol [1,25 (OH)$_2$ D_3], 0.25 to 1.0 μg/day. Although vitamins D_3 and D_2 are the least expensive forms of therapy, they have the longest duration of action and can result in prolonged toxicity. The other preparations listed all have the advantage of shorter half-lives and no requirement for renal 1-α-hydroxylation, which is impaired in hypoparathyroidism. Dihydrotachysterol is rarely used today, however, and calcitriol is probably the treatment of choice. In children, these preparations should be prescribed on a body-weight basis.

Close monitoring of urine calcium, serum calcium, and serum phosphate are required in the first month or so, but follow-up at 3- to 6-month intervals may be adequate once stable laboratory values are reached. Until recently, only patients with healthy preoperative parathyroid glands who underwent total parathyroidectomy were in a position to benefit from autotransplantation of an excised gland. However, allotransplantation has been successfully achieved by inserting semipermeable microcapsules containing cultivated parathyroid tissue in the brachioradialis muscle of a few patients. This could be a new alternative to life-long medication for some forms of hypoparathyroidism.

SUGGESTED READINGS

1. Bergada I, Schiffrin A, Abu Srair H, et al. Kenny syndrome: description of additional abnormalities and molecular studies. *Hum Genet* 1988;80:39–42.
2. Cohen MM Jr, Cole DEC. Origins of recognizable syndromes: etiologic and pathogenetic mechanisms and the process of syndrome delineation. *J Pediatr* 1989;115:161–164.
3. Daw SCM, Taylor C, Kraman M, et al. A common region of 10p deleted in diGeorge and velocardiofacial syndromes. *Nat Genet* 1996;13:458–460.
4. Gidding SS, Minciotti AL, Langman CB. Unmasking of hypoparathyroidism in familial partial DiGeorge syndrome by challenge with disodium edetate. *N Engl J Med* 1988;319:1589–1591.
5. Glover TW. CATCHing a break on 22. *Nat Genet* 1995;10:257–258.
6. Gottlieb S, Driscoll DA, Punnett HH, Sellinger B, Emanuel BS, Budarf ML. Characterization of 10p deletions suggests two nonoverlapping regions contribute to the DiGeorge syndrome phenotype. *Am J Hum Genet* 1998;62:495–498.
7. Harvey JN, Barnett D. Endocrine dysfunction in Kearns-Sayre syndrome. *Clin Endocrinol* 1992;37:97–103.
8. Hasse C, Klöck G, Schlosser A, Zimmermann U, Rothmund M. Parathyroid allotransplantation without immunosuppression. *Lancet* 1997;350:1296–1297.
9. Herrera M, Grant C, van Heerden JA, Fitzpatrick LA. Parathyroid autotransplantation. *Arch Surg* 1992;127:825–829.
10. Illum F, Dupont E. Prevalence of CT-detected calcification in the basal ganglia in idiopathic hypoparathyroidism and pseudohypoparathyroidism. *Neuroradiology* 1985;27:32–37.
11. Mallette L. Synthetic human parathyroid hormone 1-34 fragment for diagnostic testing. *Ann Intern Med* 1988;109:800–802.
12. Mumm S, Whyte MP, Thakker RV, Buetow KH, Schlessinger D. mtDNA analysis shows common ancestry in two kindreds with X-linked recessive hypoparathyroidism and reveals a heteroplasmic silent mutation. *Am J Hum Genet* 1997;60:153–159.
13. Okano O, Furukawa Y, Morii H, Fujita T. Comparative efficacy of various vitamin D metabolites in the treatment of various types of hypoparathyroidism. *J Clin Endocrinol Metab* 1982;55:238–243.
14. Parkinson DB, Thakker RV. A donor splice site mutation in the parathyroid hormone gene is associated with autosomal recessive hypoparathyroidism. *Nat Genet* 1992;1:149–152.
15. Parvari R, Hershkovitz E, Kanis A, et al. Homozygosity and linkage-disequilibrium mapping of the syndrome of congenital hypoparathyroidism, growth and mental retardation, and dysmorphism to a 1-cm interval on chromosome 1q42-43. *Am J Hum Genet* 1998;63:163–169.
16. Pollak MR, Brown EM, Estep HL, et al. Autosomal dominant hypocalcemia caused by a Ca^{2+}-sensing receptor gene mutation. *Nat Genet* 1994;8:303–307.
17. Seneca S, DeMeirleir L, DeSchepper J, et al. Pearson marrow pancreas syndrome: a molecular study and clinical management. *Clin Genet* 1997;51:338–342.
18. Sherwood LM, Santora AC. II. Hypoparathyroid states in the differential diagnosis of hypocalcemia. In: Bilezikian JP, Marcus R, Levine MA, eds. *The parathyroids*. New York: Raven Press, 1994: 747–752.

41. Parathyroid Hormone Resistance Syndromes

Michael A. Levine, M.D.

Division of Endocrinology, Department of Pediatrics, The Johns Hopkins University School of Medicine, Baltimore, Maryland

The term *pseudohypoparathyroidism* (PHP) describes a group of disorders characterized by biochemical hypoparathyroidism (i.e., hypocalcemia and hyperphosphatemia), increased secretion of parathyroid hormone (PTH), and target tissue unresponsiveness to the biological actions of PTH.

In the initial description of PHP, Fuller Albright et al. (1) focused on the failure of patients with this syndrome to show either a calcemic or a phosphaturic response to administered parathyroid extract. These observations provided the basis for the hypothesis that biochemical hypoparathyroidism in PHP was due not to a deficiency of PTH but rather to resistance of the target organs, bone and kidney, to the biologic actions of PTH. Thus the pathophysiology of PHP differs fundamentally from true hypoparathyroidism, in which PTH secretion rather than PTH responsiveness is defective.

The initial event in the expression of PTH action is binding of the hormone to specific receptors located on the plasma membrane of target cells. Because the native and cloned receptors (2) also bind PTH-related protein with equivalent affinity, they are termed PTH/PTHrP receptors. The PTH/PTHrP receptor is coupled by heterotrimeric guanine nucleotide–binding regulatory proteins (G proteins) to signal effector molecules localized to the inner surface of the plasma membrane. Hormone binding is followed rapidly by the generation of a variety of second messengers, including cyclic adenosine monophosphate (cAMP), inositol 1,4,5-trisphosphate and diacylglycerol, and cytosolic calcium, indicating that a single PTH/PTHrP receptor can couple not only to G_s to stimulate adenylyl cyclase, but also to G_q and G_{11} to stimulate phospholipase C (Fig. 1). The best-characterized mediator of PTH action is cAMP, which rapidly activates protein kinase A. The relevant target proteins that are phosphorylated by protein kinase A, and the precise

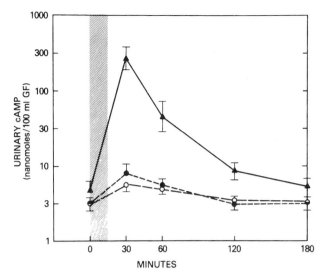

FIG. 1. cAMP excretion in urine in response to the intravenous administration of bovine parathyroid extract (300 USP units) from 9:00 a.m. to 9:15 a.m. The peak response in normals *(triangles)* is 50- to 100-fold times basal; patients with PHP type Ia *(solid circles)* or PHP type Ib *(open circles)* show only a two- to fivefold response.

actions of these proteins, have not yet been fully characterized but include enzymes, ion channels, and proteins that regulate gene expression. In contrast to the well-recognized effects of the second-messenger cAMP in bone and kidney cells, the physiological importance of the phospholipase C signaling pathway in these PTH target tissues has not yet been established. For a complete discussion, see Chapters 13 and 14.

PATHOGENESIS OF PSEUDOHYPOPARATHYROIDISM

Characterization of the molecular basis for PHP commenced with the observation that cAMP mediates many of the actions of PTH on kidney and bone and that administration of biologically active PTH to normal subjects leads to a significant increase in the urinary excretion of nephrogenous cAMP (3). The PTH-infusion test remains the most reliable test available for the diagnosis of PHP and allows distinction between the several variants of the syndrome (Fig. 1). Thus patients with PHP type I fail to show an appropriate increase in urinary excretion of both cAMP and phosphate, whereas subjects with the less common type II form show a normal increase in urinary cAMP excretion but have an impaired phosphaturic response.

Pseudohypoparathyroidism Type I

The blunted nephrogenous cAMP response to exogenous PTH in subjects with PHP type I first suggested that PTH resistance is caused by a defect in the adenylyl cyclase complex that produces cAMP in renal tubule cells (4). Recent studies (5) showed that the hormone-sensitive adenylyl cy-

clase system is far more complex than originally suspected, consisting of at least three membrane-bound components: specific receptors, adenylyl cyclase, and the heterotrimeric (α, β, γ) G proteins that couple ligand-activated receptors to stimulate (G_s) or inhibit (G_i) catalytic activity.

Pseudohypoparathyroidism Type Ia

Albright's original description of PHP emphasized PTH resistance as the biochemical hallmark of this disorder. Resistance to PTH alone would be consistent with a defect in the cell-surface receptor specific for PTH. However, some patients with PHP type I display resistance to multiple hormones, including PTH, thyroid-stimulating hormone (TSH), gonadotropins, and glucagon, whose effects are mediated by cAMP (6). Cell membranes from most of these patients have an approximately 50% reduction in expression or activity of $G_s\alpha$ protein, a property that defines this condition as PHP type Ia. The generalized deficiency of $G_s\alpha$ may impair the ability of many hormones and neurotransmitters to activate adenylyl cyclase and thereby produce hormone resistance.

In addition to hormone resistance, patients with PHP type Ia manifest a peculiar constellation of developmental and somatic defects that are collectively termed Albright's hereditary osteodystrophy (AHO) (1). The AHO phenotype consists of short stature, round facies, obesity, brachydactyly, and subcutaneous ossifications, but other sensory–neural abnormalities also may be present (7). The subsequent identification of individuals with AHO who lacked apparent hormone resistance led Albright to propose the rather awkward term *pseudopseudohypoparathyroidism* (pseudoPHP) to describe this normocalcemic variant of PHP (8). Subjects with pseudoPHP have a normal urinary cAMP response to PTH (3,9), which distinguishes them from occasional patients with PHP type Ia who maintain normal serum calcium levels without treatment (10). PseudoPHP is genetically related to PHP type Ia. Within a given kindred, some affected members will have only AHO (i.e., pseudoPHP), whereas others will have hormone resistance as well (i.e., PHP type Ia), despite equivalent functional deficiency of $G_s\alpha$ in tissues that have been analyzed (9). It therefore seems reasonable to use the term AHO to simplify description of these two variants of the same syndrome and to acknowledge the common clinical and biochemical characteristics that patients with PHP type Ia and pseudoPHP share.

$G_s\alpha$ deficiency in patients with AHO results from heterozygous inactivating mutations in the GNAS1 gene, a complex gene that maps to 20q13.2 (11). $G_s\alpha$ is encoded by 13 exons, with four forms (45 kDa and 52 kDa) generated by the inclusion or exclusion of exon 3 and by using alternative splice sites in intron 3 (12). Moreover, there appear to be additional exons upstream of the originally described exon 1 that are spliced onto exon 2 to yield alternative GNAS1 messenger RNA (mRNA) species that encode novel G proteins such as XLαs (13,14).

Molecular studies of DNA from subjects with AHO disclosed a variety of GNAS1 gene mutations (reviewed in ref. 7) that account for autosomal dominant inheritance of the disorder. Although most gene mutations impair expression of $G_s\alpha$ mRNA, in some subjects, abnormal forms of $G_s\alpha$ mRNA are produced that encode dysfunctional $G_s\alpha$ proteins (15–17). With few exceptions, distinct GNAS1 gene mutations have been found in affected individuals, implying that new and independent mutations sustain the disorder (7).

These studies confirm the molecular defect in AHO, but they do not explain the striking variability in biochemical and clinical phenotype. Why do some $G_s\alpha$-coupled pathways show reduced hormone responsiveness (e.g. PTH, TSH, gonadotropins), whereas other pathways are clinically unaffected [adrenocorticotropic hormone (ACTH) in the adrenal and vasopressin in the renal medulla]? Perhaps even more intriguing is the paradox of why some subjects with $G_s\alpha$ deficiency have hormone resistance (PHP type Ia), whereas others may lack hormone resistance (pseudoPHP) or physical features of AHO altogether (18).

The basis for the variable penetrance of these features in patients with AHO remains unknown. Analysis of published pedigrees indicated that in most cases, maternal transmission of $G_s\alpha$ deficiency leads to PHP type Ia, whereas paternal transmission of the defect leads to pseudoPHP (9,19–21), findings that implicated genomic imprinting of the GNAS1 gene as a possible mechanism (20). Although recent studies provided compelling evidence that the human GNAS1 gene is indeed imprinted, the imprinting appears to be promoter specific (14). Thus, although XLαs expression is active from only the paternal allele (14), $G_s\alpha$ expression, directed by the promoter upstream of exon 1, appears to be biallelic in fetal (22) and adult (14,18,23) human tissues. By contrast, recent analyses of heterozygous Gnas knockout mice suggest that $G_s\alpha$ expression may derive from only the maternal allele in some tissues (e.g., renal cortex) and from both alleles in other tissues (e.g., renal medulla) (24). Accordingly, mice that inherit the defective Gnas gene maternally express only that allele in imprinted tissues, such as the PTH-sensitive renal proximal tubule, in which there is no functional $G_s\alpha$ protein. By contrast, the 50% reduction in $G_s\alpha$ expression that occurs in nonimprinted tissues, which express both Gnas alleles, may account for more variable and moderate hormone resistance in these sites. Confirmation of this proposed mechanism in patients with AHO will require demonstration that the human $G_s\alpha$ transcript is paternally imprinted in the renal cortex.

In AHO, inherited $G_s\alpha$ gene mutations reduce expression or function of $G_s\alpha$ protein. By contrast, in the McCune–Albright syndrome, somatic mutations in the $G_s\alpha$ gene enhance activity of the protein (25). These mutations lead to constitutive activation of adenylyl cyclase and produce proliferation and autonomous hyperfunction of hormonally responsive cells. The clinical significance of $G_s\alpha$ activity as a determinant of hormone action is emphasized by the recent description by Iiri et al. (26) of two boys with both precocious puberty and PHP type Ia. These two unrelated boys had identical GNAS1 gene mutations that resulted in a temperature-sensitive $G_s\alpha$ that is constitutively activated in the cooler environment of the testis, while being rapidly degraded in other tissues at normal body temperature. Thus different tissues in these two individuals could show hormone resistance (to PTH and TSH), hormone responsiveness (to ACTH), or hormone independence [to luteinizing hormone (LH)].

Pseudohypoparathyroidism Type Ib

Subjects with PHP type I who lack features of AHO typically show hormone resistance that is limited to PTH target tissues and have normal $G_s\alpha$ activity (6). This variant is termed PHP type Ib. Although most cases of PHP type Ib appear to be sporadic, familial cases have been described in which transmission of the defect is most consistent with an autosomal dominant pattern (27).

As in PHP type Ia, subjects with PHP type Ib have a defective nephrogenous cAMP response to PTH (Fig. 1). However, subjects with PHP type Ib who have elevated levels of PTH often manifest skeletal lesions similar to those that occur in patients with hyperparathyroidism (28). These observations suggested that at least one intracellular signaling pathway coupled to the PTH receptor may be intact in patients with PHP type Ib.

Specific resistance of target tissues to PTH, and normal activity of $G_s\alpha$, implicated decreased expression or function of the PTH/PTHrP receptor (type 1 PTH receptor) as the cause for hormone resistance. Fibroblasts from some, but not all, PHP type Ib patients accumulate less cAMP in response to PTH (29) and contain decreased levels of mRNA encoding the PTH/PTHrP receptor (30). Furthermore, in most cases, pretreatment of the cultured fibroblasts with dexamethasone normalized the PTH-induced cAMP response and increased expression of PTH/PTHrP receptor mRNA (30). Several lines of evidence suggest that the primary defect in PHP type Ib is not in the gene encoding the PTH/PTHrP receptor, however. First, molecular studies failed to disclose mutations in the coding exons (31) and promoter regions (32) of the PTH/PTHrP receptor gene or its mRNA (33). Second, mice (34) and humans (35) that are heterozygous for inactivation of the gene encoding the PTH/PTHrP receptor do not manifest PTH resistance or hypocalcemia. Third, inheritance of two defective type PTH/PTHrP receptor genes results in Blomstrand chondrodysplasia, a lethal genetic disorder characterized by advanced endochondral bone maturation (35). Thus it is likely that the molecular defect in PHP type Ib resides in other gene(s) that regulate expression or activity of the PTH/PTHrP receptor. One potential candidate has been mapped to a region near the GNAS1 gene (36).

Pseudohypoparathyroidism Type Ic

In a few patients with PHP type I, resistance to multiple hormones occurs in the absence of a demonstrable defect in G_s or G_i (6). The nature of the lesion in such patients is unclear, but it could be related to some other general component of the receptor–adenylyl cyclase system, such as the catalytic unit (37). Alternatively, these patients could have functional defects of G_s (or G_i) that do not become apparent in the assays presently available.

Pseudohypoparathyroidism Type II

Pseudohypoparathyroidism type II is a heterogeneous disorder without a clear genetic or familial basis. In these patients renal resistance to PTH is manifested by a reduced phosphaturic response to administration of PTH, despite a normal increase in urinary cAMP excretion (4). These observations suggest that the PTH receptor–adenylyl cyclase complex functions normally to increase cAMP in response to PTH and are consistent with a model in which PTH resistance arises from an inability of intracellular cAMP to activate downstream targets. Although no supportive data are yet available, a defective cAMP-dependent protein kinase has been proposed as a potential candidate (4). Alternatively, disruption of another PTH-sensitive signal-transduction pathway might be responsible for PTH resistance in subjects with PHP type II.

A PTH Inhibitor as a Cause of PTH Resistance

Several studies reported an apparent dissociation between circulating levels of immunoreactive and bioactive PTH in patients with PHP type 1. Despite high levels of immunoreactive PTH, the levels of bioactive PTH in many patients with PHP type I have been found to be within the normal range when measured *in vitro* with highly sensitive cytochemical bioassay systems. Furthermore, plasma from many of these patients was shown to diminish the biologic activity of exogenous PTH in these *in vitro* bioassays (38). The identity of this putative inhibitor or antagonist is unknown, and its relation to PTH action *in vivo* remains unsubstantiated. Although it is conceivable that a circulating factor may cause PTH resistance in some patients with PHP, it is more likely that these circulating antagonists arise as a consequence of the sustained secondary hyperparathyroidism that results from the primary biochemical defect.

DIAGNOSIS OF PSEUDOHYPOPARATHYROIDISM

A diagnosis of PHP should be considered in an individual who has functional hypoparathyroidism (i.e., hypocalcemia and hyperphosphatemia) and an elevated plasma concentration of immunoreactive PTH. Because hypomagnesemia is associated with reduced responsiveness to PTH, it is important to measure serum concentrations of magnesium in these subjects. Moreover, similar biochemical features may occur in some patients who have severe vitamin D deficiency (39). Although hypocalcemia is usually the presenting feature of PHP, unusual initial manifestations of PHP include neonatal hypothyroidism, unexplained cardiac failure, Parkinson's disease, and spinal cord compression (7).

The diagnosis of PHP (or pseudoPHP) also may be suspected on the basis of clinical features of AHO. However, several features of AHO (e.g., obesity, round face, brachydactyly, and mental retardation) are common to other disorders (Prader–Willi syndrome, acrodysostosis, Ullrich–Turner syndrome) that are often associated with chromosomal defects. A growing number of reports described small terminal deletions of chromosome 2q in patients with variable AHO-like phenotypes. Terminal deletion of 2q37 [del(2)(q37.3)] is the first consistent karyotypic abnormality that has been documented in patients with an AHO-like syndrome (40,41). These patients have normal endocrine function and normal $G_s\alpha$ activity, however (41).

Thus high-resolution chromosome analysis, biochemical/molecular analysis, and careful physical and radiologic examination are essential in discriminating between these phenocopies and AHO.

The classic tests for PHP, the Ellsworth–Howard test, and later modifications by Chase et al. (3), involved the administration of 200 to 300 USP units of purified bovine PTH or parathyroid extract. Although these preparations are no longer available, the synthetic human PTH(1-34) peptide has been approved for human use, and several protocols for its use in the differential diagnosis of hypoparathyroidism have been developed (42,43). The patient should be fasting, supine except for voiding, and hydrated (250 mL of water hourly from 6 a.m. to noon). Two control urine specimens are collected before 9 a.m. Synthetic human PTH(1-34) peptide [5 units (0.625 μg)/kg body weight to a maximum of 200 units or 25 μg] is administered intravenously from 9 to 9:15 a.m., and experimental urine specimens are collected from 9 to 9:30, 9:30 to 10:00, 10:00 to 11:00, and 11:00 to 12:00. Blood samples should be obtained at 9 a.m. and 11 a.m. for measurement of serum creatinine and phosphorus concentrations. Urine samples are analyzed for cAMP, phosphorus, and creatinine concentrations, and results are expressed as nanomoles of cAMP per 100 mL glomerular filtrate (GF) and tubular maximum of phosphate (TmP)/glomerular filtration rate (GFR) for phosphorous. Normal subjects and patients with hormonopenic hypoparathyroidism usually display a 10- to 20-fold increase in urinary cAMP excretion, whereas patients with PHP type I (types Ia and Ib), regardless of their serum calcium concentration, will show a markedly blunted response (Fig. 1). Thus this test can distinguish patients with so-called "normocalcemic" PHP (i.e., patients with PTH resistance who are able to maintain normal serum calcium levels without treatment) from subjects with pseudoPHP (who will have a normal urinary cAMP response to PTH (3,9)). The urinary cAMP and phosphate responses to PTH are dependent on the endogenous serum PTH and calcium levels (44), and treatment with vitamin D to normalize serum calcium levels may normalize the phosphaturic response to PTH in patients with PHP type I. Recent studies indicated that measurement of plasma cAMP (45) or plasma 1,25-dihydroxyvitamin D (46) after infusion of hPTH(1-34) also may differentiate PHP type I from other causes of hypoparathyroidism.

The presence of classic features of AHO and multihormonal resistance are diagnostic of PHP type Ia, but patients who lack obvious AHO have been found to have mutations in the GNAS1 gene. Further testing (e.g., $G_s\alpha$ protein or gene analysis) may be required when it is necessary to discriminate between these two genetically distinct variants of PHP type I.

The diagnosis of PHP type II, a much rarer entity, is less straightforward. Documentation of elevated serum PTH and basal urinary (or nephrogenous) cAMP is a prerequisite for a definitive diagnosis of PHP type II (4). These subjects have a normal urinary cAMP response to infusion of PTH but characteristically fail to show a phosphaturic response. Unfortunately, interpretation of the phosphaturic response to PTH is often complicated by random variations in phosphate clearance, and it is sometimes not possible to classify a phosphaturic response as normal or subnormal regardless of the criteria used. More perplexing yet is the observation that biochemical findings that resemble PHP type II have been found in patients with various forms of vitamin D deficiency. In these patients, marked hypocalcemia is accompanied by hyperphosphatemia due presumably to an acquired dissociation between the amount of cAMP generated in the renal tubule and its effect on phosphate clearance.

TREATMENT

The basic principles of treatment of hypocalcemia in PHP are essentially those outlined for the treatment of hormonopenic hypoparathyroidism. Therapy is directed at maintaining a low- to midnormal serum calcium concentration and thereby controlling symptoms of tetany while avoiding hypercalciuria. Patients with PHP require lower doses of vitamin D and have less risk of treatment-related hypercalciuria than do patients with hypoparathyroidism. Treatment with calcium and vitamin D usually decreases the elevated serum phosphate to a high-normal level because of a favorable balance between increased urinary phosphate excretion and decreased intestinal phosphate absorption. In general, phosphate-binding gels such as aluminum hydroxide are not necessary.

Estrogen therapy and pregnancy have particularly interesting effects on the maintenance of normocalcemia in patients with PHP. Estrogen therapy may reduce serum levels of calcium in women with PHP (47) or hypoparathyroidism (48). In addition, symptomatic hypocalcemia may also occur in some women at the time of the menses, when estrogen levels are low, with the cause remaining unknown (49). Paradoxically, during the high-estrogen state of pregnancy, some patients with PHP have required less or no (50) vitamin D to maintain normal serum concentrations of calcium owing to physiologic increases in serum concentration of 1,25-dihydroxyvitamin D_3 [1,25 (OH)$_2$ D$_3$] (50). After delivery, serum calcium and 1,25 (OH)$_2$ D$_3$ levels typically decrease, and PTH rises (47). As placental synthesis of 1,25 (OH)$_2$ D$_3$ is not compromised in patients with PHP (50), it appears that the placenta may contribute to the maintenance of normocalcemia during pregnancy. By contrast, patients with hypoparathyroidism may require treatment with larger amounts of vitamin D and calcium in the latter half of pregnancy (51).

Patients with PHP type Ia will frequently manifest resistance to other hormones in addition to PTH and may display clinical evidence of hypothyroidism or gonadal dysfunction. The basic principles used in the treatment of primary hypothyroidism apply to therapy of hypothyroidism in patients with PHP type Ia, as do approaches for the evaluation and treatment of hypogonadism.

REFERENCES

1. Albright F, Burnett CH, Smith PH. Pseudohypoparathyroidism: an example of ''Seabright-Bantam syndrome.'' *Endocrinology* 1942; 30:922–932.
2. Schipani E, Karga H, Karaplis AC, et al. Identical complementary deoxyribonucleic acids encode a human renal and bone parathyroid hormone (PTH)/PTH-related peptide receptor. *Endocrinology* 1993; 132:2157–2165.
3. Chase LR, Melson GL, Aurbach GD. Pseudohypoparathyroidism: de-
fective excretion of 3',5'-AMP in response to parathyroid hormone. *J Clin Invest* 1969;48:1832–1844.
4. Drezner MK, Neelon FA, Lebovitz HE. Pseudohypoparathyroidism type II: a possible defect in the reception of the cyclic AMP signal. *N Engl J Med* 1973;280:1056–1060.
5. Neer EJ. Heterotrimeric G proteins: organizers of transmembrane signals. *Cell* 1995;80:249–257.
6. Levine MA, Downs RW Jr, Moses AM, et al. Resistance to multiple hormones in patients with pseudohypoparathyroidism: association with deficient activity of guanine nucleotide regulatory protein. *Am J Med* 1983;74:545–556.
7. Levine MA. Hypoparathyroidism and pseudohypoparathyroidism. In: Avioli LV, Krane SM, eds. *Metabolic bone disease.* San Diego: Academic Press, 1998:501–529.
8. Albright F, Forbes AP, Henneman PH. Pseudopseudohypoparathyroidism. *Trans Assoc Am Physicians* 1952;65:337–350.
9. Levine MA, Jap TS, Mauseth RS, Downs RW, Spiegel AM. Activity of the stimulatory guanine nucleotide-binding protein is reduced in erythrocytes from patients with pseudohypoparathyroidism and pseudopseudohypoparathyroidism: biochemical, endocrine, and genetic analysis of Albright's hereditary osteodystrophy in six kindreds. *J Clin Endocrinol Metab* 1986;62:497–502.
10. Drezner MK, Haussler MR. Normocalcemic pseudohypoparathyroidism. *Am J Med* 1979;66:503–508.
11. Levine MA, Modi WS, OBrien SJ. Mapping of the gene encoding the alpha subunit of the stimulatory G protein of adenylyl cyclase (GNAS1) to 20q13.2-q13.3 in human by in situ hybridization. *Genomics* 1991;11:478–479.
12. Kozasa T, Itoh H, Tsukamoto T, Kaziro Y. Isolation and characterization of the human G$_s$ alpha gene. *Proc Natl Acad Sci USA* 1988;85:2081–2085.
13. Kehlenbach RH, Matthey J, Huttner WB. XLs is a new type of G protein. *Nature* 1994;372:804–808.
14. Hayward BE, Kamiya M, Strain L, et al. The human GNAS1 gene is imprinted and encodes distinct paternally and biallelically expressed G proteins. *Proc Natl Acad Sci USA* 1998;95:10038–10043.
15. Schwindinger WF, Miric A, Zimmerman D, Levine MA. A novel G$_s$ mutant in a patient with Albright hereditary osteodystrophy uncouples cell surface receptors from adenylyl cyclase. *J Biol Chem* 1994;269:25387–25391.
16. Warner DR, Gejman PV, Collins RM, Weinstein LS. A novel mutation adjacent to the switch III domain of G(S alpha) in a patient with pseudohypoparathyroidism. *Mol Endocrinol* 1997;11:1718–1727.
17. Warner DR, Weng G, Yu S, Matalon R, Weinstein LS. A novel mutation in the switch 3 region of G$_s$alpha in a patient with Albright hereditary osteodystrophy impairs GDP binding and receptor activation. *J Biol Chem* 1998;273:23976–23983.
18. Miric A, Vechio JD, Levine MA. Heterogeneous mutations in the gene encoding the alpha subunit of the stimulatory G protein of adenylyl cyclase in Albright hereditary osteodystrophy. *J Clin Endocrinol Metab* 1993;76:1560–1568.
19. Wilson LC, Oude Luttikhuis ME, Clayton PT, Fraser WD, Trembath RC. Parental origin of G$_s$ alpha gene mutations in Albright's hereditary osteodystrophy. *J Med Genet* 1994;31:835–839.
20. Davies SJ, Hughes HE. Imprinting in Albright's hereditary osteodystrophy. *J Med Genet* 1993;30:101–103.
21. Nakamoto JM, Sandstrom AT, Brickman AS, Christenson RA, Van Dop C. Pseudohypoparathyroidism type Ia from maternal but not paternal transmission of a G$_s$alpha gene mutation. *Am J Med Genet* 1998;77:261–267.
22. Campbell R, Gosden CM, Bonthron DT. Parental origin of transcription from the human GNAS1 gene. *J Med Genet* 1994;31:607–614.
23. Namnoum AB, Merriam GR, Moses AM, Levine MA. Reproductive dysfunction in women with Albright's hereditary osteodystrophy. *J Clin Endocrinol Metab* 1998;83:824–829.
24. Yu S, Yu D, Lee E, et al. Variable and tissue-specific hormone resistance in heterotrimeric G$_s$ protein alpha-subunit (Gsalpha) knockout mice is due to tissue-specific imprinting of the G$_s$ alpha gene. *Proc Natl Acad Sci USA* 1998;95:8715–8720.
25. Schwindinger WF, Francomano CA, Levine MA. Identification of a mutation in the gene encoding the alpha subunit of the stimulatory G protein of adenylyl cyclase in McCune-Albright syndrome. *Proc Natl Acad Sci USA* 1992;89:5152–5156.
26. Iiri T, Herzmark P, Nakamoto JM, Van Dop C, Bourne HR. Rapid GDP release from G$_s$α in patients with gain and loss of function. *Nature* 1994;371:164–168.

26. Iiri T, Herzmark P, Nakamoto JM, Van Dop C, Bourne HR. Rapid GDP release from G$_s\alpha$ in patients with gain and loss of function. *Nature* 1994;371:164–168.
27. Winter JSD, Hughes IA. Familial pseudohypoparathyroidism without somatic anomalies. *Can Med Assoc J* 1980;123:26–31.
28. Kidd GS, Schaaf M, Adler RA, Lassman MN, Wray HL. Skeletal responsiveness in pseudohypoparathyroidism: a spectrum of clinical disease. *Am J Med* 1980;68:772–781.
29. Silve C, Suarez F, el Hessni A, Loiseau A, Graulet AM, Gueris J. The resistance to parathyroid hormone of fibroblasts from some patients with type Ib pseudohypoparathyroidism is reversible with dexamethasone. *J Clin Endocrinol Metab* 1990;71:631–638.
30. Suarez F, Lebrun JJ, Lecossier D, Escoubet B, Coureau C, Silve C. Expression and modulation of the parathyroid hormone (PTH)/PTH-related peptide receptor messenger ribonucleic acid in skin fibroblasts from patients with type Ib pseudohypoparathyroidism. *J Clin Endocrinol Metab* 1995;80:965–970.
31. Schipani E, Weinstein LS, Bergwitz C, et al. Pseudohypoparathyroidism type Ib is not caused by mutations in the coding exons of the human parathyroid hormone (PTH)/PTH-related peptide receptor gene. *J Clin Endocrinol Metab* 1995;80:1611–1621.
32. Bettoun JD, Minagawa M, Kwan MY, et al. Cloning and characterization of the promoter regions of the human parathyroid hormone (PTH)/PTH-related peptide receptor gene: analysis of deoxyribonucleic acid from normal subjects and patients with pseudohypoparathyroidism type 1b. *J Clin Endocrinol Metab* 1997;82:1031–1040.
33. Fukumoto S, Suzawa M, Takeuchi Y, et al. Absence of mutations in parathyroid hormone (PTH)/PTH-related protein receptor complementary deoxyribonucleic acid in patients with pseudohypoparathyroidism type Ib. *J Clin Endocrinol Metab* 1996;81:2554–2558.
34. Lanske B, Karaplis AC, Lee K, et al. PTH/PTHrP receptor in early development and Indian hedgehog-regulated bone growth. *Science* 1996;273:663–666.
35. Jobert AS, Zhang P, Couvineau A, et al. Absence of functional receptors for parathyroid hormone and parathyroid hormone-related peptide in Blomstrand chondrodysplasia. *J Clin Invest* 1998;102:34–40.
36. Juppner H, Schipani E, Bastepe M, et al. The gene responsible for pseudohypoparathyroidism type Ib is paternally imprinted and maps in four unrelated kindreds to chromosome 20q13.3. *Proc Natl Acad Sci USA* 1998;95:11798–11803.
37. Barrett D, Breslau NA, Wax MB, Molinoff PB, Downs RW Jr. New form of pseudohypoparathyroidism with abnormal catalytic adenylate cyclase. *Am J Physiol* 1989;257:E277–E283.
38. Loveridge N, Fischer JA, Nagant de Deuxchaisnes C, et al. Inhibition of cytochemical bioactivity of parathyroid hormone by plasma in pseudohypoparathyroidism type I. *J Clin Endocrinol Metab* 1982;54:1274–1275.
39. Rao DS, Parfitt AM, Kleerekoper M, Pumo BS, Frame B. Dissociation between the effects of endogenous parathyroid hormone on adenosine 3′,5′-monophosphate generation and phosphate reabsorption in hypocalcemia due to vitamin D depletion: an acquired disorder resembling pseudohypoparathyroidism type II. *J Clin Endocrinol Metab* 1985;61:285–290.
40. Wilson LC, Leverton K, Oude Luttikhuis ME, et al. Brachydactyly and mental retardation: an Albright hereditary osteodystrophy-like syndrome localized to 2q37. *Am J Hum Genet* 1995;56:400–407.
41. Phelan MC, Rogers RC, Clarkson KB, et al. Albright hereditary osteodystrophy and del(2)(q37.3) in four unrelated individuals. *Am J Med Genet* 1995;58:1–7.
42. Mallette LE, Kirkland JL, Gagel RF, Law WM Jr, Heath H III. Synthetic human parathyroid hormone-(1-34) for the study of pseudohypoparathyroidism. *J Clin Endocrinol Metab* 1988;67:964–972.
43. Bhatt B, Burns J, Flanner D, McGee J. Direct visualization of single copy genes on banded metaphase chromosomes by nonisotopic in situ hybridization. *Nucleic Acids Res* 1988;16:3951–3961.
44. Stone MD, Hosking DJ, Garcia-Himmelstine C, White DA, Rosenblum D, Worth HG. The renal response to exogenous parathyroid hormone in treated pseudohypoparathyroidism. *Bone* 1993;14:727–735.
45. Stirling HF, Darling JA, Barr DG. Plasma cyclic AMP response to intravenous parathyroid hormone in pseudohypoparathyroidism. *Acta Paediatr Scand* 1991;80:333–338.
46. Miura R, Yumita S, Yoshinaga K, Furukawa Y. Response of plasma 1,25-dihydroxyvitamin D in the human PTH(1-34) infusion test: an improved index for the diagnosis of idiopathic hypoparathyroidism and pseudohypoparathyroidism. *Calcif Tissue Int* 1990;46:309–313.
47. Breslau NA, Zerwekh JE. Relationship of estrogen and pregnancy to calcium homeostasis in pseudohypoparathyroidism. *J Clin Endocrinol Metab* 1986;62:45–51.
48. Verbeelen D, Fuss M. Hypercalcemia induced by estrogen withdrawal in vitamin D-treated hypoparathyroidism. *BMJ* 1979;1:522–523.
49. Mallette LE. Case report: hypoparathyroidism with menses-associated hypocalcemia. *Am J Med Sci* 1992;304:32–37.
50. Zerwekh JE, Breslau NA. Human placental production of 1 alpha,25-dihydroxyvitamin D$_3$: biochemical characterization and production in normal subjects and patients with pseudohypoparathyroidism. *J Clin Endocrinol Metab* 1986;62:192–196.
51. Caplan RH, Beguin EA. Hypercalcemia in a calcitriol-treated hypoparathyroid woman during lactation. *Obstet Gynecol* 1990;76:485–489.

42. Neonatal Hypocalcemia

Thomas O. Carpenter, M.D.

Department of Pediatrics, Yale University School of Medicine, and Yale-New Haven Hospital, New Haven, Connecticut

CALCIUM METABOLISM IN THE PERINATAL PERIOD

Mineralization of the fetal skeleton is provided by active calcium transport from mother to fetus across the placenta, such that the fetus is relatively hypercalcemic as compared with the mother. The rate-limiting step in calcium transport is apparently a calcium pump in the basal membrane (fetus-directed side) of the trophoblast. The net effect of this system is to maintain a 1:1.4 (mother/fetus) calcium gradient throughout gestation (1), providing ample mineral for the demands of mineralization of the skeleton, particularly late in gestation. Evidence in the pregnant ewe suggests that a midregion fragment of parathyroid hormone-related peptide (PTHrP) may play a role in the regulation of this function.

At term the fetus is hypercalcemic, is likely to have elevated circulating calcitonin, and may have low levels of parathyroid hormone (PTH) compared with maternal circulation. An abrupt transition to autonomous regulation of mineral homeostasis occurs at birth. The abundant placental supply of calcium is removed, and the circulating calcium level begins to fall, reaching a nadir within the first 4 days of life, and subsequently rising to normal adult levels in week 2 of life.

HYPOCALCEMIC SYNDROMES IN THE NEWBORN PERIOD

Manifestations of neonatal hypocalcemia are variable and may not correlate with the magnitude of depression in the circulating ionized calcium level. As in older people, increased neuromuscular excitability (tetany) is a cardinal feature of newborn hypocalcemia. Generalized or focal clonic seizures, jitteriness, irritability, and frequent twitches or jerking of limbs are seen. Hyperacusis and laryngospasm may occur. Nonspecific signs include apnea, tachycardia, tachypnea, cyanosis, and edema; vomiting also has been reported. Neonatal hypocalcemia may be classified by its time of onset; differences in etiology are suggested by "early" occurring hypocalcemia as contrasted with that occurring "late" (2) (Table 1).

Early Neonatal Hypocalcemia

Early neonatal hypocalcemia occurs during the first 3 days of life, usually between 24 and 48 hours, and characteristically is seen in premature infants, infants of diabetic mothers, and asphyxiated infants. The premature infant normally has an exaggerated postnatal depression in circulating calcium, dropping lower and earlier than that in the term infant. Total calcium levels may drop below 7.0 mg/dL, but the proportional drop in ionized calcium is less, and may explain the lack of symptoms in many prematures with total calcium in this range.

Prematures have been variably reported to show normal, elevated, or impaired secretion of PTH during citrate-induced hypocalcemia. Conflict also exists regarding the action of PTH in the newborn. A several-day delay in the phosphaturic effect of PTH in both term and preterm infants has been described; resultant hyperphosphatemia may decrease serum calcium. The premature infant's exaggerated rise in calcitonin may provoke hypocalcemia. A role for vitamin D and its metabolites in early neonatal hypocalcemia is less convincing.

The infant of the diabetic mother (IDM) also demonstrates an exaggerated postnatal drop in the circulating calcium level when compared with other infants of comparable maturity. As in premature infants, the decrease is not entirely explained by a fall in ionized calcium concentrations. The pregnant diabetic tends to have lower circulating PTH and magnesium levels; the IDM has lower circulating magnesium and PTH, but normal calcitonin. Abnormalities in vitamin D metabolism do not appear to play a role in the development of hypocalcemia in the IDM. Strict maternal glycemic control during pregnancy results in a decreased incidence of hypocalcemia in the IDM.

Early hypocalcemia occurs in asphyxiated infants; calcitonin response is augmented, and PTH levels are elevated. Infants of preeclamptic mothers and postmature infants with growth retardation develop early hypocalcemia and are prone to hypomagnesemia.

Late Neonatal Hypocalcemia

The presentation of hypocalcemic tetany between 5 and 10 days of life is termed "late" neonatal hypocalcemia. The incidence of this disorder is greater in full term than in premature infants and is not correlated with birth trauma or asphyxia. Affected children may have received cow's milk or cow's milk formula, which may have considerably more phosphate than has human milk. Hyperphosphatemia is associated with late neonatal hypocalcemia and may reflect (a) inability of the immature kidney to efficiently excrete phosphate; (b) dietary phosphate load; or (c) transiently low levels of circulating PTH. Others noted an association between late neonatal hypocalcemia and modest maternal vitamin D insufficiency. An increased occurrence of late neonatal hypocalcemia in winter also was noted.

Hypocalcemia associated with magnesium deficiency may present as late neonatal hypocalcemia. Severe hypomagnesemia (circulating levels less than 0.8 mg/dL) may occur in congenital defects of intestinal magnesium absorption or renal tubular reabsorption. Transient hypomagnesemia of unknown etiology is associated with a less severe decrease in circulating magnesium (between 0.8 and 1.4 mg/dL). Hypocalcemia frequently complicates hypomagnesemic states because of impaired secretion of PTH. Impaired PTH responsiveness also was demonstrated as an inconsistent finding in magnesium deficiency.

Other Causes of Neonatal Hypocalcemia

Symptomatic neonatal hypocalcemia may occur within the first 3 weeks of life in infants born to mothers with

---

TABLE 1. Neonatal hypocalcemia

	Characteristics	Mechanism
Early	Onset within first 3–4 days of life; seen in infants of diabetic mother, perinatal asphyxia, pre-eclampsia	Uncertain; possible exaggerated postnatal calcitonin surge, possible decrease in parathyroid response
Late	Onset days 5–10 of life, seen in winter, in infants of mother with marginal vitamin D intake; associated with dietary phosphate load	Possible transient parathyroid dysfunction; hypomagnesemia in some cases; calcium malabsorption
Other		
Congenital hypoparathyroidism	Usually present after first 5 days of life with overt tetany	
"Late-late" hypocalcemia	Seen in premature at 2–4 months; associated with skeletal hypomineralization and inadequate dietary mineral or vitamin D intake	
Infants of hyperparathyroid mother	May appear as late as 1 year of age; mother possibly undiagnosed	
Ionized hypocalcemia	In exchange transfusion with citrated blood products, lipid infusions, or alkalosis	

hyperparathyroidism. Presentation at age 1 year also was reported. Serum phosphate is often greater than 8 mg/dL; symptoms may be exacerbated by feeding cow's milk or other high-phosphate formulas. The proposed mechanism for the development of neonatal hypocalcemia in the infant of the hyperparathyroid mother is as follows: maternal hypercalcemia occurs secondary to hyperparathyroidism, resulting in increased calcium delivery to the fetus and fetal hypercalcemia, which inhibits fetal parathyroid secretion. The infant's oversuppressed parathyroid is not able to maintain normal calcium levels after birth. Hypomagnesemia may be observed in the infant of the hyperparathyroid mother. Maternal hyperparathyroidism has been diagnosed after hypocalcemic infants have been identified.

"Late-late" neonatal hypocalcemia has been used in reference to premature infants who develop hypocalcemia with poor bone mineralization within the first 3 to 4 months of life. These infants tend to have an inadequate dietary supply of mineral and/or vitamin D.

The previously discussed forms of neonatal hypocalcemia are generally found to be of a transient nature. More rarely, permanent hypocalcemia is detected in the newborn period caused by congenital hypoparathyroidism (see Chapter 40). Isolated absence of the parathyroids may be inherited in X-linked or autosomal recessive fashion. Hypocalcemia may occur secondary to activating mutations of the parathyroid calcium-sensing receptor (3). Congenital hypoparathyroidism also occurs as the DiGeorge anomaly, classically the triad of hypoparathyroidism, T-cell incompetence due to a partial or absent thymus, and conotruncal heart defects (e.g., tetralogy of Fallot, truncus arteriosus) or aortic-arch abnormalities. These structures are derived from the embryologic third and fourth pharyngeal pouches; the usual sporadic occurrence reflects developmental abnormalities of these structures, which can be seen in association with microdeletions of chromosome 22q11.2 (4). Other defects may variably occur in this broad-spectrum field defect, including other midline anomalies such as cleft palate and facial dysmorphism. Individuals with various phenotypic features of this syndrome have come to attention in late childhood or in adolescence with the onset of symptomatic hypocalcemia (5). Presumably partial hypoparathyroidism in these individuals was not apparent early in life because of the mild nature of the partial defect. On the other hand, at least one of these individuals had transient hypocalcemia in the newborn period.

The Kenny–Caffey syndrome is another congenital anomaly associated with hypoparathyroidism, growth retardation, and medullary stenosis of tubular bones. Several reports of mitochondrial and fatty acid–oxidation disorders described hypoparathyroidism as a rare associated feature. Such disorders include the Kearns–Sayre syndrome, mitochondrial trifunctional protein deficiency, and long-chain fatty acyl Co-A dehydrogenase (LCHAD) deficiency (6,7). No mechanism for the hypoparathyroidism in any of these metabolic conditions has been clearly identified. Resistance to PTH in infancy also was described in association with proprionic acidemia (8).

Decreases in the ionized fraction of the circulating calcium occur in infants undergoing exchange transfusions with citrated blood products or receiving lipid infusions. Citrate and fatty acids form complexes with ionized calcium, reducing the free calcium compartment. Alkalosis secondary to adjustments in ventilatory assistance may provoke a shift of ionized calcium to the protein-bound compartment. It should be pointed out that appropriate collection of sample for determination of ionized calcium levels may require anaerobic collection from a free-flowing vessel and prompt sample handling for accurate results; given these requirements, measurement of ionized calcium may be difficult to obtain under routine circumstances in small children.

TREATMENT OF NEONATAL HYPOCALCEMIA

Early neonatal hypocalcemia may be asymptomatic, and the necessity of therapy may be questioned in such infants. Most authors recommended that early neonatal hypocalcemia be treated when the circulating concentration of total serum calcium is less than 5 to 6 mg/dL (1.25 to 1.50 mmol/L) or of ionized calcium less than 2.5 to 3 mg/dL (0.62 to 0.72 mmol/L) in the premature infant and when total serum calcium is less than 6 to 7 mg/dL (1.50 to 1.75 mmol/L) in the term infant. Emergency therapy of acute tetany consists of intravenous (never intramuscular) calcium gluconate (10% solution) given slowly (less than 1 mL/min). A dose of 1 to 3 mL will usually arrest convulsions. Doses should generally not exceed 20 mg/kg body weight and may be repeated up to 4 times per 24 hours. After successful management of acute emergencies, maintenance therapy may be achieved by intravenous administration of 20 to 50 mg of elemental calcium per kg body weight per 24 hours. Calcium gluconate is a commonly used oral supplement. Management of late neonatal tetany should include low-phosphate formula such as Similac PM 60/40, in addition to calcium supplements. A calcium/phosphate ratio of 4 : 1 has been recommended. Generally therapy can be discontinued after several weeks.

When hypomagnesemia is a causal feature of the hypocalcemia, magnesium administration may be indicated. Magnesium sulfate is given intravenously by using cardiac monitoring or intramuscularly as a 50% solution at a dose of 0.1 to 0.2 mL/kg. One or two doses may treat transient hypomagnesemia: a dose may be repeated after 12 to 24 hours. Patients with primary defects in magnesium metabolism require long-term oral magnesium supplements.

The place of vitamin D in the management of transient hypocalcemia is less clear. Daily supplementation of 400 to 800 units of vitamin D has been suggested for all premature infants as a preventive measure. Patients with normal intestinal absorption who develop "late-late" hypocalcemia with vitamin D–deficiency rickets should respond within 4 weeks to 1000 to 2000 units of daily oral vitamin D. Such patients should receive a total of at least 40 mg of elemental calcium/kg body weight/day. In the various forms of persistent congenital hypoparathyroidism, long-term treatment with vitamin D (or its therapeutic metabolites) is used; at our center the preferred agent is calcitriol for these purposes.

REFERENCES

1. Kovacs CS, Kronenberg HM. Maternal-fetal calcium and bone metabolism during pregnancy, puerperium, and lactation. *Endocr Rev* 1997; 18:832–872.

2. Hillman LS, Haddad JG. Hypocalcemia and other abnormalities of mineral homeostasis during the neonatal period. In: Heath DA, Marx SJ, eds. *Calcium disorders: clinical endocrinology.* London: Butterworths International Medical Reviews, 1982:248–276.
3. Watanabe T, Bai M, Lane CR, et al. Familial hypoparathyroidism: identification of a novel gain of function mutation in transmembrane domain 5 of the calcium-sensing receptor. *J Clin Endocrinol Metab* 1998;83:2497–2502.
4. Webber SA, Hatchwell E, Barber JC, et al. Importance of microdeletions of chromosomal region 22q11 as a cause of selected malformations of the ventricular outflow tracts and aortic arch: a three-year prospective study. *J Pediatr* 1996;129:26–32.

5. Sykes KS, Bachrach LK, Siegel-Bartelt J, Ipp M, Kooh SW, Cytrynbaum C. Velocardiofacial syndrome presenting as hypocalcemia in early adolescence. *Arch Pediatr Adolesc Med* 1997;151:745–747.
6. Tyni T, Rapola J, Palotie A, Pihko H. Hypoparathyroidism in a patient with long-chain 3-hydroxyacyl-coenzyme A dehydrogenase deficiency caused by the G1528C mutation. *J Pediatr* 1997;131:766–768.
7. Dionisi-Vici C, Garavaglia B, Burlina AB, et al. Hypoparathyroidism in mitochondrial trifunctional protein deficiency. *J Pediatr* 1996;129:159–162.
8. Griffin TA, Hostoffer RW, Tserng KY, et al. Parathyroid hormone resistance and B cell lymphopenia in propionic acidemia. *Acta Paediatr* 1996;85:875–878.

43. Miscellaneous Causes of Hypocalcemia

Michael F. Holick, Ph.D., M.D. and *Andrew F. Stewart, M.D.

*Department of Medicine and Section of Endocrinology, Nutrition, and Diabetes, Boston University Medical Center, Boston, Massachusetts; and *Department of Medicine, University of Pittsburgh School of Medicine and Division of Endocrinology, University of Pittsburgh Medical Center, Pittsburgh, Pennsylvania*

The list of disorders that may cause hypocalcemia is a long one. Several of these disorders (hypoparathyroidism, pseudohypoparathyroidism, hypocalcemic syndromes encountered in infants, and the hypocalcemia seen in patients with hyper- and hypomagnesemia) are described in the chapters that immediately precede or follow this chapter.

"FACTITIOUS" HYPOCALCEMIA DUE TO HYPOALBUMINEMIA

In the reverse of events described in Chapter 37 for "factitious" hypercalcemia, reductions in serum albumin encountered in patients with nephrotic syndrome, chronic illness, malnutrition, cirrhosis, and volume overexpansion will result in a reduction in the total, but not the ionized fraction, of the serum calcium. Such patients display none of the signs or symptoms of hypocalcemia (QT interval changes on electrocardiogram, paresthesiae, tetany, cramping, or Chvostek or Trousseau signs). The degree of hypocalcemia correlates roughly with the degree of hypoalbuminemia, and a variety of formulae permit one to calculate a total serum calcium corrected for the serum albumin. In general, however, these formulae are imprecise. If a question arises as to the "real" serum calcium in a given case, the ionized calcium should be measured.

HYPOCALCEMIA RESULTING FROM DISORDERS INVOLVING VITAMIN D

Although it is often assumed that one of the first manifestations of vitamin D deficiency is hypocalcemia, in fact, hypocalcemia is rarely observed in vitamin D deficiency unless it is prolonged or associated with dietary calcium deficiency. However, hypocalcemia is common in disorders that mimic vitamin D deficiency (i.e., an acquired or inherited defect in the metabolism of vitamin D to 1,25-dihydroxyvitamin D [1,25 (OH)$_2$ D] or an inherited disorder in which there is either a defective or absent vitamin D receptor (VDR) for

1,25 (OH)$_2$ D). Details about vitamin D metabolism and inherited and acquired disorders in vitamin D metabolism and recognition are discussed in Chapters 15 and 61 to 63.

Vitamin D deficiency is rarely found in children or young and middle-aged adults in the United States in part because of the fortification of milk, some cereals, and breads with vitamin D. Vitamin D deficiency, however, continues to plague children in countries that either do not fortify foods with vitamin D or are incapable of providing an adequate supply of vitamin D to the general population. In addition, vitamin D deficiency is becoming recognized as a significant worldwide health problem for older adults. Vitamin D deficiency is especially prevalent in patients who are infirm and not exposed to solar ultraviolet B radiation or in patients who have intestinal fat malabsorption syndromes due to diseases of the small intestine or have hepatic failure. Because there is very little vitamin D in human milk, breast-fed infants from strictly vegetarian mothers are at risk for vitamin D deficiency. Members of cultures that practice and immigrants who continue the practice of wearing traditional dress, including long garments, hoods, and veils, also are prone to vitamin D deficiency.

The reason that hypocalcemia is not usually observed in vitamin D deficiency is because the compensatory increase in parathyroid hormone (PTH) secretion leads to an increase in tubular reabsorption of calcium in the kidney and mobilization of calcium stores from the bone. It is only when calcium stores from the skeleton are quite depleted that hypocalcemia is observed in vitamin D deficiency. The usual blood biochemistries observed in vitamin D deficiency are low-normal calcium, hypophosphatemia due to secondary hyperparathyroidism, and elevated alkaline phosphatase and PTH. The hallmark of vitamin D deficiency is low or undetectable serum 25-hydroxyvitamin D [25 (OH) D] levels.

Severe chronic vitamin D deficiency, especially in an individual who has poor skeletal calcium stores in his or her skeleton, can result in persistent hypocalcemia. In addition, acquired and inherited abnormalities in vitamin D metabolism or recognition (defective vitamin D receptor) mimic chronic vitamin D deficiency and are associated with hypocalcemia. Patients with severe chronic parenchymal and cholestatic liver disease can develop vitamin D deficiency due to associated intestinal fat malabsorption. In addition, with substantial destruction of liver tissue, the hepatic reserve of the vitamin D-25-hydroxylase enzyme can be compromised to such a degree that inadequate amounts of 25 (OH) D are produced. Similarly, patients with mild to moderate renal failure and associated hyperphosphatemia may display suppression in the production of 1,25 (OH)$_2$ D that mimics vitamin D deficiency. Resolution of the hyperphosphatemia usually corrects this abnormality. However, when more than two thirds of renal function is compromised, the kidney is unable to make sufficient amounts of 1,25 (OH)$_2$ D to satisfy the body's requirement for this active metabolite, resulting in hypocalcemia, secondary hyperparathyroidism, and renal osteodystrophy.

Several drugs can alter the bioavailability and/or processing of vitamin D and its metabolites, as discussed in Chapter 68. The most notable are the antiseizure medications, phenytoin (Dilantin) and phenobarbital. However, vitamin D deficiency is rarely observed if patients receive adequate exposure to sunlight and dietary vitamin D.

The inherited disorder, vitamin D–dependent rickets type I (DDR I), which is caused by a defective 25 (OH) D-1α-hydroxylase gene, results in insufficient production of 1,25 (OH)$_2$ D. This causes a chronic vitamin D–deficiency state that is associated with skeletal abnormalities (rickets), hypocalcemia, hypophosphatemia, secondary hyperparathyroidism, and an elevated alkaline phosphatase. Similarly, in patients with the very rare disorder, vitamin D–dependent rickets type II, there is a disruption in the production or function of the vitamin D receptor. These patients are functionally vitamin D deficient because of their inability to recognize 1,25 (OH)$_2$ D. The resulting end-organ resistance to 1,25 (OH)$_2$ D causes severe hypocalcemia, hypophosphatemia, secondary hyperparathyroidism, elevated alkaline phosphatase, and rickets. The most reliable means of distinguishing these two inherited disorders from each other is by measuring the serum 1,25 (OH)$_2$ D level: in the DDR I, the inability to produce adequate amounts of 1,25 (OH)$_2$ D results in low or undetectable circulating levels of 1,25 (OH)$_2$ D, whereas in DDR II, the constant stimulation of the renal 1α-hydroxylase by chronic hypocalcemia, hypophosphatemia, and secondary hyperparathyroidism results in markedly elevated levels of 1,25 (OH)$_2$ D in the circulation.

HYPOCALCEMIA RESULTING FROM HYPERPHOSPHATEMIA

Hypocalcemia can result from hyperphosphatemia. The causes of hyperphosphatemia and mechanisms responsible for hypocalcemia are discussed in detail in Chapter 45. In general, for hypocalcemia to occur, the increase in serum phosphorus must be very significant (i.e., greater than 6 mg/dL). This syndrome can result from delivery of endogenous and exogenous phosphorus loads into the extracellular space, as illustrated below. *Exogenous phosphorus administration* can lead to hyperphosphatemia and hypocalcemia. Settings include oral phosphorus administration in the form of exces-

sive dietary phosphorus (e.g., milk or phosphoric acid-containing soft drinks), overaggressive administration of phosphorus supplements (such as neutral phosphate), and colonoscopy preparation (by using oral phosphate-containing laxatives such as phosphosoda), particularly in subjects with renal failure. Parenteral phosphorus administration in the form of potassium phosphate to patients with diabetic ketoacidosis, or phosphate-containing parenteral nutrition solutions, particularly in the setting of renal failure, may lead to hypocalcemia. Another example of exogenous phosphorus administration occurs in subjects receiving rectal enemas containing phosphosoda. Perforation of the rectum or colon may result in peritoneal delivery and rapid systemic absorption of large amounts of phosphorus, with severe hypocalcemia, tetany, convulsions, and death. Excessive colonic absorption of phosphate in patients with megacolon also has occurred. Accidental oral ingestion of phosphosoda enemas has been described as well, resulting in very severe hyperphosphatemia (40 mg/dL) and hypocalcemia (4 mg/dL). Phosphate enema–induced hypocalcemia, although recognized for many years, appears to be occurring with increasing frequency, judging from the number of recent literature citations. Because most phosphate in the body is in intracellular locations, very significant rates of *endogenous phosphate delivery* into the extracellular fluid may occur with tissue injury or lysis. This is seen, for example, in patients with the tumor-lysis syndrome who receive effective chemotherapy for large bulky tumors. Typically these are acute leukemias or lymphomas, such as Burkitt's lymphoma. Crush injury and rhabdomyolysis, particularly in the setting of acute renal failure, may lead to severe hyperphosphatemia and hypocalcemia. Severe intravascular hemolysis may lead to a similar syndrome of hypocalcemia and hyperphosphatemia.

HYPOCALCEMIA RESULTING FROM HYPER- AND HYPOMAGNESEMIA

These subjects are covered thoroughly in Chapter 44. Hypomagnesemia deserves special mention here, however, because it is, in the authors' experience, the most common cause of hypocalcemia encountered in hospitalized patients. It should be rigorously sought and excluded in every patient with unexplained hypocalcemia.

HYPOCALCEMIA RESULTING FROM PANCREATITIS

Hypocalcemia and tetany were first recorded in patients with pancreatitis in the early 1940s. Langerhans had observed in 1890 that the white deposits in the retroperitoneum ("fat necrosis") associated with pancreatitis were, in fact, insoluble calcium soaps or complexes of calcium and free fatty acids (FFAs). It is now believed that FFAs are generated by the action of pancreatic lipase, released from the damaged pancreas, on retroperitoneal and omental fat (triglyceride) to release their component FFAs into the peritoneum. These in turn avidly chelate calcium, removing it from extracellular fluid. Other mechanisms may be responsible for hypocalcemia in individual instances of pancreatitis-induced hypocalcemia. Hypoalbuminemia regularly occurs in patients with pancreatitis and leads to a reduction in total (but not ionized) serum calcium. Hypomagnesemia resulting from poor oral intake, alcohol use, vomiting, or a combination of these is common in pancreatitis and may lead to hypocalcemia. It also has been postulated that hypocalcemia may result from excessive calcitonin secretion, resulting in turn from excessive pancreatic glucagon release. Support for this possibility is weak. Finally, it has been suggested that pancreatitis may liberate systemic factors, such as proteases, that inhibit PTH secretion and/or degrade circulating PTH. There is no support for this possibility.

Clinically, patients with pancreatitis-induced hypocalcemia have severe pancreatitis, and hypocalcemia portends a poor outcome. Hypocalcemia is treated with parenteral calcium and magnesium replacement when indicated. Hypocalcemia due to vitamin D deficiency/malabsorption should be considered and excluded.

HYPOCALCEMIA DUE TO ACCELERATED SKELETAL MINERALIZATION

Hypocalcemia occurs in settings in which the rate of skeletal mineralization significantly outpaces the rate of osteoclastic bone resorption. Three examples of this type of hypocalcemia occur. The first is the hypocalcemia that follows the surgical correction of primary or secondary hyperparathyroidism. The abrupt cessation of PTH-mediated osteoclastic skeletal resorption in concert with continued mineralization of large quantities of osteoid leads to a hypocalcemic syndrome termed the *hungry-bones syndrome.* The syndrome also has been described after thyroidectomy for hyperthyroidism. The key clinical issue is distinguishing postoperative hungry-bones syndrome from postoperative hypoparathyroidism, a distinction not always easy. Hypocalcemia also occurs in patients with extensive osteoblastic metastases. As might be anticipated, this type of hypocalcemia occurs primarily in patients with prostate cancer and breast cancer with extensive osteoblastic metastases, but it also has been reported to occur in patients with acute leukemia and osteosarcomatosis. Finally, hypocalcemia may worsen in patients with vitamin D deficiency following the institution of therapy with vitamin D. This type of hypocalcemia is confusing and alarming, for one would expect the serum calcium to rise with vitamin D replacement in patients with rickets or osteomalacia. Hypocalcemia occurs in the early phases of vitamin D therapy as the large amounts of unmineralized osteoid are permitted to mineralize when vitamin D is provided.

HYPOCALCEMIA ENCOUNTERED IN ACUTE ILLNESSES

Hypocalcemia in the setting of acute illness most often is multifactorial, reflecting combinations of hypoalbuminemia, hypomagnesemia, pancreatitis, chronic and/or acute renal failure, treatment with medications or transfusions that lower serum calcium, or cancer with osteoblastic metastases. However, a specific acute sepsis–hypocalcemia syndrome appears to exist. In one series, 12 of 60 patients with acute bacterial sepsis were hypocalcemic (displaying reductions in ionized serum calcium), and six of the 12 hypocalcemic patients died of their septic episode. In contrast, only 14 of 48 normocalcemic patients died, leading the authors to suggest that hypocalcemia confers an even graver prognosis on patients with sepsis. All of the patients had gram-negative sepsis. In contrast, none of 20 patients with staphylococcal sepsis became hypocalcemic. In addition, a reduction in total and ionized serum calcium was reported to be a feature of the toxic shock syndrome. The mechanism responsible for hypocalcemia in gram-negative sepsis and in toxic shock syndrome is unknown. It has been suggested that hypocalcemia may result from interleukin-1 production during septic episodes because interleukin-1 injections cause hypocalcemia in mice. It also was suggested that parathyroid "reserve" is subnormal in patients with acquired immunodeficiency syndrome (AIDS).

HYPOCALCEMIA ASSOCIATED WITH MEDICATIONS, TOXINS, AND OVERDOSAGE

Hypocalcemia may occur as the result of overzealous treatment with medications intended to reverse hypercalcemia and/or excessive bone resorption. Thus *mithramycin* (plicamycin), *calcitonin, bisphosphonates,* and oral or parenteral *phosphate* preparations have all been reported to cause hypocalcemia. Hypocalcemia and osteomalacia may occur as the result of prolonged therapy with anticonvulsants such as *diphenylhydantoin (phenytoin)* or *phenobarbital.* Transfusion, apheresis and plasmapheresis with *citrated blood* was reported to cause hypocalcemia, particularly in patients receiving exchange transfusions. A recent addition to the list of drugs that may cause hypocalcemia is *radiographic contrast dyes* that may contain the calcium chelator, ethylenediaminetetraacetic acid (EDTA), in conjunction with citrate. Chelation of calcium plus dilutional/osmotic effects of these agents are believed to be responsible for the mild hypocalcemia that has been observed. *Fluoride* overdosage in dialysis units, in the setting of overfluoridated public water supplies, and following ingestion of fluoride-containing cleaning agents or hydrofluoric acid has been associated with hypocalcemia, possibly because of excessive rates of skeletal mineralization and complexing of calcium by fluoride. Recently mild hypocalcemia was reported in patients receiving the chemotherapeutic combination of *5-fluorouracil and leucovorin.* The mechanisms responsible are unknown. *Cisplatin,* through its induction of hypomagnesemia, induces hypocalcemia on a regular basis. Finally, *foscarnet* (trisodium phosphonoformate), used in the treatment of patients with AIDS, has been reported to cause reductions in total and ionized serum calcium concentrations, perhaps through chelation or complexing of calcium in extracellular fluid.

SELECTED READING

Factitious Hypocalcemia

1. Ladenson JH, Lewis JH, McDonald JM, Slatopolsky E, Boyd JC. Relationship of free and total calcium in hypercalcemic conditions. *J Clin Endocrinol Metab* 1978;48:393–397.

Disorders of Vitamin D

2. Holick MF. Vitamin D. Photobiology, metabolism, and clinical applications. In: DeGroot L, Besuer M, Burger HG, et al., eds. *Endocrinology.* 3rd ed. Philadelphia: WB Saunders, 1995:990–1013.
3. Kitanaka S, Takeyama KI, Murayama A, et al. Inactivating mutations in the human 25-hydroxyvitamin D$_3$ 1-alpha-hydroxylase gene in patients with pseudovitamin D-deficient rickets. *N Engl J Med* 1998;338: 653–661.
4. Malloy PJ, Eccleshall TR, Gross C, Van Maldergem L, Bouillon R, Feldman D. Hereditary vitamin D resistant rickets caused by a novel mutation in the vitamin D receptor that results in decreased affinity for hormone and cellular hyporesponsiveness. *J Clin Invest* 1997; 99:297–304.

Hyperphosphatemia

5. Dunlay R, Camp M, Allon M, Fanti P, Malluche H, Llach F. Calcitriol in prolonged hypocalcemia due to the tumor lysis syndrome. *Ann Intern Med* 1989;110:162–164.
6. Helickson MA, Parham WA, Tobias JD. Hypocalcemia and hyperphosphatemia after phosphate enema use in a child. *J Pediatr Surg* 1997;32:1244–1246.
7. Kirschbaum B. The acidosis of exogenous phosphate administration. *Arch Intern Med* 1998;158:405–408.
8. Llach F, Felsenfeld A, Haussler M. The pathophysiology of altered calcium metabolism in rhabdomyolysis-induced acute renal failure. *N Engl J Med* 1981;305:117–123.
9. Mazariegos E, Guerrero-Romero F, Rodriguez-Moran M, Lazcano-Burciaga G, Paniagua R, Amato D. Consumption of soft drinks with phosphoric acid as a risk factor for the development of hypocalcemia in children: a case-control study. *J Pediatr* 1995;126:940–942.
10. Zusman T, Brown D, Nesbit M. Hyperphosphatemia, hyperphosphaturia and hypocalcemia in acute lymphoblastic leukemia. *N Engl J Med* 1973;289:1335–1340.

Pancreatitis

11. Dettelbach MA, Deftos LJ, Stewart AF. Intraperitoneal free fatty acids induce severe hypocalcemia in rats. *J Bone Miner Res* 1990;5:1249–1255.
12. Stewart AF, Longo W, Kreutter D, Jacob R, Burtis WJ. Hypocalcemia due to calcium soap formation in a patient with a pancreatic fistula. *N Engl J Med* 1986;315:496–498.

Accelerated Skeletal Mineralization

13. Chap LI, Mirra J, Ippolito V, Rentschler R, Rosen P. Miliary osteosarcomatosis with associated hypocalcemia. *Am J Clin Oncol* 1997;20: 505–508.

14. Cruz D, Perazella MA. Biochemical aberrations in a dialysis patient following parathyroidectomy. *Am J Kidney Dis* 1997;29:759–762.
15. Szentirmai M, Constantinou C, Rainey JM, Lowenstein JE. Hypocalcemia due to avid calcium uptake by osteoblastic metastases. *West J Med* 1995;163:577–578.

Acute Illness and Sepsis

16. Boyce BF, Yates AJP, Mundy GR. Bolus injections of recombinant human interleukin-1 cause transient hypocalcemia in normal mice. *Endocrinology* 1989;125:2780–2783.
17. Chesney RW, McCarron DM, Haddad JG, Hawker CD, DiBella FP, Chesney PJ, Davis JP. Pathogenic mechanisms of the hypocalcemia of the staphylococcal toxic-shock syndrome. *J Lab Clin Med* 1983;101:576–585.
18. Jaeger P, Otto S, Speck RF, et al. Altered parathyroid gland function in severely immunocompromised patients infected with human immunodeficiency virus. *J Clin Endocrinol Metab* 1994;79:1701–1705.
19. Zaloga GP, Chernow B. The multifactorial basis for hypocalcemia during sepsis: studies of the parathyroid hormone-vitamin D axis. *Ann Intern Med* 1987;107:36–41.

Medications and Toxins

20. Arnow PM, Bland LA, Garcia-Houchins S, Fridkin S, Fellner SK. An outbreak of fatal fluoride intoxication in a long-term hemodialysis unit. *Ann Intern Med* 1994;121:339–344.
21. Gessner BD, Beller M, Middaugh JP, Whitford GM. Acute fluoride poisoning from a public water system. *N Engl J Med* 1994;330:95–99.
22. Guillame MP, Karmali R, Pergmann P, Cogan E. Unusual prolonged hypocalcemia due to foscarnet in a patient with AIDS. *Clin Infect Dis* 1997;25:932–933.
23. Jacobson MA, Gambertoglio JG, Aweeka FT, Causey DM, Portale AA. Foscarnet-induced hypocalcemia and effects of foscarnet on calcium metabolism. *J Clin Endocrinol Metab* 1991;72:1130–1135.
24. Kido Y, Okamura T, Tomikawa M, et al. Hypocalcemia associated with 5-fluorouracil and low dose leucovorin in patients with advanced colorectal or gastric carcinomas. *Cancer* 1996;78:1794–1797.
25. Klasner AE, Scalzo AJ, Blume C, Johnson P, Thompson MW. Marked hypocalcemia and ventricular fibrillation in two pediatric patients exposed to a fluoride wheel cleaner. *Ann Emerg Med* 1996;28:713–718.
26. Mallette LE, Gomez LS. Systemic hypocalcemia after clinical injection of radiographic contrast media: amelioration by omission of calcium chelating agents. *Radiology* 1982;147:677–679.
27. Tofalletti J, Nissenson RA, Endres D, McGarry E, Mogollon G. Influence of continuous infusion of citrate on responses of immunoreactive PTH, calcium, magnesium components, and other electrolytes in normal adults during plasmapheresis. *J Clin Endocrinol Metab* 1985;60: 874–879.

44. Magnesium Depletion and Hypermagnesemia

Robert K. Rude, M.D.

Department of Medicine, University of Southern California, Los Angeles, California

HYPOMAGNESEMIA/MAGNESIUM DEPLETION

Magnesium (Mg) depletion appears to be more common than previously thought. Of patients admitted to city hospitals, 10% are hypomagnesemic, and as many as 65% of patients in an intensive care unit have been reported to be hypomagnesemic. Hypomagnesemia and/or Mg depletion is usually due to losses of Mg from either the gastrointestinal tract or the kidney, as outlined in Table 1.

Causes of Magnesium Depletion

The Mg content of upper intestinal tract fluids is approximately 1 mEq/L. Vomiting and nasogastric suction therefore

TABLE 1. *Common causes of Mg deficiency*

Gastrointestinal disorders
  Prolonged nasogastric suction/vomiting
  Acute and chronic diarrheal states
  Intestinal and biliary fistulas
  Malabsorption syndromes
  Extensive bowel resection or bypass
  Acute hemorrhagic pancreatitis
Renal loss
  Chronic parenteral fluid therapy
  Osmotic diuresis (glucose, urea)
  Hypercalcemia
  Alcohol
  Diuretics (furosemide, ethacrynic acid)
  Aminoglycosides
  Cisplatin
  Cyclosporin
  Amphotericin B
  Pentamidine
  Metabolic acidosis
  Renal disease with Mg wasting
Endocrine and metabolic
  Diabetes mellitus
  Phosphate depletion
  Primary hyperparathyroidism
  Hypoparathyroidism
  Primary aldosteronism
  Hungry-bone syndrome

may contribute to Mg depletion. The Mg content of diarrheal fluids and fistulous drainage are much higher (up to 15 mEq/L), and consequently Mg depletion is common in acute and chronic diarrhea, regional enteritis, ulcerative colitis, and intestinal and biliary fistulas. Malabsorption syndromes due to nontropical sprue, radiation injury resulting from therapy for disorders such as carcinoma of the cervix, and intestinal lymphangiectasia also may result in Mg deficiency. Steatorrhea and resection or bypass of the small bowel, particularly the ileum, often results in intestinal Mg loss or malabsorption. Last, acute severe pancreatitis is associated with hypomagnesemia, which may be due to the clinical problem causing the pancreatitis, such as alcoholism, or to saponification of Mg in necrotic parapancreatic fat.

Excessive excretion of Mg into the urine may be the basis of Mg depletion. Renal Mg reabsorption is proportional to tubular fluid flow as well as to sodium and calcium excretion. Therefore chronic parenteral fluid therapy, particularly with saline, and volume-expansion states, such as primary aldosteronism, may result in Mg depletion. Hypercalcemia and hypercalciuria have been shown to decrease renal Mg reabsorption and probably are the cause of renal Mg wasting and hypomagnesemia observed in many hypercalcemic states as well as in hypoparathyroid patients receiving vitamin D and calcium therapy. Osmotic diuresis due to glucosuria will result in urinary Mg wasting. Diabetes mellitus is probably the most common clinical disorder associated with Mg depletion.

An increasing list of drugs is becoming recognized as causing renal Mg wasting and Mg depletion. The major site of renal Mg reabsorption is at the loop of Henle; therefore diuretics such as furosemide and ethacrynic acid have been shown to result in marked Mg wasting. Aminoglycosides have been shown to cause a reversible renal lesion that results in hypermagnesuria and hypomagnesemia. Similarly, amphotericin B therapy has been reported to result in renal Mg wasting. Other renal Mg-wasting agents include cisplatin, cyclosporin, and pentamidine. A rising blood alcohol level has been associated with hypermagnesuria and is one factor contributing to Mg depletion in chronic alcoholism. Metabolic acidosis due to diabetic ketoacidosis, starvation, or alcoholism may also result in renal Mg wasting.

Hypomagnesemia may accompany a number of other disorders. Phosphate depletion was shown experimentally to result in urinary Mg wasting and hypomagnesemia. Hypomagnesemia also may accompany the "hungry bone" syndrome, a phase of rapid bone mineral accretion in subjects with hyperparathyroidism or hyperthyroidism following surgical treatment. Finally, chronic renal tubular, glomerular, or interstitial diseases may be associated with renal Mg wasting.

Manifestations of Magnesium Depletion

Because Mg depletion is usually secondary to another disease process or to a therapeutic agent, the features of the primary disease process may complicate or mask Mg depletion. A high index of suspicion is therefore warranted.

Neuromuscular hyperexcitability may be the presenting complaint. Latent tetany, as elicited by positive Chvostek's and Trousseau's signs, or spontaneous carpal-pedal spasm may be present. Frank generalized seizures also may occur. Although hypocalcemia often contributes to the neurologic signs, hypomagnesemia without hypocalcemia has been reported to result in neuromuscular hyperexcitability. Other signs may include vertigo, ataxia, nystagmus, and athetoid and choreiform movements, as well as muscular tremor, fasciculation, wasting, and weakness.

Electrocardiographic abnormalities of Mg depletion in humans include prolonged PR and QT intervals. Mg depletion also may result in cardiac arrhythmias. Supraventricular arrhythmias including premature atrial complexes, atrial tachycardia, atrial fibrillation, and junctional arrhythmias have been described. Ventricular premature complexes, ventricular tachycardia, and ventricular fibrillation are more serious complications. Recently Mg administration to patients with acute myocardial infarction was shown to decrease the mortality rate.

A common laboratory feature of Mg depletion is hypokalemia. During Mg depletion, there is loss of potassium from the cell with intracellular potassium depletion as well as an inability of the kidney to conserve potassium. Attempts to replete the potassium deficit with potassium therapy alone are not successful without simultaneous Mg therapy. This biochemical feature may be a contributing cause of the electrocardiologic findings and cardiac arrhythmias discussed earlier.

Hypocalcemia is (see Chapter 39) a common manifestation of moderate to severe Mg depletion. The hypocalcemia may be a major contributing factor to the increased neuromuscular excitability often present in Mg-depleted patients. The pathogenesis of hypocalcemia is multifactorial. In normal subjects, acute changes in the serum Mg concentration will influence parathyroid hormone (PTH) secretion in a manner similar to calcium. That is, an acute fall in serum Mg stimulates PTH secretion, whereas hypermagnesemia inhibits PTH secretion. During chronic and severe Mg depletion, however, PTH secretion is impaired. The majority of patients will have serum PTH concentrations that are undetectable or inappropriately normal for the degree of hypocalcemia. Some patients, however, may have serum PTH levels above the normal range that may reflect early magnesium depletion. Regardless of the basal circulating PTH concentration, an acute injection of Mg stimulates PTH secretion, as illustrated in Fig. 1. Impaired PTH secretion therefore appears to be a major factor in hypomagnesemia-induced hypocalcemia. Hypocalcemia in the presence of normal or elevated serum PTH concentrations also suggests end-organ resistance to PTH. Patients with hypocalcemia due to Mg depletion have both renal and skeletal resistance to exogenously administered PTH, as manifested by subnormal uri-

nary cyclic adenosine monophosphate (cAMP) and phosphate excretion and diminished calcemic response. This renal and skeletal resistance to PTH is reversed after several days of Mg therapy. The basis for the defect in PTH secretion and PTH end-organ resistance is not known. Because cAMP appears to be important in PTH secretion and mediating PTH effects in kidney and bone, it has been postulated that there may be a defect in the adenylyl cyclase complex. Magnesium is necessary for cAMP formation as substrate [Mg-adenosine triphosphate (ATP)] as well as being an allosteric activator of adenylate cyclase.

Clinically, patients with hypocalcemia due to Mg depletion are resistant not only to PTH, but also to calcium and vitamin D therapy. The vitamin D resistance may be due to impaired metabolism of vitamin D, as serum concentrations of 1,25-dihydroxyvitamin D are low.

Diagnosis of Magnesium Depletion

Measurement of the serum Mg concentration is the most commonly used test to assess Mg status. The normal serum Mg concentration ranges from 1.5 to 1.9 mEq/L (1.8 to 2.2 mg/dL) and a value less than 1.5 mEq/L usually indicates Mg depletion. Mg is principally an intracellular cation and only approximately 1% of the body Mg content is in the extracellular fluid compartments. The serum Mg concentration therefore may not reflect the intracellular Mg content. Because vitamin D and calcium therapy are relatively ineffective in correcting the hypocalcemia, there must be a high index of suspicion for the presence of Mg depletion. Patients with Mg depletion severe enough to result in hypocalcemia are usually significantly hypomagnesemic. However, occasionally, patients may have normal serum Mg concentrations. Magnesium deficiency in the presence of a normal serum Mg concentration has been demonstrated by measuring intracellular Mg (in lymphocytes or muscle biopsy), or by whole-body retention of infused Mg. Therefore hypocalcemic patients who are at risk for Mg depletion, but who have normal serum Mg levels, should receive a trial of Mg therapy. The Mg-tolerance test (or retention test) appears to be an accurate means of assessing Mg status. Correlations with skeletal muscle Mg content and Mg-balance studies have been shown. A suggested protocol for the Mg-tolerance test is shown in Table 2.

Therapy

Patients who present with signs and symptoms of Mg depletion should be treated with Mg. These patients will usually be hypomagnesemic and/or have an abnormal Mg-tolerance test. The extent of the total-body Mg deficit is impossible to predict, but it may be as high as 200 to 400 mEq. Under these circumstances, parenteral Mg administration is usually indicated. An effective treatment regimen is the administration of 2 g $MgSO_4 \cdot 7H_2O$ (16.2 mEq Mg) as a 50% solution every 8 hours intramuscularly. These injections can be painful; a continuous intravenous infusion of 48 mEq over 24 hours may therefore be preferred and is better tolerated. Either regimen will usually result in a normal to slightly increased serum Mg concentration. Despite the

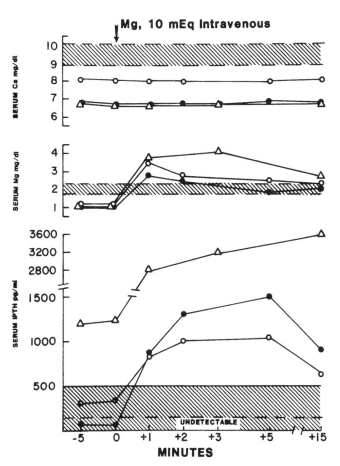

FIG. 1. Effect of an intravenous injection of 10 mEq magnesium on the serum concentration of calcium, magnesium, and immunoreactive parathyroid hormone (iPTH) in hypocalcemic magnesium-deficient patients with undetectable *(open circles)*, normal *(solid circles)*, or elevated *(triangles)*, levels of iPTH. Shaded area represents the range of normal for assay. Broken line for the iPTH assay represents the level of detectability. The magnesium injection resulted in a marked increase in PTH secretion within 1 minute in all three patients.

TABLE 2. *Suggested protocol for use of magnesium-tolerance test*

I. Collect baseline 24-hour urine for magnesium/creatinine ratio[a]
II. Infuse 0.2 mEq (2.4 mg) elemental magnesium per kg lean body weight in 50 mL 5% dextrose over a 4-hour period
III. Collect urine (starting with infusion) for magnesium and creatinine for 24 hours
IV. Percentage magnesium retained is calculated by the following formula

$$\%Mg\ retained = 1 - \left[\frac{\text{Postinfusion 24-hr urine Mg} - \text{Preinfusion urine Mg/creatinine} \times \text{Postinfusion urine creatinine}}{\text{Total elemental Mg infused}}\right] \times 100$$

V. Criteria for Mg deficiency
    >50% retention at 24 h = definite deficiency
    >25% retention at 24 h = probable deficiency

[a] A fasting 2-h spot urine may be used.

fact that PTH secretion increases within minutes after beginning Mg administration, the serum calcium concentration may not return to normal for 3 to 7 days. This probably reflects slow restoration of intracellular Mg. During this period of therapy, serum Mg concentration may be normal, but the total-body deficit may not yet be corrected. Magnesium should be continued until the clinical and biochemical manifestations (hypocalcemia and hypokalemia) of Mg depletion are resolved.

Patients who are hypomagnesemic and have seizures or an acute arrhythmia may be given 8 to 16 mEq of Mg as an intravenous injection over a 5- to 10-minute period followed by 48 mEq intravenously per day. Ongoing Mg losses should be monitored during therapy. If the patient continues to lose Mg from the intestine or kidney, therapy may have to be continued for a longer duration. Once repletion has been accomplished, patients usually can maintain a normal Mg status on a regular diet. If repletion is accomplished and the patient cannot eat, a maintenance dose of 8 mEq should be given daily. Patients who have chronic Mg loss from the intestine or kidney may require continued oral Mg supplementation. A daily dose of 300 to 600 mg of elemental Mg may be given in divided doses to avoid the cathartic effect of Mg.

Caution should be taken during Mg therapy in patients with any degree of renal failure. If a decrease in glomerular filtration rate exists, the dose of Mg should be halved, and the serum Mg concentration must be monitored daily. If hypermagnesemia ensues, therapy must be stopped.

HYPERMAGNESEMIA

Magnesium intoxication is not a frequently encountered clinical problem, although mild to moderate elevations in the serum Mg concentration may be seen in as many as 12% of hospitalized patients.

Symptomatic hypermagnesemia is virtually always due to excessive intake or administration of Mg salts. The majority of patients with hypermagnesemia have concomitant renal failure. Hypermagnesemia is usually seen in patients with renal failure who are receiving Mg as an antacid, enema, or infusion. Hypermagnesemia also is sometimes seen in acute renal failure in the setting of rhabomyolysis.

Large amounts of oral Mg have rarely been reported to cause symptomatic hypermagnesemia in patients with normal renal function. The rectal administration of Mg for purgation may result in hypermagnesemia. Mg is a standard form of therapy for pregnancy-induced hypertension (preeclampsia and eclampsia) and may cause Mg intoxication in the mother as well as in the neonate. Ureteral irrigation with hemiacidrin (Renacidin) was reported to cause symptomatic hypermagnesemia in patients with and without renal failure. Modest elevations in the serum Mg concentration may be seen in familial hypocalcemic hypercalcemia, lithium ingestion, and during volume depletion.

Signs and Symptoms

Neuromuscular symptoms are the most common presenting problem of Mg intoxication. One of the earliest demonstrable effects of hypermagnesemia is the disappearance of the deep tendon reflexes. This is reached at serum Mg concentrations of 4 to 7 mEq/L. Depressed respiration and apnea due to paralysis of the voluntary musculature may be seen at serum Mg concentrations in excess of 8 to 10 mEq/L. Somnolence may be observed at levels as low as 3 mEq/L and above.

Moderate elevations in the serum Mg concentration of 3 to 5 mEq/L result in a mild reduction in blood pressure. High concentrations may result in severe symptomatic hypotension. Mg also can be cardiotoxic. At serum Mg concentrations greater than 5 mEq/L, electrocardiographic findings of prolonged PR intervals as well as increased QRS duration and QT interval are seen. Complete heart block, as well as cardiac arrest, may occur at concentrations greater than 15 mEq/L.

Hypermagnesemia causes a fall in the serum calcium concentration. The hypocalcemia may be related to the suppressive effect of hypermagnesemia on PTH secretion or to hypermagnesemia-induced parathyroid hormone end-organ resistance. A direct effect of Mg on decreasing the serum calcium is suggested by the observation that hypermagnesemia causes hypocalcemia in hypoparathyroid subjects as well.

Other nonspecific manifestations of Mg intoxication include nausea, vomiting, and cutaneous flushing at serum levels of 3 to 9 mEq/L.

Therapy

The possibility of Mg intoxication should be anticipated in any patient receiving Mg, especially if the patient has a reduction in renal function. Mg therapy should merely be discontinued in patients with mild to moderate increases in the serum Mg level. Excess Mg will be excreted by the kidney, and any symptoms or signs of Mg intoxication will resolve. Patients with severe Mg intoxication may be treated with intravenous calcium. Calcium will antagonize the toxic effects of Mg. This antagonism is immediate, but transient. The usual dose is an infusion of 100 to 200 mg of elemental calcium over a period of 5 to 10 minutes. If the patient is in renal failure, peritoneal dialysis or hemodialysis against a low-dialysis Mg bath will rapidly and effectively lower the serum Mg concentration.

SUGGESTED READING

1. Cholst IN, Steinberg SF, Trooper PJ, Fox HE, Segre GV, Bilezikian JP. The influence of hypermagnesemia on serum calcium and parathyroid hormone levels in human subjects. *N Engl J Med* 1984;310:1221–1225.
2. Fassler CA, Rodriguez RM, Badesch DB, Stone WJ, Marini JJ. Magnesium toxicity as a cause of hypotension and hypoventilation: occurrence in patients with normal renal function. *Arch Intern Med* 1985; 145:1604–1606.
3. Flink EB. Magnesium deficiency in human subjects: a personal historical perspective. *J Am Coll Nutr* 1985;4:17–31.
4. Kafka H, Langevin L, Armstrong PW. Serum magnesium and potassium in acute myocardial infarction: influence on ventricular arrhythmias. *Arch Intern Med* 1987;147:465–469.
5. Mordes JP. Excess magnesium. *Pharmacol Rev* 1978;29:273–300.
6. Rasmussen HS, McNair P, Norregard P, Backer V, Lindeneg O, Balslev S. Intravenous magnesium in acute myocardial infarction. *Lancet* 1986;1:234–235.
7. Rude RK. Magnesium deficiency in parathyroid function. In: Bilezikian JP, ed. *The parathyroids.* New York: Raven Press, 1994:829–842.
8. Rude RK. Magnesium disorders. In: Kokko JP, Tannen RL, eds. *Fluids and electrolytes.* 3rd ed. Philadelphia: WB Saunders, 1996:421–445.
9. Rude RK. Magnesium metabolism In: Becker KL, ed. *Principles and practice of endocrinology and metabolism.* Philadelphia: JB Lippincott, 1995:616–622.
10. Rude RK, Oldham SB. Hypocalcemia of Mg deficiency: altered modulation of adenylate cyclase by Mg^{++} and Ca^{++} may result in impaired PTH secretion and PTH end-organ resistance. In: Altura BM, Aurbach J, Seelig JS, eds. *Magnesium in cellular processes and medicine.* Basel: Karger, 1987:183–195.
11. Shah GM, Hirschenbaum MA. Renal magnesium wasting associated with therapeutic agents. *Miner Electrolyte Metab* 1991;17:58–64.
12. Woods KL, Fletcher S. Long-term outcome after intravenous magnesium sulphate in suspected acute myocardial infarction: the second Leicester intravenous magnesium intervention trial (Limit-2). *Lancet* 1994;343:816–819.

45. Hyperphosphatemia and Hypophosphatemia

Keith A. Hruska, M.D. and *Eleanor D. Lederer, M.D., Ph.D.

*Renal Division, Barnes-Jewish Hospital, St. Louis, Missouri; and *Department of Medicine/Nephrology, University of Louisville, and Renal Department, University of Louisville Affiliated Hospitals, Louisville, Kentucky*

HYPERPHOSPHATEMIA

Serum inorganic phosphorus (P_i) concentrations are generally maintained at 2.5 to 4.5 mg/dL or 0.75 to 1.45 mM in adults, whereas hyperphosphatemia is not present in children unless serum P_i levels are greater than 6 mg/dL. Hyperphosphatemia may be the consequence of an increased intake of P_i, a decreased excretion of P_i, or translocation of P_i from tissue breakdown into the extracellular fluid (Table 1). Because the kidneys are able to excrete phosphate very efficiently over a wide range of dietary intake, hyperphosphatemia most frequently results from renal insufficiency and the attendant inability to excrete P_i.

Etiology and Pathogenesis

Increased Intake

Hyperphosphatemia can be the consequence of an *increased intake* or administration of P_i. Intravenous administration of 1 to 2 g of P_i during the treatment of P_i depletion or hypercalcemia can cause hyperphosphatemia, especially in patients with underlying renal insufficiency. Hyperphosphatemia also may result from overzealous use of oral phosphates or of phosphate-containing enemas, as phosphate can be absorbed passively from the colon through paracellular pathways (1,2) (see also Chapter 43). Administration of vitamin D and its metabolites in pharmacologic doses may be responsible for the development of hyperphosphatemia. Suppression of parathyroid hormone (PTH) and hypercalcemia-induced renal failure are important pathogenetic factors in this setting.

Impaired Excretion

Clinically, hyperphosphatemia occurs most commonly as a result of impaired excretion due to renal failure. During the early and middle stages of *chronic renal insufficiency,* phosphate balance is maintained by a progressive reduction in tubular P_i transport, leading to increased P_i excretion by the remaining nephrons and a maintenance of normal renal P_i clearance (3). In advanced renal insufficiency, the fractional excretion of P_i may be as high as 60% to 90% of the filtered load of phosphate. However, when the number of functional nephrons becomes too diminished (glomerular filtration rate usually less than 20 mL/min) and dietary intake is constant, P_i balance can no longer be maintained by reductions of tubular reabsorption, and hyperphosphatemia develops (3).

TABLE 1. *Causes of hyperphosphatemia*

Increased intake
    Oral administration: NeutraPhos
    Rectal: Fleet phosphosoda enemas
    Intravenous: sodium or potassium phosphate
Decreased renal excretion
    Childhood
    Renal insufficiency/failure: acute or chronic
    Hypoparathyroidism
    Pseudohypoparathyroidism
    Acromegaly
    Bisphosphonates
    Tumoral calcinosis
Transcellular shift from intracellular to extracellular spaces
    Catabolic states
    Fulminant hepatitis
    Hyperthermia
    Rhabdomyolysis: crush injuries or nontraumatic
    Cytotoxic therapy: tumor lysis
    Hemolytic anemia
    Acute leukemia
    Acidosis: metabolic or respiratory
Artifactual

When hyperphosphatemia develops, the filtered load of P_i per nephron increases, and P_i excretion rises. As a result, P_i balance and renal excretory rate is reestablished, but at a higher serum P_i level.

Defects in renal excretion of P_i in the absence of renal failure may be primary, as in *pseudohypoparathyroidism* (see Chapter 41) or *tumoral calcinosis* (4,5). The latter is usually seen in young black men with ectopic calcification around large joints and is characterized by increased tubular reabsorption of calcium, P_i, and normal responses to PTH (6). Secondary tubular defects include *hypoparathyroidism* (see Chapter 40) (7) and high blood levels of growth hormone (8). Serum phosphorus values are normally elevated in children as compared with adults. Bisphosphonates, particularly Didronel (disodium etidronate), may cause hyperphosphatemia secondary to cellular phosphate redistribution and decreased renal excretion. More commonly, however, newer bisphosphonates cause hypophosphatemia because of stimulation of secondary hyperparathyroidism (9).

Transcellular Shift

Transcellular shift of P_i from cells into the extracellular fluid compartment may lead to hyperphosphatemia, as seen in conditions associated with increased catabolism or tissue destruction (e.g., systemic infections, fulminant hepatitis, severe hyperthermia, crush injuries, nontraumatic rhabdomyolysis, and cytotoxic therapy for hematologic malignancies such as acute lymphoblastic leukemia and Burkitt's lymphoma). In this *tumor-lysis syndrome,* serum P_i levels typically rise within 1 to 2 days after initiation of treatment. The rising serum P_i concentration often is accompanied by hypocalcemia, hyperuricemia, hyperkalemia, and renal failure.

Patients with *diabetic ketoacidosis* commonly present with hyperphosphatemia despite total body P_i depletion secondary to ketone-induced urinary losses (10). Correction of the hyperglycemia, volume depletion, and acidosis with insulin and fluids causes a shift of P_i back into cells, often resulting in the development of mild, transient hypophosphatemia.

In lactic acidosis, hyperphosphatemia likely results from tissue hypoxia with a breakdown of adenosine triphosphate (ATP) to adenosine monophosphate (AMP) and P_i (11).

Artifactual Hyperphosphatemia

Hyperphosphatemia may be *artifactual* when hemolysis occurs during the collection, storage, or processing of blood samples.

Clinical Consequences of Hyperphosphatemia

The most important short-term consequences of hyperphosphatemia are hypocalcemia and tetany, which occur most commonly in patients with an increased P_i load from any source, exogenous or endogenous. By contrast, soft-tissue calcification and secondary hyperparathyroidism are long-term consequences of hyperphosphatemia that occur mainly in patients with renal insufficiency and decreased renal P_i excretion.

Hypocalcemia and Tetany

With rapid elevations of serum P_i, hypocalcemia and tetany may occur with serum P_i concentrations as low as 6 mg/dL, a level that, if reached more slowly, has no detectable effect on serum calcium. Hyperphosphatemia, in addition to its effect on the calcium $\times$ phosphate ion product with resultant calcium deposition in soft tissues, also inhibits the activity of 1α-hydroxylase in the kidney, resulting in a lower circulating level of 1,25-dihydroxyvitamin D_3 [1,25 $(OH)_2$ D_3]. This further aggravates hypocalcemia by impairing intestinal absorption of calcium and inducing a state of skeletal resistance to the action of PTH.

Phosphate-induced hypocalcemia (Chapter 43) is common in patients with acute or chronic renal failure and usually develops slowly. Tetany is uncommon unless a superimposed acid–base disorder produces an abrupt rise in plasma pH that acutely lowers the serum ionized calcium concentration. Profound hypocalcemia and tetany are occasionally observed during the early phase of the tumor-lysis syndrome and rhabdomyolysis.

Soft-Tissue Calcification

Ectopic calcification is usually seen in patients with chronic renal failure. Occasionally, an acute rise in serum P_i (e.g., during P_i treatment for hypercalcemia) may lead to ectopic calcification, especially when the calcium phosphate product exceeds 70. The blood vessels, skin, cornea (band keratopathy), and periarticular tissues are common sites of calcium precipitation.

Secondary Hyperparathyroidism and Renal Osteodystrophy

Hyperphosphatemia due to renal failure also plays a critical role in development of secondary hyperparathyroidism and renal osteodystrophy. Several mechanisms contribute to these complications including hyperphosphatemia-induced hypocalcemia through physical–chemical interactions, hyperphosphatemia-induced hypocalcemia through inhibition of vitamin D synthesis, and hyperphosphatemia-stimulated PTH secretion (Chapter 69). In patients with advanced renal failure, the enhanced phosphate load from PTH-mediated osteolysis may ultimately become the dominant influence on serum phosphorus levels. This phenomenon may account for the correlation between serum phosphorus levels and the severity of osteitis fibrosa cystica in patients maintained on chronic hemodialysis.

Treatment

Correction of the pathogenetic defect should be the primary aim in the treatment of hyperphosphatemia. When hyperphosphatemia is due solely to increased intake, discontinuation of supplemental phosphate and maintenance of adequate volume for diuresis is generally sufficient, as the kidneys will promptly excrete the excess. In the uncommon circumstance of significant hyperphosphatemia due to transcellular shift, treatment should be dictated by the underlying cause. For example, hyperphosphatemia that accompanies diabetic ketoacidosis will resolve with insulin therapy, as insulin stimulates cellular uptake of phosphate. On the other hand, hyperphosphatemia seen with tumor lysis, rhabdomyolysis, or other conditions characterized by massive cell death or injury should be treated as an excess phosphate load, albeit endogenous instead of exogenous. Limitation of phosphate intake and enhanced diuresis will generally resolve this cause of hyperphosphatemia, provided renal function is adequate.

When renal insufficiency is present, however, the most effective way to treat hyperphosphatemia is to reduce dietary P_i intake and to add phosphate-binding agents. Because P_i is present in almost all foodstuffs, rigid dietary phosphate restriction requires a barely palatable diet that few patients can accept. However, dietary P_i can be reduced to 600 to 1000 mg/day with modest protein restriction. A predialysis level of 4.5 to 5.0 mg/dL is reasonable and allows some room for removal of phosphorus with dialysis while avoiding severe postdialysis hypophosphatemia. To achieve this, most patients require the addition of phosphate binders to reduce intestinal absorption of dietary P_i. Aluminum hydroxide or aluminum carbonate, when administered to patients with renal failure over the long term, has been shown to result in aluminum toxicity with encephalopathy, osteomalacia, proximal myopathy, and anemia. Therefore calcium salts have replaced aluminum salts as first-line P_i binders (12–14). Calcium acetate and aluminum carbonate are equally potent and bind more P_i than equivalent amounts of calcium carbonate or citrate. In general, treatment is started with 1 g of calcium carbonate (two 500-mg tablets) or 1334 mg calcium acetate (two 667-mg tablets) with each meal and gradually increased up to 8 to 12 g daily. This regimen effectively controls serum P_i in about two thirds of patients on chronic dialysis (13). Calcium salts tend to increase serum calcium levels, and if hypercalcemia (more than 11 mg/dL) develops, calcium carbonate should not be increased further, and reduction in dialysate calcium should be considered. Because

citrate markedly increases the absorption of aluminum, the use of calcium citrate as a phosphate binder should probably be avoided, and particularly if the patient is concomitantly taking aluminum. Maximal P_i binding occurs when phosphate binder is taken with a meal rather than 2 hours afterward. Magnesium-containing antacids also are effective phosphate binders; however, their use in renal failure is limited because intestinal absorption of magnesium can lead to magnesium toxicity.

The treatment of chronic hyperphosphatemia secondary to hypoparathyroidism occasionally requires that phosphate binders be added to the other therapeutic agents.

HYPOPHOSPHATEMIA

Hypophosphatemia is defined as an abnormally low concentration of P_i in serum or plasma. Hypophosphatemia does not necessarily indicate total body P_i depletion because only 1% of the total body P_i is found in extracellular fluids. Conversely, serious P_i depletion may exist in the presence of a normal or even elevated serum P_i concentration. Moderate hypophosphatemia, defined as a serum P_i concentration between 2.5 and 1 mg/dL, is not uncommon and is usually not associated with signs or symptoms. Severe hypophosphatemia, defined as serum phosphorus levels below 1.0 mg/dL, is often associated with clinical signs and symptoms that require therapy. Approximately 3% of hospital patients have levels of serum P_i below 2 mg/dL, according to some estimates, with up to 0.43% of patients developing severe hypophosphatemia (15). In critically ill patients, the incidence of hypophosphatemia rises dramatically, with reported incidences up to 77% in selected populations (16–20). Hypophosphatemia is encountered more frequently among alcoholic patients, and up to 10% of patients admitted to hospitals because of chronic alcoholism are hypophosphatemic.

Etiology and Pathogenesis

Three types of pathophysiologic abnormalities can cause hypophosphatemia and total body P_i depletion: decreased intestinal absorption of P_i, increased urinary losses of this ion, and a shift of P_i from extracellular to intracellular compartments. Combinations of these disturbances are common (15,21). The causes and mechanisms of moderate hypophosphatemia are shown in Table 2; the clinical conditions associated with severe hypophosphatemia are shown in Table 3.

Decreased Intake

Impaired Gastrointestinal Absorption

Severe hypophosphatemia and phosphate depletion may result from vigorous use of oral antacids that bind phosphate, usually for peptic ulcer disease (22). Patients so treated may develop osteomalacia and severe skeletal symptoms because of phosphorus deficiency. Intestinal malabsorption syndromes can cause hypophosphatemia and phosphate depletion through malabsorption of P_i and vitamin D and through increased urinary P_i losses resulting from secondary hyper-

TABLE 2. *Causes of moderate hypophosphatemia, phosphate depletion, or both*

Decreased intestinal absorption
    Antacid abuse
    Vitamin D deficiency
    Malabsorption
    Starvation: famine, anorexia nervosa, alcoholism
Increased urinary losses
    Hyperparathyroidism
    Renal tubular defects: Fanconi, posttransplant, hypomagnesemia, fructose intolerance
    Abnormalities of Vitamin D metabolism
        X-linked hypophosphatemic rickets
        Vitamin D–dependent rickets
        Vitamin D deficiency
    Oncogenic osteomalacia
    Alcoholism
    Diabetic ketoacidosis
    Metabolic or respiratory acidosis
    Drugs: calcitonin, diuretics, glucocorticoids, bicarbonate, β agonists
    Extracellular fluid volume expansion
Transcellular shift from the extracellular to the intracellular space
    Nutritional repletion–refeeding syndrome
    Respiratory alkalosis
    Recovery from metabolic acidosis, commonly diabetic ketoacidosis
    Recovery from hypothermia
    Sepsis, especially gram-negative bacteremia
    Salicylate intoxication
    Sugars: glucose, fructose, glycerol
    Insulin therapy
    Blast crisis in leukemia
    "Hungry-bone" syndrome after parathyroidectomy

parathyroidism induced by calcium malabsorption. Primary vitamin D deficiency in the absence of a malabsorption syndrome, especially superimposed on poor oral P_i intake, also can lead to hypophosphatemia. Vitamin D–deficiency rickets (when the deficiency occurs in children) or osteomalacia (when the deficiency occurs in adults) may result in severe deformities of the skeleton (see Chapter 61). Hypophosphatemia is the most frequent biochemical alteration associated with this metabolic abnormality.

TABLE 3. *Risk factors for severe hypophosphatemia, phosphate depletion, or both*

Alcohol withdrawal
Nutritional repletion in at-risk patients
    Anorexia nervosa and other eating disorders
    Starvation due to famine, neglect, alcoholism, malabsorption, prisoners of war
    Acquired immunodeficiency syndrome (AIDS) and other chronic infections
    Massive weight loss for morbid obesity
Treatment of diabetic ketoacidosis
Critical illness
    Sepsis
    After trauma
    Extensive burns

Alcohol and Alcohol Withdrawal

Alcohol abuse is a common cause of severe hypophosphatemia (Table 3) (23,24) due to both poor intake and excessive losses. Poor intake results from dietary deficiencies, the use of antacids, and vomiting. Patients with alcoholism also have been shown to have a variety of defects in renal tubular function, including a decrease in threshold for phosphate excretion, which are reversible with abstinence. Ethanol enhances urinary P_i excretion, and marked phosphaturia tends to occur during episodes of alcoholic ketoacidosis. Because such patients often eat poorly, ketonuria is common. Repeated episodes of ketoacidosis catabolize organic phosphates within cells and cause phosphaturia by mechanisms analogous to those seen in diabetic ketoacidosis. Chronic alcoholism also may cause magnesium deficiency and hypomagnesemia, which may, in turn, cause phosphaturia and P_i depletion, especially in skeletal muscle (see Chapter 44).

Nutritional Repletion: Oral, Enteral, and Parenteral Nutrition

Nutritional repletion of the malnourished patient implies the provision of sufficient calories, protein, and other nutrients to allow accelerated tissue accretion. In the course of this process, cellular uptake and utilization of P_i increase. When insufficient amounts of P_i are provided, an acute state of severe hypophosphatemia and intracellular P_i depletion with serious clinical and metabolic consequences can occur (25). Patients at risk include those with acquired immunodeficiency syndrome or other chronic infections, eating disorders (anorexia nervosa, bulimia, alcoholism), prolonged starvation (famine, prisoners of war, abuse, and neglect), massive weight loss for morbid obesity, Crohn's disease, cystic fibrosis, thermal injury, cancer, or prolonged parenteral therapy.

Increased Losses

Primary Hyperparathyroidism

This is a common entity in clinical medicine. PTH is secreted in excess of the physiologic needs for mineral homeostasis owing either to adenoma or hyperplasia of the parathyroid glands (see Chapter 30). This results in decreased phosphorus reabsorption by the kidney, and the urinary losses of phosphorus result in hypophosphatemia. The degree of hypophosphatemia varies considerably because mobilization of phosphorus from stimulation of skeletal remodeling in part mitigates the hypophosphatemia. Secondary hyperparathyroidism associated with normal renal function has been observed in patients with gastrointestinal abnormalities, resulting in calcium malabsorption. Such patients may have low levels of serum calcium and phosphorus (see Chapter 43). In these patients, the hypocalcemia is responsible for increased release of PTH. Decreased intestinal absorption of phosphorus as a result of the primary gastrointestinal disease may contribute to the decrement in the levels of the serum phosphorus. Patients with hypophos-

46. Epidemiology of Osteoporosis

Richard D. Wasnich, M.D., F.A.C.P.

Department of Medicine, University of Hawaii, and Radiant Research-Honolulu, Honolulu, Hawaii

A recent consensus conference defined osteoporosis as a metabolic bone disease characterized by low bone mass and microarchitectural deterioration of bone tissue, leading to enhanced bone fragility and a consequent increase in fracture risk (1). Another distinguishing characteristic of osteoporosis is a normal mineral/collagen ratio, which distinguishes it from osteomalacia, a disease characterized by relative deficiency of mineral in relation to collagen.

Osteoporosis is the most prevalent metabolic bone disease in the United States and other developed countries. Fracture prevalence refers to the number of people in the population who at a given time have already had fractures related to osteoporosis. Vertebral fracture prevalence among women aged 65 years has been estimated to be 27% in Minnesota (2) and 21% among Danish women at age 70 years (3).

Incidence refers to the number of new fracture cases in a population within a specified time. For example, among Japanese American women in Hawaii, 5% of 80-year-old women will experience a new vertebral fracture each year. In general, data concerning the prevalence and incidence of hip, wrist, and other nonvertebral fractures are more reliable than are vertebral fracture data. That is because many vertebral fractures are not clinically evident; therefore only populations that have been surveyed by periodic spine radiographs yield accurate prevalence data. Vertebral fracture data are further hampered by the absence of a clear radiographic definition of vertebral fracture (4).

Osteoporotic fractures increase with age; wrist fractures show a rising incidence in the 50s, vertebral fractures in the 60s, and hip fractures in the 70s (Fig. 1). There is at least a twofold higher incidence among women compared with men for all age-related fracture sites. Because life expectancy is longer for women, there are proportionately more older women than men, resulting in a greater fracture prevalence among women than would be predicted from the age-adjusted incidence ratio.

Interesting geographic and ethnic differences exist. For example, hip-fracture rates are higher in white populations regardless of geographic location (5). In contrast, hip-fracture rates are lower among blacks in the United States and South Africa and also among Japanese in both Japan and the United States (6,7).

Frequently, but not always, ethnic and geographic differences in fracture prevalence can be explained by differences in bone density. The strong relation between diminishing bone density and the risk of fragility fractures is well established. The risk of new vertebral fractures increases by a factor of 2.0 to 2.4 for each standard deviation (SD) decrease of bone density, irrespective of the site of bone density measurement (8). Similar findings have been found for hip and other nonvertebral fractures. It has therefore been proposed by a World Health Organization (WHO) expert panel that women with bone density values more than 2.5 SD below the young adult mean value be considered osteoporotic (9). If they also have one or more fragility fractures, they would be classified as severe or established osteoporosis. Those women with bone density values between 1 and 2.5 SD below the young adult mean values would be classified as osteopenic.

Because surveys of bone density are easier to obtain than are accurate fracture-incidence data, they may provide better estimates of osteoporosis prevalence. Based on the WHO diagnostic categories, Melton (10) estimated that 54% of postmenopausal white women in the United States have osteopenia, and another 30% have osteoporosis. Thus white women alone account for 26 million people who are at risk for fracture. The addition of men and nonwhite women would increase the total considerably. This number compares with 30 to 54 million Americans who have hypertension.

The aging of the world population, when combined with the exponential, age-related increases in fracture incidence, portend drastic increases in the costs of osteoporosis. Cummings et al. (11) estimated that the cost of hip fractures alone in the United States could reach $240 billion within 50 years. Although there is an increased mortality rate following both hip and vertebral fractures, the worst consequence of osteoporosis might not be the increased mortality but rather the fact that most patients must live with the disease for many years, with its associated loss of independence and impaired quality of life (12). This is particularly true for vertebral fractures, which begin at an earlier age than hip fractures and affect many more women and men.

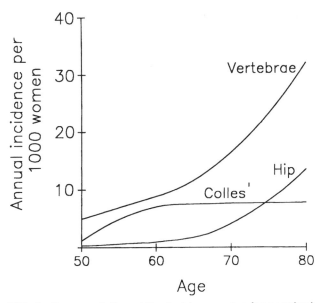

FIG. 1. Representation of the incidence rates for vertebral, Colles', and hip fractures in women.

RISK FACTORS

Major risk factors for osteoporosis, such as age and bone density, have been established by virtue of their direct and strong relation to fracture incidence. These more potent risk factors might be categorized as clinical risk indicators (8). However, a majority of the suspected or established risk factors for osteoporosis are based on their relation to bone density as a surrogate indicator of disease presence and are therefore only as valid as the surrogate indicator. This category of risk factors might be categorized as etiologic; the utility of these risk factors is more likely to be in the realm of public health than in the management of individual clinical patients.

Most risk factors are in five major categories: age, or age-related; genetic; environmental; endogenous hormones and chronic diseases; and physical characteristics of bone (Table 1).

The relative contribution of individual risk factors is much influenced by the age at which they are expressed. For example, estrogen deficiency during the adolescent years can be catastrophic to the growing skeleton. It also has a significant impact at age 50 years, but for some women, the impact is negligible. After age 70 or 80 years, estrogen deficiency may be overshadowed by other risk factors. This concept is illustrated in Fig. 2. The clinical utility of bone density is derived from the fact that it is a composite, cumulative index of multiple other risk factors, both past and present, and including both genetic and lifestyle influences. This concept has been reinforced by recent data relating high bone density to higher breast cancer risk; the basis for this relation is probably lifetime estrogen exposure, both endogenous and exogenous (13,14).

HETEROGENEITY

Because of its multifactorial etiology, it is not surprising that osteoporosis is a heterogeneous disorder. The relative

TABLE 1. *Risk factors for osteoporosis*

Age, or Age-Related
    Each decade associated with 1.4–1.8-fold increased risk
Genetic
    Ethnicity: Caucasians and Oriental > blacks and Polynesians
    Gender: Female > male
    Family history
Environmental
    Nutrition; calcium deficiency
    Physical activity and mechanical loading
    Medications, e.g., corticosteroids
    Smoking
    Alcohol
    Falls (trauma)
Endogenous Hormones and Chronic Diseases
    Estrogen deficiency
    Androgen deficiency
    Chronic diseases, e.g., gastrectomy, cirrhosis, hyperthyroidism, hypercortisolism
Physical Characteristics of Bone
    Density (mass)
    Size and geometry
    Microarchitecture
    Composition

contributions of age and estrogen deficiency have been emphasized in the past, but it is difficult to differentiate these two factors in most patients. It is also increasingly apparent that there are multiple other contributing etiologies, including those that are unknown or poorly understood. Furthermore, the predominant etiology may vary substantially from patient to patient. The major contribution of peak bone mass to ultimate fracture risk indicates that risk factors that are expressed during childhood and adolescence may contribute as much to lifetime fracture risk as do aging and menopause. In any case, *treatable* (and preventable) etiologies are of

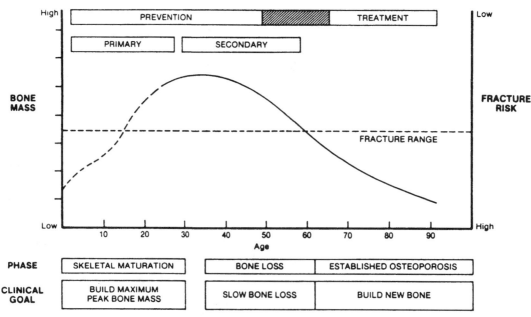

FIG. 2. Schematic lifetime representation of bone mass and fracture risk.

greater clinical and public health importance, particularly if they are also common, such as low bone density.

CLINICAL IMPLICATIONS

Ultimately, knowledge gained from epidemiologic studies should influence public health practice and clinical management of individual patients. These two applications are different and are sometimes confused, perhaps because the correct interpretation and application of epidemiologic findings to clinical practice is not always intuitively apparent. For example, estrogen deficiency following menopause is a consistently demonstrated risk factor in population studies. However, many women do not show significant bone loss in the years soon after menopause, and a minority, perhaps 25% to 30% of women, never experience a fracture in their lifetimes. These women generally have high bone density before the age of menopause and/or show less bone loss after menopause. For these women, estrogen deficiency is not a major risk factor, and providing estrogen replacement to these women provides no demonstrable skeletal benefit. Thus risk factors that apply to population groups may not necessarily apply to every (or any) individual. For example, black men have an increased risk of hypertension; however, it would not be considered prudent to treat all black men for hypertension in the absence of an objective indicator of disease.

THE MEANING OF A FRACTURE

Aside from the clinical and socioeconomic consequences of a fracture, there is another, crucial implication of a fragility fracture in an individual patient. The very presence of a fracture is a potent risk factor for future fractures, independent of bone density (15,16). Although the explanation for this finding is uncertain, in the spine it may be partially explained by altered load distribution on neighboring vertebral bodies. This also would help explain why vertebral fractures tend to cluster in the midthoracic and lower thoracic/upper lumbar spine.

However, one important implication is that the clinical goal of fracture-risk management should be prevention of the first fracture. It is considered prudent to manage hypertension prior to the onset of complications, such as stroke or renal failure. Likewise, early identification of high fracture risk offers greater opportunities to prevent future fractures. Hip fractures occur at older ages than other osteoporotic fractures. More emphasis should be placed on early identification of women at high fracture risk, and preventive measures initiated well prior to any fracture.

FUTURE FRACTURE RISK

The concept of lifetime fracture risk has typically been applied to populations. An average 50-year-old white woman has an approximate 17% lifetime risk of hip fracture (17). However, depending on levels of bone density and other risk factors, this figure will vary substantially between individuals.

The term "remaining lifetime fracture probability" (RLFP) has been used to describe an individual's fracture risk. RLFP is calculated from age, bone density, life expectancy, and anticipated future bone loss (18). The concept of cumulative fracture risk is important when deciding whether to use pharmacologic agents to prevent future fractures. For such clinical decisions, measures of bone density alone are insufficient; current age must also be considered. The reason is that a woman whose bone density value is −1 SD (*T* score, −1.0, and therefore osteopenic) at age 80 years may not benefit from drug treatment because of her limited life expectancy and future bone loss. However, a 50-year-old with a similar, but normal, bone density, say −0.9 SD (*T* score, −0.9), may gain a substantial benefit from drug intervention.

For this reason, the concept of RLFP is a useful means of incorporating multiple risk factors into a single index of risk severity, which can better guide clinical decision making.

REFERENCES

1. Consensus Development Conference V, 1993. Diagnosis, prophylaxis, and treatment of osteoporosis. *Am J Med* 1994;90:646–650.
2. Melton LJ III. Epidemiology of vertebral fractures in women. *Am J Epidemiol* 1989;129:1000–1011.
3. Jensen GF, Christiansen C, Boesen J, Hegedus V, Transbol I. Epidemiology of postmenopausal spinal and long bone fractures. *Clin Orthop* 1982;166:75–81.
4. Cooper C, O Neill T, Silman A, on behalf of the European Vertebral Osteoporosis Study Group. The epidemiology of vertebral fractures. *Bone* 1993;14:589–597.
5. Melton LJ, Riggs BL. Epidemiology of age-related fractures. In: Avioli LV, ed. *The osteoporotic syndrome: detection, prevention, and treatment.* New York: Grune & Stratton, 1983:45–72.
6. Solomon L. Osteoporosis and fracture of the femoral neck in the South African Bantu. *J Bone Joint Surg Br* 1968;50:2–13.
7. Ross PD, Norimatsu H, Davis JW, et al. A comparison of hip fracture incidence among native Japanese, Japanese-Americans, and American-Caucasians. *Am J Epidemiol* 1991;133:801–809.
8. Wasnich R. Bone mass measurement: prediction of risk. *Am J Med* 1993;95:65–105.
9. Kanis JA, Melton LJ III, Christiansen C, Johnston CC, Khaltaev N. The diagnosis of osteoporosis. *J Bone Miner Res* 1994;9:1137–1141.
10. Melton LJ III. How many women have osteoporosis now? *J Bone Miner Res* 1995;10:175–177.
11. Cummings SR, Rubin SM, Black D. The future of hip fractures in the United States. *Clin Orthop* 1990;252:163–166.
12. Barrett-Connor E. The economics and human costs of osteoporotic fracture. *Am J Med* 1995;98:3–8.
13. Cauley JA, Lucas FL, Kuller LH, et al. Bone mineral density and risk of breast cancer in older women. *JAMA* 1996;276:1404–1408.
14. Zhang Y, Kiel DP, Kreger BE, et al. Bone mass and the risk of breast cancer among postmenopausal women. *N Engl J Med* 1997;336:611–617.
15. Ross PD, Davis JW, Epstein R, Wasnich RD. Pre-existing fractures and bone mass predict vertebral fracture incidence in women. *Ann Intern Med* 1991;114:919–923.
16. Wasnich RD, Davis JW, Ross PD. Spine fracture risk is predicted by non-spine fractures. *Osteoporos Int* 1995;4:1–5.
17. Black D, Cummings S, Melton LJ. Appendicular bone mineral and a woman's lifetime risk of hip fracture. *J Bone Miner Res* 1992;7:639–646.
18. Wasnich RD, Ross PD, Vogel JM, Davis JW. *Osteoporosis: critique and practicum.* Honolulu: Banyan Press, 1989.

47. Pathogenesis of Postmenopausal Osteoporosis

Richard Eastell, M.D., F.R.C.P.

Division of Clinical Sciences, University of Sheffield and Department of Medicine, Northern General Hospital, Sheffield, England

Osteoporosis-related fractures result from a combination of decreased bone mineral density (BMD) and a deterioration in bone microarchitecture. A BMD below average for age can be considered a consequence of inadequate accumulation of bone in young adult life (low peak bone mass) or of excessive rates of bone loss. The microarchitectural changes occur with the bone loss but will be considered separately.

DETERMINANTS OF PEAK BONE MASS

The increase in bone mass that occurs during childhood and puberty results from a combination of bone growth at the end plates (endochondral bone formation) and of change in bone shape (modeling). The rapid increase in bone mass at puberty is associated with an increase in sex hormone levels and the closure of the growth plates. Within 3 years of menarche, there is little further increase in bone mass. The small increase in BMD over the next 5 to 15 years is referred to as *consolidation.* The resulting peak bone mass is achieved by age 20 to 30 years.

Genetic factors are the main determinants of peak bone mass (1). This was shown by studies made on twins or on mother–daughter pairs. Heritability appears to account for about 50% to 85% of the variance in bone mass, depending on the skeletal site. It is likely that several genes regulate bone mass, each with a modest effect, and likely candidates include the genes for type I collagen (COL1A1) and for the vitamin D receptor (1). The nongenetic factors include low calcium intake during childhood, low body weight at maturity and at 1 year of life, sedentary lifestyle, and delayed puberty. Each of these results in decreased bone mass.

BONE LOSS

Mechanisms

Bone loss occurs in the postmenopausal woman as a result of an increase in the rate of bone remodeling and an imbalance between the activity of osteoclasts and osteoblasts. Bone remodeling occurs at discrete sites within the skeleton and proceeds in an orderly fashion, with bone resorption always being followed by bone formation, a phenomenon referred to as *coupling.* In cortical and cancellous bone, the sequence of bone remodeling is similar (2). The quiescent bone surface is converted to activity (*origination*), and the osteoclasts resorb bone (*progression*), forming a cutting cone (cortical bone) or a trench (cancellous bone). The osteoblasts synthesize bone matrix that subsequently mineralizes. The sequence takes up to 8 months. If the processes of bone resorption and bone formation are not matched, then there is *remodeling imbalance.* In postmenopausal women, this imbalance is magnified by the increase in the rate of initiation of new bone-remodeling cycles (*activation frequency*).

Remodeling imbalance results in irreversible bone loss. There are two other causes of irreversible bone loss, referred to as *remodeling errors.* First is excavation of overlarge haversian spaces in cortical bone (3). Radial infilling is regulated by signals from the outermost osteocytes and is generally no more than 90 μm. Hence large external diameters, which may simply occur randomly, lead to large central haversian canals, which then accumulate with age, leading to increased cortical porosity. In a similar way, osteoclast penetration of trabecular plates, or severing of trabecular beams, removes the scaffolding needed for osteoblastic replacement of resorbed bone. In both ways, random remodeling errors tend to reduce both cancellous and cortical bone density and structural integrity.

Causes

Estrogen Deficiency

Bone loss in the postmenopausal woman occurs in two phases (4). There is a phase of rapid bone loss that lasts for 5 years (about 3%/year in the spine). Subsequently there is lower bone loss that is more generalized (about 0.5%/year at many sites). This slower phase of bone loss affects men, starting at about age 55 years.

The major mechanism of the rapid phase of bone loss in women is estrogen deficiency. The circulating level of estradiol decreases by 90% at the time of the menopause. This bone loss can be prevented by the administration of estrogen and progestins to the postmenopausal woman. It has been estimated that this rapid phase of bone loss contributes 50% to the spinal bone loss across life in women.

The major effect of estrogen deficiency is on bone, where it increases activation frequency and may contribute to the remodeling imbalance. The exact mechanism of action of estrogen on bone is unclear. Estrogen may act partly through the osteoblast (e.g. increased synthesis of insulin-like growth factor I and transforming growth factor-β) and partly through monocytes in the bone marrow environment (e.g., decreased synthesis of interleukin 1 and tumor necrosis factor-α). This modulation of locally active growth factors and cytokines mediates the effects of estrogen on osteoblasts and osteoclasts. Thus a greater increase in cytokines (e.g., interleukin 1) in response to estrogen deficiency may account for the more rapid bone loss in some women.

Aging

The slow phase of bone loss is attributed to age-related factors such as an increase in PTH levels and to osteoblast senescence (Fig. 1). An increase in PTH levels (and action) occurs in both men and women with aging (5). PTH levels correlate with biochemical markers of bone turnover, and both may be returned to those found in young adults by the intravenous infusion of calcium (4). The increase in PTH results from decreased renal calcium reabsorption and decreased intestinal calcium absorption. The latter may result

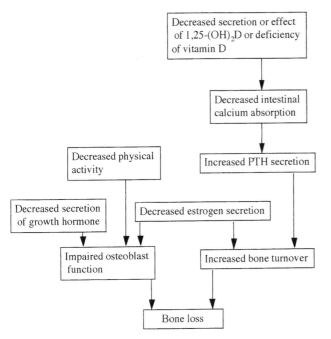

FIG. 1. Proposed mechanism for age-related bone loss in women. Note how estrogen deficiency probably results in both increased bone turnover and remodeling imbalance. (Reproduced from Blumsohn A, Eastell R. Pathophysiology of osteoporosis: age-related factors. In: Riggs BL, Melton LJ III, eds. *Osteoporosis, etiology, diagnosis and management.* Philadelphia: Lippincott-Raven, 1995:161–182 and Riggs BL, Khosla S, Melton LJ III. A unitary model for involutional osteoporosis: estrogen deficiency causes both type I and type II osteoporosis in postmenopausal women and contributes to bone loss in aging men. *J Bone Miner Res* 1998;13:763–773 with permission of the American Society for Bone and Mineral Research.)

from vitamin D deficiency (e.g., in the housebound elderly), decreased 1α-hydroxylase activity in the kidney, resulting in decreased synthesis of 1,25-dihydroxyvitamin D [1,25 $(OH)_2$ D], or resistance to vitamin D. Whatever the cause, a diet high in calcium returns both PTH and bone-turnover markers to levels found in healthy young adults.

It has been proposed that the age-related increase in PTH could result from indirect effects of estrogen deficiency (4). This proposal is based on the following evidence. In older women treated with estrogen, (a) there is a decrease in bone-turnover markers and PTH levels, (b) there is an increase in calcium absorption, possibly mediated by an increase in 1,25 $(OH)_2$ D, (c) there is an increase in the PTH-independent calcium reabsorption in the kidney, and (d) there is a decrease in the parathyroid secretory reserve.

Accelerating Factors

A number of diseases and drugs are clearly related to accelerated bone loss, and these are described elsewhere (see Chapters 55, 58, and 60). Their effects are superimposed on those described earlier. Thus a patient starting on corticosteroid therapy is more likely to have an osteoporosis-related fracture if she has low BMD resulting from low peak bone mass and the accelerated bone loss of the menopause.

Identification of Mechanism of Bone Loss in an Individual

In a woman with presenting osteoporosis at age 65 years, it is often possible to identify several reasons for the low BMD (Fig. 2). Some of these may be identified from history taking (early menopause, drugs that accelerate bone loss), but some cannot be identified in retrospect (low peak bone mass, rapid losers).

OTHER DETERMINANTS OF BONE STRENGTH

Bone Geometry

Bone geometry has a major effect on fracture risk (3). One example is hip-axis length, the distance from the lateral surface of the trochanter to the inner surface of the pelvis, along the axis of the femoral neck. Short hip-axis length results in an architecturally stronger structure for any given bone density. This is probably the reason that Japanese and other Asian populations have about half the hip-fracture rate of whites, despite similar bone density values. Likewise,

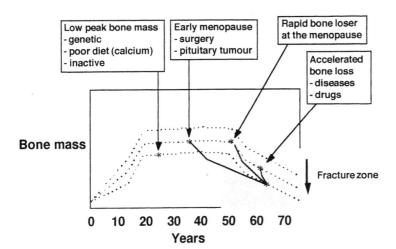

FIG. 2. Causes of low bone mineral density (BMD) in postmenopausal women. BMD reaches a peak between ages 20 and 30 years and then is followed by a rapid phase of bone loss at the menopause lasting 5 years, followed by a slower phase of bone loss. Bone loss in a 65-year-old woman may have a single cause (as shown here), or there may be several causes contributing to the low BMD.

large vertebral body end-plate areas result in lower spine-pressure values for individuals of the same body size. Those with small vertebral bodies are thus more likely to fracture. Such geometric factors both contribute to individual fracture risk and explain a substantial portion of the population-level variance in fracture rate. In each situation, however, the ultimate pathogenesis of the fracture is the fall and the force sustained by the bone on impact.

Fatigue Damage

Fatigue damage consists of ultramicroscopic rents in the basic bony material, resulting from the inevitable bending that occurs when a structural member is loaded (3). Fatigue damage is the principal cause of failure in mechanical engineering structures; its prevention is the responsibility of the remodeling apparatus, which detects and removes fatigue-damaged bone. Fractures related to fatigue damage occur whenever the damage occurs faster than remodeling can repair it or whenever the remodeling apparatus is defective. March fractures and the fractures of radiation necrosis are well-recognized examples of fractures due to these two mechanisms. Fatigue damage definitely occurs in normal bone, under ordinary use, although it is less certain precisely what role it may play in predisposing to osteoporotic fracture. Furthermore, there is suggestive evidence for certain fractures (notably hip) that remodeling repair may be defective specifically at the site that ultimately fractures. Why remodeling surveillance or effectiveness might fail locally is not known. Nevertheless, it is clear that such failure would lead to accumulation of fatigue damage and, therefore, to local weakening of bone (6).

Loss of Trabecular Connectivity

Bone structures loaded vertically, such as the vertebral bodies and femoral and tibial metaphyses, derive a substantial portion of their structural strength from a system of horizontal, cross-bracing trabeculae, which support the verti-cal elements and limit lateral bowing and consequent snapping under vertical loading. Severance of such trabecular connections is known to occur preferentially in postmenopausal women and is considered to be a major reason for the large female/male preponderance of vertebral osteoporosis. That long, unsupported vertical trabeculae are susceptible to fracture is reflected in the extraordinarily high prevalence of trabecular fracture callus sites in vertebral bodies examined at autopsy, typically 200 to 450 healing or healed fractures per vertebral body. Whereas many of these will be well enough healed at any given time to be structurally competent, others will be fresh and structurally weak. Such fractures are asymptomatic, and their accumulation both reflects the impact of lost trabecular connections and greatly weakens the cancellous structure of the vertebral body. The incident fracture-prediction ability of prior vertebral fractures is probably due in part to the presence of such otherwise undetected trabecular defects. That is why prior fracture seems to predict future fracture even when bone density is relatively high. The reason for preferential osteoclastic severance of horizontal trabeculae is not known. It is sometimes attributed to overaggressive osteoclastic resorption, but that seems more descriptive than explanatory (6).

REFERENCES

1. Ralston SH. Science, medicine and the future: osteoporosis. *BMJ* 1997; 315:469–472.
2. Parfitt AM, Mundy GR, Roodman GD, Hughes DE, Boyce BF. A new model for the regulation of bone resorption, with particular reference to the effects of bisphosphonates. *J Bone Miner Res* 1996;11:150–159.
3. Marcus R. The nature of osteoporosis. *J Clin Endocrinol Metab* 1996; 81:1–5.
4. Riggs BL, Khosla S, Melton LJ III. A unitary model for involutional osteoporosis: estrogen deficiency causes both type I and type II osteoporosis in postmenopausal women and contributes to bone loss in aging men. *J Bone Miner Res* 1998;13:763–773.
5. Blumsohn A, Eastell R. Pathophysiology of osteoporosis: age-related factors. In: Riggs BL, Melton LJ III, eds. *Osteoporosis, etiology, diagnosis and management*. Philadelphia: Lippincott-Raven, 1995:161–182.
6. Heaney RP. Pathogenesis of postmenopausal osteoporosis. In: Favus MJ, ed. *Primer on the metabolic bone diseases and disorders of mineral metabolism*, 3rd ed. Philadelphia: Lippincott-Raven, 1996:253–254.

48. Physical Activity and Regulation of Bone Mass

Robert Marcus, M.D.

Department of Medicine, Stanford University, and Aging Study Unit, Geriatrics Research, Education and Clinical Center, Veterans Affairs Medical Center, Palo Alto, California

The primary function of bone is to provide a strong and resilient structure that permits resistance against gravitational and other forces while providing structural rigidity for locomotion. To accommodate both requirements, bone adapts to the mechanical demands that are placed on it. This principle, known as Wolff's law, may be paraphrased to state that bone accommodates the loads imposed on it by altering its mass and distribution of mass. When habitual loading increases, bone is gained; when loading decreases, bone is lost. What appears to be optimized by this adaptive response is the distribution of load-related strain, or deformation, within bones. As an example of how effective and broadly applicable this process is, it is remarkable that when animals with diverse loading patterns engage in typical activities (running, jumping, and so forth), peak long-bone strains consistently fall within a fairly narrow range of 2000 to 3500 microstrain (1 strain = 1% deformation; 3000 microstrain = 0.12% deformation) (1).

Habitual loading can be described as the sum of all individual daily loading events, with each event further characterized by its intensity and number of repetitions. Load magnitude seems to outweigh load repetitions as an influence on bone mass (2). The relation between mechanical loading and bone mass is curvilinear, with a much steeper slope at very low levels of loading. Thus the most easily demonstrable interaction between physical activity and bone mass is the substantial loss of bone that occurs with immobilization. Completely immobilized patients may lose 40% of their original bone mass in 1 year, whereas standing upright with postural shifting for 30 minutes each day may completely prevent the deleterious skeletal effects of bed rest. By contrast, the amount of bone that can be gained by active people who increase their level of exercise is very limited, accounting for only a few percentage increase over a year's time.

BONE MASS IN ATHLETES

Trained athletes have higher bone mass than do nonathletes (3), with the largest effect seen when the regimen includes strength training (4). Much of this literature may be confounded by the possibility that the musculoskeletal characteristics of athletes may differ from those of the general population even prior to training. This may explain why the results of exercise-intervention studies have been relatively meager compared with differences reported in comparative studies. That there is certainly some skeletal effect of training emerges from the exaggerated increases in bone mineral density (BMD) that are observed in the racquet versus the nonracquet forearms of elite tennis players (5).

PHYSICAL ACTIVITY AND BONE MASS IN NONATHLETES

A critical issue is whether the skeletal benefits enjoyed by elite athletes also extend to ordinary mortals. Bone ''acquisition'' by children (6), adolescents (7), and young women (8) seems clearly to reflect habitual physical activity. In contrast, a few (9,10), but certainly not all (11,12) cross-sectional studies in adults have shown a positive relation of BMD to current or previous self-reported levels of physical activity. The validity of such studies is severely constrained by major difficulties in assessing a person's true physical activity level but is hampered even more in attempting to extrapolate rough indices of overall physical exertion to estimate skeletal loading. It may be that some of the most important daily loading events for the skeleton are not even recognized by a person who maintains an exercise record. This would be particularly true for such activities as pushing against a heavy door, lifting a box of canned goods, or some other occupational activity.

RESPONSE OF BONE TO EXERCISE

With one notable exception (13), well-controlled randomized exercise trials using strength (14–17) and endurance (15,16) activities reported significant but modest positive effects of exercise on lumbar spine BMD of young women.

Increases averaged 1% to 3% and were achieved during the first year, with few if any gains thereafter (16,17). Improvement in hip BMD was found in only one study, which continued for 2 years (17). Another study showed that strength training maintains lumbar spine BMD of recently menopausal women, but no such protection was found at other skeletal sites (18).

In older individuals, walking exercise has been correlated to BMD, but intervention studies have not found brisk walking either to increase BMD or to protect against loss (19). Some, but not all, intervention trials using resistance or mixed endurance/resistance exercise showed significant gains in bone mass in older men and women (20–23). Other studies of older people, although not reporting significant gains in bone mass, do indicate that exercise may constrain the rate of bone loss (24).

SPECIAL ASPECTS OF EXERCISE AND BONE: AMENORRHEA, GYMNASTS, AND SWIMMERS

Optimal skeletal maintenance requires an adequate hormonal, mechanical, and nutritional milieu. Deficits in one sphere are not adequately compensated by overzealous attention to the others. Amenorrheic women athletes lose bone and have increased risk for fracture despite herculean training schedules (25,26). Despite initial views that cortical bone is spared in these women, recent data show significant deficits at all appendicular sites except the radius (27).

Competitive women gymnasts have a high prevalence of oligo- and amenorrhea. It would be expected that they would also suffer deficits in BMD. However, these athletes actually show higher than predicted BMD at all sites (28). One aspect of gymnastics training may explain this finding: whereas runners load their lumbar vertebrae with 3–5 body weights with each step, dismounting from parallel bars or other high-impact gymnastics activities gives vertebral loading of 15–20 body weights. Thus the experience in gymnasts may provide insight into the type of mechanical loads that are most osteotrophic. By contrast, even though collegiate swimmers also participate in muscle strength training, they have lower bone mass than do other athletes or even sedentary individuals of similar age (29). This may be explained by the fact that elite swimmers spend ~25 buoyant hours per week, time taken from their possible weight-bearing activity.

CONTRIBUTION OF EXERCISE TO BONE HEALTH OF OLDER PEOPLE

The modest BMD results with strength training should not trivialize the importance of exercise for protecting older people against falls. More than 90% of hip fractures are the immediate consequence of a fall onto the hip. Among the important risk factors for falls, muscle strength is perhaps most susceptible to improvement with strength training (30). Many older patients and their physicians ask which exercise is best for the skeleton. One must realize that only one of five adult Americans exercises as little as once each week and that the 6-month attrition rate for people who start exercising is >50%. Thus it serves no purpose to recommend a rigorous program to most people. Most important is to stimulate them to participate safely in any activity in a frequent, regular, and sustained manner. Therefore for sedentary and/or frail elderly, a program of walking, low-impact or water aerobics, or other pleasant, nonthreatening, and safe activity is recommended. If after several months the patient wishes to do more rigorous activity, a referral to a physical therapy department for initiation of muscle strength exercise is warranted.

REFERENCES

1. Rubin CT, Lanyon LE. Dynamic strain similarity in vertebrates: an alternative to allometric limb bone scaling. *J Theoret Biol* 1994; 107:321–327.
2. Whalen RT, Carter DR, Steele CR. The relationship between physical activity and bone density. *Trans Orthop Res Soc 33rd Mtg* 1987;12: 464–470.
3. Snow-Harter C, Marcus R. Exercise, bone mineral density, and osteoporosis. *Exerc Sport Sci Rev* 1991;19:351–388.
4. Block JE, Genant HK, Black D. Greater vertebral bone mineral mass in exercising young men. *West J Med* 1992;145:39–42.
5. Huddleston AL, Rockwell D, Kulund DN, et al. Bone mass in lifetime tennis players. *JAMA* 1980;244:1107–1109.
6. Slemenda CW, Miller JZ, Hui SL, Reister TK, Johnston CC Jr. Role of physical activity in the development of skeletal mass in children. *J Bone Miner Res* 1991;6:1227–1233.
7. Ruiz JC, Mandel C, Garabedian M. Influence of spontaneous calcium intake and physical exercise on the vertebral and femoral bone mineral density of children and adolescents. *J Bone Miner Res* 1995;10: 675–682.
8. Recker RR, Davies KM, Hinders SM, Heaney RP, Stegman MR, Kimmel DB. Bone gain in young adult women. *JAMA* 1992;268:2403– 2408.
9. Aloia JF, Vaswani AN, Yeh JK, Cohn SH. Premenopausal bone mass is related to physical activity. *Arch Intern Med* 1988;148:121–123.
10. Snow-Harter C, Whalen R, Myburgh K, Arnaud S, Marcus R. Bone mineral density, muscle strength, and recreational exercise in men. *J Bone Miner Res* 1992;7:1291–1296.
11. Sowers MR, Wallace RB, Lemke JH. Correlates of mid-radius bone density among postmenopausal women: a community study. *Am J Clin Nutr* 1985;41:1045–1053.
12. Mazess RB, Bardin HS. Bone density in premenopausal women: effects of age, dietary intake, physical activity, smoking, and birth-control pills. *Am J Clin Nutr* 1991;53:132–142.
13. Rockwell J, Sorensen A, Baker S, et al. Weight training decreases vertebral bone density in premenopausal women: a prospective study. *J Clin Endocrinol Metab* 1990;71:988–993.
14. Gleeson PB, Protas EJ, LeBlanc AD, Schneider VS, Evans HJ. Effects of weight lifting on bone mineral density in premenopausal women. *J Bone Miner Res* 1990;5:153–158.
15. Snow-Harter C, Bouxsein ML, Lewis BT, Carter DR, Marcus R. Effects of resistance and endurance exercise on bone mineral status of young women: a randomized exercise intervention trial. *J Bone Miner Res* 1992;7:761–769.
16. Friedlander AL, Genant HK, Sadowsky S, Byl NN, Glüer C-C. A two year program of aerobics and weight training enhances bone mineral density of young women. *J Bone Miner Res* 1995;10:574–585.
17. Lohman T, Going S, Pamenter R, et al. Effects of resistance training on regional and total bone mineral density in premenopausal women: a randomized prospective study. *J Bone Miner Res* 1995;10:1015–1024.
18. Pruitt LA, Jackson RD, Bartels RL, Lehnhard HJ. Weight-training effects on bone mineral density in early postmenopausal women. *J Bone Miner Res* 1992;7:179–185.
19. Cavanaugh DJ, Cann CE. Brisk walking does not stop bone loss in postmenopausal women. *Bone* 1988;9:201–204.
20. Simkin A, Ayalon J, Leichter I. Increased trabecular bone density due to bone-loading exercises on postmenopausal osteoporotic women. *Calcif Tissue Int* 1987;40:59–63.
21. Dalsky G, Stocke KS, Eshani AA, et al. Weight-bearing exercise training and lumbar bone mineral content in postmenopausal women. *Ann Intern Med* 1988;108:824–828.
22. Menkes A, Mazel S, Redmond RA, et al. Strength training increases regional bone mineral density and bone remodeling in middle-aged and older men. *J Appl Physiol* 1993;74:2478–2484.
23. Notelovitz M, Martin D, Tesar R, et al. Estrogen therapy and variable-resistance weight training increase bone mineral in surgically menopausal women. *J Bone Miner Res* 1991;6:583–590.
24. Prince RL, Devine A, Dick I, et al. The effects of calcium supplementation (milk powder or tablets) and exercise on bone density in postmenopausal women. *J Bone Miner Res* 1995;10:1068–1075.
25. Drinkwater BL, Nilson K, Chesnut CH III, Bremner WJ, Shainholtz S, Southworth MB. Bone mineral content of amenorrheic and eumenorrheic athletes. *N Engl J Med* 1984;311:277–281.
26. Marcus R, Cann C, Madvig P, et al. Menstrual function and bone mass in elite women distance runners: endocrine and metabolic features. *Ann Intern Med* 1985;102:158–163.
27. Myburgh KH, Bachrach LK, Lewis B, Kent K, Marcus R. Low bone mineral density at axial and appendicular sites in amenorrheic athletes. *Med Sci Sports Exerc* 1993;25:1197–1202.
28. Robinson TL, Snow-Harter C, Taaffe DR, Gillis D, Shaw J, Marcus R. Gymnasts exhibit higher bone mass than runners despite similar prevalence of amenorrhea. *J Bone Miner Res* 1995;10:26–35.
29. Taaffe DR, Snow-Harter C, Connolly DA, Robinson TL, Brown MD, Marcus R. Differential effects of swimming versus weight-bearing activity on bone mineral status of eumenorrheic athletes. *J Bone Miner Res* 1995;10:586–593.
30. Cummings SR, Nevitt MC, Browner WS, et al. Risk factors for hip fracture in white women. *N Engl J Med* 1995;332:767–773.

49. Prevention of Osteoporosis

Robert Lindsay, Ph.D., M.B.Ch.B., F.R.C.P. and *Felicia Cosman, M.D.

*Internal Medicine, Helen Hayes Hospital and *Department of Clinical Medicine, and Clinical Research Center, Columbia University, Helen Hayes Hospital, West Haverstraw, New York*

An ounce of prevention is worth more than any amount of treatment.

Osteoporosis is defined as a skeletal disease in which bone mass is reduced, accompanied by microarchitectural changes in the skeleton, such that there is a significant increase in the risk of fracture. Although it is clear that even in the young population, a lower bone mass is associated with some amount of increase in fracture risk, it is the phenomenon of loss of bone tissue that results in both reduced mass and the architectural changes that create the unique relation between declining bone mass and fracture risk that has been seen in major epidemiologic studies. The consequence is that a *loss* of tissue that equates to approximately 10% to 12% of bone mineral density (BMD) results in a doubling in the risk of fracture. Given that osteoporosis requires both low bone mass and a preexisting loss of bone tissue, the operational definition created for the World Health Organization (WHO), which is based solely on the measurement of bone density, seems a reasonable and pragmatic one (1). That definition that provides a diagnostic label requires that BMD be reduced below the normal range for young adult (a *T* score of −2.5 or less). However, this diagnostic definition is less helpful when considering intervention for prevention of osteoporosis.

In most circumstances, prevention of osteoporosis means prevention of fractures, which are the only clinical sequelae of importance. However, for the purposes of this chapter, prevention means intervention to prevent declining bone mass. The assumption is that prevention of bone loss will reduce fracture risk, which is the only benefit of intervention that is important to the patient. Strategies to prevent fracture in someone who already has osteoporotic fractures, whether directed at maintenance or rebuilding of skeletal mass or at interventions of other kinds to reduce fracture risk, are beyond the scope of this chapter and are dealt with elsewhere in this volume (see Chapters 52 and 53).

Because the phenomenon of bone loss produces (within cancellous bone) the loss of trabecular elements, a process that is considered virtually irreversible, the most efficient method of tackling these skeletal changes would appear to be effective prevention. However, because all individuals lose bone mass with age, and bone loss is asymptomatic, an intervention strategy that is associated with a high risk of side effects or high cost would not be considered appropriate on a population basis. Correspondingly, those strategies that are effective, and with low cost and minimal side effects, might be instituted as public health priorities. The level of bone density at which pharmacologic intervention would be recommended depends on an individual's risk of fracture, which in part is independent of BMD. Consequently the first priority is an assessment of risk with an attempt to utilize pharmacologic intervention in only those at greatest risk of fracture. In many ways, this approach to osteoporosis is similar to that for hypertension or hypercholesterolemia.

IDENTIFICATION OF AT-RISK INDIVIDUALS

As in many other disorders of aging, a large number of factors (Table 1) have been incriminated in the pathogenesis of fractures among the elderly (2). Some clearly change the onset, duration, or rate of bone loss in individuals, whereas others increase fracture risk by modifying the risk of injury. Some of these risk factors are linked by association without any demonstrable cause-and-effect relation. Some are sufficiently rare among the population that their utility as risk factors is modest. Consequently a rough clinical evaluation of risk can be obtained by assessment of comparatively few such factors, most of which can be obtained during adequate history taking. These general factors include being a female subject, white or Asian, and becoming postmenopausal (with surgical or early natural menopause probably conferring greater risk). For those fulfilling these criteria, a personal history of fracture after age 45 years or a history of an osteoporotic fracture in a first-degree relative, low body weight, cigarette consumption, and excess alcohol intake add to the risk (with each conferring additional risk).

TABLE 1. *Proposed risk factors for osteoporosis*

Genetic
  Race
  Sex
  Familial prevalence
Nutritional
  Low calcium intake
  High alcohol
  High caffeine
  High sodium
  High animal protein
Lifestyle
  Cigarette use
  Low physical activity
Endocrine
  Menopausal age (oophorectomy)
  Obesity

Superimposed on these simple features are a wide variety of factors, including chronic illness, disuse, and drugs [steroids, diuretics, thyroid hormone, gonadotropin-releasing hormone agonists, phenytoin (Dilantin), tetracyclines, aluminum, and methotrexate].

Others are sufficiently endemic in the population that they can almost be assumed. These include inadequate calcium intake and physical activity. Because these contribute to other diseases of aging and are relatively inexpensive and safe to correct, approaches to improve calcium intake and physical activity can be considered to be important public health strategies for prevention of osteoporosis. In general, for each patient, the more risk factors present (2) and the longer the duration of their presence, the greater the risk of future fracture (2,3). For example, a 55-year-old postmenopausal woman who has a family history, a prior fracture, is thin, and smokes has a relative risk of further fracture that is about 16 times the average for the 55-year-old postmenopausal population. Physicians can use the presence of these factors in two ways. First, they can be used to sensitize the patient and the physician to the likelihood of osteoporosis and to target these individuals for further investigation and/or treatment. Second, those risk factors that are amenable to elimination or alteration should be discussed with the patient. Many risk factors (e.g., smoking, poor calcium intake, physical inactivity, and alcohol excess) also contribute to development of diseases in organ systems other than bone and should be discussed in those terms. Risk factors cannot be used clinically to determine BMD, which should be measured if it is to guide intervention. Again, the clinical analogy is hypertension for which there is also a list of risk factors, but no assemblage of these predicts an individual patient's blood pressure (although they may be predictive of risk of stroke). Practically, menopause is the most common time when evaluation of the patient for osteoporosis begins, although nutritional and lifestyle habits should be changed as early in life as possible. Consequently, in outpatients, risk-factor review is a useful initial approach to the patient.

Bone Mineral Density Testing

The best-documented risk factor for fracture is BMD. Although on a population basis, both the starting bone mass and the subsequent rate of loss of bone tissue contribute to risk of fracture, for any individual, we usually use bone mass at the time of consultation as the principal determinant of fracture risk. Fracture prevalence and future fracture incidence have been shown to be greater in those with low BMD at any age. Several studies in elderly populations indicated that low BMD is particularly predictive of an increased fracture risk (4,5). On a population basis, measurement of bone density at any skeletal site can be used to predict the overall risk of fracture. However, measurements of the hip are better predictors of the risk of hip fracture and are equally good at predicting the risk of fractures at other skeletal sites. Consequently in most populations, measurements of the hip are probably preferable. However, when bone density is required for clinical management of an individual patient, most would agree that any measurement is better than none. For a complete review of the techniques available for bone-mass measurement and their interpretation, the reader is referred to Chapter 25. The clinician should learn about the use of these techniques available in his or her geographic area. The analogies in clinical practice are the measurement of blood pressure for the assessment for cardiovascular risk and cholesterol or lipoprotein fractionation as risk factors for coronary heart disease.

In individual patients, there is no absolute value of bone mass or density that indicates a need for treatment. The results of BMD testing should be incorporated into the entire clinical profile of any individual to establish the urgency for intervention. The presence of one or more risk factors would, for example, influence the decision to treat, as would the benefits, risks, and cost of intervention. *Guidelines established by the National Osteoporosis Foundation suggest that BMD determination should be performed in all women by the age of 60 to 65 years and in postmenopausal estrogen-deficient women younger than that age who have more than one risk factor (in addition to being estrogen deficient) (6).*

CLINICAL PROTOCOL

Prevention of bone loss in asymptomatic women is generally achieved by using two complementary approaches: behavior modification (public health approach) and pharmacologic intervention. Again, this is similar to the management of hypertension and hypercholesterolemia. The initial approach to the patient is based on modification of the risk-factor profile. Evaluation for and elimination of secondary causes of osteoporosis is a mandatory part of this initial evaluation. For prevention of primary (postmenopausal) osteoporosis, alterations in nutrition and lifestyle form the primary approach, on the assumption that a reduction in risk-factor profile will be beneficial. Reductions in alcohol consumption and elimination of cigarette use also are amenable to intervention and are particularly important because those modifications are both beneficial to the patient's general health.

Calcium Supplementation

Although calcium is a nutrient and adequate intake should preferably be obtained from nutritional sources (7), in prac-

tice, it is difficult for many people to achieve a dietary intake of more than the advisable intake for adults. Self-imposed calorie restrictions and the avoidance of cholesterol results in limitation of dairy products, the major source of dietary calcium in the western world. Other sources of calcium include green vegetables, nuts, and certain fish. Bioavailability of calcium from foods is ~30%, with high individual variability (calcium in spinach is unavailable for absorption).

In providing advice about calcium intake, the intent is to ensure that the majority of the population obtain sufficient calcium to maintain calcium balance. Recommendations include an intake of calcium of 500 mg/day for children aged 1 to 3 years; 800 mg/day for those 4 to 8 years; 1300 mg/day for those 9 to 18 years; 1000 mg/day from 19 to 50 years; and for those older than 50 years, 1200 mg/day. To achieve such intakes, it is commonly necessary to resort to calcium supplementation. Most individuals require only 500 to 1000 mg/day as a supplement to dietary sources to realize these intakes. Many forms of calcium are available as supplements, and the advice to the patient should be as simple as possible. The least expensive calcium supplements are usually carbonate salts. Because calcium absorption is better in an acid environment for the carbonate, we recommend that the supplement be taken with food, although one school of thought argues for the supplement to be taken at night to reduce the nocturnal surge in bone remodeling. The addition of a modest calcium supplement at the end of each meal is a regimen to which the patient can easily adhere. Calcium carbonate offers the highest calcium content per unit tablet weight (40%), with calcium citrate being second at 30%. Absorption of calcium as a citrate is slightly more efficient and not dependent on gastric acidity. Because citrate is more expensive, it should be recommended mostly for those with hypochlorhydria or achlorhydria or those who experience side effects by using the carbonate. At the recommended dietary intakes, calcium supplementation has a low incidence of side effects. If eructation, intestinal colic, and constipation occur with the carbonate, then citrate may be used. Care should be taken in prescribing calcium supplements to patients with a history of renal stones. If urine calcium excretion is not increased, the citrate salt may be used.

Clinical trials indicate that calcium supplementation to prepubertal children increases bone mass. It is, however, not entirely established as yet whether that results in achievement of a higher peak skeletal mass in the late teens or early third decade. Clinical trials demonstrated the effect of calcium supplementation on bone mass in older populations. In general, the results confirm a weak antiresorptive effect with evidence for prevention of bone loss. The effects are most obvious in the elderly but can be seen in some premenopausal populations. The effect is more modest in the years immediately following menopause, when estrogen loss is driving bone loss. Increased calcium intake has been shown to reduce the risk of fracture in the aging population. The risk of vertebral fracture may be lowered by as much as 50% and risk of hip fracture by about 20%. The effects are sufficiently great that calcium supplementation may be considered a public health priority. Evidence suggests that bone loss among the elderly is associated with secondary hyperparathyroidism, which in part may be driven by inadequate supply of vitamin D. Some studies indicate a modest effect of supplemental vitamin D on bone mass in at-risk populations such as the elderly, the institutionalized, and those with disorders likely to impair vitamin D supply or metabolism. It is not yet clear whether vitamin D supplementation by itself can reduce the risk of fracture. Combinations of vitamin D supplementation with calcium have been shown to reduce the risk of hip fracture. For those who do not get sun exposure, and all individuals older than 70 years, vitamin D intake should be in the range of 400 to 800 IU/day. Vitamin D metabolites and analogues are currently not recommended for prevention of osteoporosis.

Physical Activity

It has long been assumed that adequate physical activity is associated with the prevention of osteoporotic fractures, but the evidence is sparse, largely because of the difficulty in conducting good-quality controlled clinical trials in this area (see Chapter 48). There is no doubt that at the extremes of activity, effects on bone and fracture are evident, but it is within the range of normal activity that the doubts persist. However, because physical activity is associated with a number of health benefits and well-being, it remains an important feature of osteoporosis prevention.

Changing the pattern of physical activity may be difficult, especially for patients who are less than positively motivated. This is especially true when discussing prevention with patients, who are, by definition, asymptomatic. Most of the patients seen in our clinic are at a relatively low level of fitness and may require formal cardiovascular evaluation before beginning an exercise program. We suggest that the exercise activity chosen be pleasurable to improve adherence. In the absence of proven benefit for any specific exercise for prevention of osteoporosis, any weight-bearing activity suffices (8). Recreational therapy that has a social component may serve to improve patient adherence. However, even simple activities such as walking are useful and can be added to the daily routine with minimal difficulty. Back-strengthening exercise is probably also of value, and patients may be referred to a trainer or therapist for specific instructions because there may be limitations, particularly with exercises that force spinal flexion. In addition to any potential beneficial effects on the skeleton, continued activity in patients' daily lives reduces the risk of falls, trauma from falls, and fracture.

Pharmacologic Therapy to Prevent Bone Loss

A considerable body of data supports the concept that estrogen administration to postmenopausal women reduces skeletal turnover and the rate of bone loss (9). Epidemiologic data indicate that estrogen use is associated with a reduction in the risk of fracture, particularly fractures of the hip and wrist (Colles' fracture). Risk reduction averaged over several studies appears to be on the order of 50%. However, recent data suggest that the effects are maximized when hormone-replacement therapy (HRT) is begun early in the postmenopause and continued into old age, because the maximal reduction in hip fracture appears to occur in patients who are still currently receiving HRT (10). For vertebral frac-tures, only one controlled clinical trial of primary prevention has been completed, suggesting about a 75% reduction in the risk. Epidemiologic data suggest that the reduction in the risk overall may be approximately the same as that seen for hip fracture. Several general principals govern the use of HRT for prevention of osteoporosis. Because estrogens primarily reduce the rate of bone loss, in general, the earlier therapy is begun, the more likely the bone mass and structure will be preserved. However, estrogen therapy also reduces the rate of bone loss in estrogen-deficient women independent of age, with reduction in bone loss among older individuals, at least up to the eighth decade (11). The minimal effective dose of estrogen is commonly stated to be 0.625 mg of conjugated equine estrogen or its equivalent (12). However, some recent data suggest that lower doses may be effective in many individuals (13). This may be related to the utilization of calcium supplementation in the more recent clinical trials, because we have shown that there is a significantly smaller response, at least in terms of bone density, when estrogens are given alone (14). Efficacy has been demonstrated for several other estrogens, including estradiol, esterified estrogens, estrone sulfate, and ethinylestradiol. It also is apparent that the route of administration is not important, and several studies demonstrated that transdermal estrogen effectively prevents bone loss (15). Some recent data suggested that the estrogen effect also may be magnified by the addition of small doses of androgen. Such combinations are as yet not Food and Drug Administration (FDA) approved for osteoporosis prevention.

The effects of estrogen continue for as long as treatment is provided, whereas bone loss ensues when treatment is discontinued at a rate comparable to the rate that occurs immediately after ovariectomy. Prospective controlled clinical trials confirmed the long-term efficacy of estrogen for bone-loss prevention for at least 10 years. However, as noted earlier, long-term administration (possibly lifelong) is required to produce the maximal reduction of fracture risk, perhaps because of the bone loss that occurs when treatment is stopped (10). Some data from observational studies suggest that in the more elderly population, estrogen by itself may be insufficient to totally prevent bone loss, especially in the hip, which may at that age be being driven by secondary hyperparathyroidism.

Practical Aspects of Estrogen Administration

Although menopausal symptoms remain the most frequent indication for estrogen therapy, prevention of osteoporosis is becoming a more widely recognized indication for HRT in the postmenopausal population. Treatment of menopause is accompanied by an excellent symptomatic response to therapy. For the long-term prevention of osteoporosis, however, the physician always faces the problems of acceptance and compliance in providing therapy for an asymptomatic phase of a disease. Epidemiologic data suggest that estrogens may reduce the risk of ischemic heart disease, which if proven in controlled clinical trials, adds another larger health benefit for estrogen use. The recent suggestion that estrogens improve cognitive function and reduce the risk of Alzheimer's disease among aging women, again if proven in clinical trials, will add yet another benefit. Finally, estrogens also improve atrophy of the urogenital system, a common problem among postmenopausal women. It is perhaps not surprising, therefore, that estrogens have been associated with improvement in premature mortality. Consequently it has been suggested that the use of HRT among large segments of the postmenopausal population is a cost-effective approach to the health of the postmenopausal population. Because HRT remains the gold standard for prevention and treatment of osteoporosis when patients present already on HRT, there is usually little requirement to consider any other intervention.

When therapy is being considered specifically for osteoporosis prevention, consideration should be given to performing bone density measurements. This is especially true in the early postmenopausal years if other risk factors are present and should be considered clinically appropriate in all women older than 60 years. A combination of risk-factor analysis and BMD allows determination of the future risk of fracture for the individual patient (16). When considering intervention for osteoporosis alone, HRT should be begun in women who have no other risk factors if bone density falls more than 2 standard deviation units below the average for young adults (T score <-2), and if patients have risk factors, then intervention should be offered at a T score of -1.5. Some general recommendations can be made regarding the protocol for HRT intervention. All patients require a history and physical, including gynecologic, examination. All patients should have a mammogram and be taught breast self-examination before therapy is initiated. The guidelines for mammography in this age range should be based on the National Cancer Institute guidelines and be independent of the decision to treat, but treatment certainly mandates regular mammography. If the patient has gone through natural menopause, combination or sequential therapy with a progestin is used to protect the endometrium (17). There is no rationale at present for progestin in patients who have undergone hysterectomy. There is no evidence that the addition of a progestin will modify the estrogen effect in the skeleton, although one study with norethindrone acetate, a 19-nortestosterone derivative, suggested that there may be an additive effect on bone when it is given along with estrogens (18). For younger women just after menopause, we favor a sequential regimen. Estrogen is given every day with a progestin initiated on the first of each calendar month for at least 12 days (2 weeks is often simpler). Most patients will have some endometrial shedding, which may be fairly light between days 11 and 21 of each month. Recurrent bleeding, not on that schedule, requires investigation. The progestin dose should be the minimum required for endometrial protection. For medroxyprogesterone acetate, the most commonly used progestin in the United States, 5 mg/day is the minimum.

Sequential therapy in which estrogen and progestin are combined in a single tablet is now available in the United States. If there are progestin-precipitated symptoms with medroxyprogesterone acetate, norethindrone [one-half tablet a day (2.5 mg)] may be tried, or two tablets a day of a progestin-only oral contraceptive containing 0.35 mg norethindrone per tablet. The latter is an expensive regimen even when used for only 2 weeks each month. Older women and those who wish to avoid monthly vaginal bleeding may consider a combined continuous regimen. In this regimen, the estrogen and progestin are both given each day of the month. The estrogen dose is similar to that noted earlier, but the progestin dose is reduced by half. This regimen is associated with some irregular, unheralded bleeding in the first 2 to 6 months of treatment in ~50% of patients, but close to 80% who remain on therapy will become amenorrheic thereafter. Because the early bleeding is often light and may just be spotting, many patients will have this temporary inconvenience in return for the promise of no further bleeding. One combined continuous preparation is available in the United States as a single tablet.

Side effects of therapy include occasional weight gain and, rarely, an idiosyncratic increase in blood pressure. Blood pressure should be measured in all patients after 3 months of therapy. Progestin side effects include irritability and mood swings (often described as being premenstrual), which may become sufficiently troublesome to require the progestin dose to be reduced to the minimum. Increased risks of deep vein thrombosis and gallstones are recorded as side effects but clinically are unusual.

For prevention of osteoporosis, treatment should probably be continued for as long as feasible, perhaps lifelong. As a practical issue, we review each patient on at least an annual basis and evaluate with her the benefits and her concerns regarding treatment. We now use repeated measurements of bone mass by dual-energy x-ray absorptiometry (DXA) to monitor patients to ensure that bone loss is not progressing. Repeated measurements of bone mass are allowed on a two-yearly basis by Medicare, but many clinicians prefer more frequent measurements. An alternative to the use of bone mass is the measurement of biochemical markers of bone turnover (see Chapter 22), which if measured before and 6 months after initiating HRT, may provide evidence that there is reduced bone turnover. The major purpose in the use of either bone-mass measurement or biochemical markers is to improve compliance with HRT because it is well known that there is relatively poor long-term compliance not dissimilar to that seen in the treatment of other asymptomatic conditions. Poor compliance may be associated with failure to educate the patient adequately about the expected results of therapy and the potential problems. However, discontinuation of HRT is also often related to an increased awareness of the problem of breast cancer in the aging population. Breast cancer is common in the age group in whom HRT is being used for prevention of osteoporosis. Breast cancer also often is commonly discussed in the popular press, especially in relation to HRT. A current suggestion that long-term use of HRT (more than 10 years) may be associated with a modest 10% to 30% increase in the risk of breast cancer (19). This often is sufficient to discourage patients from initiating HRT, or if a friend or relative develops breast cancer, is sufficient to provoke discontinuation. The introduction recently of the tissue-selective estrogens (or selective estrogen-receptor modulators) offers an alternative to HRT for patients who are concerned about breast cancer and perhaps also for those who have a personal history of breast cancer. The first of these agents, raloxifene, is described in detail in Chapter 52. The main contraindication to estrogen therapy is the presence or history of an estrogen-dependent tumor, especially breast malignancy. Other relative contraindications include undiagnosed vaginal bleeding, a history of endometrial malignancy (4 years after hysterectomy), active thromboembolic disease, and grossly abnormal liver or renal function. Hypertension and diabetes are not contraindications but must be controlled before therapy is begun.

Alternatives to Estrogen

Bisphosphonates

These agents are derivatives of pyrophosphate but are not metabolized by the body (20). The bisphosphonates are potent inhibitors of bone remodeling; however, the mode of action of these drugs is still not entirely clear, and each of the bisphosphonates may affect remodeling with subtle but important differences. The major advantages of bisphosphonates include the oral route of administration and their specificity for the skeleton. One bisphosphonate, alendronate, is approved by the FDA for both prevention and treatment of osteoporosis. Controlled clinical trials have demonstrated that 5 mg of alendronate (the prevention dose) prevents bone loss in the hip, spine, radius, and total body about as effectively as the recommended dose of estrogen in standard HRT regimen (21). Most of the evidence that alendronate reduces the risk of fractures comes from controlled clinical trials of patients with osteoporosis. However, in many of these studies, for the majority of the duration of the period of observation, 5 mg was the dose used (22). Consequently, it is perhaps a reasonably logical jump to suggest that 5 mg will produce reduction in fracture when used for prevention. Alendronate appears to produce about a 50% reduction in the risk of vertebral fractures and perhaps a similar reduction in the risk of fractures of the hip. Curiously, other peripheral fractures appear significantly less affected. Recent data suggest that the maximal benefit of alendronate is achieved when it is used for the treatment of those who are at highest risk (those who already have osteoporosis; i.e., a T score of -2.5 or below). Alendronate is generally well tolerated. However, some patients experience upper gastrointestinal distress probably related to the irritant effect of the drug on esophageal mucosa caused by failure to transport the tablet into the stomach or reflux of the tablet into the esophagus. Rarely esophageal ulceration and perforation can result. The 10-mg dose (used for treatment) appears more likely to produce these effects than does 5 mg.

Because of their ease of use and their low level of side effects, particularly at low dose, bisphosphonates may become important therapies in the prevention of osteoporosis of all types. The concerns with these agents is their poor intestinal absorption (generally less than 1% of ingested dose) and their long residence time in bone. Alendronate dosing recommendations include that it should be given first thing in the morning with 6 to 8 ounces of water (not coffee or juice) and that a minimum of one-half hour be allowed before any additional food or drink is taken. The patient also must be cautioned not to assume a recumbent position to avoid reflux. Long-term data will be required to determine if the residence time in bone is a problem.

Selective Estrogen-Receptor Modulators

In the United States, raloxifene, 60 mg/day, is a novel agent approved for prevention of osteoporosis. This drug appears to act through the estrogen receptors and produces estrogen-agonist effects on bone and low-density lipoprotein (LDL) cholesterol but estrogen-antagonist effects on breast, endometrium, and the hypothalamus. Raloxifene use in the prevention of osteoporosis is discussed in detail in Chapter 52. Long-term data will be required to determine the effects of raloxifene on diseases in other organ systems.

Calcitonin

Salmon calcitonin is an FDA-approved alternative to estrogen for the treatment but not prevention of osteoporosis (23). Salmon calcitonin can be delivered by an intranasal spray, which obviates the problems of parenteral administration. The indication for its use is osteoporosis, as a second-line therapy for those who cannot or should not take estrogens. The recommended dose is 200 U/day as a single nasal administration. It is possible that larger doses may be required for prevention, especially in the immediate postmenopausal period. Controlled data documenting the effect of calcitonin on fractures are somewhat sparse, although recent data suggest that 200 U/day is associated with approximately a 40% reduction in the risk of vertebral fractures. Side effects of nasal administration are usually mild, with local nasal irritation being the most frequent. Flushing and nausea are more usually associated with parenteral administration but may occur especially with higher doses by the intranasal route. With long-term use, antibody formation occurs in a significant proportion of patients and has been suggested to be responsible for reduced long-term efficacy, without definitive proof that this is so. The major advantages to calcitonin are its safety, its specificity to bone, and the fact that it can be used in men.

Other Agents

Certain progestins by themselves also appear to have bone-sparing effects but are unlikely to be used by themselves in prevention. The addition of a progestin to estrogen, as previously noted, does not negatively affect the skeletal effect of the estrogen, and certain progestins may enhance the bone-sparing effects of estrogens. Currently tibolone, a progestin with some estrogenic and androgenic effects, is in clinical trials in the United States for osteoporosis prevention. For postmenopausal patients with a history of breast cancer, there is some evidence that the so-called antiestrogen tamoxifen in doses usually used to prevent cancer recurrence (20 to 30 mg/day) (24,25) may reduce the rate of bone loss and prevent osteoporosis, a potentially serious problem for this group of patients. Tamoxifen is not FDA approved for osteoporosis prevention, and patients who are taking tamoxifen should have bone mass carefully monitored so that a bone-specific agent can be added early, should bone loss occur.

CONCLUSIONS

The initial approach to osteoporosis prevention consists of identification of those subjects likely to be at risk; behavior modification to eliminate risk factors and improved nutrition and lifestyle; and estrogen intervention, which remains the cornerstone of prevention for the postmenopausal patient. Calcitonin (nasal spray) and oral bisphosphonates are alternatives available for those at greatest risk or those who cannot or will not take HRT.

Because both calcitonin and bisphosphonates are agents that affect the skeleton specifically and are more expensive than estrogens (cost of drug), guidelines for their use differ, and both at present should probably be reserved for the highest-risk groups.

REFERENCES

1. Report of a WHO Study Group. *Assessment of fracture risk and its application to screening for postmenopausal osteoporosis.* Geneva: WHO Technical Report Series 843: World Health Organization, 1994.
2. Riggs BL, Melton LJ III. Involutional osteoporosis. *N Engl J Med* 1986;314:1676–1686.
3. Consensus Development Conference. Prophylaxis and treatment of osteoporosis. *Osteoporos Int* 1991;1:114–126.
4. Hui SL, Slemenda CW, Johnston CC Jr. Baseline measurement of bone mass predicts fracture in white women. *Ann Intern Med* 1989;111:355–361.
5. Johnston CC Jr, Melton LJ III, Lindsay R, et al. Clinical indications for bone mass measurement. *J Bone Miner Res* 1989;4:128.
6. Eddy DM, Johnston CC Jr., for the Development Committee. Status report, Osteoporosis: review of the evidence for prevention, diagnosis and treatment, and cost-effectiveness analysis. *Osteoporos Int* 1998;8: S1–S88.
7. Heaney RP. Effect of calcium on skeletal development, bone loss, and risk of fractures. *Am J Med* 1991;91:23S–28S.
8. Dalsky GP, Stocke KS, Ehsani AA, et al. Weight-bearing exercise training and lumbar bone mineral content in postmenopausal women. *Ann Intern Med* 1988;108:824–828.
9. Lindsay R. Sex steroids in the pathogenesis and prevention of osteoporosis. In: Riggs BL, ed. *Osteoporosis: etiology, diagnosis and management.* New York: Raven Press, 1988:333–358.
10. Cauley JA, Seeley DG, Ensrud K, Ettinger B, Black D, Cummings SR. Estrogen replacement therapy and fractures in older women. *Ann Intern Med* 1995;122:9–16.
11. Lindsay R, Tohme J. Estrogen treatment of patients with established postmenopausal osteoporosis. *Obstet Gynecol* 1990;76:290–295.
12. Lindsay R, Hart DM, Clark DM. The minimum effective dose of estrogen for prevention of postmenopausal bone loss. *Obstet Gynecol* 1994;63:759–763.
13. Genant HK, Lucas J, Weiss S, et al. for the Estratab/Osteoporosis Study Group. Low-dose esterified estrogen therapy. *Arch Intern Med* 1997;157:2609–2615.
14. Nieves JW, Komar L, Cosman F, Lindsay R. Calcium potentiates the effect of estrogen and calcitonin on bone mass: review and analysis. *Am J Clin Nutr* 1998;67:18–24.
15. Stevenson JC, Cust MP, Gangar KF, Hillard TC, Lees B, Whitehead MI. Effects of transdermal versus oral hormone replacement therapy on bone density in spine and proximal femur in postmenopausal women *Lancet* 1990;336:265–269.
16. Cummings SR, Nevitt MC, Browner WS, et al., Study of Osteoporotic Fractures Research Group. Risk factors for hip fracture in white women. *N Engl J Med* 1995;332:767–773.
17. Padwick ML, Pryse-Davies J, Whitehead MI. A simple method for determining the optimal dosage of progestin in postmenopausal women receiving estrogen. *N Engl J Med* 1986;315:930–934.
18. Christiansen C, Riis BJ. 17β-Estradiol and continuous norethisterone: a unique treatment for established osteoporosis in elderly women. *J Clin Endocrinol Metab* 1990;71:836–841.
19. Hulka BS. Hormone-replacement therapy and the risk of breast cancer. *Cancer* 1990;40:289–296.
20. Fleisch H. The possible use of bisphosphonates in osteoporosis. In: DeLuca HF, Mazess R, eds. *Osteoporosis: physiological basis, assessment and treatment.* New York: Elsevier, 1990:323–330.
21. Liberman UA, Weiss SR, Bruil I, et al. Effect of oral alendronate on bone mineral density and the incidence of fracture in postmenopausal osteoporosis. *N Engl J Med* 1995;333:1437–1443.
22. Black DM, Cummings SR, Karpf DB, et al. Randomized trial of effect of alendronate on risk of fracture in women with existing vertebral fracture: Fracture intervention trial research group. *Lancet* 1996;348: 1535–1541.
23. Overgaard K, Hansen MA, Jensen SB, Christiansen C. Effect of calcitonin given intranasally on bone mass and fracture rates in established osteoporosis: a dose response study. *Br Med J* 1992;305:556–561.
24. Turken S, Siris E, Seldin D, Lindsay R. Effects of tamoxifen on spinal bone density. *JNCI* 1989;81:1086–1088.
25. Love RR, Mazess RB, Barden HS, et al. Effects of tamoxifen on bone mineral density in postmenopausal women with breast cancer. *N Engl J Med* 1992;852–856.

50. Nutrition and Osteoporosis

Robert P. Heaney, M.D., F.A.C.P., F.A.I.N.

Creighton University, Omaha, Nebraska

Nutrition plays a role in pathogenesis, prevention, and treatment of osteoporosis (1). The nutrients known with certainty to be important are calcium, vitamin D, protein, and calories. Phosphorus, certain trace minerals (manganese, copper, and zinc), and vitamins C and K, although involved in bone health generally, are less certainly involved in osteoporosis. Bone cells, of course, are as dependent on total nutrition, including all the vitamins and trace minerals, as are any other cell or tissue types. However, current bone mass and bone strength are dependent on cell activity over a many-year period, and thus acute nutrient deficiencies, although they undoubtedly impair current cellular competence, tend to have little effect on overall bone strength, which is our concern. The major exceptions to this generalization are the nutrients calcium and vitamin D.

CALCIUM

Calcium is the principal cation of bone mineral. Bone constitutes a very large nutrient reserve for calcium, which, over the course of evolution, acquired a secondary, structural function that explains its importance with respect to osteoporosis. Bone strength varies as the approximate second power

10. Aloia JF, Vaswani A, Yeh JK, Ross PL, Flaster E, Dilmanian FA. Calcium supplementation with and without hormone replacement therapy to prevent postmenopausal bone loss. *Ann Intern Med* 1994; 120:97–103.

11. Dawson-Hughes B, Harris SS, Krall EA, Dallal GE. Effect of calcium and vitamin D supplementation on bone density in men and women 65 years of age or older. *N Engl J Med* 1997;337:670–676.

12. Dawson-Hughes B, Dallal GE, Krall EA, Sadowski L, Sahyoun N, Tannenbaum S. A controlled trial of the effect of calcium supplementation on bone density in postmenopausal women. *N Engl J Med* 1990;323:878–883.

13. McKane WR, Khosla S, O'Fallon WM, Robins SP, Burritt MF, Riggs BL. Role of calcium intake in modulating age-related increases in parathyroid function and bone resorption. *J Clin Endocrinol Metab* 1996;81:1699–1703.

14. Heaney RP, Recker RR, Weaver CM. Absorbability of calcium sources: the limited role of solubility. *Calcif Tissue Int* 1990;46:300–304.

15. Heaney RP, Dowell MS, Barger-Lux MJ. Absorption of calcium as the carbonate and citrate salts, with some observations on method. *Osteoporosis Int* 1999;9:19–23.

16. Davis JW, Ross PD, Johnson NE, Wasnich RD. Estrogen and calcium supplement use amone Japanese-American women: effects upon bone loss when used singly and in combination. *Bone* 1995;17:369–373.

17. Nieves JW, Komar L, Cosman F, Lindsay R. Calcium potentiates the effect of estrogen and calcitonin on bone mass: review and analysis. *Am J Clin Nutr* 1998;67:18–24.

18. Chapuy M-C, Preziosi P, Maamer M, et al. Prevalence of vitamin D insufficiency in an adult normal population. *Osteoporosis Int* 1997; 7:439–443.

19. Heikinheimo RJ, Inkovaara JA, Harju EJ, et al. Annual injection of vitamin D and fractures of aged bones. *Calcif Tissue Int* 1992; 51:105–110.

20. Thomas MK, Lloyd-Jones DM, Thadhani RI, et al. Hypovitaminosis D in medical inpatients. *N Engl J Med* 1998;338:777–783.

21. Delmi M, Rapin CH, Bengoa JM, Delmas PD, Vasey H, Bonjour JP. Dietary supplementation in elderly patients with fractured neck of the femur. *Lancet* 1990;335:1013–1016.

22. Rico H, Revilla M, Villa LF, Hernandez ER, Fernandez JP. Crush fracture syndrome in senile osteoporosis: a nutritional consequence. *J Bone Miner Res* 1992;7:317–319.

23. Bastow MD, Rawlings J, Allison SP. Benefits of supplementary tube feeding after fractured neck of femur. *Br Med J* 1983;287:1589–1592.

24. Heaney RP. Nutritional factors in osteoporosis. *Annu Rev Nutr* 1993;13:287–316.

25. Strause L, Saltman P, Smith K, Andon M. The role of trace elements in bone metabolism. In: Burckhardt P, Heaney RP, eds. *Nutritional aspects of osteoporosis*. New York: Raven Press, 1991:223–233.

26. Vermeer C, Jie K-SG, Knapen MHJ. Role of vitamin K in bone metabolism. *Annu Rev Nutr* 1995;15:1–22.

51. Evaluation of Postmenopausal Osteoporosis

Marjorie M. Luckey, M.D.

Mount Sinai Medical Center, New York, New York and Osteoporosis and Metabolic Bone Disease Center, Saint Barnabas Medical Center, Livingston, New Jersey

The pathogenesis of osteoporosis is multifactorial, with inadequate peak bone mass and bone loss due to age and cessation of gonadal function being the most important determinants. Many other medical and surgical conditions, dietary habits, lifestyle factors, and medications also can accelerate bone loss and increase the risk of fragility fractures. The onset and progression of osteoporosis is asymptomatic until its advanced stages when fractures occur. As with other chronic diseases with long latent periods, such as hypertension and hyperlipidemia, early identification of osteoporosis requires vigilance from all healthcare providers and, often, the use of diagnostic testing before overt signs of the disease. Although there is no universally accepted algorithm for the assessment of women who are at risk for or already have osteoporosis, the aims of the evaluation of every postmenopausal woman should be to

1. identify women at high risk for osteoporosis and fractures;
2. establish the correct diagnosis and identify correctable causes of bone loss;
3. determine the severity, extent, and activity of the disease; and
4. select and monitor therapy.

IDENTIFICATION OF WOMEN AT HIGH RISK FOR OSTEOPOROSIS

Compared with men, women are at higher risk for osteoporosis because of somewhat lower peak bone mass, smaller skeletal size, and accelerated postmenopausal bone loss (see Chapter 47). Among women, the incidence of osteoporotic fractures is significantly higher in whites and Asians than in African-Americans, whereas women of Hispanic heritage appear to have an intermediate level of risk (1). Within each ethnic group, however, the risk of osteoporotic fractures varies widely among individuals. In fact, the variability of bone density in each race is much greater than the differences between races. Therefore no estrogen-deficient postmenopausal woman can be assumed, *a priori*, to be at low risk for osteoporosis without an individualized assessment.

Risk Factors for Osteoporosis

A large number of genetic, medical, pharmacologic, and lifestyle factors are associated with low bone mass and a heightened risk of osteoporotic fractures in women (Table 1). Some of these are related to inadequate peak bone mass, whereas others cause or accelerate bone loss. Unfortunately, many studies have demonstrated that risk factors, alone or in combination, are inadequate to predict an individual's bone mass or the future risk for fractures (2,3). The presence of one or more of these risk factors, however, should alert clinicians to the heightened possibility of osteoporosis and lead to bone density testing, which can diagnose osteoporosis, assess its severity, and monitor therapy.

TABLE 1. *Risk factors for osteoporosis and fractures in women*

Age
Genetic
  White or Asian ethnicity
  Family history of osteoporosis
  Small body size/weight
Hormonal
  Late menarche (>15 years)
  Prolonged amenorrhea
  Premature or surgical menopause
Lifestyle/nutrition
  Inadequate calcium intake
  Smoking
  Alcoholism
  Eating disorders
Medical diseases
  Hyperthyroidism
  Hyperparathyroidism
  Glucocorticoid excess
  Malabsorption
  Liver disease
  Rheumatoid arthritis
  Depression
Medications
  Anticonvulsants
  Glucocorticoids
  Heparin
  Chemotherapeutics

Independent Risk Factors for Fractures

Although low bone density is the major determinant of fracture risk, other factors (Table 2) independently increase the risk of hip fractures even after adjustment for bone mass (4–6). Some of these risk factors, such as poor vision, lower-

TABLE 2. *Independent risk factors for fractures*

Prior fragility fracture
Age
Maternal history of hip fracture
Low body weight (<127 lb)
Weight loss since age 25
Hyperthyroidism (ever)
Low sunlight exposure/vitamin D deficiency
Poor health
Impaired neuromuscular function
Decreased visual acuity
Sedative/hypnotic drug use
Frequent falls
Resting pulse >80 beats/min
Hip geometry (longer hip-axis length)
Increased levels of biochemical markers of bone turnover

Adapted from Grisso JA, Kelsey JL, Strom BL, et al. Risk factors for falls as a cause of hip fracture in women. *N Engl J Med* 1991;324:1326–1331; Kelsey JL, Browner WS, Seeley DG, Nevitt MC, Cummings SR. Risk factors for fractures of the distal forearm and proximal humerus. *Am J Epidemiol* 1992;135:477–489; and Ross PD, Davis JW, Epstein RS, Wasnich RD. Pre-existing fractures and bone mass predict vertebral fracture incidence in women. *Ann Intern Med* 1991;114:919–923.

extremity weakness, sedative medications, and general frailty, probably increase fracture risk by increasing the likelihood of falling. Others, such as advanced age, a maternal history of hip fracture, high bone turnover, a previous adult fracture, and vitamin D deficiency, may be indicative of other abnormalities in bone quality that enhance its fragility (e.g., fatigue fractures, loss of trabecular connectivity, or subclinical osteomalacia). Anatomic risk factors, such as low body weight and hip geometry, also increase the risk of hip fractures, perhaps by influencing the force, direction, or distribution of impact during a fall.

The relationship of risk factors to the incidence of other fractures has been less well studied. It appears, however, that low bone density, a preexisting fracture, high levels of biochemical markers of bone turnover, and age are among the primary determinants of the risk of vertebral fractures (7–9).

Bone Density Measurements

Bone mass accounts for approximately 80% of bone strength *in vitro* and *in vivo* (10) and is the single best predictor of osteoporotic fractures in postmenopausal women. Numerous prospective studies have shown that the risk for future fractures increases exponentially as bone density declines (11,12). The availability of safe, simple, and accurate methods for measuring bone density have now made it possible to detect osteoporosis in its earliest stages, quantitate an individual's risk for future fractures, and monitor the effectiveness of treatment. As expected, bone density measurements also appear to increase women's willingness to undertake nutritional modifications, exercise, and pharmacologic therapy for osteoporosis (13). For a detailed discussion of bone densitometry techniques, appropriate use, and interpretation, see Chapter 25.

Who Should Be Measured?

If cost containment were not an issue, bone densitometry, like blood pressure and lipid-profile measurements, would be readily available to almost all postmenopausal women needing to make informed decisions about therapy to prevent and treat osteoporosis. Medicare now covers densitometry for estrogen-deficient women older than 65 years, but many private insurers continue to limit its use in younger women. Although the specific indications for testing remain somewhat controversial, several professional organizations have published guidelines for the use of bone densitometry. A recent cost-effectiveness analysis, supported by the National Osteoporosis Foundation, concluded that it is worthwhile to measure bone density in any woman with a vertebral fracture and in all white women older than 60 to 65 years, regardless of risk factors (13a). In otherwise healthy, postmenopausal women between ages 50 and 60 years, indications for bone-densitometry testing include a history of low-trauma fracture, weight under 127 pounds, smoking, or a family history of an osteoporotic fracture (14). Most experts would also recommend bone-density testing for any woman with known secondary causes of bone loss (Table 3) if the results of the measurement will influence treatment decisions. Guidelines for bone-mass measurements in other ethnic groups have

TABLE 3. *Differential diagnosis of low bone mass, fractures, or both*

Primary osteoporosis	Connective tissue diseases
Postmenopausal	Osteogenesis imperfecta
Senile	Marfan's syndrome
Osteomalacia	Homocystinuria
Vitamin D deficiency/resistance	Ankylosing spondylitis
Hypophosphatemia	Rheumatoid arthritis
Hypophosphatasia	Gastrointestinal (GI) diseases
Endocrine disorders	Cholestatic liver disease
Hypogonadism (primary and secondary)	Gluten-sensitive enteropathy
Hyperparathyroidism	Inflammatory bowel disease
Hyperthyroidism	Hemochromatosis
Hypercortisolemia	Parenteral nutrition
Marrow dysplasia/infiltration	After gastrectomy
Mastocytosis	Renal disorders
Myeloma/leukemia/lymphoma	Renal tubular acidosis
Gaucher disease	Renal osteodystrophy
Acquired immunodeficiency syndrome (AIDS)	Hypercalciuria

not been established because of insufficient data. Until data become available, however, it seems prudent to measure bone density in any woman with a history of low-trauma fractures, major risk factors for osteoporosis, or diseases known to accelerate bone loss.

MAKING THE CORRECT DIAGNOSIS AND IDENTIFYING TREATABLE CAUSES OF BONE LOSS

Postmenopausal and age-related bone loss are, by far, the most common causes of osteoporosis in women, but other diseases also can present as low bone density or fractures (Table 3). Although many of these disorders can be identified in the medical history, others may be undiagnosed. Starting treatment for osteoporosis without a search for underlying disease processes may result in missed opportunities to treat modifiable conditions or lead to the initiation of inappropriate therapy. In osteoporotic men, the incidence of secondary osteoporosis is high, ranging from 30% to 64% in published studies (15). The incidence of secondary causes of bone loss in women in the general population has not been established. In 180 osteoporotic women attending an osteoporosis clinic, 46% had a history of at least one condition known to accelerate bone loss, whereas a new, unsuspected diagnosis was identified in 11% (16). The proportion of women with previously unidentified, contributing conditions may be even higher in osteoporotic women without major risk factors for osteoporosis. In a recent study, 31% of these women were found to have disorders with possible effects on skeletal health that had not been previously identified (17). The most frequent new diagnoses were hypercalciuria, calcium malabsorption, vitamin D deficiency, and exogenous hyperthyroidism. However, previously unsuspected cases of gluten-sensitive enteropathy, primary hyperparathyroidism, multiple myeloma, Cushing's syndrome, Paget's disease, and hypervitaminosis D also were identified.

No signs, symptoms, or diagnostic tests are specific for osteoporosis; therefore the diagnosis must be made by excluding other diseases. This process begins with a careful history and physical examination, keeping the differential diagnoses (Table 3) in mind. Table 4 lists some of the important issues to be assessed during this evaluation. The medical history will identify diseases and/or medications that have contributed to the development of osteoporosis. Risk-factor assessment detects correctable causes of bone loss, such as smoking, inadequate nutrition, or excessive thyroid hormone replacement, and identifies other factors that increase fracture risk (Table 2). At this stage of the evaluation, the presence or absence of major risk factors will determine the level of suspicion of other pathologic processes and help decide the extent of laboratory testing. For example, vigorous pursuit of other diagnoses is appropriate for an osteoporotic woman with no major risk factors, but may not be indicated for the woman in whom severe osteoporosis is expected because of her medical history.

Careful attention also should be given to the presence of physical symptoms. Osteoporosis is asymptomatic and causes symptoms only when fractures occur. Although chronic back pain sometimes develops from disordered biomechanics after vertebral compression fractures, the presence of severe pain, bone tenderness unrelated to an acute fracture, or persistence of severe pain for more than 10 to 12 weeks following a fracture suggests another etiology. In addition, localized or diffuse muscle weakness, weight loss, or other systemic symptoms and/or the presence of abnormal laboratory tests should prompt additional evaluation in search of other underlying pathology.

Routine Laboratory Testing

There is no established algorithm for the evaluation of women with low bone density, but some simple screening studies, such as chemistry profile, complete blood count (CBC), and 24-hour urine calcium are appropriate for all osteoporotic women prior to the start of therapy. Thyroid function tests [T_4 and ultrasensitive thyroid-stimulating hormone (TSH)] are indicated for any patient receiving thyroid hormone replacement or in those with signs or symptoms

TABLE 4. *Important elements of the medical history and physical examination in postmenopausal osteoporosis*

Skeletal history	Fractures, pain, deformity, reduced mobility, height loss
Risk-factor assessment	
Family history	Osteoporosis, fractures, renal stones
Medical history	Age, ethnicity, weight
Reproductive	Menarche > age 15 years, oligo/amenorrhea, menopause
Medical disease	Renal, GI, endocrine, rheumatic, or neurologic diseases; eating disorder, depression, prolonged immobilization
Surgery	Gastrectomy, small-bowel resection, intestinal bypass, organ transplant
Medications	Glucocorticoids, anticonvulsants, cytotoxic agents, GnRH agonists, heparin, lithium
Lifestyle and exercise	Smoking, ETOH intake, frequent dieting, poor nutrition and exercise
Diet and supplements	Calcium, protein, vitamins D and A, caffeine
Current medications	Nonprescription drugs, hormones (estrogen, thyroid, glucocorticoids), sedatives or narcotics, antihypertensives, diuretics
Review of systems/physical examination (findings that suggest other diseases)	
Weight loss, diarrhea	Thyrotoxicosis, malabsorption
Weight gain, hirsutism	Cushing's syndrome
Muscle weakness	Cushing's syndrome, osteomalacia
Bone pain	Osteomalacia, hyperparathyroidism, malignancy, fractures
Tooth loss	Hypophosphatasia
Joint or lens dislocation	Abnormalities of collagen
Skin rash/pigmentation/stria	Mastocytosis, hemochromatosis, Cushing's syndrome
Nephrolithiasis	Hypercalciuria, hyperparathyroidism

GI, gastrointestinal; GnRH, gonadotropin-releasing hormone; ETOH, ethyl alcohol.

of hyperthyroidism. The results of these studies are usually normal in osteoporosis, whereas abnormalities may indicate the presence of other pathology. A biochemical profile provides information on renal and hepatic function, primary hyperparathyroidism ($\uparrow$ Ca), and possible malnutrition ($\downarrow$ Ca, $\downarrow$ phosphorus, or $\downarrow$ albumin). A hematologic profile may give evidence of bone marrow malignancy or infiltrative processes (anemia, $\downarrow$ WBC, or $\downarrow$ platelets) or of malabsorption (anemia, microcytosis, or macrocytosis). Measurement of 24-hour urinary calcium excretion on a high calcium intake (1000 to 1500 mg/day) screens simultaneously for malabsorption and hypercalciuria, frequently silent but potentially correctable causes of bone loss. Low 24-hour urine calcium (<50 mg/24 hours) suggests vitamin D deficiency, osteomalacia, or malabsorption due to small bowel diseases such as celiac sprue. Values over 300 mg/day represent hypercalciuria, which should prompt further evaluation to define its etiology. Possibilities include (a) renal tubular leak of calcium, for which a thiazide diuretic could be beneficial; (b) absorptive hypercalciuria (either idiopathic or related to granulomatous or hematologic diseases), which would require caution in prescribing calcium supplementation; or (c) excessive bone resorption, which could be a clue to the presence of an underlying malignancy, hyperparathyroidism, or another bone disease (i.e., hyperthyroidism, Paget's disease), any of which could influence the choice of appropriate treatment.

Additional laboratory studies are indicated in patients with unusual signs or symptoms or abnormal baseline laboratory results. They also are appropriate when the severity of osteoporosis is unexplained or more advanced than expected for age [e.g., bone mineral density (BMD) is more than 1.5 to 2.0 SD below the age-matched mean]. Serum and urine protein electrophoreses help to rule out multiple myeloma, whereas 24-hour urine free cortisol or an overnight dexa-

methasone-suppression test will detect occult Cushing's disease. Parathyroid hormone (PTH) and vitamin D metabolites are used to evaluate hypercalcemia and hypercalciuria. Measurements of vitamin D levels [25 (OH) D and/or 1,25 $(OH)_2$ D], serum ferritin, carotene, and anti-gliadin or anti-endomyseal antibodies are useful in evaluating calcium malabsorption. If these antibodies are positive, a small-bowel biopsy is needed to confirm the diagnosis of celiac sprue. If suspicion is high, a bone marrow biopsy may be required to make the diagnosis of diseases affecting the bone marrow such as mastocytosis, multiple myeloma, Gaucher disease or leukemia.

Bone biopsy has been used clinically to diagnose osteomalacia, to detect causes of osteoporosis involving the bone marrow, and to assess bone-remodeling rates. Today, however, bone biopsy is rarely required in the evaluation of women with postmenopausal osteoporosis. Accurate measures of serum and urine chemistry, vitamin D metabolites, and biochemical markers of bone turnover now make it possible to diagnose most cases of osteomalacia and to identify high bone turnover without an invasive procedure. In unusual cases of osteoporosis (e.g., premenopausal or early perimenopausal women) in which the diagnosis remains unexplained after other evaluation, a biopsy may be helpful to detect occult osteomalacia or to reveal unusual causes of osteoporosis such as mastocytosis.

DETERMINE THE SEVERITY, EXTENT, AND ACTIVITY OF DISEASE

Radiology

Bone densitometry (discussed earlier) is the single most helpful radiographic tool to assess the extent and severity of osteoporosis. Other radiographic studies, however, may be needed to evaluate bone or back pain, determine the etiology of height loss, detect undiagnosed vertebral fractures, and rule out other bone diseases.

In a patient with osteoporosis, loss of height and/or back pain suggest the presence of vertebral fractures that, if present, indicate the need for aggressive therapy. However, height loss and back pain also may result from degenerative disc disease, worsening of a developmental scoliosis or kyphosis, or other bone, joint, or soft-tissue pathology. The distinction between these conditions has important implications for both evaluation and treatment. In these patients, routine posteroanterior (PA) and lateral spine radiographs are required to make the correct diagnosis and establish a baseline for follow-up. Additional radiographic studies should be pursued in patients who experience (a) persistent pain for more than 10 to 12 weeks after an acute fracture; (b) fragility fractures despite normal bone density; (c) fractures with minimal trauma in unusual locations (ribs); or (d) in patients who have a history of malignancy. In these cases, the suspicion of nonosteoporotic causes of fractures, particularly malignant or infiltrative diseases, should be high. Appropriate evaluation may include a radionuclide bone scan, computerized tomography, and/or magnetic resonance imaging (MRI).

Biochemical Indices of Bone Turnover

Bone is constantly being remodeled in a cyclic process by which packets of old bone tissue are resorbed by osteoclasts and replaced by new bone matrix produced by osteoblasts. The rate at which this process is occurring can be assessed either by measuring the enzymatic activity of bone cells (alkaline or acid phosphatase levels) or by measuring the breakdown products of bone matrix (osteocalcin or pyridinoline crosslinks of type 1 collagen. In postmenopausal women, biochemical markers of bone remodeling correlate with histomorphometric indices of bone turnover, rates of bone loss, and fracture risk. At present, the most practical uses for these markers are (a) as an adjunct to bone densitometry in the evaluation of fracture risk, (b) to assist in the evaluation of unexplained osteoporosis, and (c) to monitor the response to therapy. When used in the evaluation of osteoporotic patients, markers of bone remodeling also make it possible to detect high bone turnover which may influence treatment decisions and/or direct the differential diagnosis toward certain conditions which are associated with excess bone resorption such as occult hyperparathyroidism, hyperthyroidism, or malignancy. (For a detailed discussion of the use and interpretation of biochemical bone markers, see Chapter 22.)

SUMMARY

The appropriate evaluation of postmenopausal osteoporosis requires the assessment of risk factors, quantification of bone mass, documentation of fractures, and a diligent search for other diseases and treatable causes of bone loss. The process begins with a careful assessment of the medical history, physical examination, bone density measurements, routine laboratory tests, and bone radiographs as needed. Suggestive findings should be pursued with additional, targeted laboratory and radiologic procedures until the correct diagnosis is established and appropriate treatment is begun.

REFERENCES

1. Farmer ME, White LR, Brody JA. Race and sex differences in hip fracture incidence. *Am J Public Health* 1984;44:1374–1380.
2. Slemenda CW, Hui SL, Longcope C, Wellman H, Johnston CC Jr. Predictors of bone mass in perimenopausal women: a prospective study of clinical data using photon absorptiometry. *Ann Intern Med* 1990;112:96–101.
3. Bauer DC, Browner WS, Cauley JA, et al. Factors associated with appendicular bone mass in older women. *Ann Intern Med* 1993;118:657–665.
4. Cummings SR, Nevitt MC, Browner WS, et al., for the Study of Osteoporotic Fractures Research Group. Risk factors for hip fracture in white women. *N Engl J Med* 1995;332:767–773.
5. Johnell O, Gullberg B, Kanis JA, et al. Risk factors for hip fracture in European women: the MEDOS study. *J Bone Miner Res* 1995;10:1802–1815.
6. Grisso JA, Kelsey JL, Strom BL, et al. Risk factors for falls as a cause of hip fracture in women. *N Engl J Med* 1991;324:1326–1331.
7. Kelsey JL, Browner WS, Seeley DG, Nevitt MC, Cummings SR. Risk factors for fractures of the distal forearm and proximal humerus. *Am J Epidemiol* 1992;135:477–489.
8. Ross PD, Davis JW, Epstein RS, Wasnich RD. Pre-existing fractures and bone mass predict vertebral fracture incidence in women. *Ann Intern Med* 1991;114:919–923.
9. Wasnich RD, Davis JW, Ross PD. Spine fracture risk is predicted by nonspine fractures. *Osteoporos Int* 1994;4:1–5.
10. Melton LJ III, Chao EYS, Lane J. Biomechanical aspects of fractures. In: Riggs BL, Melton LJ III, eds. *Osteoporosis: etiology, diagnosis, and management.* New York: Raven Press, 1988:111–131.
11. Hui SL, Slemenda CW, Johnston CC Jr. Age and bone mass as predictors of fracture in a prospective study. *J Clin Invest* 1988;81:1804–1809.
12. Black DM, Cummings SR, Genant HK, Nevitt MC, Palermo L, Browner W. Axial and appendicular bone density predict fractures in older women. *J Bone Miner Res* 1992;7:633–638.
13. Rubin SM, Cummings SR. Results of bone densitometry affect women's decisions about taking measures to prevent fractures. *Ann Intern Med* 1992;116(12 Pt 1):990–995.
13a. *Physician's Guide to Prevention and Treatment of Osteoporosis.* New Jersey: Excerpta Media, Inc., 1988.
14. Eddy DM, Cummings SR, Johnston CC, et al. Osteoporosis: review of the evidence for prevention, diagnosis and treatment and cost-effectiveness analysis. *Osteoporos Int* 1998;8:S1–S88.
15. Orwoll ES, Klein RF. Osteoporosis in men. *Endocr Rev* 1995;16:87–116.
16. Johnson BE, Lucasey B, Tobinson RG, Lukert BP. Contributing diagnosis in osteoporosis. *Arch Intern Med* 1989;149:1069.
17. Clark J, Tamenbaum C, Posnett K, Meier D, Luckey M. Laboratory testing in healthy, osteopenic women. *J Bone Miner Res* 1997;12:S141.

52. Pharmacology of Agents to Treat Osteoporosis

Nelson B. Watts, M.D.

Department of Medicine, Emory University School of Medicine, and Osteoporosis and Metabolic Bone Diseases Program,
The Emory Clinic, Atlanta, Georgia

ESTROGEN

General

Estrogen is the agent of choice for both prevention and treatment of postmenopausal osteoporosis. Estrogen relieves symptoms such as hot flashes and vaginal dryness. It also reduces the risk of myocardial infarction, which, from a public health viewpoint, is more important than the benefits it affords for osteoporosis. Estrogen prevents bone loss when begun at menopause (1) and increases spine bone mineral density (BMD) by 5% to 10% when started after age 65 years (2). Once estrogen is stopped, BMD decreases quickly, which means that estrogen must be continued for the benefits to be maintained (3). Despite well-documented benefits, long-term compliance is low.

Various estrogen preparations are available. A progestin is usually added for a woman with an intact uterus, but progestins do not add anything to the bone effects of estrogen (except perhaps for norethisterone acetate, an androgenic progestin commonly used in Europe).

Mechanism(s) of Action

Although estrogen has been linked to skeletal health and disease for over 50 years, the understanding of its mechanisms of action on bone is still being developed. Estrogens bind with receptors in nuclei of target cells and activate responsive genes (4). One clear result is suppression of osteoclastic bone resorption, likely through multiple pathways (4). Estrogen has important effects on cytokine and growth-factor production and action in both osteoclasts and osteoblasts (4). Estrogen also affects calcium homeostasis through actions on bone, kidney, and bowel; may affect regulation of calcitropic hormones; and may affect tissue responsiveness to these hormones (5). Estrogen appears to sensitize remodeling units to respond to electrical and mechanical forces by altering the "mechanistat" (6).

The optimal dose, method of delivery, or blood level of estrogen for optimal bone effect is not clear. For years it was thought that 0.625 mg daily of conjugated equine estrogens was the minimally effective dose. A recent study of esterified estrogens showed a typical dose response, with 0.3 mg daily effective for prevention of bone loss, gains in BMD with 0.625 mg daily, and further gains with 1.25 mg daily (7). At least one study suggested that a serum estradiol level of 60 pg/mL is needed for maximal effect (8), but lower serum estradiol levels do have some effect (7).

Absorption and Elimination

Estrogens are well absorbed through skin, mucous membranes (e.g., vagina), and gastrointestinal tract. After oral administration, absorption (t_{max}, 5 to 9 hours) and elimination are slow (half-life, 10 to 18 hours), and the mean residence time is long (13 to 28 hours) (9). Orally administered synthetic estrogens (e.g., ethinyl estradiol) are degraded very slowly by the liver and other tissues.

Transdermal estradiol achieves adequate levels with $\frac{1}{20}$ the oral dose (a transdermal dose of 0.1 mg daily is equivalent to approximately 2 mg oral micronized estradiol). A variety of patches, applied once or twice weekly, are available in a wide dose range.

The parenteral absorption of estrogens conjugated with aryl groups (valerate or cypionate) is quite slow, with a single intramuscular injection being absorbed over several weeks. Pellets inserted subcutaneously deliver steady levels of estradiol for up to 6 months.

Orally administered estrogens undergo extensive metabolism by the liver ("first pass"), but systemically administered estrogens also are metabolized by the liver and peripheral tissues. Regardless of the type of estrogen administered, there is a stable equilibrium between estrone (the dominant form) and estradiol (the more active form) and conjugated and esterified forms. For example, orally administered micronized estradiol is well absorbed but is rapidly converted to estrone (10).

Estrogens circulate largely bound to sex hormone–binding globulin (SHBG) and albumin, with only the unbound fraction being biologically active. Because estrogen itself raises levels of SHBG, measurements of total estrogens or estradiol are of limited clinical importance.

Estrogens are excreted in bile and reabsorbed in the small intestine (enterohepatic circulation). During this phase they are metabolized to less active and more polar compounds that are excreted in the urine. Estrogen activity is significantly reduced by smoking.

Adverse Events and Contraindications

Estrogens are usually well tolerated but may cause dose-dependent side effects including breast tenderness, fluid retention, and weight gain. There is a small but significant risk of deep vein thrombosis and pulmonary emboli. The possibility that long-term estrogen use increases the risk of breast cancer discourages many women from even considering estrogen treatment. Recent data suggest that this risk may be limited to women who consume alcohol regularly (11).

Estrogens should not be used in women who are or might be pregnant, women with undiagnosed genital bleeding, known or suspected cancer of the breast, known or suspected estrogen-dependent neoplasm, or with active thrombophlebitis or thromboembolic disorder.

SELECTIVE ESTROGEN-RECEPTOR MODULATORS

General

The only selective estrogen-receptor modulator (SERM) currently approved by the Food and Drug Administration (FDA) for use in osteoporosis is raloxifene (Evista), which is approved for prevention of bone loss in recently menopausal women (12). Other FDA-approved agents in this category are used for other purposes (e.g., tamoxifen and torimifene for treatment of breast cancer) or are used for osteoporosis in other countries (e.g., tibolone).

Mechanism(s) of Action

The actions of raloxifene are mediated through binding to estrogen receptors. After binding, raloxifene produces different expression of estrogen-regulated genes in different tissues, activating some and inhibiting others (13,14). Raloxifene has been shown to prevent bone loss in recently menopausal women (15). The recommended dose for prevention of bone loss is 60 mg daily (12). Raloxifene has some of the effects of estrogen on lipids (16), but does not stimulate the endometrium and does not increase the risk of breast cancer.

Absorption and Elimination

Approximately 60% of an oral dose of raloxifene is absorbed and then undergoes extensive first-pass metabolism in the liver, resulting in about 2% bioavailability (17). Food does not appreciably affect bioavailability. Raloxifene is avidly bound to plasma proteins but does not interact with binding of warfarin or phenytoin (18). Final elimination is through hepatic metabolism and fecal excretion, with minimal renal clearance (19). Safety in patients with severe liver disease has not been established. Other than interference of cholestyramine with absorption, no significant drug–drug interactions have been identified.

Concurrent use of raloxifene with estrogens has not been studied, nor has use in men or premenopausal women.

Adverse Effects and Contraindications

In clinical trials, hot flashes occurred more frequently with raloxifene than with placebo (24% with raloxifene vs. 18% with placebo) but were generally mild and did not result in discontinuation. Raloxifene is associated with a low but statistically significant increased risk of thrombophlebitis and pulmonary emboli (similar to estrogen). It is contraindicated in women with active or past history of venous thrombosis or embolism. If a patient taking raloxifene is immobilized (for example, after surgery), the drug should be stopped 72 hours in advance, if possible, and held until the patient is fully ambulatory. In clinical trials, leg cramps (usually mild), occurred approximately 2 to 3 times more often with raloxifene than with placebo (5.9% with raloxifene vs. 1.9% with placebo). Raloxifene may cause fetal harm and is contraindicated in women who are or may become pregnant.

CALCITONIN

General

Calcitonin is a peptide hormone secreted by specialized cells in the thyroid. Salmon calcitonin is more potent and has a longer duration of action than human calcitonin (20). In some countries, eel calcitonin is used (21).

Mechanism(s) of Action

Calcitonin has actions on the kidneys and gastrointestinal tract, but its primary action is on bone to reduce osteoclastic bone resorption (22). Calcitonin causes a diminution in the number of osteoclasts, changes in their appearance (shrinkage of cells, loss of ruffled border) (23), a reduction of resorptive activity, movement away from bone, and a shortening of life span (increased apoptosis). These changes are mediated by binding of calcitonin to specific receptors of the osteoclast (20).

Calcitonin treatment results in slight gains in spinal BMD, somewhat less than those with estrogen or bisphosphonates (24). The greatest effect appears to be in patients with rapid bone turnover (25). No increases have been shown at peripheral bone sites. Nasal calcitonin appears to reduce the risk of new vertebral fractures (26). The results of a 5-year multicenter study, soon to be complete, should better define the role for calcitonin. An important side benefit of calcitonin is an analgesic effect (27), unrelated to its effect on bone (possibly mediated by increased levels of endorphins). This analgesic effect makes calcitonin the first drug to consider for osteoporotic patients who have acute or chronic pain.

Absorption and Elimination

Calcitonin is effective when given by injection (subcutaneous or intramuscular) and by nasal spray (28). Other routes of administration also have been investigated. Bioavailability of nasal calcitonin is less than 10% of that given by injection (29). Plasma levels peak about 20 to 30 minutes after nasal administration (somewhat faster after injection) (30). The half-life is about 40 minutes. The recommended dose of salmon calcitonin for treatment of postmenopausal osteoporosis is 50 to 100 IU daily by injection or 200 IU (one puff) daily intranasally.

Calcitonin is rapidly metabolized, primarily by the kidneys (30). Unchanged hormone and inactive metabolites are excreted in the urine (30).

Adverse Events and Contraindications

Salmon calcitonin by injection has been available since 1984 but saw limited use because of the discomfort of injections, relatively high cost, and limited tolerance. In December 1995, nasal calcitonin was introduced. It is better tolerated than the subcutaneous form (31). The recommended dose of nasal calcitonin is 200 IU (one spray) daily. Nausea, vomiting, and flushing occur in about 10% of patients treated with parenteral calcitonin (32). Local reactions at the injection site may occur. Prolonged use of the nasal spray may cause local irritation and occasionally severe epistaxis and nasal ulcerations.

Circulating antibodies develop in about half of patients treated with calcitonin for 6 months or more. Occasionally these antibodies can neutralize the effect of calcitonin (32). Tachyphylaxis through downregulation of calcitonin receptors also may occur. Although uncommon, serious systemic allergic reactions to calcitonin have been reported. Because of this, skin testing should be considered prior to treatment.

BISPHOSPHONATES

General

Bisphosphonates are analogues of pyrophosphates, consisting of two phosphonic acids joined to a carbon (Fig. 1) (33). The two phosphonic acids cause bisphosphonates to be avidly adsorbed to bone surfaces. The central carbon renders the compound impervious to enzymatic degradation. Side chains R_1 and R_2 affect the avidity of adsorption to bone and the antiresorptive potency (34,35) (see Table 1).

Mechanism(s) of Action

Bisphosphonates reduce bone resorption. After binding to bone surfaces, bisphosphonates are released locally and interfere with resorption by reducing the production of protons and lysosomal enzymes beneath the osteoclast (36). Some bisphosphonates interfere with activation of osteoclast precursors, differentiation of precursor cells into mature osteoclasts, chemotaxis, and attachment of osteoclasts to bone (37). Bisphosphonates may shorten the life span of osteoclasts (apoptosis) (36).

Bisphosphonates also may have indirect effects, causing osteoblasts to produce substances that inhibit osteoclasts (38) and decreasing levels of osteoclast stimulators. Bisphosphonates also may increase osteoblast differentiation and number (39).

Through actions on osteoclasts, bisphosphonates reduce activation frequency (the rate at which new bone-remodeling

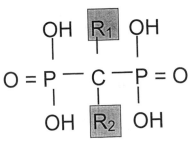

FIG. 1. General structure of bisphosphonates; side chains (R_1 and R_2) can be modified to alter the potency and the side-effect profile. (From Watts NB. Bisphosphonate therapy for postmenopausal osteoporosis. *South Med J* 1992;85:2S–31, with permission.)

units are formed). At least with etidronate, the reduction of activation frequency is transient, with a return toward baseline after about 5 years of treatment (40). Perhaps an even more important effect of bisphosphonates is a positive bone balance at individual remodeling units (41). The positive bone balance explains the continued increase of bone mass with long-term use (42).

The molecular mechanism of bisphosphonate action appears to involve, at least in part, inhibition of the mevalonate pathway and prevention of posttranslation prenylation of guanosine triphosphate (GTP)-binding proteins (43).

Absorption and Elimination

Orally administered bisphosphonates are absorbed in the upper small intestine. Absorption is extremely poor after oral administration. Typically, less than 5% of an oral dose is absorbed (it varies from 6% for tiludronate, 3.5% for etidronate, to 0.7% for alendronate). The amount absorbed is dose dependent. Absorption is significantly reduced or eliminated if the drug is taken with calcium, other divalent cations, or with foods or beverages other than plain water. Bisphosphonates should be taken with water, ideally first thing in the morning, after an overnight fast, with nothing by mouth for at least 30 minutes (and possibly longer).

TABLE 1. *Generations of bisphosphonates*

Chemical modification	Examples	Relative antiresorptive potency
First generation Short alkyl or halide side chain	Etidronate	1
	Clodronate	10
Second generation Amino-terminal group	Tiludronate[a]	10
	Pamidronate	100
	Alendronate	100–1000
Third generation Cyclic side chain	Risedronate	1000–10,000
	Ibandronate	1000–10,000
	Zoledronate	10,000+

[a] Tiludronate has a cyclic side chain, not an amino-terminal group, but is generally classified as a second-generation compound based on its time of development and its potency.

Because absorption of etidronate is less effected by food than is that of other bisphosphonates, etidronate may be taken 2 hours before or 2 hours after eating.

Between 20% and 50% of administered bisphosphonate binds to bone surfaces within 12 to 24 hours. After binding to bone and acting on osteoclasts, the drug is buried in bone, where it is retained for months or years but is no longer active (44). [It is estimated that after 10 years of treatment, approximately 25% of the amount absorbed from a daily dose would be released from skeletal sites each day (44)]. Bisphosphonates are not metabolized; drug that does not bind to skeletal sites is excreted unchanged in the urine. Because of the renal route of elimination, bisphosphonates should be given with caution to patients with renal insufficiency.

Adverse Events and Contraindications

Etidronate (but not other bisphosphonates) given continuously in doses used to treat Paget's disease (10 to 20 mg/kg/day for 3 to 6 months) may cause impaired mineralization of bone with accumulation of unmineralized osteoid and other histologic findings similar to osteomalacia. Clinical manifestations are bone pain and fractures (45). An intermittent cyclic regimen of etidronate has been used that has only rarely been associated with this problem. There has also been concern that potent bisphosphonates might turn off remodeling completely, leading to "frozen bone," but there has been no evidence that this actually occurs.

In dogs, healing of fractures is impaired in bones that show gross histologic abnormalities caused by high doses of etidronate. Fracture healing does not appear to be a problem with low doses of etidronate, tiludronate, alendronate (46), or the newer bisphosphonates in clinical use.

Nausea and diarrhea occur in 20% to 30% of patients treated with high doses of etidronate but are rarely seen with doses used for treatment of osteoporosis. Upper gastrointestinal side effects are seen with oral administration of aminobisphosphonates (pamidronate and alendronate) because aminobisphosphonates can chemically irritate the esophagus (47) and may cause erosive esophagitis. Gastrointestinal side effects were infrequent in the Phase III trials of alendronate, but appear to be higher in general use, perhaps as a result of errors in administration or in patient selection, and may be as high as 10% to 15%. To minimize esophageal irritation, alendronate should be taken with 6 to 8 ounces of water (to be certain the tablet passes through the esophagus and into the stomach), and the patient should remain upright (seated or standing) until after eating, to avoid reflux. Alendronate should not be given to patients who cannot remain upright, or who have active upper gastrointestinal symptoms, or who have abnormal esophageal emptying (e.g., strictures, achalasia, or severe dysmotility), and it should be discontinued if such problems develop during its use. Most patients who have side effects from alendronate develop them soon after starting treatment. Tolerability does not appear to be affected by age.

Acute-phase reactions (fever and lymphopenia) may occur with parenteral use of bisphosphonates (48) but usually do not recur with repeated administration. Hypocalcemia with parenteral administration is infrequent and usually mild.

Possible side effects or idiosyncratic reactions to bisphosphonates include acute renal failure (caused by too rapid intravenous infusions), bronchoconstriction in aspirin-sensitive asthmatic patients, hearing loss in patients with otosclerosis, severe toxic skin reactions, aseptic peritonitis, and a variety of eye complications (35). Thus far, risedronate, ibandronate, and zoledronate have been remarkably nontoxic.

SODIUM FLUORIDE

General

Sodium fluoride is not approved by the U.S. FDA but is widely used in other countries to treat osteoporosis. Of all current agents, only fluoride works by increasing bone formation. A slow-release fluoride regimen for postmenopausal osteoporosis was endorsed by the FDA advisory committee in 1995 but is still under review because of questions about its effectiveness in strengthening bone (49).

Fluoride can be given as the sodium salt (in enteric-coated capsules), as a slow-release preparation, and as monofluorophosphate. Two hundred mg of disodium monofluorophosphate is equivalent to 36 mg sodium fluoride or 16.4 mg of fluoride ion (50). Although there is debate about the optimal dose, most studies show increases in bone mass with doses of 20 to 30 mg fluoride ion daily (51). By comparison, fluoride for prevention of dental caries is 2 to 4 mg daily.

Mechanism(s) of Action

Fluoride is mitogenic for osteoblasts, perhaps through alteration of G protein–dependent tyrosine phosphorylation (52,53) and possibly other signaling pathways (52). Fluoride action requires the presence of growth factors (53). In contrast to antiresorptive agents, which produce early gains in BMD that either plateau or slow, fluoride produces dramatic, sustained, linear increases in spinal BMD, averaging 9% per year for 4 years (54). In some studies, peripheral (cortical) bone density decreased in fluoride-treated patients, inversely proportional to the gain in bone mass in the spine (trabecular bone) (54,55). This "shifting" of bone from cortical to trabecular sites, which could result in increase in peripheral fractures, may be reduced or eliminated by the administration of calcium and vitamin D or by fluoride-free periods.

Absorption and Elimination

Fluoride is rapidly absorbed from the stomach, with a maximal serum level reached in 30 minutes (50). Most of an oral dose is absorbed when taken on an empty stomach, but bioavailability (except from monofluorophosphate) is reduced by 20% to 50% in the presence of food or calcium or in the absence of gastric acid. Slow-release and monofluorophosphate are absorbed less rapidly, with lower peak levels and areas under the curve (50). The kidneys eliminate about 50% (initial half-life approximately 3 hours), and the remainder is stored in bone. When creatinine clearance is below 40 to 50 mL/min, decreased fluoride clearance by the kidneys may be significant (50). Based on limited data (56), serum fluoride levels between 0.1 and 0.25 mg/L (5 to 10 μmol/L) have been considered "therapeutic." Sodium fluoride doses below 30 or 40 mg daily (13 or 18 mg fluoride ion) do not have measurable effects on bone, whereas doses above 75 or 80 mg daily (34 or 36 mg fluoride ion) produce grossly abnormal bone (55).

Fluoride alters the crystallization sequence leading to formation of hydroxyapatite, and replaces hydroxyl groups, forming fluoroapatite, a compound with less structural stability and more resistance to resorption (57).

Adverse Events and Contraindications

Orally administered sodium fluoride may irritate the stomach (through formation of hydrofluoric acid) (54). Gastrointestinal side effects are infrequent with enteric-coated and slow-release formulations and with monofluorophosphate. High doses may cause arthralgias, typically in the ankles, knees, and feet, perhaps caused by stress microfractures or by rapid bone remodeling (54,58).

The main problem with fluoride is the narrow therapeutic window, with toxic doses leading to production of bone that is histologically abnormal, undermineralized, more dense, but less strong than normal (54,59). Cortical bone loss may result in an increased risk of peripheral fractures and hip fractures (60). Until issues of safety, optimal dose, and best schedule are answered, sodium fluoride should not be used for routine treatment of postmenopausal osteoporosis.

REFERENCES

1. Bush TL, Wells HB, James MK, et al. Effects of hormone therapy on bone mineral density: results from the postmenopausal estrogen/progestin interventions (PEPI) trial. *JAMA* 1996;276:1389–1396.
2. Lindsay R, Thome JF. Estrogen treatment of patients with established osteoporosis. *Obstet Gynecol* 1990;76:290–295.
3. Lindsay R, Hart DM, MacLean A, Clark AC, Kraszewski A, Garwood J. Bone response to termination of oestrogen treatment. *Lancet* 1978;1:1325–1327.
4. Turner RT, Riggs BL, Spelsberg TC. Skeletal effects of estrogen. *Endocr Rev* 1994;15:275–300.
5. Prince RL. Estrogen effects on calcitropic hormones and calcium homeostasis. *J Clin Endocrinol Metab* 1994;15:301–308.
6. Schiessl H, Frost HM, Jee WSS. Estrogen and bone-muscle strength and mass relationships. *Bone* 1998;22:1–6.
7. Genant HK, Lucas J, Weiss S, et al., for the Estratab/Osteoporosis Study Group. Low-dose esterified estrogen therapy: effects on bone, plasma estradiol concentrations, endometrium, and lipid levels. *Arch Intern Med* 1997;157:2609–2615.
8. Reginster JY, Sarlet N, Deroisy R, Albert A, Gaspard U, Franchimont P. Minimal levels of serum estradiol prevent postmenopausal bone loss. *Calcif Tissue Int* 1992;51:340–343.
9. Bhavnani BR. Pharmacokinetics and pharmacodynamics of conjugated equine estrogens: chemistry and metabolism. *Proc Soc Exp Biol Med* 1998;217:6–16.
10. Lobo RA, Cassidenti DL. Pharmacokinetics of oral 17 beta-estradiol. *J Reprod Med* 1992;37:77–84.
11. Zumoff B. The critical role of alcohol consumption in determining the risk of breast cancer with postmenopausal estrogen administration. *J Clin Endocrinol Metab* 1997;82:1656–1657.
12. Anonymous. Raloxifene for postmenopausal osteoporosis. *Med Lett Drugs Ther* 1998;40:29–30.
13. Brzozowski AM, Pike AC, Dauder Z, et al. Molecular basis of agonism and antagonism in the oestrogen receptor. *Nature* 1997;389:753–758.
14. Paech K, Webb P, Kuiper GG, et al. Differential ligand activation of estrogen receptors ERalpha and ERbeta at AP1 sites. *Science* 1997;277:1508–1510.
15. Delmas PD, Bjarnason NH, Mitlak BH, et al. Effects of raloxifene on bone mineral density, serum cholesterol concentrations, and uterine endometrium in postmenopausal women. *N Engl J Med* 1997;337:1641–1647.
16. Walsh BW, Kuller LH, Wild RA, et al. Effects of raloxifene on serum lipids and coagulation factors in healthy postmenopausal women. *JAMA* 1998;279:1445–1451.
17. Grese TA, Pennington LD, Sluka JP, et al. Synthesis and pharmacology of conformationally restricted raloxifene analogues: highly potent selective estrogen receptor modulators. *J Med Chem* 1998;41:1272–1283.
18. Lindstrom TD, Whitaker NG, Whitaker GW. Disposition and metabolism of a new benzothiophene antiestrogen in rats, dogs and monkeys. *Xenobiotica* 1984;14:841–847.
19. Balfour JA, Goa KL. Raloxifene. *Drugs Aging* 1998;12:335–341.
20. Azria M, Copp DH, Zanelli JM. 25 years of salmon calcitonin: from synthesis to therapeutic use. *Calcif Tissue Int* 1995;57:1–4.
21. Orimo H, Morii H, Inoue T, et al. Effect of elcatonin on involutional osteoporosis. *J Bone Miner Res* 1996;14:73–78.
22. Singer FR, Melvin KEW, Mills BG. Acute effects of calcitonin on osteoclasts in man. *Clin Endocrinol* 1976;5(suppl):333s–340s.
23. Chambers TJ, Moore A. The sensitivity of isolated osteoclasts to morphological transformation by calcitonin. *J Clin Endocrinol Metab* 1983;57:819–824.
24. Overgaard K, Riis BJ, Christiansen C, Podenphant J, Johansen JS. Nasal calcitonin for treatment of established osteoporosis. *Clin Endocrinol (Oxf)* 1989;30:435–442.
25. Civitelli R, Gonnelli S, Zacchei F, et al. Bone turnover in postmenopausal osteoporosis: effect of calcitonin treatment. *J Clin Invest* 1988;82:1268–1274.
26. Stock JL, Avioli LV, Baylink DJ, et al., for the PROOF Study Group. Calcitonin-salmon nasal spray reduces the incidence of new vertebral fractures in postmenopausal women: three-year interim results of the PROOF study [Abstract]. *J Bone Miner Res* 1997;12:S149.
27. Pun KK, Chan LW. Analgesic effect of intranasal salmon calcitonin in the treatment of osteoporotic vertebral fractures. *Clin Ther* 1989;11:205–209.
28. Patel S, Lyons AR, Hosking DJ. Drugs used in the treatment of metabolic bone disease: clinical pharmacology and therapeutic use. *Drugs* 1993;46:594–617.
29. Kurose H, Seino Y, Shima M, et al. Intranasal absorption of salmon calcitonin. *Calcif Tissue Int* 1987;41:249–251.
30. Huwyler R, Born W, Ohnhaus EE, Fischer JA. Plasma kinetics and urinary excretion of exogenous human and salmon calcitonin in man. *Am J Physiol* 1979;236:E15–E19.
31. Carstens JH Jr, Feinblatt JD. Future horizons for calcitonin: a U.S. perspective. *Calcif Tissue Int* 1991;49(suppl 2):S2–S6.
32. Grauer A, Reinel HH, Ziegler R, Raue F. Neutralizing antibodies against calcitonin. *Horm Metab Res* 1993;25:486–488.
33. Watts NB. Bisphosphonate therapy for postmenopausal osteoporosis. *South Med J* 1992;85:2S31–2S33.
34. Fleisch H. Bisphosphonates: mechanisms of action. *J Clin Endocrinol Metab* 1998;19:80–100.
35. Watts NB. Treatment of osteoporosis with bisphosphonates. *Endocrinol Metab Clin North Am* 1998;27:419–439.
36. Rodan GA, Fleisch HA. Bisphosphonates: mechanisms of action. *J Clin Invest* 1996;97:2692–2696.
37. Lowik CW, Boonekamp PM, van de Pluym G, et al. Bisphosphonates can reduce osteoclastic bone resorption by two different mechanisms. *Adv Exp Med Biol* 1986;208:275–281.
38. Vitte C, Fleisch H, Guenther HL. Bisphosphonates induce osteoblasts to secrete an inhibitor of osteoclast-mediated resorption. *Endocrinology* 1996;137:2324–2333.
39. Giuliani N, Pedrazzoni M, Negri G, Passeri G, Impicciatore M, Girasole G. Bisphosphonates stimulate formation of osteoblast precursors and mineralized nodules in murine and human bone marrow cultures in vitro and promote early osteoblastogenesis in young and aged mice in vivo. *Bone* 1998;22:455–461.
40. Storm T, Steiniche T, Thamsborg G, Melsen F. Changes in bone histomorphometry after long-term treatment with intermittent, cyclic etidronate for postmenopausal osteoporosis. *J Bone Miner Res* 1993;8:199–208.

41. Heaney RP, Yates AJ, Santora AC II. Bisphosphonate effects and the bone remodeling transient. *J Bone Miner Res* 1997;12:1143–1151.
42. Miller PD, Watts NB, Licata AA, et al. Cyclical etidronate in the treatment of postmenopausal osteoporosis: efficacy and safety after 7 years of treatment. *Am J Med* 1997;103:468–476.
43. Luckman SP, Hughes DE, Coxon FP, Russell RGG, Rogers MJ. Nitrogen-containing bisphosphonates inhibit the mevalonate pathway and prevent post-translational prenylation of GTP-binding proteins, including Ras. *J Bone Miner Res* 1998;13:581–589.
44. Kasting GB, Francis MD. Retention of etidronate in human, dog, and rat. *J Bone Miner Res* 1992;7:513–522.
45. Eyres KS, Marshall P, McCloskey E, Douglas DL, Kanis JA. Spontaneous fractures in a patient treated with low doses of etidronic acid (disodium etidronate). *Drug Safety* 1992;7:162–165.
46. Peter CP, Cook WO, Nunamaker DM, Provost MT, Seedor JG, Rodan GA. Effect of alendronate on fracture healing and bone remodeling in dogs. *J Orthop Res* 1996;14:74–79.
47. Graham EM, Malaty HM, Goodgame R. Primary amino-bisphosphonates: a new class of gastrotoxic drugs—comparison of alendronate and aspirin. *Am J Gastroenterol* 1997;92:1322–1325.
48. Gallacher SJ, Ralston SH, Patel U, Boyle IT. Side-effects of pamidronate. *Lancet* 1989;2:42–43.
49. Pak CYC, Zerwekh JE, Antich PP, Bell NH, Singer FR. Perspective: slow-release sodium fluoride in osteoporosis. *J Bone Miner Res* 1996;11:561–567.
50. Kanis JA. Treatment of symptomatic osteoporosis with fluoride. *Am J Med* 1993;95(suppl 5A):53S–61S.
51. Dure-Smith BA, Kraenzlin ME, Farley SM, Libanti CR, Schulz EE, Baylink DJ. Fluoride therapy for osteoporosis: a review of dose response, duration of treatment, and skeletal sites of action. *Calcif Tissue Int* 1991;49(suppl):S64–S67.
52. Caverzasio J, Palmer G, Bonjour JP. Fluoride: mode of action. *Bone* 1998;22:585–603.
53. Libanti CR, Lau K-HW, Baylink DJ. Fluoride therapy for osteoporosis. In: Marcus R, Feldman D, Kelsey J, eds. *Osteoporosis.* San Diego: Academic Press, 1996:1259–1277.
54. Riggs BL, Hodgson SF, O'Fallon WM, et al. Effect of fluoride treatment on the fracture rate in postmenopausal women with osteoporosis. *N Engl J Med* 1990;322:802–809.
55. Riggs BL, O'Fallon WM, Lane A, et al. Clinical trial of fluoride therapy in postmenopausal osteoporotic women: extended observations and additional analysis. *J Bone Miner Res* 1994;9:265–275.
56. Johansen E, Taves DA, Olson T, eds. *Continuing evaluation of the use of fluorides.* Boulder, CO: Westview, 1979:149–156.
57. Eanes ED, Reddi AH. The effect of fluoride on bone mineral apatite. *Metab Bone Dis Relat Res* 1979;2:3–10.
58. O'Duffy JD, Wahner HW, O'Fallon WM, et al. Mechanism of acute lower extremity pain syndrome in fluoride-treated osteoporotic patients. *Am J Med* 1986;80:561–566.
59. Sogaard CH, Mosekilde Li, Richards A, Mosekilde LE. Marked decrease in trabecular bone quality after five years of sodium fluoride therapy—assessed by biomechanical testing of iliac crest biopsies in osteoporotic patients. *Bone* 1994;15:393–399.
60. Hedlund LR, Gallagher JC. Increased incidence of hip fracture in osteoporotic women treated with sodium fluoride. *J Bone Miner Res* 1989;4:223–225.

53. Pharmacologic Treatment of Postmenopausal Osteoporosis

Bess Dawson-Hughes, M.D.

Division of Endocrinology, New England Medical Center, and Calcium and Bone Metabolism Laboratory, U.S.D.A. Human Nutrition Research Center on Aging, Tufts University, Boston, Massachusetts

This chapter reviews the drugs currently available for the treatment and/or prevention of osteoporosis (estrogen, alendronate, calcitonin, and raloxifene) and considers who should be treated, and how patients receiving treatment should be monitored. The criteria for establishing efficacy of treatments for osteoporosis have changed. The Food and Drug Administration (FDA) currently requires demonstration of antifracture efficacy for treatments of established osteoporosis, whereas demonstration of a reduction in the rate of bone loss is sufficient for a prevention indication. Of the currently available drugs, estrogen and calcitonin were approved before antifracture efficacy was required, and alendronate was approved after the change. This explains the variability in the quality and quantity of fracture data on these three treatments. Raloxifene has at this time been approved for prevention only.

Each of the available drugs works by reducing bone resorption. The resulting decline in bone-turnover rate causes a one-time increase in bone mineral density (BMD) in the first year of treatment. The magnitude of the increase, called the "bone remodeling transient," varies inversely with the initial bone-remodeling rate. BMD change after the first year of treatment reflects a rate of change that can be expected over the ensuing several years and possibly longer. Recent evidence indicates that lowering the bone-turnover rate may lower fracture risk, independent of the effects on BMD (1).

APPROVED THERAPIES

Hormone-Replacement Therapy

Hormone-replacement therapy (HRT) usually consists of estrogen and progesterone in postmenopausal women with an intact uterus and estrogen only in women who have had a hysterectomy. Commonly prescribed estrogens and their replacement dosages are as follows: oral conjugated equine estrogens, 0.625 mg/day; oral ethinyl estradiol, 0.2 mg/day; and transdermal estradiol, 0.05 mg/day (1 patch twice per week). Oral preparations are most widely used, but transdermal estrogen may be more effective for smokers because smokers have an increased hepatic metabolism of oral estrogens. Progesterone may be given cyclically (as medroxyprogesterone, 10 mg/day, for 10 to 12 days each month) or continuously (2.5 mg/day). The latter is associated with less withdrawal bleeding.

Nonskeletal Effects

Estrogen affects many tissues. The beneficial effect of estrogen on the cardiovascular system (i.e., the 50% reduction in risk of fatal myocardial infarction) justifies its serious consideration in all eligible women at menopause (2). Estrogen also appears to have a favorable effect on cognitive function in women with (3) and without Alzheimer's disease.

Of particular concern to many women, however, estrogen use may increase breast cancer risk by 30% or so (4). Use of estrogen alone is known to increase endometrial cancer risk about fourfold [relative risk (RR) = 4], whereas use of estrogen with cyclic progesterone for at least 10 days per month or with continuous low-dose progesterone essentially eliminates this risk (5). The RR of endometrial cancer with shorter cycles of progesterone is higher than 1.3.

HRT use increases risk of venous thromboembolism two- or threefold, and the strongest association is present in the first year of therapy (6). This increase would result in one or two additional cases of thromboembolism per year for every 10,000 women taking HRT.

Women taking estrogen can expect relief of menopausal symptoms. Many women, however, will experience return of menstrual bleeding, breast tenderness, headaches, and rarely, worsening hypertension. Symptoms, concern about breast cancer, and other factors have contributed to generally poor compliance with HRT. Hormone replacement should not be given to women with thrombophlebitis or thromboembolic disorders; to women with breast, uterine, or other estrogen-sensitive cancers; or to women with postmenopausal bleeding of undetermined cause. Some physicians consider breast cancer in a first-degree relative to be a contraindication to HRT use. Women taking estrogen should be monitored with annual pelvic examinations, mammograms, and regular breast examinations.

Skeletal Effects

Several controlled studies have examined the effect of HRT on fracture incidence. One 10-year intervention study in 100 oophorectomized women found that estrogen reduced height loss and vertebral compression-fracture incidence (7). Another controlled study in 164 women found no fractures in the HRT group and 7 fractures in the placebo group during 10 years of treatment (8). In a short-term study of 75 women with prior vertebral fracture(s), transdermal estrogen and oral progesterone significantly reduced the incidence of clinical fractures (9). Seven women in the estrogen group and 12 in the placebo group had one or more new fractures during the 1-year intervention (9). These studies provide evidence that estrogen is effective in both primary and secondary prevention of osteoporotic fractures.

There is additional evidence from large, longitudinal cohort studies that supports the antifracture efficacy of HRT. Among 9704 postmenopausal women age 65 and older, current estrogen use was associated with a significant decrease in risk of wrist fracture (RR, 0.39) and of all nonspinal fractures (RR, 0.66) (10). Estrogen also appears to reduce risk of hip fractures by 20% to 60%. Larger reductions were generally seen with durations of estrogen use longer than 5 years.

HRT not only prevents bone loss in early and late postmenopausal women but causes some BMD gain. The effect of estrogen, with and without calcium, on change in BMD was examined in a recent meta-analysis (11). Of the 31 controlled estrogen trials in the analysis, 20 added calcium from either food or supplement sources to the estrogen and control groups, and 11 did not. The mean calcium intake in the trials that added calcium was 1183 mg/day and 563 mg/day in those that did not. As shown in Fig. 1, HRT alone increased BMD by 1% to 2%, depending on skeletal site. Concomitant calcium use was associated with greater gains in BMD of the lumbar spine, femoral neck, and forearm, on the order of 2% to 3% (Fig. 1). This analysis underscores not only the effectiveness of HRT but also the importance of an adequate calcium intake in women taking HRT.

Loss of estrogen at menopause is associated with an increase in bone turnover and treatment with HRT lowers the turnover rate to premenopausal levels. In women between 6 months and 3 years after menopause, oral and transdermal HRT lowered mean levels of bone-resorption markers by about 25% to 50% after 1 year of treatment (9,12). Oral and transdermal estrogen also lowered markers of bone formation, by 15% to 25% (9).

Rapid bone loss occurs in women after discontinuation of estrogen treatment. In a randomized, 2-year controlled trial in early postmenopausal women, HRT increased BMD at the distal forearm (13). After 2 years, the women were randomized to placebo or estrogen and followed for another year. The women who discontinued HRT lost BMD rapidly. Because of the rapid bone loss that occurs after stopping HRT, this treatment for osteoporosis should be considered a long-term therapy, preferably for 8 to 10 years or longer.

Alendronate

Alendronate is the most comprehensively studied drug currently approved for the treatment of osteoporosis. It is a bisphosphonate, or pyrophosphate derivative, with antiresorptive effects on the skeleton. Like other bisphosphonates,

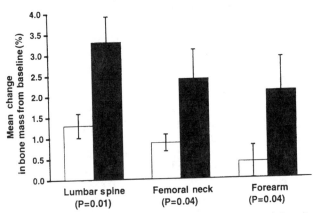

FIG. 1. Mean (SEM) annual change in bone mineral density (BMD) in women treated with estrogen alone (*open bars;* mean calcium intake, 563 mg/day) and with estrogen and calcium (*solid bars;* mean calcium intake, 1183 mg/day). (From Nieves JW, Komar L, Cosman F, Lindsay R. Calcium potentiates the effects of estrogen and calcitonin on bone mass: review and analysis. *Am J Clin Nutr* 1998;67:18–24, with permission.)

alendronate is poorly absorbed and must be taken without food. Once absorbed, it is either deposited in bone or excreted in the urine.

Alendronate can irritate the esophagus, particularly in patients with gastric reflux. On rare occasion, it has caused esophageal perforation (14). To minimize this risk, patients must be instructed to take the single daily dose with at least 8 oz of water, 30 to 60 minutes before breakfast. They must remain upright (sitting or standing) for 30 to 60 minutes after taking the pill.

Alendronate affects BMD, bone turnover, and fracture risk. The Fracture Intervention Trial (FIT) in 2027 postmenopausal women demonstrated that alendronate (5 mg per day for 2 years and 10 mg per day for a third year) increased BMD and reduced the incidence of fractures of the spine, hip, and wrist by about 50% (Fig. 2) (15). At entry, the women, mean age 71 years, had at least one vertebral fracture. On the basis of this and an earlier study (16), alendronate, in a dosage of 10 mg/day, was approved for the treatment of osteoporosis.

The effects of alendronate and HRT on BMD change were recently compared in healthy postmenopausal women younger than 60 years (17). Over a period of 2 years of treatment, alendronate, in the 5-mg dosage, and HRT significantly increased BMD at the spine (Fig. 3) and hip (not shown). The BMD increase in women taking alendronate was less than that in women taking HRT (Fig. 3). Effects of the two treatments on fracture incidence have not been compared in the same study. In a second prevention study in 447 women who were between 6 and 36 months after menopause, 5 mg per day of alendronate over a 3-year period resulted in a 2% mean gain in spinal BMD and a 1% mean gain in femoral neck BMD (18). These studies establish the efficacy of alendronate in preventing the rapid bone loss that follows the menopause.

The effect of alendronate on bone turnover has been evaluated. In early postmenopausal women, 5 mg alendronate per day lowered excretion of deoxypyridinoline, a marker of bone resorption, by about 40% and serum bone-specific alkaline phosphatase, a marker of bone formation, by about 30% (18). In older women taking the 5-mg dose, the declines were somewhat greater, averaging 50% and 40%, respectively (19). With the higher alendronate dose of 10 mg per day, levels of these markers declined by an additional 10% to 20% (19). As expected for a drug that interferes with osteoclast function, the maximal effect of alendronate on indices of bone resorption occurred earlier (after 1 to 3 months) than the maximal effect on bone formation markers (6 to 12 months).

There appears to be a residual effect of alendronate on BMD and bone turnover after the drug is discontinued (20). When women taking 5 to 10 mg/day of alendronate stopped taking the drug, bone loss occurred, but the rate of loss was not accelerated (compared with women who had taken placebo) during a 1-year follow-up period. Two-year followup in women who discontinued higher alendronate doses (20 to 40 mg) also revealed a persistent treatment effect. Longer-term studies are needed to confirm and determine the duration of the residual effect of this drug.

It should be noted that none of the treatments for osteoporosis is approved for premenopausal women. The sustained

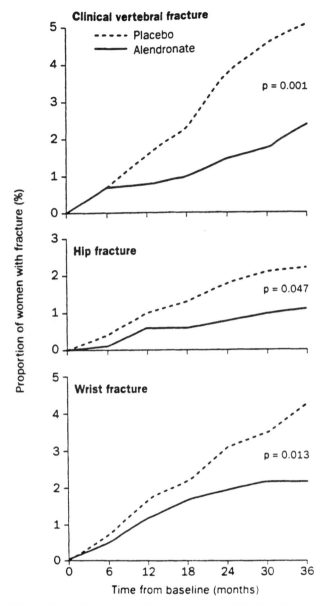

FIG. 2. Cumulative proportions of women with clinical vertebral, hip, and wrist fractures in postmenopausal women treated with placebo and alendronate. (From Black DM, Cummings SR, Karpf DB, et al. Randomized trial of effect of alendronate on risk of fracture in women with existing vertebral fractures: Fracture Intervention Trial research group. *Lancet* 1996;348:1535–1541, with permission.)

presence in bone and the residual BMD effect after discontinuing alendronate are of particular concern in view of the childbearing potential of this population.

Raloxifene

Raloxifene is the first selective estrogen-receptor modulator (SERM) to be approved for the prevention of postmenopausal osteoporosis. Raloxifene is a nonsteroidal benzothiophene compound with tissue-specific agonist and antagonist actions. It prevents bone loss and lowers serum low-density

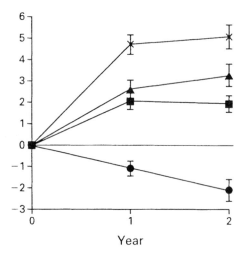

FIG. 3. Mean (SEM) change in spinal bone mineral density (BMD) in European women treated for 2 years with placebo, alendronate (2.5 and 5.0 mg), and estrogen/progestin. Change was significantly greater with each treatment (*x*, estrogen/progestin; *triangle*, alendronate, 5 mg; *square*, alendronate, 2.5 mg) compared with placebo *(circle)*. The response to estrogen/progestin was significantly greater than the response to alendronate (5 mg/day). (From Hosking D, Chilvers CED, Christiansen C, et al. Prevention of bone loss with alendronate in postmenopausal women under 60 years of age. *N Engl J Med* 1998;338:485–492, with permission.)

lipoprotein (LDL) cholesterol concentrations but does not stimulate breast or uterine tissue. The clinical effects of raloxifene have been assessed in a large randomized trial in 601 European women (21).

Nonskeletal Effects

Raloxifene, in the approved dosage of 60 mg/day, lowers serum LDL cholesterol by 8% to 10% and total cholesterol by about 6% but, unlike estrogen, it does not alter high-density lipoprotein (HDL) cholesterol or triglyceride levels (21). The effects on cardiovascular disease risk are not yet defined. Preliminary evidence indicates that raloxifene reduces the incidence of breast cancer, but more time is needed to establish and confirm this important observation. As expected, the drug does not cause breast tenderness or pain. Raloxifene does not induce endometrial thickening, as determined by intrauterine ultrasound, or uterine bleeding. Although an increased incidence of phlebitis was not reported in the European study (21), raloxifene should not be used during periods of immobilization, pending more extensive evaluation. There was no increase in the incidence of hot flashes in the European study, but the manufacturer reported hot flashes in 24.6% of women taking raloxifene compared with 18.3% of women taking placebo.

Skeletal Effects

Raloxifene prevented bone loss in early postmenopausal women and induced a 1% to 2% gain in BMD of the spine,

femoral neck, and total body in the European study (21) (Table 1). Both the treatment and placebo arms received 400 to 600 mg/day of supplemental calcium. Compared with the estrogen plus calcium responses shown in Fig. 1, the effects of raloxifene on BMD are modest. The effect of raloxifene on fracture incidence is not yet known.

Raloxifene, at 60 mg per day, lowered urinary type 1 collagen C-telopeptide, a marker of bone resorption, by about 25% and serum osteocalcin, a marker of bone formation, by about 20% (21). These reductions are smaller than those observed with HRT and alendronate. Residual effects of raloxifene are presently unknown.

In summary, raloxifene is well tolerated but has weaker effects on BMD and bone turnover than do HRT and alendronate. The role of raloxifene in the treatment of osteoporosis will ultimately depend on its effects on fracture rates, cardiovascular disease incidence, and breast cancer risk.

Salmon Calcitonin

Calcitonin is a synthetic peptide with antiresorptive properties. The drug, administered as a nasal spray, is well tolerated. The only established side effect is rhinitis (23% vs. 7% for placebo) (22). The drug also is available in the original form, as a subcutaneous injection. Calcitonin has an analgesic effect in some patients when injected daily but not when administered as a nasal spray.

Nasal calcitonin reduces bone loss from the spine in older postmenopausal women (22). The effect of calcitonin on hip BMD is more modest. Studies published to date have not been large enough to provide meaningful fracture data. Biochemical markers of bone turnover decline with calcitonin treatment by up to 40%. In summary, calcitonin is well tolerated and is a reasonable choice for women who cannot take approved drugs with established antifracture efficacy.

WHO SHOULD BE TREATED?

The most extensive evaluation of this issue to date was carried out by the National Osteoporosis Foundation. The NOF used a combination of evidence-based methods and expert clinical judgment to develop a reference document for clinical decision making (23). The recommendations

TABLE 1. *Mean percentage changes from baseline in bone mineral density in postmenopausal women given raloxifene (60 mg/day) or placebo for 2 years*

Site	Placebo	Raloxifene[a]
Lumbar spine	−0.8 ± 0.3	1.6 ± 0.3
Hip	−0.8 ± 0.3	1.6 ± 0.2
Femoral neck	−1.3 ± 0.3	1.2 ± 0.3
Total body	−0.6 ± 0.2	1.4 ± 0.2

Values expressed as mean ± SEM.
[a] All values are significantly different from those for placebo ($p < 0.03$). From Delmas PD, Bjarnason NH, Mitlak BH, et al. Effects of raloxifene on bone mineral density, serum cholesterol concentrations, and uterine endometrium in postmenopausal women. *N Engl J Med* 1997;337:1641–1647, with permission.

pertain to healthy postmenopausal white women, the population in whom the effects of treatment have been evaluated. They do not directly apply to men or to patients with secondary causes of osteoporosis.

The NOF analysis evaluated the effectiveness and cost of several treatments to prevent fractures over a 5-year horizon, a period selected to align with available evidence from randomized controlled trials. The treatments analyzed included HRT, alendronate, calcitonin, calcium, and vitamin D, and the results are summarized in Table 2. The risk factors considered in the analysis included smoking, thinness, a fracture after age 40 years, and osteoporosis in a first-degree relative. It would be reasonable to consider additional risk factors including lifelong low calcium intake, limited physical activity, alcoholism, recurrent falls, and frailty. The BMD thresholds for treatment derived from this analysis are expressed as T scores. A T score is defined as the number of standard deviations between an individual's BMD and the mean BMD of the young, same-sex white reference population. For example, a woman with a T score of -1 has BMD that is 1 standard deviation, or about 10% to 12%, below the mean value of the young female white reference population. Hip BMD values were used in the NOF analysis, but a T score from other skeletal sites may be used to identify the treatment threshold.

Because of the broad-based health benefits it provides, HRT should be offered to all eligible women at menopause. Calcium and vitamin D were found to be cost-effective and are generally recommended. Postmenopausal women up to age 65 years, and not on HRT, should have bone-density testing if they have one or more risk factors for osteoporosis and should be treated if their T score is -1.5 or less. The T-score thresholds presented in the table were based on the effectiveness and cost of HRT. Although the T scores needed to warrant treatment with alendronate and calcitonin were lower, it seems appropriate that if a woman meets the BMD criteria for treatment with HRT and cannot take or tolerate it, then she should be considered a candidate for treatment with the next most cost-effective alternative, currently alendronate (followed by calcitonin). As indicated in Table 2,

the NOF analysis calls for universal BMD screening of women age 65 and older. As with the younger postmenopausal women, their treatment threshold is dependent on the presence or absence of risk factors. All postmenopausal women who have had a vertebral or hip fracture are at high risk for subsequent fractures and should be treated. Raloxifene was not included in the analysis because fracture data were not available. It and other new drugs may be evaluated in this model in the future. Moreover, new evidence and/or price changes on currently approved treatments would be likely to change their treatment thresholds.

MANAGEMENT OF PATIENTS DURING TREATMENT

Evaluating Response

The optimal measure of response to treatment is change in fracture rate, but this is difficult to assess in individual patients. Currently the most common method of tracking treatment response is serial bone-mass measurements. The minimal change that can be detected is intimately related to the *in vivo* reproducibility of the measurements. Spine dual-energy x-ray absorptiometry (DXA) scans have a coefficient of variation (CV) of about 1%. From Table 3, it is apparent that a woman would have to lose at least 2.8% of her BMD for her physician to have confidence (at the 95% level) that she had in fact lost bone. But clinical decisions must often be based on less certain evidence and a confidence level of 80% seems reasonable. In that case, the minimal detectable difference in two spine scans would be 1.8% (Table 3). Untreated women lose BMD at an average rate of 3% per year in the first few years after menopause and at a rate of about 1% per year thereafter. In general, serial DXA scans of the spine and hip to monitor response to treatment should be performed at intervals of no less than about 2 years. Exceptions would be situations in which accelerated bone loss is expected, such as in patients taking glucocorticoids. Peripheral scanning devices often have CVs in the range of 2% to 3%. These instruments are useful in identifying patients with low T scores but are less useful for monitoring therapy because large changes must occur before they can be detected (Table 3).

Biochemical markers of bone turnover are valuable research tools, and their usefulness in monitoring response to treatment in individuals is currently being evaluated (see

---

TABLE 2. *Postmenopausal women: who should be treated?[a]*

- At menopause, all eligible women should be offered HRT
- All women should consume adequate calcium (1200 mg/day) and vitamin D (400–800 IU/day)
- Up to age 65 and not receiving HRT
    If one risk factor, measure bone density
    If T score is -1.5 or less, treat
- Age 65+, and not receiving HRT
    Assess risk factors and measure bone density
    If no risk factor and T score is -2.0 or less, treat
    If risk factor(s) and T score is -1.5 or less, treat
- All women with vertebral or hip fracture, treat

HRT, hormone-replacement therapy
[a] Derived from the National Osteoporosis Foundation evidence-based analysis, Eddy DM, Johnston CC Jr., for the Development Committee. Status report, Osteoporosis: review of the evidence for prevention, diagnosis, and treatment and cost-effectiveness analysis. *Osteoporosis Int* 1998;8:S1–S88.

TABLE 3. *Impact of measurement variability on ability to detect change over time in individuals*

Within-subject coefficient of variation (%CV)	Percentage difference that would have to be observed to reject the hypothesis of no change at two significance levels	
	$p < 0.05$	$p < 0.20$
1	2.38	1.81
3	8.32	5.43
20	55.4	36.2

Chapter 22). There is clearly a need to assess the efficacy of treatment in individual patients sooner than the 2-year interval required for serial DXA scans. As with DXA scans, the usefulness of markers is linked to their *in vivo* reproducibility or biologic variability. CVs of around 20% are commonly observed over intervals of 6 to 9 months (24,25), and larger CVs are observed over longer intervals. In general, variability is greater in urine than in serum markers of turnover. With a CV of 20%, the minimal detectable changes, with confidence levels of 80% and 95%, are 36% and 55%, respectively (Table 3). A recent report discussed factors that influence the ability of currently available markers to detect treatment responses of individual patients (24). At this time, the role of biochemical markers in patient monitoring is not clearly defined.

Patient Management

Single-drug treatment together with adequate nutrition and exercise will stabilize bone mass in most patients. Unfortunately, there will be patients in whom the initial treatment does not stabilize BMD or lower the fracture rate. In these patients, it may be necessary to use a different drug or empirically to add a second drug. Evidence for the efficacy of combined drug therapy, however, is not available at this time. Reevaluation for secondary causes should also be considered in unresponsive patients.

REFERENCES

1. Riggs BL, Melton LJ III, O'Fallon WM. Drug therapy for vertebral fractures in osteoporosis: evidence that decreases in bone turnover and increases in bone mass both determine antifracture efficacy. *Bone* 1996;18:197S–301S.
2. Grodstein F, Stampfer MJ, Manson JE, et al. Postmenopausal estrogen and progestin use and the risk of cardiovascular disease. *N Engl J Med* 1996;335:453–461.
3. Tang MX, Jacobs D, Stern Y, et al. Effect of oestrogen during menopause on risk and age at onset of Alzheimer's disease. *Lancet* 1996;348:429–432.
4. Colditz GA, Hankinson SE, Hunter DJ, et al. The use of estrogens and progestins and the risk of breast cancer in postmenopausal women. *N Engl J Med* 1995;332:1589–1593.
5. Beresford SAA, Weiss NS, Voigt LF, McKnight B. Risk of endometrial cancer in relation to use of oestrogen combined with cyclic progestagen therapy in postmenopausal women. *Lancet* 1997;349:458–461.
6. Jick H, Derby LE, Myers MW, Vasilakis C, Newton KM. Risk of hospital admission for idiopathic venous thromboembolism among users of postmenopausal oestrogens. *Lancet* 1996;348:981–983.
7. Lindsay R, Hart DM, Forrest C, Baird C. Prevention of spinal osteoporosis in oophorectomised women. *Lancet* 1980;2:1151–1154.
8. Nachtigall LE, Nachtigall RH, Nachtigall RD, Beckman EM. Estrogen replacement therapy I: a 10-year prospective study in the relationship to osteoporosis. *J Am Coll Obstet Gynecol* 1979;53:277–281.
9. Lufkin EG, Wahner HW, O'Fallon WM, et al. Treatment of postmenopausal osteoporosis with transdermal estrogen. *Ann Intern Med* 1992;117:1–9.
10. Cauley JA, Seeley DG, Ensrud K, Ettinger B, Black D, Cummings SR. Estrogen replacement therapy and fractures in older women: study of Osteoporosis Research Group. *Ann Intern Med* 1995;122:9–16.
11. Nieves JW, Komar L, Cosman F, Lindsay R. Calcium potentiates the effects of estrogen and calcitonin on bone mass: review and analysis. *Am J Clin Nutr* 1998;67:18–24.
12. Chesnut CH III, Bell NH, Clark GS, et al. Hormone replacement therapy in postmenopausal women: urinary *N*-telopeptide of type I collagen monitors therapeutic effect and predicts response of bone mineral density. *Am J Med* 1997;102:29–37.
13. Christiansen C, Christensen MS, Transbol I. Bone mass in postmenopausal women after withdrawal of oestrogen/gestagen replacement therapy. *Lancet* 1981;2:459–461.
14. de Groen PC, Lubbe DF, Hirsch LJ, et al. Esophagitis associated with the use of alendronate. *N Engl J Med* 1996;335:1016–1021.
15. Black DM, Cummings SR, Karpf DB, et al. Randomized trial of effect of alendronate on risk of fracture in women with existing vertebral fractures: Fracture Intervention Trial research group. *Lancet* 1996;348:1535–1541.
16. Liberman UA, Weiss SR, Broll J, et al. Effect of oral alendronate on bone mineral density and the incidence of fractures in postmenopausal osteoporosis. *N Engl J Med* 1995;333:1437–1443.
17. Hosking D, Chilvers CED, Christiansen C, et al. Prevention of bone loss with alendronate in postmenopausal women under 60 years of age. *N Engl J Med* 1998;338:485–492.
18. McClung M, Clemmesen B, Daifotis A, et al. Alendronate prevents postmenopausal bone loss in women without osteoporosis. *Ann Intern Med* 1998;128:253–261.
19. Chesnut CH III, McClung MR, Ensrud KE, et al. Alendronate treatment of the postmenopausal osteoporotic woman: effect of multiple dosages on bone mass and bone remodeling. *Am J Med* 1995;99:144–152.
20. Stock JL, Bell NH, Chesnut CH III, et al. Increments in bone mineral density of the lumbar spine and hip and suppression of bone turnover are maintained after discontinuation of alendronate in postmenopausal women. *Am J Med* 1997;103:291–297.
21. Delmas PD, Bjarnason NH, Mitlak BH, et al. Effects of raloxifene on bone mineral density, serum cholesterol concentrations, and uterine endometrium in postmenopausal women. *N Engl J Med* 1997;337:1641–1647.
22. Ellerington MC, Hillard TC, Whitcroft SIJ, et al. Intranasal salmon calcitonin for the prevention and treatment of postmenopausal osteoporosis. *Calcif Tissue Int* 1996;59:6–11.
23. National Osteoporosis Foundation. Osteoporosis: review of the evidence for the prevention, diagnosis, and treatment: and cost-effectiveness analysis. *Osteoporos Int* 1998;8:1–88.
24. Hannon R, Blumsohn A, Naylor K, Eastell R. Response of biochemical markers of bone turnover to hormone replacement therapy: impact of biological variability. *J Bone Miner Res* 1998;13:1124–1133.
25. Gertz BJ, Shao P, Hanson DA, et al. Monitoring bone resorption in early postmenopausal women by an immunoassay for cross-linked collagen peptides in urine. *J Bone Miner Res* 1994;9:135–142.

may provide an alternative therapy for transplantation osteoporosis.

CONCLUSIONS

Candidates for all types of transplantation have risk factors for osteoporosis and many have low BMD, fractures, or abnormal mineral metabolism. With the exception of cholestatic liver disease, biochemical markers of bone turnover are elevated before transplantation. After transplantation, there is exposure to high doses of GC, CsA, and tacrolimus, all of which may have deleterious effects on the skeleton. The majority of patients experience rapid bone loss, and fragility fractures also are common, particularly during the first posttransplant year. Early posttransplantation bone loss is associated with biochemical evidence of uncoupled bone turnover, with increases in markers of resorption, and with decreases in markers of formation. Most of the evidence favors the notion that, after the first 6 months, transplantation-related bone loss is a form of high-turnover osteoporosis. Because significant bone disease frequently antedates transplantation, all patients awaiting transplantation should have a BMD determination, spine radiographs, and pertinent biochemistries. Those with osteoporosis and abnormal mineral metabolism can be identified and treated, and any potentially reversible causes of bone loss can be corrected. Because no pretransplant parameter reliably predicts fracture in the individual patient, most patients should be given appropriate pharmacologic therapy immediately after transplantation to prevent bone loss and fractures. Although few data are available from randomized, controlled clinical trials, both bisphosphonates and calcitriol show promise in the prevention of transplantation osteoporosis.

ACKNOWLEDGMENT

This work was supported in part by grants AR-41391 and RR-006645 from the National Institutes of Health.

REFERENCES

1. United Network of Organ Sharing (UNOS), Richmond, VA, and the Division of Transplantation, Office of Special Programs, Health Resources and Services Administration, U.S. Department of Health and Human Services, Rockville, MD. *1997 Annual report of the U.S. scientific registry for transplant recipients and the organ procurement and transplantation network—transplant data: 1988–1996.* 1997 OPTN/SR AR 1988–1996. UNOS; DOT/HRSA/DHHS.
2. Rodino MA, Shane E. Osteoporosis after organ transplantation. *Am J Med* 1998;104:459–469.
3. Epstein S. Post-transplantation bone disease: the role of immunosuppressive agents on the skeleton. *J Bone Miner Res* 1996;11:1–7.
4. Stein MS, Packham DK, Ebeling PR, Wark JD, Becker GJ. Prevalence and risk factors for osteopoenia in dialysis patients. *Am J Kidney Dis* 1996;28:515–522.
5. Addesso V, Elmer D, Gaber AO, Shane E. Bone mass in patients with type I diabetes mellitus awaiting simultaneous pancreas-kidney transplantation. *Bone* 1998;23:5(Suppl):588.
6. Pichette V, Bonnardeaux A, Prudhomme L, Gagne M, Cardinal J, Ouimet D. Long-term bone loss in kidney transplant recipients: a cross-sectional and longitudinal study. *Am J Kidney Dis* 1996;28:105–114.
7. Nisbeth U, Lindh E, Ljunghall S, Backman U, Fellstrom B. Fracture frequency after kidney transplantation. *Transplant Proc* 1994;26:1764.
8. Moreira Kulak C, Shane E. Bone turnover in transplantation osteoporosis. In: Seibel MJ, Robins SP, Bilezikian JP, eds. *Dynamics of bone*

and cartilage metabolism: principles and clinical applications San Diego: Academic Press, 1999 (in press).

9. Rambausek M, Ritz E, Pomer S, Mohring K, Rohl L. Alkaline phosphatase levels in renal transplant recipients receiving cyclosporine or azathioprine/steroids. *Lancet* 1988;1:247.
10. Aubia J, Masramon J, Serrano S, Lloveras J, Marinoso LL. Bone histology in renal transplant patients receiving cyclosporin. *Lancet* 1988;1:1048.
11. Wilmink JM, Bras J, Surachno S, Heyst JLAM, Horst JM. Bone repair in cyclosporin-treated renal transplant patients. *Transplant Proc* 1989;21:1492–1494.
12. Shane E, Mancini D, Aaronson K, et al. Bone mass, vitamin D deficiency, and hyperparathyroidism in congestive heart failure. *Am J Med* 1997;103:197–207.
13. Sambrook PN, Kelly PJ, Keogh A, et al. Bone loss after cardiac transplantation: a prospective study. *J Heart Lung Transplant* 1994;13:116–121.
14. Shane E, Rivas M, McMahon DJ, et al. Bone loss and turnover after cardiac transplantation. *J Clin Endocrinol Metab* 1997;82:1497–1506.
15. Shane E, Rivas M, Staron RB, et al. Fracture after cardiac transplantation: a prospective longitudinal study. *J Clin Endocrinol Metab* 1996;81:1740–1746.
16. Leidig-Bruckner G, Eberwein S, Czeczatka D, et al. Incidence of osteoporosis fractures after liver and heart transplantation. *J Bone Miner Res* 1997;12(suppl 1):S145.
17. Monegal A, Navasa M, Guanabens N, et al. Osteoporosis and bone mineral metabolism in cirrhotic patients referred for liver transplantation. *Calcif Tissue Int* 1997;60:148–154.
18. Guanabens N, Pares A, Alvarez L, et al. Collagen-related markers of bone turnover reflect the severity of liver fibrosis in patients with primary biliary cirrhosis. *J Bone Miner Res* 1998;13:731–738.
19. Donovan DS, Papadopoulos A, Staron RB, et al. Bone mass and vitamin d deficiency in adults with advanced cystic fibrosis lung disease. *Am J Respir Crit Care Med* 1998;157:1892–1899.
20. Aris RM, Neuringer IP, Weiner MA, Egan TM, Ontjes D. Severe osteoporosis before and after lung transplantation. *Chest* 1996;109:1176–1183.
21. Shane E, Silverberg SJ, Donovan D, et al. Osteoporosis in lung transplantation candidates with end-stage pulmonary disease. *Am J Med* 1996;101:262–269.
22. Ferrari SL, Nicod LP, Hamacher J, et al. Osteoporosis in patients undergoing lung transplantation. *Eur Respir J* 1996;9:2378–2382.
23. Stern JM, Chesnut CH III, Bruemmer B, et al. Bone density loss during treatment of chronic GVHD. *Bone Marrow Transplant* 1996;17:395–400.
24. Adachi JD, Bensen WG, Brown J, et al. Intermittent etidronate therapy to prevent corticosteroid-induced osteoporosis. *N Engl J Med* 1997;337:382–387.
25. Saag KG, Emkey R, Schnitzer TJ, et al. Alendronate for the prevention and treatment of glucocorticoid-induced osteoporosis. *N Engl J Med* 1998;339:292–299.
26. Fan S, Almond MK, Ball E, Evans K, Cunningham J. Randomized prospective study demonstrating prevention of bone loss by pamidronate during the first year after renal transplantation [Abstract]. *J Am Soc Nephrol* 1996;7:A2714.
27. Shane E, Rodino M, McMahon DJ, et al. Prevention of bone loss after cardiac transplantation with antiresorptive therapy: a pilot study. *J Heart Lung Transplant* 1998;17:1089–1096.
28. Riemens SC, Oostdijk A, van Doormaal J, et al. Bone loss after liver transplantation is not prevented by cyclical etidronate, calcium and alpha calcidiol. *Osteoporos Int* 1996;6:213–218.
29. Valero MA, Loinaz C, Larrodera L, Leon M, Moreno E, Hawkins F. Calcitonin and bisphosphonate treatment and bone loss after liver transplantation. *Calcif Tissue Int* 1995;57:15–19.
30. Sambrook P, Birmingham J, Kelly P, et al. Prevention of corticosteroid osteoporosis: a comparison of calcium, calcitriol and calcitonin. *N Engl J Med* 1993;328:1747–1752.
31. Sambrook P, Marshall G, Henderson K, et al. Effect of calcitriol in the prevention of bone loss after cardiac or lung transplantation. *J Bone Miner Res* 1997;12(suppl 1):S400.
32. Henderson NK, Marshall G, Sambrook PN, Keogh A, Eisman JA. Prevention of bone loss after heart of lung transplantation. *J Bone Miner Res* 1997;12(suppl 1):S400.
33. Meunier PJ, Brancon D, Chavassieux P, et al. Treatment with fluoride. In: Johansen JS, Christiansen C, Riis BJ, eds. *Osteoporosis.* Copenhagen: Osteopress, 1987:824–828.

57.   Juvenile Osteoporosis

Michael E. Norman, M.D.

Department of Pediatrics, University of North Carolina, Chapel Hill and Carolinas Medical Center,
Charlotte, North Carolina

The diagnosis of osteoporosis in children is usually made when skeletal radiographs reveal a generalized decrease in mineralized bone (e.g., osteopenia) in the absence of rickets or excessive bone resorption (e.g., osteitis fibrosa). Juvenile osteoporosis occurs typically before the onset of puberty, but it also may be seen in younger children, especially when they are growing rapidly. It may be due to an inherited condition that is clinically evident from birth or early infancy, or it may be acquired during childhood. There are a primary or idiopathic form and a number of secondary forms of juvenile osteoporosis. The condition is uncommon; between 1939 and 1991, ~60 cases of idiopathic juvenile osteoporosis (IJO) were reported in the literature. However, the onset of osteoporosis just before or after the onset of puberty can have far-reaching effects, because one half of skeletal mass is acquired during the adolescent years.

PATHOPHYSIOLOGY

True osteoporosis is defined histomorphometrically by a decreased total amount of normally formed bone. During bone formation (modeling) and bone remodeling, two fundamental defects may occur, singly or in combination: (a) a defect in bone-forming cells leading to decreased or defective matrix formation; and (b) abnormalities in the coupling of bone formation and resorption, in which an imbalance develops between matrix formation (mineralization) and bone resorption. An inherited group of disorders known as osteogenesis imperfecta usually represents defects in bone-forming cells, in which mutations in one of the two genes encoding type I procollagen produce defective matrix (see Chapter 72). IJO and the secondary causes of osteoporosis represent various expressions of the latter type of defect. IJO and chronic corticosteroid therapy are the most important forms of acquired juvenile osteoporosis. Early reports of calcium balance suggested that IJO changes, with initially negative or inappropriately neutral balances (1,2), progressing to positive balance during the healing phase (2,3) and in response to vitamin D administration. Preexisting calcium deficiency for any reason, but particularly in adolescence and in pregnancy may lead to especially severe forms of IJO (4). Jowsey and Johnson (5) and Hoekman et al. (6) presented histologic evidence of increased bone resorption, whereas Smith (7) and Reed et al. (8) found decreased bone formation as the major pathophysiologic event in IJO. Evans et al. (9) and Marder et al. (10) suggested a role for 1,25-dihydroxyvitamin D [1,25 (OH)$_2$ D] deficiency in the pathogenesis of IJO. Several reports also suggested a role for calcitonin deficiency in some patients (11,12). The bone loss noted in astronauts undergoing prolonged periods of weightlessness in space may be analogous to IJO, with rapid resorption of weight-bearing bones and suppressed bone formation. Both weightlessness and IJO appear to be reversible (7). Some have speculated that IJO, like weightlessness, consists of some fundamental disturbance in the mechanical forces that stimulate new bone formation in the growing and young adult skeleton. Finally, recent data in adult osteoporotic patients suggest impaired bone formation related in part to reduced insulin-like growth factor I secretion (8).

CLINICAL FEATURES

The typical child with IJO is immediately prepubertal and healthy. A recent series of 21 children with IJO indicated a mean age at onset of 7 years with a range of 1 to 13 years and no gender differences (13). Symptoms begin with an insidious onset of pain in the lower back, hips, and feet, and difficulty walking. Knee and ankle pain and fractures of the lower extremities may be present. IJO affects both sexes equally; family and dietary histories are negative. Physical examination may be entirely normal or may reveal thoracolumbar kyphosis or kyphoscoliosis, pigeon-chest deformity, crown/pubis to pubis/heel ratio of less than 1.0, loss of height, deformities of the long bones, and limp. Generally, these physical abnormalities are reversible, and spontaneous recovery is noted in most patients (12), although several of the original patients subsequently developed crippling deformities that left them wheelchair bound with cardio-respiratory abnormalities (1). The history and physical examination of children with secondary forms of osteoporosis reflect the primary disease more than the osteoporosis (Table 1). There is usually a family history of osteoporosis or of the primary disease, evidence of failure to thrive, immobilization, or administration of corticosteroid or anticonvulsant drugs.

BIOCHEMICAL FEATURES

No known biochemical abnormalities are characteristic of IJO, and no known endocrine disorder has been identified. In some children (1,2,6), calcium balance is markedly negative or inappropriately neutral, and serum calcium levels are normal. Urine calcium excretion may be normal or elevated. Serum phosphorus, bicarbonate, magnesium, and alkaline phosphatase levels also are normal. The disease eventually resolves with time and the onset of puberty and can be detected by improvement in calcium balance. Increased urinary hydroxyproline excretion, an indirect indicator of increased bone resorption, as well as hypercalcemia and suppressed parathyroid hormone secretion have been observed in some patients. Suppression of parathyroid hormone secretion reduces 1,25 (OH)$_2$ D synthesis and decreases intestinal calcium absorption, contributing to the negative calcium balance (6). In secondary forms of osteoporosis, biochemical

TABLE 1. *Differential diagnosis of juvenile osteoporosis*

I. Primary
    Calcium deficiency
    Idiopathic juvenile osteoporosis
    Osteogenesis imperfecta
        Multiple subtypes
II. Secondary
    Endocrine
        Cushing syndrome
        Diabetes mellitus
        Glucocorticoid therapy
        Thyrotoxicosis
    Gastrointestinal
        Biliary atresia
        Glycogen storage disease, type I
        Hepatitis
        Malabsorption
    Inborn errors of metabolism
        Homocystinuria
        Lysinuric protein intolerance
    Miscellaneous
        Acute lymphoblastic leukemia
        Anticonvulsant therapy
        Cyanotic congenital heart disease
        Immobilization

and clinical clues to diagnosis depend on the underlying primary disease (2,9).

RADIOLOGIC FEATURES

Conventional radiography is a relatively insensitive method for detecting bone loss; ~30% of skeletal mineral must be lost before osteopenia can be appreciated. In the absence of fractures or rickets, osteomalacia may be difficult to distinguish from osteoporosis as the cause of osteopenia. Looser lines or changes of secondary hyperparathyroidism favor rickets or osteomalacia, whereas biconcave vertebral deformities favor osteoporosis (see Chapter 26). Children with fully expressed IJO present with generalized osteopenia, fractures of the weight-bearing bones, and collapsed or misshapen vertebrae. Disc spaces may be widened asymmetrically because of wedging of the vertebral bodies (Fig. 1). Sclerosis may be noted. Long bones are usually normal in length and cortical width, unlike the thin, gracile bones of children with osteogenesis imperfecta (see Chapter 72). The pathognomonic radiographic finding of IJO is neoosseous osteoporosis, an impaction-type fracture occurring at sites of newly formed weight-bearing metaphyseal bone. Typically such fractures are seen at the distal tibiae, adjacent to the ankle joint and adjacent to the knee and hip joints (2,7). By using photon absorptiometry and computed tomography for detection of decreased bone mineral density, childhood osteoporosis may be diagnosed much earlier.

BONE BIOPSY

Few qualitative or quantitative studies of bone tissue have been performed in childhood osteoporosis. From micro-radiographs of bone, Cloutier et al. (3) and Jowsey and Johnson (5) reported increased bone resorption in IJO. They speculated that excessive dietary phosphorus intake may have stimulated parathyroid-mediated bone resorption. In contrast, Smith (7), by using quantitative static histology of iliac bone, found indirect evidence of decreased bone formation. Evans et al. (9) found no abnormalities of endosteal bone formation by histomorphometry (by using double tetracycline labeling) in a 12-year-old boy with severe IJO. They suggested that the major evidence for impaired periosteal new bone formation in IJO would come from careful study of skeletal radiographs and not from bone-biopsy material.

DIFFERENTIAL DIAGNOSIS

Osteogenesis imperfecta is the most important entity to consider in the differential diagnosis of IJO (14). Comparisons with IJO are listed in Table 2 (see Chapter 72). Osteogenesis imperfecta can usually be differentiated from IJO by clinical characteristics, radiologic findings, and a positive family history. Diseases resulting in osteoporosis in childhood that must be differentiated from IJO are outlined in Table 1. Secondary causes of osteoporosis must be excluded in those children without the typical features of IJO. As a result, the diagnosis of IJO is reached by excluding secondary causes of osteoporosis and osteogenesis imperfecta.

THERAPY

Prompt and definitive diagnosis early in the course of the disease is important, although there is no specific medical or surgical therapy. Supportive care is instituted promptly (non–weight-bearing, crutch walking, and physical therapy) in anticipation of spontaneous recovery with the onset of puberty. There may be a role for supplemental calcitriol therapy in selected patients (9,10). Sodium fluoride increases bone mass and has been reported to reduce fracture rates in primary vertebral osteoporosis (15). Fluoride treatment has been associated with a number of toxicity symptoms and musculoskeletal complaints in adults, and it remains unclear whether the hyperosteoidosis associated with this therapy produces increased bone strength. I have used long-term fluoride therapy with a positive clinical response in one patient with IJO. Based on findings of decreased bone resorption on bone biopsy in one child, Hoekman et al. (6) reported dramatic clinical, biochemical, and radiologic responses with bisphosphonate, which inhibits bone resorption. Osteoporosis in most patients is reversible. Treatment of secondary causes of osteoporosis requires careful management of the underlying disease to minimize bone loss.

PROGNOSIS

With the exception of a few patients who develop progressive lower-extremity, spine, and chest-wall deformities and require confinement to wheelchairs or bed, the prognosis of IJO is generally excellent. Distinguishing features have been

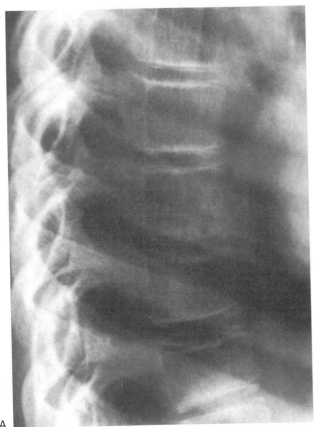
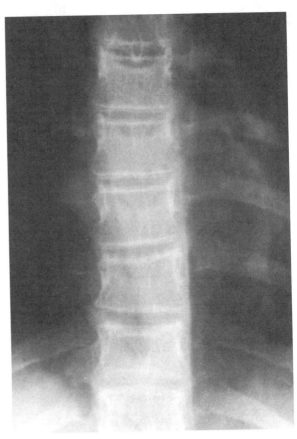

A

B

FIG. 1. A 10-year-old white girl with back pain. **A:** Lateral view of thoracolumbar spine reveals wedge compression fracture of T8 and T9 with patchy sclerosis of T7. There was generalized osteopenia of the skeleton, confirmed by computed tomography. **B:** Anterior view of the same patient reveals loss of height of T8 on the right side. The vertebral bodies are osteopenic.

recognized that identify the subgroup of children with poor prognosis. The prognosis of osteogenesis imperfecta is dependent on the inherited subtype and is discussed in Chapter 72. The most effective treatment of secondary osteoporosis is successful therapy of the underlying disease. Failing this, supportive care should be provided as with IJO.

REFERENCES

1. Dent CE, Friedman M. Idiopathic juvenile osteoporosis. *Q J Med* 1965;34:177–210.
2. Brenton DP, Dent CE. Idiopathic juvenile osteoporosis. In: Bickel JH, Stern J, eds. *Inborn errors of calcium and bone metabolism.* Baltimore: University Park Press, 1976:223–238.

TABLE 2. *Differential diagnosis: osteogenesis imperfecta (OI) vs. idiopathic juvenile osteoporosis (IJO)*

Characteristic	OI	IJO
Family history	Often positive	Negative
Age at onset	Birth	2–3 yr before puberty
Duration of signs/symptoms	Lifelong (intermittent)	1–4 yr
Physical findings	Thin gracile bones, short stature	Upper-lower segment ratio <1.0
	Multiple deformities and contractures	Dorsal kyphoscoliosis
	Blue sclerae[a], deafness	Pectus carinatum
	Lax joints, hernias	Abnormal gait
	Abnormal dentition	
Calcium balance	Positive	Negative in acute phase
Radiologic findings	Narrow long bones	Long bones with thin cortices
	Thin ribs	Wedge compression fractures of spine
	Pathologic fractures, rarely metaphyseal in location	Metaphyseal fractures common
	Wormian skull bones	
Molecular studies (dermal fibroblasts)	Abnormal collagen	Normal collagen

[a] Classic dominant inherited form, with associated nerve deafness.

3. Cloutier MD, Hayles AB, Riggs BL, Jowsey J, Bickel WH. Juvenile osteoporosis: report of a case including a description of some metabolic and microradiographic studies. *Pediatrics* 1967;40:649–655.
4. Koo WW, Chesney RW, Mitchell N. Case report: effect of pregnancy on idiopathic juvenile osteoporosis. *Am J Med Sci* 1995;309:223–225.
5. Jowsey J, Johnson KA. Juvenile osteoporosis: bone findings in seven patients. *J Pediatr* 1972;81:511–517.
6. Hoekman K, Papapoulos SE, Peters ACB, Bijvoet OL. Characteristics and bisphosphonate treatment of a patient with juvenile osteoporosis. *J Clin Endocrinol Metab* 1985;61:952–956.
7. Smith R. Idiopathic osteoporosis in the young. *J Bone Joint Surg Br* 1980;62:417–427.
8. Reed BY, Zeswekh JE, Sakhaee K, Breslau N, Gottschalk F, Pak CYC. Serum IGF-I is low and correlated with osteoblastic surface in idiopathic osteoporosis. *J Bone Miner Res* 1995;10:1218–1224.
9. Evans RA, Dunstan CR, Hills E. Bone metabolism in idiopathic juvenile osteoporosis: a case report. *Calcif Tissue Int* 1983;35:58.
10. Marder HK, Tsang RC, Hug G, Crawford AC. Calcitriol deficiency in idiopathic juvenile osteoporosis. *Am J Dis Child* 1982;136:914–917.
11. Saggese G, Bertelloni S, Baroncelli GI, Perri G, Calderazzi A. Mineral metabolism and calcitriol therapy in idiopathic juvenile osteoporosis. *Am J Dis Child* 1991;145:457–461.
12. Jackson EC, Strife CF, Tsang RC, Marder HK. Effect of calcitonin replacement therapy in idiopathic juvenile osteoporosis. *Am J Dis Child* 1988;142:1237–1239.
13. Smith R. Idiopathic juvenile osteoporosis: experience of twenty-one patients. *Br J Rheum* 1995;34:68–77.
14. Teotia M, Teotia SPS, Singh RK. Idiopathic juvenile osteoporosis. *Am J Dis Child* 1979;133:894–900.
15. Harrison JE. Fluoride treatment for osteoporosis. *Calcif Tissue Int* 1990;46:287–288.

58. Secondary Causes of Osteoporosis: Thyrotoxicosis and Lack of Weight Bearing

Daniel T. Baran, M.D.

Departments of Orthopedics and Medicine, University of Massachusetts Medical School, Worcester, Massachusetts

THYROTOXICOSIS

Thyroid hormone increases bone remodeling (1). Although both osteoblast and osteoclast activities are increased by elevated levels of thyroid hormone, osteoclast activity predominates, with a resultant loss of bone mass. It appears that thyroid hormones stimulate osteoclastic bone resorption by an indirect effect mediated by osteoblasts. The presence of osteoblasts is required for thyroid hormones to increase bone resorption (2,3).

Thyroid hormone directly stimulates osteoblast production of alkaline phosphatase (4), osteocalcin (5), and insulin-like growth factor (6). Thyrotoxicosis is associated with increased serum levels of osteocalcin (7) and alkaline phosphatase (8). Despite increased osteoblastic activity, the enhanced bone formation cannot compensate for thyroid hormone–induced increments in bone resorption. The increased bone resorption is detected by increased urinary levels of hydroxyproline and collagen cross-links in thyrotoxic patients (1,9,10). The levels of these biochemical markers of bone turnover appear to correlate with circulating levels of thyroid hormone.

In thyrotoxicosis, the surface area of unmineralized matrix (osteoid) is increased. In contrast to osteomalacia, mineralization rates are increased. The increased bone turnover in the presence of excessive levels of thyroid hormone is characterized by an increase in the number of osteoclasts, the number of resorption sites, and the ratio of resorptive to formative surfaces. In contrast to the normal bone-remodeling cycle, which lasts about 200 days, in hyperthyroid patients, the cycle is shortened, primarily because of a decrease in the length of the formation period, with failure to replace resorbed bone completely (1) (Fig. 1). The histologic changes in cortical bone in hyperthyroidism are characterized by increased porosity (1). In hyperthyroidism, there are also changes in the gene-expression markers in cortical bone.

In summary, thyroid hormone effects on osteoblasts and osteoclasts result in alterations in mineral metabolism and in the remodeling cycle, manifested by histologic and molecular changes in bone. These changes appear to be reflected in altered bone mineral density (BMD).

Bone mass is reduced in patients with thyrotoxicosis (11,12). The detrimental effects of thyroid hormone on the skeleton appear to occur more frequently in female patients. As a result of the decrease in bone density, individuals with a history of thyrotoxicosis have an increased risk of fracture (13) and sustain fractures at an earlier age than individuals who have never been thyrotoxic (14).

The decreased bone density noted in thyrotoxic patients is reversible after effective treatment. Normalization of the thyroid-function tests results in significant increases in axial and appendicular bone density compared with pretreatment values (11,12). If the detrimental skeletal effects of supraphysiologic levels of thyroid hormone were restricted to individuals with thyrotoxicosis, therapy would be expected to prevent any further skeletal damage and in fact restore at least a portion of the bone mass that was lost before effective treatment.

Administration of high doses of thyroid hormone to suppress thyroid-stimulating hormone (TSH) secretion in patients with differentiated thyroid carcinoma and nontoxic goiter is considered appropriate therapy for those conditions. In patients prone to osteoporosis, however, this therapy may aggravate fracture risk. TSH-suppressive doses of thyroid hormone have been reported to decrease or to have no effect on BMD in women. A meta-analysis of the reports in which BMD was assessed in women receiving TSH-suppressive doses of thyroxine concluded that treatment led to a 1% increase in annual bone loss in postmenopausal women (15). In contrast, thyroid hormone replacement therapy in the absence of TSH suppression does not appear to be associated with detrimental effects on BMD (16).

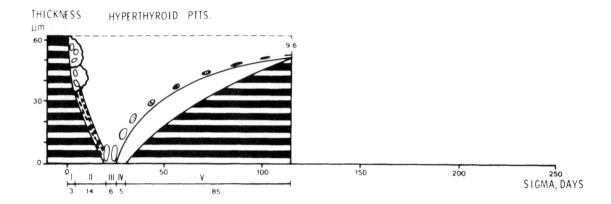

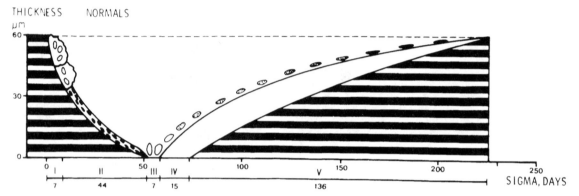

FIG. 1. Smoothed resorption and formation curves in hyperthyroid patients and their controls. The durations of the different resorption and formation periods are given below the curves. I, osteoclastic function period; II, mononuclear function period; III, preosteoblast-like cell function period; IV, initial mineralization lag time; V, mineralization period. For the hyperthyroid group, the negative balance between resorption depth and formation thickness is indicated ($-9.6\ \mu m$). (Reprinted from Eriksen EF, Mosekilde L, Melsen F. Trabecular bone remodeling and bone balance in hyperthyroidism. *Bone* 1985;6:421–428, with permission from Elsevier Science, Ltd., Kidlington, United Kingdom.)

LACK OF WEIGHT BEARING

Numerous studies documented the beneficial effects of weight-bearing forces on the skeleton. Increased physical activity is associated with increased bone mass in individuals of all ages (17). Conversely, lack of weight bearing whether due to paralysis (18), space flight (19), immobilization (20), or stress shielding adjacent to prosthetic implants (21) is associated with a decrease in bone mass. Immobilization of the upper extremity following surgery is attended by a decrease in BMD. Interestingly, while one extremity is immobilized, there is an increase in BMD in the contralateral extremity, perhaps the result of greater forces placed on the nonimmobilized extremity (22). The rapidity and extent of bone loss in the absence of normal weight-bearing forces is exemplified by stress shielding adjacent to femoral prostheses and the natural history of bone loss following paralysis. Within 2 months of surgery, there is a 12% decrease in BMD adjacent to the prosthesis, and by 24 months, there is a 25.5% decrease (21). Similarly, much of the decrease in bone mass following paralysis occurs within the first year (23). These observational studies indicate the importance of limiting inactivity and immobilization when possible. The

potential utility of inhibitors of bone resorption in the maintenance of BMD in the absence of normal mechanical forces has yet to be determined.

REFERENCES

1. Mosekilde L, Eriksen EF, Charles P. Effects of thyroid hormone on bone and mineral metabolism. *Endocrinol Metab Clin North Am* 1990;19:3563.
2. Allain TJ, Chambers TJ, Flanagan AM, McGregor AM. Tri-iodothyronine stimulates rat osteoclastic bone resorption by an indirect effect. *J Endocrinol* 1992;133:327–331.
3. Britto JM, Fenton AJ, Holloway WR, Nicholson GC. Osteoblasts mediate thyroid hormone stimulation of osteoclastic bone resorption. *Endocrinology* 1994;134:169–176.
4. Sato K, Han DC, Fujii Y, Tsushima T, Shizume K. Thyroid hormone stimulates alkaline phosphatase activity in cultured rat osteoblastic cells (ROS 17/2.8) through 3,5,3-triiodo-L-thyronine nuclear receptors. *Endocrinology* 197;120:1873–1881.
5. Rizzoli R, Poser J, Burgi U. Nuclear thyroid hormone receptors in cultured bone cells. *Metabolism* 1986;35:71–74.
6. Milne M, Kang M-I, Quail, JM, Baran DT. Thyroid hormone excess increases insulin-like growth factor I transcripts in bone marrow cell cultures: divergent effects on vertebral and femoral cell cultures. *Endocrinology* 1998;139:2527–2534.
7. Garrel DR, Delmas PD, Malaval L, Tourniaire J. Serum bone Gla

protein: a marker of bone turnover in hyperthyroidism. *Clin Endocrinol Metab* 1986;62:1052–1055.

8. Cooper DS, Kaplan MM, Ridgway EC, Maloof F, Daniels GH. Alkaline phosphatase isoenzyme patterns in hyperthyroidism. *Ann Intern Med* 1979;90:164–168.

9. Harvey RD, McHardy KC, Reid IW, et al. Measurement of bone collagen degradation in hyperthyroidism and during thyroxine replacement therapy using pyridinium cross-links as specific urinary markers. *J Clin Endocrinol Metab* 1991;72:1189–1194.

10. Krakerauer JC, Kleerekoper M. Borderline low serum thyrotropin level is correlated with increased fasting urinary hydroxyproline excretion. *Arch Intern Med* 1992;152:360–364.

11. Rosen CJ, Alder RA. Longitudinal changes in lumbar bone density among thyrotoxic patients after attainment of euthyroidism. *J Clin Endocrinol Metab* 1992;75:1531–1534.

12. Diamond T, Vine J, Smart R, Butler P. Thyrotoxic bone disease in women: a potentially reversible disorder. *Ann Intern Med* 1994; 120:811.

13. Cummings SR, Nevitt MC, Browner WS, et al. Risk factors for hip fracture in white women: study of osteoporotic fractures research group. *N Engl J Med* 1995;332:767–773.

14. Solomon BL, Wartofsky L, Burman KD. Prevalence of fractures in postmenopausal women with thyroid disease. *Thyroid* 1993;3:1723.

15. Faber J, Galloe AM. Changes in bone mass during prolonged subclinical hyperthyroidism due to L-thyroxine treatment: a meta-analysis. *Eur J Endocrinol* 1994;130:350–356.

16. Duncan WE, Chung A, Solomon B, Wartofsky L. Influence of clinical characteristics and parameters associated with thyroid hormone therapy on the bone mineral density of women treated with thyroid hormone. *Thyroid* 1994;4:183–190.

17. Snow CM, Shaw JM, Matkin CC. Physical activity and risk for osteoporosis. In: Marcus R, Feldman D, Kelsey J, eds. *Osteoporosis.* San Diego: Academic Press, 1996:511–528.

18. Elias AN, Gwinup G. Immobilization osteoporosis in paraplegia. *J Am Paraplegia Soc* 1992;15:163–170.

19. Rambaut PC, Goode AW. Skeletal changes during space flight. *Lancet* 1985;2:1050–1052.

20. Marchetti ME, Houde JP, Steinberg GG, Crane GK, Goss TP, Baran DT. Humeral bone density losses after shoulder surgery and immobilization. *J Shoulder Elbow Surg* 1996;5:471–476.

21. Marchetti ME, Steinberg GG, Greene JM, Jenis LG, Baran DT. A prospective study of proximal femur bone mass following cemented and uncemented hip arthroplasty. *J Bone Miner Res* 1996;11:1033–1039.

22. Houde JP, Schulz LA, Morgan WJ, et al. Bone mineral density changes in the forearm after immobilization. *Clin Orthop* 1995;317:199–205.

23. Biering-Sorensen F, Bohr H, Schaadt O. Longitudinal study of bone mineral content in the lumbar spine, the forearm, and the lower extremities after spinal cord injury. *Eur J Clin Invest* 1990;20:330–335.

59. Orthopedic Complications of Osteoporosis

Thomas A. Einhorn, M.D.

Department of Orthopaedic Surgery, Boston University School of Medicine, and Boston Medical Center, Boston, Massachusetts

Most osteoporosis-related complications in orthopedics relate to problems associated with fractures and fracture management, and how the osteoporotic skeleton responds to joint reconstructive procedures. Specific attention to the quality of fracture fixation and the use of implants in weak bone is required. Control of the metabolic condition, including treatment of the underlying cause of the osteoporosis (if known), and pharmaceutical management of the condition may improve surgical results. It may be necessary to alter the surgeon's usual preference for specific fixation devices to meet the anatomic and physiologic needs of the deformed or qualitatively impaired bone. In certain osteoporotic conditions in which bone remodeling is affected, a prolonged period of fracture healing may be anticipated, and this period of healing may exceed the rate of healing in normal non-osteoporotic bone.

The orthopedist must be aware that the osteoporotic skeleton may have unusual types of injuries because of the fragile quality of the bone. For example, patients with osteoporosis who are engaged in athletic events may experience injuries in which their soft-tissue structures have a greater ability to withstand mechanical loads than the bones that support them. As an example, a common skiing injury, rupture of the anterior cruciate of the knee, usually occurs when an anterior-displacement force is applied to the knee and the ligament becomes stretched, rupturing in its midsubstance. However, because the ligament is anchored in the joint to the bone of the femur and tibial plateau, if the cross-sectional area and strength of the ligament exceeds the bone's resistance to tensile loading, an avulsion fracture may occur in osteoporotic bone instead of a failure (tear)

occurring in the ligament. Not only must the orthopedist be aware of the possibility of this type of problem, but the method of operative repair and the rehabilitation program must take into consideration the limited capacity of the bone to support a tensile force in the ligament. Other complications of osteoporosis relate to the reconstruction of the diseased or deformed skeleton during treatments such as osteotomy, arthrodesis, and arthroplasty. In each case, the ability of the osteoporotic skeleton to respond to mechanical conditions, implant devices, or cementation techniques must be recognized and addressed.

MANAGEMENT OF FRACTURES IN PATIENTS WITH OSTEOPOROSIS

Skeletal fractures are the most common orthopedic condition associated with osteoporosis. The goals of treatment are rapid mobilization and a return to normal activities; prolonged immobilization through the use of conservative fracture management is generally discouraged because it places the patient at risk of pulmonary decompensation, thromboembolic disease, decubitus formation, and further skeletal deterioration from disuse. Although the treatment of each fracture must be addressed individually, the following are general guidelines for the management of osteoporotic fractures:

1. Elderly patients are best treated by rapid, definitive fracture management aimed at early restoration of mobility and function. In general, these patients are considered to be at their healthiest on the initial day of injury and thus

are in the best condition to undergo an operation at that time (1). In some cases, survival is benefited by judicious preoperative management to reverse medical decompensation causing or resulting from the injury. In addition, the extent and scope of the operative intervention should be minimized in order to reduce operative time, blood loss, and physiologic stress to the patient. A recent study prospectively examined outcomes of hip fractures in cognitively intact, ambulatory patients living at home prior to injury. It concluded that an operative delay of more than two calendar days is an important predictor of mortality within one year of the time of the fracture (2).

2. The goal of operative intervention is to achieve stable fracture fixation and permit early return of function. For the lower extremity, this is dictated by the ability of the patient to return to full weight-bearing status early in the treatment period. Although anatomic restoration is important for intraarticular fractures, metaphyseal and diaphyseal fractures require early stabilization, and perfect anatomic reduction is less important.

3. The primary mode of failure of internal fixation is the inability of the osteoporotic bone to support fixation devices. Because the strength of bone is directly related to the square of its mineral density (3), osteoporotic bone may lack the strength to support rigid fixation devices such as plates and screws. Moreover, comminution is generally more extensive in osteoporotic fractures, and fixation devices should be chosen to allow compaction and settling of fracture fragments into stable patterns that minimize stresses at the bone–implant interface. Finally, implants should be chosen that minimize stress shielding to avoid further regional bone loss. For these reasons, sliding nail–plate devices, intramedullary systems, and tension-band wiring constructs that allow load sharing and compaction are generally preferred to rigid systems.

4. Although the events of fracture healing proceed normally in almost all osteoporotic patients, an inadequate calcium intake could result in deficits in callus mineralization or remodeling (4). Because it has been shown that many elderly patients are malnourished, fracture healing may be enhanced when nutritional deficiencies are corrected (4,5). Therefore for optimal results, nutritional assessment should be included in patient evaluation, and in certain cases, protein supplementation, physiologic doses of vitamin D (400 to 800 IU/day), and calcium (1.5 g elemental calcium/day) should be administered in the perioperative and postoperative periods.

Hip Fractures

A number of factors influence the occurrence of hip fractures. Although hip fractures have been classified according to several systems, patients with osteoporosis generally sustain one of two types of hip fractures, intracapsular or intertrochanteric. In intracapsular fractures, the fracture occurs within the hip capsule and frequently results in an interruption of the blood supply to the femoral head. These fractures also are known as cervical fractures, transcervical fractures, or femoral neck fractures (Fig. 1). Intertrochanteric fractures are extracapsular fractures that occur in an area in which

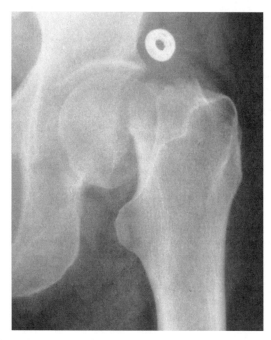

FIG. 1. Anteroposterior view of a typical intracapsular (femoral neck) fracture. Because the hip capsule inserts just above the greater and lesser trochanters of the femur, this fracture is anatomically located within the hip joint. As such, it is referred to as an intracapsular fracture.

biomechanical forces are only moderately high. The name ''intertrochanteric'' is derived from the fact that the fracture is anatomically propagated between the greater and lesser trochanters of the femur (Fig. 2).

Intracapsular fractures are problematic because of the high incidence of nonunion and avascular necrosis that occurs in spite of adequate treatment. These complications are related to the retrograde blood supply to the femoral head and the fact that the branches of the medial femoral circumflex artery, which nourish the femoral head within the hip capsule, are apposed to the femoral neck and are usually interrupted when intracapsular fractures are displaced. Closed reduction and pin-and-screw fixation with a variety of implants are consistently associated with a 14% incidence of nonunion and a 15% incidence of avascular necrosis (Fig. 3) (2).

The treatment options for intracapsular fractures are reduction and internal fixation versus hemiarthroplasty. Because the degree of displacement of an intracapsular fracture may predict its prognosis, the decision of operative treatment is dictated by the extent of displacement of the fracture. The classification system used to help make these assessments is known as the Garden classification (Fig. 4). This is a four-stage classification system in which stage I fractures are those that are incomplete, nondisplaced, and frequently angled into a valgus position; stage II fractures are those that are complete, nondisplaced, but potentially unstable; stage III fractures are completely displaced, but a portion of the capsule remains intact; and in stage IV fractures, the fracture is completely displaced, and the capsule is completely disrupted. Studies have shown that stage III and IV fractures have the highest rates of nonunion. Therefore reduction and fixation with pins is generally preferred in

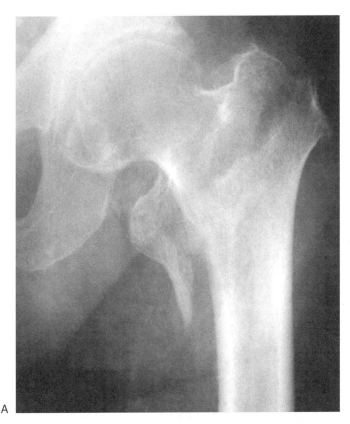

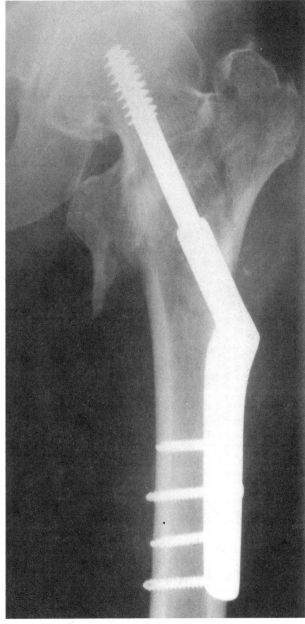

FIG. 2. A: Anteroposterior view of a typical intertrochanteric fracture. Note that the fracture line is propagated between the greater and lesser trochanters, and the lesser trochanter is actually displaced from the femur being pulled medially by the iliopsoas muscle insertion. **B:** Anteroposterior view of the same fracture 2 months after operative treatment. Note that with the use of a sliding hip screw, the fracture fragments have settled or compacted into a stable configuration.

stage I and II fractures, whereas hemiarthroplasty is often used in the treatment of stage III and IV injuries (Fig. 5). The advantages of internal fixation are that the anatomy is restored, the patient undergoes a normal period of fracture healing, and if the joint has not been injured, the patient can expect normal service from the hip after the fracture has healed. The advantage of hemiarthroplasty is the immediate return to function because the replaced joint does not need to undergo a period of healing. However, hemiarthroplasty is associated with its own set of complications including loosening and breakage of implants and the risk of infection. Most authors agree that treatment with hemiarthroplasty is associated with a higher perioperative morbidity.

Intertrochanteric fractures have received less attention than femoral neck fractures because nonunion and avascular necrosis are uncommon in intertrochanteric fractures. However, the prevalence of malunion with resulting varus, shortening, and external rotational deformity is significant and can be disabling. In addition, when bone quality is particularly poor, the use of fixation devices may be beset with problems such as loss of fixation and screw penetration into the hip joint (2). Telescoping or sliding hip screw devices are an improvement over fixed nail devices in that they allow controlled compaction of the fracture until a stable fracture pattern is achieved. However, it is still necessary for the surgeon to obtain an adequate reduction before using such a device. When used properly, a load-sharing device will result in a decrease in the stresses between the implant and the bone and a more favorable biomechanical situation (Fig. 2B).

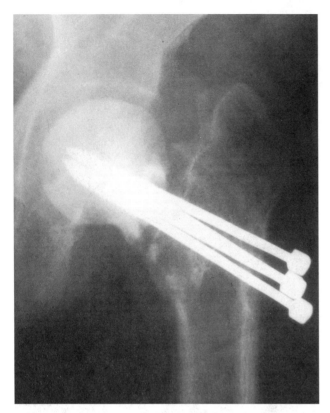

FIG. 3. Anteroposterior view of the proximal femur of a patient 3 months after open reduction and internal fixation of a displaced intracapsular fracture. Note that there is a diastasis at the fracture site, the pins have begun to migrate laterally, and the femoral head is radiodense, suggesting osteonecrosis.

In some situations, the bone in the trochanteric region of the femur is so osteoporotic that any type of fixation system is at risk of failure. In these situations, orthopedists have resorted to the use of methyl methacrylate cement to enhance the purchase of implant devices in the bone and prevent penetration or cutting out of the device. More recently, a calcium phosphate–based material was developed that may prove effective when injected into the site of a fracture or used with a fixation device at the time of fracture management (6). The use of this material in the treatment of hip fractures has yielded encouraging results (6,7).

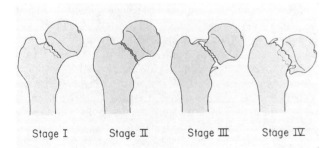

FIG. 4. Schematic of the Garden classification of intracapsular hip fractures.

Stage I   Stage II   Stage III   Stage IV

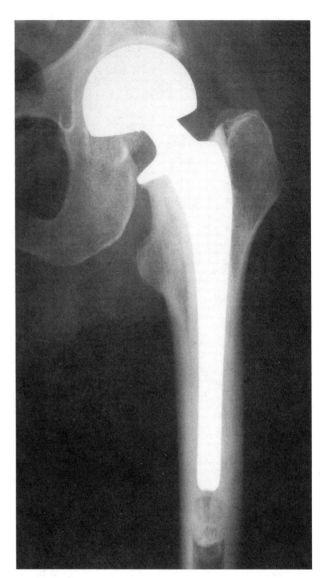

FIG. 5. Anteroposterior view of the hip in a patient who has undergone a hemiarthroplasty for the treatment of a displaced (stage IV) intracapsular hip fracture.

Fractures About the Knee

Osteoporotic bone that supports the knee joint is susceptible to supracondylar fractures of the distal femur and fractures of the tibial plateau. Because both of these fractures may be associated with comminution and intraarticular extension, they carry a high risk for postoperative degenerative joint disease and arthrofibrosis. Treatment protocols are therefore aimed at early knee rehabilitation and strengthening of the quadriceps mechanism.

Management of fractures about the knee in patients with osteoporosis can be difficult. Frequently the degree of comminution is so extensive that choices of internal fixation are limited. Occasionally, special imaging techniques such as computed tomography (CT) scanning and plain tomography can help delineate the size and position of the fracture fragments. Because these fractures can be immobilized in a well-padded long-leg cast or brace, the urgency for operative treatment is usually not so great as for the hip or the femoral shaft. However, long-term immobilization of these fractures not only limits a patient's activity but also can lead to joint stiffness, particularly in the elderly population.

In supracondylar fractures, the objectives of operative treatment are anatomic restoration and rigid fixation to allow immediate rehabilitation. Although good results have been obtained with one-piece blade plates and 90-degree telescoping screw plates, the use of locked intramedullary retrograde nails are preferred in the management of these injuries. The advantage of this type of fixation is that the patient's knee can be immediately moved in rehabilitation protocols.

Tibial plateau fractures generally result from a valgus stress to the knee in conjunction with falling and twisting. The degree of compromise that occurs as a result of tibial plateau fractures depends on the degree of instability and angular deformity. Minimally displaced fractures (i.e., those with less than 5 mm of depression) can be treated with immobilization of the knee followed by active motion. Non–weight bearing of the injured limb should be maintained until fracture healing has occurred at approximately 6 to 8 weeks. The use of continuous passive motion (CPM) has been found to be extremely helpful, and the use of a hinged knee brace between CPM sessions enhances recovery. Fractures displaced by more than 8 mm, or those with associated varus or valgus instability of 5 to 10 degrees or greater, require open reduction and internal fixation. After surgery, a varus molded cast brace followed by CPM is used. Weight bearing is delayed for a period of 8 to 10 weeks after treatment. Where there is loss of trabecular bone due to crushing, such defects may be filled with autogenous bone graft; bone graft substitutes composed of calcium phosphate, calcium sulfate, or coralline hydroxyapatite; or calcium-based bone cement.

Fractures of the Humerus

Three types of humeral fractures occur in osteoporotic patients: fractures of the proximal humerus, the humeral diaphysis, and the supracondylar region of the elbow. Generally, these fractures result from minor falls and usually occur with minimal displacement.

Fractures of the proximal humerus are common and account for approximately 5% of fractures in this patient population. Eighty percent of these fractures occur through the cancellous bone of the surgical neck and are impacted without significant displacement (2). These fractures are considered stable and can be treated with immobilization in a sling or sling-like system. Range-of-motion activities including pendulum exercises can be started to avoid shoulder stiffness. Generally, 3 to 4 weeks is sufficient to allow early healing before full passive range of motion, with active range of motion taking place by 5 to 6 weeks. Unimpacted fractures can be treated with a sling or sling-like device. Occasionally, closed reduction and percutaneous pin fixation are required to achieve stable reduction. Comminuted fractures involving three- or four-part displacement are best treated by prosthetic replacement followed by early vigorous physical therapy. Open reduction and internal fixation can be used when the fragments are sufficiently large and there

is less than extensive comminution. Open reduction and internal fixation by using screws and tension-band wires have been shown to work well. However, if difficulty is encountered in obtaining adequate purchase of screws, pins, or wires in bone, hemiarthroplasty is recommended.

Humeral shaft fractures in most cases are treated with nonoperative means. Occasionally, intramedullary nailing is needed to control angulation; however, because of the large amount of soft tissue in the arm, more angulation is acceptable with humeral shaft fractures than with fractures of other long bones.

Fractures of the distal humerus, especially those with an intraarticular component, present a particular challenge to orthopedic treatment. The potential for chronic disability is high, and so anatomic reduction and stable fixation is required. These fractures are associated with a high degree of morbidity, and elbow stiffness is not uncommon. Early operative intervention followed by carefully planned physical therapy is needed.

Fractures of the Distal Radius

Fractures of the distal radius, most notably Colles' fractures, are a common complication of osteoporosis. Although it is generally held that substantial deformity of the distal radius can be acceptable when associated with relatively normal function, complications arising from this injury include loss of reduction, radial shortening, and painful prominence of the ulna (2). Many of these complications can be avoided by accurate reduction that restores the normal length and orientation of the distal radioulnar joint followed by early mobilization of the hand and upper extremity. Closed reduction and casting under local or regional anesthesia are generally successful in restoring the length of the distal radius. Healing is usually rapid, and return to function occurs in about 6 weeks. Adequate reduction implies no radial shortening and at least a neutral angulation of the distal radial articular surface in the anteroposterior plane. Unstable and severely comminuted fractures are best treated with internal or external fixation. External fixation is frequently difficult in osteopenic bone because of loosening of the pins in bone of poor quality. Therefore the goal of treatment in these types of injuries is to obtain adequate reduction and control over the fracture fragments and immobilization long enough for early healing to take place. Once this has occurred, conversion to a cast or a splint is recommended. Current investigations with a calcium-based bone cement paste suggest that this material may enhance the fixation of these fragments and allow early conversion from a long-arm cast to a short-arm volar splint (8).

Spinal Fractures

Fractures of the spinal column are common in patients with osteoporotic bone. Vertebral fractures are grouped according to fracture type (wedge, biconcavity, or compression) and by degree of deformity (9). However, the vast majority of fractures of the osteoporotic spine are considered stable because the posterior spinal elements remain intact.

Therefore operative intervention is rarely required in spinal osteoporosis.

Symptomatic relief of spinal pain is often difficult to achieve because the causes are related not only to microcracks or fractures within the bone but also to stresses placed on the interspinous ligaments, facet-joint capsules, and paraspinal muscles. Although narcotic medications are sometimes effective, their use should be discouraged or at least limited because the abuse potential is high. In many instances, significant symptomatic relief can be achieved through physical therapy, rehabilitation, and bracing. External support in the form of a bivalved custom polypropylene body jacket is useful during the acute painful phase of a fracture but should be discontinued when symptoms subside. These devices may cause paraspinal muscles to undergo atrophy with prolonged use, and those paraspinal muscles are ultimately needed for support in maintaining the integrity of the spinal column complex. In those patients who, on careful evaluation, are deemed able to withstand some low-level spinal stresses, a program of back extension and deep-breathing exercises should be prescribed (10). In addition, counseling and instruction should be provided to all patients on the subjects of correct posture and body mechanics to prevent further pathologic fractures and the propensity to fall.

Operative management of osteoporotic spinal fractures is rarely indicated and should be reserved for the patient who has a fracture that is causing gross deformity, resulting in pulmonary or neurologic impairment. The ability of the surgeon to obtain adequate purchase in bone is the main problem affecting any type of spinal-fixation system. The recent development of the calcium-based cements may lead to the availability of new, fast-setting materials that could be effective in this application.

PROBLEMS ASSOCIATED WITH RECONSTRUCTIVE OPERATIVE PROCEDURES

Patients with osteoporosis are more prone to develop skeletal deformities as a result of physiologic bowing of qualitatively impaired bone or malunions of previous fractures. Correction of these deformities involves osteotomy, fixation, and bone healing. Planning of the osteotomy site and the placement of the bone cuts follow the same principles used in reconstructive surgery of the normal skeleton. Fixation, however, follows the principles outlined earlier for fracture management. In general, load-sharing devices such as intramedullary nails are preferred to rigid fixation systems. In addition, a very popular and effective method of osteotomy correction, small-pin external fixation, is not suitable for patients with severe osteoporosis because of the propensity of small pins to cut out of qualitatively impaired bone.

Patients with diseased joints such as those with degenerative osteoarthritis are candidates for arthrodeses or total joint arthroplasties. Although no special problems are associated with arthrodeses in patients with osteoporosis, the types of fixation systems used in conjunction with these procedures follow the same principles described for fractures. With respect to total joint arthroplasty, surgeons should follow the same principles used in the management of joints sup-ported by normal bone; however, special care should be taken during reaming and component insertion. In reaming the acetabular socket, reamers should be used at lower speeds, and the results of the reaming should be checked more frequently so that penetration of the acetabulum does not occur. This is particularly relevant in patients who use corticosteroids. In reaming the femoral canal, special attention should be paid to the positioning of all reamers and guide-wire systems because it is easy to penetrate the cortex.

Insertion of cement under pressure in patients with osteoporotic bone can lead to unusual complications. For example, even when there are no breaks in the cortices of the femoral canal, highly pressurized cement and implant insertion can result in a blowout of the cortical wall. Similarly, once an implant has been seated in the joint and the cement cured, settling or subsidence of the implant–cement composite may occur leading to increased joint laxity.

Fractures occur more frequently around total joint prostheses in osteoporotic bone, and the surgeon must be prepared to handle these complications. A common example occurs in the patient who has a total knee replacement and subsequent supracondylar fracture. Although controversy exists concerning the management of these injuries in patients with normal bone, the prolonged period of healing associated with osteoporotic bone and the limited amount of trabecular bone in this area dictates that the best method of management is fixation. A short intramedullary nail can be very useful in this setting. Finally, although most fractures occur from traumatic events, the surgeon must be aware that resistance encountered intraoperatively in the process of reduction or dislocation of the joint can lead to an increased risk of iatrogenic fracture. For this reason, particular care must be taken in the gentle intraoperative manipulation of the limbs of osteoporotic patients who are undergoing total joint arthroplasty.

SUMMARY

Patients with osteoporosis present a special challenge to the orthopedist. Although most issues relate to the management of fractures sustained in fragile bone, special problems associated with reconstructive orthopedic procedures also must be addressed. The goal of any treatment is the rapid restoration of mobility and function and a return of patients to a level of activity that supports their general health. Long-term immobilization should be avoided. In situations in which it is possible to reduce the effects of an offending agent, such as corticosteroids, all efforts should be made to do so. In the past three years, several new pharmacologic agents, including bisphosphonates and estrogen receptor modulators, were approved by the U.S. Food and Drug Administration for the treatment of osteoporosis. These agents carry the hope of reducing the morbidity of this disease. We hope they also will lead to an improvement in bone quality such that the response of the skeleton to operative interventions will be improved. Although concern has been expressed about the potential effects of these drugs on a fracture-healing process, at least one study with alendronate failed to show any negative effect (11). The effects of other bisphosphonates or selective estrogen-receptor modulators on fracture healing are unknown. The combined approach of general health maintenance, the judicious use of pharmacologic agents, and a program of regular exercise should reduce the orthopedic complications associated with this disease.

REFERENCES

1. Cornell CN. Management of fractures in patients with osteoporosis. *Orthop Clin North Am* 1990;21:121–141.
2. Zuckerman JD, Skovron ML, Koval KJ, Aharonoff G, Frankel VH. Postoperative complications and mortality associated with operative delay in older patients who have a fracture of the hip. *J Bone Joint Surg* 1995;77:1551–1556.
3. Carter DR, Hayes WC. The compressive behavior of bone as a two-phase porous structure. *J Bone Joint Surg* 1977;59:954–962.
4. Einhorn TA, Bonnarens F, Burstein AH. The contributions of dietary protein and mineral to the healing of experimental fractures: a biomechanical study. *J Bone Joint Surg Am* 1986;68:1389–1395.
5. Jensen JE, Jensen TG, Smith TK, Johnston DA, Dudrick SJ. Nutrition in orthopaedic surgery. *J Bone Joint Surg Am* 1982;64:1263–1272.
6. Constantz BR, Ison IC, Fulmer MT, et al. Skeletal repair by in situ formation of the mineral phase of bone. *Science* 1995;267:1796–1799.
7. Stankewich CJ, Swiontkowski MF, Tencer AF, Yetkinler DN, Poser RD. Augmentation of femoral neck fracture fixation with an injectable calcium-phosphate bone mineral cement. *J Orthop Res* 1996;14: 786–793.
8. Jupiter JB, Winter S, Sigman S, et al. Repair of 5 distal radius fractures with an investigational cancellous bone cement: a preliminary report. *J Orthop Trauma* 1997;11:110–116.
9. Eastell R, Cedel SI, Wahner HW, Riggs BL, Melton LJ III. Classification of vertebral fractures. *J Bone Miner Res* 1991;6:207–214.
10. Sinaki M, Mikkelesen BA. Postmenopausal spinal osteoporosis: flexion versus extension exercises. *Arch Phys Med Rehabil* 1984;65:593–596.
11. Peter CP, Cook WO, Nunamaker DM, Provost MT, Seedor JG, Rodan GA. Effect of alendronate on fracture healing and bone remodeling in dogs. *J Orthop Res* 1996;14:74–79.

60. Osteoporosis and Rheumatic Diseases

Steven R. Goldring, M.D.

Division of Rheumatology, Beth Israel Deaconess Medical Center, Harvard Medical School, Boston, Massachusetts

The rheumatic diseases include a diverse group of disorders that share in common their propensity to affect articular structures. The most commonly involved joints are the so-called diarthrodial joints which consist of two articulating surfaces lined by hyaline cartilage. Arthritic processes most often affect the cartilage surfaces and the synovial lining but also may involve the subchondral bone and joint capsule. Amphiarthroses, which are characterized by fibrocartilaginous union (e.g., the intervertebral discs), also are frequently affected in rheumatic disorders.

Osteoarthritis is a prototypical example of a rheumatic disease in which the pathologic events are restricted almost entirely to the joint structures. Many of the rheumatic diseases, however, may affect extraarticular organ systems, and these conditions are often accompanied by significant systemic symptoms that may dominate the clinical picture. These illnesses, which include, for example, conditions such as rheumatoid arthritis (RA), systemic lupus erythematosus (SLE) and the spondyloarthropathies, are believed to be initiated by disturbances in immune regulation that involve complex interactions between unique host genetic susceptibility and specific environmental factor(s). In these disorders, skeletal tissues may be involved not only at juxtaarticular and subchondral sites, but in addition, there is evidence that many of these conditions may produce generalized effects on bone remodeling that affect the entire skeleton.

Among the rheumatic disorders, RA is an excellent model for gaining insights into the effects of local as well as systemic consequences of inflammatory processes on skeletal tissue remodeling. Three principal forms of bone disease have been described in RA. The first is that characterized by a focal process that affects the immediate subchondral and juxtaarticular bone. The synovial lesion of RA is charac-terized by the proliferation of the synovial lining cells and infiltration of the tissue by inflammatory cells, including lymphocytes, plasma cells, endothelial cells, and activated macrophages. The proliferative synovial tissue (pannus) invades the immediately adjacent bone, resulting in progressive focal osteolysis that gives rise to the characteristic cystic bone "erosions" that can be detected radiographically. Analysis of the immediate bone–pannus interface reveals the frequent presence of multinucleated cells with phenotypic features of osteoclasts (1,2) suggesting that the focal osteolytic lesions of RA are mediated at least in part by authentic osteoclasts. The recent demonstration of calcitonin receptors on these multinucleated cells provides further direct evidence that they are authentic osteoclasts (2). The origin of the resorbing osteoclast-like multinucleated cells has not been firmly established, but they likely are derived from mononuclear cell precursors present within the inflamed synovium. These cells are induced to differentiate into osteoclasts by the cytokines that are produced locally within the inflamed synovial tissue (2). There is evidence that the macrophages and macrophage polykaryons associated with this lesion also can contribute to the bone resorption.

A second form of bone disease observed in patients with RA is the presence of juxtaarticular osteopenia adjacent to inflamed joints. Histologic examination of this bone tissue reveals the presence of frequent osteoclasts and increased osteoid and resorptive surfaces consistent with increased bone turnover (1,3). Local aggregates of inflammatory cells, including macrophages and lymphocytes, are often detected in the marrow space. It has been suggested that these cells are derived from the synovial lining and that they migrate into the marrow, where they release local products that affect bone remodeling (1). Decreased joint motion and immobilization in response to the joint inflammation likely represent additional contributing factors to this local bone loss.

The third form of bone disease associated with RA is the presence of generalized axial and appendicular osteopenia at sites that are distant from inflamed joints (4,5). Although there are conflicting data concerning the effects of RA on skeletal mass, the presence of a generalized reduction in bone mass has been confirmed by using multiple different techniques, and there is compelling evidence that this reduction is associated with an increased risk of hip and vertebral fracture (6). The conflicting data are in part related to the fact that most observations have been based on cross-sectional studies and have focused on patients late in the evolution of their disease when factors such as disability, corticosteroids, and other treatments may confound the analyses. Histomorphometric analysis of bone biopsies from patients with RA indicate that, in the absence of corticosteroid use, the cellular basis of the generalized reduction in bone mass is related to a decrease in bone formation rather than an increase in bone resorption (7,8). However, more recently, biochemical markers of bone turnover have been used to evaluate individuals with RA, and the results of these studies indicate that in patients with early RA, an increase in bone resorption (rather than decreased bone formation) is the dominant process leading to bone loss (9).

Several factors have emerged as important determinants of bone mass in patients with RA, and these include age and menopausal status, reduced mobility, disease activity, the influence of antirheumatic therapy (especially corticosteroids), and disease duration (10–13). A recent, large longitudinal prospective study by Gough et al. (10) concluded that significant amounts of generalized skeletal bone were lost early in RA and that this loss was associated with disease activity. These findings support the observations of Als (14), who also noted a significant decrease in bone mass during the early phases of RA.

There is still considerable controversy regarding the effects of corticosteroids in affecting the progression of bone loss in RA. In part, this is related to the tendency to use these medications in patients with more severe disease. Some authors suggested that if steroids satisfactorily suppress inflammation and maintain mobility, their deleterious effects may be outweighed (10,11). It is premature, however, generally to advocate the use of corticosteroids in patients with RA because there is considerable evidence that their prolonged use is associated with many potentially serious extraskeletal complications (15). This cautionary note is supported by the recent findings of Saag et al. (16), who noted that low-dose long-term prednisone use, ≥5 g/day, was correlated in a dose-dependent fashion with the development of several adverse reactions, including fracture (16).

Although not associated with focal bone erosions, generalized bone loss also is a significant clinical problem in patients with SLE. Reductions in both cortical and trabecular bone mass have been reported, even in the absence of corticosteroid treatment. As in patients with RA, the effects of systemic inflammation, decreased physical activity, nutritional factors, sex steroid influences, and drug treatments all likely contribute to the adverse effects on generalized bone mass. Similar factors contribute to the reduced bone mass, delayed skeletal linear growth, and increased incidence of fractures in patients with a history of juvenile chronic (rheumatoid) arthritis.

Ankylosing spondylitis is characterized by inflammation at the entheses in the spine and peripheral skeleton. Although local bone erosions may be detected early in the course of the disease, new-bone formation and ankylosis of the spine eventually develop in many patients. Several studies documented an increased incidence of spinal compression fractures in patients with this disorder (17). Because of the chronic back pain experienced by many patients with ankylosing spondylitis and the high incidence of paraspinal calcifications and syndesmophytes, many of these fractures are not detected. Although not well studied, the decrease in axial bone density has been attributed to the effects of immobilization of the spine associated with the progressive ankylosis. Of interest, appendicular bone mass appears to be normal in these individuals.

Osteoarthritis (OA) is the most common form of joint disease. In contrast to RA and other forms of inflammatory arthritis, in individuals with OA, there is an absence of systemic disease manifestations, and the pathologic changes are limited to the joint structures. OA is characterized by progressive loss of articular cartilage, thickening of the trabeculae of the subchondral bone, and formation of new bone and cartilage at the joint margins, giving rise to osteophytes that are the radiologic hallmark of OA. Despite the well-established evidence of increased periarticular bone mass, there remains considerable controversy concerning the relation between OA and systemic osteoporosis. Several recent studies examined the relation between OA of the hand, knee, and spine and bone density by using dual x-ray absorptiometry (18,19). Results from these studies suggest that there is a reduced frequency of osteoporosis in patients with OA. Dequeker et al. (20) suggested that individuals with OA tend to produce increased levels of anabolic bone-growth factors at skeletal sites, and this may contribute to the generalized increase in bone mass. Further studies are needed, however, firmly to establish the relation between OA and osteoporosis.

REFERENCES

1. Bromley M, Woolley DE. Chondroclasts and osteoclasts at subchondral sites of erosion in the rheumatoid joint. *Arthritis Rheum* 1984;27:968–975.
2. Gravallese EM, Harada Y, Wang JT, Gorn AH, Thornhill TS, Goldring SR. Identification of the cell types responsible for bone resorption in rheumatoid arthritis and juvenile arthritis. *Am J Pathol* 1998;152:943–951.
3. Shimizo S, Shiozawa S, Shiozawa K, Imura S, Fujita T. Quantitative histological studies on the pathogenesis of peri-articular osteoporosis in rheumatoid arthritis. *Arthritis Rheum* 1985;28:25–31.
4. Peel NF, Eastell R, Russell RG. Osteoporosis in rheumatoid arthritis: the laboratory perspective. *Br J Rheum* 1991;30:84–85.
5. Woolf AD. Osteoporosis in rheumatoid arthritis: the clinical viewpoint. *Br J Rheum* 1991;30:82–84.
6. Spector TD, Hall GM, McCloskey EV, Kanis JA. Risk of vertebral fracture in women with rheumatoid arthritis. *BMJ* 1993;306:558.
7. Kroger H, Arnala I, Alhava EM. Bone remodeling in osteoporosis associated with rheumatoid arthritis. *Calcif Tissue Int* 1991;49:S90.
8. Compston JE, Vedi S, Croucher PI, Garrahan NJ, O'Sullivan MM. Bone turnover in non-steroid treated rheumatoid arthritis. *Ann Rheum Dis* 1994;53:163–166.
9. Gough A, Sambrook P, Devlin J, et al. Osteoclastic activation is the

principal mechanism leading to secondary osteoporosis in rheumatoid arthritis. *J Rheumatol* 1998;7:1282–1289.

10. Gough AK, Lilley J, Eyre S, Holder RL, Emergy P. Generalized bone loss in patients with early rheumatoid arthritis. *Lancet* 1994;344:23–27.

11. Kirwan JR. The effect of glucocorticoids on joint destruction in rheumatoid arthritis. *N Engl J Med* 1995;333:142–146.

12. Sambrook P, Birmingham J, Champion D, et al. Postmenopausal bone loss in rheumatoid arthritis: effect of estrogens and androgens. *J Rheum* 1992;19:357–361.

13. Sambrook P, Nguyen T. Vertebral osteoporosis in rheumatoid arthritis patients: effect of low dose prednisone therapy. *Br J Rheum* 1992; 31:573–574.

14. Als OS, Gotfredsen A, Riis BJ, Christiansen C. Are disease duration and degree of functional impairment determinants of bone loss in rheumatoid arthritis? *Ann Rheum Dis* 1985;44:406–411.

15. Lane NE, Goldring SR. Bone loss in rheumatoid arthritis: what role does inflammation play? *J Rheumatol* 1998;7:1251–1253.

16. Saag KG, Koehnke R, Caldwell JR, et al. Low dose long-term corticosteroid therapy in rheumatoid arthritis: an analysis of serious adverse events. *Am J Med* 1994;6:115–123.

17. Ralston SH, Urquhart GD, Brzeski M, Sturrock RD. Prevalence of vertebral compression fractures due to osteoporosis in ankylosing spondylitis. *BMJ* 1990;300:563–565.

18. Nevitt MC, Lane NE, Scott JC, et al. Radiographic osteoarthritis of the hip and bone mineral density. *Arthritis Rheum* 1995;38:907–916.

19. Hannan MT, Anderson JJ, Zhang Y, Levy D, Felson DT. Bone mineral density and knee osteoarthritis in elderly men and women: the Framingham study. *Arthritis Rheum* 1993;36:1671–1680.

20. Dequeker J, Mohan S, Finkelman RD, Aerssens J, Baylink DJ. Generalized osteoarthritis associated with increased insulin-like growth factor types I and II and transforming growth factor β in cortical bone from the iliac crest; possible mechanism of increased bone density and protection against osteoporosis. *Arthritis Rheum* 1993;36:1702–1708.

61. Nutritional Rickets and Osteomalacia

Gordon L. Klein, M.D., M.P.H.

Departments of Pediatrics and Preventive Medicine, University of Texas Medical Branch, Galveston, Texas

Recommended dietary intakes of vitamin D and minerals for infants, children, and adults are discussed in Chapter 50. Intakes of vitamin D, calcium, or phosphorus substantially below these recommendations may result in rickets or osteomalacia. Rickets is a disorder of mineralization of the bone matrix, or osteoid, in growing bone; it involves both the growth plate (epiphysis) and newly formed trabecular and cortical bone. Osteomalacia also is a defect in bone matrix mineralization, but it occurs after the cessation of growth and involves only the bone and not the growth plate. The mineralization defects in rickets, resulting from inadequate calcium and/or phosphate deposition in the matrix, has an uncertain etiology. However, there is a common finding of low calcium and phosphate concentration in the extracellular fluid surrounding rachitic cartilage and bone, suggesting that local factors may be responsible for the undermineralization (1).

Deficiencies of vitamin D, calcium, or phosphorus due to inadequate nutritional intake (Table 1) can result in defective bone mineralization. We consider each separately.

VITAMIN D DEFICIENCY

The main natural sources of vitamin D in foods are the fish liver foods. Otherwise, fortification of foods such as milk and eggs has been necessary to prevent the occurrence of vitamin D deficiency in the United States (2,3). However, consumption of unfortified foods in an environment with reduced exposure to sunlight can lead to vitamin D deficiency in many developing countries (2,3). This is especially true of Asian women who wear veils, consume unfortified foods when pregnant, and nurse their infants. Another group at risk for vitamin D deficiency is breast-fed infants who do not receive vitamin D supplementation. Breast milk has been shown to be low in vitamin D, and cases of rickets in breast-fed infants have been reported (3).

Rickets also can develop in infants receiving total parenteral nutrition (TPN) solution exclusively, from which vitamin D and calcium were inadvertently omitted (4).

However, it is unclear whether absence of vitamin D alone would have been sufficient to produce bone disease. Adults who received TPN devoid of vitamin D for up to 1 year did not develop osteomalacia although their serum levels of 25-hydroxyvitamin D [25 (OH) D] were very low (5).

Pathogenesis

A diagram illustrating the steps in the pathogenesis of vitamin D–deficient rickets is shown in Fig. 1. The most biologically active vitamin D metabolite, 1,25-dihydroxyvitamin D [1,25 (OH)$_2$ D], is made in the kidney by hydroxylation of 25 (OH) D that comes from the liver (see Chapter 15). 1,25-Dihydroxyvitamin D enhances calcium and phosphate absorption from the small intestine. During vitamin D deficiency, intestinal calcium and phosphate absorption are reduced, causing hypocalcemia. The hypocalcemia in turn stimulates the parathyroid glands to secrete increased quantities of parathyroid hormone (PTH). Parathyroid hormone acts indirectly on osteoclasts to promote bone resorption and increase calcium and phosphorus available to the blood. In addition, PTH acts on the kidney to promote tubular calcium reabsorption and increase phosphate excretion. Parathyroid hormone also stimulates the renal conversion of 25 (OH) D to 1,25 (OH)$_2$ D. 1,25-Dihydroxyvitamin D stimulates the small intestine to absorb more calcium and phosphorus (3).

Clinical and Laboratory Manifestations

Clinical manifestations of rickets include hypotonia, muscle weakness, and, in severe cases, tetany. Weight bearing produces a bowing deformity of the long bones.

TABLE 1. *Causes and recommended management of nutritional rickets and osteomalacia*

Condition	Causes	Recommended management (ref.)
Vitamin D deficiency	Lack of adequate sunlight	Ultraviolet lamp or increased sunlight exposure (2)
	Consumption of diet low in fortified foods	Vitamin D_2 treatment. Variable: usually 1500–5000 IU/day orally (3); 10,000–50,000 IU/month intramuscular (3); 600,000 IU (15 mg) in 6 doses orally (7) in 1–2 hours
	Unsupplemented breast-fed infant	Prevention: vitamin D_2 400 IU/day orally (3) for premature infants
	Total parenteral nutrition	400–800 IU/day orally (10, 14); 20–25 IU/kg/day in total parenteral nutrition (9)
Calcium deficiency	Lack of dietary calcium	Treatment: 700 mg/day orally (11); 1–2 g/day orally (13)
	High phytate diet	
	Inadequate calcium in total parenteral nutrition	30 mg/kg/day orally in breast-fed infants (17)
		Prevention: in premature infants, 200 mg/kg/day orally (14); 20–60 mg/dl (5–15 mM) in parenteral nutrition (9)
Phosphate deficiency	Breast-fed infants, inadequate phosphate in total parenteral nutrition-premature infants	Treatment: 25 mg/kg/day in breast-fed infants (17); withdrawal of aluminum-containing antacids (18); 115–120 mg/kg/day orally in premature infants (14); 15–47 mg/dl (5–15 mM) in parenteral nutrition (9)

Prominence of the costochondral junction, the so-called rachitic rosary, also can be seen (Fig. 2), as can an indentation of the lower ribs, Harrison's groove, due to softening. Occasionally there is indentation of the sternum in response to the force exerted by the diaphragm and intercostal muscles. There is an increased incidence of pneumonia in rachitic patients (6). Deformities of the back, including kyphosis and lordosis, along with limb bowing, can contribute to a waddling gait. There also is an increased frequency of fractures.

Abnormalities of the skull, especially in younger infants, include a softened calvarium (craniotabes), parietal flattening, and frontal bossing. There is delayed eruption of permanent dentition, and enamel defects can occur (3).

Diffuse bone pain is the most common manifestation of osteomalacia, although there is some tendency for localization of pain in the hip area. Pelvic deformities and a waddling gait also may be present.

Roentgenographically the long bones are the earliest and most common sites of change. Typically there is thinning of the cortex and rarefaction of the shaft with widening, fraying, and cupping of the distal ends of the shaft and disappearance of the zone of provisional cartilaginous calcification (Fig. 3). Thin cortical radiolucent lines (stress fractures) at right angles to the bone shaft may be seen in osteomalacia as well as in other metabolic bone disorders. These are most often symmetric and bilateral. Decreased bone density also is seen. The pelvis and ribs are the most frequently affected areas (3).

Biochemical findings, as expected, include low or normal serum levels of calcium, low serum levels of phosphorus, and markedly elevated serum alkaline phosphatase levels.

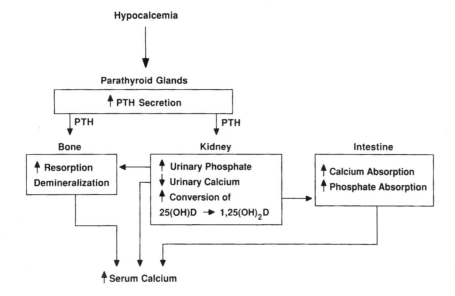

FIG. 1. Body's reaction to hypocalcemia with the consequent resorption of bone.

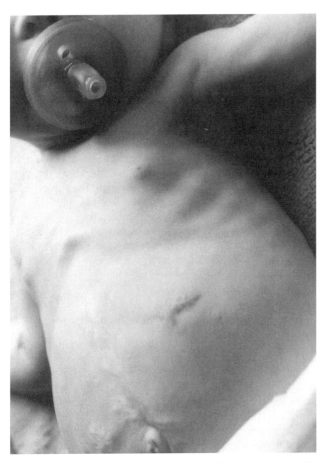

FIG. 2. An infant with nutritional rickets displaying a rachitic rosary at the costochondral junction.

This enzyme elevation probably reflects increased bone turnover. Serum PTH levels are elevated when hypocalcemia is present. Serum levels of 25 (OH) D are low in vitamin D deficiency; secondary hyperparathyroidism and low serum phosphorus stimulate renal production of 1,25 (OH)$_2$ D so that levels of this hormone are either normal or high if adequate vitamin D is present (3). Serum osteocalcin concentrations are within the normal range, although insufficient data are available to be definitive. Iliac crest bone biopsies of two Indian children, ages 36 and 69 months, revealed increased osteoid seams and reduced mineralization when compared with normal, although only semiquantitative data were published (7).

Treatment and Prevention

Recommended doses of vitamin D for treatment and prevention of vitamin D–deficiency rickets are given in Table 1. In vitamin D deficiency due to fat malabsorption, use of a more polar compound, such as 25 (OH) D, 20 to 30 μg/day, or 1,25 (OH)$_2$ D, 0.15 to 0.5 μg/day, may be more efficacious. Alternatively, ergocalciferol (vitamin D$_2$ in oil) given intramuscularly may be effective (4). The dose and frequency of administration must be adjusted depending on the serum levels of calcium, phosphorus, alkaline phosphatase, and 25 (OH) D. In infants, doses have ranged from

10,000 to 50,000 IU (250 to 1250 μg) per month. Complications of vitamin D$_2$ therapy include hypercalcemia and hypercalciuria (3). Alternatively, for patients whose rickets or osteomalacia results from lack of exposure to sunlight, either increased exposure to sunlight or ultraviolet-lamp treatment may prove beneficial (2). Alternatively, recent data suggested that single-day large-dose therapy with vitamin D (600,000 IU, 15 mg) will result in improvement in nutritional rickets within 4 to 7 days and can serve as a useful diagnostic test to differentiate nutritional rickets from other forms (8).

Rickets of prematurity is generally considered a disease of calcium and/or phosphate deficiency rather than vitamin D deficiency. When long-term TPN therapy is involved, aluminum accumulation also may be a contributing factor (9). Currently, doses of vitamin D$_2$ for parenteral use in TPN-fed infants are 20 to 25 IU (0.5 μg/kg/day) (10). The oral dose of vitamin D$_2$ is between 400 and 800 IU (10 and 20 μg) daily (11–15).

For prevention of vitamin D deficiency not due to malabsorption or prematurity, daily exposure to adequate sunlight, consumption of fortified milk, or dietary supplementation of 400 IU (10 μg) is recommended.

CALCIUM DEFICIENCY

Decreased calcium intake or intestinal absorption has been associated with rickets. Kooh et al. (12) described rickets in an infant receiving prolonged nutrition with lamb-based formula, which provided adequate phosphorus but only 180 mg/day of calcium. Vitamin D supplements were provided to give this child up to 800 IU (20 μg) per day. With

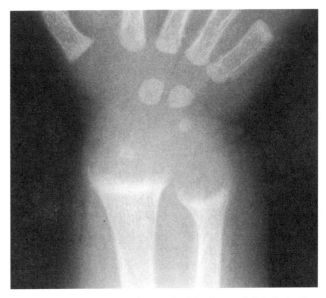

FIG. 3. Wrist demonstrating typical findings of rickets in the radius and ulna. Note widening of the metaphyses, irregularity of the metaphyses, widening of the epiphyseal line, and cupping of the metaphyses. In addition, note that the bones in general are demineralized. (Radiograph and interpretation provided courtesy of Leonard Swischuk, M.D., Department of Radiology, University of Texas Medical Branch, Galveston, Texas.)

the provision of 700 mg calcium/day, there was marked biochemical and roentgenographic improvement after 1 month (12).

Similarly, Pettifor et al. (13) identified a population of children in South Africa who consumed no milk or dairy products and whose daily calcium intake was estimated to be only 125 mg, whereas phosphate intake was adequate. Biochemical and roentgenographic evidence of rickets was present. Moreover, bone histology in three children revealed increased unmineralized osteoid (matrix) and decreased bone turnover, diagnostic of osteomalacia (13,14). Calcium supplementation led to both biochemical and histologic improvement (14).

Reduction in calcium absorption may contribute to calcium-deficiency rickets. Consumption of cereals and other grain products high in phytate could lead to intraluminal calcium phytate complexation and consequent calcium malabsorption. This was postulated by Stamp et al. (2) in Asian populations living in London. However, they subsequently demonstrated in two children that, despite continued consumption of a high-phytate diet, rickets improved with ultraviolet-light therapy (2). Thus it is possible that lack of sunlight rather than phytate-induced calcium malabsorption was responsible for the rickets in these children.

Another source of calcium deficiency–induced bone disease is TPN. Early in the development of TPN therapy, inadvertent omission of calcium led to rickets that was reversed by addition of calcium (4). Today relative lack of calcium in the TPN solutions may be in part responsible for the osteopenia and rickets of prematurity (11).

Pathogenesis

The pathogenesis of calcium-deficiency rickets is similar to that of vitamin D–deficiency rickets in that hypocalcemia causes secondary hyperparathyroidism. Parathyroid hormone increases bone resorption and enhances the renal conversion of 25 (OH) D to 1,25 (OH)$_2$ D to increase intestinal calcium and phosphorus absorption. Alkaline phosphatase also reflects elevated osteoblastic bone cell activity. Both the patients of Kooh et al. (12) and those of Pettifor et al. (13,14) had normal serum 25 (OH) D levels, demonstrating that they were not vitamin D deficient. The patients of Kooh et al. were hypophosphatemic, whereas those from South Africa were not.

Clinical manifestations of calcium-deficiency rickets are similar to those described for vitamin D deficiency.

Treatment and Prevention

In the cases described from Canada and South Africa, oral calcium treatment was given (12–14), as shown in Table 1. Response to treatment was assessed by reduction in serum alkaline phosphatase levels and improvement in roentgenographic and histologic abnormalities. Special premature baby formulas now contain 75 to 150 mg calcium/dL. Currently approximately 200 mg/kg/day is the goal for daily oral calcium intake (15). Parenteral solutions contain from 20 to 60 mg calcium/dL (10). Use of solutions containing 20 mg/dL of calcium resulted in a 20% incidence of rickets

and osteopenia among premature infants in an intensive care nursery (16). Experience with 60 mg calcium/dL has been too limited to determine whether it reduces the incidence of rickets.

PHOSPHATE DEFICIENCY

Phosphate deficiency has been reported to cause rickets and osteomalacia. During the early development of TPN, omission of phosphate resulted in rickets that resolved with appropriate phosphate supplementation (4). However, premature infants may still receive inadequate phosphate relative to their needs (11). The calcium and phosphate added to parenteral nutrition solutions are limited by the possibility of calcium phosphate precipitation. According to Mierzwa (17), the following equation may serve as a guide to determining whether calcium and phosphate will precipitate in solutions:

$$\text{Phosphate (mmol)} \times 1.8/\text{Volume (L)} = A \qquad [1]$$

$$\text{Calcium gluconate (mg)} \times (4.6/1000)/\text{Volume (L)} = B \qquad [2]$$

If A × B is <300, the parenteral nutrition solution is not likely to precipitate. Preliminary reports indicate that newer amino acid formulations supplemented with the sulfur-containing amino acids taurine and cysteine allow greater quantities of calcium and phosphate to remain in solution in TPN formulations (17).

Nutritional hypophosphatemic rickets has also been reported in a premature infant who was breast-fed without calcium or phosphate supplements (18).

Others at risk for hypophosphatemic osteomalacia include those who have been taking antacids for long periods (19) and those patients receiving dialysis who have osteomalacia (see Chapter 69). Antacid-induced osteomalacia results from aluminum complexation with dietary phosphate in the intestinal lumen, which prevents phosphate absorption. Aluminum itself does not become deposited in bone in significant quantities (19).

Pathogenesis

The pathogenesis of phosphate-deficiency rickets differs from that of vitamin D and calcium deficiency in that neither hyperparathyroidism nor vitamin D deficiency is present. Patients become phosphate deficient, causing a reduction in serum phosphorus. Phosphate deficiency and hypophosphatemia increase renal production of 1,25 (OH)$_2$ D. 1,25-Dihydroxyvitamin D increases bone resorption *in vitro*, and it is possible but not proven that elevated serum levels of 1,25 (OH)$_2$ D cause bone resorption in these patients (18), although there is evidence that it may do so in adults (20).

Treatment and Prevention

Recommended parenteral phosphate intake for premature infants and phosphate and calcium supplementation regimens for breast-fed prematures are given in Table 1. Roentgenographic changes of rickets resolved in one breast-fed infant after 3 months of calcium and phosphate supplementation (18). However, these recommendations may not be sufficient to ensure optimal bone mineral content (15). The phosphate available in specialized premature infant formulas is approximately 75 mg/dL (15). Long-term evaluation must be completed before we can conclude that this supplementation is effective in reducing the incidence of osteopenia and rickets in prematures.

For patients requiring long-term antiulcer therapy, use of non–aluminum-containing medications such as histamine-receptor antagonists should be considered.

REFERENCES

1. Klein GL, Simmons DJ. Nutritional rickets: thoughts on pathogenesis. *Ann Med* 1993;25:379–386.
2. Stamp TCB. Factors in human vitamin D nutrition and in the production and cure of classical rickets. *Proc Nutr Soc* 1975;34:119–130.
3. Sandstead HH. Clinical manifestations of certain classical deficiency diseases. In: Goodhart RS, Shils ME, eds. *Modern nutrition in health and disease.* 6th ed. Philadelphia: Lea & Febiger, 1980:693–696.
4. Klein GL, Chesney RW. Metabolic bone disease associated with total parenteral nutrition. In: Lebenthal E, ed. *Total parenteral nutrition: indication, utilization, complications, and pathophysiological considerations.* 1st ed. New York: Raven Press, 1986:431–443.
5. Shike M, Sturtridge WC, Tam CS, et al. A possible role of vitamin D in the genesis of parenteral nutrition, induced metabolic bone disease. *Ann Intern Med* 1981;95:560–568.
6. Muhe L, Lulseged S, Mason KE, Simoes EA. Case-control study of the role of nutritional rickets in the risk of developing pneumonia in Ethiopian children. *Lancet* 1997;349:1801–1804.
7. Mukherjee A, Battacharyya AIG, Barkar PC. Kwashiorkor, marasmus syndrome and nutritional rickets: a bone biopsy study. *Trans R Soc Trop Med Hyg* 1991;85:688–689.
8. Shah BR, Finberg L. Single day therapy for vitamin D-deficiency rickets: a preferred method. *J Pediatr* 1994;125:487–490.
9. Sedman AB, Klein GL, Merritt RJ, et al. Evidence of aluminum loading in infants receiving intravenous therapy. *N Engl J Med* 1985;312:1337–1343.
10. Koo WWK, Kaplan LA, Bendon R, et al. Response to aluminum in parenteral nutrition during infancy. *J Pediatr* 1986;109:877–883.
11. Hillman LS. Neonatal osteopenia: diagnosis and management. In: Frame B, Potts JT Jr, eds. *Clinical disorders of bone and mineral metabolism.* Amsterdam: Excerpta Medica, 1983:427–430.
12. Kooh SW, Fraser D, Reilly BJ, Hamilton JR, Gall DG, Bell L. Rickets due to calcium deficiency. *N Engl J Med* 1977;297:1264–1266.
13. Pettifor JM, Ross FP, Travers R, Glorieux FH, DeLuca HF. Dietary calcium deficiency: a syndrome associated with bone deformities and elevated serum 1,25-dihydroxyvitamin D concentrations. *Metab Bone Dis Rel Res* 1981;2:301–306.
14. Marie PJ, Pettifor JM, Ross FP, Glorieux FH. Histological osteomalacia due to dietary calcium deficiency in children. *N Engl J Med* 1982; 307:584–588.
15. Greer FR, Steichen JJ, Tsang RC. Effects of increased calcium, phosphorus and vitamin D intake on bone mineralization in very low birth weight infants fed formulas with polycose and medium chain triglycerides. *J Pediatr* 1982;100:951–955.
16. Koo WWK, Oestreich A, Tsang RC, Sherman R, Steichen J. Natural history of rickets and fractures in very low birth weight (VLBW) infants during infancy [Abstract 255]. *J Bone Miner Res* 1986;1:123.
17. Mierzwa MW. Stability and compatibility in preparing TPN solution. In: Lebenthal E, ed. *Total parenteral nutrition: indications, utilization, complications, and pathophysiological considerations.* 1st ed. New York: Raven Press, 1986:219–230.
18. Rowe JC, Wood DH, Rowe DW, Raisz LG. Nutritional hypophosphatemic rickets in a premature infant fed breast milk. *N Engl J Med* 1979;300:293–296.
19. Carmichael KA, Fallon MD, Dalinka M, Kaplan FS, Axel L, Haddad JG. Osteomalacia and osteitis fibrosa in a man ingesting aluminum hydroxide antacid. *Am J Med* 1984;76:1137–1143.
20. Maierhofer WJ, Gray RW, Cheung H, Lemann J Jr. Bone resorption stimulated by elevated serum 1,25(OH)$_2$-vitamin D concentrations in healthy men. *Kidney Int* 1983;24:555–560.

62. Metabolic Bone Disease of Total Parenteral Nutrition

Gordon L. Klein, M.D., M.P.H.

Departments of Pediatrics and Preventive Medicine, University of Texas Medical Branch, Galveston, Texas

Total parenteral nutrition (TPN) is a therapeutic regimen designed to provide for the administration of all nutritional requirements in a concentrated solution infused into either a central or a peripheral vein. This method of treatment is generally used in patients with gastrointestinal disease severe enough to prevent adequate oral or enteral nutrition. Because parenteral requirements for various nutrients are unknown and because the purity of individual intravenous solutions is variable, TPN therapy may be subject to the inadequate provision of certain nutrients as well as to the inadvertent contamination of solutions with toxic substances. Bone disease may be a manifestation of the various deficiencies or toxicities.

Bone disease resulting from inadequate provision of calcium or phosphate in the TPN solution was discussed in Chapter 61. This chapter deals with bone disease brought about by aluminum toxicity in adults. It also covers the role of aluminum in the metabolic bone disease in infants and children receiving long-term TPN therapy.

BONE DISEASE IN ADULTS

Clinical Presentation

The initial and, in many cases, only clinical presentation of bone disease in a group of patients studied in Los Angeles and Seattle was periarticular bone pain, especially in weight-bearing bones, lower back, or ribs. The pain presented from 2 to 36 months after initiation of TPN therapy, increased in intensity, and did not respond to narcotic analgesics. In some instances, movement was so painful that patients confined

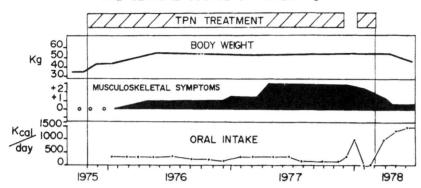

THE CLINICAL COURSE OF PATIENT #1

FIG. 1. Changes in bone pain in relation to total parenteral nutrition (TPN) therapy in the index case with TPN bone disease. (Modified from Klein GL, Targoff CM, Ament ME, et al. Bone disease associated with total parenteral nutrition. *Lancet* 1980;2:1041–1044.)

themselves to bed. Improvement occurred only when TPN treatment was discontinued (1; Fig. 1). However, only about 20% of the patients evaluated prospectively were symptomatic.

Roentgenographic Findings

Approximately 80% of patients evaluated had diffuse osteopenia (1). Photon absorptiometry of the radius in one patient revealed decreased bone mineral content. Neutron-activation studies in a similar series of patients in Toronto revealed that bone mass decreased to the level seen in osteoporosis in 60% of the subjects, whereas 40% had intermediate values between normal and osteoporotic (2).

Histologic Evaluation

Within 4 months of initiating TPN treatment, hyperkinetic, rapidly turning-over bone (increased formation and resorption) was described, which changed to low-turnover osteomalacia after at least 1 year of therapy (3). Patchy osteomalacia was found in patients from Los Angeles and Seattle who had bone biopsies performed after at least 1 year of TPN. Increased unmineralized osteoid and decreased bone formation were seen (Fig. 2).

Biochemical Features

In both the Canadian and American reports, serum calcium and phosphorus levels were normal or mildly elevated. Serum levels of alkaline phosphatase were often elevated, but the cholestatic complications of TPN treatment interfered with interpretation. A striking hypercalciuria, often with negative calcium balance, was found in most TPN patients. Because the hypercalciuria resolved when TPN was stopped, and because the urinary calcium excretion was not related to serum levels of immunoreactive parathyroid hormone (iPTH), the hypercalciuria was thought to be due to increased filtered load of calcium from the exogenously administered calcium and possibly the protein load in the TPN solutions (1,4).

Serum levels of iPTH were in the low-normal range, whereas serum levels of 1,25-dihydroxyvitamin D [1,25 (OH)₂ D] were very low, giving rise to the possibility of TPN-induced hypoparathyroidism. However, when calcium was removed from the TPN solution in two patients, serum PTH levels rose without any detectable rise in serum levels of 1,25 (OH)₂ D. Serum levels of 25-hydroxyvitamin D [25 (OH) D] and 24,25-dihydroxyvitamin D were normal (5). Cessation of TPN treatment in one patient with low serum levels of 1,25 (OH)₂ D resulted in a rise in serum levels to normal within 6 weeks after discontinuing TPN treatment (5), thus raising the possibility that a component of the TPN solution was acting as a toxin.

Aluminum

Because osteomalacia with decreased bone formation had been observed in patients with renal failure undergoing hemodialysis and because aluminum accumulation in bone had been previously observed (6), bone biopsies were obtained from TPN patients. Aluminum content in biopsy specimens was elevated, up to 30 times normal, and elevated aluminum levels also were found in plasma and urine (7). Analysis of the TPN solutions revealed that casein hydrolysate was found to contain large quantities of aluminum, up to 1 mg/L, which provided a parenteral aluminum intake of 2000 to 3000 μg/day (7). Substitution for casein hydrolysate of a synthetic amino acid mixture containing only about 2% of the aluminum in casein resulted in an acute decline in plasma aluminum concentration and urinary aluminum excretion. However, aluminum retention by tissues such as bone persisted for up to 3 years after discontinuation of casein (4,8).

The primary route of aluminum excretion is urinary. However, patients receiving TPN have relatively normal renal function (7). One possibility for the accumulation of aluminum in patients with normal renal function is the fact that plasma ultrafilterable aluminum is only about 5% of total plasma aluminum (8). Therefore most circulating aluminum is protein bound and not filtered. We suggested that there are at least two pools of aluminum in the body: a rapidly exchangeable pool that is quickly depleted on reduction or cessation of aluminum loading and a slowly exchangeable pool, which may represent a tissue pool in equilibrium with plasma.

Proposed Pathogenesis of the Adult Form of TPN Bone Disease

Aluminum has been localized by aurin tricarboxylic acid stain to the mineralization front of bone, both in patients

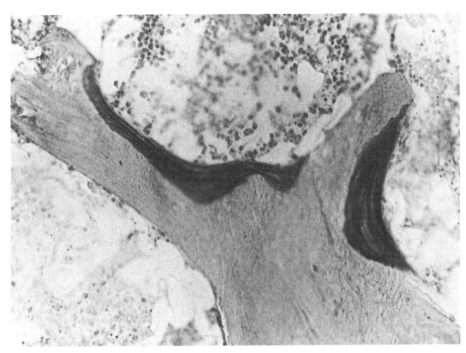

FIG. 2. Goldner's trichrome stain of an iliac crest bone biopsy of a patient with total parenteral nutrition (TPN) bone disease, magnification ×160. Mineralized bone is shown in gray; unmineralized osteoid is shown in black. This patient has patchy areas of excessive unmineralized osteoid, one of the diagnostic features of osteomalacia. (Photograph courtesy of Dr. D.J. Sherrard, VA Medical Center, Seattle, WA.)

with TPN bone disease and in those with dialysis osteomalacia (see Chapters 27 and 69). Under conditions of chronic aluminum loading, the extent of surface-stainable aluminum in bone correlates very closely with quantitative bone aluminum determined by flameless atomic absorption spectroscopy. However, surface-stainable bone aluminum was inversely correlated with rate of bone formation (6; Fig. 3).

FIG. 3. Correlation between bone formation rate and stainable aluminum in patients receiving total parenteral nutrition who had received casein hydrolysate. The values for bone aluminum are plotted on a logarithmic scale. (From Ott SM, Maloney NA, Klein GL, et al. Aluminum is associated with low bone formation in patients receiving chronic parenteral nutrition. *Ann Intern Med* 1983;98:910–914, with permission.)

It remains unknown whether aluminum impairs bone formation directly by affecting bone, indirectly by accumulating in the parathyroid glands and interfering with PTH secretion (6), by altering vitamin D metabolism (6), or by a combination of these mechanisms.

Role of Vitamin D

Removal of vitamin D from the TPN solutions resulted in low serum levels of 25 (OH) D but no clinical or histologic manifestations of bone disease (3). In another study patients receiving chronic parenteral nutrition failed to develop osteomalacia even though they received amounts of vitamin D comparable to the quantities postulated to produce osteomalacia in aluminum-loaded patients (9). Although vitamin D is in standard multivitamin mixes for parenteral use, the role of vitamin D in the pathogenesis of TPN bone disease remains open to question.

Treatment and Prevention

Replacement of casein hydrolysate, the chief source of aluminum from the TPN solutions, with a synthetic amino acid solution resulted in reduction of bone pain and hypercalciuria, improvement in bone-formation rate, and return of serum levels of 1,25 (OH)$_2$ D to normal (4). Whether aluminum reduction was the only factor resulting in improvement is not certain because the amounts of protein and vitamin D$_2$ in the TPN solution also were reduced (4). The reduction in protein content may have corrected the hypercalciuria, although it was probably not responsible for the increase in bone-formation rate (4). It also is unlikely that the reduction in vitamin D content played a major role in the increased bone-formation rate.

At least one report showed that bone histology in TPN patients is heterogeneous in the absence of stainable bone aluminum (10). Bone-formation rate was not lower than in normal subjects but was higher than that in aluminum-toxic TPN patients (10). Another study described low-turnover TPN bone disease in the absence of stainable bone aluminum but with elevated serum aluminum levels (11).

Bone biopsies in aluminum-loaded patients who had casein hydrolysate removed from their TPN solutions showed inverse relations between bone-formation rate and surface-stainable aluminum and between bone-formation rate and plasma aluminum (4). This latter relation suggests that plasma aluminum, even before it accumulates in bone, reduces bone formation. It would appear that TPN bone disease can be reduced or eliminated if care is taken to avoid contamination of the solution with calcium-containing additives. Because the current aluminum content of TPN solutions is highly variable, measurements of aluminum in blood, urine, and TPN solution is advisable in patients who develop bone disease while receiving TPN therapy.

Two concerns remain. First, the attribution of metabolic bone disease to TPN therapy may be mistaken if preexisting bone disease is not excluded. Malabsorption of vitamin D, calcium, or phosphorus, for example, could result in osteomalacia caused by gastrointestinal disease. Elderly women requiring TPN treatment may have postmenopausal osteoporosis. Therefore evaluation of bone density, histology, and biochemistry early in the course of TPN therapy can help to determine the presence of preexisting metabolic bone disease.

Second, the recent report of long-term persistence of low bone density in TPN patients (12) suggests that either TPN treatment fails to improve osteopenia produced by a preexisting condition or TPN treatment itself contributes to the persistence of this problem in a still-unspecified way.

BONE DISEASE IN INFANTS

Long-term treatment with TPN has been associated with rickets or osteopenia in premature infants (13). Although insufficient provision of calcium or phosphate may be primarily responsible for the rickets, aluminum loading may be a complicating factor. Evidence supporting this is as follows.

Significant quantities of aluminum may still be found in TPN solutions, mainly in calcium and phosphate salts, heparin, and albumin (13). These sources can result in aluminum concentrations of some TPN solutions from 30 to 306 μg/L (14,15) (see Table 1).

This concentration of aluminum can result in aluminum administration to premature infants of 15 to 30 μg/kg/day (15). Adult patients with normal renal function receiving TPN who were loaded with aluminum to the point of bone toxicity received 60 μg/kg/day, whereas others receiving long-term TPN therapy with crystalline amino acids instead of casein hydrolysate received only 1 μg/kg/day. The latter groups had no evidence of elevated serum, urine, or bone content of aluminum (15). Thus premature infants receive aluminum in TPN solutions intermediate between known safe and known toxic amounts.

Because renal function in premature infants is developmentally reduced, the risk of aluminum retention is increased. Older term infants receiving chronic TPN treatment retain approximately 75% of the intravenous aluminum load (13).

In premature infants, aluminum has been observed to accumulate in bone, blood, and urine, occasionally to high levels (13,14). Autopsy specimens of vertebrae from two infants who died while receiving TPN revealed a positive aurin tricarboxylic acid stain for aluminum at the level of the mineralization front (14). Thus premature infants receiving TPN therapy may accumulate aluminum in bone at the mineralization front in a manner similar to that of adults.

Although accumulation of aluminum at the mineralization front in premature infants is not by itself evidence of aluminum toxicity, aluminum accumulation in bone has been associated with decreased bone formation and osteomalacia in adults (6).

In addition, long-term TPN therapy in three infants led to rickets despite the provision of 1000 IU (25 μg daily vitamin D_2 in the TPN solution. The rickets finally resolved after high-dose vitamin D_2 (ergocalciferol in oil) was given (16). The reason for vitamin D–dependent rickets with long-term TPN therapy is unclear. However, all three patients were subsequently found to have accumulated large quantities of aluminum.

Treatment and Prevention

Every attempt should be made to provide, especially to premature infants, as much calcium and phosphate as permit-

TABLE 1. *Sources of aluminum in common intravenously administered products*[a]

Solution	Number of lots tested	Aluminum content, μg/L	Ref.
Potassium phosphate	3	16,598 $\pm$ 1801	13
Sodium phosphate	1	5977	13
10% Calcium	5	5056 $\pm$ 335	13
Heparin (1000 $\pm$ gm/ml)	3	684 $\pm$ 761	13
25% Normal serum albumin	4	1822 $\pm$ 2503	13
Trace metal solution	7	972 $\pm$ 108	11

[a] Values are given as mean $\pm$ SD.

ted by the TPN solution. Although the United States Food and Drug Administration recently proposed standards for the aluminum content of parenteral-solution components (17), until manufacturers reduce the aluminum content of these products, periodic monitoring of infants receiving TPN for roentgenographic evidence of bone disease is recommended. Furthermore, until aluminum content of intravenous solutions is regulated, other groups of patients receiving aluminum-contaminated parenteral solutions, such as burn patients (18), also may develop the osteopenia of low bone formation. Periodic determinations of serum levels of calcium, phosphorus, PTH, 25 (OH) D, and 1,25 $(OH)_2$ D can identify associated hyperparathyroidism and vitamin D deficiency [low 25 (OH) D]. If bone disease persists despite maximal calcium and phosphate supplementation, and if 24-hour urine excretion of calcium and phosphorus does not exceed intake, then aluminum in plasma, urine, and the TPN solution should be obtained. Specimens must be collected in plastic containers and sent to a specialized laboratory for analysis.

Plasma aluminum concentration exceeding 100 μg/L and/or urine aluminum/creatinine (μg/mg) greater than 0.3 (normal, <0.05) requires analysis of the components of the TPN solution for aluminum content: Inform the hospital pharmacy of the source(s) of the high levels of aluminum so that they may inform the manufacturer and possibly stop or reduce TPN. Although deferoxamine therapy has been useful in chelating aluminum from the bones of adults with dialysis osteomalacia, there has been insufficient experience with this drug in infants to recommend its general use. Moreover, use of deferoxamine in one infant was reported to be associated with sustained hypocalcemia (19), raising concerns about its safety in this age group.

REFERENCES

1. Klein GL, Targoff CM, Ament ME, et al. Bone disease associated with total parenteral nutrition. *Lancet* 1980;2:1041–1044.
2. Harrison JE, Jeejeebhoy KN, Track NS. The effect of total parenteral nutrition (TPN) on bone mass. In: Coburn JW, Klein GL, eds. *Metabolic bone disease in total parenteral nutrition.* Baltimore: Urban & Schwarzenberg, 1985:53–61.
3. Jeejeebhoy KN, Shike M, Sturtridge WC, et al. TPN bone disease at Toronto. In: Coburn JW, Klein GL, eds. *Metabolic bone disease in total parenteral nutrition.* Baltimore: Urban & Schwarzenberg, 1985:17–29.
4. Vargas JH, Klein GL, Ament ME, et al. Metabolic bone disease of total parenteral nutrition: course after changing from casein to amino acids in parenteral solutions with reduced aluminum content. *Am J Clin Nutr* 1988;48:1070–1078.
5. Klein GL, Horst RL, Norman AW, Ament ME, Slatopolsky E, Coburn JW. Reduced serum levels of 1,25-dihydroxyvitamin D during long term parenteral nutrition. *Ann Intern Med* 1981;94:638–643.
6. Ott SM, Maloney NA, Klein GL, et al. Aluminum is associated with low bone formation in patients receiving chronic parenteral nutrition. *Ann Intern Med* 1983;98:910–914.
7. Klein GL, Alfrey AC, Miller NL, et al. Aluminum loading during total parenteral nutrition. *Am J Clin Nutr* 1982;35:1425–1429.
8. Klein GL, Ott SM, Alfrey AC, et al. Aluminum as a factor in the bone disease of long-term parenteral nutrition. *Trans Assoc Am Physicians* 1982;95:155–164.
9. Shike M, Shils ME, Heller A, et al. Bone disease in prolonged parenteral nutrition: osteopenia without mineralization defect. *Am J Clin Nutr* 1986;44:89–98.
10. Lipkin EW, Ott SM, Klein GL. Heterogeneity of bone histology in parenteral nutrition patients. *Am J Clin Nutr* 1987;46:673–680.
11. DeVernejoul MC, Messing B, Modrowski D, Bielakoff J, Buisine A, Miravet L. Multifactorial low remodeling bone disease during cyclic total parenteral nutrition. *J Clin Endocrinol Metab* 1985;60:109–113.
12. Saitta JC, Ott SM, Sherrard DJ, et al. Metabolic bone disease in adults in long-term parenteral nutrition: longitudinal study with regional densitometry and bone biopsy. *J Parenter Enter Nutr* 1993;17:214–219.
13. Sedman AB, Klein GL, Merritt RJ, et al. Evidence of aluminum loading in infants receiving intravenous therapy. *N Engl J Med* 1985;312:1337–1343.
14. Koo WWK, Kaplan LA, Bendon R, et al. Response to aluminum in parenteral nutrition during infancy. *J Pediatr* 1986;109:877–883.
15. Klein GL. Unusual sources of aluminum. In: DeBroe ME, Coburn JW, eds. *Aluminum and renal failure.* Boston: Kluwer Academic, 1990:203–211.
16. Klein GL, Cannon RA, Diament M, et al. Infantile vitamin D-resistant rickets associated with total parenteral nutrition. *Am J Dis Child* 1982;136:74–76.
17. Food and Drug Administration. Aluminum in large and small volume parenterals used in total parenteral nutrition: proposed rule. *Fed Reg* 1998;63:176–185.
18. Klein GL, Rutan TC, Herndon DN, et al. Bone disease in burn patients. *J Bone Miner Res* 1993;8:337–345.
19. Klein GL, Snodgrass WR, Griffin MP, Miller NL, Alfrey AC. Hypocalcemia complicating deferoxamine therapy in an infant with parenteral nutrition-associated aluminum overload: evidence for a role of aluminum in the bone disease of infants. *J Pediatr Gastroenterol Nutr* 1989;9:400–403.

63. Vitamin D-Dependent Rickets

Uri A. Liberman, M.D., Ph.D. and *Stephen J. Marx, M.D.

*Division of Endocrinology and Metabolism, Rabin Medical Center, Beilinson Campus, Sackler Faculty of Medicine, Tel Aviv University, Petach-Tikva, Israel; and *Genetics and Endocrinology Section, National Institute of Diabetes and Digestive and Kidney Diseases, National Institutes of Health, Bethesda, Maryland*

Vitamin D-dependent rickets (VDDR), types I and II, are rare inborn errors of vitamin D metabolism, characterized by all of the classic clinical, radiologic, biochemical, and histologic features of vitamin D deficiency (see Chapter 61) despite adequate vitamin D intake and without a therapeutic response to an accepted vitamin D–replacement therapy. The two syndromes differ (Table 1) in the circulating concentration of 1,25-dihydroxyvitamin D [1,25 $(OH)_2$ D], the

therapeutic response to 1-hydroxylated active vitamin D metabolites, and obviously in the primary defect in vitamin D metabolism.

VITAMIN D-DEPENDENT RICKETS TYPE I

Prader et al. (1) in 1961 were the first to report two young children with VDDR-I and coined the phrase "pseudovita-

TABLE 1. *Vitamin D-dependent rickets (VDDR)*

	Serum concentrations				
	Calcium	25 (OH) D	1,25 (OH)$_2$ D	iPTH	Presumed defect
VDDR I	↓	N- ↓	↓ ↓	↑	Renal 25 (OH) D 1-hydroxylase
VDDR II	↓	N- ↓	N- ↑	↑	Intracellular 1,25 (OH)$_2$ D receptor

iPTH, immunoreactive parathyroid hormone.

min D deficiency'' to describe this syndrome. The disease manifests itself before age 2 years and often during the first 6 months of life. Complete remission could be obtained but was dependent on continuous therapy with high doses of vitamin D. Family studies revealed this to be a genetic disorder with a pattern suggestive of autosomal recessive inheritance (2), and linkage analysis assigned the gene responsible for the disease to chromosome 12q14. It was shown very recently that decidua cells isolated from term placenta of two patients with VDDR-I were unable to synthesize calcitriol, in contrast to control decidual cells (3). This may imply that there is a defect in the renal tubular 25-hydroxyvitamin D [25 (OH) D] 1-hydroxylase as well. Several indirect measurements support this notion. First, serum concentrations of 25 (OH) D were normal or markedly elevated in patients treated with high doses of vitamin D or 25 (OH) D$_3$. Second, blood levels of 1,25 (OH)$_2$ D were very low in several studies of children with VDDR-I. Finally, whereas massive doses of vitamin D and 25 (OH) D$_3$ (1000 to 3000 μg/day and 200 to 900 μg/day, respectively, 100 to 300 times the recommended daily dose) are required to maintain remission of rickets in VDDR-I, 0.25 to 1.0 μg/day of 1,25 (OH)$_2$ D$_3$ (a normal physiologic dose) are sufficient to achieve the same effect. Taken together, these observations support the thesis that many if not all patients with VDDR-I have a hereditary defect in the renal tubular 25 (OH) D-1-hydroxylase. The beneficial therapeutic effect of high circulating levels of 25 (OH) D in patients with VDDR-I treated with vitamin D or 25 (OH) D$_3$, where 1,25 (OH)$_2$ D concentrations remain low, has several possible explanations. First, 25 (OH) D at high concentrations may activate the specific intracellular receptor for 1,25 (OH)$_2$ D whose affinity of 25 (OH) D is about two orders of magnitude lower than for the active hormone (see Chapter 15). Second, high concentrations of the substrate 25 (OH) D may drive the local production of 1,25 (OH)$_2$ D in some tissues in a paracrine or autocrine manner. Finally, a metabolite of 25 (OH) D may act directly on target tissues (4).

VITAMIN D-DEPENDENT RICKETS TYPE II

In 1978, Brooks et al. (5) described a patient with hypocalcemia, osteomalacia, and elevated circulating levels of 1,25 (OH)$_2$ D. Treatment with vitamin D$_3$ resulted in a further increase in serum 1,25 (OH)$_2$ D levels and corrected the hypocalcemia of the patient. The term "vitamin D-dependent rickets type II'' was suggested to describe this disorder. Based on additional case reports, in which about half of the patients with this disorder did not respond to any form of vitamin D therapy and therefore were not dependent on the vitamin, and some *in vivo* and *in vitro* studies to be

discussed, the term VDDR-II seems to be a misnomer. We therefore suggest the term "hereditary resistance to 1,25 (OH)$_2$ D'' as more appropriate to describe this syndrome. However, because of convention and convenience, the term VDDR-II is retained in this chapter.

Clinical Manifestations

The clinical, radiologic, histologic, and biochemical characteristics common to all patients with VDDR-II are rickets and/or osteomalacia of varying severity; no history or biochemical evidence of vitamin D or calcium deficiency; hypocalcemia and/or secondary hyperparathyroidism; no remission with physiologic doses of vitamin D or its active metabolites; and increased serum levels of 1,25 (OH)$_2$ D before or during treatment with calciferol preparations (6).

Patients with VDDR-II show the highest serum levels of 1,25 (OH)$_2$ D found in any living system. These levels could represent the result of synergistic action of three potential stimulators of the 25 (OH) D-1-hydroxylase: hypocalcemia, secondary hyperparathyroidism, and hypophosphatemia; or they might also reflect an additional defect in regulation of the renal hydroxylase.

There are fewer than 50 known kindreds with this syndrome (a partial list in references 6–31). Contrary to the homogeneity of the clinical and biochemical presentation of VDDR-I, a marked heterogeneity exists in VDDR-II.

Affected children appear normal at birth, and the metabolic bone disease presents early, usually before age 2 years. However, late onset of the disease was reported in several sporadic cases, presenting in some patients in their teens (5); in one patient, the onset of osteomalacia was at age 45 years (10). All cases with late presentation have been normocalcemic, and they represent the mildest form of the disease.

A peculiar feature of the syndrome that appears in about two thirds of the kindreds is alopecia, which varies from sparse hair to total alopecia without eyelashes (Fig. 1). In some patients, additional ectodermal anomalies, such as multiple milia, epidermal cysts (Fig. 1), and oligodontia, appear as well (9). The alopecia may be obvious at birth but usually develops during the first months of life. Alopecia seems to be a marker of a more severe form of the disease, as judged by the earlier age of the presentation of the disease, the marked clinical aberrations, the number of patients who did not respond to treatment with high doses of vitamin D and metabolites (in contrast to the complete remission achieved in almost all patients with normal hair), and the high levels of serum 1,25 (OH)$_2$ D recorded during successful and unsuccessful therapy (6,32). Although some patients with alopecia have a satisfactory calcemic response to high doses of vita-

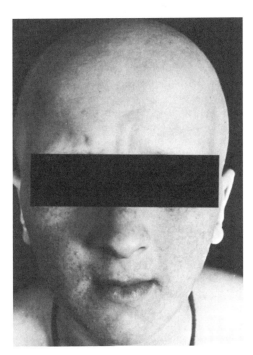

FIG. 1. A patient with vitamin D-dependent rickets type II (VDDR-II): total alopecia, multiple milia, and epidermal cysts.

min D and metabolites, none has shown improvement of hair growth.

The notion that total alopecia is probably a direct consequence of resistance to 1,25 (OH)$_2$ D is supported by the following observations: (a) alopecia is present in kindreds with different biochemical and molecular defects in the 1,25 (OH)$_2$ D receptor–effector system; (b) high-affinity uptake of [^{3}H]1,25 (OH)$_2$ D$_3$ occurred in the nucleus of the outer root-sheath cells of the hair follicle of rodents; and (c) the epidermis and hair follicles contain a calcium-binding protein that is at least partially vitamin D dependent. Alopecia has been observed only with end-organ resistance to 1,25 (OH)$_2$ D and has not been noted with hereditary or acquired states associated with low circulating levels of 1,25 (OH)$_2$ D. Thus either the deficiency in vitamin D action is more severe in VDDR-II or, alternatively, 1,25 (OH)$_2$ D may have an effect on differentiation of the hair follicle in the fetus that is unrelated to mineral homeostasis.

Parental consanguinity and multiple siblings with the same defect occur in about half of the reported kindreds with VDDR-II, suggesting an autosomal recessive mode of inheritance in these and perhaps all kindreds. Parents of patients appear phenotypically normal. However, *in vitro* studies of cultured cells (see the following discussion) from parents of some kindreds with VDDR-II revealed heterogeneity of their 1,25 (OH)$_2$ D$_3$ receptor (VDR; i.e., expression of both a normal and an abnormal VDR allele). The affected children expressed only the abnormal allele (23,24). There is a striking clustering of patients close to the Mediterranean, and most of the patients reported from Europe and North America are descendants of families originating from around the Mediterranean as well. Notable exceptions are several kindreds reported from Japan (10,11,22).

Classification by Cellular Defect

Studies on the nature of the intracellular defect in the 1,25 (OH)$_2$ D receptor–effector system of patients with VDDR-II became possible with demonstration that cells originating from tissues easily accessible for biopsy contain receptors for the hormone that are similar if not identical to those of classic target tissues. The cells used are mainly dermal fibroblasts, but keratinocytes, cells derived from bone, and, recently, peripheral blood mononuclear (PBM) cells [mitogen-stimulated T lymphocytes and Epstein–Barr (EB) virus–transformed lymphocytes] have been used as well (6,12–16,24,25,33–35). These cells are used to assess most of the steps in 1,25 (OH)$_2$ D action from cellular uptake to bioresponse and to elucidate the molecular aberrations in the hormone-receptor protein and the nuclear DNA that encodes for it (23,24). The latter became feasible with the recent cloning and sequencing of the human VDR chromosomal gene.

Several methods have been used to characterize the hormone–receptor interaction, including binding capacity and affinity of [^{3}H]1,25 (OH)$_2$ D$_3$ to intact cells, nuclei, or high-salt-soluble extract (cytosol) (6,12,13,16); measurements of receptor content by monoclonal antibodies (23,36,37); and characterization of the hormone–receptor complex on continuous sucrose gradient and heterologous DNA-cellulose columns (6,13,19,38). For studies on the molecular defects, isolation, amplification, and sequencing of genomic VDR DNA, as well as cloning and sequencing of VDR complementary DNA (cDNA) and recreation of the mutant VDR *in vitro*, have been used. *In vitro* bioeffects of 1,25 (OH)$_2$ D on the various cells have been assayed by induction of the 25 (OH) D-24-hydroxylase in skin- and bone-derived cells (17,39–41), osteocalcin synthesis in cells derived from bone (41), inhibition of cell proliferation in PBM cells (34,35) and dermal fibroblasts (15,42), a mitogenic effect on dermal fibroblasts (42), and stimulation of cyclic guanosine monophosphate (cGMP) production in cultured skin fibroblasts (43).

Heterogeneity of the cellular and molecular defects of the vitamin D receptor–effector system had been revealed in studies of different kindreds with VDDR-II. However, based on the hormone–receptor nuclear interaction, three different classes of intracellular defects have been identified.

1. Hormone-binding defects. These include:
   a. Markedly decreased capacity (number of binding sites was about 10% of controls) in one patient, who did not respond to prolonged treatment with high doses of active calciferol metabolites (14).
   b. Decreased hormone-binding affinity. [^{3}H]1,25 (OH)$_2$ D$_3$ binding affinity is reduced 20- to 30-fold with normal binding capacity of soluble (cytosolic) dermal fibroblasts extract. A complete remission of the disease in these patients could be achieved by high doses of vitamin D or its active metabolites (21,30). An additional patient, recently described, had a modest decrease of the affinity of the receptor for 1,25 (OH)$_2$ D$_3$ when measured at 0°C and a substantial decrease in affinity of approximately eightfold when the binding was measured at 24°C. A missense point mutation in the VDR gene encoding the hormone-binding domain was elucidated (30).

c. No hormone binding. Unmeasurable specific binding of [³H]1,25 (OH)₂ D₃ to either high-salt-soluble cell extract and/or intact cells or nuclei. This is the most common abnormality observed. In the majority of these patients, high concentrations of 1,25 (OH)₂ D in serum or culture medium did not evoke a biologic or biochemical response in vivo or in vitro. Recently different point mutations in the DNA region transcribing the hormone-binding domain of VDR were described (26,36,37). In five affected kindreds, the nucleotide substitution resulted in a stop codon in the coding sequence (which was different for each kindred), thus causing a truncated receptor having no or only a nonfunctional part of the hormone-binding site of the VDR. In an additional patient, a missense mutation resulted in the substitution of arginine by leucine (26). It is of interest that in a cotransfection assay, normal transcription could be induced in the presence of 1000-fold higher levels of the hormone than were needed for the wild-type VDR. This may indicate that the mutation caused an extreme decrease in the affinity of the receptor to 1,25 (OH)₂ D₃.

2. Deficient nuclear localization. Normal or near-normal binding affinity and capacity of [³H]1,25 (OH)₂ D₃ binding to soluble cell extract was seen with normal binding to heterologous DNA but unmeasurable localization of [³H]1,25 (OH)₂ D₃ to nuclei in intact cells (12,16,27,31). An identical defect was demonstrated with cells cultured from a bone biopsy of one patient (12) and in mitogen-stimulated PBM cells from several kindreds (22). These patients were treated successfully with high doses of vitamin D and its active metabolites (7,12,27,31). No mutation was found on sequencing VDR cDNA of some of these patients (37). However, recently two VDDR unrelated patients were described with a lowered 1,25 (OH)₂ D₃ retention in intact cells incubated at 37°C. Two different point mutations leading to impaired heterodimerization with a retinoid X receptor (RXR), the magnitude of the defect, the response in vivo to the hormone, and in vitro to 1,25 (OH)₂ D₃ and RXR were different between these two missense mutations (31).

3. Normal or near-normal [³H]1,25 (OH)₂ D₃ binding to soluble cell extract and to nuclei of intact cells, but decreased affinity of the hormone–receptor complex to heterologous DNA (19,24,38). No biologic response to high doses of vitamin D or its active metabolites either in vivo or in vitro was documented in almost all patients with this type of defect (9,19,38). Recently a single nucleotide missense mutation within exon 2 or 3 encoding the DNA-binding domain of the VDR was demonstrated in genomic DNA isolated from fibroblasts and/or EB virus–transformed lymphocytes from members from eight unrelated kindreds with this defect (24,25,28,29,44). Different single-nucleotide mutations were found, with the exception of two unrelated patients that share the same defect. All mutations caused a single amino acid substitution localized to the region of the two zinc fingers of the VDR protein. This region is essential for DNA binding of the hormone–receptor complex. The DNA-binding domain of the VDR is evolutionarily highly conserved throughout all members of the v-ERB-A–related proteins that include the receptors for steroid hormones, thyroid hormones, and retinoic acid.

Measurements of an in vitro bioresponse of cells to 1,25 (OH)₂ D₃ were carried out in less than half of the kindreds with VDDR-II. Induction of 25 (OH) D-24-hydroxylase by 1,25 (OH)₂ D₃ in cultured dermal fibroblasts showed an invariable correlation to the therapeutic response to vitamin D and metabolites in vivo (17,27,39,40,44).

A mouse model of the disease was created by targeted ablation of the second zinc finger of the VDR-DNA binding domain. Homozygous mice who were phenotypically normal at birth developed hypocalcemia, secondary hyperparathyroidism, rickets, osteomalacia, and alopecia with normal survival to at least 6 months (45).

Treatment

If the predictive therapeutic value of the in vitro bioresponse to 1,25 (OH)₂ D₃ could be substantiated, it may eliminate the need for expensive and time-consuming therapy trials with vitamin D and metabolites. In the meantime, it is mandatory to treat every patient with VDDR-II, regardless of the type of receptor defect. An adequate therapeutic trial must include (a) vitamin D alone for the mildest cases, though in more severe typical cases, therapy should be initiated with high doses of vitamin D analogs that will ensure maintenance of high serum concentrations of 1,25 (OH)₂ D (this can be accomplished by treatment with 1,25 (OH)₂ D₃ or 1α (OH) D₃ at daily doses in the range of up to 6 μg/kg body weight or a total of 30 to 60 μg); (b) supplemental calcium of up to 3 g elementary calcium per day; and (c) a duration of therapy (about 3 to 5 months) sufficient to mineralize depleted bones and thus allow recovery from the hypocalcemia of hungry bones. Close follow-up is essential and consists of clinical signs and symptoms; bone radiographs; serum levels of calcium, phosphorus, alkaline phosphatase, and creatinine; urinary excretion of calcium, phosphorus, and creatinine; parameters of parathyroid function; and serum 1,25 (OH)₂ D levels. Failure of therapy may be considered if no change in any of these parameters occurs during the treatment period while 1,25 (OH)₂ D serum levels are maintained above 100 times the mean normal range. It was reported recently that remarkable clinical and biochemical remission, including catch-up growth and histologic healing of defective osteoid mineralization, was achieved by long-term therapy with high-dose oral calcium in one patient (46) or long-term intracaval infusion of calcium in several unusual patients with VDDR-II who did not respond to adequate trial with active vitamin D metabolites (41,47,48). These important studies imply that clinical remission could be achieved by calcium administration even in the most resistant patients with VDDR-II.

CONCLUSION

In summary, two inborn errors in vitamin D metabolism are presented and discussed. The important message is not just the description of a rare curiosity of nature but rather the finding that rare aberrations of natural metabolic processes are important to unveil basic physiologic, biochemical, and molecular mechanisms in general and in human beings in particular.

REFERENCES

1. Prader A, Illig R, Heierli E. Eline besondere Form der primaren vitamin D-resistenten Rachitis mit Hypocalcemie und autoso- mal-dominanten Erbgang: Die hereditare Psuedo-Mangelrachi tis. *Helv Paediatr Acta* 1961;16:452–468.

2. Scriver CR, Fraser D, Kooh SW. Hereditary rickets. In: Heath D, Marx SJ, eds. *Calcium disorders.* London: Butterworth, 1982:1–46.

3. Glorieux FH, Azabian A, Delvin EE. Pseudo-vitamin D deficiency: absence of 25-hydroxyvitamin D 1-hydroxylase activity in human placenta decidual cells. *J Clin Endocrinol Metab* 1995;80:2255–2258.

4. Harmeyer JV, Grabe C, Winkley I. Pseudovitamin D deficiency rickets in pigs: an animal model for the study of familial vitamin D dependency. *Exp Biol Med* 1982;7:117–125.

5. Brooks MH, Bell NH, Love L, et al. Vitamin D dependent rickets type II, resistance of target organs to 1,25-dihydroxyvitamin D. *N Engl J Med* 1978;293:996–999.

6. Marx SJ, Liberman UA, Eil C, Gamblin GT, DeGrange DA, Balsan S. Hereditary resistance to 1,25-dihydroxyvitamin D. *Recent Prog Horm Res* 1984;40:589–620.

7. Marx SJ, Spiegel AM, Brown EM, et al. A familial syndrome of decrease in sensitivity of 1,25-dihydroxyvitamin D. *J Clin Endocrinol Metab* 1978;47:1303–1310.

8. Rosen JF, Fleischman AR, Finberg L, Hamstra A, DeLuca HF. Rickets with alopecia: an inborn error of vitamin D metabolism. *J Pediatr* 1979;94:729–735.

9. Liberman UA, Samuel R, Halabe A, et al. End-organ resistance to 1,25-dihydroxy cholecalciferol. *Lancet* 1980;1:504–506.

10. Fujita T, Nomura M, Okajima S, Suzuya H. Adult-onset vitamin D-resistant osteomalacia with unresponsiveness to parathyroid hormone. *J Clin Endocrinol Metab* 1980;50:927–931.

11. Tsuchiya Y, Matsuo N, Cho H, et al. An unusual form of vitamin D-dependent rickets in a child: alopecia and marked end-organ hyposensitivity to biological active vitamin D. *J Clin Endocrinol Metab* 1980;51:685–690.

12. Eil C, Liberman UA, Rosen JF, Marx SJ. A cellular defect in hereditary vitamin D-dependent rickets type II: defective nuclear uptake of 1,25-dihydroxyvitamin D in cultured skin fibroblasts. *N Engl J Med* 1981;304:1588–1591.

13. Feldman D, Chen T, Cone C, et al. Vitamin D resistant rickets with alopecia: cultured skin fibroblasts exhibit defective cytoplasmic receptors and un- responsiveness to 1,25(OH)$_2$D$_3$. *J Clin Endocrinol Metab* 1982;55:1020–1025.

14. Balsan A, Garabedian M, Liberman UA, et al. Rickets and alopecia with resistance to 1,25-dihydroxyvitamin D: two different clinical courses with two different cellular defects. *J Clin Endocrinol Metab* 1983;57:803–811.

15. Clemems TL, Adams JC, Horiuchi N, et al. Interaction of 1,25-dihydroxyvitamin D$_3$ with keratinocytes and fibroblasts from skin of a subject with vitamin D-dependent rickets type II: a model for the study of action of 1,25-dihydroxyvitamin D$_3$. *J Clin Endocrinol Metab* 1983;56:824–830.

16. Liberman UA, Eil C, Marx SJ. Resistance of 1,25-dihydroxyvitamin D: association with heterogeneous defects in cultured skin fibroblasts. *J Clin Invest* 1983;71:192–200.

17. Chen TL, Hirst MA, Cone CM, Hochberg Z, Tietze HU, Feldman D. 1,25-dihydroxyvitamin D resistance, rickets and alopecia: analysis of receptors and bioresponse in cultured skin fibroblasts from patients and parents. *J Clin Endocrinol Metab* 1984;59:383–388.

18. Hochberg Z, Benderli Z, Levy J, Weisman Y, Chen T, Feldman D. 1,25-dihydroxyvitamin D resistance, rickets, and alopecia. *Am J Med* 1984;77:805–811.

19. Hirst MA, Hochman HI, Feldman D. Vitamin D resistance and alopecia: a kindred with normal 1,25-dihydroxyvitamin D$_3$ binding, but decreased receptor affinity for deoxyribonucleic acid. *J Clin Endocrinol Metab* 1985;60:490–495.

20. Fraher LJ, Karmali R, Hinde FRJ, et al. Vitamin D-dependent rickets type II: extreme end organ resistance to 1,25-dihydroxyvitamin D$_3$ in a patient without alopecia. *Eur J Pediatr* 1986;145:389–395.

21. Castells S, Greig F, Fusi MA, et al. Severely deficient binding of 1,25-dihydroxyvitamin D to its receptor in a patient responsive to high doses of this hormone. *J Clin Endocrinol Metab* 1986;63:252–256.

22. Tajkeda E, Kuroda Y, Saijo T, et al. 1-Hydroxyvitamin D$_3$ treatment of three patients with 1,25-dihydroxyvitamin D-receptor-defect rickets and alopecia. *Pediatrics* 1987;80:97–101.

23. Malloy PJ, Hochberg Z, Pike JW, Feldman D. Abnormal binding of vitamin D receptors to deoxyribonucleic acid in a kindred with D dependent rickets, type II. *J Clin Endocrinol Metab* 1989;68:263–269.

24. Hughes MR, Malloy PJ, Kieback DG, et al. Point mutations in the human vitamin D receptor gene associated with hypocalcemia rickets. *Science* 1988;242:1702–1705.

25. Stone T, Marx SJ, Liberman UA, Pike JW. A unique point mutation in the human vitamin D receptor chromosomal gene confers hereditary resistance to 1,25-dihydroxyvitamin D$_3$. *Mol Cell Endocrinol* 1990;4:623–631.

26. Kristjansson K, Rut AR, Hewison M, O'Riordan JLF, Hughes MR. Two mutations in the hormone binding domain of the vitamin D receptor cause tissue resistance to 1,25 dihydroxyvitamin D$_3$. *J Clin Invest* 1993;92:12–16.

27. Hewison M, Rut AR, Kristjansson K, et al. Tissue resistance to 1,25-dihydroxyvitamin D without a mutation in the vitamin D receptor gene. *Clin Endocrinol* 1993;39:663–670.

28. Yagi H, Ozono K, Miyake H, Nagashima K, Kuraum T, Pike JW. A new point mutation in the deoxyribonucleic acid-binding domain of the vitamin D receptor in a kindred with hereditary 1,25-dihydroxyvitamin D resistant rickets. *J Clin Endocrinol Metab* 1993;76:509–512.

29. Saijjo T, Ito M, Takeda E, et al. A unique mutation in the vitamin D receptor gene in three Japanese patients with vitamin D-dependent rickets type II: utility of single-strand conformation polymorphism analysis for heterozygous carrier detection. *Am J Hum Genet* 1991;49:668–673.

30. Malloy PJ, Eccleshall TR, Gross C, Van Maldergem L, Bouillon R, Feldman D. Hereditary vitamin D resistant rickets caused by a novel mutation in the vitamin D receptor that results in decreased affinity for hormone and cellular hyporesponsiveness. *J Clin Invest* 1997;99:297–304.

31. Whitfield GK, Selznick SH, Haussler CA, et al. Vitamin D receptors from patients with resistance to 1,25-dihydroxyvitamin D$_3$: point mutations confer reduced transactivation in response to ligand and impaired interaction with the retinoid X receptor heterodimeric partner. *Mol Endocrinol* 1996;10:1617–1631.

32. Marx SJ, Bliziotes MM, Nanes M. Analysis of the relation between alopecia and resistance to 1,25-dihydroxyvitamin D. *Clin Endocrinol* 1986;25:373–381.

33. Liberman UA, Eil C, Holst P, Rosen JF, Marx JS. Hereditary resistance to 1,25-dihydroxyvitamin D: defective function of receptors for 1,25-dihydroxyvitamin D in cells cultured from bone. *J Clin Endocrinol Metab* 1983;57:958–962.

34. Koren R, Ravid A, Liberman UA, Hochberg Z, Weisman J, Novogrodsky A. Defective binding and function of 1,25-dihydroxyvitamin D$_3$ receptors in peripheral mononuclear cells of patients with end-organ resistance to 1,25-dihydroxyvitamin D. *J Clin Invest* 1985;76:2012–2015.

35. Takeda E, Kuzoda Y, Saijo T, et al. Rapid diagnosis of vitamin D-dependent rickets type II by use of phytohemagglutinin-stimulated lymphocytes. *Clin Chim Acta* 1986;155:245–250.

36. Malloy PJ, Hochberg Z, Tiosano D, Pike JW, Hughes MR, Feldman D. The molecular basis of hereditary 1,25-dihydroxyvitamin D$_3$ resistant rickets in seven related families. *J Clin Invest* 1990;86:2017–2079.

37. Weise RJ, Goto H, Prahl JM, et al. Vitamin D-dependency rickets type II: truncated vitamin D receptor in three kindreds. *Mol Cell Endocrinol* 1993;90:197–201.

38. Liberman UA, Eil C, Marx SJ. Receptor positive hereditary resistance to 1,25-dihydroxyvitamin D: chromatography of hormone-receptor complexes on DNA-cellulose shows two classes of mutation. *J Clin Endocrinol Metab* 1986;62:122–126.

39. Griffin JE, Zerwekh JE. Impaired stimulation of 25-hydroxyvitamin D-24-hydroxylase in fibroblasts from a patient with vitamin D-dependent rickets, type II. *J Clin Invest* 1983;72:1190–1199.

40. Gamblin GT, Liberman UA, Eil C, Downs RW Jr, DeGrange DA, Marx SJ. Vitamin D-dependent rickets type II, defective induction of 25-hydroxyvitamin D$_3$24-hydroxylase by 1,25-dihydroxyvitamin D$_3$ in cultured skin fibroblasts. *J Clin Invest* 1985;75:954–960.

41. Balsan S, Garabedian M, Larchet M, et al. Long-term nocturnal calcium

infusions can cure rickets and promote normal mineralization in hereditary resistance to 1,25-dihydroxyvitamin D. *J Clin Invest* 1986;77:1661–1667.

42. Barsony J, McKoy W, DeGrange DA, Liberman UA, Marx SJ. Selective expression of a normal action of 1,25-dihydroxyvitamin D₃ receptor in human skin fibroblasts with hereditary severe defects in multiple action of this receptor. *J Clin Invest* 1989;83:2093–2101.

43. Barsony J, Marx SJ. Receptor-mediated rapid action of 1-25-dihydroxycholecalciferol: increase of intracellular cGMP in human skin fibroblasts. *Proc Natl Acad Sci USA* 1988;85:1223–1226.

44. Rut AR, Hewison K, Kristjansson K, Luisi B, Hughes MR, O'Riordan JLH. Two mutations causing vitamin D resistant rickets: modelling on the basis of steroid hormone receptor DNA-binding domain crystal structures. *Clin Endocrinol* 1994;41:581–590.

45. Li YC, Pirro AE, Amling M, et al. Targeted ablation of the vitamin D receptor: an animal model of vitamin D-dependent rickets type II with alopecia. *Proc Natl Acad Sci USA* 1997;94:9831–9835.

46. Sakati N, Woodhouse NTY, Niles N, Harji H, DeGrange DA, Marx SJ. Hereditary resistance to 1,25-dihydroxyvitamin D: clinical and radiological improvement during high-dose oral calcium therapy. *Horm Res* 1986;24:280–287.

47. Weisman Y, Bab I, Gazit D, Spirer Z, Jaffe M, Hochberg Z. Long-term intracaval calcium infusion therapy in end-organ resistance to 1,25-dihydroxyvitamin D. *Am J Med* 1987;83:984–990.

48. Bliziotes M, Yergey AL, Nanes MS, et al. Absent intestinal response to calciferols in hereditary resistance to 1,25-dihydroxyvitamin D: documentation and effective therapy with high dose intravenous calcium infusions. *J Clin Endocrinol Metab* 1988;66:294–300.

64. Hypophosphatemic Vitamin D-Resistant Rickets

Francis H. Glorieux, M.D., Ph.D.

Departments of Surgery and Pediatrics, McGill University, and Shriners Hospital, Montreal, Quebec, Canada

Bone growth and mineralization require adequate availability of calcium and phosphate, the two major constituents of hydroxyapatite, which is the crystalline part of bone tissue. Defective supply of either calcium or phosphate will result in impaired mineralization, which will cause rickets at the growth-plate level and osteomalacia at the corticoendosteal level. Thus in growing individuals, both lesions will be present, whereas by definition, only osteomalacia can possibly develop in adults.

Deficiency in calcium, as a consequence of either insufficient intake (1) or vitamin D simple deficiency or abnormal metabolism (2), will induce hypocalcemia, rickets, and osteomalacia. The latter will be characterized by osteopenia, as a consequence of the increased resorption induced by hyperparathyroidism secondary to hypocalcemia.

In chronic hypophosphatemia, although clinical and radiologic manifestations of rickets are similar to those seen in calcium deficiency, osteomalacia is characterized by an accumulation of unmineralized osteoid along the trabeculae. Because calcemia is normal, there is no secondary hyperparathyroidism and therefore no increased osteoclast activity or excessive resorption. Consequently, bone mass is not decreased. It is, in fact, often measured above normal values for age.

CLASSIFICATION OF HYPOPHOSPHATEMIC SYNDROMES

There are acquired and congenital forms of hypophosphatemia. In most instances, the acquired forms can be controlled by acting on the underlying causes (insufficient phosphate intake, increased renal loss secondary to a mesenchymal tumor or an altered tubular function). However, the inherited syndromes present a challenge sometimes for diagnosis and always for management. The most frequent of the hypophosphatemic syndromes was described more than 50 years ago by Albright (3), who coined the term "hypophosphatemic vitamin D–resistant rickets." It is inherited as an X-linked dominant trait (4) with the mutant gene being located in the distal part of the short arm of the X chromosome (5); thus it is often referred to as X-linked hypophosphatemia (XLH or HYP). In 1976, a homologous mutation was discovered in the mouse (Hyp) (6). The high degree of conservatism of the mammalian X chromosome and comparative mapping of the human and mouse gonosomes (7) support the contention of a close analogy between the human and murine mutations. Active studies have thus been pursued in parallel in the two species to better understand the phenotypic expression of the abnormal genes.

CLINICAL EXPRESSION

The classic triad, fully expressed in hemizygous male patients, consists of (a) hypophosphatemia, (b) lower limb deformities, and (c) stunted growth rate. Although low serum phosphate (P) is evident early after birth, it is only at the time of weight bearing that leg deformities and progressive departure from normal growth rate become sufficiently striking to attract attention and make parents seek medical opinion. An often overlooked clinical sign is the appearance of the teeth. There is no enamel hypoplasia in XLH, as opposed to what is seen in hypocalcemic rickets. Hypophosphatemic rickets rather presents with dentin defects not apparent on examination but that may cause dental abscesses and early decay in the young adult. In several families, isolated hypophosphatemia can be found in some heterozygous female subjects. Thus this trait is considered the marker for the mutation (4). These healthy trait carriers provide evidence that hypophosphatemia and renal P waste cannot solely explain the abnormal phenotype.

BASIC DEFECT

Several studies based on genetic linkage and multilocus analysis have allowed fine mapping of the HYP gene to the

Xp22.1-22.2 region of the X chromosome between markers DXS41 and DXS43. There is, however, accumulating evidence for possible locus heterogeneity in X-linked hypophosphatemic rickets (8). The question will be resolved by the identification of the mutant gene(s) by positional cloning. A major step in that direction has been made by the isolation of a candidate gene in the HYP region (9). This gene, first called *PEX* and subsequently *PHEX,* codes for a membrane-bound endopeptidase. Further characterization of its full sequence and tissue expression will be needed to dissect its role in phosphate homeostasis. *PHEX* mutations have been identified in a large number of XLH kindreds as well as in patients with no family history (9,10). The latter point indicates that familial and sporadic cases share a similar etiology.

The most intriguing question regarding XLH concerns the primary lesion causing the disease. It has long been accepted that hypophosphatemia is the consequence of a primary inborn error of phosphate transport, probably located in the proximal nephron. It is noteworthy that the defect is less severe in female heterozygotes than it is in male hemizygotes (11). This gene–dose effect indicates that the observed defect is close to the abnormal gene product. The abnormality in the Hyp mouse has been localized to the brush border of the proximal tubular cells (12). The possibility that it would be secondary to the presence of a humoral hypophosphatemic factor (13) has received experimental support from kidney cross-transplantation studies in the mouse model (14).

Because of the close link between the phosphate-repletion status and 1,25-dihydroxyvitamin D [1,25 (OH)$_2$ D] synthesis, the metabolism of this hormone has been extensively studied in mutant individuals. It is important to point out that there is no simple 1,25 D deficiency (as seen in vitamin D pseudodeficiency) and that there is no close correlation between extracellular P concentration and 1,25 D synthesis. Rather the reported inappropriate response of 1,25 D synthesis to a low phosphate challenge (15), although there is no abnormality in the response to a low calcium challenge (16), points to the vitamin D metabolism abnormality being secondary to the primary P transport defect and its consequences on intracellular P economy.

Studies both in human and mouse indicate that defective bone formation in X-linked hypophosphatemia is linked to an intrinsic osteoblast defect. The hypomineralized periosteocytic lesions (HPLs), which are a hallmark of XLH, never completely disappear, even after active mineralization has been restored at the endosteal surfaces. After more than 2 years of efficient therapy, HPLs are still present around 20% of the osteocytes in the newly formed osteons (17). As HPLs are never present in other chronic hypophosphatemic states, this observation gives substance to the early proposal that there may be an osteoblast primary metabolic defect in XLH (18). The lesions are also present in the Hyp mouse (19), in which an abnormal osteoblast response to 1,25 D has been demonstrated (20). Studies conducted with osteoblasts isolated from mouse calvaria have provided morphologic evidence that Hyp osteoblasts, even when transplanted in a normal environment, are unable to produce adequate amounts of mineralized matrix (21). Deletions in the *Phex* gene have been reported in the Hyp mouse, which confirms definitely its validity as a model for XLH (22). It is interesting that *Phex* is predominantly expressed in normal osteo-blasts, whereas the transcript is not detectable in Hyp osteoblasts (23). This suggests that a bone gene product may be part of a pathway that regulates phosphate homeostasis and underscores the central role of an osteoblast defect in the etiology of XLH. Unraveling this mechanism must await the identification of the putative circulating factor, which may be a natural substrate for the PHEX protein.

RESPONSE TO TREATMENT

Based on the established renal P waste, therapy has centered on often aggressive P replacement (1 to 3 g elemental P/day in four to five doses). To offset the hypocalcemic effect of P supplementation, which has sometimes caused severe secondary hyperparathyroidism, large (20 to 75,000 IU/day) amounts of vitamin D were added to the regimen. With adequate compliance to such a combined treatment, growth rate improved markedly, and there was radiologic evidence of healed rickets (24,25). The early observation that heterozygous girls responded better to treatment than hemizygous boys (24) was substantiated, supporting the concept of a gene–dose effect in this X-linked dominant disorder (26). However, histologic studies of iliac crest bone biopsies showed that the osteomalacic component of the bone disease was hardly improved (27). It was only by substituting 1,25 D to vitamin D at the dose of 30 to 70 ng/kg/day that improvement and sometimes healing of the mineralization defect was observed on the trabecular surfaces (28–31).

LONG-TERM EFFECTS OF TREATMENT

Except for occasional osmotic diarrhea, P supplementation has not caused any harmful effects. Coated tablets should be preferred to liquid forms, as they provide a slower rate of absorption. Tablets are also made of a mixture of sodium and potassium salts, avoiding the high sodium load so frequent with the solutions.

Before 1978, large amounts of vitamin D were administered to offset the hypocalcemic effect of P supplementation and the ensuing iatrogenic hyperparathyroidism. This was often difficult to control, and several cases of autonomous hyperparathyroidism were encountered that could only be treated surgically (24). The substitution of 1,25 D for vitamin D has now allowed a more precise control of parathyroid hormone (PTH) secretion throughout the treatment period. It thus appears that 1,25 D, through its direct effect on PTH release, is able to maintain PTH levels within acceptable limits, together with ensuring adequate bone modeling and remodeling (30–32). Interestingly, this may also be the case for 24,25 (OH)$_2$ D$_3$. A placebo-controlled trial based on the addition of the metabolite (10 μg/day) to the standard protocol (1,25 D and phosphate) showed that better control of the therapy-induced hyperparathyroidism was achieved over a 2-year period (33).

One major concern with long-term administration of 1,25 D is a possible deterioration of renal function through interstitial nephrocalcinosis. Frequent ultrasound observations of echodense renal pyramids have been reported (34). Histologic studies confirmed that they correspond to mineral deposits exclusively made of calcium phosphate (35). Whether the induction of such deposits is primarily related to the phosphate load or to the long-term use of 1,25 D is not clear. Such findings are, however, not directly related to evidence of decreased renal function. Our experience with 18 patients treated for an average of 8 years indicates that two thirds of them present with profiles of increased echogenicity of the renal pyramids (too quickly labeled nephrocalcinosis), but no alteration of renal function (unpublished data). Thus long-term use of 1,25 D associated with supplemental P and with frequent monitoring of urinary calcium excretion to avoid episodes of hypercalciuria should be considered a safe and efficient way to control the clinical expression of the PHEX mutation. When hypercalciuria develops, adjustment of the 1,25 D dosage is necessary.

Because stunted growth is a major consequence of the XLH phenotype, the use of recombinant human growth hormone (rhGH), as a third therapeutic component, also was advocated (36). The hormone increased serum P levels, and over a 24-week period, appeared to positively affect growth rate, in 11 XLH children. These results have been substantiated by long-term (2 to 3 years) studies showing that adding rhGH to phosphate and 1,25 D had a significant positive effect on growth in young XLH patients (37,38). These studies have not been extended through the completion of the growth process (closure of the epiphysis), so it is premature to conclude that the basic treatment protocol should be uniformly modified.

TREATMENT OF ADULT PATIENTS

With early initiation of therapy and good compliance throughout the growing period, clinical results are usually satisfactory in terms of stature achieved and prevention of lower-limb deformities. An important question is whether one should maintain the demanding treatment schedule combining 1,25 D and phosphate, after fusion of the epiphyseal plates. Because growth has ceased and bone turnover is reduced, the appropriateness of maintaining a high phosphate intake can rightly be questioned. The demonstration that in 18 symptomatic XLH adult patients, who received P + 1,25 D for 4 years, the treatment resulted in significant clinical and histomorphometric improvement (39), suggests that such an approach is worthwhile. Its optimal duration, however, remains unresolved. Because strict compliance to P supplements on a five-dose per day schedule is difficult, one may envisage that continuing 1,25 D alone, through its stimulation of bone turnover and intestinal phosphate absorption, would maintain the good results obtained with the combined therapy. Preliminary observations in six XLH patients indicated that 1,25 D alone (at a dose of 1 to 2 μg/day) positively influenced the parameters of bone mineralization over an 11- to 17-month period (unpublished data). Such studies should allow better definition of a long-term strategy for metabolic and clinical control of adult XLH patients.

CONCLUSION

Despite the persistent questions about the pathogenesis of XLH, medical control of its clinical expression has greatly improved over the past 15 years. The combination of large amounts of phosphate salts and supraphysiologic doses of 1,25 D has allowed normal growth and adequate bone-matrix mineralization. With close and careful follow-up, the regimen is safe, and no deleterious effects on renal function are to be expected. Uncertainty continues with regard to the treatment of asymptomatic adult subjects.

REFERENCES

1. Marie PJ, Pettifor JM, Ross FP, Glorieux FH. Histologic osteomalacia due to dietary calcium deficiency in children. *N Engl J Med* 1982;307:584.
2. Glorieux FH, Pettifor JM. Metabolic bone disease. In: Kelly VC, ed. *Practice of pediatrics*. Vol 7. New York: Harper & Row, 1984:34.
3. Albright F, Butler AM, Bloomberg E. Rickets resistant to vitamin D therapy. *Am J Dis Child* 1937;54:529.
4. Winters RW, Graham JB, Williams TF, McFalls VW, Burnett CH. A genetic study of familial hypophosphatemia and vitamin D-resistant rickets with a review of the literature. *Medicine* 1958;37:97.
5. Thakker RV, Read AP, Davies KE, et al. Bridging markers defining the map position of X-linked hypophosphatemic rickets. *J Med Genet* 1987;24:756.
6. Eicher EM, Southard JL, Scriver CR, Glorieux FH. Hypophosphatemia: mouse model for human familial hypophosphatemic (vitamin D-resistant) rickets. *Proc Natl Acad Sci USA* 1976;73:4667.
7. Davisson MT. X-linked genetic homologies between mouse and man. *Genomics* 1987;1:213.
8. Rowe PSN. Molecular biology of hypophosphatemic rickets and oncogenic osteomalacia. *Hum Genet* 1994;94:457.
9. Francis F, Henning S, Korn B, et al. A gene (PEX) with homologies to endopeptidases is mutated in patients with X-linked hypophosphatemic rickets. *Nat Genet* 1995;11:150.
10. Dixon PH, Christie PT, Wooding C, et al. Mutational analysis of the PHEX gene in X-linked hypophosphatemia. *J Clin Endocrinol Metab* 1998;33:3615.
11. Glorieux F, Scriver CR. Loss of a PTH sensitive component of phosphate transport in X-linked hypophosphatemia. *Science* 1972;175:997.
12. Tenenhouse HS, Scriver CR, McInnes RR, Glorieux FH. Renal handling of phosphate in vivo and in vitro by the X-linked hypophosphatemic male mouse (Hyp/Y): evidence for a defect in the brush border membrane. *Kidney Int* 1978;14:236.
13. Bonjour J-P, Caverzasio J, Muhlbauer R, Trechsel U, Troechler U. Are 1,25(OH)$_2$D$_3$ production and tubular phosphate transport regulated by one common mechanism which would be defective in X-linked hypophosphatemic rickets? In: Norman AW, Schaefer K, Herrath D, Grigoleit H-G, eds. *Vitamin D: chemical, biochemical and clinical endocrinology of calcium metabolism.* New York: Walter de Gruyter, 1982:427–433.
14. Nesbitt T, Coffman TM, Griffiths R, Drezner MK. Cross-transplantation of kidneys in normal and Hyp mice: evidence that the Hyp mouse phenotype is unrelated to an intrinsic renal defect. *J Clin Invest* 1992;89:1453.
15. Lobaugh B, Drezner MK. Abnormal regulation of renal 25-dihydroxyvitamin D-1 α-hydroxylase activity in the X-linked hypophosphatemic mouse. *J Clin Invest* 1983;71:400.
16. Meyer RA Jr, Gray RW, Roos BA, Kiebzak GM. Increased plasma 1,25-dihydroxyvitamin D after low calcium challenge in X-linked hypophosphatemic mice. *Endocrinology* 1982;111:174.
17. Marie PJ, Glorieux FH. Relation between hypomineralized periosteocytic lesions and bone mineralization in vitamin D-resistant rickets. *Calcif Tissue Int* 1983;35:443.
18. Frost HM. Some observations on bone mineral in a case of vitamin D resistant rickets. *Henry Ford Hosp Med Bull* 1958;6:300.
19. Glorieux FH, Ecarot-Charrier B. X-linked vitamin D-resistant rickets: is osteoblast activity defective? In: Cohn DV, Martin TJ, Meunier PJ, eds. *Calcium regulation and bone metabolism.* Vol 9. Amsterdam: Excerpta Medica, 1987:227–231.
20. Yamamoto T, Ecarot B, Glorieux FH. Abnormal response of osteoblasts from Hyp mice to 1,25-dihydroxyvitamin D$_3$. *Bone* 1992;13:209.
21. Ecarot-Charrier E, Glorieux FH, Travers R, Desbarats M, Bouchard F, Hinek A. Defective bone formation by transplanted Hyp mouse bone cells into normal mice. *Endocrinology* 1988;123:768.

22. Strom TM, Francis F, Lorenz B, et al. *Pex* gene deletions in Gy and Hyp mice provide mouse models for X-linked hypophosphatemia. *Hum Mol Genet* 1997;6:165.
23. Du L, Desbarats M, Viel J, Glorieux FH, Cawthorn C, Ecarot B. cDNA cloning of the murine *pex* gene implicated in X-linked hypophosphatemia and evidence for expression in bone. *Genomics* 1996;36:22.
24. Glorieux FH, Scriver CR, Reade TM, Goldman H, Roseborough A. The use of phosphate and vitamin D to prevent dwarfism and rickets in X-linked hypophosphatemia. *N Engl J Med* 1972;281:481.
25. Verge CF, Lam A, Simpson JM, Cowell CR, Howard NJ, Silink M. Effects of therapy in X-linked hypophosphatemic rickets. *N Engl J Med* 1991;325:1843.
26. Petersen DJ, Boniface AM, Schranck FW, Rupich RC, Whyte MP. X-linked hypophosphatemic rickets: a study (with literature review) of linear growth response to calcitriol and phosphate therapy. *J Bone Miner Res* 1992;7:583.
27. Glorieux FH, Bordier PJ, Marie P, Delvin EE, Travers R. Inadequate bone response to phosphate and vitamin D in familial hypophosphatemic rickets. In: Massry S, Ritz E, Rapada A, eds. *Homeostasis of phosphate and other minerals.* New York: Plenum Press, 1980:227–232.
28. Glorieux FH, Marie PJ, Pettifor JM, Delvin EE. Bone response to phosphate salts, ergocalciferol and calcitriol in hypophosphatemic vitamin-D resistant rickets. *N Engl J Med* 1980;303:1023.
29. Costa T, Marie PJ, Scriver CR, et al. X-linked hypophosphatemia: effect of calcitriol on renal handling of phosphate, serum phosphate, and bone mineralization. *J Clin Endocrinol Metab* 1981;52:463.
30. Drezner MK, Lyles KW, Haussler MR, Harrelson JM. Evaluation of a role for 1,25-dihydroxyvitamin D in the pathogenesis and treatment of X-linked hypophosphatemic rickets and osteomalacia. *J Clin Invest* 1980;66:1020.
31. Harrell RM, Lyles KW, Harrelson JM, Friedman NE, Drezner MK. Healing of bone disease in X-linked hypophosphatemic rickets/osteomalacia: induction and maintenance with phosphorus and calcitriol. *J Clin Invest* 1985;75:1858.
32. Bettinelli A, Bianchi ML, Mazazucchi E, Gandolini G, Appliani AC. Acute effects of calcitriol and phosphate salts on mineral metabolism in children with hypophosphatemic rickets. *J Pediatr* 1991;118:373.
33. Carpenter TO, Keller M, Schwartz D, et al. 24,25-Dihydroxyvitamin D supplementation corrects hyperparathyroidism and improves skeletal abnormalities in X-linked hypophosphatemic rickets: a clinical research center study. *J Clin Endocrinol Metab* 1996;81:2381.
34. Goodyer PR, Kronick JB, Jequier S, Reade TM, Scriver CR. Nephrocalcinosis and its relationship to treatment of hereditary rickets. *J Pediatr* 1987;111:700.
35. Alon U, Donaldson DL, Hellerstein S, Warady BA, Harris DJ. Metabolic and histologic investigation of the nature of nephrocalcinosis in children with hypophosphatemic rickets and in the Hyp mouse. *J Pediatr* 1992;120:899.
36. Wilson DM, Lee PDK, Morris AH, et al. Growth hormone therapy in hypophosphatemic rickets. *Am J Dis Child* 1991;145:1165.
37. Saggese G, Baroncelli GI, Bertelloni S, Perri G. Long-term growth hormone treatment in children with renal hypophosphatemic rickets: effects on growth, mineral metabolism, and bone density. *J Pediatr* 1995;127:395.
38. Seikaly MG, Brown R, Baum M. The effect of recombinant human growth hormone in children with X-linked hypophosphatemia. *Pediatrics* 1997;100:879.
39. Sullivan W, Carpenter T, Glorieux FH, Travers R, Insogna K. A prospective trial of phosphate and 1,25-dihydroxyvitamin D₃ therapy in symptomatic adults with X-linked hypophosphatemic rickets. *J Clin Endocrinol Metab* 1992;75:879.

65. Tumor-Induced Osteomalacia

Marc K. Drezner, M.D.

Department of Medicine, Duke University Medical Center, Durham, North Carolina

TUMOR-INDUCED OSTEOMALACIA

Although McCance described the first case of oncogenic osteomalacia–rickets in 1947, Prader et al. first recognized the causal role of a tumor in this syndrome in 1959. Since that time there have been reports of approximately 120 patients in whom rickets and/or osteomalacia have been induced with various types of tumors (Table 1). With time, the name of the syndrome has varied and included oncogenous osteomalacia, oncogenic osteomalacia, and tumor-induced osteomalacia. In at least 58 cases, a tumor was clearly documented as causing the osteomalacia–rickets, because the metabolic disturbances improved or completely disappeared on removal of the tumor. In the remainder of cases, patients had inoperable lesions, and investigators could not determine the effects of tumor removal on the syndrome, incomplete data are available to judge the effectiveness of a surgical intervention, or surgery did not result in complete resolution of the syndrome during the period of observation. In any case, with greater awareness of the disease, physician-scientists have recognized >50% of known affected subjects within the past decade. The syndrome is characterized, in general, by remission of the unexplained bone disease after resection of the coexisting tumor. Patients usually present with vague symptoms that are of long standing but that generally include bone and muscle pain and muscle weakness, and less often, recurrent fractures of long bones. Additional symptoms manifest in younger patients are fatigue, gait disturbances, slow growth, and skeletal abnormalities, including bowing of the lower extremities. The duration of symptoms before diagnosis ranges from 2.5 months to 19 years, with an average of more than 2.5 years. The age at diagnosis is generally the sixth decade, with a range of 1 to 74 years. Approximately 15% of the patients are younger than 20 years at presentation.

The biochemical findings characterizing this disorder prior to tumor removal include hypophosphatemia and an abnormally low renal tubular maximum for the reabsorption of phosphorus per liter of glomerular filtrate (TmP/GFR), indicative of renal phosphate wasting. The serum phosphorus values average from 0.7 to 2.4 mg/dL in adults and somewhat higher in children, in whom the normal level is considerably higher. After removal of the tumor, the concentration returns to normal. Additional abnormalities include gastrointestinal malabsorption of phosphorus, which coupled with renal phosphorus wasting, results in a negative phosphorus

TABLE 1. *Tumor-induced osteomalacia*

Age/Sex	Symptom duration (yr)	Serum phosphorus		Tumor type
		Preop (mg/dL)	Postop (mg/dL)	
15/F	9.0	2.1	4.7	Degenerated osteoid
11/F	1.0	1.9	4.1	Giant-cell granuloma
55/M	—	2.1	4.7	Malignant neuroma
54/F	6.0	0.9	5.4	Cavernous hemangioma
56/M	3.0	1.4	3.2	Giant-cell tumor
38/M	4.0	1.4	4.6	Sclerosing hemangioma
30/M	3.0	1.2	3.3	Sclerosing hemangioma
47/F	1.5	1.7	3.6	Primary bone tumor (type ?)
40/M	10.0	1.1	3.5	Ossifying mesenchymal tumor
9/F	1.5	1.7	4.8	Nonossifying fibroma
54/M	1.0	1.7	—	Nonossifying fibroma
11/F	3.5	1.7	4.4	Ossifying mesenchymal tumor
36/M	9.0	1.4	4.0	Hemangiopericytoma
51/M	4.0	0.9	1.6	Hemangioma
53/F	5.0	1.2	—	Hemangiopericytoma
58/M	14.0	1.6	—	Hemangiopericytoma
43/F	2.0	1.5	1.8	Hemangiopericytoma
30/M	5.0	0.7	3.5	Fibrous xanthoma
12/M	7.0	1.0	3.9	Fibroangioma
42/F	8.0	1.3	3.2	Giant-cell tumor of bone
18/M	5.0	1.5	4.0	Benign osteoblastoma
18/F	5.0	1.2	5.0	Benign osteoblastoma
44/M	5.0	1.2	3.5	Sarcoma
50/M	—	—	—	Hemangiofibroma
?	—	2.0	4.1	Sclerosing hemangioma
?	—	1.9	—	Atypical chondroma
56/F	8.0	—	—	Cavernous hemangioma
49/F	4.0	1.5	1.5	Mesenchymoma
34/M	0.8	1.8	—	Hemangioma
27/F	—	1.5	3.1	Osteoblastoma
62/F	2.5	1.8	3.6	Benign connective tissue
37/M	6.0	1.7	3.4	Hemangiopericytoma
37/F	1.0	2.2	3.2	Hemangioma
37/M	9.0	1.6	3.4	Hemangiopericytoma
72/M	0.5	1.8	3.4	Neuroma
25/F	1.0	1.5	2.7	Hemangiopericytoma
61/M	0.5	1.4	—	Prostatic carcinoma
74/M	4.0	1.7	—	Prostatic carcinoma
26/M	2.0	1.5	3.1	Brown tumor
14/F	1.0	1.7	3.8	Nonossifying fibroma
15/M	1.0	2.1	4.2	Nonossifying fibroma
56/M	5.0	1.7	1.2	Hemangiopericytoma
65/F	—	—	—	Cavernous hemangioma
44/F	3.0	1.3		Fibroangioma
29/M	2.0	1.3	3.6	Osteosarcoma
64/M	4.0	1.8	2.1	Primary bone tumor (type?)
66/F	2.5	1.3	—	Type?
44/M	1.0	1.2	2.4	Malignant chondroblastoma
57/M	0.3	1.5		Oat cell carcinoma
20/M	1.0	1.6	3.5	Nonossifying fibroma
73/M	—	1.7	—	Giant-cell tumor
40/F	—	1.1	—	Hemangiopericytoma
14/M	—	2.2	—	Odontogenic fibroma
44/M	1.0	1.2	2.4	Malignant chondroblastoma
4 Patients	—	2.0	—	Prostatic carcinoma
44/F	0.3	1.4	2.6	Hemangiopericytoma
48/F	3.0	1.2	3.8	Mesenchymal tumor (type ?)
31/M	9.0	0.9	4.7	Giant-cell fibrous malignant histiocytoma
7/M	5.0	2.6	—	Epidermal nevi
23/F	14.0	1.2	—	Epidermal nevi
44/M	2.0	2.1	3.5	Vascular mesenchymoma

continued

TABLE 1. *Continued.*

Age/Sex	Symptom duration (yr)	Serum phosphorus Preop (mg/dL)	Postop (mg/dL)	Tumor type
57/F	16.0	1.1	2.7	Mixed mesenchymal tumor
73/M	1.0	1.6	3.4	Diffuse giant-cell tumor
19/M	0.5	1.6	3.9	Ossifying fibroma
50/M	3.0	1.8	3.7	Low-grade fibrosarcoma
69/F	—	2.4	3.1	Myelomatosis
70/F	—	2.4	3.0	Chronic lymphocytic leukemia
60/F	2.0	1.2	—	Hemangiopericytoma
54/M	7.0	1.0	3.9	Hemangiopericytoma
40/F	10.0	1.0	—	Neurofibromatosis
53/M	19.0	2.0	6.0	Fibrosarcoma
34/F	1.0	1.3	4.1	Mesenchymal tumor
51/M	6.0	2.1	3.8	Hemangiopericytoma
34/F	2.0	1.2	4.0	Synovial sarcoma
53/F	17.0	1.5	6.0	Benign ossifying mesenchymal tumor of bone
62/M	2.0	1.6	—	Hemangiopericytoma
24/W	1.8	1.6	—	Chondroid, giant-cell tumor
38/W	2.0	1.2	—	Hemangiopericytoma
52/M	—	2.1	—	Polyostotic fibrous dysplasia
8/F	—	2.1	—	Polyostotic fibrous dysplasia
55/M	0.6	2.2	—	Neurofibromatosis
18/M	0.3	—	—	Osteoblastoma
53/M	6.0	1.4	—	Giant-cell tumor
60/F	3.0	—	—	Hemangiopericytoma
70/M	0.3	1.8	—	Prostatic carcinoma
10/M	2.5	1.6	4.4	Nonossifying fibroma
69/M	1.0	1.9	2.7	Transitional cell carcinoma
57/M	7.0	1.2	2.5	Mesenchymal tumor
66/F	3.0	1.8	—	Giant-cell granuloma
32/F	12.0	1.8	—	Mesenchymal chrondrosarcoma
46/M	3.0	1.1	Normal	Osteochondroblastoma
24/M	4.0	1.3	4.2	Mesenchymal tumor
46/M	—	1.2–1.9	—	Small-cell carcinoma
58/F	—	—	—	Mesenchymal spindle cell tumor
54/F	0.5	1.8	—	Angiofibroma
13/F	0.2	1.7	4.1	Nonossifying fibroma
9/M	0.5	1.9	3.2	Hemangiopericytoma
56/F	—	—	—	Hemangioendothelioma
39/F	7.0	2.3	—	Neurofibromatosis
66/M	0.5	1.4	—	Prostatic carcinoma
37/F	1.5	1.6	4.8	Primitive mesenchymal tumor
34/M	1.0	1.6	4.2	Giant-cell chondroma
47/F	7.0	1.4	4.4	Sclerosing hemangioma
41/M	4.0	1.5	4.9	Giant-cell granuloma
32/F	8.0	<2.5	4.6	Ossifying fibroma
60/F	2.0	1.4	2.7	Mesenchymal tumor: mixed connective tissue variant
55/M	2.0	1.5	4.3	Paraganglioma
69/M	1.0	0.5	—	Prostate carcinoma
65/M	—	1.3	—	Prostate carcinoma
1/F	—	2.7	5.0	Epidermal nevi
34/M	2.0	Low	Normal	Vascular tumor
21/M	6.0	0.9	3.5	Extraskeletal chondroma
62/M	8.0	1.0	2.6	Neurinoma
44/F	3.0	0.8	3.0	Hemangiopericytoma
69/F	17.0	Low	—	Mesenchymal tumor
54/M	1.5	1.6	Normal	Hemangiopericytoma
10/M	2.0	1.3	Normal	Benign mesenchymal tumor

balance. The serum levels of 25-hydroxyvitamin D [25 (OH) D] and 24,25-dihydroxyvitamin D [24,25 (OH)$_2$ D] are normal, and the serum 1,25 (OH)$_2$ D concentration generally overtly low or inappropriately normal relative to the hypophosphatemia. Alkaline phosphatase is commonly high, and aminoaciduria, most frequently glycinuria and glucosuria, is occasionally present. Radiographic abnormalities include generalized osteopenia, pseudofractures, and coarsened trabeculae, as well as widened epiphyseal plates in children.

TUMORS

The tumors in patients with tumor-induced osteomalacia have been of mesenchymal origin in the large majority of patients (Table 1). However, the frequent occurrence of Looser zones in the radiographs of moribund patients with carcinomas of epidermal and endodermal derivation (1) indicates that the disease may be secondary to a variety of tumor types. Indeed the recent observation of tumor-induced osteomalacia concurrent with breast carcinoma (2), prostate carcinoma (3–5), oat cell carcinoma (6), small-cell carcinoma (7), multiple myeloma, and chronic lymphocytic leukemia (8) supports this conclusion. The occurrence of osteomalacia in patients with widespread fibrous dysplasia of bone (2,9), neurofibromatosis (10,11) and linear nevus sebaceous syndrome (12,13) could also be tumor induced. Proof of a causal relation has been precluded by the multiplicity of lesions and the consequent inability to effect surgical cure in most patients. However, in one case of fibrous dysplasia (9) and linear nevus sebaceous syndrome (13), removal of virtually all of the abnormal bone or skin lesions, respectively, did result in appropriate biochemical and radiographic improvement.

The mesenchymal tumors associated with this osteomalacia syndrome have been variably described as sclerosing angioma, benign angiofibroma, hemangiopericytoma, chondrosarcoma, primitive mesenchymal tumor, soft-parts chondroma-like tumor, and giant-cell tumor of bone. The diversity of these diagnostic labels underscores the morphologic complexity of these tumors. However, Weidner and Cruz (11) recently established that the histologically polymorphous mesenchymal tumors can be subdivided into four distinct morphologic patterns: (a) primitive-appearing, mixed connective tissue tumors; (b) osteoblastoma-like tumors; (c) nonossifying fibroma-like tumors; and (d) ossifying fibroma-like tumors. The most common of these, the mixed connective tissue variant, occurs in soft tissue, behaves in a benign fashion, and is characterized by variable numbers of primitive-appearing stromal cells growing in poorly defined sheets and punctuated by clusters of osteoclast-like giant cells. Often vascularity also is prominent, but in less-vascular areas, poorly developed cartilage or foci of osteoid or bone are commonly present. The cartilage-like areas sometimes exhibit considerable dystrophic calcification. Likely the primitive stromal cells are the source of the hormonal factor(s) that causes the syndrome. However, immunohistochemical studies have shown no evidence of epithelial, neural, vascular, or neuroendocrine differentiation in these cells. Indeed, these cells are organelle poor and do not have neurosecretory granules. This, of course, does not preclude them from secreting hormonally active substances (probably protein in nature). Whether similar mesenchymal elements exist in the epidermal and endodermal tumors associated with the syndrome remains unknown. However, fibrous mesenchymal components are present in many neural tumors, and metastatic carcinoma of the prostate is frequently associated with an osteoblastic lesion marked by varying degrees of fibrous tissue proliferation. Thus it is possible that the expression of tumor-induced osteomalacia, concurrent with the presence of epidermal or endodermal tumors, depends on the presence and activity of such mesenchymal elements in many cases.

Regardless of the cell type responsible for the syndrome, the tumors at fault often are small, slow-growing, difficult to locate, and present in obscure areas. In this regard, many of the reported lesions have been located in a relatively inaccessible area within bone, such as within the femur or tibia, the nasopharynx, mandible, or a sinus. Alternatively, small lesions have been found in the popliteal region, the groin, the suprapatellar area, and in the brain. In any case, a careful and thorough examination is necessary to document/ exclude the presence of such a tumor. Indeed, computed tomography (CT) and/or magnetic resonance imaging (MRI) scan of any clinically suggestive area should be undertaken. In addition, a technetium-labeled blood pool also has been used successfully to locate tumors. Despite a diligent search, the tumor may elude localization. However, continued follow-up is essential, including repeated periodic attempts at identification of a tumor, because documentation of a tumor often does not happen until the disease has progressed over several years.

PATHOPHYSIOLOGY

The pathophysiologic basis underlying tumor-induced osteomalacia remains unknown. Such incomplete understanding of the disorder undoubtedly relates to its infrequent occurrence and, consequently, the few physiologic studies of the disease. Nevertheless, most investigators agree that tumor production of a humoral factor(s) that may affect multiple functions of the proximal renal tubule, particularly phosphate reabsorption (and result in hypophosphatemia), is the probable pathogenesis of the syndrome. This possibility has been supported by (a) the presence of phosphaturic activity in tumor extracts from three of four patients with tumor-induced osteomalacia (14–16), (b) the occurrence of hypophosphatemia and increased urinary phosphate excretion in heterotransplanted tumor-bearing athymic nude mice (17–19), (c) the inhibition of phosphate uptake in opossum kidney cells by conditioned medium collected from cultured tumor cells obtained from affected patients (20–23), (d) the demonstration that extracts of the heterotransplanted tumor inhibited renal 25-hydroxyvitamin D-1α-hydroxylase activity in cultured kidney cells (17), and (e) the coincidence of aminoaciduria and glycosuria with renal phosphate wasting in some affected subjects, indicative of complex alterations in proximal renal tubular function (24). Indeed, partial purification of ''phosphatonin'' from a cell culture derived from a sclerosing hemangioma causing tumor-induced osteomalacia reaffirmed this possibility (20). These studies reveal that the putative phosphatonin may be a peptide with molecular mass of 8 to 25 kDa, which does not alter glucose or alanine transport but inhibits sodium-dependent phosphate transport. However, recent studies that documented the presence in various disease states of additional phosphate-transport inhibitors (25) indicated that the tumor-induced osteomalacia syndrome is heterogeneous, and phosphatonin may be a family of hormones. In this regard, Rowe et al. (21) reported that screening of conditioned medium from the tumor cells of an affected patient, by using an antiserum raised preoperatively, and subsequent Western analysis revealed the presence of two proteins of 56 and 58 kDa. However, no further characterization or functional studies of these proteins has yet been reported. Thus the pathogenesis of the disorder may be more complicated than currently appreciated.

In any case, abnormal vitamin D metabolism is an additional factor that likely contributes to the pathogenesis of the tumor-induced osteomalacia. Several observations support this possibility including (a) the decreased circulating $1,25 (OH)_2 D$ level observed in virtually all patients who manifest the characteristic syndrome; (b) normalization of the serum $1,25 (OH)_2 D$ concentration rapidly after surgical removal of the coincident tumor, and in association with resolution of the biochemical abnormalities of the syndrome; and (c) diminished renal 25 (OH) D-1α-hydroxylase activity in heterotransplanted tumor-bearing athymic nude mice (26) and in kidney cell cultures exposed to tumor extracts (17). To date, however, no reduction in enzyme activity has been documented in response to tumor cell-conditioned medium (21).

The interrelation between the abnormal renal phosphate transport and the defect in vitamin D metabolism evident in affected subjects remains unknown. An innate heterogeneity in the pathogenesis of the syndrome cannot be excluded. However, an interplay between these abnormalities likely contributes to the phenotypic expression of the disorder in the majority of patients.

Regardless, the mechanism by which the tumor-derived factors function remains unknown. Immunoassay of conditioned medium (20,27) and Northern blot analysis of RNA (22) prepared from cultured tumor cells provided no evidence that the factor is either parathyroid hormone (PTH), PTH-related protein (PTHrP), or the recently described phosphate regulator, human stanniocalcin. However, stimulation of cyclic adenosine monophosphate (AMP) in response to tumor extracts from three affected patients has been demonstrated in a PTH-sensitive renal membrane adenylyl cyclase system (28) and elevated urinary cyclic AMP in a single patient with the syndrome (29), suggesting the involvement of PTH/PTHrP receptors in the activity of the factor. Although two additional studies (20,22) revealed no evidence of cyclic AMP involvement in the renal effects of the putative factor, the inability of these investigators to suppress phosphate inhibitory activity with the PTH analog, [Nle8.18, Tyr34]-3-34 bPTH, does not exclude PTH/PTHrP receptors in the activity of the factor, because such suppression has proven difficult in OK cells (30). Indeed, confirmation of this possibility derives from the observations that the tumor-extract stimulation of renal membrane adenylyl cyclase activity is suppressed by 3-34 bPTH (28), as is the cyclic AMP

stimulation evoked by conditioned medium in an osteosarcoma cell line (22). Further, the inability of Nitzan et al. (18) to detect inhibition of phosphate-uptake inhibitory activity, in response to conditioned medium of tumor cells, by using the JTC-12 cell line that is insensitive to PTH, and the contrasting success of several investigators with PTH-sensitive renal cell lines also are consistent with the hypothesis that PTH/PTHrP receptors may be involved in mediating the activity of the factor.

In any case, in contrast to these observations, patients with tumor-induced osteomalacia secondary to hematogenous malignancy manifest abnormalities of the syndrome caused by a distinctly different mechanism. In these subjects, the nephropathy induced with light-chain proteinuria results in the decreased renal tubular reabsorption of phosphate characteristic of the disease. To date at least 15 patients potentially manifest this form of the disorder (8). In many instances, however, the diagnosis of tumor-induced osteomalacia was not considered. Nevertheless, at least in some cases of this syndrome, renal tubular damage may be mediated by tissue deposition of light chains or of some other immunoglobulin derivative with similar toxic effects on the kidney. Thus light-chain nephropathy must be considered one possible mechanism for the tumor-induced osteomalacia syndrome.

DIFFERENTIAL DIAGNOSIS

The tumor-induced osteomalacia syndrome has all the classic biochemical and radiologic criteria of the hypophosphatemic osteomalacias. Diagnosis is dependent, therefore, on a diligent search for tumors in all patients with hypophosphatemic vitamin D–resistant rachitic/osteomalacic disease. Tumors may range from small to large and benign to malignant. Moreover, the tumor may be present for many years before the clinical appearance of bone disease. Thus regardless of the temporal association between the onset of the osteomalacia and the clinical awareness of tumor, tumor-induced osteomalacia should be considered. Indeed, where possible, resection of any induced tumor should be attempted both to confirm the diagnosis and possibly to induce resolution of the syndrome.

When the tumor cannot be totally resected, diagnosis remains inferential. However, several observations can support the diagnosis: (a) a normal serum 25 (OH) D level; (b) a selective deficiency of $1,25 (OH)_2 D$, manifest by a decreased serum concentration; (c) presence of light-chain proteinuria; (d) demonstration of phosphaturic activity in tumor extracts or the conditioned medium from cultured tumor cells; and/or (e) induction of the tumor-induced osteomalacia syndrome in athymic nude mice on heterotransplantation of tumor tissue from affected subjects.

In the absence of tumor and/or family history of disease, and after exclusion of common causes of osteomalacia, the possibility of adult-onset hypophosphatemic osteomalacia with or without Fanconi's syndrome must be considered. This syndrome may result from acquired or genetic causes, and age of onset is extremely variable. Biochemical abnormalities are indistinguishable from those in patients with tumor-induced osteomalacia. Thus in the absence of genetic transmission of the disorder, careful long-term follow-up for tumor occurrence must be maintained in all patients with hypophosphatemic osteomalacia.

TREATMENT

The first and foremost treatment of tumor-induced osteomalacia is complete resection of the induced tumor. However, recurrence of mesenchymal tumors, such as giant-cell tumors of bone, or inability to resect completely certain malignancies, such as prostatic carcinoma, has resulted in the need for developing effective therapeutic intervention for the tumor-induced osteomalacia syndrome. Historically, pharmacologic doses of vitamin D have been used in an effort to heal the bone disease. For the most part, the trials have been short, and the results have not been assessed in detail. Nevertheless, it appears certain that this treatment does not cure the rachitic or osteomalacic components of the syndrome. Moreover, no resolution of the abnormal biochemistries ensues.

More recently, administration of 1,25 (OH)$_2$ D alone or in combination with phosphorus supplementation served as effective therapy for the tumor-induced osteomalacia. In this regard, Drezner and Feinglos (24) and Lobaugh et al. (31) noted striking improvement of the biochemical and bone abnormalities of the syndrome in response to calcitriol (2.0 to 3.0 μg/day). In two such patients, the serum phosphorus level increased from pretreatment levels of 1.5 $\pm$ 0.7 mg/dL and 2.2 $\pm$ 0.1 mg/dL to normal values of 3.7 $\pm$ 0.03 mg/dL and 2.8 $\pm$ 0.08 mg/dL, respectively. Similarly, the renal TmP/GFR rose from an abnormally low level, 0.8 $\pm$ 0.03 mg/dL and 1.9 $\pm$ 0.03 mg/dL, to normal 3.0 $\pm$ 0.01 mg/dL and 2.8 $\pm$ 0.09 mg/dL. Commensurately, evidence of bone healing was present in bone biopsies from these subjects.

In contrast, several investigators observed only modest symptomatic, biochemical, and histologic improvement in response to calcitriol. However, in general, such patients responded well to combination therapy with pharmacologic amounts of 1,25 (OH)$_2$ D and phosphorus (32). Phosphorus supplementation (2 to 4 g/day) directly replaces the ongoing renal loss of inorganic phosphorus, whereas calcitriol (1.5 to 3 μg/day) serves to replace insufficient renal production of the sterol and to enhance renal phosphate reabsorption. Such therapy normalizes the biochemical abnormalities of the syndrome and results in healing of the osteomalacia. These data indicate that patients with tumor-induced osteomalacia may benefit from a combination drug regimen.

COMPLICATIONS OF THERAPY

Little information is available regarding the long-term consequences of therapy in patients with tumor-induced osteomalacia. The doses of medicines used, however, increase the possibility that nephrolithiasis, nephrocalcinosis, and hypercalcemia may frequently complicate the therapeutic course. Indeed, hypercalcemia secondary to parathyroid hyperfunction was documented in five affected subjects, representing approximately 5% of the reported cases. All of these patients had received phosphorus [as part of a combination regimen with vitamin D$_2$ or 1,25 (OH)$_2$ D], which may have stimulated PTH secretion and ultimately led to parathyroid autonomy. Thus careful assessment of parathyroid function, serum and urinary calcium, and renal function are essential to ensure safe and efficacious therapy.

REFERENCES

1. Dent CE, Stamp TCB. Vitamin D rickets and osteomalacia. In: Avioli LV, Krane S, eds. *Metabolic bone disease.* Vol 1. New York: Academic Press, 1978:237.
2. Dent CE, Gertner JM. Hypophosphatemic osteomalacia in fibrous dysplasia. *Q J Med* 1976;45:411–420.
3. Lyles KW, Berry WR, Haussler M, Harrelson JM, Drezner MK. Hypophosphatemic osteomalacia: association with prostatic carcinoma. *Ann Intern Med* 1980;93:275–278.
4. Murphy P, Wright G, Rai GS. Hypophosphatemic osteomalacia induced with prostatic carcinoma. *Br Med J* 1985;290:1945.
5. Hosking DJ, Chamberlain MJ, Whortland-Webb WR. Osteomalacia and carcinoma of prostate with major redistribution of skeletal calcium. *Br J Radiol* 1975;48:451–456.
6. Leehey DJ, Ing TS, Daugirdas JT. Fanconi syndrome induced with a non-ossifying fibroma of bone. *Am J Med* 1985;78:708–710.
7. Shaker JL, Brickner RC, Divgi AB, Raff H, Findling JW. Case report: renal phosphate wasting, syndrome of inappropriate antidiuretic hormone and ectopic corticotropin production in small cell carcinoma. *Am J Med Sci* 1995;310:38–41.
8. McClure J, Smith PS. Oncogenic osteomalacia. *J Clin Pathol* 1987;40:446–453.
9. Saville PD, Nassim JR, Stevenson FH. Osteomalacia in von Recklinghausen's neurofibromatosis: metabolic study of a case. *Br Med J* 1955;1:1311–1313.
10. Konishi K, Nakamura M, Yamakawa H, et al. Case report: hypophosphatemic osteomalacia in von Recklinghausen neurofibromatosis. *Am J Med Sci* 1991;301:322–328.
11. Weidner N, Cruz DS. Phosphaturic mesenchymal tumors: a polymorphous group causing osteomalacia or rickets. *Cancer* 1987;59:1442–1454.
12. Carey DE, Drezner MK, Hamdan JA, et al. Hypophosphatemic rickets/osteomalacia in linear sebaceous nevus syndrome: a variant of tumor-induced osteomalacia. *J Pediatr* 1986;109:994–1000.
13. Ivker R, Resnick SD, Skidmore RA. Hypophosphatemic vitamin D-resistant rickets, precocious puberty and the epidermal nevus syndrome. *Arch Dermatol* 1997;133:1557–1561.
14. Aschinberg LC, Soloman LM, Zeis PM, Justice P, Rosenthal IM. Vitamin D-resistant rickets induced with epidermal nevus syndrome: demonstration of a phosphaturic substance in the dermal lesions. *J Pediatr* 1977;91:56–60.
15. Yoshikawa S, Nakamura T, Takagi M, Imamura T, Okano K, and Sasaki S. Benign osteoblastoma as a cause of osteomalacia: a report of two cases. *J Bone Joint Surg Br* 1977;59:279–289.
16. Lau K, Strom MC, Goldberg M, et al. Evidence for a humoral phosphaturic factor in oncogenic hypophosphatemic osteomalacia [Abstract]. *Clin Res* 1979;27:421A.
17. Miyauchi A, Fukase M, Tsutsumi M, Fujita T. Hemangiopericytoma-induced osteomalacia: tumor transplantation in nude mice causes hypophosphatemia and tumor extracts inhibit renal 25-hydroxyvitamin D-1-hydroxylase activity. *J Clin Endocrinol Metab* 1988;67:46–53.
18. Nitzan DW, Horowitz AT, Darmon D, et al. Oncogenous osteomalacia: a case study. *Bone Miner Res* 1989;6:191–197.
19. Drezner MK, Lobaugh B, Lyles KW, Carey DE, Paulson DF, Harrelson JM. The pathogenesis and treatment of tumor-induced osteomalacia. In: Norman AW, Schaefer K, Errath DV, Grigoleit HG, eds. *Vitamin D, chemical, biochemical and clinical endocrinology of calcium metabolism.* Berlin: De Gruyter, 1982:949–954.
20. Cai Q, Hodgson SF, Kao PC, et al. Brief report: inhibition of renal phosphate transport by a tumor product in a patient with oncogenic osteomalacia. *N Engl J Med* 1994;330:1645–1649.
21. Rowe PSN, Ong ACM, Cockerill FJ, Goulding JN, Hewison M. Candi-

date 56 and 58 kDA protein(s) responsible for the mediating the renal defects in oncogenic hypophosphatemic osteomalacia. *Bone* 1996;18: 159–169.

22. Nelson AE, Namkung HJ, Patava J, et al. Characteristics of tumor cell bioactivity in oncogenic osteomalacia. *Mol Cell Endocrinol* 1996; 124:17–23.

23. Chalew SA, Lovchik JC, Brown CM, Sun C-CJ. Hypophosphatemia induced in mice by transplantation of a tumor-derived cell line from a patient with oncogenic rickets. *J Pediatr Endocrinol Metab* 1996; 9:593–597.

24. Drezner MK, Feinglos MN. Osteomalacia due to 1,25-dihydroxychole-calciferol deficiency: association with a giant cell tumor of bone. *J Clin Invest* 1977;60:1046–1053.

25. Kumar R, Haugen JD, Wieben ED, Londowski JM, Cai Q. Inhibitors of renal epithelial phosphate transport in tumor induced osteomalacia and uremia. *Proc Am Assoc Physicians* 1995;107:296–305.

26. Boriani S, Campanacci. Osteoblastoma associated with osteomalacia (presentation of a case and review of the literature). *Ital J Orthop Traumatol* 1978;4:379–382.

27. Wilkins GE, Granleese S, Hegele RG, Holden J, Anderson DW, Bondy GP. Oncogenic osteomalacia: evidence for a humoral phosphaturic factor. *J Clin Endocrinol Metab* 1995;80:1628–1634.

28. Seshadri MS, Cornish CJ, Mason RS, Posen S. Parathyroid hormone-like bioactivity in tumours from patients with oncogenic osteomalacia. *Clin Endocrinol* 1985;23:689–697.

29. Shane E, Parisien M, Henderson JE, et al. Tumor-induced osteomalacia: clinical and basic studies. *J Bone Miner Res* 1997;12:1502–1511.

30. Muff R, Caulfield MP, Fischer JA. Dissociation of cAMP accumulation and phosphate uptake in opossum kidney (OK) cells with parathyroid hormone (PTH) and parathyroid related protein (PTHrP). *Peptides* 1990;11:945–949.

31. Lobaugh B, Burch WM Jr, Drezner MK. Abnormalities of vitamin D metabolism and action in the vitamin D resistant rachitic and osteo-malacic diseases. In: Kumar R, ed. *Vitamin D*. Boston: Martinus Nij-hoff, 1984:665–720.

32. Leicht E, Biro G, Langer H-J. Tumor-induced osteomalacia: pre- and postoperative biochemical findings. *Horm Metab Res* 1990;22: 640–643.

66. Hypophosphatasia

Michael P. Whyte, M.D.

Division of Bone and Mineral Diseases, Washington University School of Medicine at Barnes–Jewish Hospital, and Metabolic Research Unit, Shriners Hospital for Children, St. Louis, Missouri

Hypophosphatasia is a rare heritable type of rickets or osteomalacia that occurs in all races with an incidence of about one per 100,000 live births for the severe forms; the mild forms seem to be more common (1,2). Approximately 300 cases have been described. It is an inborn error of metabolism characterized biochemically by subnormal activity of the tissue-nonspecific (bone/liver/kidney) isoenzyme of alkaline phosphatase (TNSALP). Activity of the tissue-specific intestinal, placental, and germ-cell ALP isoenzymes is not diminished (3).

Although there is overlap in disease severity among them, four principal clinical forms of hypophosphatasia are reported, depending on the age at which skeletal lesions are discovered: perinatal, infantile, childhood, and adult. When dental manifestations alone are present, the condition is called odontohypophosphatasia. In general, the earlier the onset of skeletal problems, the more severe the clinical course (1,2).

CLINICAL PRESENTATION

Although some TNSALP is normally present in all tissues, hypophosphatasia affects predominantly the skeleton and dentition. The severity of clinical expression is, however, remarkably variable [e.g., death may occur *in utero* or symptoms may never appear (1,2)].

Perinatal hypophosphatasia manifests during gestation. The pregnancy may be complicated by polyhydramnios. Typically, extreme skeletal hypomineralization (causing short and deformed limbs and caput membranaceum) is apparent at birth. Rarely, unusual bony spurs appear on long bones. Some of these newborns survive briefly but suffer increasing respiratory compromise, unexplained fever, ane-mia (perhaps from encroachment on the marrow space by excessive osteoid), failure to gain weight, irritability, periodic apnea with cyanosis and bradycardia, intracranial hemorrhage, and seizures. This is almost always a lethal condition (1,2).

Infantile hypophosphatasia becomes clinically apparent before age 6 months. Developmental milestones often seem normal until poor feeding, inadequate weight gain, hypotonia, and wide fontanelles are noted. Rachitic deformities then manifest. Hypercalcemia and hypercalciuria can cause recurrent vomiting, nephrocalcinosis, and occasionally renal compromise. Despite widely ''open'' fontanelles (actually hypomineralized areas of calvarium), functional cranio-synostosis is common. Raised intracranial pressure can cause bulging of the anterior fontanelle, proptosis, and papilledema. Mild hypertelorism and brachycephaly can occur. A flail chest predisposes to pneumonia. During the months after diagnosis, there may be spontaneous improvement or progressive deterioration in the skeleton; this form is fatal in about 50% of patients. Prognosis seems to improve if there is survival beyond infancy (1,2).

Childhood hypophosphatasia varies greatly in severity. Premature loss of deciduous teeth (before age 5 years) from hypoplasia or aplasia of dental cementum is a clinical hallmark. Odontohypophosphatasia is diagnosed when radiographs show no evidence of skeletal disease. The incisors are typically lost first, but in severe cases, the entire dentition can be affected. Exfoliation occurs despite minimal tooth-root resorption. Dental radiographs often show enlarged pulp chambers and root canals, forming shell teeth. When rickets is present, delayed walking with a waddling gait, short stature, and a dolichocephalic skull with frontal bossing are often present. A static myopathy is a poorly understood complication. Childhood hypophosphatasia may improve spontaneously during puberty, but recurrence of skeletal symptoms during adult life is likely (1,2).

Adult hypophosphatasia usually presents during middle age, often with painful and poorly healing recurrent metatarsal stress fractures. Pain in the thighs or hips can originate from femoral pseudofractures. About 50% of affected adults will have a history of rickets and/or premature loss of deciduous teeth during childhood. The prognosis for the permanent dentition is more favorable. Chondrocalcinosis occurs frequently, and calcium pyrophosphate dihydrate crystal deposition disease and calcific periarthritis trouble some patients (see later) (4). Femoral pseudofractures will mend following intramedullary rodding (5).

LABORATORY FINDINGS

Hypophosphatasia is diagnosed from a consistent clinical history and physical findings, radiologic or histopathologic evidence of rickets or osteomalacia, and the presence of low serum ALP activity (hypophosphatasemia) (1). Diagnosticians must recognize that there are changes in the normal range for serum ALP activity with age, and that rarely other conditions and treatments can cause hypophosphatasemia (6).

The rickets/osteomalacia of hypophosphatasia is unusual in that serum levels of calcium and inorganic phosphate (P_i) are not reduced. In fact, hypercalcemia and hypercalciuria occur frequently in perinatal and infantile hypophosphatasia, apparently from dyssynergy between gut absorption of calcium and defective skeletal growth and mineralization (severely affected patients also may show progressive skeletal demineralization). Children and adults with hypophosphatasia have serum P_i levels that are above mean levels for age-matched controls, and about 50% of these patients are hyperphosphatemic. Enhanced renal reclamation of P_i (increased TmP/GFR) accounts for this abnormality. In serum, vitamin D metabolite concentrations are usually normal (1). Parathyroid hormone levels may be low (unpublished observation).

Three phosphocompounds accumulate endogenously in hypophosphatasia (1): phosphoethanolamine (PEA), inorganic pyrophosphate (PP_i), and pyridoxal 5'-phosphate (PLP). Demonstration of phosphoethanolaminuria supports the diagnosis, but is not specific. Urinary PEA levels can be modestly increased in a variety of other disorders, and normal levels can occur in mild cases of hypophosphatasia. Assay of PP_i in plasma and urine remains a research technique. The elevated plasma level of PLP is the most sensitive and specific test among these markers for hypophosphatasia (subjects should not be taking vitamin B_6 supplements when studied). In general, the lower the serum level of ALP activity for age and the greater the plasma PLP level, the more severe the clinical manifestations of hypophosphatasia (1,3).

RADIOLOGIC FINDINGS

Perinatal hypophosphatasia has pathognomonic features (7). Marked skeletal undermineralization occurs with severe rachitic changes. In extreme cases, the skeleton may be so poorly calcified that only the base of the skull is visualized.

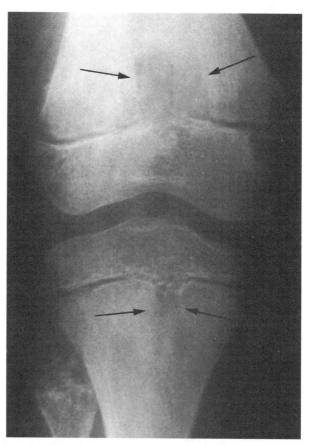

FIG. 1. The metaphysis of the proximal tibia of this 10-year-old boy with mild childhood hypophosphatasia shows a subtle but characteristic "tongue" of radiolucency (*arrows*). Note, however, that his rickets does not manifest with widening of the growth plate.

Segments of the spinal column may appear to be missing. In less remarkable cases, the calvarium may be ossified at central portions of the membranous bones and thereby give the illusion that the sutures are open and widely separated. Fractures also are common.

Infantile hypophosphatasia causes characteristic but less severe changes. Abrupt transition from relatively normal-appearing diaphyses to hypomineralized metaphyses may suggest a sudden metabolic deterioration. Worsening rickets with progressive skeletal demineralization heralds a lethal outcome. Skeletal scintigraphy may help to show premature closure of cranial sutures that appear widened radiographically.

Childhood hypophosphatasia often features tongues of radiolucency that project from rachitic growth plates into metaphyses (Fig. 1). True premature fusion of cranial sutures can cause a "beaten-copper" appearance of the skull.

Adult hypophosphatasia is associated with osteopenia, metatarsal stress fractures, chondrocalcinosis, and proximal femoral pseudofractures.

HISTOPATHOLOGIC FINDINGS

Nondecalcified sections of bone reveal typical histologic features of rickets or osteomalacia in all clinical forms of hypophosphatasia except odontohypophosphatasia. However, biochemical or histochemical detection of low ALP activity in bone distinguishes hypophosphatasia from other disorders. Open cranial sutures are actually uncalcified osteoid. Dental histopathology shows aplasia or hypoplasia of cementum. Enlarged pulp chambers indicate impaired dentinogenesis. These changes vary from tooth to tooth.

INHERITANCE

Perinatal and infantile hypophosphatasia are inherited as autosomal recessive traits. Parents of severely affected patients may have low or low-normal serum ALP activity, mildly elevated plasma PLP levels, and modest phosphoethanolaminuria. Challenge with vitamin B_6 (pyridoxine) orally is followed by a distinctly abnormal increment in plasma PLP levels in patients and perhaps in most carriers (3).

The mode of inheritance for the milder forms of hypophosphatasia is less clear. Some cases of odontohypophosphatasia and adult-onset disease may reflect clinical expression in heterozygotes for whom the disorder was transmitted as an autosomal dominant trait (see later) (1,2).

BIOCHEMICAL/GENETIC DEFECT

In keeping with an inborn error of metabolism that selectively affects the TNSALP isoenzyme, autopsy studies of perinatal and infantile hypophosphatasia patients demonstrate profound deficiency of ALP activity in bone, liver, and kidney, but not in the intestine or placenta. An increasing number of molecular defects are being identified in the TNSALP gene in severe forms of hypophosphatasia (8). Some exceptional patients may reflect a regulatory abnormality involving TNSALP biosynthesis (1). Childhood and adult hypophosphatasia can be due to compound heterozygosity for TNSALP gene missense mutations (8).

PATHOGENESIS

Studies of vitamin B_6 metabolism in hypophosphatasia indicate that TNSALP acts to regulate the extracellular concentration of a variety of phosphocompounds (3). Accumulation of PP_i, an inhibitor of hydroxyapatite crystal growth, may account for the impaired skeletal mineralization (3). Development of a knockout mouse model for hypophosphatasia should help to clarify further the physiologic role of TNSALP (9).

TREATMENT

There is no established medical therapy for hypophosphatasia. Unless there is a well-documented deficiency, it is important to avoid traditional treatments for rickets or osteomalacia (e.g., vitamin D sterols and mineral supplementation) because circulating levels of calcium, P_i, 25-hydroxyvitamin D, and 1,25-dihydroxyvitamin D are usually not reduced (1). Furthermore, traditional regimens may exacerbate any predisposition to hypercalcemia or hypercalciuria.

The hypercalcemia of perinatal or infantile hypophosphatasia may respond to restriction of dietary calcium and to salmon calcitonin and/or glucocorticoid therapy (10). Fractures in children and adults do mend; however, this process may be slow, and delayed healing after osteotomy with casting has been observed. Placement of load-sharing intramedullary rods, rather than load-sparing plates, is best for the acute or prophylactic treatment of fractures and pseudofractures in adults (5). Expert dental care is important. Dentures may be necessary even for pediatric patients.

PRENATAL DIAGNOSIS

Perinatal hypophosphatasia can be detected prenatally. Combined use of serial ultrasonography (with attention to the limbs as well as to the skull), assay of ALP activity in amniotic fluid cells by an experienced laboratory, and radiographic study of the fetus have been used successfully in the second trimester (11). First-trimester diagnosis has been achieved by using chorionic villus samples and a monoclonal antibody–based TNSALP assay (12). Recently DNA-based techniques have also proven informative (11).

REFERENCES

1. Whyte MP. Hypophosphatasia. In: Scriver CR, Beaudet AL, Sly WS, Valle D, eds. *The metabolic and molecular bases of inherited disease.* 8th ed. New York: McGraw-Hill, 1999 (in press).
2. Caswell AM, Whyte MP, Russell RGG. Hypophosphatasia and the extracellular metabolism of inorganic pyrophosphate: clinical and laboratory aspects. *Crit Rev Clin Lab Sci* 1992;28:175–232.
3. Whyte MP. Hypophosphatasia: nature's window on alkaline phosphatase function in man. In: Bilezikian J, Raisz L, Rodan G, eds. *Principles of bone biology.* San Diego: Academic Press, 1996:951–968.
4. Chuck AJ, Pattrick MG, Hamilton E, Wilson R, Doherty M. Crystal deposition in hypophosphatasia: a reappraisal. *Ann Rheum Dis* 1989;48:571–576.
5. Coe JD, Murphy WA, Whyte MP. Management of femoral fractures and pseudofractures in adult hypophosphatasia. *J Bone Joint Surg Am* 1986;68A:981–990.
6. Weinstein RS, Whyte MP. Heterogeneity of adult hypophosphatasia: report of severe and mild cases. *Arch Intern Med* 1981;141:727–731.
7. Shohat M, Rimoin DL, Gerber HE, Lachman RS. Perinatal hypophosphatasia: clinical, radiologic, and morphologic findings. *Pediatr Radiol* 1991;21:421–427.
8. Henthorn PS, Raducha M, Fedde KN, Lafferty MA, Whyte MP. Different missense mutations at the tissue-nonspecific alkaline phosphatase gene locus in autosomal recessively inherited forms of mild and severe hypophosphatasia. *Proc Natl Acad Sci U S A* 1992;89:9924–9928.
9. Waymire KG, Mahuren JD, Jaje JM, Guilarte TR, Coburn SP, MacGregor GR. Mice lacking tissue non-specific alkaline phosphatase die from seizures due to defective metabolism of vitamin B-6. *Nat Genet* 1995;11:45–51.
10. Barcia JP, Strife CF, Langman CB. Infantile hypophosphatasia: treatment options to control hypercalcemia, hypercalciuria, and chronic bone demineralization. *J Pediatr* 1997;130:825–828.
11. Henthorn PS, Whyte MP. Infantile hypophosphatasia: successful prenatal assessment by testing for tissue-nonspecific alkaline phosphatase gene mutations. *Prenat Diagn* 1995;15:1001–1006.
12. Brock DJH, Barron L. First-trimester prenatal diagnosis of hypophosphatasia: experience with 16 cases. *Prenat Diagn* 1991;11:387.

67. Fanconi Syndrome and Renal Tubular Acidosis

Russell W. Chesney, M.D.

Department of Pediatrics, University of Tennessee and Le Bonheur Children's Medical Center, Memphis, Tennessee

FANCONI SYNDROME

Osteomalacia with or without rickets is a common feature of Fanconi syndrome. The renal aspects of Fanconi syndrome are characterized by a generalized defect in renal proximal tubule transport capacity including impaired reabsorption of glucose, phosphate, amino acids, bicarbonate, uric acid, citrate and other organic acids, and low-molecular-weight proteins (less than 50,000 kDa). Calcium, magnesium, sodium, potassium, and water also are excreted in excess (1).

Fanconi syndrome is often the ultimate expression of toxic and/or metabolic injury to the proximal tubule; thus the syndrome has many associated disorders (Tables 1 and 2). The occurrence of the syndrome in patients with disorders of mitochondrial respiration and myopathy stresses the importance of intact energy production in proximal tubular function (1). Abnormal intracellular metabolism could result in either a reduction in high-energy phosphate compounds necessary for active transport processes or defective membrane biosynthesis or epithelial integrity (2). The syndrome also has been seen in association with vitamin D deficiency (3), although autosomal recessive cystine storage disease (cystinosis) and light-chain myeloma are the most common causes in children and adults, respectively (4). Some cases of Fanconi syndrome are not linked to any of the known associations, and these idiopathic cases can be seen in both children and adults by a sporadic, recessive, dominant, or sex-linked hereditary pattern (4).

Pathogenesis

Fanconi syndrome represents a global tubulopathy with a large number of associated disorders, suggesting that the most likely pathogenic sequence involves deranged intracellular metabolic regulation rather than a defect in individual solute or ion-transport sites.

TABLE 1. *Hereditary disorders associated with Fanconi syndrome*

Cystinosis (Lignac–Fanconi disease)
Lowe syndrome
Hereditary fructose intolerance
Tyrosinemia, type I (tyrosinosis)
Galactosemia
Glycogen storage disease
Wilson's disease
Hereditary mitochondrial myopathy with lactic acidemia
Metachromatic leukodystrophy
Subacute necrotizing encephalomyelopathy (Leigh syndrome)
Hereditary nephritis (Alport syndrome)
Medullary cystic disease
Pseudovitamin D–deficiency rickets

TABLE 2. *Acquired disorders associated with Fanconi syndrome*

Disorders of protein metabolism/excretion
  Multiple myeloma
  Benign monoclonal gammopathy
  Light-chain nephropathy
  Amyloidosis
  Sjögren syndrome
  Nephrotic syndrome
Immunologic disorders
  Interstitial nephritis with anti-Tubular basement membrane antibody
  Renal transplantation
  Malignancy
Other renal disorders
  Balkan nephropathy
  Paroxysmal nocturnal hemoglobinuria
  Renal vein thrombosis in newborn infant
Vitamin D disorders with secondary hyperparathyroidism
  Vitamin D deficiency
  Vitamin D–dependent rickets
  Pseudovitamin D–deficiency rickets
Disorders linked with drug, heavy metal, or other toxin exposure
  Drug-related causes
    Outdated, degraded tetracycline
    Methyl-3-chromone
    6-Mercaptopurine
    Gentamicin and aminoglycoside antibiotics
    Valproic acid
    Streptozotocin
    Isophthalanilide
    Ifosfamide
  Heavy metal exposure
    Cadmium
    Lead
    Mercury
    Uranium
    cis-Platinum
  Other toxin exposure
    Paraquat poisoning
    Lysol burn
    Toluene inhalation (glue sniffing)

Both rickets and osteomalacia are common in many forms of Fanconi syndrome (Table 3). Ascribed mechanisms for the metabolic bone disorder include hypophosphatemia due to phosphaturia, increased urinary calcium excretion, abnormal vitamin D metabolism, and renal insufficiency (5). Because 85% to 90% of filtered phosphate is reabsorbed by the S1 and S2 segments of the proximal tubule, the global defect in proximal tubule transport capacity limits phosphate reclamation. Despite any other alterations in mineral or hormone regulation in Fanconi syndrome, this persistent phosphaturia is a major factor in the development and maintenance of rickets and/or osteomalacia because phosphate levels in the extracellular fluid are diminished. This hypophosphatemic osteomalacia can result in osteonecrosis as a

340

TABLE 3. *Factors contributing to osteomalacia and rickets in Fanconi syndrome*

Hypophosphatemia
Hypercalciuria
Vitamin D deficiency
Reduced 1α-hydroxylation of 25 (OH) D
Mesenchymal tumor-elaborating substances, causing hypophosphatemia

result of microfractures (6) and may be a late feature of lifelong Fanconi syndrome (7).

Abnormalities of Vitamin D Metabolism

As indicated, vitamin D deficiency can result in a proximal tubulopathy resembling Fanconi syndrome that is reversed by vitamin D treatment (3). Galactosemia, Wilson's disease, tyrosinemia, Fanconi–Bickel syndrome, and fructose intolerance may result in sufficient hepatic damage and cirrhosis to impair the 25-hydroxylation of vitamin D (8). The circulating values of 1,25-dihydroxyvitamin D [1,25 $(OH)_2$ D] are either low or normal but are not elevated, as would be anticipated in the face of hypophosphatemia and secondary hyperparathyroidism (9). Whenever 1,25 $(OH)_2$ D values are reduced, bone demineralization appears to be more pronounced (10). This reduction in 1,25 $(OH)_2$ D circulating values may be related to impaired proximal tubule cell metabolism or to structural changes in this tissue, because the 25 (OH) D-1α-hydroxylase is localized to proximal tubule cell mitochondria (2). Other researchers, however, have shown reduced production of 1,25 $(OH)_2$ D only when renal insufficiency is demonstrable (11), especially in cystinosis, a disorder associated with progressive renal insufficiency (5).

Light-chain nephropathy may result in bone disease due to defective vitamin D metabolism [reflected in low serum 1,25 $(OH)_2$ D values] and hypophosphatemic osteomalacia (12).

Tumor-Induced Abnormalities

Osteomalacia related to the presence of a tumor that possibly produced a tubulopathic substance, phosphate regulatory protein (now termed phosphotonin or PEX) has been reported and results in the features of Fanconi syndrome (13). As in oncogenous rickets (see Chapter 65), removal of the bone tumor reverses all signs of Fanconi syndrome, including metabolic bone disease, because removal of the tumor removes the source of PEX.

Renal Transplant–Induced Abnormalities

Bone disease may occur in association with Fanconi syndrome found in patients with chronic rejection of a renal transplant (14). Presumably the bone disease is due to phosphaturic hypophosphatemia and steroid-induced osteopenia related to the use of glucocorticoids as part of immunosuppressive therapy associated with transplantation (see Chapter 56).

Genetic Causes

A variety of genetic defects are now known to cause several forms of Fanconi syndrome. A defective lysosomal cystine afflux transporter is defective in cystinosis (1,4). The facultative hepatic-form diffusional glucose (and galactose) transporter is defective in the Fanconi–Bickel syndrome (Table 1) (1,4). Several variants are due to defects in mitochondrial DNA that affect mitochondrial enzymes responsible for energy metabolism (1,4). How these mutations affect bone metabolism is unclear, but osteopenia is a feature of each of these disorders.

In functional assays using COS-1 cells, patients with pseudovitamin D–deficiency rickets and Fanconi syndrome have been shown to have mutations of the gene for renal 25 (OH) D_3-1-hydroxylase (15), the key enzyme in the synthesis of calcitriol. The gene for hydroxylase has been mapped to chromosome 12q13.3, the locus for pseudovitamin D–deficiency rickets by linkage analysis.

Therapy

The therapy of osteomalacia/rickets in Fanconi syndrome is predicated on the cause of the bone disease. In general, oral phosphate supplements, in the form of either neutral phosphate or Joulie's solution, are provided at doses between 1 and 4 g daily, given in four to six daily divided doses (4). In patients with vitamin D deficiency, treatment with appropriate doses may reverse the bone disease (3,5). Many patients with Fanconi syndrome and osteomalacia will benefit from therapy with the 1Y-hydroxylated vitamin D analogues or dihydrotachysterol (DHT) in appropriate doses (4,7–11). In patients with myeloma, therapy for the underlying monoclonal gammopathy is often curative, but oral phosphate and vitamin D also may be required. Finally, in patients with the unexpected occurrence of osteomalacia and Fanconi syndrome, a bone scan may be indicated to seek a nonossifying fibroma that we hope can then be fully extirpated.

RENAL TUBULAR ACIDOSIS

Renal tubular acidosis (RTA) is a disorder in which the kidney is incapable of conserving bicarbonate; thus patients develop a decline in plasma bicarbonate concentrations and systemic metabolic acidosis (16). The underlying renal defect consists of a reduction in tubular bicarbonate reabsorption, the inability to secrete protons (H^+) so that a pH gradient between blood and the lumen cannot be formed, or the back-diffusion of previously secreted hydrogen ions across a cell membrane that cannot sustain a pH gradient (16). A current classification of the types of RTA considers a distal tubular hydrogen ion gradient limited form (type I), a proximal tubular bicarbonate wasting form (type II), and a hyperkalemic form (type IV). The term type III is no longer used and is thought to have represented a hybrid of types I and II. The magnitude of bicarbonate wasting into the urine is greatest in type II and least in type IV (2). Some patients with RTA will have a limited gradient defect and demonstrate renal bicarbonate wasting and a low plasma bicarbonate concentration but no systemic metabolic acidosis; this type is difficult to classify.

Type IV RTA has been divided into several subtypes. Subtype 1 is related to aldosterone deficiency in the absence of overt intrinsic renal insufficiency, and subtype 2 arises from hyporeninemic hypoaldosteronism. Another subtype is associated with partial or total end-organ resistance to aldosterone. If these patients have total lack of responsiveness to the hormone, with high circulating values of aldosterone, this disorder is termed pseudohypoaldosteronism.

Whenever type IV RTA is associated with renal insufficiency, renal osteodystrophy may be expected to occur as renal failure progresses (2).

A rare form of RTA is associated with osteopetrosis (2). This is discussed elsewhere but clearly does not result in bone demineralization.

Pathogenesis

Metabolic bone disease is a feature of RTA (1–4,16); osteomalacia and/or rickets in RTA also has several causes. Rickets is rare in children with RTA type I, as is osteomalacia in adults with the same condition (2,15). Nevertheless, these patients have erosion of bone as a result of systemic metabolic acidosis and release of calcium from bone as calcium carbonate is used as a buffer (2). This additional calcium is excreted into the urine, and many of these patients are hypercalciuric by any criteria used, with a urine calcium level greater than 4 mg/kg/day or a urine calcium/creatinine ratio greater than 0.2. Calcium excretion decreases with correction of metabolic acidosis (17), so oral NaHCO₃ or Shohl's solution will reverse this bone demineralization. As noted by numerous groups, nephrocalcinosis may persist long after correction of systemic metabolic acidosis (2). Hypercalciuria and nephrocalcinosis are especially common in Wilson disease, in which both a proximal and a distal RTA are present; hence the finding of calcium deposition in the renal interstitium. Nevertheless, the serum calcium concentration is not reduced, and hypocalcemia probably does not cause metabolic bone disease.

Rickets and osteomalacia are common features of RTA type II, particularly if the proximal tubular bicarbonaturia is a component of a more global tubulopathy. The mechanisms and therapy for metabolic bone disease in RTA type II are covered in the previous section on the Fanconi syndrome. Nephrocalcinosis and hypercalciuria are not so common, because the final urine pH in proximal RTA is often acidic, and thus the deposition of calcium phosphate complexes is not favored (16).

In type II RTA, which is isolated, systemic metabolic acidosis presumably results in demineralization; however, this has not been systematically evaluated.

Certain patients with nutritional vitamin D deficiency show evidence of bicarbonate wasting, although this is not usually an isolated event (2). In view of experimental studies in animals, an impaired conversion of 25 (OH) D to 1,25 (OH)₂ D may be a consequence of systemic metabolic acido-

sis (18). A somewhat similar study in normal men who were made acidotic by an ammonium chloride challenge indicated impaired conversion of vitamin D to its active metabolite (19). However, this effect was seen only acutely. Chronic acidosis did not impair conversion of 25 (OH) D to 1,25 (OH)₂ D in a study in children with RTA types I and II. Several had never been treated with bicarbonate therapy and had normal values of 1,25 (OH)₂ D in serum (20). There is little evidence for the role of impaired metabolic conversion in bone demineralization.

Therapy

The therapy for RTA includes correction of systemic metabolic acidemia by oral NaHCO₃; the doses vary according to the nephron segment affected. Type I RTA is generally treated with 1 to 2 mEq/kg/24 h of oral NaHCO₃, but higher doses may be needed in young children (17). Type II RTA requires 10 to 15 mEq/kg/24 h or slightly lower doses if thiazides are used in addition (2). Thiazides reduce plasma volume and thereby enhance tubule bicarbonate reabsorption. Patients with type IV disease also may require fluorinated glucocorticoids in supraphysiologic doses that augment potassium secretion (2). Hypercalciuria and bone resorption are reversed by NaHCO₃ therapy.

REFERENCES

1. Chesney RW, Novello AC. Defects of renal tubular transport. In: Massry SG, Glassock RJ, eds. *Textbook of nephrology.* 4th ed. Baltimore: Williams & Wilkins, 1998:513–529.
2. Baum M. The cellular basis of Fanconi syndrome. *Hosp Pract* 1994; Nov 15:137–148.
3. Chesney RW, Harrison HE. Fanconi syndrome following bowel surgery and hepatitis reversed by 25-hydroxycholecalciferol. *J Pediatr* 1975; 86:857–861.
4. Chesney RW. Noncystic inherited renal disease. In: Brady HF, Wilcox CM, eds. *Therapy in nephrology and hypertension.* Philadelphia: WB Saunders (in press).
5. Chesney RW. Metabolic bone disease. In: Behrman RE, Kliegman R, Jensen HB, eds. *Nelson textbook of pediatrics.* 16th ed. Philadelphia: WB Saunders (in press).
6. Gaucher A, Thomas JL, Netter P, Faure G. Osteomalacia, pseudosacroiliitis and necrosis of the femoral heads in Fanconi syndrome in an adult. *J Rheumatol* 1981;8:512–515.
7. Brenton DP, Isenberg DA, Ainsworth DC, Garrod P, Krywawych S, Stamp TC. The adult presenting idiopathic Fanconi syndrome. *J Inherit Metab Dis* 1981;4:211–215.
8. Kitagawa T, Akatsuka A, Owada M, Mano T. Biologic and therapeutic effects of 1-alpha-hydroxycholecalciferol in different types of Fanconi syndrome. *Contrib Nephrol* 1980;22:107–119.
9. Baran DT, March TW. Evidence for a defect in vitamin D metabolism in a patient with incomplete Fanconi syndrome. *J Clin Endocrinol Metab* 1984;59:998–1001.
10. Colussi G, DeFerrari ME, Surean M, et al. Vitamin D metabolites and osteomalacia in the human Fanconi syndrome. *Proc Eur Dial Transplant Assoc* 1985;21:756–760.
11. Steinberg R, Chesney RW, Schulman J, DeLuca HF, Phelps M. Circulating vitamin D metabolites in nephropathic cystinosis. *J Pediatr* 1983;120:592–594.
12. Rao DS, Parfitt AM, Villanueva AR, Dorman PJ, Kleerekoper M. Hypophosphatemic osteomalacia and adult Fanconi syndrome due to light chain nephropathy: another form of oncogenous osteomalacia. *Am J Med* 1987;82:333–338.
13. Cai Q, Hodgson SF, Kao PC. Inhibition of renal phosphate transport

by a tumor product in a patient with oncogenic osteomalacia. *N Engl J Med* 1994;330:1645–1647.

14. Friedman AL, Chesney RW. Fanconi syndrome in renal transplantation. *Am J Nephrol* 1981;1:45–47.

15. Kitanaka S, Takeyama KI, Murayama A, et al. Inactivating mutations in the 25-hydroxyvitamin D₃ 1$_a$-hydroxylase gene in patients with pseudovitamin D-deficiency rickets. *N Engl J Med* 1998;338:653–661.

16. Battle DC, Kurtzman NA. The defect in distal tubular acidosis. In: Gonick HC, Buckalew VM, eds. *Renal tubular disorders.* New York: Marcel Dekker, 1985:281–306.

17. Brenner RJ, Spring DB, Sebastian A. Incidence of radiographically evident bone disease, nephrocalcinosis and nephrolithiasis in various types of renal tubular acidosis. *N Engl J Med* 1982;307:217–221.

18. Rodriguez-Soriano J, Vallo A, Vastillo G. Natural history of primary distal renal tubular acidosis treated since infancy. *J Pediatr* 1982; 101:669–676.

19. Lee SW, Russell J, Avioli LV. 25-Hydroxycholecalciferol to 1,25-dihydroxycholecalciferol: conversion impaired by systemic metabolic acidosis. *Science* 1977;195:994.

20. Kraut JF, Gordon EM, Ranson JC. Effect of chronic metabolic acidosis on vitamin D metabolism in humans. *Kidney Int* 1983;24:644–648.

68. Drug-Induced Osteomalacia

Daniel D. Bikle, M.D., Ph.D.

Departments of Medicine and Dermatology, University of California, San Francisco and Department of Medicine, Veterans Affairs Medical Center, San Francisco, California

Bone formation requires calcium and phosphate. Vitamin D through its active metabolites provides for adequate amounts of calcium and phosphate in addition to regulating the differentiation and function of the bone cells involved. Osteomalacia results from the reduction in mineralization of the matrix, demonstrated histomorphometrically as increased osteoid thickness and osteoid surface area coupled with decreased mineral apposition rate and active mineralizing surface area. Drugs that result in deficiencies in calcium, phosphate, and the active vitamin D metabolites or that interfere with their deposition in or action on bone could lead to osteomalacia. Drugs affecting the vitamin D endocrine system include blockers of vitamin D production (sunscreens could play this role in an otherwise marginally deficient individual), inhibitors of vitamin D absorption (e.g., cholestyramine), modifiers of vitamin D metabolism (anticonvulsants such as phenytoin, antituberculous agents such as rifampicin, proximal renal tubule toxins such as cadmium), or antagonists of vitamin D action at the target tissue (e.g., glucocorticoids). Phosphate deficiency can be induced by ingestion of aluminum-containing antacids that prevent its absorption from the intestine or by proximal renal tubule toxins that result in renal phosphate wasting. Calcium deficiency as a cause of osteomalacia has been demonstrated conclusively only in children ingesting a very low calcium diet, although theoretically drugs that interfere with intestinal calcium absorption or accelerate its excretion by the kidney could lead to osteomalacia. Even in the presence of adequate levels of vitamin D, calcium, and phosphate, direct inhibitors of bone mineralization such as bisphosphonates, aluminum, and fluoride can lead to osteomalacia. Thus drugs can cause osteomalacia by several mechanisms, and any one drug may do so by several mechanisms, as summarized in Table 1. This chapter focuses on those drugs for which clinical evidence linking them to the development of osteomalacia is reasonably secure.

BLOCKERS OF VITAMIN D PRODUCTION

Lack of sunlight is a well-appreciated risk factor for the development of osteomalacia in adults and rickets in chil-

dren. The elderly and/or institutionalized with limited nutrition and access to sunlight are at particular risk. The association of sunlight exposure with the development of skin cancer has led some authorities to claim that all sunlight exposure is harmful and that sunscreens should be used to protect against the harmful rays. The degree to which this recent campaign to eliminate solar exposure will increase the incidence of vitamin D deficiency and osteomalacia remains for future investigation.

INHIBITORS OF VITAMIN D ABSORPTION

Vitamin D, like other fat-soluble vitamins, is absorbed in the jejunum and ileum by a process facilitated by bile acids. Bile acid–binding resins such as cholestyramine and colestipol have the potential to interfere with vitamin D absorption. The development of osteomalacia has been described after ileal resection in a patient with Crohn's disease who was treated with cholestyramine (1). This patient was successfully treated with 25 hydroxyvitamin D [25 (OH) D] (calcifediol). The relative contribution of cholestyramine to the onset of osteomalacia is difficult to assess in this patient predisposed to vitamin D deficiency on the basis of the underlying disease. However, this case report indicates that in the marginally vitamin D–deficient patient, bile acid–binding resins may suffice to precipitate osteomalacia, and their impact on vitamin D absorption should be monitored with serum 25 (OH) D levels.

INTERFERENCE WITH VITAMIN D METABOLISM

Vitamin D must be metabolized first in the liver to 25 (OH) D and then in the kidney to 1,25-dihydroxyvitamin D [1,25 (OH)₂ D] and other metabolites to be active. Drugs that induce the drug-metabolizing enzymes in the liver can accelerate the catabolism of vitamin D and its metabolites. Anticonvulsants are the best studied of these drugs with respect to their ability to induce osteomalacia or rickets.

TABLE 1. *Drugs causing osteomalacia*

Disruption of vitamin D endocrine system
  Block vitamin D production
    ? Sun screens
  Inhibit vitamin D absorption
    Cholestyramine
  Interfere with vitamin D metabolism
    25 (OH) D production
      Phenytoin
      Phenobarbital
      Rifampicin
    1,25 (OH)$_2$ D production
      Cadmium
  Antagonize vitamin D action
    Glucocorticoids
Disruption of phosphate homeostasis
  Inhibit phosphate absorption
    Aluminum-containing antacid
  Induce renal phosphate wasting
    Cadmium
    Lead
  Disruption of bone mineralization
    Aluminum
    Fluoride
    Bisphosphonates

Rifampicin also may accelerate vitamin D metabolite catabolism, but the link between rifampicin and osteomalacia is less well established (2).

Early reports suggested that 20% to 65% of those with epilepsy receiving anticonvulsants developed signs of rickets or osteomalacia, especially if they were institutionalized (3–8). Such patients are at increased risk of fractures during their epileptic seizures, and the low serum calcium may aggravate the seizure disorder. Outpatient populations appear to be at much lower risk of developing clinically significant bone disease (9–16), although biochemical abnormalities [reduced serum and urine calcium and serum 25 (OH) D, elevated serum parathyroid hormone (PTH) and alkaline phosphatase], reduced bone density, and increased osteoid on bone biopsy are observed in 10% to 40% of patients receiving long-term anticonvulsant therapy (11–19). In ambulatory subjects, definitive histomorphometric evidence of osteomalacia is seldom found.

The high rate of bone disease in institutionalized patients, regardless of anticonvulsant therapy, emphasizes the importance of nutrition and sunlight, which can be lacking in this setting. However, anticonvulsant therapy clearly compounds this problem. Two of the most frequently used anticonvulsants, phenobarbital and phenytoin, induce liver drug-metabolizing enzymes and increase the metabolism and clearance of vitamin D (20,21). Anticonvulsants such as sodium valproate, which do not induce the hepatic drug-metabolizing enzymes, have little or no impact on serum calcium and 25 (OH) D levels (22,23). *In vitro* studies suggest that phenobarbital and phenytoin have direct inhibitory effects on PTH-stimulated bone resorption (24) and intestinal calcium absorption (25), but the relevance of these studies to the *in vivo* situation is unclear.

Numerous studies pointed out that the well-nourished patient exposed to adequate amounts of sunlight will seldom develop clinically significant bone disease as a result of anticonvulsant therapy. However, patients taking anticonvulsants require higher intakes of vitamin D to achieve positive calcium balance (26), with doses up to 4000 units (100 μg) per day sometimes being required to normalize 25 (OH) D levels (27).

ANTAGONISTS OF VITAMIN D ACTION

Glucocorticoids interfere with intestinal calcium absorption by a little-understood mechanism. As such, they provide one means of treating vitamin D toxicity. However, as discussed elsewhere, glucocorticoids cause osteoporosis but not osteomalacia and are not direct antagonists of vitamin D at the receptor level. There are no known drugs in clinical use that directly interfere with the actions of 1,25 (OH)$_2$ D at the target-tissue level.

INHIBITORS OF PHOSPHATE ABSORPTION

Hypophosphatemia is a central feature of a number of diseases presenting as osteomalacia or rickets including X-linked hypophosphatemic rickets, oncogenic hypophosphatemic osteomalacia (see Chapter 65), and various forms of Fanconi syndrome (see Chapter 67). These feature renal phosphate wasting and reduced 1,25 (OH)$_2$ D production. In contrast, the major drug-induced form of hypophosphatemic osteomalacia is caused by excessive ingestion of aluminum-containing antacids, which inhibit intestinal phosphate absorption. Such patients present with little or no urine phosphate excretion and increased 1,25 (OH)$_2$ D levels (28–30). Serum and urine calcium levels tend to be high. This syndrome is uncommon and must be distinguished from that in patients with renal failure given aluminum-containing antacids to normalize serum phosphate who develop osteomalacia because of the aluminum-induced inhibition of bone mineralization (see later). The absence of aluminum in the bone-biopsy sample helps identify those patients who develop osteomalacia on the basis of the antacid-induced hypophosphatemia rather than aluminum-induced inhibition of mineralization (31). Treatment consists of discontinuing the aluminum-containing antacid; healing of the bone lesions may be expedited with supplemental vitamin D and phosphate.

INHIBITORS OF BONE MINERALIZATION

Aluminum

The two principal situations in which aluminum-induced osteomalacia is found are hemodialysis and total parenteral nutrition (32). The sources of aluminum include antacids used to control serum phosphate levels in patients with renal failure, nondeionized water used during dialysis, and aluminum contamination of various components used during total parenteral nutrition. Unlike patients with antacid-induced hypophosphatemia, patients with aluminum-induced osteomalacia generally have normal or even high serum phosphate levels and low 1,25 (OH)$_2$ D levels. Patients with renal failure have a lower than expected PTH level and often become hypercalcemic at low doses of 1,25 (OH)$_2$ D, which generally fail to treat the osteomalacia. Awareness of this complication of aluminum and reduction of the aluminum exposure of the patients has reduced if not totally eliminated the incidence of aluminum-induced osteomalacia. Deferoxamine is currently being used with success to reduce the body load of aluminum and reverse the osteomalacia (33). This form of drug-induced osteomalacia is covered in greater depth in the chapters concerned with renal osteodystrophy and total parenteral nutrition.

Bisphosphonates

Etidronate is the first bisphosphonate approved for clinical use, initially for the treatment of Paget's disease and more recently for the treatment of hypercalcemia of malignancy. The bisphosphonates are nonhydrolyzable analogues of pyrophosphate, an inhibitor of mineralization. The original experimental applications of the bisphosphonates were to prevent ectopic calcification. Therefore it was no surprise when the early studies with etidronate as therapy for Paget's disease resulted in a patchy, hypocellular form of osteomalacia (34). This effect appeared to be direct, in that no changes in serum calcium and vitamin D metabolite levels were observed, and phosphate levels tended to be increased at least early in treatment (34,35). These early studies used 20-mg/kg doses. Subsequent studies with lower doses indicated that most of the reduction in alkaline phosphatase and urinary hydroxyproline levels observed at 20-mg/kg doses could be achieved with 6 months of treatment with a 5-mg/kg dose (the current recommended therapy for Paget's disease) without increasing the risk of nontraumatic fractures or mineralization defects on bone biopsy (36). However, even this lower dose (effectively 400 mg/day because the tablets each contain 200 mg) proved capable of inducing a patchy form of osteomalacia in some subjects (37). Fractures, when they occur, tend to involve lytic lesions of Paget's disease, so that the presence of such lesions is a relative contraindication to the use of etidronate.

Etidronate is the first-generation bisphosphonate. Pamidronate, a second-generation bisphosphonate, has been approved for treatment of hypercalcemia of malignancy. However, it also is effective therapy for Paget's disease. Pamidronate is given intravenously because of its poor oral absorption and gastric side effects. Pamidronate appears to have a less inhibitory effect on bone mineralization than does etidronate (38,39). However, one recent study of 20 patients with Paget's disease treated with pamidronate showed a patchy form of osteomalacia (focal areas of increased osteoid) in several of the subjects treated with 180- to 360-mg doses over a 6- to 9-week period (40). Alendronate is the first of the third-generation bisphosphonates to be approved for clinical use, and it is being widely used for treatment of osteoporosis. At this point, no reports of osteomalacia caused by alendronate have been published, and bone biopsies of subjects treated for several years with alendronate have shown no evidence of a mineralization disorder (41).

Fluoride

Fluoride has attracted attention as a therapeutic agent for osteoporosis because it is an effective stimulator of new bone growth (42). How fluoride stimulates new bone formation is not clear. Fluoride is rapidly and extensively accumulated into bone and teeth, where x-ray crystallographic data show stabilization by fluoride of the hydroxyapatite crystal (43). Numerous clinical studies have demonstrated increased bone mineral density in subjects treated with fluoride, especially in bones with a high cancellous bone component, yet decreased fracture risk has been hard to document in carefully performed, double-blind, placebo-controlled trials (44,45). At least part of the problem is that the new bone stimulated by fluoride often shows evidence of abnormal mineralization (46–48). This mineralization defect is aggravated by conditions of low calcium intake but is not completely prevented by the coadministration of adequate amounts of calcium and vitamin D (49). Conceivably, the painful lower extremity syndrome seen in some subjects treated with fluoride is the consequence of the imbalance between matrix production and mineralization, leading to microfractures (50). More controversial is the possibility that fluoride treatment increases the risk of hip fracture, again hypothesized to involve the imbalance between matrix formation and mineralization (51,52). A slow-release form of fluoride may circumvent some or all of the problems associated with the usual formulation of NaF, but this formulation remains under investigation (53).

REFERENCES

1. Compston JE, Horton LW. Oral 25-hydroxyvitamin D$_3$ in treatment of osteomalacia associated with ileal resection and cholestyramine therapy. *Gastroenterology* 1978;74:900–902.
2. Perry W, Erooga MA, Brown J, Stamp TC. Calcium metabolism during rifampicin and isoniazid therapy for tuberculosis. *J R Soc Med* 1982;75:533–536.
3. Dent CE, Richens A, Rowe DJ, Stamp TC. Osteomalacia with long-term anticonvulsant therapy in epilepsy. *Br Med J* 1970;4:69–72.
4. Richens A, Rowe DJ. Disturbance of calcium metabolism by anticonvulsant drugs. *Br Med J* 1970;4:73–76.
5. Hunter J, Maxwell JD, Stewart DA, Parsons V, Williams R. Altered calcium metabolism in epileptic children on anticonvulsants. *Br Med J* 1971;4:202–204.
6. Tolman KG, Jubiz W, Sannella JJ, et al. Osteomalacia associated with anticonvulsant drug therapy in mentally retarded children. *Pediatrics* 1975;56:45–50.
7. Hunt PA, Wu-Chen ML, Handal NJ, et al. Bone disease induced by anticonvulsant therapy and treatment with calcitriol (1,25-dihydroxyvitamin D$_3$). *Am J Dis Child* 1986;140:715–718.
8. Offermann G, Pinto V, Kruse R. Antiepileptic drugs and vitamin D supplementation. *Epilepsia* 1979;20:3–15.
9. Livingston S, Berman W, Pauli LL. Anticonvulsant drugs and vitamin D metabolism. *JAMA* 1973;224:1634–1635.
10. Fogelman I, Gray JM, Gardner MD, et al. Do anticonvulsant drugs commonly induce osteomalacia? *Scot Med J* 1982;27:136–142.
11. Pylypchuk G, Oreopoulos DG, Wilson DR, et al. Calcium metabolism in adult outpatients with epilepsy receiving long-term anticonvulsant therapy. *Can Med Assoc J* 1978;118:635–638.
12. Keck E, Gollnick B, Reinhardt D, Karch D, Peerenboom H, Kruskemper HL. Calcium metabolism and vitamin D metabolite levels in children receiving anticonvulsant drugs. *Eur J Pediatr* 1982;139:52–55.
13. Ashworth B, Horn DB. Evidence of osteomalacia in an outpatient group of adult epileptics. *Epilepsia* 1977;18:37–43.
14. Hoikka V, Savolainen K, Alhava EM, Sivenius J, Karjalainen P, Parvia-

ninen M. Anticonvulsant osteomalacia in epileptic outpatients. *Ann Clin Res* 1982;14:129–132.

15. Bogliun G, Beghi E, Crespi V, Delodovici L, d'Amico P. Anticonvulsant drugs and bone metabolism. *Acta Neurol Scand* 1986;74:284–288.

16. Weinstein RS, Bryce GF, Sappington LJ, King DW, Gallagher BB. Decreased serum ionized calcium and normal vitamin D metabolite levels with anticonvulsant drug treatment. *J Clin Endocrinol Metab* 1984;58:1003–1009.

17. Hahn TJ, Hendin BA, Scharp CR, Haddad JGJ. Effect of chronic anticonvulsant therapy on serum 25-hydroxycalciferol levels in adults. *N Engl J Med* 1972;287:900–904.

18. Hahn TJ, Hendin BA, Scharp CR, Boisscau VC, Haddad JG Jr. Serum 25-hydroxycalciferol levels and bone mass in children on chronic anticonvulsant therapy. *N Engl J Med* 1975;292:550–554.

19. Christiansen C, Rodbro P. Treatment of anticonvulsant osteomalacia with vitamin D. *Calcif Tissue Res* 1976;21(suppl):252–259.

20. Matheson RT, Herbst JJ, Jubiz W, Freston JW, Tolman KG. Absorption and biotransformation of cholecalciferol in drug-induced osteomalacia. *J Clin Pharmacol* 1976;16:426–432.

21. Hahn TJ, Birge SJ, Scharp CR, Avioli LV. Phenobarbital-induced alterations in vitamin D metabolism. *J Clin Invest* 1972;51:741–748.

22. Gough H, Goggin T, Bissessar A, Baker M, Crowley M, Callaghan N. A comparative study of the relative influence of different anticonvulsant drugs, UV exposure and diet on vitamin D and calcium metabolism in out-patients with epilepsy. *Q J Med* 1986;59:569–577.

23. Davie MW, Emberson CE, Lawson DE, et al. Low plasma 25-hydroxyvitamin D and serum calcium levels in institutionalized epileptic subjects: associated risk factors, consequences and response to treatment with vitamin D. *Q J Med* 1983;52:79–91.

24. Hahn TJ, Scharp CR, Richardson CA, Halstead LR, Kahn AJ, Teitelbaum SL. Interaction of diphenylhydantoin (phenytoin) and phenobarbital with hormonal mediation of fetal rat bone resorption in vitro. *J Clin Invest* 1978;62:406–414.

25. Corradino RA. Diphenylhydantoin: direct inhibition of the vitamin D_3-mediated calcium absorptive mechanism in organ-cultured duodenum. *Biochem Pharmacol* 1976;25:863–864.

26. Peterson P, Gray P, Tolman KG. Calcium balance in drug-induced osteomalacia: response to vitamin D. *Clin Pharmacol Ther* 1976;19:63–67.

27. Collins N, Maher J, Cole M, Baker M, Callaghan N. A prospective study to evaluate the dose of vitamin D required to correct low 25-hydroxyvitamin D levels, calcium, and alkaline phosphatase in patients at risk of developing antiepileptic drug-induced osteomalacia. *Q J Med* 1991;78:113–122.

28. Godsall JW, Baron R, Insogna KL. Vitamin D metabolism and bone histomorphometry in a patient with antacid-induced osteomalacia. *Am J Med* 1984;77:747–750.

29. Carmichael KA, Fallon MD, Dalinka M, Kaplan FS, Axel L, Haddad JG. Osteomalacia and osteitis fibrosa in a man ingesting aluminum hydroxide antacid. *Am J Med* 1984;76:1137–1143.

30. Pivnick EK, Kerr NC, Kaufman RA, Jones DP, Chesney RW. Rickets secondary to phosphate depletion: a sequela of antacid use in infancy. *Clin Pediatr* 1995;34:73–78.

31. Kassem M, Eriksen EF, Melsen F, Mosekilde L. Antacid-induced osteomalacia: a case report with a histomorphometric analysis. *J Intern Med* 1991;229:275–279.

32. Nebeker HG, Coburn JW. Aluminum and renal osteodystrophy. *Annu Rev Med* 1986;37:79–95.

33. Felsenfeld AJ, Rodriguez M, Coleman M, Ross D, Llach F. Desferrioxamine therapy in hemodialysis patients with aluminum-associated bone disease. *Kidney Int* 1989;35:1371–1378.

34. Smith R, Russell RG, Bishop MC, Woods CG, Bishop M. Paget's disease of bone: experience with a diphosphonate (disodium etidronate) in treatment. *Q J Med* 1973;42:235–256.

35. Gibbs CJ, Aaron JE, Peacock M. Osteomalacia in Paget's disease treated with short term, high dose sodium etidronate. *Br Med J* 1986;292:1227–1229.

36. Khairi MR, Altman RD, DeRosa GP, Zimmermann J, Schenk RK, Johnston CC. Sodium etidronate in the treatment of Paget's disease of bone: a study of long-term results. *Ann Intern Med* 1977;87:656–663.

37. Boyce BF, Smith L, Fogelman I, Johnston E, Ralston S, Boyle IT. Focal osteomalacia due to low-dose diphosphonate therapy in Paget's disease. *Lancet* 1984;1:821–824.

38. Fenton AJ, Gutteridge DH, Kent GN, et al. Intravenous aminobisphosphonate in Paget's disease: clinical, biochemical, histomorphometric and radiological responses. *Clin Endocrinol* 1991;34:197–204.

39. Harinck HI, Bijvoet OL, Blanksma HJ, Dahlinghaus-Nienhuys PJ. Efficacious management with aminobisphosphonate (APD) in Paget's disease of bone. *Clin Orthop* 1987;217:79–98.

40. Adamson BB, Gallacher SJ, Byars J, Ralston SH, Boyle IT, Boyce BF. Mineralisation defects with pamidronate therapy for Paget's disease. *Lancet* 1993;342:1459–1460.

41. Chavassieux PM, Arlot ME, Reda C, Wei L, Yates AJ, Meunier PJ. Histomorphometric assessment of the long-term effects of alendronate on bone quality and remodeling in patients with osteoporosis. *J Clin Invest* 1997;100:1475–1480.

42. Farley JR, Wergedal JE, Baylink DJ. Fluoride directly stimulates proliferation and alkaline phosphatase activity of bone-forming cells. *Science* 1983;222:330–332.

43. Eanes ED, Reddi AH. The effect of fluoride on bone mineral apatite. *Metab Bone Dis Relat Res* 1979;2:3–10.

44. Riggs BL, Hodgson SF, O'Fallon WM, et al. Effect of fluoride treatment on the fracture rate in postmenopausal women with osteoporosis. *N Engl J Med* 1990;322:802–809.

45. Kleerekoper M, Mendlovic DB. Sodium fluoride therapy of postmenopausal osteoporosis. *Endocr Rev* 1993;14:312–323.

46. Jowsey J, Riggs BL, Kelly PJ, Hoffmann DL. Effect of combined therapy with sodium fluoride, vitamin D and calcium in osteoporosis. *Am J Med* 1972;53:43–49.

47. Briancon D, Meunier PJ. Treatment of osteoporosis with fluoride, calcium, and vitamin D. *Orthop Clin North Am* 1981;12:629–648.

48. Baylink DJ, Bernstein DS. The effects of fluoride therapy on metabolic bone disease: a histologic study. *Clin Orthop* 1967;55:51–85.

49. Compston JE, Chadha S, Merrett AL. Osteomalacia developing during treatment of osteoporosis with sodium fluoride and vitamin D. *Br Med J* 1980;281:910–911.

50. Schnitzler CM, Solomon L. Histomorphometric analysis of a calcaneal stress fracture: a possible complication of fluoride therapy for osteoporosis. *Bone* 1986;7:193–198.

51. Gutteridge DH, Price RI, Kent GN, Prince RL, Michell PA. Spontaneous hip fractures in fluoride-treated patients: potential causative factors. *J Bone Miner Res* 1990;5(suppl 1):S205–S215.

52. Bayley TA, Harrison JE, Murray TM, et al. Fluoride-induced fractures: relation to osteogenic effect. *J Bone Miner Res* 1990;5(suppl 1):S217–S222.

53. Pak CYC, Zerwekh JE, Antich PP, Bell NH, Singer FR. Slow-release sodium fluoride in osteoporosis. *J Bone Miner Res* 1996;11:561–564.

69. Renal Osteodystrophy in Adults and Children

William G. Goodman, M.D., *Jack W. Coburn, M.D., †Eduardo Slatopolsky, M.D., and ‡Isidro B. Salusky, M.D.

*Departments of Medicine, Division of Nephrology, and ‡Pediatrics, Pediatric Dialysis Program, UCLA School of Medicine, Los Angeles, California; and *Department of Medicine, UCLA School of Medicine, and Nephrology Section, West Los Angeles VA Medical Center, Los Angeles, California; and †Department of Medicine, Washington University School of Medicine, and Barnes–Jewish Hospital, St. Louis, Missouri*

INTRODUCTION

Mineral metabolism is a closely integrated process involving the kidneys, intestine, parathyroid glands, and bone. When renal disease develops, mineral homeostasis is disrupted, resulting in diverse manifestations in bone and other tissues. In the broadest sense, the term renal osteodystrophy encompasses all of the disorders of bone and mineral metabolism associated with chronic renal disease.

Both the excretory and the metabolic components of renal function participate in the regulation of mineral metabolism. The total body balances for calcium, phosphorus, magnesium, and numerous other minerals are modulated by adjusting the amount of each ion excreted in the urine. Reduced net acid excretion by the kidney leads to systemic acidosis, which not only affects the mineral composition of bone but also alters bone cell metabolism. Substances such as aluminum and β_2-microglobulin may be retained in patients with impaired renal function, leading to specific disorders of the bones and joints (1).

As regards renal metabolism, the kidney is a major target organ for the actions of parathyroid hormone (PTH), and it also serves as an important site for the degradation of PTH. Calcitriol, or 1,25-dihydroxyvitamin D [1,25 (OH)$_2$ D], which is the biologically most active form of vitamin D, is synthesized predominantly by epithelial cells of the proximal tubule of the nephron. This hormone has diverse actions in many tissues, serving as a key determinant of intestinal calcium absorption and an important regulator of pre-pro-PTH gene transcription; it also acts as a potent modifier of cell proliferation and differentiated cellular function in a variety of tissues including bone, cartilage, and the parathyroid glands. Because even modest reductions in renal function substantially alter the excretory and metabolic capacities of the kidney, mineral homeostasis becomes increasingly compromised in patients with progressive renal failure.

Disturbances in the regulation of PTH secretion, parathyroid gland hyperplasia, and alterations in calcium and vitamin D metabolism represent key elements in the pathogenesis of renal bone disease. Together with other factors such as systemic acidosis and the retention of either aluminum or β_2-microglobulin, the skeletal lesions that develop in patients with renal failure reflect complex interactions among these pathogenic considerations.

THE RENAL BONE DISEASES

The renal bone diseases represent a spectrum of skeletal disorders ranging from high-turnover lesions arising predominantly from excess PTH secretion to low-turnover lesions of diverse etiology that are most often associated with normal or reduced serum PTH levels (Fig. 1). The transition from one histologic subtype to another is determined by one or more dominant pathogenic factors, and such changes can be documented in individual patients by periodically obtaining bone biopsies for quantitative histology. Because the serum level of PTH represents the major regulator of bone formation and turnover in patients with chronic renal disease, alterations in parathyroid gland function associated with renal failure play a pivotal role in the pathogenesis and evolution of renal osteodystrophy (2).

Regulation of PTH Synthesis and Secretion

Parathyroid hormone is synthesized in the parathyroid cell, and it is stored in secretory granules, providing a reservoir of hormone that is available for immediate release into the blood. Pre-pro-PTH gene transcription is negatively regulated by 1,25 (OH)$_2$ D through binding of the vitamin D receptor (VDR) to a response element located 100 to 125 base pairs upstream from the transcriptional start site. A calcium-response element located approximately 3.5 kilobases upstream from the gene for pre-pro-PTH confers additional negative regulatory transcriptional control. As such, decreases in the availability of either 1,25 (OH)$_2$ D or calcium promote pre-pro-PTH gene transcription, whereas PTH synthesis diminishes when 1,25 (OH)$_2$ D and calcium are abundant.

Recent work has delineated a key molecular mechanism that regulates PTH release from the parathyroid cell (3). The calcium-sensing receptor (CaSR) is a 1078-amino acid protein composed of seven membrane-spanning segments and a long extracellular domain that contains clusters of

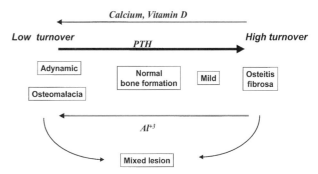

FIG. 1. The Spectrum of renal osteodystrophy. (From Salusky IB, Goodman WG. Growth hormone and calcitriol as modifiers of bone formation in renal osteodystrophy. *Kidney Int* 1995;48:657–665, with permission of Blackwell Science, Inc.)

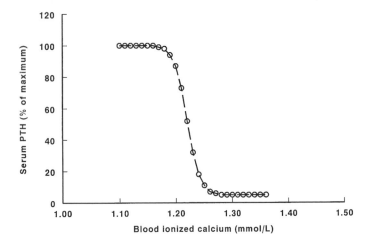

FIG. 2. The inverse sigmoidal relation between blood ionized calcium concentrations and serum parathyroid hormone (PTH) levels in subjects with normal renal and parathyroid gland function. PTH values are expressed as a percentage of the maximal concentration achieved during hypocalcemia. (Adapted with permission from Ramirez JA, Goodman WG, Gornbein J, et al. Direct *in vivo* comparison of calcium-regulated parathyroid hormone secretion in normal volunteers and patients with secondary hyperparathyroidism. *J Clin Endocrinol Metab* 1993;76:1489–1494, © The Endocrine Society.)

acidic amino acids that are likely to serve as binding sites for calcium and other cations. The receptor is coupled to G proteins, and it is abundantly expressed in the plasma membrane of parathyroid cells. Increases in blood ionized calcium concentration activate the CaSR, triggering a rise in cytosolic calcium concentration through the release of calcium from the endoplasmic reticulum. This rapid intracellular calcium transient diminishes PTH release, whereas inactivation of the CaSR enhances PTH secretion (4,5).

Although minute-to-minute variations in PTH secretion are regulated by the CaSR, a component of PTH release from the parathyroid glands cannot be suppressed by calcium; thus basal amounts of hormone are discharged into the circulation even at high blood calcium concentrations (Fig. 2). The peptide fragments released from the parathyroid cell also vary according to the prevailing calcium level in blood, probably reflecting changes in intracellular hormone degradation. When calcium levels are reduced, the secretion of intact 1–84 PTH predominates. In contrast, the secretion of intact hormone decreases, whereas the release of metabolically inactive peptide fragments increases, when blood calcium levels are elevated.

Pathogenesis of High-Turnover Bone Disease (Secondary Hyperparathyroidism)

Several factors contribute to sustained increases in PTH secretion and, ultimately, to the development of high-turnover lesions of bone in patients with chronic renal failure. Among these are hypocalcemia, impaired renal calcitriol production, skeletal resistance to the calcemic actions of PTH, alterations in the regulation of pre-pro-PTH gene transcription, reductions in CaSR expression in the parathyroids, and hyperphosphatemia due to diminished renal phosphorus excretion.

Because the level of ionized calcium in blood represents the most immediate stimulus for PTH secretion, factors that contribute to the development of hypocalcemia in patients with renal disease indirectly promote excess PTH secretion. The production of 1,25 $(OH)_2$ D by the kidney plays a pivotal physiological role in maintaining serum calcium levels by modulating active intestinal calcium absorption, by facilitat-

ing the release of calcium from bone, and by enhancing renal tubular calcium reabsorption. Serum 1,25 $(OH)_2$ D levels decline progressively, however, as renal function diminishes (Fig. 3), and this abnormality has wide-ranging effects on mineral homeostasis. Although serum 1,25 $(OH)_2$ D levels vary considerably at any given level of renal function, the proportion of patients with subnormal values increases as renal function declines. This change accounts, at least in part, for impaired intestinal calcium absorption and for moderate decreases in serum calcium concentrations in patients with moderate to advanced renal failure (6). Diminished VDR expression in intestinal epithelial cells also may contribute to reductions in active intestinal calcium transport.

Skeletal resistance to the calcemic actions of PTH further compromises the ability to maintain normal serum calcium levels in those with renal disease. During infusions of parathyroid extract, the magnitude of the increase in serum calcium is less in patients with moderate to advanced renal failure than in normal subjects, and the correction of hypocalcemia occurs more slowly than normal in those with renal failure (7); thus higher serum PTH levels are required to elicit equivalent biologic responses in patients with chronic renal failure (8). Abnormalities in vitamin D metabolism have been reported to account for these changes, but alterations in VDR expression also could contribute. In addition, expression of the receptor for PTH/PTH-related protein (PTHrP) is reduced in renal failure; this abnormality is probably attributable to renal failure per se rather than to PTH-mediated downregulation of its own receptor because receptor expression is low in uremic animals regardless of the prevailing serum level of PTH (9). Decreases in PTH/PTHrP-receptor expression may contribute, therefore, to tissue resistance to the actions of PTH in renal failure.

Reductions in VDR expression are well documented in the parathyroid glands of humans and experimental animals with secondary hyperparathyroidism due to renal failure (10); this change disrupts the normal feedback inhibition of pre-pro-PTH gene transcription by 1,25 $(OH)_2$ D. Abnormalities in binding of the VDR to DNA response elements may further impede the regulation of pre-pro-PTH gene transcription by vitamin D sterols. Because calcitriol upregulates its own receptor (11), reductions in VDR expression

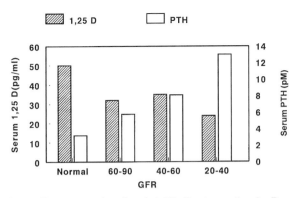

FIG. 3. The serum levels of 1,25-dihydroxyvitamin D and parathyroid hormone (PTH) in patients with varying degrees of renal insufficiency. (Adapted from Reichel et al. *Nephrol Dialysis Transplant* 1991;6:162–169, with permission.)

in renal failure may simply reflect the low serum levels of calcitriol that result from impaired renal 1,25 (OH)$_2$ D production. Differences in gene expression in hyperplastic parathyroid tissues and metabolic changes attributable to uremia per se represent additional mechanisms by which VDR expression in the parathyroid glands may be altered in renal failure.

Because 1,25 (OH)$_2$ D is a potent inhibitor of cell proliferation, disturbances in renal calcitriol production and/or changes in VDR expression may be particularly important determinants of the degree of parathyroid hyperplasia and the extent of parathyroid gland enlargement in chronic renal failure (12). VDR expression is markedly reduced in parathyroid tissues that exhibit a nodular pattern of tissue hyperplasia, whereas lesser reductions in VDR expression are seen in glands with a diffuse pattern of hyperplasia (13). Interestingly, the extent of glandular enlargement is generally greater in nodular parathyroid hyperplasia. The clonal expansion of subpopulations of parathyroid cells and selected chromosomal deletions represent additional mechanisms that may influence the extent of parathyroid gland enlargement in end-stage renal disease (14).

The development and progression of parathyroid gland hyperplasia is a particularly important aspect of renal secondary hyperparathyroidism (15). Once established, parathy-

roid enlargement is difficult to reverse because the rate of apoptosis in parathyroid glands is quite low, and the half-life of parathyroid cells has been estimated to be approximately 30 years. Clinical assessments of parathyroid gland function suggest that differences in functional parathyroid gland size contribute substantially to the wide variation in serum PTH levels in patients with chronic renal failure. Excess PTH secretion may become uncontrollable clinically if the parathyroid glands become greatly enlarged, because the nonsuppressible component of PTH release from a very large number of parathyroid cells can be sufficient to produce hypercalcemia and progressive bone disease in patients with end-stage renal disease.

Expression of the CaSR is reduced by 30% to 70%, as judged by immunohistochemical methods in hyperplastic parathyroid tissues obtained from human subjects with renal failure (16). As such, the primary mechanism by which parathyroid cells detect and respond to changes in blood ionized calcium is abnormal in advanced renal secondary hyperparathyroidism, possibly rendering parathyroid tissues less sensitive to the inhibitory effect of calcium on PTH release. In this regard, CaSR messenger RNA (mRNA) levels in the parathyroid gland have been reported to increase in vitamin D–deficient rats given exogenous 1,25 (OH)$_2$ D, suggesting that alterations in vitamin D metabolism in renal failure could account for changes in calcium sensing by the parathyroids. Reductions in CaSR expression have not been a consistent finding, however, in animals with renal failure, and further work is needed to clarify the role of 1,25 (OH)$_2$ D as a modifier of CaSR expression in parathyroid tissue.

The temporal relation between the duration and/or the severity of renal failure and the decrease in parathyroid CaSR expression has yet to be determined. *In vivo* studies of parathyroid gland function in patients with end-stage renal disease indicated that calcium sensing by the parathyroid glands is altered in advanced but not in mild to moderate secondary hyperparathyroidism (Table 1) (17). Such findings are consistent with *in vitro* assessments, which demonstrated that calcium-regulated PTH release is altered in dispersed parathyroid cells obtained from hyperplastic tissues removed from patients undergoing parathyroidectomy for severe secondary hyperparathyroidism. In contrast, evidence of a calcium sensing defect is not found in patients with moderate

TABLE 1. *Biochemical features and set-point estimates in normal subjects, patients with moderate secondary hyperparathyroidism documented by bone biopsy, patients with advanced secondary hyperparathyroidism studied several days before undergoing subtotal parathyroidectomy, and patients with primary hyperparathyroidism*

	Normal (n = 20)	2°HPT (n = 31)	Pre-PTX (n = 8)	1°HPT (n = 3)
Blood ionized calcium (mM)	1.22 ± 0.04	1.22 ± 0.07	1.27 ± 0.08[ab]	1.38 ± 0.08[abc]
Basal serum PTH level (pg/ml)	26 ± 6	536 ± 395[a]	1026 ± 324[ab]	88 ± 25[a]
Set point for calcium-regulated PTH release (mM)	1.21 ± 0.04	1.22 ± 0.05	1.28 ± 0.08[ab]	1.35 ± 0.06[abc]

Values expressed as mean ± SD.

[a] Differs significantly from normal.

[b] Differs significantly from 2°HPT (patients with moderate secondary hyperparathyroidism).

[c] Differs significantly from Pre-PTX (patients with advanced secondary hyperparathyroidism studied several days before undergoing subtotal parathyroidectomy). From Goodman WG, Veldhuis JD, Belin TR, Van Herle AJ, Jüppner H, Salusky IB. Calcium-sensing by parathyroid glands in secondary hyperparathyroidism. *J Clin Endocrinol Metab* 1998;81:1–2.

renal insufficiency who do not require dialysis, as judged by *in vivo* studies of parathyroid gland function. These *in vivo* findings in mild to moderate secondary hyperparathyroidism have yet to be confirmed by *in vitro* assessments of either calcium-regulated PTH release or CaSR expression, because parathyroid tissues from such individuals are not available for study. It remains uncertain, therefore, whether alterations in CaSR expression fully account for disturbances in PTH secretion in mild to moderate chronic renal failure.

Phosphorus retention and hyperphosphatemia have been recognized for many years as important factors in the pathogenesis of secondary hyperparathyroidism. The development of secondary hyperparathyroidism is prevented in experimental animals with chronic renal failure when dietary phosphorus intake is lowered in proportion to the glomerular filtration rate (GFR), and dietary phosphate restriction can reduce previously elevated serum PTH levels in patients with moderate renal failure. Phosphorus retention and hyperphosphatemia indirectly promote the secretion of PTH in several ways. First, hyperphosphatemia lowers blood ionized calcium levels and stimulates PTH release as free calcium ions form complexes with excess amounts of inorganic phosphate. Second, phosphorus impairs renal 1α-hydroxylase activity, which diminishes the conversion of 25-hydroxyvitamin D [25 (OH) D] to 1,25 $(OH)_2$ D; high rates of transepithelial phosphate transport in the proximal tubule when GFR is reduced may account for this change, thereby contributing to reductions in renal calcitriol production. In addition, recent evidence suggests that phosphorus can directly enhance PTH synthesis by the parathyroid cell. The amount of PTH released from parathyroid glands maintained in tissue culture increases at high medium phosphorus concentrations; this response appears to be mediated by a posttranscriptional mechanism because the rate of pre-pro-PTH gene transcription is not affected by the level of phosphorus in the culture medium (18).

In summary, a number of factors contribute to excess PTH secretion in patients with chronic renal failure. Persistently high serum PTH levels activate both osteoblastic and osteoclastic activity in bone, resulting in increases in bone formation and turnover. Overall, serum PTH values generally correspond to the histologic severity of secondary hyperparathyroidism, as assessed by iliac crest bone biopsy in patients with end-stage renal disease who are not receiving active vitamin D sterols and in those given small daily oral doses of 1,25 $(OH)_2$ D.

The osseous changes in renal secondary hyperparathyroidism are usually more pronounced than those of primary hyperparathyroidism, probably due to the higher serum levels of PTH. Serum PTH values are typically fivefold to 10-fold above the upper limit of normal in patients with secondary hyperparathyroidism due to end-stage renal disease, and they may reach levels 20 to 40 times higher than normal. In contrast, serum PTH levels in most patients with primary hyperparathyroidism fall within a range that is only twofold to fourfold above the upper limit of normal.

Unlike patients with end-stage renal disease, those with moderate renal failure who do not require dialysis often exhibit overt histologic evidence of secondary hyperparathyroidism when serum PTH levels are only 1 to 2 times higher than normal (19). The discordance in the skeletal changes of secondary hyperparathyroidism between patients with moderate renal failure and those with end-stage renal disease is probably attributable to differences in tissue resistance to the actions of PTH and to variations in the extent to which vitamin D metabolism is disrupted.

Pathogenesis of Low-Turnover Bone Disease (Adynamic Bone and Osteomalacia)

In the past, secondary hyperparathyroidism was an almost invariable consequence of chronic renal failure, and it was the most common skeletal lesion of renal osteodystrophy. Currently, a substantial proportion of patients do not have markedly elevated serum PTH levels when regular dialysis is begun, and many have biopsy evidence of adynamic bone. The prevalence of adynamic renal osteodystrophy also has increased substantially in recent years in adult patients receiving regular dialysis. Approximately 40% of those treated with hemodialysis and more than half of adult patients undergoing peritoneal dialysis have serum PTH levels that are only minimally elevated or fall within the normal range; such values are typically associated with normal or reduced rates of bone formation and turnover.

The adynamic lesion of renal osteodystrophy currently accounts for most cases of low-turnover bone disease in patients with end-stage renal disease, whereas osteomalacia is seen much less frequently. Bone formation and turnover are reduced in both disorders, but osteomalacia is characterized by an additional defect in skeletal mineralization.

In the 1970s and 1980s, aluminum intoxication was largely responsible for the development of adynamic bone and osteomalacia in patients with chronic renal failure, and two distinct patterns of aluminum exposure were identified. Epidemic, or clustered outbreaks, of aluminum-related bone disease most often resulted from technical errors in the preparation of dialysis solutions or from the use of inadequate methods of water purification in dialysis facilities (20). Failure to remove aluminum from municipal water sources during the preparation of dialysate led to intense parenteral aluminum exposure over short periods. In contrast, other patients developed aluminum-related bone disease by ingesting large amounts of aluminum-containing, phosphate-binding agents over many months to control serum phosphorus levels. Bone aluminum deposition was a prominent finding both in patients with adynamic lesions and in those with osteomalacia, and severe bone and muscle pain, proximal myopathy, and skeletal fractures were prominent clinical manifestations (20). Bone histology and bone formation improved when aluminum overload was effectively treated.

Aluminum has diverse effects on bone and mineral metabolism (21). It adversely influences the proliferation and the differentiated function of osteoblasts, reduces collagen synthesis, and suppresses PTH secretion; thus adynamic lesions can develop both from direct inhibitory actions of aluminum on bone cells and from indirect effects mediated through PTH (21). The causes of adynamic renal osteodystrophy include:

- Aluminum toxicity
- Diabetes
- Corticosteroid therapy

- Hyperparathyroidism
  Surgical
  Medical
- Immobilization
- Malnutrition
- Advanced age-osteoporosis
- Excess doses of vitamin D sterols
- Calcium supplementation
  Oral calcium salts
  Dialysate

In addition, aluminum impairs skeletal mineralization, and it may impede renal calcitriol production. Both disturbances can contribute to the development of osteomalacia.

Factors that increase the risk of aluminum-related bone disease in patients with renal failure include previous parathyroidectomy, a history of renal transplantation and graft failure, bilateral nephrectomy, and diabetes mellitus. Moreover, citrate anions, unlike carbonate, form soluble complexes with aluminum in aqueous solutions, and they markedly enhance intestinal aluminum absorption. The concurrent administration of citrate and aluminum-containing medications can lead to acute aluminum intoxication, and this combination of agents must be avoided. Persistently high serum PTH levels appear partially to offset the adverse skeletal effects of aluminum, and this phenomenon may account for the increased risk of aluminum-related bone disease in diabetics and patients who have undergone parathyroidectomy, because serum PTH levels are generally low in both conditions.

Aluminum-related bone disease is much less common now that adequate water-purification methods have become widely used and the use of aluminum-containing medications has been curtailed in patients with end-stage renal disease; thus aluminum is currently an infrequent cause of adynamic renal osteodystrophy. Diabetes, corticosteroid therapy, and increasing age account for adynamic skeletal findings in many patients (see bulleted list above). In this regard, the proportion of diabetic and elderly patients in the dialysis population in the United States continues to increase. Diabetics often have only modestly elevated serum PTH levels even when renal failure is advanced, and insulin deficiency diminishes osteoblastic activity and bone collagen synthesis. Corticosteroids directly suppress osteoblastic activity and bone formation, and their use in large doses and for sustained periods can result in low-turnover osteoporosis.

The histologic features of adynamic renal osteodystrophy, in the absence of bone aluminum deposition, cannot be distinguished from those of corticosteroid-induced osteoporosis or either age-related or postmenopausal osteoporosis. It is not possible to determine whether osteoporosis accounts for decreases in osteoblastic activity and bone formation in patients with adynamic renal osteodystrophy unless the amount of trabecular bone is reduced. Decreases in bone mass and histologic evidence of trabecular bone loss are not, however, integral features of the adynamic lesion of renal osteodystrophy when other causes of osteoporosis can be excluded.

The widespread use of large doses of oral calcium carbonate to control hyperphosphatemia and treatment with active vitamin D sterols to lower serum PTH levels have probably contributed to the increased prevalence of adynamic bone in patients with end-stage renal disease. High concentrations of calcium in dialysis solutions also may play a role. As discussed previously, both calcium and vitamin D diminish PTH secretion by lowering pre-pro-PTH gene transcription. Because PTH is the major determinant of bone formation and skeletal remodeling in renal failure, oversuppression of PTH secretion can result in adynamic renal osteodystrophy. Calcitriol may also directly suppress osteoblastic activity when given intermittently in large doses to patients receiving regular dialysis (22).

The long-term consequences of adynamic renal osteodystrophy when not attributable to aluminum toxicity remain to be determined, but concerns have been raised about increases in the risk of skeletal fracture and delayed fracture healing due to low rates of bone remodeling. The development of soft-tissue and vascular calcifications may be facilitated because of frequent episodes of hypercalcemia. Recent work suggested that calcification of the coronary arteries and cardiac valves is common in patients undergoing long-term dialysis, but the relation between these changes and the presence of adynamic renal osteodystrophy is uncertain (23). In children, adynamic renal osteodystrophy has been associated with a reduction in linear growth in prepubertal patients (24).

Although low serum PTH levels diminish bone formation and turnover, they do not explain the mineralization defect of osteomalacia; thus other pathogenic factors must be considered in patients with renal osteomalacia. Aluminum intoxication must be excluded by meticulous and thorough investigation. Evidence of vitamin D deficiency, as judged by low serum levels of 25 (OH) D, was noted in some dialysis patients with osteomalacia in England, but this has been considered an uncommon finding in the United States. Differences in sunlight exposure and in the amounts of vitamin D provided in fortified foods and nutritional supplements probably account for this disparity, but the prevalence of reduced serum 25 (OH) D levels in the United States may be greater than previously thought. Long-term therapy with phenytoin and/or phenobarbital has been associated with osteomalacia in nonuremic patients, and a higher incidence of symptomatic bone disease was reported in dialysis patients receiving these drugs. Persistent hypocalcemia and/or hypophosphatemia can cause osteomalacia in some patients. In infants and small children, excess dietary phosphorus restriction must be avoided because serum phosphorus levels are normally higher in this age group, and the skeletal requirements for phosphorus are greater than those in older children or adults because of high rates of bone mineral accretion. Overall, better nutritional management and the less frequent use of aluminum-containing medications have diminished the prevalence of osteomalacia in patients with end-stage renal disease.

HISTOLOGIC FEATURES OF RENAL OSTEODYSTROPHY

The use of bone biopsy has contributed substantially to our understanding of renal bone disease. Quantitative histomorphometry of bone provides information about the status

TABLE 2. *Histologic features of high-turnover renal osteodystrophy*

	Mild lesion of 2°HPT	Osteitis fibrosa
Bone formation		
Trabecular bone volume	Normal	Normal–High
Osteoid volume	Normal–High	Normal–High
Osteoid seam thickness	Normal	Normal–High
No. of osteoblasts	High	Very high
Bone-formation rate	High	Very high
Mineralization lag time	Normal	Normal
Bone resorption		
Eroded bone perimeter	High	Very high
No. of osteoclasts	High	Very high
Marrow fibrosis	Absent	Present

of skeletal mineralization, the structural characteristics of cancellous and cortical bone, the levels of osteoblastic and osteoclastic activity, and the presence or absence of marrow fibrosis. Measurements of bone formation also can be obtained by using the technique of double tetracycline labeling. The tetracyclines are deposited in bone at sites of active mineralization, and their presence can be demonstrated in tissue sections examined by fluorescence microscopy. Where new bone has been formed, double bands of tetracycline fluorescence are seen. The amount of mineralized tissue deposited during the labeling interval is demarcated by the two labels, and the rate of bone formation can be measured directly. Such information is often essential for the correct diagnostic interpretation of biopsy material from patients with renal osteodystrophy.

Methods for achieving double tetracycline labeling of bone differ among laboratories, but the following approach is suitable for patients with chronic renal failure. Patients are given either demeclocycline, 300 mg orally twice a day, or tetracycline HCl, 500 mg orally twice daily, for 2 days, followed by a 10- to 20-day interval during which no tetracycline is given. A second course of oral tetracycline HCl, 500 mg twice a day, is then given for another 2 days. Bone biopsy should be obtained 3 to 7 days after finishing of the second course of oral tetracycline. For pediatric patients, doses of tetracycline should not exceed 10 mg/kg/day.

In addition to standard histologic assessments, special staining procedures can be used to demonstrate deposits of aluminum, iron, and amyloid in bone, and the bone aluminum content can be measured by atomic absorption spectroscopy in separate samples obtained at the time of biopsy. Iliac crest bone biopsy can be done safely in the outpatient setting with little morbidity both in adults and in children.

High-Turnover Bone Disease

Osteitis fibrosa is the most common high-turnover lesion of renal osteodystrophy both in adults and in children. The disorder represents the response of bone to persistently high serum levels of PTH. There is histologic evidence of active bone resorption with increases in the number and size of osteoclasts and in the number of resorption bays, or Howship's lacunae, within cancellous bone (Table 2). Fibrous tissue is found immediately adjacent to bony trabeculae, or it may accumulate more extensively within the mar-

row space (Fig. 4). Partial or complete fibrous replacement of bony trabeculae occurs in advanced cases.

Osteoblastic activity is increased in patients with osteitis fibrosa, and the combined increase in osteoblastic and osteoclastic activity accounts for the high rates of bone remodeling and turnover in secondary hyperparathyroidism. Bone formation is elevated, and values are often 2 to 4 times higher than normal (Table 2). The number of osteoblasts is substantially increased, and a greater proportion of the surface of cancellous bone is covered with newly formed osteoid. Overall, the amount of osteoid is moderately elevated, and many osteoid seams have a woven, or hatched, appearance similar to that of a straw basket; this is a characteristic feature of skeletal disorders in which the rates of collagen synthesis and deposition are markedly increased, and it reflects the disordered arrangement of collagen fibrils within osteoid seams when bone formation proceeds rapidly.

Patients with only moderate increases in osteoclastic activity and bone formation and in whom there is little or no evidence of peritrabecular fibrosis are classified as mild lesions of renal osteodystrophy (Table 2). The disorder is a

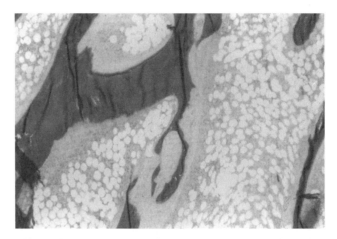

FIG. 4. Photomicrograph of a section of undecalcified bone obtained by iliac crest biopsy from a patient with osteitis fibrosa cystica; magnification, ×50. The dark structures represent mineralized bone. Pale regions adjacent to individual trabeculae represent fibrous tissue, which has partially replaced a portion of one trabeculum. The scalloped or eroded bone margins represent sites of osteoclastic bone resorption.

less severe manifestation of hyperparathyroid bone disease. Serum PTH levels are elevated, but values are substantially lower than those in patients with overt osteitis fibrosa (25,26). Other biochemical and radiographic manifestations of secondary hyperparathyroidism may be present. Because the histologic changes of the mild lesion are less striking than those of overt osteitis fibrosa, tetracycline-based measurements of bone formation are useful for distinguishing this subgroup from those with either normal rates of bone formation and turnover or patients with adynamic lesions (Table 2).

Low-Turnover Bone Disease

Osteomalacia is the most striking histologic manifestation of low-turnover bone disease (Fig. 5). Excess osteoid, or unmineralized bone collagen, accumulates in bone because of a primary defect in mineralization. Osteoid seams are wide, and they have multiple lamellae (Table 3); the extent of trabecular bone surfaces covered with osteoid also is increased. In contrast, osteoblastic activity is markedly reduced, and bone formation often cannot be measured because of the lack of tetracycline uptake into bone (Table 3). In patients with aluminum-related osteomalacia, the bone aluminum content is elevated. Deposits of aluminum can be seen along trabecular bone surfaces by using histochemical staining methods, and the histologic severity of osteomalacia in such cases corresponds to the amount of surface-stainable aluminum in trabecular bone (27).

Bone biopsies from patients with the adynamic lesion of renal osteodystrophy exhibit normal or reduced amounts of osteoid, no tissue fibrosis, diminished numbers of osteoblasts and osteoclasts, and low or unmeasurable rates of bone formation (Table 3; Fig. 6). This disorder was originally described in patients with evidence of aluminum toxicity, and aluminum deposition along trabecular bone surfaces was a prominent finding. *In vivo* studies in experimental animals suggest the disorder is a forerunner of overt histologic osteomalacia when bone aluminum deposition is the underlying

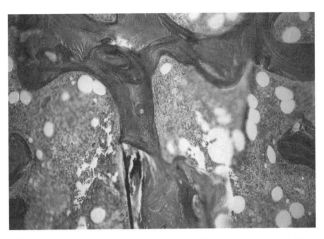

FIG. 5. The histologic appearance of cancellous bone in a patient with osteomalacia; magnification, ×50. Osteoid seams are wide, and they exhibit multiple lamellae. The total amount of osteoid is markedly increased, but few osteoblasts can be identified.

cause; thus bone aluminum levels are not so high in this subgroup of patients compared with those with aluminum-related osteomalacia.

Currently the majority of adult and pediatric dialysis patients with adynamic lesions of renal osteodystrophy do not have evidence of bone aluminum deposition. Other factors are now more common causes of adynamic bone (see bulleted list above).

Mixed Lesion of Renal Osteodystrophy

Some patients demonstrate histologic features of both osteitis fibrosa and osteomalacia. This combination of findings is called the mixed lesion of renal osteodystrophy. Patients have biochemical evidence of secondary hyperparathyroidism, but other factors account for impaired mineral-

TABLE 3. *Histologic features of low-turnover renal osteodystrophy*

	Adynamic	Osteomalacia
Bone formation		
Trabecular bone volume	Normal, low	Variable Low, normal or high
Osteoid volume	Normal, low	High–very high
Osteoid seam thickness	Normal, low	High–very high
No. of osteoblasts	Low	Low
Bone-formation rate	Low–very low	Low–very low
Mineralization lag time	Normal[a]	Prolonged
Bone resorption		
Eroded bone perimeter	Normal, low	Variable Often low; may be high
No. of osteoclasts	Low	Low; may be normal or high
Marrow fibrosis	Absent	Absent

[a] As measured by conventional histomorphometry, the mineralization lag time (Mlt) reflects the average value for all osteoid seams, and it is often prolonged in adynamic renal osteodystrophy. In contrast, the osteoid maturation time (O.mt) represents the average only for osteoid seams that are undergoing active mineralization, and it is usually normal in the adynamic lesion. The disparity in values for Mlt and O.mt between adynamic bone and osteomalacia is due to differences in the proportion of osteoid seams undergoing active mineralization at any given time.

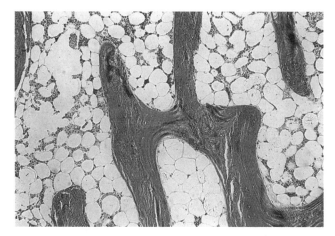

FIG. 6. The histologic appearance of adynamic renal osteodystrophy. There is little, if any, osteoid, and resorption lacunae are not seen along the trabecular margins. Note the paucity of cells along trabecular bone surfaces.

ization. Persistent hypocalcemia and/or hypophosphatemia are found in some patients; nutritional vitamin D deficiency is present in others. Mixed lesions of renal osteodystrophy can be seen in patients with osteitis fibrosa who are in the process of developing aluminum-related bone disease or in those with aluminum-related osteomalacia who are responding favorably to treatment with deferoxamine (DFO) with increases in bone formation; thus mixed renal osteodystrophy can represent a transitional state between the high-turnover lesions of secondary hyperparathyroidism and the low-turnover disorders of osteomalacia or adynamic bone (21).

CLINICAL MANIFESTATIONS

The signs and symptoms of renal osteodystrophy are rather nonspecific, and various laboratory and roentgenographic abnormalities often fail to correspond to the severity of the clinical manifestations. Common features include bone pain, muscle weakness, skeletal deformities, and extraskeletal calcifications. In children, growth retardation is a prominent feature.

Bone Pain

Bone pain is often present in patients with renal osteodystrophy; its onset is insidious, and symptoms progress gradually over many months. The pain is frequently diffuse and nonspecific, but it is often aggravated by weightbearing or by changes in posture. When it is localized, the lower back, hips, and legs are most often affected. Pain in the heels or ankles may be a presenting complaint. Occasionally the initial manifestation is an acute arthritis or periarthritis that is not relieved by massage or by the application of heat locally. Severe bone pain is more common in patients with aluminum-related bone disease than in those with osteitis fibrosa, and it is a prominent clinical feature of this disorder. There is marked variation among patients, however, and some with advanced secondary hyperparathyroidism are se-

verely incapacitated. The physical examination is generally unremarkable unless fractures or skeletal deformities are present.

Muscle Weakness

Proximal myopathy develops in some patients with advanced renal failure. Symptoms appear very slowly, and weakness and aching are the most common manifestations both in adults and in children. The physiological basis of this disorder is not understood. Favorable clinical responses have been noted in some patients after treatment with calcitriol or 25 (OH) D, after parathyroidectomy, after successful renal transplantation, or during treatment of aluminum-related bone disease with DFO. The role of abnormal vitamin D metabolism in the pathogenesis of uremic myopathy remains uncertain, but a careful evaluation must be done to exclude severe secondary hyperparathyroidism or bone aluminum toxicity. In those with prominent symptoms of muscle pain and weakness, an empiric therapeutic trial of calcitriol or 25 (OH) D is warranted.

Skeletal Deformities

Bone deformities are a prominent manifestation of renal osteodystrophy, particularly in children with long-standing renal failure. The frequency of skeletal deformity in pediatric patients is probably related to high rates of linear bone growth and skeletal modeling during endochondral bone formation in the immature skeleton. Bone deformities can affect both the axial and appendicular skeleton.

The pattern of deformity varies with age in children with chronic renal failure. In patients younger than 4 years, the changes of secondary hyperparathyroidism most often resemble those of vitamin D–deficiency rickets; characteristic features include rachitic rosary, Harrison's grooves, and enlargement of the wrists and ankles due to widening of the metaphysis beneath the growth plate of long bones. Craniotabes and frontal bossing of the skull occur in children who develop renal failure in the first 2 years of life.

The onset of overt renal failure before age 10 years is often associated with deformities of long bones; bowing is the most frequent change. Genu valgum is a common manifestation at any age, and ulnar deviation of hands, pes varus, "swelling" of the wrists, ankles, or medial ends of clavicles due to metaphyseal widening and pseudoclubbing are frequently observed. Despite regular treatment with vitamin D sterols, 20% to 25% of pediatric patients undergoing long-term dialysis require orthopedic procedures to correct skeletal deformities.

Slipped epiphyses are another serious complication of renal bone disease in pediatric patients. The disorder typically occurs in those with severe secondary hyperparathyroidism, and the femoral epiphysis is most often affected. Dental abnormalities, including enamel defects and malformations of the teeth, are typical in children with congenital renal disease because mineral metabolism is disturbed early in life.

In adults with aluminum-related bone disease, skeletal deformities are confined predominantly to the axial skeleton;

changes include lumbar scoliosis, kyphosis, and distortion of the thoracic cage. Adult patients with severe osteitis fibrosa may develop rib deformities and pseudoclubbing.

Growth Retardation

Children with chronic renal failure almost invariably exhibit growth retardation; contributing factors include metabolic acidosis, malnutrition, renal bone disease, and disturbances in the growth hormone insulin-like growth factor I (IGF-I) axis. Treatment with calcitriol has been reported to improve linear growth in children with advanced secondary hyperparathyroidism, but increases in growth during treatment with vitamin D, 25 (OH) D, or calcitriol have not been consistently observed in children undergoing maintenance dialysis. Indeed, linear growth may be less in prepubertal children with adynamic renal osteodystrophy (24).

Extraskeletal Manifestations

Several types of soft-tissue calcification can be detected by radiographic examination. Most frequent are tumoral or periarticular calcifications; these are sometimes associated with acute periarticular inflammation, and the clinical presentation may suggest acute arthritis. Soft-tissue calcifications are common when serum phosphorus levels are greater than 8 to 9 mg/dL or when the calcium/phosphorus ion product exceeds a value of 70 to 75. Indeed, high serum phosphorus levels have been identified as an independent risk factor for death in adults undergoing regular hemodialysis (28). Soft-tissue calcifications can regress if sustained reductions in serum phosphorus levels are achieved. Although extraskeletal calcifications are more common with advancing age, they also occur in children with end-stage renal disease.

The most frequent form of vascular calcification in patients with renal failure is localized to the medial layer of small and medium-sized arteries (Mockerberg's sclerosis); it is diffuse and continuous along the vessel wall. Medial vascular calcifications are most common in diabetic patients, and the radiographic appearance differs from the irregular pattern of calcified intimal plaques. Medial calcifications are usually asymptomatic, but palpation of the peripheral pulses and blood pressure measurements may be difficult in affected limbs. Vascular calcifications are best detected by lateral views of the ankle or anteroposterior views of the hands or feet by using magnification techniques with macroradioscopy. The importance of a high serum calcium/phosphorus ion product in the development of vascular calcifications has been questioned, but a concerted effort should be made to avoid values above 65 to 70. Newer radiographic imaging techniques such as electron beam computed tomography can detect calcifications in coronary arteries and cardiac valves, and these methods may prove useful in future assessments of vascular calcification in subjects with renal failure (23).

In extreme cases, there may be ischemic necrosis of the skin, muscle, and/or subcutaneous tissues, a syndrome known as ''calciphylaxis''; its pathogenesis is not understood (29). Some patients have advanced secondary hyperparathyroidism, and parathyroidectomy may provide significant clinical improvement. Calciphylaxis can be seen in patients with advanced renal failure, in those receiving regular dialysis, and in patients with functioning renal allografts (29). The tendency for patients with adynamic renal osteodystrophy to develop hypercalcemia may be a risk factor, but the evidence currently available is insufficient to implicate adynamic renal osteodystrophy as a distinct pathogenic cause of vascular calcification.

Visceral calcifications are rather infrequent, and they may differ in chemical composition from vascular calcifications; the lungs, heart, kidneys, skeletal muscle, and stomach mainly are involved. Pulmonary calcifications result in restrictive lung disease that may be progressive, and the disorder often persists even after successful kidney transplantation or parathyroidectomy.

AMYLOIDOSIS IN PATIENTS WITH CHRONIC RENAL FAILURE

Many adults whose end-stage renal disease is managed with dialysis for longer than 10 to 15 years develop dialysis-related amyloidosis (DRA), a unique type of amyloidosis with amyloid fibrils that contain β_2-microglobulin (β_2M), a normal plasma constituent. Patients with DRA exhibit the carpal tunnel syndrome, multiple bone cysts, scapulohumeral arthritis, spondyloarthropathy, and fractures (1,30). The predilection for DRA to affect the musculoskeletal system and to cause significant articular and skeletal symptoms necessitates its differentiation from other forms of renal osteodystrophy.

β_2-Microglobulin is a protein of approximately 12,000 daltons that is produced by many cells, particularly lymphoid cells and other cells with high rates of turnover. In cells of this type, β_2M stabilizes the structure of the major histocompatibility complex (MHC) class I antigen on the cell surface, but β_2M is released when the complexes are shed from the cell membrane. Approximately 180 to 250 mg of β_2M is normally generated each day. Almost all available β_2M is filtered at the glomerulus, and it is then catabolized by cells of the renal tubules (1,30). With advanced renal failure, β_2M accumulates in plasma, and levels increase to values 50 times greater than normal in anuric dialysis patients (30).

Histologically, β_2M amyloid fibrils are similar in appearance to those of amyloid AA; however, β_2M amyloid deposits are predominantly osteoarticular, leading to musculoskeletal manifestations. The slow rate of appearance and the predilection for bone and articular structures both suggest that elevated serum β_2M levels do not fully account for the clinical syndrome observed in patients with chronic renal failure. Increased age-related glycosylation products, certain specific proteases, and inhibitors of other proteases have been suggested as factors that lead to the deposition of β_2M amyloid in bony structures and in synovial tissues. In rare cases, systemic deposits occur, and these may be fatal.

The clinical features of amyloid deposition rarely appear before 5 years of dialysis therapy, and the disorder is more common in patients who start regular dialysis after age 50 years (31). Carpal tunnel syndrome is the most frequent clinical feature, but shoulder pain, other arthritic complaints, and cystic bone lesions are common. Deposits of β_2M are found in periarticular structures, joints, bone, and tendon sheaths. Far less commonly, the liver, spleen, rectal mucosa, or blood vessels are involved.

Skeletal manifestations include generalized arthritis, erosive arthritis, and joint effusions. Scapulohumeral involvement with shoulder pain is a common clinical presentation. Generalized arthritis can lead to pain and stiffness, decreased joint mobility, joint effusions, and deformities. Characteristically, pain is worse at night or when the patient must sit quietly for several hours during dialysis sessions; joint motion or activity can provide temporary relief. Erosive arthritis can involve the metacarpophalangeal joints, the interphalangeal joints, the shoulders, wrists, and knees; effusions sometimes occur at these sites. The cervical spine is the most common site of destructive spondyloarthropathy.

Roentgenographically, bone cysts are most common at the ends of long bones, particularly the femoral head and proximal humerus, and they also may be found in the metacarpal and carpal bones. Multiple cystic lesions are common, and serial radiographs often demonstrate cyst enlargement with time. Cystic deposits of β_2M may resemble brown tumors of osteitis fibrosa; however, their location and the presence of multiple rather than solitary cysts suggest that amyloid deposition is responsible. Cystic changes most commonly occur at sites of tendinous insertions, and pathologically these may represent ''amyloidomas'' that have replaced trabecular bone (Fig. 7). Fractures sometimes occur at these sites, and hip fractures in dialysis patients commonly arise at sites of β_2M deposition. Ultrasound examinations of the shoulder are a simple noninvasive method to assess progressive tendinous involvement with β_2M amyloid deposits.

The fraction of patients afflicted with amyloidosis increases progressively with the duration of dialysis therapy; thus 70% to 80% of adult patients treated with hemodialysis

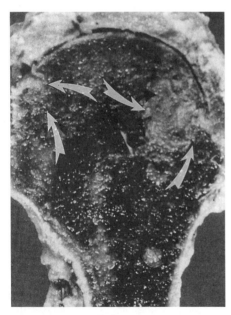

FIG. 7. Postmortem photograph showing extensive deposits of amyloid in the head of the femur *(white arrows)*. Such areas appear as cystic lesions on radiographs. (From Broucke JM, et al. *Kidney Int* 1988;33:S35–S36, with permission of Blackwell Science, Inc.)

for 10 years or more will have clinical features of β_2M amyloidosis. The distinction between this disorder and either severe secondary hyperparathyroidism or aluminum-related bone disease can be difficult, and thorough clinical, biochemical, and radiographic evaluations are required; β_2M amyloidosis can coexist with either high-turnover or low-turnover lesions of renal osteodystrophy.

The overall clinical management of amyloidosis in patients with end-stage renal disease has thus far proven unsatisfactory. The carpal tunnel syndrome may respond to surgical correction, but it often recurs. The use of highly permeable dialysis membranes can achieve slightly lower serum levels of β_2M, but there is no evidence that this intervention alters the progression of established disease. There is some evidence that patients treated from the onset of long-term dialysis with polyacrilonitrile (PAN) membranes have a delayed appearance of certain clinical features of dialysis amyloidosis compared with those treated with conventional cellulosic dialyzers. Successful renal transplantation is followed by symptomatic relief in most patients, but there is no evidence that bony or soft-tissue lesions actually regress after renal transplantation.

BIOCHEMICAL FEATURES OF RENAL OSTEODYSTROPHY

Serum calcium levels are often subnormal in patients with advanced renal failure. With the initiation of hemodialysis, values usually increase, and they may return to normal. The magnitude of the rise in serum calcium is partly related to the calcium concentration in dialysis solutions. In patients treated with continuous ambulatory peritoneal dialysis (CAPD) who are not receiving vitamin D supplements, serum calcium levels can often be maintained within the normal range.

The development of hypercalcemia in patients undergoing regular dialysis warrants prompt and thorough investigation. Conditions associated with hypercalcemia include marked hyperplasia of the parathyroid glands due to severe secondary hyperparathyroidism, aluminum-related bone disease, adynamic renal osteodystrophy, therapy with calcitriol or other vitamin D sterols, the administration of large doses of calcium carbonate or other calcium-containing compounds, immobilization, malignancy, and granulomatous disorders such as sarcoidosis or tuberculosis, in which there is extrarenal production of $1,25 (OH)_2 D$. Basal serum calcium levels are higher in patients with adynamic bone than in subjects with other lesions of renal osteodystrophy, and episodes of hypercalcemia are common (25). Because skeletal calcium uptake is limited in the adynamic lesion, calcium entering the extracellular fluid from dialysate or after intestinal absorption cannot adequately be buffered in bone, and serum calcium levels rise (32). Reducing the dose of calcium-containing, phosphate-binding agents and decreasing dialysate calcium concentrations usually corrects the hypercalcemia.

When the GFR falls below 25% to 30% of normal, hyperphosphatemia is common, and phosphate-binding agents and dietary phosphorus restriction are required to avoid phosphate retention. Although hemodialysis and CAPD remove substantial amounts of phosphorus, additional measures are usually needed to control hyperphosphatemia in patients ingesting adequate amounts of dietary protein.

In advanced renal failure, serum magnesium levels rise as a result of diminished renal magnesium excretion. Values are normal or slightly elevated when the concentration of magnesium in dialysate is kept between 0.5 and 0.8 mEq/L. The use of magnesium-containing laxatives or antacids can abruptly raise serum magnesium levels in patients with renal failure, and these medications should be avoided. Serum magnesium levels should be measured frequently and regularly if magnesium-containing medications are used.

Serum alkaline phosphatase values are fair markers of the severity of secondary hyperparathyroidism in patients with renal failure. Osteoblasts normally express large amounts of the bone isoenzyme of alkaline phosphatase, and serum levels are usually elevated when osteoblastic activity and bone-formation rates are increased. High levels generally reflect the extent of histologic change in patients with high-turnover lesions of renal osteodystrophy, and values frequently correlate with serum PTH levels. Serum total alkaline phosphatase measurements also are useful for monitoring the skeletal response to treatment with vitamin D sterols in patients with osteitis fibrosa; values that decrease over several months usually indicate histologic improvement. Serum alkaline phosphatase levels may increase early in the course of treating aluminum-related bone disease with the chelating agent DFO.

Newer assays for bone-specific alkaline phosphatase and measurements of serum osteocalcin levels provide additional information about the level of osteoblastic activity in patients with chronic renal failure. Osteocalcin levels are generally elevated in renal failure, but values may help to distinguish between patients with high-turnover or low-turnover skeletal lesions. If these assays are not unavailable, measurements of the heat-stable and heat-labile fractions of alkaline phosphatase help to separate skeletal from hepatic causes of elevated total alkaline phosphatase levels.

Serum PTH levels vary widely in patients with advanced renal failure, but currently available assays are reliable and useful for assessing patients with renal osteodystrophy. Assays that use double antibody methods to measure intact 1–84 PTH are highly recommended. The interpretation of serum PTH values in patients with renal failure must be done with knowledge about the relation between the levels in serum that correspond to specific histologic findings in bone, as documented by bone biopsy.

Double-antibody immunoradiometric serum PTH assays are generally better than other methods for separating patients with secondary hyperparathyroidism from those with adynamic lesions of bone (25). In untreated patients and in those receiving small daily oral doses of calcitriol, bone-biopsy evidence of secondary hyperparathyroidism is found when serum-intact PTH levels are above 250 to 300 pg/mL, or 25 to 30 pM (Fig. 8). In contrast, values in patients with adynamic lesions are usually below 150 pg/mL, or 15 pM, and levels frequently fall below 100 pg/mL, or 10 pM (Fig. 8). Both in children and in adults with chronic renal failure, intact serum PTH levels that are 2 to 3 times the upper limit of normal generally correspond to normal rates of bone formation, as documented by bone biopsy.

Plasma aluminum levels may be elevated in patients with chronic renal failure and in those treated with maintenance dialysis if there is ongoing exposure to aluminum-containing medications or to inadequately purified dialysate. Electrothermal atomic absorption spectrometry is an accurate and reproducible method for measuring aluminum in tissues and plasma, and values from reliable reference laboratories in normal subjects are usually less than 10 μg/L. Levels of 15 to 40 μg/L are common in patients undergoing regular dialysis who have previously ingested aluminum-containing medications, whereas values above 50 μg/L suggest some degree of aluminum loading. Aluminum levels in plasma reflect recent exposure to aluminum by either contaminated dialysate or aluminum-containing medications. Accordingly, plasma aluminum levels should be monitored at regular intervals in patients undergoing maintenance dialysis, particularly in those who continue to use aluminum-containing, phosphate-binding antacids.

Although plasma aluminum levels often correspond to the amount of aluminum ingested orally, they do not accurately reflect tissue stores of aluminum. Bone and liver represent major sites of aluminum deposition within the body, but tissue aluminum levels do not correspond to plasma values. Serum aluminum levels fall substantially after aluminum-containing medications have been discontinued despite persistent aluminum retention in tissues.

Deferoxamine is a chelating agent that binds to aluminum, and infusions of DFO can mobilize aluminum from tissues, markedly increasing plasma aluminum levels in patients with

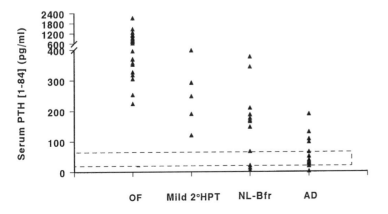

FIG. 8. Serum parathyroid hormone (PTH) levels in various subtypes of renal osteodystrophy as documented by iliac crest biopsy in patients undergoing regular dialysis. Subjects were either untreated or they had been maintained on small daily doses of oral calcitriol. Serum PTH values were measured using an immunoradiometric assay for intact 1–84 PTH. Dashed line, limits of normal for subjects with normal renal and parathyroid gland function. (From Salusky IB, Ramirez JA, Oppenheim WL, Gales B, Segre GV, Goodman WG. Biochemical markers of renal osteodystrophy in pediatric patients undergoing CAPD/CCPD. *Kidney Int* 1994;45:253–258, with permission of Blackwell Science, Inc.)

aluminum-related bone disease. It is used to treat some patients with severe aluminum intoxication (33). Infusions of DFO can be used as a diagnostic test for the noninvasive assessment of aluminum loading in patients with chronic renal failure.

The DFO-infusion test is completed as follows: standard intravenous doses of DFO, 40 mg/kg in 100 mL of 5% dextrose solution, are given over a 2-hour period immediately after a hemodialysis procedure; plasma aluminum levels are measured before and 24 to 48 hours after the infusion. An increase in plasma aluminum greater than 300 μg/L above preinfusion levels is a better predictor of bone aluminum deposition in symptomatic patients than measurements of basal plasma aluminum.

Unfortunately, the magnitude of the rise in plasma aluminum after DFO infusions is not specific when applied to unselected groups of patients. Dialysis patients with secondary hyperparathyroidism may exhibit substantial increases in plasma aluminum after infusions of DFO despite little evidence of stainable aluminum in bone-biopsy specimens. Thus some patients with osteitis fibrosa have high tissue levels of aluminum and a positive DFO-infusion test but no histologic evidence of bone aluminum toxicity. Such patients may be at risk, however, for developing aluminum-related bone disease if parathyroidectomy is done or if aluminum-containing medications are continued.

RADIOGRAPHIC FEATURES OF RENAL OSTEODYSTROPHY

Osteitis Fibrosa

Subperiosteal erosions are among the most consistent radiographic findings in patients with secondary hyperparathyroidism, and the extent of these changes corresponds to serum PTH and alkaline phosphatase levels. Patchy osteosclerosis also is common, and this feature accounts for the classic "rugger jersey" appearance of the spine on lateral views of the thoracic vertebrae and for the "salt and pepper" appearance of the skull. Skeletal roentgenographs may be normal, however, in patients with mild to moderate secondary hyperparathyroidism. Subperiosteal erosions are seen in some patients with aluminum-related osteomalacia, emphasizing the need for independent biochemical or histologic confirmation of the diagnosis of secondary hyperparathyroidism.

Subperiosteal erosions are detected at the margins of the digital phalanges, at the distal ends of the clavicles, beneath the surfaces of the ischium and pubis, at the sacroiliac joints, and at the junction of the metaphysis and diaphysis of long bones. Fine-grain films and a hand lens of ×6 to 7 magnification can help to detect erosions in radiographs of the hands. In pediatric patients, metaphyseal changes, or growth-zone lesions, are common, and these have been described as "rickets-like lesions." This radiographic finding of secondary hyperparathyroidism differs from that of true vitamin D deficiency. Both subperiosteal erosions of the digits and growth-zone lesions are best demonstrated by examining x-ray films of the hands. In children, the presence of growth-zone changes is a reliable indicator of the severity of secondary hyperparathyroidism, as judged by the serum levels of PTH and alkaline phosphatase.

Slipped epiphyses are among the most striking clinical and radiographic manifestations of renal osteodystrophy in children, and they are usually a consequence of advanced osteitis fibrosa in uremic children. The age of patients often determines the site affected. In preschool children, epiphyseal slippage occurs in either the upper or lower femoral region or in the distal tibial epiphysis, but not in the distal radius or distal ulna. In contrast, the upper femoral epiphysis and the distal epiphyses of the forearm are affected most often in older children. Severe epiphyseal slippage can lead to gross deformities of the skeleton with ulnar deviation of the hands and abnormalities in gait.

Osteomalacia

The roentgenographic features of osteomalacia are less specific than those of secondary hyperparathyroidism; indeed, pseudofractures are the only pathognomonic finding in adults. These are straight, wide radiolucent bands in the cortex oriented perpendicular to the long axis of the bone. Fractures of the ribs and hips and compression fractures of the vertebral bodies are more common in dialysis patients with osteomalacia than in those with osteitis fibrosa.

Rickets-like lesions have been described in pediatric patients with aluminum-related bone disease and osteomalacia, and these changes can resolve after treatment with DFO. Rachitic changes in children are not specific, however, and bone biopsy is usually required to determine the specific type of bone disease in pediatric patients with end-stage renal failure.

Amyloidosis

Cystic changes in bone, particularly if they are large, suggest amyloid deposits. Cysts most commonly involve the metacarpals and regions immediately adjacent to large joints near the site of tendon insertions; the hip, wrist, proximal humerus, pubic ramus, and proximal tibia are affected most often, but the carpal and tarsal bones also may be involved. Radiographs may reveal fractures at the site of cyst formation. Multiple bone cysts suggest the presence of amyloidosis, whereas brown tumors more often occur as isolated cystic lesions, usually in the ribs or the jaw.

Bone Scan

The compounds used most frequently for skeletal scintigraphy are technetium-labeled bisphosphonates, mainly ^{99}Tc-methylene diphosphonate. Bone scintigraphy may reveal fractures, pseudofractures, or extraskeletal calcifications, and local increases in tracer uptake occur in areas of amyloid deposition. Patients with osteitis fibrosa often exhibit symmetric increases in isotope activity in the skull, mandible, sternum, shoulders, vertebral bodies, and distal portions of the femur and tibia; collectively, these findings have been termed the "super scan." In contrast, the skeletal uptake of isotopic tracers is less in patients with aluminum-related osteomalacia than in those with osteitis fibrosa. Despite such general trends, findings on bone scan often do not agree closely with data obtained by bone biopsy; bone scans provide supportive information, but they are of limited diagnostic value in the assessment of patients with renal bone disease.

TREATMENT OF RENAL OSTEODYSTROPHY

The successful clinical management of patients with renal osteodystrophy includes measures to counteract or correct several different pathogenic factors. Key objectives include (a) maintenance of normal serum calcium and phosphorus levels; (b) prevention of extraskeletal calcifications; (c) avoidance of exposure to toxic agents such as aluminum and excess iron; (d) judicious use of vitamin D sterols and phosphate-binding agents; and (e) selective use of chelating agents such as DFO to manage aluminum intoxication.

Dietary Adjustments

Adequate control of serum phosphorus levels is important for preventing soft-tissue calcifications and for managing secondary hyperparathyroidism in patients with advanced renal failure. The intake of phosphorus in the diet normally ranges from 1.0 to 1.8 g/day in adults, but it must be lowered to 400 to 800 mg/day to prevent hyperphosphatemia in patients with renal failure. Such diets are generally unpalatable, and long-term compliance is difficult to achieve. Consequently phosphate-binding antacids are usually required to control hyperphosphatemia adequately when the GFR decreases to 25% to 30% of normal.

Phosphate-Binding Agents

Phosphate-binding antacids diminish intestinal phosphate absorption by forming poorly soluble complexes with phosphorus in the intestinal lumen. In the past, aluminum-containing medications were widely used, but these should be used sparingly, if at all, to avoid aluminum loading and aluminum toxicity. If they are used, the duration of treatment should be limited, and doses must be kept as low as possible. The concurrent administration of citrate-containing compounds must be avoided, and plasma aluminum levels should be monitored regularly.

Several calcium-containing compounds have been used to reduce intestinal phosphorus absorption, but calcium carbonate is used most often. Calcium carbonate can adequately control serum phosphorus levels in most patients undergoing maintenance dialysis, although hypercalcemia remains a major side effect (34). The use of dialysis solutions containing 2.5 mEq/L rather than 3.5 mEq/L of calcium reduces the frequency of hypercalcemic episodes in patients ingesting calcium carbonate (35). Phosphate-binding agents that contain neither calcium nor aluminum will soon be available, and their use should enhance the ability of clinicians to control serum phosphorus levels with fewer adverse effects (36).

Calcium carbonate should be ingested with meals to increase the efficiency of phosphate binding and to minimize intestinal calcium absorption. Doses range from 1 to 12 to 15 g/day. Some patients require combined therapy with aluminum hydroxide and calcium carbonate to achieve adequate control of serum phosphorus levels. The long-term adverse effects associated with the ingestion of very large doses of calcium in patients with renal failure remain to be determined; no increase in the prevalence of vascular calcification was reported, however, in adult patients treated for 3 years.

Calcium acetate has also been used to control hyperphosphatemia in patients with chronic renal failure. In vitro studies and short-term in vivo studies indicated that calcium acetate binds more phosphorus than do equivalent doses of either calcium carbonate or aluminum hydroxide. The frequency of hypercalcemic episodes was no less, however, in patients given calcium acetate than in those receiving calcium carbonate (37).

Calcium citrate is an effective phosphate-binding agent, but the role of citrate in enhancing intestinal aluminum absorption is a major concern for patients who may be given other medications that contain aluminum. Magnesium carbonate was found to be effective when used together with magnesium-free dialysate in patients undergoing regular hemodialysis.

Vitamin D Sterols

Despite dietary phosphate restriction, maintenance of an adequate dietary calcium intake, the use of appropriate levels of calcium in dialysate, and the regular ingestion of phosphate-binding agents, a substantial proportion of patients receiving regular dialysis develop secondary hyperparathyroidism. Consequently treatment with active vitamin D sterols is required in many patients. Although calcifediol, or 25 (OH) D, 1α-hydroxyvitamin D, and dihydrotachysterol have all proven to be effective in the management secondary hyperparathyroidism, calcitriol is by far the most widely used agent in the United States.

The efficacy of daily oral doses of calcitriol for the treatment of patients with symptomatic renal osteodystrophy has been documented in several clinical trials (38). Bone pain diminishes, muscle strength and gaitposture improve, and osteitis fibrosa frequently resolves either partially or completely. When measured with reliable assays, serum PTH levels decrease in patients who respond favorably to treatment. Growth velocity has been reported to increase during calcitriol therapy in some children with severe bone disease.

Similar findings have been reported in patients treated with daily doses of oral 1α-hydroxyvitamin D which undergoes 25-hydroxylation in the liver to form calcitriol; this agent is widely used in Europe and Japan. Calcitriol and 1α-hydroxyvitamin D are similarly effective for the treatment of secondary hyperparathyroidism in patients with chronic renal failure. Doses of oral calcitriol in most clinical trials have ranged from 0.25 to 1.5 μg/day. Hypercalcemia is the most common side effect, but most adult patients tolerate daily doses of 0.25 to 0.50 μg without marked increases in serum calcium levels; children may require somewhat larger daily oral doses of calcitriol.

Treatment is started by using small doses, and these are periodically adjusted to maintain serum calcium levels between 10.0 and 10.5 mg/dL; such an approach lowers serum PTH levels in many patients. Because the biologic half-life of calcitriol is relatively short, episodes of hypercalcemia resolve within several days after treatment is withheld.

The development of hypercalcemia during calcitriol therapy may predict the underlying type of skeletal lesion. When hypercalcemia occurs after several months of treatment and previously elevated serum PTH and alkaline phosphatase levels have returned toward normal, it is likely that osteitis fibrosa has substantially resolved. In contrast, hypercalcemia that occurs within the first several weeks of treatment suggests the presence of either low-turnover bone disease, which in some cases is due to bone aluminum deposition, or severe secondary hyperparathyroidism. Bone biopsy and measurements of bone aluminum content are needed to exclude aluminum-related bone disease. If there is evidence of autonomous hyperparathyroidism, parathyroidectomy may be required.

Large intermittent doses of oral calcitriol also have been used to treat secondary hyperparathyroidism in patients undergoing regular dialysis (39). This approach is particularly useful for those receiving peritoneal dialysis in whom parenteral therapy is not practical. When given 2 or 3 times per week, the cumulative weekly dose of calcitriol is greater, and higher peak serum levels of 1,25 (OH)$_2$ D are achieved after each dose. Large intermittent oral doses of calcitriol may be more effective than smaller daily oral doses for reducing PTH gene transcription and reducing serum PTH levels in patients with secondary hyperparathyroidism. Dosage regimens have ranged from 0.5 to 1.0 μg to 3.5 to 4.0 μg thrice weekly or 2.0 to 5.0 μg twice weekly; low doses should be used initially, and dosage adjustments must be based on frequent measurements of serum calcium and phosphorus levels.

In adult hemodialysis patients, the intravenous administration of calcitriol thrice weekly effectively lowers serum PTH levels (40). A portion of this response appears to be independent of changes in serum ionized calcium, suggesting that calcitriol directly reduces PTH synthesis and/or release (40). Intravenous calcitriol is now the most widely used approach for the treatment of secondary hyperparathyroidism in patients undergoing regular hemodialysis. Advantages of intravenous calcitriol include assured patient compliance, convenience of therapy because doses are given during regularly scheduled hemodialysis treatments, and the ability to achieve high serum levels of 1,25 (OH)$_2$ D after bolus intravenous injections. As with intermittent oral calcitriol therapy, the rise in serum calcium levels during treatment with thrice weekly doses of intravenous calcitriol appears to be less than with daily oral doses of calcitriol; thus larger amounts of 1,25 (OH)$_2$ D can be given each week. This may enhance delivery of calcitriol to the parathyroid glands and promote the suppressive effect of 1,25 (OH)$_2$ D on PTH secretion.

Most clinical trials have used reductions in serum PTH levels as an index of efficacy during treatment with active vitamin D sterols in patients with secondary hyperparathyroidism. Although serum PTH levels generally correspond to the severity of osseous changes of secondary hyperpara-

thyroidism in untreated patients and in those receiving small daily oral doses of calcitriol, similar relations may not apply during treatment with larger intermittent doses of vitamin D sterols given twice or thrice weekly (22). Bone formation and turnover may fall dramatically during intermittent calcitriol therapy, and a substantial proportion of patients develop adynamic renal osteodystrophy (22). In some, adynamic lesions are seen with marked reductions in basal serum PTH levels, but PTH values remain substantially elevated in others despite substantial decreases in bone formation (22). Such findings suggest that large intermittent doses of calcitriol diminish osteoblastic activity directly and reduce bone formation and turnover by PTH-independent mechanisms. Accordingly, serum PTH levels should be monitored regularly during intermittent calcitriol therapy, and the dose of calcitriol should be lowered when serum PTH levels fall to values 4 to 5 times the upper limit of normal to reduce the risk of developing adynamic bone.

Increases in serum calcium and phosphorus levels often limit the dose of calcitriol that can be given to patients with end-stage renal disease. Several newer vitamin D analogues have been shown, however, to lower serum PTH levels effectively with only minor increases in serum calcium concentration in patients with renal secondary hyperparathyroidism (41). 1α (OH) D$_2$ and 19-nor-1α,25 (OH)$_2$ D$_2$ may provide wider margins of safety than calcitriol when treating patients with overt renal secondary hyperparathyroidism. Whether these compounds diminish osteoblastic activity and reduce bone formation in a manner similar to that observed during intermittent calcitriol therapy remains to be determined.

Novel therapeutic agents called calcimimetics also are being developed; these compounds activate the CaSR, resulting in prompt reductions in PTH release from the parathyroid glands. Serum PTH levels fall within 1 to 2 hours after drug administration (42,43). In contrast to the response to most vitamin D sterols, serum calcium concentrations decline rather than increase as PTH-mediated calcium release from bone diminishes. Although not yet available for clinical use, calcimimetic agents may permit clinicians in the future to more reliably diminish PTH secretion and to more precisely regulate serum PTH levels in patients with secondary hyperparathyroidism due to chronic renal failure.

Parathyroidectomy

Certain events indicate the need to consider parathyroid surgery in patients with advanced secondary hyperparathyroidism. In all instances, the diagnosis of aluminum-related bone disease must be considered and excluded before parathyroidectomy, and evidence of severe secondary hyperparathyroidism should be thoroughly documented by biochemical, radiographic, and if necessary, bone histologic criteria. Specific indications for parathyroidectomy include (a) persistent hypercalcemia with serum calcium levels above 11.0 to 11.5 mg/dL; (b) intractable pruritus that does not respond to intensive dialysis or to other medical interventions; (c) progressive extraskeletal calcifications and/or persistent hyperphosphatemia despite the continued use of dietary phosphorus restriction and phosphate-binding agents; (d) severe bone pain or fractures; and (e) the development of calciphylaxis (44). Other causes of hypercalcemia such as sarcoidosis, malignancy, or the intake of excess amounts of calcium or vitamin D also must be considered and excluded. Because the risk of aluminum toxicity is greater after parathyroidectomy, aluminum hydroxide should be avoided, and calcium carbonate should be used as the sole phosphate-binding agent after parathyroid surgery.

There is ongoing disagreement about the use of subtotal versus total parathyroidectomy in patients with chronic renal failure (45). The 15% to 30% incidence of recurrent secondary hyperparathyroidism in patients undergoing subtotal parathyroidectomy is a legitimate concern, and the availability of calcitriol and other active vitamin D sterols greatly facilitates the management of hypocalcemia after total parathyroidectomy. For patients who may subsequently undergo renal transplantation, the preservation of residual parathyroid tissue after subtotal parathyroidectomy helps to maintain calcium homeostasis when renal function is restored.

It is generally not advisable to implant remnants of parathyroid tissue removed at parathyroidectomy subcutaneously into the forearm or other sites in an effort to preserve parathyroid function after surgery. Such grafts may exhibit autonomous secretory behavior, and they occasionally spread locally into surrounding tissues, leading to recurrent hyperparathyroidism. Adequate surgical resection may be difficult.

Management of Aluminum Intoxication

The clinical manifestations and histologic features of aluminum-related bone disease improve during DFO therapy in patients undergoing regular dialysis (33), and aluminum removal during hemodialysis and peritoneal dialysis increases substantially after intravenous or subcutaneous doses of DFO. After 4 to 10 months of therapy, clinical benefit was observed in a large proportion of patients with severe bone disease (20,33). Analgesic use decreased, and patients who were confined to bed or a wheelchair were able to resume walking without assistance.

Typical biochemical changes after DFO treatment include reductions in serum calcium levels and increases in serum alkaline phosphatase, findings consistent with improvements in skeletal mineralization and osteoblastic activity. Serum PTH levels rise modestly in most patients, but it is not known whether this change is due to aluminum removal from the parathyroid glands or to a fall in serum calcium concentrations. Serial bone biopsies generally show an increase in bone formation and improvements in mineralization; indeed, some patients with low-turnover lesions of bone may develop osteitis fibrosa (33). The amount of surface-stainable aluminum in bone decreases in most patients who improve with treatment, but patients who have undergone previous parathyroidectomy respond less well or not at all (33). Adequate residual parathyroid gland function may be important for skeletal recovery from bone aluminum intoxication.

Serious and often lethal infections with *Rhizopus* and *Yersinia* species may develop in dialysis patients given DFO. In one series, six of 131 patients treated with DFO over a 3-year period were affected. The chelation of iron by DFO enhances iron delivery to certain organisms, increasing their pathogenic potential. These observations emphasize the need to use DFO judiciously for treating aluminum intoxication in patients undergoing regular dialysis.

Deferoxamine should be given only to patients with symptomatic aluminum intoxication, and evidence of tissue toxicity should be fully documented before therapy is begun. Doses of DFO should not exceed 0.5 to 1.0 g/week, and plasma aluminum levels should be measured regularly. Subcutaneous administration avoids the high serum levels of feroxamine that can occur after intravenous doses; this approach may reduce the risk of opportunistic infection. In asymptomatic patients with aluminum deposition in bone, bone histology and bone formation can improve solely by discontinuing aluminum-containing medications and using calcium carbonate to control serum phosphorus levels (46).

BONE AND MINERAL METABOLISM IN RENAL TRANSPLANT RECIPIENTS

Although the restoration of kidney function after successful renal transplantation corrects many of the disturbances that lead to renal osteodystrophy, disorders of bone and mineral metabolism remain a major clinical problem in renal transplant recipients. Indeed, as many as 80% to 90% of patients have histologic evidence of bone disease 5 years after transplantation. In such patients, alterations in bone and mineral homeostasis can be a manifestation of preexisting renal osteodystrophy or the result of changes peculiar to the posttransplant setting.

Hypercalcemia is not uncommon after renal transplantation; its frequency corresponds to the duration of dialysis, and probably to the degree of parathyroid gland hyperplasia, before transplantation. Several other factors also contribute. The presence of a functioning renal allograft rapidly corrects the deficit in renal $1,25(OH)_2 D$ production that characterizes chronic renal failure, and calcitriol synthesis is further enhanced by the resolution of hyperphosphatemia. Because the reversal of parathyroid gland hyperplasia takes many months or years, most patients exhibit persistently high serum PTH levels in the immediate posttransplant period, and this abnormality further promotes renal calcitriol production. Together, these changes increase intestinal calcium absorption, calcium mobilization from bone, and renal tubular calcium reabsorption, each of which contributes to the development of hypercalcemia.

Hypercalcemia during the first several months after renal transplantation can be quite severe, and serum calcium levels may reach 15 mg/dL. Hypercalcemia can lead to allograft dysfunction, and peripheral ischemia occasionally develops because of extensive vascular calcification (i.e., calciphylaxis). Those with advanced secondary hyperparathyroidism before transplantation are at greatest risk.

More often, the degree of hypercalcemia after renal transplantation is less severe. Serum calcium levels usually range from 10.5 to 12.0 mg/dL in such cases, and episodes of hypercalcemia are intermittent and of short duration; the disorder usually resolves within 12 months. In 4% to 10% of patients, mild to moderate hypercalcemia may persist for more than a year and as long as 5 years. Serum calcium levels between 10.5 and 12.0 mg/dL are tolerated in many patients without adverse effects on renal allograft function, but elective parathyroidectomy should be considered when serum calcium levels persistently exceed 11.5 to 12.0 mg/dL more than 1 year after renal transplantation.

Hypophosphatemia is common in the early postoperative period after renal transplantation. Persistent secondary hyperparathyroidism is the major contributor, leading to reduced renal tubular phosphate reabsorption and increased renal phosphate excretion. Defects in renal tubular phosphorus reabsorption occasionally develop, and some patients excrete large amounts of phosphorus in the urine despite normal levels of PTH in serum. Pharmacologic doses of glucocorticoids increase renal phosphorus excretion, and this may further aggravate renal phosphate wasting in the immediate posttransplant period.

The clinical manifestations of hypophosphatemia are quite variable; some patients complain of malaise, fatigue, and proximal muscle weakness. Although hypophosphatemia can persist for many months, osteomalacia rarely develops. Symptomatic patients with serum phosphorus levels below 1.0 mg/dL should be given oral phosphorus supplements, and serum phosphorus levels should be monitored regularly. In those who require supplemental phosphorus, potassium rather than sodium salts should be used to avoid extracellular volume expansion, which increases renal phosphate excretion by lowering phosphate reabsorption in the proximal nephron.

Bone loss is common after renal transplantation, and evidence of reduced bone mass is found in nearly all patients after 5 years. Bone mass decreases substantially within the first 6 to 18 months after renal transplantation. These changes are associated with histologic evidence of diminished bone formation and turnover, findings consistent with the known effects of glucocorticoids on bone and rapidly falling serum PTH levels [47]. Osteoporosis also is common in other types of organ transplantation.

The use of large, immunosuppressive doses of corticosteroids is generally considered to be a major contributor to the development of osteoporosis in transplant recipients. Glucocorticoids directly inhibit osteoblastic activity and collagen synthesis, and they impede the differentiation of progenitor cells into fully mature osteoblasts. The rate of programed cell death, or apoptosis, in osteoblasts may also increase. In addition, glucocorticoids accelerate bone resorption by lowering intestinal calcium absorption, thereby contributing to mild secondary hyperparathyroidism.

The effects of cyclosporine on human bone have not been well characterized. Increases in bone remodeling with reductions in cancellous bone volume have been reported in rats given cyclosporine without changes in the serum levels of calcium, magnesium, 1,25 $(OH)_2$ D, or PTH. Cyclosporine inhibits *in vitro* bone resorption in a dose-dependent manner during incubations with PTH, 1,25 $(OH)_2$ D, and interleukin-1. Although preliminary data in humans suggest that cyclosporine decreases the incidence of osteonecrosis in renal transplant recipients by lowering the dose of prednisone required for adequate immunosuppression, the effects of this immunosuppressive agent on bone and mineral metabolism require further investigation.

Measures that are effective for the prevention of bone loss in transplant recipients have yet to be identified, but few studies have been done. Newer synthetic derivatives of prednisolone, such as deflazacort, are effective immunosuppressive agents, and they appear to have fewer adverse effects on bone and mineral metabolism. Bisphosphonates such as pamidronate and alendronate diminish bone resorption by lowering osteoclastic activity, but their efficacy in preserving bone mass after renal transplantation awaits further clinical evaluation [48].

Osteonecrosis, or avascular necrosis, is by far the most debilitating skeletal complication associated with organ transplantation. Approximately 15% of patients will develop osteonecrosis within 3 years of renal transplantation. The occurrence of osteonecrosis in patients undergoing cardiac, hepatic, and bone marrow transplantation, as well as in those with systemic lupus erythematosus given high doses of corticosteroids, strongly suggests that glucocorticoids play a critical pathogenic role.

The mechanism by which corticosteroids contribute to the development of osteonecrosis has not been established. These agents may promote the accumulation of adipocytes within the marrow space, thereby increasing intraosseous hydrostatic pressure and altering blood flow within bone. Alternatively, corticosteroids may interfere with the process of microfracture repair, leading to a loss of the structural integrity of bone. Increased apoptotic rates in osteocytes also may play a role.

Osteonecrosis usually begins in weight-bearing areas; the femoral head and femoral neck are commonly affected in adults, but the distal femur, proximal tibia, and humeral head also may be involved. Osteonecrosis can occur at multiple sites in individual patients. In one report, two skeletal sites were involved in 85% of renal transplant recipients, whereas three or more sites were affected in 27%. Risk factors for osteonecrosis include the cumulative dose of corticosteroids, advanced age, and the duration of dialysis before transplantation.

REFERENCES

1. Koch KM. Dialysis-related amyloidosis. *Kidney Int* 1992;41:1416–1429.
2. Salusky IB, Goodman WG. Growth hormone and calcitriol as modifiers of bone formation in renal osteodystrophy. *Kidney Int* 1995;48:657–665.
3. Brown EM, Pollak M, Seidman CE, et al. Calcium-ion-sensing cell-surface receptors. *N Engl J Med* 1995;333:234–240.
4. Brown EM. Extracellular Ca^{2+} sensing, regulation of parathyroid cell function, and the role of Ca^{2+} and other ions as extracellular (first) messengers. *Physiol Rev* 1991;71:371–411.
5. Brown EM. Mechanisms underlying the regulation of parathyroid hormone secretion in vivo and in vitro. *Curr Opin Nephrol Hypertens* 1993;2:541–551.
6. Coburn JW, Kopple JD, Brickman AS. Study of intestinal absorption of calcium in patients with renal failure. *Kidney Int* 1973;3:264–272.
7. Massry SG, Coburn JW, Lee DBN, Jowsey J, Kleeman CR. Skeletal resistance to parathyroid hormone in renal failure. *Ann Intern Med* 1973;78:357–364.
8. Cohen-Solal ME, Sebert JL, Boudailliez B, et al. Comparison of intact, midregion, and carboxy-terminal assays of parathyroid hormone for the diagnosis of bone disease in hemodialyzed patients. *J Clin Endocrinol Metab* 1991;73:516–524.
9. Urena P, Mannstadt M, Hruby M, et al. Parathyroidectomy does not

prevent the renal PTH/PTHrP receptor down-regulation in uremic rats. *Kidney Int* 1995;47:1797–1805.

10. Korkor AB. Reduced binding of ³H-1,25-dihydroxyvitamin D in the parathyroid glands of patients with renal failure. *N Engl J Med* 1987;316:1573–1577.

11. Strom M, Sandgren ME, Brown TA, DeLuca HF. 1,25-Dihydroxyvitamin D₃ up-regulates the 1,25-dihydroxyvitamin D₃ receptor in vivo. *Proc Natl Acad Sci U S A* 1989;86:9770–9773.

12. Szabo A, Merke J, Beier E, Mall G, Ritz E. 1,25(OH)₂ vitamin D₃ inhibits parathyroid cell proliferation in experimental uremia. *Kidney Int* 1989;35:1049–1056.

13. Fukuda N, Tanaka H, Tominaga Y, Fukagawa M, Kurokawa K, Seino Y. Decreased 1,25-dihydroxyvitamin D₃ receptor density is associated with a more severe form of parathyroid hyperplasia in chronic uremic patients. *J Clin Invest* 1993;92:1436–1443.

14. Arnold A, Brown MF, Uren~a P, Gaz RD, Sarfati E, Drüeke TB. Monoclonality of parathyroid tumors in chronic renal failure and in primary parathyroid hyperplasia. *J Clin Invest* 1995;95:2047–2053.

15. Parfitt AM. The hyperparathyroidism of chronic renal failure: a disorder of growth. *Kidney Int* 1997;52:3–9.

16. Kifor O, Moore FD Jr, Wang P, et al. Reduced immunostaining for the extracellular Ca²⁺-sensing receptor in primary and uremic secondary hyperparathyroidism. *J Clin Endocrinol Metab* 1996;81:1598–1606.

17. Goodman WG, Veldhuis JD, Belin TR, Van Herle AJ, Jüppner H, Salusky IB. Calcium-sensing by parathyroid glands in secondary hyperparathyroidism. *J Clin Endocrinol Metab* 1998;81:1–2.

18. Denda M, Finch J, Slatopolsky E. Phosphorus accelerates the development of parathyroid hyperplasia and secondary hyperparathyroidism in rats with renal failure. *Am J Kidney Dis* 1996;28:596–602.

19. Hamdy NA, Kanis JA, Beneton MNC, et al. Effect of alfacalcidol on natural course of renal bone disease in mild to moderate renal failure. *Br Med J* 1995;310:358–363.

20. Coburn JW, Norris KC, Nebeker HG. Osteomalacia and bone disease arising from aluminum. *Semin Nephrol* 1986;6:68–89.

21. Goodman WG, Leite Duarte ME. Aluminum: effects on bone and role in the pathogenesis of renal osteodystrophy. *Miner Electrolyte Metab* 1991;17:221–232.

22. Goodman WG, Ramirez JA, Belin TR, et al. Development of adynamic bone in patients with secondary hyperparathyroidism after intermittent calcitriol therapy. *Kidney Int* 1994;46:1160–1166.

23. Braun J, Oldendorf M, Moshage W, Heidler R, Zeitler E, Luft FC. Electron beam computed tomography in the evaluation of cardiac calcifications in chronic dialysis patients. *Am J Kidney Dis* 1996;27:394–401.

24. Kuizon BD, Goodman WG, Jüppner H, et al. Diminished linear growth during treatment with intermittent calcitriol and dialysis in children with chronic renal failure. *Kidney Int* 1998;53:205–211.

25. Salusky IB, Ramirez JA, Oppenheim WL, Gales B, Segre GV, Goodman WG. Biochemical markers of renal osteodystrophy in pediatric patients undergoing CAPD/CCPD. *Kidney Int* 1994;45:253–258.

26. Sherrard DJ, Hercz G, Pei Y, et al. The spectrum of bone disease in end-stage renal failure: an evolving disorder. *Kidney Int* 1993;43:436–442.

27. Hodsman AB, Sherrard DJ, Alfrey AC, et al. Bone aluminum and histomorphometric features of renal osteodystrophy. *J Clin Endocrinol Metab* 1982;54:539–546.

28. Block GA, Hulbert-Shearon TE, Levin NW, Port FK. Association of serum phosphorus and calcium × phosphorus product with mortality risk in chronic hemodialysis patients: a national study. *Am J Kidney Dis* 1998;31:607–617.

29. Gipstein RM, Coburn JW, Adams JA, et al. Calciphylaxis in man: a syndrome of tissue necrosis and vascular calcification in 11 patients with chronic renal failure. *Arch Intern Med* 1976;136:1273–1280.

30. Bardin T, Kuntz D, Zingraff J, Voisin MC, Zelmar A, Lansaman J.

31. van Ypersele de Strihou C, Jadoul M, Malghem J, Maldague B, Jamart J, the Working party on Dialysis Amyloidosis. Effect of dialysis membrane and patient's age on signs of dialysis-related amyloidosis. *Kidney Int* 1991;39:1012–1019.

Synovial amyloidosis in patients undergoing long-term hemodialysis. *Arthritis Rheum* 1985;28:1052–1058.

32. Kurz P, Monier-Faugere MC, Bognar B, et al. Evidence for abnormal calcium homeostasis in patients with adynamic bone disease. *Kidney Int* 1994;46:855–861.

33. Ott SM, Andress DL, Nebeker HG, et al. Changes in bone histology after treatment with desferrioxamine. *Kidney Int* 1986;29(suppl 18):S108–S113.

34. Slatopolsky E, Weerts C, Lopez-Hilker S, et al. Calcium carbonate is an effective phosphate binder in patients with chronic renal failure undergoing dialysis. *N Engl J Med* 1986;315:157–161.

35. Mactier RA, Van Stone J, Cox A, Van Stone M, Twardowski Z. Calcium carbonate is an effective phosphate binder when dialysate calcium concentration is adjusted to control hypercalcemia. *Clin Nephrol* 1987;28:222–226.

36. Chertow GM, Burke SK, Lazarus JM, et al. Poly[allylamine hydrochloride] (RenaGel): a noncalcemic phosphate binder for the treatment of hyperphosphatemia in chronic renal failure. *Am J Kidney Dis* 1997;29:66–71.

37. Schaefer K, Scheer J, Asmus G, Umlauf E, Hagemann J, von Herrath D. The treatment uraemic hyperphosphataemia with calcium acetate and calcium carbonate: a comparative study. *Nephrol Dial Transplant* 1991;6:171–175.

38. Berl T, Berns AS, Huffer WE, et al. 1,25-dihydroxycholecalciferol effects in chronic dialysis: a double-blind controlled study. *Ann Intern Med* 1978;88:774–780.

39. Martin KJ, Bullal HS, Domoto DT, Blalock S, Weindel M. Pulse oral calcitriol for the treatment of hyperparathyroidism in patients on continuous ambulatory peritoneal dialysis: preliminary observations. *Am J Kidney Dis* 1992;19:540–545.

40. Slatopolsky E, Weerts C, Thielan J, Horst RL, Harter H, Martin KJ. Marked suppression of secondary hyperparathyroidism by intravenous administration of 1,25-dihydroxycholecalciferol in uremic patients. *J Clin Invest* 1984;74:2136–2143.

41. Tan AU Jr, Levine BS, Mazess RB, et al. Effective suppression of parathyroid hormone by 1 alpha-hydroxy-vitamin D₂ in hemodialysis patients with moderate to severe secondary hyperparathyroidism. *Kidney Int* 1997;51:317–323.

42. Silverberg SJ, Bone HG III, Marriott TB, et al. Short-term inhibition of parathyroid hormone secretion by a calcium-receptor agonist in patients with primary hyperparathyroidism. *N Engl J Med* 1997;337:1506–1510.

43. Antonsen JE, Sherrard DJ, Andress DL. A calcimimetic agent acutely suppresses parathyroid hormone levels in patients with chronic renal failure: rapid communication. *Kidney Int* 1998;53:223–227.

44. Llach F. Parathyroidectomy in chronic renal failure: indications, surgical approach, and the use of calcitriol. *Kidney Int* 1990;38(suppl 29):S29.

45. Kaye M, D'Amour P, Henderson J. Elective total parathyroidectomy without autotransplant in end-stage renal disease. *Kidney Int* 1989;35:1390–1399.

46. Hercz G, Andress DL, Nebeker HG, Shinaberger JH, Sherrard DJ, Coburn JW. Reversal of aluminum-related bone disease after substituting calcium carbonate for aluminum hydroxide. *Am J Kidney Dis* 1988;11:70–75.

47. Julian BA, Laskow DA, Dubovsky J, Dubovsky EV, Curtis JJ, Quarles LD. Rapid loss of vertebral mineral density after renal transplantation. *N Engl J Med* 1991;325:544–550.

48. Rodino MA, Shane E. Osteoporosis after transplantation. *Am J Med* 1998;104:459–469.

SECTION VII

Genetic, Developmental, and Dysplastic Skeletal Disorders

Introduction

Michael P. Whyte, M.D.

Division of Bone and Mineral Diseases, Washington University School of Medicine at Barnes–Jewish Hospital, and Metabolic Research Unit, Shriners Hospital for Children, St. Louis, Missouri

Physicians are confronted with a great diversity of rare genetic, developmental, and dysplastic skeletal disorders (1–5). Some are simply radiologic curiosities; others are challenging clinical problems. Some cause focal bony abnormalities; others result in generalized disturbances of skeletal growth, modeling, or remodeling and cause osteosclerosis, hyperostosis, or osteoporosis. A few of these conditions are associated with overt derangements in mineral homeostasis. Several are important because they are heritable and therefore offer clues concerning factors and mechanisms that regulate mineral metabolism and skeletal homeostasis. Cumulatively, the number of such patients is substantial (1–5).

This section provides a concise overview of a number of the more common or more revealing of the genetic, developmental, and dysplastic skeletal disorders beginning with a description of some that are traditionally grouped together as sclerosing bone dysplasias (2–4). Subsequently there is a discussion of several additional important heritable or sporadic developmental and dysplastic disorders.

REFERENCES

1. McKusick VA. *Mendelian inheritance in man: a catalog of human genes and genetic disorders.* 12th ed. Baltimore: The Johns Hopkins University Press, 1998.
2. Whyte MP. Skeletal disorders characterized by osteosclerosis or hyperostosis. In: Avioli LV, Krane SM, eds. *Metabolic bone disease.* San Diego: Academic Press, 1997:697–738.
3. Scriver CR, Beaudet AL, Sly WS, Valle D. *The metabolic and molecular bases of inherited disease.* 7th ed. New York: McGraw-Hill, 1995.
4. Royce PM, Steinmann B, eds. *Connective tissue and its heritable disorders.* New York: Wiley-Liss, 1993.
5. Beighton P, ed. *McKusick's heritable disorders of connective tissue.* St Louis: Mosby-Year Book, 1993.

70. Sclerosing Bone Disorders

Michael P. Whyte, M.D.

Division of Bone and Mineral Diseases, Washington University School of Medicine at Barnes–Jewish Hospital, and Metabolic Research Unit, Shriners Hospital for Children, St. Louis, Missouri

Osteosclerosis and *hyperostosis* refer to trabecular and cortical bone thickening, respectively (1). Increased bone mass is caused by many rare (often hereditary) dysplastic conditions (2), as well as by a variety of dietary, metabolic, endocrine, hematologic, infectious, and neoplastic problems (Table 1) (1). The following sections describe the principal disorders among the bone dysplasias and several other unusual conditions associated with localized or generalized osteosclerosis and/or hyperostosis.

OSTEOPETROSIS

Osteopetrosis (marble bone disease) was characterized in 1904 by Albers-Schönberg (3). More than 300 cases have been reported. Two major clinical forms are well delineated: the autosomal dominant adult (benign) type that is associated with few or no symptoms (4) and the autosomal recessive infantile (malignant) type that, if untreated, is typically fatal during infancy or early childhood (5). A rarer autosomal recessive (intermediate) form presents during childhood with some of the symptoms and signs of malignant osteopetrosis, but its impact on life expectancy is not known (6). A fourth clinical type, inherited as an autosomal recessive trait, was formerly called the syndrome of osteopetrosis with renal tubular acidosis and cerebral calcification, but it is now understood to be an inborn error of metabolism, carbonic anhydrase II (CA II) deficiency (1). Neuronal storage disease with malignant osteopetrosis has been reported in several patients and seems to reflect a distinct entity (7). There also appear to be especially rare forms of osteopetrosis, called lethal, transient infantile, and postinfectious (8).

Although the diversity of clinical and hereditary types makes it apparent that defects in several different genes and disturbances in a variety of biologic events cause osteopetrosis in humans, the pathogenesis of all true forms is expressed through a failure of osteoclast-mediated resorption of the skeleton. Consequently primary spongiosa (calcified cartilage deposited during endochondral bone formation) persists and serves as histopathologic marker for these disorders (see later) (9). For some other conditions, the term *osteopetrosis* has been incorrectly used to refer generically to a radiodense skeleton that is without this hallmark. Accordingly, it is important to recognize that therapeutic approaches for true forms of osteopetrosis, for which the pathogenesis is partly elucidated, may be inappropriate for these other, typically enigmatic, disorders.

Clinical Presentation

Infantile osteopetrosis manifests during infancy (5). Recurrence within sibships and an increased incidence of parental consanguinity indicate that this condition is transmitted as an autosomal recessive trait. Nasal stuffiness resulting from malformation of the mastoid and paranasal sinuses is

an early symptom. Cranial foramina do not widen fully, and this problem can gradually cause palsies of the optic, oculomotor, and facial nerves. There is also failure to thrive. Eruption of the dentition is delayed. Bones may appear to be dense on radiographic study, but they are actually fragile. Some patients develop hydrocephalus; sleep apnea may oc-

TABLE 1. *Disorders that cause osteosclerosis*

Dysplasias
   Craniodiaphyseal dysplasia
   Craniometaphyseal dysplasia
   Dysosteosclerosis
   Endosteal hyperostosis
   van Buchem disease
   Sclerosteosis
   Frontometaphyseal dysplasia
   Infantile cortical hyperostosis (Caffey's disease)
   Melorheostosis
   Metaphyseal dysplasia (Pyle's disease)
   Mixed sclerosing bone dystrophy
   Oculodentoosseous dysplasia
   Osteodysplasia of Melnick and Needles
   Osteoectasia with hyperphosphatasia (hyperostosis corticalis)
   Osteopathia striata
   Osteopetrosis
   Osteopoikilosis
   Progressive diaphyseal dysplasia (Engelmann's disease)
   Pycnodysostosis
Metabolic
   Carbonic anhydrase II deficiency
   Fluorosis
   Heavy metal poisoning
   Hypervitaminosis A, D
   Hyper-, hypo-, and pseudohypoparathyroidism
   Hypophosphatemic osteomalacia
   Milk-alkali syndrome
   Renal osteodystrophy
Other
   Axial osteomalacia
   Fibrogenesis imperfecta ossium
   Intravenous drug abuse (hepatitis C–associated osteosclerosis)
   Ionizing radiation
   Lymphomas
   Mastocytosis
   Multiple myeloma
   Myelofibrosis
   Osteomyelitis
   Osteonecrosis
   Paget's disease
   Sarcoidosis
   Skeletal metastases
   Tuberous sclerosis

Updated and reproduced from Whyte MP, Murphy WA. Osteopetrosis and other sclerosing bone disorders. In: Avioli LV, Krane SM, eds. *Metabolic bone disease.* 2nd ed. Philadelphia: WB Saunders, 1990:616–658, with permission.

367

cur. Retinal degeneration is an additional cause of blindness. Recurrent infection and spontaneous bruising and bleeding are common problems that appear to be partly due to myelophthisis from excessive bone, abundant osteoclasts, and fibrous tissue crowding the marrow spaces. Hypersplenism and hemolysis can exacerbate severe anemia. Physical examination shows short stature, frontal bossing, a large head, an "adenoid" appearance, nystagmus, hepatosplenomegaly, and genu valgum. Untreated children usually die during the first decade of life from hemorrhage, pneumonia, severe anemia, or sepsis (5).

Intermediate osteopetrosis causes short stature. Some patients develop cranial nerve deficits, macrocephaly, ankylosed teeth that predispose to osteomyelitis of the jaw, mild or occasionally moderately severe anemia, and recurrent fractures (6). CA II deficiency is described in the next section.

Adult osteopetrosis is a developmental disorder in which radiographic abnormalities become apparent during childhood. In some kindreds, generations are skipped, and carriers show no radiographic disturbances. Although most patients are asymptomatic (4), the long bones are brittle, and fractures can occur. Facial palsy, deafness, osteomyelitis of the mandible, compromised vision or hearing, psychomotor delay, carpal tunnel syndrome, and osteoarthritis can be additional clinical problems. Studies from Denmark proposed that there are two types of adult osteopetrosis (10).

Neuronal storage disease with osteopetrosis features severe skeletal disease and is characterized by the additional complications of epilepsy and neurodegenerative disease (7). Lethal osteopetrosis manifests *in utero* and results in stillbirth (8). Transient infantile osteopetrosis resolves during the first few years of life (8).

Radiologic Features

Generalized symmetric increase in bone mass is the principal radiographic finding in osteopetrosis (11). Trabecular and cortical bone appear thickened. In the severe forms, all three principal components of skeletal development are disturbed, causing diminished bone growth, modeling, and remodeling. Most of the skeleton can be uniformly dense, but alternating sclerotic and lucent bands are commonly noted in the iliac wings and near the ends of the long bones. Diaphyses and metaphyses are typically broadened and may have an "Erlenmeyer flask" deformity (Fig. 1). Rarely the distal phalanges in the hands are eroded (a finding more typical of pycnodysostosis). Pathologic fracture of long bones is not uncommon. Rachitic-like changes in growth plates may occur (12). In the axial skeleton, the cranium is usually thickened and dense, especially at the base, and the paranasal and mastoid sinuses are underpneumatized (Fig. 2). Vertebrae may show, on lateral view, a "bone-in-bone" (endobone) configuration.

Albers-Schönberg disease, the adult form of osteopetrosis, manifests with progressive osteosclerosis beginning in childhood, with selective thickening of the base of the skull together with typical vertebral end-plate accentuation that causes an endobone, or "rugger jersey," appearance of the spine (10). Skeletal-modeling defects are absent.

In the various forms of osteopetrosis, scintigraphic study

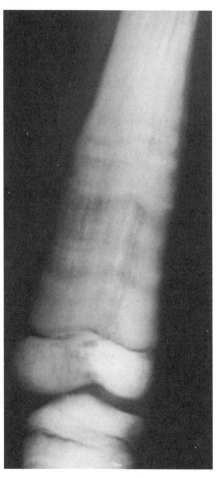

FIG. 1. Osteopetrosis. Anteroposterior radiograph of the distal femur of a 10-year-old boy shows a widened metadiaphyseal region with characteristic alternating dense and lucent bands. (From Whyte MP, Murphy WA. Osteopetrosis and other sclerosing bone disorders. In: Avioli LV, Krane SM, eds. *Metabolic bone disease.* 2nd ed. Philadelphia: WB Saunders, 1990:616–658.)

of the skeleton reveals fractures and osteomyelitis (13). Magnetic resonance imaging (MRI) may help to monitor patients with severe disease who undergo bone marrow transplantation, because successful engraftment will enlarge medullary spaces (14) (see later). Computed tomography (CT) and MRI findings on examination of the heads of infants and children have been described (15).

Laboratory Findings

In infantile osteopetrosis, serum calcium levels generally reflect the dietary intake (16). Hypocalcemia can occur and may be severe enough to cause rachitic changes in growth plates. Secondary hyperparathyroidism with elevated serum levels of calcitriol is commonly present (17). Acid phosphatase (ACP) activity is often increased in serum. Presence of the brain isoenzyme of creatine kinase (BB-CK) in serum is a biochemical marker for genuine forms of osteopetrosis (18). Both ACP and BB-CK appear to originate from patient,

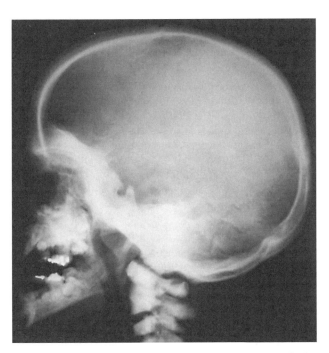

FIG. 2. Osteopetrosis. Lateral radiograph of the skull of a 13-year-old boy shows osteosclerosis, especially apparent at the base. (From Whyte MP, Murphy WA. Osteopetrosis and other sclerosing bone disorders. In: Avioli LV, Krane SM, eds. *Metabolic bone disease.* 2nd ed. Philadelphia: WB Saunders, 1990:616–658.)

osteoclasts (18). In adult osteopetrosis, standard biochemical indices of mineral homeostasis are usually described as unremarkable. However, recent studies indicated that immunoreactive parathyroid hormone (PTH) levels in serum are often increased (10).

Histopathologic Findings

The radiographic features of the osteopetroses can be diagnostic (11). Nevertheless, failure of osteoclasts to resorb skeletal tissue provides a histologic finding that is pathognomonic (19) [i.e., remnants of mineralized primary spongiosa persist as islands or bars of calcified cartilage within mature bone (Fig. 3)].

In the human osteopetroses, osteoclasts may be increased, normal, or decreased in number. In the infantile form, these cells are usually abundant and are found at bone surfaces. Their nuclei are especially numerous, yet the ruffled borders or clear zones that characterize normal osteoclasts are absent (20). Fibrous tissue often crowds the marrow spaces (20). Adult osteopetrosis may show increased amounts of osteoid, and osteoclasts can be few and lack ruffled borders or can be especially numerous and large (21). A common histologic finding is "woven" bone (19).

Etiology and Pathogenesis

Although most forms of human osteopetrosis appear to be transmitted as autosomal traits, the molecular bases remain largely unknown (8). CA II deficiency is caused by defects in the CA II gene (see later). In 1997, the gene for adult osteopetrosis was mapped to chromosome 1p21 (22). The pathogenesis of all true forms, however, involves diminished osteoclast-mediated skeletal resorption (23,24). The potential causes of osteoclast failure, however, are complex (24). Abnormalities in the osteoclast stem cell or its microenvironment, in the osteoclast precursor cell or the mature heterokaryon itself, or in the bone matrix could be at fault (8,9). Furthermore, in 1996, an osteoblast defect was reported in two severely affected patients (25). Cases of osteopetrosis with neuronal storage disease (characterized by accumula-

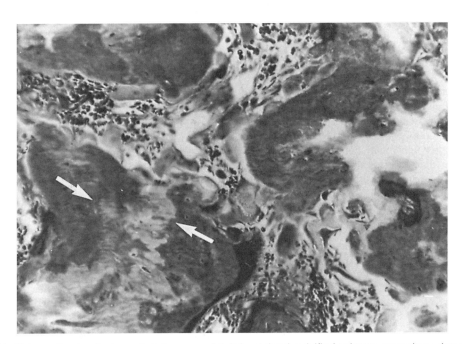

FIG. 3. Osteopetrosis. A characteristic area of lightly stained calcified primary spongiosa *(arrows)* is found within darkly stained mineralized bone (×150).

tion of ceroid lipofuscin) may involve a defect centered in lysosomes (7). Virus-like inclusions have been found in the osteoclasts of a few sporadic cases of benign osteopetrosis, but their significance is uncertain (26). Synthesis of an abnormal PTH (27) or defective production of interleukin-2 (IL-2) (28) or superoxide (29)—factors necessary for bone resorption—may also be pathogenetic defects. In fact, leukocyte-function studies in the infantile form have revealed abnormalities in circulating monocytes and granulocytes (29,30). Ultimately, impaired bone resorption causes skeletal fragility because fewer collagen fibrils properly connect osteons, and there is defective remodeling of woven bone to compact bone (9).

Treatment

Because the etiology, precise pathogenesis, pattern of inheritance, and prognosis for the various forms of osteopetrosis can differ, a correct diagnosis is critical before therapy is attempted. Intermediate osteopetrosis is relatively benign compared with the infantile type. Infants or young children with CA II deficiency may have radiographic features consistent with malignant osteopetrosis, yet serial radiographic studies show spontaneous gradual resolution of their bony sclerosis. A precise diagnosis from among the various forms of osteopetrosis may require investigation of the family and careful evaluation of the patient's disease severity and progression.

Bone Marrow Transplantation

Bone marrow transplantation (BMT) has remarkably improved some patients with infantile osteopetrosis (31). Transplanted osteoclasts, but not osteoblasts, were shown to be of donor origin in 1980 (32). These observations supported the hypothesis that osteopetrosis is caused by defective osteoclast-mediated bone resorption, and that the progenitor cell for the osteoclast is derived from marrow (32). However, patients with severely crowded marrow spaces appear less likely to engraft after BMT. Early intervention seems to be more successful. Accordingly, histomorphometric studies of bone may help to assess the outcome of this procedure. Use of marrow from human leukocyte antigen (HLA)-nonidentical donors warrants continued study (33). It is understandable that BMT may not benefit all patients (8), because a variety of defects (not all of which are intrinsic to marrow) could cause osteopetrosis. Successful BMT can result in hypercalcemia as osteoclast function begins (34).

Hormonal and Dietary Treatments

Some success in the treatment of osteopetrosis has been reported with a calcium-deficient diet alone. However, supplementation of dietary calcium may be necessary for symptomatic hypocalcemia in severely affected infants or children (12). Large oral doses of calcitriol, together with limited dietary calcium intake to prevent hypercalciuria/hypercalcemia, has been reported to improve infantile osteopetrosis occasionally (35). Calcitriol seems to be helpful by stimulating dormant osteoclasts. Some patients appear, however, to become resistant to this treatment (23,29). Long-term infusion of PTH was helpful for one infant (27), perhaps by stimulating calcitriol synthesis. The observation that leukocytes from severely affected individuals have diminished production of superoxide has led to recombinant human interferon gamma-1b therapy and clinical, laboratory, and histopathologic evidence of a successful response (23,29).

High-dose glucocorticoid treatment stabilizes pediatric patients with pancytopenia and hepatomegaly. Prednisone and a low-calcium/high-phosphate diet may be an alternative to BMT (36).

Supportive

Hyperbaric oxygenation can be an important adjunctive treatment for osteomyelitis of the jaw. Surgical decompression of the optic and facial nerves may benefit some patients.

Early prenatal diagnosis of osteopetrosis by ultrasound has generally been unsuccessful. Conventional radiographic studies occasionally diagnose malignant osteopetrosis late in pregnancy (37).

CARBONIC ANHYDRASE II DEFICIENCY

In 1983, the autosomal recessive syndrome of osteopetrosis with renal tubular acidosis (RTA) and cerebral calcification was discovered to be an inborn error of metabolism caused by deficiency of the CA II isoenzyme (38).

Clinical Presentation

Description of more than 50 cases of CA II deficiency revealed considerable clinical variability among affected families (39). The perinatal history is typically unremarkable, but then in infancy or early childhood, patients may sustain a fracture or manifest failure to thrive, developmental delay, or short stature. Mental subnormality is common but not invariable. Compression of the optic nerves and dental malocclusion are additional complications. RTA may explain the hypotonia, apathy, and muscle weakness that trouble some patients. Periodic hypokalemic paralysis has been described. Although fracture is unusual, recurrent breaks in long bones can cause significant morbidity (38). Life expectancy does not seem to be shortened, but to date the oldest published cases have been young adults (40,41).

Radiologic Features

CA II deficiency resembles other forms of osteopetrosis on radiographic study, except that cerebral calcification develops during childhood, and the osteosclerosis and the defects in skeletal modeling diminish spontaneously (rather than increase) over years (42). Abnormalities in skeletal radiographs are typically present at diagnosis, although findings can be subtle at birth. CT has demonstrated that the cerebral calcification appears between ages 2 and 5 years, increases during childhood, affects gray matter of the cortex and basal ganglia, and is similar if not identical to that of idiopathic hypoparathyroidism or pseudohypoparathyroidism.

Laboratory Findings

Bone marrow examination is unremarkable. If anemia is present, it is generally mild and of nutritional origin. Metabolic acidosis occurs as early as the neonatal period. Both proximal and distal RTA have been described (43); distal (type I) RTA seems to be better documented. Additional studies, however, are required (43). Aminoaciduria and glycosuria are absent (40).

Autopsy studies have not been reported (40). Histopathologic examination of bone from four individuals, who represented two affected families, revealed characteristic areas of unresorbed calcified primary spongiosa (42).

Etiology and Pathogenesis

The CA isoenzymes accelerate the first step in the reaction $CO_2 + H_2O \rightarrow H_2CO_3 \rightarrow H^+ + HCO_3^-$. Accordingly, they function importantly in acid–base regulation. CA II is present in many tissues, such as brain, kidney, erythrocytes, cartilage, lung, and gastric mucosa (44). The other CA isoenzymes have a more limited tissue distribution.

All of 21 patients from 12 unrelated kindreds of diverse ethnic and geographic origin were shown to have selective deficiency of CA II in erythrocytes (40). Red cell CA II levels are approximately half normal in carriers (40,41). Although deficiency of CA II remains to be shown in tissues other than erythrocytes, the presence of osteopetrosis, RTA, and cerebral calcification in patients predicted a global deficiency of CA II and important function in bone, kidney, and perhaps brain (38,40). In fact, a variety of mutations in the CA II gene have now been documented in patients worldwide (44).

Treatment

RTA in CA II deficiency has been treated with HCO_3^- supplementation, but the long-term impact is unknown. Transfusion of CA II–replete erythrocytes to one patient did not correct the systemic acidosis (45).

PYCNODYSOSTOSIS

Pycnodysostosis is the skeletal dysplasia that is believed to have troubled the French impressionist painter Henri de Toulouse-Lautrec (1864–1901) (46). More than 100 cases from 50 kindreds have been described since the condition was delineated in 1962 (47). The disorder is transmitted as an autosomal recessive trait; parental consanguinity has been reported for about 30% of patients. Most case descriptions have come from Europe or the United States, but the dysplasia has been found in Israelis, Indonesians, Asian Indians, and Africans. Pycnodysostosis appears to be especially common in the Japanese (48). In 1996, the genetic defect was discovered (see later).

Clinical Presentation

Pycnodysostosis is generally diagnosed during infancy or early childhood because of disproportionate short stature associated with a relatively large cranium and dysmorphic features that include frontooccipital prominence, obtuse mandibular angle, small facies and chin, high-arched palate, dental malocclusion with retained deciduous teeth, proptosis, bluish sclerae, and a beaked and pointed nose (49). The anterior fontanel and other cranial sutures are usually open. Fingers are short and clubbed from acroosteolysis or aplasia of terminal phalanges, fingernails are hypoplastic, and hands are small and square. The thorax is narrow, and there may be pectus excavatum, kyphoscoliosis, and increased lumbar lordosis. Recurrent fractures typically involve the lower limbs and cause genu valgum deformity. Patients are, however, usually able to walk independently. Visceral manifestations and rickets have been described. Mental retardation affects about 10% of cases (49). Adult height ranges from 4 feet 3 inches to 4 feet 11 inches. Recurrent respiratory infections and right heart failure from chronic upper airway obstruction due to micrognathia occur in some patients.

Radiographic Features

Pycnodysostosis shares many radiographic features with osteopetrosis. For example, both conditions cause generalized osteosclerosis and are associated with recurrent fractures. Furthermore, the osteosclerosis is developmental and uniform, first becomes apparent in childhood, and increases with age. However, the marked modeling defects of the severe forms of osteopetrosis do not occur in pycnodysostosis, although long bones manifest hyperostosis and narrow medullary canals. Additional findings that help to differentiate pycnodysostosis include delayed closure of cranial sutures and fontanels (prominently the anterior; Fig. 4), obtuse mandibular angle, wormian bones, gracile clavicles that are hypoplastic at their lateral segments, hypoplasia or aplasia of the distal phalanges and ribs, and partial absence of the hyoid bone (50). Endobones and radiodense striations are absent (11). However, the calvarium and base of the skull are sclerotic, and the orbital ridges are radiodense. Hypoplasia of facial bones, sinuses, and terminal phalanges are characteristic. Vertebrae are dense, yet their transverse processes are uninvolved; anterior and posterior concavities occur. Lumbosacral spondylolisthesis is not uncommon, and lack of segmentation of the atlas and axis may be present. Madelung deformity can affect the forearms.

Laboratory Findings

Serum calcium and inorganic phosphate levels and alkaline phosphatase activity are usually unremarkable. Anemia is not a problem. Histopathologic study of bone shows cortical bone structure that seems normal despite the appearance of diminished osteoclastic and osteoblastic activity (51). Electron microscopy of bone from two patients suggested that degradation of collagen might be defective, perhaps from an abnormality in the bone matrix or in the osteoclast

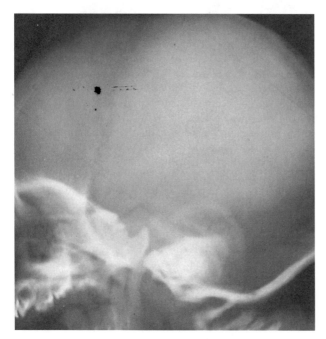

FIG. 4. Pycnodysostosis. Lateral radiograph of the skull of an infant shows that the cranial sutures are markedly widened. The base is sclerotic. (From Whyte MP, Murphy WA. Osteopetrosis and other sclerosing bone disorders. In: Avioli LV, Krane SM, eds. *Metabolic bone disease.* 2nd ed. Philadelphia: WB Saunders, 1990:616–658.)

itself (52). In chondrocytes, abnormal inclusions have been described.

Etiology and Pathogenesis

In 1996, the molecular basis for pycnodysostosis was discovered to be defects within the cathepsin K gene (53). Cathepsin K, a lysosomal cysteine protease, is highly expressed in osteoclasts. Impaired collagen degradation appears to be a fundamental pathogenetic defect.

Absorption of dietary calcium may be increased. Both the rate of bone accretion and the size of the exchangeable calcium pool can be reduced (54). Accordingly, diminished rates of bone resorption may explain the osteosclerosis. Virus-like inclusions were found in the osteoclasts of two affected brothers (55). In 1993, the killing activity and IL-1 secretion of circulating monocytes were found to be low (56). In 1996, defective growth hormone secretion and low serum insulin-like growth factor-I (IGF-I) levels were reported in five of six affected children (57).

Treatment

There is no effective medical therapy for pycnodysostosis. Bone marrow transplantation has not been reported. Fractures of the long bones are typically transverse. They usually heal at a satisfactory rate, although delayed union and massive callus formation have been described. Internal fixation of long bones is formidable because of their hardness. Extraction of teeth is similarly difficult; fracture of the jaw has

occurred (49). Osteomyelitis of the mandible may require treatment with a combined antibiotic and surgical approach. The orthopedic problems have been briefly reviewed (58).

PROGRESSIVE DIAPHYSEAL DYSPLASIA (CAMURATI–ENGELMANN DISEASE)

Progressive diaphyseal dysplasia was characterized by Cockayne in 1920 (59). Camurati found that the condition is heritable. Engelmann described the severe typical form in 1929 (60). This disorder is transmitted as an autosomal dominant trait. Descriptions of more than 100 cases show that the clinical and radiologic penetrance is quite variable (61). The characteristic feature is hyperostosis that occurs gradually on both the periosteal and endosteal surfaces of long bones. All races are affected. In severe cases, the skull and axial skeleton also are involved, and osteosclerosis is widespread. Some carriers have no radiographic changes, but bone scintigraphy is abnormal.

Clinical Presentation

Progressive diaphyseal dysplasia typically presents during childhood with limping or a broad-based and waddling gait, leg pain, muscle wasting, and decreased subcutaneous fat in the extremities. These features can be mistaken for a form of muscular dystrophy (62). Severely affected patients have a characteristic body habitus that includes an enlarged head with prominent forehead, proptosis, and thin limbs with thickened bones and little muscle mass. Cranial nerve palsies may develop when the skull is affected. Puberty is sometimes delayed. Raised intracranial pressure can occur. Physical findings include palpable bony thickening and skeletal tenderness. Some patients have hepatosplenomegaly, Raynaud's phenomenon, and other findings suggestive of vasculitis (63). Although radiologic studies typically show progressive disease, the clinical course is variable, and remission of symptoms seems to occur in some patients during adult life (64).

Radiologic Features

The principal radiographic feature of progressive diaphyseal dysplasia is hyperostosis of major long bone diaphyses from proliferation of new bone on both the periosteal and the endosteal surfaces (11). The sclerosis is fairly symmetric and gradually spreads to involve metaphyses; however, the epiphyses are characteristically spared (Fig. 5). The tibiae and femora are most commonly involved; less frequently, the radii, ulnae, humeri, and occasionally the short tubular bones are affected. The scapulae, clavicles, and pelvis also may become thickened. Typically, the shafts of long bones gradually widen and develop irregular surfaces. The age of onset, rate of progression, and degree of bony involvement are highly variable. With relatively mild disease, especially in adolescents or young adults, radiographic and scintigraphic abnormalities may be confined to the long bones of the lower limbs. Maturation of the new bone increases the

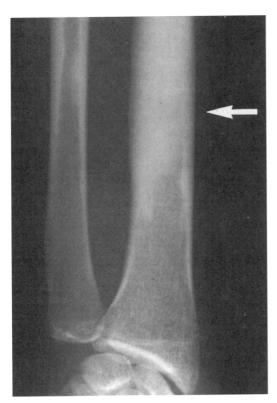

FIG. 5. Progressive diaphyseal dysplasia (Camurati–Engelmann disease). The distal radius of this 20-year-old woman has a characteristic area of patchy thickening *(arrow)* of the periosteal and endosteal surfaces of the diaphysis.

degree of hyperostosis. However, in severely affected children, some areas of the skeleton can appear osteopenic.

Bone scanning typically reveals focally increased radionuclide accumulation in affected areas (65). Clinical, radiographic, and scintigraphic findings are generally concordant. In some patients, however, bone scans are unremarkable despite considerable radiographic abnormality. This association seems to reflect advanced but quiescent disease (65). Markedly increased radioisotope accumulation with minimal radiographic findings can reflect early and active skeletal disease (65). MRI and CT findings delineating cranial involvement have been reported (66).

Laboratory Findings

Routine biochemical parameters of bone and mineral metabolism are typically normal, although serum alkaline phosphatase activity, urinary hydroxyproline levels, and the erythrocyte sedimentation rate are elevated in some patients. Modest hypocalcemia and significant hypocalciuria occur in some affected individuals who have severe disease and appear to reflect positive calcium balance (64). Mild anemia and leukopenia also may be present (63).

New bone formation along diaphyses is the characteristic feature of progressive diaphyseal dysplasia. Peripheral to the original bony cortex, there is disorganized, newly formed, woven bone undergoing centripetal maturation and then incorporation into the cortex (61). Electron microscopy of muscle has shown myopathic changes and vascular abnormalities (62).

Etiology and Pathogenesis

Progressive diaphyseal dysplasia is caused by an autosomal gene defect that has not been mapped and characterized. Some especially mild cases were reported to represent an autosomal recessive condition known as Ribbing's disease (67). However, sporadic cases of progressive diaphyseal dysplasia do occur, and mild clinical forms can be transmitted as an autosomal dominant trait with variable penetrance.

The clinical and laboratory features of severe disease and its responsiveness to glucocorticoid treatment have led some investigators to suggest that progressive diaphyseal dysplasia is a systemic condition (i.e., an inflammatory connective tissue disease) (63).

Aberrant differentiation of monocytes/macrophages to fibroblasts, and hence to osteoblasts, has been discussed as a fundamental pathogenetic feature (68).

Treatment

Progressive diaphyseal dysplasia is a chronic and somewhat unpredictable disorder (69). Symptoms may remit during adolescence or adult life. Subsequent to its initial use in 1967 for this disorder, glucocorticoid therapy (typically prednisone given in small doses on an alternate-day schedule) has become a well-documented effective treatment that can relieve bone pain and also normalize histologic abnormalities in affected bone (70). Complete relief of localized pain has followed surgical removal of diseased diaphyseal bone, forming a cortical window (71).

ENDOSTEAL HYPEROSTOSIS

In 1955, van Buchem et al. (72) first described the condition *hyperostosis corticalis generalisata*. Their report led to characterization of the disorders that are considered endosteal hyperostoses.

VAN BUCHEM DISEASE

This is an autosomal recessive, clinically severe condition (72) that is differentiated from an autosomal dominant, more mild, benign form of endosteal hyperostosis (Worth type) (72,73). Van Buchem disease is considerably less common than the cumulative number of reports in the literature might suggest (74).

Clinical Presentation

Van Buchem disease has been described in children and adults; sex distribution seems to be equal. Progressive asymmetric enlargement of the jaw occurs during puberty. The adult mandible is markedly thickened with a wide angle, but there is no prognathism, and dental malocclusion is uncommon. Patients may be symptom free; however, recurrent facial nerve palsy, deafness, and optic atrophy from narrowing of cranial foramina are common and can begin as early as infancy. Long bones may become painful with applied pressure, but they are not fragile, and joint range of motion is generally normal. Sclerosteosis had been differentiated from van Buchem disease because these patients are excessively tall and have syndactyly (75) (see later).

Radiologic Features

Endosteal cortical thickening that produces a dense and homogeneous diaphyseal cortex and narrows the medullary canal is the major radiographic feature of van Buchem disease. The hyperostosis is selectively endosteal; long bones are properly modeled. However, generalized osteosclerosis affects the base of the skull, facial bones, vertebrae, pelvis, and ribs. The mandible becomes enlarged (Fig. 6). Cranial CT features have been reported (76).

Laboratory Findings

Alkaline phosphatase activity in serum is primarily of skeletal origin and may be increased; calcium and inorganic phosphate levels are unremarkable. Van Buchem and colleagues suggested that the excessive bone was essentially of normal quality.

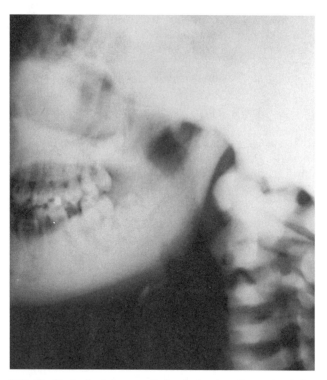

FIG. 6. Endosteal hyperostosis. Lateral radiograph of the mandible and facial bones of a 9-year-old boy with van Buchem disease shows dense sclerosis of all osseous structures. (From Whyte MP, Murphy WA. Osteopetrosis and other sclerosing bone disorders. In: Avioli LV, Krane SM, eds. *Metabolic bone disease*. 2nd ed. Philadelphia: WB Saunders, 1990:616–658.)

Etiology and Pathogenesis

Van Buchem disease and sclerosteosis seem to be allelic disorders; their clinical/radiographic differences are likely explained by the epistatic effects of modifying genes (75).

Treatment

There is no specific medical therapy. Surgical decompression of narrowed foramina may help to alleviate cranial nerve palsies (77). Surgery also has been used to recontour the mandible (78).

SCLEROSTEOSIS

Sclerosteosis (cortical hyperostosis with syndactyly), like van Buchem disease (see earlier), is an autosomal recessive form of endosteal hyperostosis. It occurs primarily in Afrikaners or others of Dutch ancestry (75). Initially, sclerosteosis was distinguished from van Buchem disease by some radiographic differences and the presence of syndactyly, but clinical studies suggest that both disorders are caused by a defect in the same gene (75).

Clinical Presentation

At birth, only syndactyly may be noted (79). During early childhood, there is overgrowth and sclerosis of the skeleton, involving especially the skull and causing facial disfigurement. Patients are tall and heavy beginning in childhood. Understandably, the term *gigantism* has been used to refer to their appearance. Deafness and facial palsy due to nerve entrapment also are prominent problems. The mandible has a rather square configuration. Raised intracranial pressure and headache may be sequelae of a small cranial cavity. The brainstem can become compressed. Syndactyly from either cutaneous or bony fusion of the middle and index fingers is typical, but of variable severity. The fingernails are dysplastic. Patients are not prone to fracture, and their intelligence is normal. Life expectancy may be shortened (80).

Radiologic Features

Except when syndactyly is present, the skeleton is normal in early childhood. The principal radiographic feature is progressive bony thickening that causes widening of the skull and prognathism (81). In the long bones, modeling defects occur, and the cortices are thickened. The vertebral pedicles, ribs, pelvis, and tubular bones also may become somewhat dense. CT has shown fusion of the ossicles and narrowing of the internal auditory canals and cochlear aqueducts (75).

Histopathologic Findings

In an American kindred with sclerosteosis, dynamic histomorphometry of the skull of one patient showed thickened trabeculae and osteoidosis where the rate of bone formation was increased; osteoclastic bone resorption appeared to be quiescent (82).

Etiology and Pathogenesis

In 1998, van Buchem disease was mapped to chromosome 17q12-q21 (83).

Enhanced osteoblast activity with failure of osteoclasts to compensate for increased bone formation seems to explain the dense bone of sclerosteosis (82). No abnormality of calcium homeostasis or of pituitary gland function has been documented (84). The pathogenesis of the neurologic defects has been described in detail (82).

Treatment

There is no specific medical treatment for sclerosteosis. Surgical correction of syndactyly is especially difficult if there is bony fusion. Repairing prognathism is complicated by dense mandibular bone. Management of associated neurologic dysfunction has been reviewed (82).

OSTEOPOIKILOSIS

Osteopoikilosis literally translated means spotted bones. This condition is a radiologic curiosity that is transmitted as an autosomal dominant trait with a high degree of penetrance (85). Patients in some kindreds may also have a form of connective tissue nevus called *dermatofibrosis lenticularis disseminata;* the disorder is then called the Buschke–Ollendorff syndrome (86). The bony lesions are not symptomatic, but incorrectly diagnosed patients may undergo rigorous and expensive studies for other important conditions, including metastatic disease to the skeleton (87). Family members at risk should be screened with a radiograph of the hand/wrist and knee after childhood.

Clinical Presentation

Osteopoikilosis is typically an incidental finding. Musculoskeletal pain, described in many cases, is probably coincidental. The nevi usually involve the lower trunk or extremities and are present before puberty, sometimes congenitally. This dermatosis characteristically appears as small asymptomatic papules; however, they are sometimes yellow or white discs or plaques, deep nodules, or streaks (86).

Radiologic Features

The characteristic radiographic finding is numerous small foci of osteosclerosis of variable shape (usually round or oval) (11). Commonly affected sites are the ends of the short tubular bones, the metaepiphyseal regions of the long bones, and the tarsal, carpal, and pelvic bones (Fig. 7). These foci do not change shape and size for decades, but they may

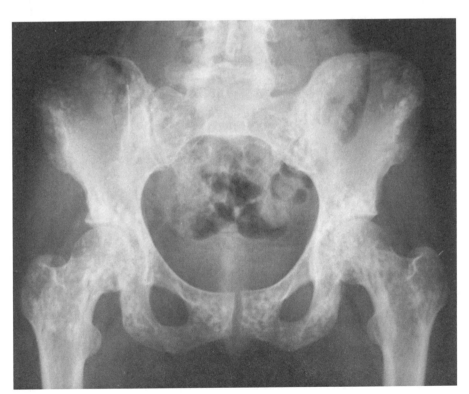

FIG. 7. Osteopoikilosis. Characteristic features shown here include the spotted appearance of the pelvis and metaepiphyseal regions of the femora. (From Whyte MP. Rare disorders of skeletal formation and homeostasis. In: Becker KN, ed. *Principles and practice of endocrinology and metabolism.* 2nd ed. Philadelphia: Lippincott-Raven Publishers, 1995:594–606.)

mimic metastatic lesions. Radionuclide accumulation is not increased on bone scanning (87).

Histopathologic Studies

Dermatofibrosis lenticularis disseminata is characterized by excessive amounts of unusually broad, markedly branched, interlacing elastin fibers in the dermis; the epidermis is normal (86).

The foci of osteosclerosis are thickened trabeculae that merge with surrounding normal bone or islands of cortical bone that include haversian systems. Mature lesions seem to be remodeling slowly (88).

OSTEOPATHIA STRIATA

Osteopathia striata is characterized by linear striations at the ends of long bones and in the ilium (11). Like osteopoikilosis, it is a radiographic curiosity when the skeletal findings occur alone. However, osteopathia striata also is a feature of a variety of clinically important syndromes, including osteopathia striata with cranial sclerosis (89) and osteopathia striata with focal dermal hypoplasia (90).

Clinical Presentation

Isolated osteopathia striata is transmitted as an autosomal dominant trait. The musculoskeletal symptoms that may have led to the radiographic studies are probably unrelated. However, when there is sclerosis of the skull, cranial nerve palsies are common (89). This condition also is inherited as an autosomal dominant trait. Osteopathia striata with focal dermal hypoplasia (Goltz syndrome) is a serious X-linked recessive disorder in which affected boys have widespread linear areas of dermal hypoplasia through which adipose tissue can herniate. They also have a variety of additional bony defects in their limbs (90). Histopathologic studies of bone have not been described.

Radiologic Features

Gracile linear striations in the cancellous regions of the skeleton, particularly in metaepiphyses of major long bones and in the periphery of the iliac bones, is the characteristic radiographic finding (Fig. 8) (11). The carpal, tarsal, and tubular bones of the hands and feet are less commonly and more subtly affected. The striations appear unchanged for years. Radionuclide accumulation is not increased during bone scanning (87).

Treatment

The bone lesions are benign. Although the characteristic skeletal findings are unlikely to be misdiagnosed, radiographic screening after childhood of family members at risk would seem prudent. In one family with osteopathia striata and cranial sclerosis, the diagnosis was reportedly made prenatally by ultrasound examination (91).

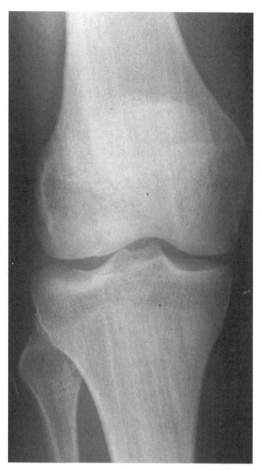

FIG. 8. Osteopathia striata. Characteristic longitudinal striations are present in the femur and tibia of this 17-year-old girl.

MELORHEOSTOSIS

Melorheostosis, from the Greek, refers to flowing hyperostosis of the limbs. The skeletal radiographic findings have been likened to wax that has dripped down the side of a candle. Since its initial description in 1922 (92), about 200 cases have been reported (93,94). No mendelian pattern of inheritance has been found; the disorder occurs sporadically.

Clinical Presentation

Melorheostosis typically manifests during childhood. Usually there is monomelic involvement; bilateral disease, when it occurs, is generally asymmetric. Cutaneous changes that overlie affected skeletal sites are not uncommon. Of 131 patients reported in one investigation, 17% had linear scleroderma-like patches and hypertrichosis. Fibromas, fibrolipomas, capillary hemangiomas, lymphangiectasia, and arterial aneurysms also occur (95,96). Soft-tissue abnormalities are often noted before the hyperostosis is discovered. Pain and stiffness are the major symptoms. Affected joints may become contracted and deformed. In affected children, leg-length inequality occurs from soft-tissue contractures and premature fusion of epiphyses. The skeletal lesions appear to progress most rapidly during childhood. During the adult years, melorheostosis may or may not gradually extend (97). Nevertheless, pain is a more frequent symptom in adults because of subperiosteal new bone formation.

Radiologic Features

Irregular, dense, eccentric hyperostosis of both the cortex and the adjacent medullary canal of a single bone, or several adjacent bones, is the characteristic radiographic finding in melorheostosis (Fig. 9) (11,94). Any anatomic region or bone may be affected, but the lower extremities are most commonly involved. Bone also can develop in soft tissues near affected skeletal areas, particularly near joints. Melorheostotic bone has increased blood flow and avidly accumulates radionuclide during bone scanning (98).

Laboratory Findings

Routine laboratory studies (e.g., serum calcium and inorganic phosphate levels and alkaline phosphatase activity) are normal in melorheostosis.

Histopathologic Findings

The skeletal lesion in melorheostosis features endosteal thickening during infancy and childhood and then periosteal new bone formation during adult life (94). Bony lesions are sclerotic with thickened irregular lamellae that may occlude

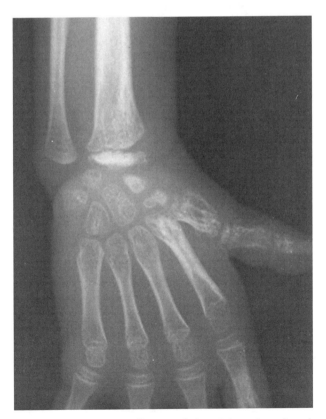

FIG. 9. Melorheostosis. Characteristic patchy osteosclerosis is most apparent in the radius and second metacarpal of this 8-year-old girl.

haversian systems. Marrow fibrosis also may be present (94). Unlike in true scleroderma, the collagen of the sclerodermatous lesions of melorheostosis appears normal. Thus, this dermatosis has been called linear melorheostotic scleroderma (95,99).

Etiology and Pathogenesis

The distribution of melorheostosis and its associated soft-tissue lesions in sclerotomes, myotomes, and dermatomes suggests that a segmentary embryogenetic defect explains this sporadic condition (95,99). The linear scleroderma may reflect the primary abnormality that extends into the skeleton to cause the hyperostosis.

Treatment

Surgical correction of contractures can be difficult; recurrent deformity is common. Distraction techniques, however, have been associated with promising outcomes (100).

MIXED SCLEROSING BONE DYSTROPHY

Mixed sclerosing bone dystrophy is a rare skeletal dysplasia in which features of osteopoikilosis, osteopathia striata, melorheostosis, cranial sclerosis, or additional skeletal defects occur together in various combinations in one individual (101).

Clinical Presentation

Patients may experience the problems typically associated with the individual patterns of osteosclerosis; for example, cranial sclerosis may result in cranial nerve palsy, and melorheostosis can cause localized bone pain (101).

Radiologic Features

Two or more dense bone patterns are noted (osteopoikilosis, osteopathia striata, melorheostosis, cranial sclerosis, generalized cortical hyperostosis, focal osteosclerosis, or progressive diaphyseal dysplasia). However, just one portion of the skeleton may be affected.

Bone scanning shows increased radionuclide uptake in the areas of greatest skeletal sclerosis (101,102).

Histopathologic Findings

Although the term *osteopetrosis* has been used to describe the generalized osteosclerosis that occurs in some patients, histopathologic study has failed to show remnants of calcified primary spongiosa (see osteopetrosis) (101,102).

Etiology and Pathogenesis

Delineation of mixed sclerosing bone dystrophy suggests a common etiology and pathogenesis for its individual osteosclerotic patterns. However, osteopoikilosis and most forms of osteopathia striata are heritable, whereas mixed sclerosing bone dystrophy, like melorheostosis, seems to be a sporadic disorder (101,102).

Treatment

There is no specific medical treatment. Contractures or neurovascular compression by osteosclerotic lesions can require surgical intervention.

AXIAL OSTEOMALACIA

Axial osteomalacia is characterized radiographically by coarsening of the trabecular pattern of the axial but not the appendicular skeleton (103). Fewer than 20 patients have been described. Most affected individuals have been sporadic cases, but dominant transmission has been reported (104); thus additional family studies are necessary.

Clinical Presentation

Most patients with axial osteomalacia have been middle-aged or elderly men; a few middle-aged women have been described. Radiographic manifestations, however, are likely to be detectable much earlier (104). The majority of cases have presented with dull, vague, and chronic axial bone pain (often in the cervical region) that prompted radiographic study. Family histories are usually negative for skeletal disease.

Radiologic Features

Abnormalities are essentially confined to the spine and pelvis, where trabeculae are coarsened and form a pattern like that found in other types of osteomalacia (105). However, Looser's zones (a radiologic hallmark of osteomalacia) have not been reported. The cervical spine and ribs seem to be the most severely affected; the lumbar spine is abnormal to a lesser degree. Two patients also had features of ankylosing spondylitis (106). Radiographic survey of the appendicular skeleton is unremarkable.

Laboratory Studies

In four patients, serum inorganic phosphate levels tended to be low (106). In others, osteomalacia occurred despite normal serum levels of calcium, inorganic phosphate, 25-hydroxyvitamin D [25 (OH) D] and 1,25-dihydroxyvitamin D [1,25 (OH)$_2$ D]. Serum alkaline phosphatase activity (bone isoenzyme) may be increased.

Histopathologic Findings

Iliac crest specimens have distinct corticomedullary junctions, but the cortices can be especially wide and porous. Trabeculae are of variable thickness; total bone volume may be increased. Collagen has a normal lamellar pattern on polarized-light microscopy. There is increased width and extent of osteoid seams on trabecular bone surfaces and in cortical bone spaces. Tetracycline labeling confirms the defective skeletal mineralization and results in fluorescent "labels" that are single, irregular, and wide (104). Osteoblasts are flat and inactive-appearing "lining" cells, with reduced Golgi zones and rough endoplasmic reticulum and increased amounts of cytoplasmic glycogen, but these cells do stain intensely for alkaline phosphatase activity. Changes of secondary hyperparathyroidism are absent (104).

Etiology and Pathogenesis

Axial osteomalacia possibly results from an osteoblast defect (107). Electron microscopy of iliac crest bone from one patient (104) revealed osteoblasts that had an inactive appearance but were able to form matrix vesicles within abundant osteoid.

Treatment

Effective medical therapy has not been reported. The natural history for axial osteomalacia, however, seems relatively benign. Methyltestosterone and stilbestrol have been tested unsuccessfully (107). Vitamin D$_2$ (as much as 20,000 U/day for 3 years) was similarly without beneficial effect (107). Slight improvement in skeletal histology, but not in symptoms, was reported for calcium and vitamin D$_2$ therapy in a study of four cases (106). Long-term follow-up of one patient showed that symptoms and radiographic findings did not change (107).

FIBROGENESIS IMPERFECTA OSSIUM

Fibrogenesis imperfecta ossium was first described in 1950 (105). Fewer than 10 cases have been reported (108,109). Although radiographic studies suggest that there is generalized osteopenia, the coarse and dense appearance of trabecular bone explains why this condition is included among the osteosclerotic disorders. The clinical, biochemical, radiologic, and histopathologic features of fibrogenesis imperfecta ossium and axial osteomalacia have been carefully contrasted (105).

Clinical Presentation

Fibrogenesis imperfecta ossium typically presents during middle age or later. Both sexes are affected. Gradual onset of intractable skeletal pain that rapidly progresses is the characteristic symptom. Subsequently there is a debilitating course with progressive immobility. Spontaneous fractures also are a prominent clinical feature. Patients generally become bedridden. Physical examination typically shows marked bony tenderness.

Radiologic Features

Radiographic changes are noted throughout the skeleton, except in the skull. Initially there may be only osteopenia and a slightly abnormal appearance of trabecular bone (109). Subsequently the changes become more consistent with osteomalacia (i.e., further alterations of the trabecular bone pattern, heterogeneous bone density, and thinning of cortical bone). The corticomedullary junctions become indistinct as cortices are replaced by an abnormal pattern of trabecular bone. Areas of the skeleton may have a mixed lytic and sclerotic appearance (105,109). The generalized osteopenia causes remaining trabeculae to appear coarse and dense in a fish-net pattern. Pseudofractures may develop. Deformities secondary to fractures can be present, although bony contours are typically normal. Some patients have a rugger jersey spine. The shafts of long bones may show periosteal reaction. In fibrogenesis imperfecta ossium and axial osteomalacia, the distribution of the radiographic abnormalities (generalized vs. axial) helps to distinguish between the two conditions. Furthermore, the histopathologic features are clearly different (105).

Laboratory Findings

Serum calcium and inorganic phosphate concentrations are normal, but alkaline phosphatase activity is increased. Acute agranulocytosis and macroglobulinemia have been reported. Hydroxyproline levels in urine may be normal or elevated (109). Typically there is no aminoaciduria or other evidence of renal tubular dysfunction.

Histopathologic Findings

The bony lesion is a form of osteomalacia, although the amount of affected bone varies considerably from area to area (109). Aberrant collagen is found in regions with abnormal mineralization patterns, but this protein is unremarkable in other tissues. Cortical bone in the shaft of the femora and tibiae may demonstrate the least abnormality. Osteoid seams are thick. Osteoblasts and osteoclasts can be abundant. Polarized-light microscopy shows that the abnormal collagen fibrils lack birefringence. Electron microscopy reveals that the collagen fibrils are thin and randomly organized in a "tangled" pattern. In some regions, peculiar circular matrix structures of 300- to 500-nm diameter have been observed (109). Unless bone specimens are viewed with polarized light or electron microscopy, fibrogenesis imperfecta ossium can be mistaken for osteoporosis or other forms of osteomalacia (109).

Etiology and Pathogenesis

The etiology is unknown. Genetic factors have not been implicated for this sporadic condition. It seems to be an acquired disorder of collagen synthesis in lamellar bone. Subperiosteal bone formation and collagen synthesis in nonosseous tissues appears to be normal.

Treatment

There is no recognized medical therapy. Temporary clinical improvement can occur (109). Treatment with vitamin D$_2$ (or an active metabolite) together with calcium supplementation has been tried without significant benefit. Indeed, ectopic calcification complicated high-dose vitamin D$_2$ therapy in one patient. Synthetic salmon calcitonin, sodium fluoride, and 24,25 (OH)$_2$ D also have been without apparent benefit (109). Treatment with melphalan and prednisolone seemed to help one patient (110).

PACHYDERMOPERIOSTOSIS

Pachydermoperiostosis (hypertrophic osteoarthropathy: primary or idiopathic) causes clubbing of the digits, hyperhidrosis and thickening of the skin, especially of the face and forehead, and periosteal new bone formation that occurs prominently in the distal limbs. Autosomal dominant inheritance with variable expression is established (111), but autosomal recessive transmission also seems to occur (112).

Clinical Presentation

Men appear to be more severely affected than women, and blacks more commonly than whites. The age at presentation is variable, but symptoms typically first manifest during adolescence (111,112). All three principal features (pachydermia, cutis verticis gyrata, periostitis) are present in some patients; others have just one or two of these findings. Clinical expression develops during the course of a decade, but the disorder then becomes quiescent (113). Progressive gradual enlargement of the hands and feet can result in a "pawlike" appearance. Some affected individuals are described as acromegalic. Arthralgias of the ankles, knees, wrists, and elbows are common. Occasionally, the small joints are also painful. Acroosteolysis has been reported. Symptoms of pseudogout can occur. Chondrocalcinosis, with calcium pyrophosphate crystals in synovial fluid, has been found in one patient. Stiffness and limited mobility of both the appendicular and the axial skeleton can develop. Compression of cranial or spinal nerves has been described. Cutaneous changes include coarsening, thickening, furrowing, pitting, and oiliness of especially the scalp and face. Fatigue is not uncommon. Myelophthisic anemia with extramedullary hematopoiesis may occur. Life expectancy is normal (113).

Radiologic Features

Severe periostitis that thickens the distal portions of the tubular bones—typically the tibia, fibula, radius, and ulna—is the principal radiographic abnormality (Fig. 10). The metacarpals, tarsals/metatarsals, clavicles, pelvis, base of the skull, and phalanges also may be affected. Clubbing is obvious, and acroosteolysis can occur. The spine is rarely involved. Ankylosis of joints, especially in the hands and in the feet, may occur in older patients (11).

The major consideration in the differential diagnosis for pachydermoperiostosis is secondary hypertrophic osteoarthropathy (pulmonary or otherwise). The radiographic features of this condition are, however, somewhat different. In secondary hypertrophic osteoarthropathy, periosteal reaction

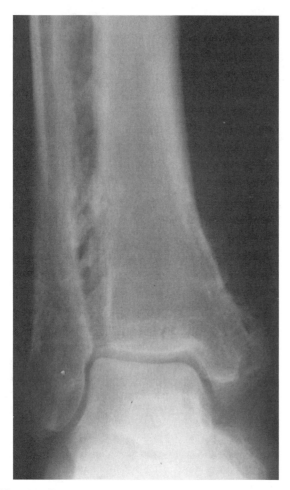

FIG. 10. Pachydermoperiostosis. Anteroposterior radiograph of the ankle shows ragged periosteal reaction along the interosseous membrane between the tibia and fibula (note also the proliferative bone formation along the medial malleolus). (From Whyte MP. Rare disorders of skeletal formation and homeostasis. In: Becker KN, ed. *Principles and practice of endocrinology and metabolism.* 2nd ed. Philadelphia: Lippincott-Raven Publishers, 1995:594–606.)

typically has a smooth, undulating appearance (114). In pachydermoperiostosis, periosteal proliferation is more exuberant, has an irregular appearance, and often involves epiphyses. Bone scanning in either condition reveals symmetric, diffuse, regular uptake along the cortical margins of long bones, especially in the legs. This feature results in a "double-stripe" sign.

Laboratory Findings

Synovial fluid examination typically does not reveal evidence of inflammation.

Periosteal new bone formation roughens the surface of cortical bone (115). This newly formed osseous tissue undergoes cancellous compaction and can accordingly be difficult to distinguish from the original cortex on histopathologic examination (115). There may also be osteopenia of trabecular bone from quiescent formation (11). Mild cellular hyper-

plasia and thickening of subsynovial blood vessels is found near synovial membranes (116). Electron microscopy demonstrates layered basement membranes.

Etiology and Pathogenesis

Pachydermoperiostosis has not been mapped within the human genome. A controversial hypothesis suggests that some unknown circulating factor acts on vasculature initially to cause hyperemia, and thus alters soft tissues, but later blood flow is reduced (112). Recently in one patient, skin fibroblasts were found to synthesize decreased amounts of collagen but increased amounts of decorin (117).

Treatment

There is no established medical treatment. Painful synovial effusions may respond to nonsteroidal antiinflammatory drugs (118). Colchicine was reported to help arthralgias, clubbing, folliculitis, and pachyderma in one patient (119). Contractures or neurovascular compression by osteosclerotic lesions may require surgical intervention.

HEPATITIS C–ASSOCIATED OSTEOSCLEROSIS

In 1992, a new syndrome was characterized that featured remarkably severe, acquired, generalized osteosclerosis and hyperostosis in former intravenous drug abusers exposed to hepatitis C virus (120). Ten cases have been reported (121).

Periosteal, endosteal, and trabecular bone thickening occurs throughout the skeleton except, apparently, in the cranium (Fig. 11). During active disease, the forearms and legs are painful. Densitometric studies show bone mass that can be 200% to 300% above mean values for age and sex. Skeletal remodeling is often abnormally rapid during active disease and may respond to pamidronate or to calcitonin therapy. Gradual spontaneous remission in pain and normalization of bone-remodeling rates may occur. Exposure to blood contaminated with hepatitis C virus is the historical feature common to all patients (121). In 1998, abnormalities in the IGF system were reported (122).

OTHER SCLEROSING BONE DYSPLASIAS

Table 1 lists the relatively large number of conditions that cause focal or generalized increases in skeletal mass (1,123). Of note, sarcoidosis characteristically causes cysts within coarsely reticulated bone; occasionally, however, sclerotic areas are found in the axial skeleton or in long tubular bones. These skeletal changes may occur well after the pulmonary disease is arrested. Although multiple myeloma typically presents with generalized osteopenia or with discrete osteolytic lesions, widespread osteosclerosis can occur. Lymphoma, myelosclerosis, and mastocytosis are additional hematologic causes of increased bone mass. Metastatic carcinoma, primarily prostatic, commonly causes dense bone. Diffuse osteosclerosis is also a relatively frequent radiologi-

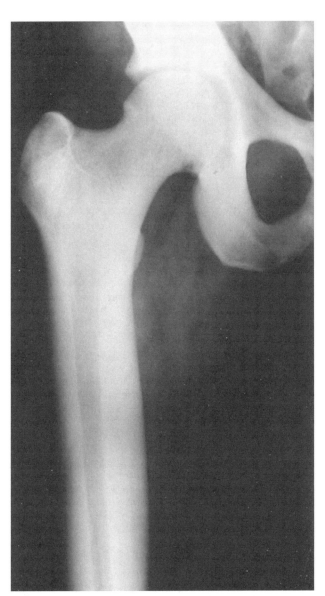

FIG. 11. Hepatitis C–associated osteosclerosis. Anteroposterior view of the proximal right femur of this middle-aged, former intravenous drug abuser shows diffuse bony sclerosis with marked cortical thickening. The medullary cavity is narrow, and the periosteal margins of the cortex are mildly convex, suggesting endosteal and periosteal bone apposition, respectively. The cortices of the greater and lesser trochanters are relatively spared. The trabecular pattern in the femoral neck is especially prominent. (From Whyte MP, Teitelbaum SL, Reinus WR. Doubling skeletal mass during adult life: the syndrome of diffuse osteosclerosis after intravenous drug abuse. *J Bone Miner Res* 1996;11:554–558, with permission of the American Society for Bone and Mineral Research.)

cal finding in secondary hyperparathyroidism (e.g., renal disease), but occurs very rarely in primary hyperparathyroidism. Intoxication with vitamin A or vitamin D, heavy metal poisoning, milk-alkali syndrome, ionizing radiation, osteomyelitis, and osteonecrosis are additional explanations for increased bone mass (1,123).

REFERENCES

1. Whyte MP. Skeletal disorders characterized by osteosclerosis or hyperostosis. In: Avioli LV, Krane SM, eds. *Metabolic bone disease,* 2nd ed. San Diego: Academic Press, 1997:697–738.
2. McKusick VA. *Mendelian inheritance in man: a catalog of human genes and genetic disorders.* 12th ed. Baltimore: Johns Hopkins University Press, 1998.
3. Albers-Schönberg H. Rontgenbilder einer seltenen, Knochenerkrankung. *Munch Med Wochenschr* 1904;51:365.
4. Johnston CC Jr, Lavy N, Lord T, et al. Osteopetrosis: a clinical, genetic, metabolic, and morphologic study of the dominantly inherited, benign form. *Medicine* 1968;47:149–167.
5. Loria-Cortes R, Quesada-Calvo E, Cordero-Chaverri E. Osteopetrosis in children: a report of 26 cases. *J Pediatr* 1977;91:43–47.
6. Kahler SG, Burns JA, Aylsworth AS. A mild autosomal recessive form of osteopetrosis. *Am J Med Genet* 1984;17:451–464.
7. Jagadha V, Halliday WC, Becker LE, Hinton D. The association of infantile osteopetrosis and neuronal storage disease in two brothers. *Acta Neuropathol* 1988;75:233–240.
8. Whyte MP. Recent advances in osteopetrosis. In: Cohn DV, Gennari C, Tashian AH, eds. *Calcium-regulating hormones and bone metabolism.* Amsterdam: Elsevier, 1992:420–430.
9. Marks SC Jr. Osteopetrosis: multiple pathways for the interception of osteoclast function. *Appl Pathol* 1987;5:172–183.
10. Bollerslev J. Autosomal dominant osteopetrosis: bone metabolism and epidemiological, clinical and hormonal aspects. *Endocr Rev* 1989;10:45–67.
11. Resnick D, Niwayama G. *Diagnosis of bone and joint disorders.* 3rd ed. Philadelphia: WB Saunders, 1995.
12. Oliveira G, Boechat MI, Amaral SM, et al. Osteopetrosis and rickets: an intriguing association. *Am J Dis Child* 1986;140:377–378.
13. Park H-M, Lambertus J. Skeletal and reticuloendothelial imaging in osteopetrosis: case report. *J Nucl Med* 1977;18:1091–1095.
14. Rao VM, Dalinka MK, Mitchell DG, et al. Osteopetrosis: MR characteristics at 1.5 T. *Radiology* 1986;161:217–220.
15. Elster AD, Theros EG, Key LL, Chen MYM. Cranial imaging in autosomal recessive osteopetrosis (parts I & II). *Radiology* 1992; 183:129–144.
16. Key LL, Carnes D, Holtrop M, et al. Treatment of congenital osteopetrosis with high dose calcitriol. *N Engl J Med* 1984;310:409–415.
17. Cournot G, Trubert-Thil CL, Petrovic M, et al. Mineral metabolism in infants with malignant osteopetrosis: heterogeneity in plasma 1,25-dihydroxyvitamin D levels and bone histology. *J Bone Miner Res* 1992;7:1–10.
18. Whyte MP, Chines A, Silva DP Jr, Landt Y, Ladenson JH. Creatine kinase brain isoenzyme (BB-CK) presence in serum distinguishes osteopetrosis among the sclerosing bone disorders. *J Bone Miner Res* 1996;11:1438–1443.
19. Revell PA. *Pathology of bone.* Berlin: Springer-Verlag, 1986.
20. Helfrich MH, Aronson DC, Everts V, et al. Morphologic features of bone in human osteopetrosis. *Bone* 1991;12:411–419.
21. Bollerslev J, Steiniche T, Melsen F, Mosekilde L. Structural and histomorphometric studies of iliac crest trabecular and cortical bone in autosomal dominant osteopetrosis: a study of two radiological types. *Bone* 1989;10:19–24.
22. Van Hul W, Bollerslev J, Gram J, et al. Localization of a gene for autosomal dominant osteopetrosis (Albers-Schönberg disease) to chromosome 1p21. *Am J Hum Genet* 1997;61:363–369.
23. Whyte MP. Chipping away at marble bone disease [Editorial]. *N Engl J Med* 1995;332:1639–1640.
24. Teitelbaum SL, Tondravi MM, Ross FP. Osteoclast biology. In: Marcus R, Feldman D, Kelsey J, eds. *Osteoporosis.* San Diego: Academic Press, 1996:61–94.
25. Lajeunesse D, Busque L, Mènard P, Brunette MG, Bonny Y. Demonstration of an osteoblast defect in two cases of human malignant osteopetrosis: correction of the phenotype after bone marrow transplant. *Bone* 1996;98:1835–1842.
26. Mills BG, Yabe H, Singer FR. Osteoclasts in human osteopetrosis contain viral-nucleocapsid-like nuclear inclusions. *J Bone Miner Res* 1988;3:101–106.
27. Glorieux FH, Pettifor JM, Marie PJ, et al. Induction of bone resorption

by parathyroid hormone in congenital malignant osteopetrosis. *Metab Bone Dis Relat Res* 1981;3:143–150.

28. Key LL, Ries WL, Schiff R. Osteopetrosis associated with interleukin-2 deficiency [Abstract]. *J Bone Miner Res* 1987;2(suppl II):85.

29. Key LL, Rodriguiz RN, Willi SM, et al. Recombinant human interferon gamma therapy for osteopetrosis. *N Engl J Med* 1995;332:1594–1599.

30. Beard CJ, Key L, Newburger PE, et al. Neutrophil defect associated with malignant infantile osteopetrosis. *J Lab Clin Med* 1986;108:498–505.

31. Kaplan FS, August CS, Fallon MD, et al. Successful treatment of infantile malignant osteopetrosis by bone-marrow transplantation: a case report. *J Bone Joint Surg Am* 1988;70:617–623.

32. Coccia PF, Krivit W, Cervenka J, et al. Successful bone-marrow transplantation for infantile malignant osteopetrosis. *N Engl J Med* 1980;302:701–708.

33. Orchard PJ, Dickerman JD, Mathews CHE, et al. Haploidentical bone marrow transplantation for osteopetrosis. *Am J Pediatr Hematol Oncol* 1987;9:335–340.

34. Rawlinson PS, Green RH, Coggins AM, Boyle IT, Gibson BE. Malignant osteopetrosis: hypercalcaemia after bone marrow transplantation. *Arch Dis Child* 1991;66:638–639.

35. Key LL Jr: Osteopetrosis: a genetic window into osteoclast function. *Cases Metab Bone Dis* 1987;2:1–12.

36. Dorantes LM, Mejia AM, Dorantes S. Juvenile osteopetrosis: effects of blood and bone of prednisone and low calcium, high phosphate diet. *Arch Dis Child* 1986;61:666–670.

37. Ogur G, Ogur E, Celasun B, et al. Prenatal diagnosis of autosomal recessive osteopetrosis, infantile type, by x-ray evaluation. *Prenat Diagn* 1995;15:477–481.

38. Sly WS, Hewett-Emmett D, Whyte MP, et al. Carbonic anhydrase II deficiency identified as the primary defect in the autosomal recessive syndrome of osteopetrosis with renal tubular acidosis and cerebral calcification. *Proc Natl Acad Sci USA* 1983;80:2752–2756.

39. Whyte MP. Carbonic anhydrase II deficiency. *Clin Orthop* 1993;294:52–63.

40. Sly WS, Whyte MP, Sundaram V, et al. Carbonic anhydrase II deficiency in 12 families with the autosomal recessive syndrome of osteopetrosis with renal tubular acidosis and cerebral calcification. *N Engl J Med* 1985;313:139–145.

41. Sly WS, Hu PY. The carbonic anhydrase II deficiency syndrome: osteopetrosis with renal tubular acidosis and cerebral calcification. In: Scriver CR, Beaudet AL, Sly WS, Valle D, eds. *The metabolic and molecular bases of inherited disease.* 7th ed. New York: McGraw-Hill, 1995:4113–4124.

42. Whyte MP, Murphy WA, Fallon MD, et al. Osteopetrosis, renal tubular acidosis and basal ganglia calcification in three sisters. *Am J Med* 1980;69:64–74.

43. Sly WS, Whyte MP, Krupin T, et al. Positive renal response to acetazolamide in carbonic anhydrase II-deficient patients. *Pediatr Res* 1985;19:1033–1036.

44. Roth DE, Venta PJ, Tashian RE, Sly WS. Molecular basis of human carbonic anhydrase II deficiency. *Proc Natl Acad Sci USA* 1992;89:1804–1808.

45. Whyte MP, Hamm LL III, Sly WS. Transfusion of carbonic anhydrase-replete erythrocytes fails to correct the acidification defect in the syndrome of osteopetrosis, renal tubular acidosis, and cerebral calcification (carbonic anhydrase II deficiency). *J Bone Miner Res* 1988;3:385–388.

46. Maroteaux P, Lamy M. The malady of Toulouse-Lautrec. *JAMA* 1965; 191:715–717.

47. Maroteaux P, Lamy M. La pycnodysostose. *Presse Med* 1962;70:999–1002.

48. Sugiura Y, Yamada Y, Koh J. Pycnodysostosis in Japan: report of six cases and a review of Japanese literature. *Birth Defects* 1974;10:78–98.

49. Elmore SM. Pycnodysostosis: a review. *J Bone Joint Surg Am* 1967;49:153–162.

50. Wolpowitz A, Matisson A. A comparative study of pycnodysostosis, cleidocranial dysostosis, osteopetrosis and acro-osteolysis. *S Afr Med J* 1974;48:1011–1118.

51. Soto TJ, Mautalen CA, Hojman D, et al. Pycnodysostosis, metabolic and histologic studies. *Birth Defects* 1969;5:109–115.

52. Everts V, Aronson DC, Beertsen W. Phagocytosis of bone collagen by osteoclasts in two cases of pycnodysostosis. *Calcif Tissue Int* 1985;37:25–31.

53. Gelb BD, Shi GP, Chapman HA, Desnick RJ. Pycnodysostosis, a lysosomal disease caused by cathepsin K deficiency. *Science* 1996;273:1236–1238.

54. Cabrejas ML, Fromm GA, Roca JF, et al. Pycnodysostosis: some aspects concerning kinetics of calcium metabolism and bone pathology. *Am J Med Sci* 1976;271:215–220.

55. Beneton MNC, Harris S, Kanis JA. Paramyxovirus-like inclusions in two cases of pycnodysostosis. *Bone* 1987;8:211–217.

56. Karkabi S, Reis ND, Linn S, et al. Pyknodysostosis: imaging and laboratory observations. *Calcif Tissue Int* 1993;53:170–173.

57. Soliman AT, Rajab A, AlSalmi I, Darwish A, Asfour M. Defective growth hormone secretion in children with pycnodysostosis and improved linear growth after growth hormone treatment. *Arch Dis Child* 1996;75:242–244.

58. Edelson JG, Obad S, Geiger R, On A, Artul HJ. Pycnodysostosis: orthopedic aspects, with a description of 14 new cases. *Clin Orthop* 1992;280:263–276.

59. Cockayne EA. A case for diagnosis. *Proc R Soc Med* 1920;13:132–136.

60. Engelmann G. Ein fall von osteopathia hyperostotica (sclerotisans) multiplex infantilis. *Fortschr Geb Rontgen* 1929;39:1101–1106.

61. Hundley JD, Wilson FC. Progressive diaphyseal dysplasia: review of the literature and report of seven cases in one family. *J Bone Joint Surg Am* 1973;55:461–474.

62. Naveh Y, Ludatshcer R, Alon U, et al. Muscle involvement in progressive diaphyseal dysplasia. *Pediatrics* 1985;76:944–949.

63. Crisp AJ, Brenton DP. Engelmann's disease of bone: a systemic disorder? *Ann Rheum Dis* 1982;41:183–188.

64. Smith R, Walton RJ, Corner BD, et al. Clinical and biochemical studies in Engelmann's disease (progressive diaphyseal dysplasia). *Q J Med* 1977;46:273–294.

65. Kumar B, Murphy WA, Whyte MP. Progressive diaphyseal dysplasia (Engelmann's disease): scintigraphic-radiologic-clinical correlations. *Radiology* 1981;140:87–92.

66. Applegate LJ, Applegate GR, Kemp SS. MR of multiple cranial neuropathies in a patient with Camurati-Engelmann disease: case report. *Am Soc Neuroradiol* 1991;12:557–559.

67. Shier CK, Krasicky GA, Ellis BI, Kottamasu SR. Ribbing's disease: radiographic-scintigraphic correlation and comparative analysis with Engelmann's disease. *J Nucl Med* 1987;28:244–248.

68. Labat ML, Bringuier AF, Seebold C, et al. Monocytic origin of fibroblasts: spontaneous transformation of blood monocytes into neo-fibroblastic structures in osteomyelosclerosis and Engelmann's disease. *Biomed Pharmacother* 1991;45:289–299.

69. Kaftori JK, Kleinhaus U, Neveh Y. Progressive diaphyseal dysplasia (Camurati-Engelmann): radiographic follow-up and CT findings. *Radiology* 1987;164:777–782.

70. Naveh Y, Alon U, Kaftori JK, et al. Progressive diaphyseal dysplasia: evaluation of corticosteroid therapy. *Pediatrics* 1985;75:321–323.

71. Fallon MD, Whyte MP, Murphy WA. Progressive diaphyseal dysplasia (Engelmann's disease): report of a sporadic case of the mild form. *J Bone Joint Surg Am* 1980;62:465–472.

72. van Buchem FSP, Prick JJG, Jaspar HHJ. *Hyperostosis corticalis generalisata familiaris* (van Buchem's disease). Amsterdam: Excerpta, 1976.

73. Perez-Vicente Jr, Rodriguez de Castro E, Lafuente J, et al. Autosomal dominant endosteal hyperostosis: report of a Spanish family with neurological involvement. *Clin Genet* 1987;31:161–169.

74. Eastman JR, Bixler D. Generalized cortical hyperostosis (van Buchem disease): nosologic considerations. *Radiology* 1977;125:297–304.

75. Beighton P, Barnard A, Hamersma H, et al. The syndromic status of sclerosteosis and van Buchem disease. *Clin Genet* 1984;25:175–181.

76. Hill SC, Stein SA, Dwyer A, Altman J, Dorwart R, Doppman J. Cranial CT findings in sclerosteosis. *Am J Neuroradiol* 1986;7:505–511.

77. Ruckert EW, Caudill RJ, McCready PJ. Surgical treatment of van Buchem disease. *J Oral Maxillofac Surg* 1985;43:801–805.

78. Schendel SA. van Buchem disease: surgical treatment of the mandible. *Ann Plast Surg* 1988;20:462–467.

79. Beighton P, Durr L, Hamersma H. The clinical features of sclerosteosis: a review of the manifestations in twenty-five affected individuals. *Ann Intern Med* 1976;84:393–397.

80. Barnard AH, Hamersma H, Kretzmar JH, et al. Sclerosteosis in old age. *S Afr Med J* 1980;58:401–403.

81. Beighton P, Cremin BJ, Hamersma H. The radiology of sclerosteosis. *Br J Radiol* 1976;49:934–939.

82. Stein SA, Witkop C, Hill S, et al. Sclerosteosis, neurogenetic and pathophysiologic analysis of an American kinship. *Neurology* 1983;33:267–277.

83. Van Hul W, Balemans W, Van Hul E, et al. Van Buchem disease (hyperostosis corticalis generalisata) maps to chromosome 17q12-q21. *Am J Hum Genet* 1998;62:391–399.

84. Epstein S, Hamersma H, Beighton P. Endocrine function in sclerosteosis. *S Afr Med J* 1979;55:1105–1110.

85. Berlin R, Hedensio B, Lilja B, et al. Osteopoikilosis: a clinical and genetic study. *Acta Med Scand* 1967;18:305–314.

86. Uitto J, Starcher BC, Santa-Cruz DJ, et al. Biochemical and ultrastructural demonstration of elastin accumulation in the skin of the Buschke-Ollendorff syndrome. *J Invest Dermatol* 1981;76:284–287.

87. Whyte MP, Murphy WA, Seigel BA. 99m Tc-pyrophosphate bone imaging in osteopoikilosis, osteopathia striata, and melorheostosis. *Radiology* 1978;127:439–443.

88. Lagier R, Mbakop A, Bigler A. Osteopoikilosis: a radiological and pathological study. *Skeletal Radiol* 1984;11:161–168.

89. Rabinow M, Unger F. Syndrome of osteopathia striata, macrocephaly, and cranial sclerosis. *Am J Dis Child* 1984;138:821–823.

90. Happle R, Lenz W. Striation of bones in focal dermal hypoplasia: manifestation of functional mosaicism? *Br J Dermatol* 1977;96:133–138.

91. Kornreich L, Grunebaum M, Ziv N, Shuper A, Mimouni M. Osteopathia striata, cranial sclerosis with cleft palate and facial nerve palsy. *Eur J Pediatr* 1988;147:101–103.

92. Léri A, Joanny J. Une affection non decrite des os. Hyperostose en coulée sur toute la longueur d un membre ou melorheostose. *Bull Mem Soc Med Hop Paris* 1922;46:1141–1145.

93. Murray RO, McCredie J. Melorheostosis and sclerotomes: a radiological correlation. *Skeletal Radiol* 1979;4:57–71.

94. Campbell CJ, Papademetriou T, Bonfiglio M. Melorheostosis: a report of the clinical, roentgenographic, and pathological findings in fourteen cases. *J Bone Joint Surg Am* 1968;50:1281–1304.

95. Miyachi Y, Horio T, Yamada A, et al. Linear melorheostotic scleroderma with hypertrichosis. *Arch Dermatol* 1979;115:1233–1234.

96. Applebaum RE, Caniano DA, Sun C-C, et al. Synchronous left subclavian and axillary artery aneurysms associated with melorheostosis. *Surgery* 1986;99:249–253.

97. Colavita N, Nicolais S, Orazi C, Falappa PG. Melorheostosis: presentation of a case followed up for 24 years. *Arch Orthop Trauma Surg* 1987;106:123–125.

98. Davis DC, Syklawer R, Cole RL. Melorheostosis on three-phase bone scintigraphy: case report. *Clin Nucl Med* 1992;17:561–564.

99. Wagers LT, Young AW Jr, Ryan SF. Linear melorheostotic scleroderma. *Br J Dermatol* 1972;86:297–301.

100. Atar D, Lehman WB, Grant AD, Strongwater AM. The Ilizarov apparatus for treatment of melorheostosis: case report and review of the literature. *Clin Orthop* 1992;281:163–167.

101. Whyte MP, Murphy WA, Fallon MD, et al. Mixed-sclerosing-bone-dystrophy: report of a case and review of the literature. *Skeletal Radiol* 1981;6:95–102.

102. Pacifici R, Murphy WA, Teitelbaum SL, Whyte MP. Mixed-sclerosing-bone-dystrophy: 42-year follow-up of a case reported as osteopetrosis. *Calcif Tissue Int* 1986;38:175–185.

103. Frame B, Frost HM, Ormond RS, et al. Atypical axial osteomalacia involving the axial skeleton. *Ann Intern Med* 1961;55:632–639.

104. Whyte MP, Fallon MD, Murphy WA, et al. Axial osteomalacia: clinical, laboratory and genetic investigation of an affected mother and son. *Am J Med* 1981;71:1041–1049.

105. Christman D, Wenger JJ, Dosch JC, et al. L'osteomalacie axiale: analyse compare avec la fibrogenese imparfaite. *J Radiol* 1981;62:37–41.

106. Nelson AM, Riggs BL, Jowsey JO. Atypical axial osteomalacia: report of four cases with two having features of ankylosing spondylitis. *Arthritis Rheum* 1978;21:715–722.

107. Condon JR, Nassim JR. Axial osteomalacia. *Postgrad Med* 1971;47:817–820.

108. Swan CHJ, Shah K, Brewer DB, et al. Fibrogenesis imperfecta ossium. *Q J Med* 1976;45:233–253.

109. Lang R, Vignery AM, Jenson PS. Fibrogenesis imperfecta ossium with early onset: observations after 20 years of illness. *Bone* 1986;7:237–246.

110. Ralphs JR, Stamp TCB, Dopping-Hepenstal PJC, Ali SY. Ultrastructural features of the osteoid of patients with fibrogenesis imperfecta ossium. *Bone* 1989;10:243–249.

111. Rimoin DL. Pachydermoperiostosis (idiopathic clubbing and periostosis): genetic and physiologic considerations. *N Engl J Med* 1965;272:923–931.

112. Matucci-Cerinic M, Lott T, Jajic IVO, Pignone A, Bussani C, Cagnoni M. The clinical spectrum of pachydermoperiostosis (primary hypertrophic osteoarthropathy). *Medicine* 1991;79:208–214.

113. Herman MA, Massaro D, Katz S. Pachydermoperiostosis: clinical spectrum. *Arch Intern Med* 1965;116:919–923.

114. Ali A, Tetalman M, Fordham EW. Distribution of hypertrophic pulmonary osteoarthropathy. *Am J Roentgenol* 1980;134:771–780.

115. Vogl A, Goldfischer S. Pachydermoperiostosis: primary or idiopathic hypertrophic osteoarthropathy. *Am J Med* 1962;33:166–187.

116. Lauter SA, Vasey FB, Huttner I, Osterland CK. Pachydermoperiostosis: studies on the synovium. *J Rheumatol* 1978;5:85–95.

117. Wegrowski Y, Gillery P, Serpier H, et al. Alteration of matrix macromolecule synthesis by fibroblasts from a patient with pachydermoperiostosis. *J Invest Dermatol* 1996;106:70–74.

118. Cooper RG, Freemont AJ, Riley M, Holt PJL, Anderson DC, Jayson MIV. Bone abnormalities and severe arthritis in pachydermoperiostosis. *Ann Rheum Dis* 1992;51:416–419.

119. Matucci-Cerinic M, Fattorini L, Gerini G, et al. Colchicine treatment in a case of pachydermoperiostosis with acroosteolysis. *Rheumatol Int* 1988;8:185–188.

120. Whyte MP, Teitelbaum SL, Reinus WR. Doubling skeletal mass during adult life: the syndrome of diffuse osteosclerosis after intravenous drug abuse. *J Bone Miner Res* 1996;11:554–558.

121. Shaker JL, Reinus WR, Whyte MP. Hepatitis C-associated osteosclerosis: late onset after blood transfusion in an elderly woman. *J Clin Endocrinol Metab* 1998;84:93–98.

122. Khosla S, Hassoun AAK, Baker BK, et al. Insulin-like growth factor system abnormalities in hepatitis C-associated osteosclerosis: a means to increase bone mass in adults? *J Clin Invest* 1998;101:2165–2173.

123. Frame B, Honasoge M, Kottamasu SR. *Osteosclerosis, hyperostosis, and related disorders*. New York: Elsevier, 1987.

71. Fibrous Dysplasia

Michael P. Whyte, M.D.

Division of Bone and Mineral Diseases, Washington University School of Medicine at Barnes–Jewish Hospital, and Metabolic Research Unit, Shriners Hospital for Children, St. Louis, Missouri

Fibrous dysplasia is a sporadic, developmental disorder characterized by a unifocal or multifocal expanding fibrous lesion of bone-forming mesenchyme that often results in pain, fracture, and/or deformity.

McCune–Albright syndrome refers to patients with fibrous dysplasia (generally polyostotic) and patches of skin pigmentation, called café-au-lait spots, who also have hyperfunction of one or more endocrine glands.

Postzygotic somatic mosaicism for "activating" mutations in the gene that encodes the Gsα subunit of the receptor/adenylate cyclase–coupling G protein [which stimulates cyclic adenosine monophosphate (cAMP) production] causes all types of fibrous dysplasia (see the following).

CLINICAL PRESENTATION

Monostotic fibrous dysplasia characteristically develops during the second or third decade of life; polyostotic disease generally manifests before age 10 years (1). The condition affects both sexes. The monostotic form is more common. Typically an expansile bony lesion causes pain, fracture, and/or deformity and may occasionally entrap nerves. The skull and long bones are involved most often. Sarcomatous degeneration of affected skeletal sites occurs with increased frequency (incidence, <1%), especially when the facial bones or femora are involved (2). Pregnancy may reactivate previously quiescent lesions (3).

In the McCune–Albright syndrome, café-au-lait spots are hyperpigmented macules with rough borders (Fig. 1) compared with the smooth borders of these lesions in neurofibromatosis (i.e., "Coast-of-Maine" versus "Coast-of-California," respectively) (4). Typically, the endocrinopathy is pseudoprecocious puberty in girls due to premature ovarian activity. Less commonly, there is thyrotoxicosis, Cushing syndrome, acromegaly, hyperprolactinemia, hyperparathyroidism, or pseudoprecocious puberty in boys (5–8). In some patients with widespread skeletal lesions, renal phosphate wasting causes hypophosphatemic bone disease. This situation resembles an oncogenic form of rickets or osteomalacia (see Chapter 65) (9).

RADIOLOGIC FEATURES

Femora, tibiae, ribs, and facial bones are involved most frequently, but any skeletal site can be affected (10). Small bones show radiographic features in about 50% of patients with polyostotic disease. In the long bones, the lesions may be found either in the metaphysis or in the diaphysis.

Typically, they are well defined and are characterized by thin cortices and a ground-glass appearance (Fig. 2). Occasionally the lesions are lobulated with trabeculated areas of radiolucency.

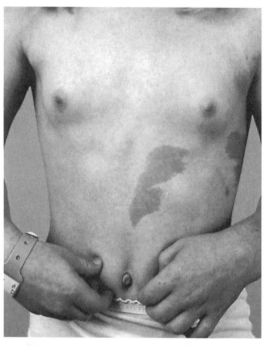

FIG. 1. McCune–Albright syndrome. Characteristic café-au-lait spots *(rough border)* are present on the left abdomen and chest of this 3 10/12-year-old girl who also has precocious breast development.

LABORATORY FINDINGS

Although serum alkaline phosphatase activity may be elevated, calcium and inorganic phosphate levels are usually normal. Biochemical markers of bone remodeling are sometimes elevated (11).

Both monostotic and polyostotic bone lesions have a similar histologic appearance. They are anatomically well defined but are not encapsulated. Characteristic spindle-shaped fibroblasts form "swirls" within marrow spaces. Haphazardly arranged trabeculae are composed of woven bone. Cartilage is found within these lesions more often when there is polyostotic involvement. Cystic regions, which are lined by multinucleated giant cells, may be present. These findings resemble the histopathologic characteristics of hyperparathyroidism (osteitis fibrosa cystica), but an important distinction is that mature osteoblasts are scarce in fibrous dysplasia rather than plentiful in hyperparathyroid bone disease (1,12).

ETIOLOGY AND PATHOGENESIS

Monostotic and polyostotic fibrous dysplasia are associated with the same activating mutations in the gene that encodes the Gsα protein discovered in 1991 (13) to cause

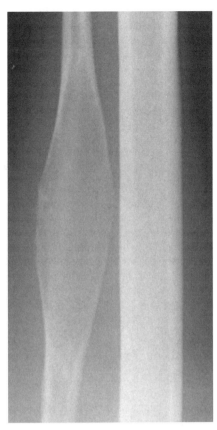

FIG. 2. Fibrous dysplasia. A characteristic expansile lesion with ground-glass appearance has caused thinning of the cortex in the middiaphyseal region of the right fibula of this young man.

the McCune–Albright syndrome (14). The skeletal lesion results from the formation of imperfect bone, because mesenchymal cells actively proliferate but do not fully differentiate to osteoblasts (15). There is increased expression of the c-*fos* protooncogene (16). Excessive production of interleukin-6 (IL-6) seems to be a pathogenetic factor (17). Endocrine hyperfunction in the McCune–Albright syndrome is generally due to end-organ overactivity (5,18). Studies of growth hormone and prolactin hypersecretion in this syndrome suggest that some patients have defective hypothalamic regulation of the pituitary gland and/or an embryologic abnormality in pituitary cell differentiation and function (18).

TREATMENT

There is no established medical treatment for the skeletal disease of fibrous dysplasia. Spontaneous healing of the bone lesions does not occur. In most patients with mild disease, the radiographic appearance of skeletal defects does not change. In more severe cases, individual lesions may progress, and new ones can appear (10). Preliminary reports describe some relief from bone pain and radiographic improvement after pamidronate therapy (11). Fractures generally mend well. Nevertheless, stress or fissure fractures can

be difficult to detect and treat. When the skull is involved, neurologic assessment and careful follow-up are necessary, because nerve compression may require surgical intervention.

In the McCune–Albright syndrome, an aromatase inhibitor, testolactone, can control the precocious puberty of affected girls, although some patients may escape the drug's effects after several years of treatment (19). Medroxyprogesterone also has been used (20). Calcitriol and inorganic phosphate supplementation have not been extensively evaluated for associated hypophosphatemic bone disease (21), but they have reversed radiographic features of rickets in some of our patients (personal observation).

REFERENCES

1. Harris WH, Dudley HR Jr, Barry RJ. The natural history of fibrous dysplasia: an orthopedic, pathological and roentgenographic study. *J Bone Joint Surg Am* 1962;44:207–233.
2. Johnson CB, Gilbert EF, Gottlieb LI. Malignant transformation of polyostotic fibrous dysplasia. *South Med J* 1979;72:353–356.
3. Kaplan FS, Fallon MD, Boden SD, Schmidt R, Senior M, Haddad JG. Estrogen receptors in bone in a patient with polyostotic fibrous dysplasia (McCune-Albright syndrome). *N Engl J Med* 1988;319:421–425.
4. Schwindinger WF, Levine MA. McCune-Albright syndrome. *Trends Endocrinol Metab* 1993;4:238–242.
5. Harris RI. Polyostotic fibrous dysplasia with acromegaly. *Am J Med* 1985;78:539–542.
6. Feuillan PP, Jones J, Ross JL. Growth hormone hypersecretion in a girl with McCune-Albright syndrome: comparison with controls and response to a dose of long-acting somatostatin analog. *J Clin Endocrinol Metab* 1995;80:1357–1360.
7. Cavanah SF, Dons RF. McCune-Albright syndrome: how many endocrinopathies can one patient have? *South Med J* 1993;86:364–367.
8. Shenker A, Weinstein LS, Moran A, et al. Severe endocrine and nonendocrine manifestations of the McCune-Albright syndrome associated with activating mutations of stimulatory G protein G$_s$. *J Pediatr* 1993;123:509–518.
9. Lever EG, Pettingale KW. Albright's syndrome associated with a soft-tissue myxoma and hypophosphatemic osteomalacia: report of a case and review of the literature. *J Bone Joint Surg Br* 1983;65:621–626.
10. Resnick D, Niwayama G. *Diagnosis of bone and joint disorders.* 3rd ed. Philadelphia: WB Saunders, 1995.
11. Chapurlat RD, Delmas PD, Liens D, Meunier PJ. Long-term effects of intravenous pamidronate in fibrous dysplasia of bone. *J Bone Miner Res* 1997;12:1746–1752.
12. Riminucci M, Fisher LW, Shenker A, Spiegel AM, Bianco P, Gehron RP. Fibrous dysplasia of bone in the McCune-Albright syndrome: abnormalities in bone formation. *Am J Pathol* 1997;151:1587–1600.
13. Weinstein LS, Shenker A, Gejman PV, Merino MJ, Friedman E, Spiegel AM. Activating mutations of the stimulatory G protein in the McCune-Albright syndrome. *N Engl J Med* 1991;325:1688–1695.
14. Ringel MD, Schwindinger WF, Levine MA. Clinical implications of genetic defects in G proteins: the molecular basis of McCune-Albright syndrome and Albright hereditary osteodystrophy. *Medicine* 1996;75:171–184.
15. Marie PJ, dePollak C, Chanson P, Lomri A. Increased proliferation of osteoblastic cells expressing the activating G$_s$ alpha mutation in monostotic and polyostotic fibrous dysplasia. *Am J Pathol* 1997;150:1059–1069.
16. Candeliere GA, Glorieux FH, Prud Homme J, St.-Arnaud R. Increased expression of the c-fos proto-oncogene in bone from patients with fibrous dysplasia. *N Engl J Med* 1995;332:1546–1551.
17. Motomura T, Kasayama S, Takagi M, et al. Increased interleukin-6 production in mouse osteoblastic MC3T3-E1 cells expressing activating mutant of the stimulatory G protein. *J Bone Miner Res* 1998;13:1084–1091.
18. Cuttler L, Jackson JA, Saeed uz-Zafar M, Levitsky LL, Mellinger RC,

Frohman LA. Hypersecretion of growth hormone and prolactin in McCune-Albright syndrome. *J Clin Endocrinol Metab* 1989;68:1148–1154.

19. Feuillan PP, Jones J, Cutler GB Jr. Long-term testolactone therapy for precocious puberty in girls with the McCune-Albright syndrome. *J Clin Endrocrinol Metab* 1993;77:647–651.

20. Escobar ME, Gryngarten M, Domene H, Ropelato G, Lopez MR, Bergada C. Persistence of autonomous ovarian activity after discontinuation of therapy for precocious puberty in McCune-Albright syndrome. *J Pediatr Adolesc Gynecol* 1997;10:147–151.

21. Feuillan PP. McCune-Albright syndrome. *Curr Ther Endocrinol Metab* 1997;6:235–239.

72. Osteogenesis Imperfecta

Michael P. Whyte, M.D.

Division of Bone and Mineral Diseases, Washington University School of Medicine at Barnes–Jewish Hospital, and Metabolic Research Unit, Shriners Hospital for Children, St. Louis, Missouri

Osteogenesis imperfecta (OI), sometimes called brittle bone disease, is a heritable disorder of connective tissue. The pathogenesis of all major types (Table 1) centers on a qualitative or quantitative abnormality of the most abundant protein in bone, type I collagen (1–3). The clinical hallmark of OI is osteopenia associated with recurrent fractures and skeletal deformity (4). However, type I collagen is also present in teeth, ligaments, skin, sclerae, and elsewhere, and many patients with OI have dental disease caused by defective formation of dentin (dentinogenesis imperfecta) as well as abnormalities of other tissues that contain this fibrous protein (1–4). Severity of OI is, however, extremely variable and ranges from stillbirth to perhaps life-long absence of symptoms. The classification system for OI devised by Sillence et al. (5), according to clinical features and apparent mode of inheritance, has been useful in providing a framework for prognostication and a foundation for further biochemical/ molecular studies. However, this nosology has limitations, and DNA-based findings have provided important insights concerning inheritance patterns, especially for the severe forms (1,6). The clinical heterogeneity of OI is now better understood because a great number of molecular defects have been characterized within the genes that encode the two types of large protein strands (the pro-α_1 and pro-α_2 chains) that combine to form type I collagen heterotrimers (1,7).

CLINICAL PRESENTATION

The differential diagnosis for OI in infants and children includes idiopathic juvenile osteoporosis, Cushing's disease, homocystinuria, congenital indifference to pain, and child abuse (see Chapter 57). However, the disturbances in type I collagen biosynthesis that cause OI usually produce signs

TABLE 1. *Clinical heterogeneity and biochemical defects in osteogenesis imperfecta (OI)*

OI type	Clinical features	Inheritance	Biochemical defects
I	Normal stature, little or no deformity, blue sclerae, hearing loss in about 50% of individuals. Dentinogenesis imperfecta is rare and may distinguish a subset	AD	Decreased production of type I procollagen. Substitution for residue other than glycine in triple helix of $\alpha_1(I)$
II	Lethal in the perinatal period, minimal calvarial mineralization, beaded ribs, compressed femurs, marked long bone deformity, platyspondyly	AD (new mutation) AR (rare)	Rearrangements in the COL1A1 and COL1A2 genes. Substitutions for glycyl residues in the triple-helical domain of the $\alpha_1(I)$ $\alpha_2(I)$ chain. Small deletion in $\alpha_2(I)$ on the background of a null allele
III	Progressively deforming bones, usually with moderate deformity at birth. Sclerae variable in hue, often lighten with age. Dentinogenesis imperfecta is common, hearing loss is common. Stature very short	AD AR	Point mutations in the $\alpha_1(I)$ or $\alpha_2(I)$ chain Frameshift mutation that prevents incorporation of pro $\alpha_2(I)$ into molecules. (Noncollagenous defects)
IV	Normal sclerae, mild to moderate bone deformity, and variable short stature. Dentinogenesis imperfecta is common, and hearing loss occurs in some	AD	Point mutations in the $\alpha_2(I)$ chain. Rarely, point mutations in the $\alpha_1(I)$ chain. Small deletions in the $\alpha_2(I)$ chain

AD, autosomal dominant; AR, autosomal recessive.
From Byers PH. Disorders of collagen biosynthesis and structure. In: Scriver CR, Beaudet AL, Sly WS, Valle D, eds. *The metabolic and molecular bases of inherited disease.* 7th ed. New York: McGraw Hill, 1995:4029–4077.

and symptoms that allow a correct diagnosis to be made easily from the patient's medical history, physical features, and radiographic findings (4). A family history is especially helpful, but many affected individuals reflect new mutations (1). Patients can manifest ligamentous laxity with joint hypermobility, diaphoresis, susceptibility to bruises, fragile and discolored teeth, and hearing loss (which occurs in about 50% of patients younger than 30 years and in nearly all patients who are older) (8). Deafness is typically from conductive or mixed pathogenesis, but sometimes results from sensorineural defects (8). Scleral discoloration ranges from a blue or gray tint that may be startling or subtle. In severe OI, signs and symptoms also include a high-pitched voice, short stature, scoliosis, herniae, disproportionately large head compared with body size, triangular face, and chest deformity. Mitral valve clicks are not uncommon, but cardiac disease is unusual. Thoracic distortion predisposes to pneumonia. Patients with even the most deformed skeletons are generally of normal intelligence. Variable severity of OI can, however, occur even among affected individuals in a single family (4).

CLINICAL TYPES

The classification scheme for OI devised in the late 1970s by Sillence and coworkers (5) (Table 1) is based on the clinical manifestations and apparent mode of inheritance (5). This nosology remains useful but has been greatly clarified by revelation of the heterogeneous genetic defects and their dominant mode of inheritance, especially for the more severe types of OI (1–3).

Type I OI features sclerae with bluish discoloration (especially apparent during childhood), relatively mild osteopenia with infrequent fractures (deformity is uncommon or slight), and deafness (30% incidence) that first manifests during early adulthood. Typically, patient height is normal. Elderly women with this most mild form of OI can be mistaken as having postmenopausal osteoporosis if they present with fracture during middle age, because radiographic findings may not distinguish between the two disorders. However, more numerous cortical osteocytes may be detected by iliac crest biopsy in OI patients compared with other osteoporoses (9,10). Type I OI has been subclassified into I-A and I-B disease depending on the absence or (more rarely) the presence, respectively, of dentinogenesis imperfecta. Type I OI is transmitted as an autosomal dominant trait. However, approximately one third of cases are new mutations.

Type II OI is often fatal within the first few days or weeks of life from respiratory complications. Affected newborns are often premature and small for gestational age and have short, bowed limbs, numerous fractures, markedly soft skulls, and small thoraces.

Type III OI is characterized by progressive skeletal deformity during childhood from recurrent fractures. Short stature results, in part, from fragmentation of growth plates (5). Dentinogenesis imperfecta is common.

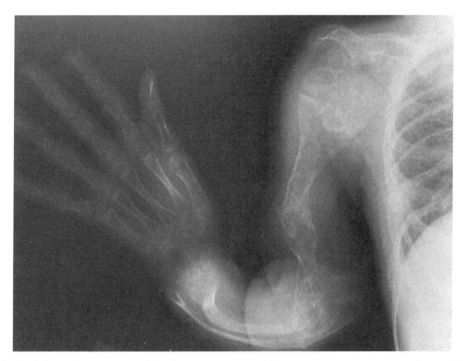

FIG. 1. Osteogenesis imperfecta (OI). Severe changes of OI are apparent in the upper limb of this 14-year-old boy, including marked osteopenia with characteristic thinning of bony cortices, evidence of old fractures, gracile ribs, and limb deformities. (From Whyte MP. Hereditary disorders of bone and mineral metabolism. In: Monolagas SC, Olefsky JM, eds. *Metabolic bone and mineral disorders.* New York: Churchill Livingston, 1988:232–248.)

Type IV OI is transmitted as an autosomal dominant trait and frequently explains multigeneration disease (1). The sclerae have normal color, but skeletal deformity, dental disease, and hearing loss are typical features.

RADIOGRAPHIC FEATURES

Characteristic findings manifest in severely affected patients (11). The cardinal features are generalized osteopenia, modeling (shaping) defects of long bones, and deformity from recurrent fractures. The modeling defects are caused by diminished rates of periosteal bone formation that retard circumferential widening of bones, so cortices appear thin. Multiple and recurrent fractures deform vertebrae as well as long bones (Fig. 1). In some severely affected infants, micromelia occurs with major long bones that are short but appear "thick" in external diameter. Wormian bones (Fig. 2) of significant number and size in the skull are a common, but not pathognomonic, feature of OI (12). Platybasia, which can progress to basilar impression, and excessive pneumatization of the frontal and mastoid sinuses are common in severely affected patients (12). The pelvis can have

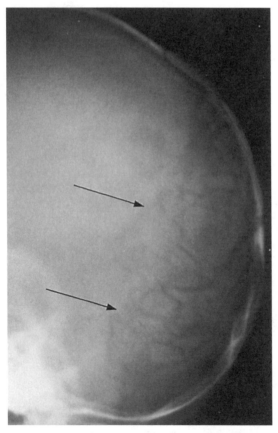

FIG. 2. Osteogenesis imperfecta (OI). Wormian bones *(arrows)*, although not pathognomonic of OI, may be found near the lambdoidal suture of the posterior occiput. (From Whyte MP. Rare disorders of skeletal formation and homeostasis. In: Becker KN, ed. *Principles and practice of endocrinology and metabolism.* 2nd ed. Philadelphia: Lippincott-Raven Publishers, 1995:594–606.)

a triradiate-shaped appearance. Osteoarthritis is a frequent problem for ambulatory adults with skeletal deformity.

Radiographic abnormalities may worsen markedly during growth, a feature that helps to define progressively deforming, type III, OI. "Popcorn" calcifications are unusual acquired defects in the regions of the epiphyses and metaphyses of major long bones (predominantly at the ankles and knees) that occur most often in type III OI (13). The finding is believed to result from traumatic fragmentation of growth-plate cartilage. The complication severely limits long-bone growth and contributes importantly to short stature. This finding is noted during childhood, but it then "resolves" during puberty when endochondral cartilage becomes fully mineralized and is then replaced by bone. When fractures occur in OI, they are often transverse but heal at normal rates. Occasionally exuberant callus has been mistaken for skeletal malignancy.

LABORATORY FINDINGS

Routine biochemical parameters of bone and mineral metabolism are typically unremarkable; however, elevations in serum alkaline phosphatase activity, urinary levels of hydroxyproline, or other markers of bone turnover occur in some patients. Hypercalciuria is common in severely affected children, but their renal function is not compromised (14).

Bone histology reflects the abnormal skeletal matrix, especially in severely affected patients. Polarized-light microscopy often shows an abundance of disorganized (woven) bone or abnormally thin collagen bundles in lamellar osseous tissue. Numerous osteocytes are found in the cortical bone of some patients. This finding seems to reflect decreased amounts of bone produced by individual osteoblasts, yet many cells that are active simultaneously. Subsequently the overall rate of skeletal turnover can be rapid, as shown by *in vivo* tetracycline labeling (15).

ETIOLOGY AND PATHOGENESIS

Table 1 summarizes the types of biochemical/molecular defects that have been identified in the various clinical forms of OI (1). The hallmark is low levels of type I collagen synthesized by skin fibroblasts (1–3). Various types of mutation occur within the pro-α_1 and pro-α_2 type I collagen genes. The large size and complex nature of type I collagen is such that nearly all OI families have unique ("private") mutations in one of these genes. The interested reader is referred elsewhere for detailed information (1–3,7).

TREATMENT

Although there has been considerable progress in the elucidation of the etiology of OI, there is no established medical therapy. Promising results have been reported for bisphosphonate treatment, especially in growing children, but the trials generally have not yet been blinded or placebo controlled (16). Preliminary reports concerning growth hormone injections mention improved linear growth rates and positive changes in bone formation in some affected children (17). Mouse models for OI provide a new way to test potential therapies (18,19). Treatment of patients is largely supportive and generally requires expert orthopedic, rehabilitative, and dental intervention to care for recurrent fractures, limb deformities, kyphoscoliosis, dental sequelae, and so on. Rodding of long bones and bracing of the lower limbs has enabled some affected children to walk. Stapes surgery has been used for hearing loss (20). The current management of OI has been reviewed (21).

National support groups (e.g., Osteogenesis Imperfecta Foundation, Inc., U.S.A.) are important sources of comfort and lay-language information for patients and their families.

Genetic counseling should be periodically updated when appropriate, because progress in this area has been considerable. Although rare patients with type II OI represent homozygosity for an autosomal recessive trait, most cases result from new dominant mutations or reflect germline mosaicism for such gene defects. The recurrence risk of this most severe OI phenotype is now estimated to be 5% to 10% (1,6). Some mildly affected patients are mosaics and have severely affected children (1).

Prenatal diagnosis of severe OI by a variety of techniques, particularly ultrasound examination at 14 to 18 weeks' gestation, has been successful (22). Biochemical and molecular studies are proving increasingly important (6).

REFERENCES

1. Byers PH. Disorders of collagen biosynthesis and structure. In: Scriver CR, Beaudet AL, Sly WS, Valle D, eds. *The metabolic and molecular bases of inherited disease.* 8th ed. Ney York: McGraw-Hill, (in press).
2. Tsipouras P. Osteogenesis imperfecta. In: *McKusick's heritable disorders of connective tissue.* 5th ed. St Louis: Mosby, 1993:281–314.
3. Rowe DW, Shapiro JR. Osteogenesis imperfecta. In: Avioli LV, Krane SM, eds. *Metabolic bone disease.* San Diego: Academic Press, 1995:651–695.
4. Albright JA, Millar EA. Osteogenesis imperfecta [Symposium]. *Clin Orthop* 1981;159:1–156.
5. Sillence D. Osteogenesis imperfecta: an expanding panorama of variants. *Clin Orthop* 1981;159:11–25.
6. Pepin M, Atkinson M, Starman BJ, Byers PH. Strategies and outcomes of prenatal diagnosis for osteogenesis imperfecta: a review of biochemical and molecular studies completed in 129 pregnancies. *Prenat Diagn* 1997;17:559–570.
7. Byers PH, Wallis GA, Willing MC. Osteogenesis imperfecta: translation of mutation to phenotype. *Med Genet* 1991;28:433–442.
8. Pedersen U. Hearing loss in patients with osteogenesis imperfecta. *Scand Audiol* 1984;13:67–74.
9. Revell PA. *Pathology of bone.* Berlin: Springer-Verlag, 1986.
10. Falvo KA, Bullough PG. Osteogenesis imperfecta: a histometric analysis. *J Bone Joint Surg Am* 1973;55:275–286.
11. Resnick D, Niwayama G. *Diagnosis of bone and joint disorders.* 3rd ed. Philadelphia: WB Saunders, 1995.
12. Cremin B, Goodman H, Prax M, Spranger J, Beighton P. Wormian bones in osteogenesis imperfecta and other disorders. *Skeletal Radiol* 1982;8:35–38.
13. Goldman AB, Davidson D, Pavlor H, Bullough PG. Popcorn calcifications: a prognostic sign in osteogenesis imperfecta. *Radiology* 1980; 136:351–358.
14. Chines A, Boniface A, McAlister W, Whyte M. Hypercalciuria in osteogenesis imperfecta: a follow-up study to assess renal effects. *Bone* 1995;16:333–339.
15. Baron R, Gertner JM, Lang R, Vighery A. Increased bone turnover with decreased bone formation by osteoblasts in children with osteogenesis imperfecta tarda. *Pediatr Res* 1983;17:204–207.
16. Glorieux FH, Bishop NJ, Plotkin H, Chabot G, Lanoue G, Travers R. Cyclic administration of pamidronate in children with severe osteogenesis imperfecta. *N Engl J Med* 1998;339:947–942.
17. Hopkins E, Chrousos GP, Glorieux FH, Reing CM, Gundberg CM, Marini JC. Growth hormone treatment trial of children with types III and IV osteogenesis imperfecta. *Am J Hum Genet* 1997;61:A356.
18. McBride DJ Jr, Choe V, Shapiro JR, Brodsky B. Altered collagen structure in mouse tail tendon lacking the alpha 2(I) chain. *J Mol Biol* 1997;170:275–284.
19. Pereira RF, Hume EL, Halford KW, Prockop DJ. Bone fragility in transgenic mice expressing a mutated gene for type I procollagen (COL1A1) parallels the age-dependent phenotype of human osteogenesis imperfecta. *J Bone Miner Res* 1995;10:1837–1843.
20. Garretsen TJ, Cremers CW. Stapes surgery in osteogenesis imperfecta: analysis of postoperative hearing loss. *Ann Otol Rhinol Laryngol* 1991;100:120–130.
21. Binder H, Conway A, Hason S, Gerber LH, Marini J, Weintrob J. Comprehensive rehabilitation of the child with osteogenesis imperfecta. *Am J Med Genet* 1993;45:265–269.
22. Thompson EM. Non-invasive prenatal diagnosis of osteogenesis imperfecta. *Am J Med Genet* 1993;45:201–206.

73. Chondrodystrophies and Mucopolysaccharidoses

Michael P. Whyte, M.D.

Division of Bone and Mineral Diseases, Washington University School of Medicine at Barnes–Jewish Hospital, and Metabolic Research Unit, Shriners Hospital for Children, St. Louis, Missouri

Beginning in the 1960s, concerted efforts to classify the skeletal dysplasias led to recognition of more than 80 such entities (1). Most appeared to be heritable; however, the resulting nosology at that time was essentially descriptive because the biochemical basis was unknown for nearly all of these conditions, and the molecular/genetic defects were largely unapproachable. The nomenclature for the bone dysplasias traditionally is based on the parts of the skeleton that are most involved on radiographic study (1–4). As reviewed subsequently, however, positional cloning of genes has revealed the molecular basis of many of these conditions and greatly widened the spectrum of disorders that can now be considered "metabolic bone diseases" (Table 1) (5,6).

OSTEOCHONDRODYSPLASIAS

The term *osteochondrodysplasia* comprises a group of conditions among the skeletal dysplasias (7,8). Each is characterized by abnormal growth or development of cartilage

TABLE 1. *Gene and protein defects involved in the osteochondrodysplasias*

Disorder	Gene	Protein
1. *Achondroplasia group*		
Thanatophoric dysplasia, type I	FGFR3	Fibroblast growth factor receptor 3
Thanatophoric dysplasia, type II	"	"
Achondroplasia	"	"
Hypochondroplasia	"	"
2. *Diastrophic dysplasia group*		
Diastrophic dysplasia	DTDST	Sulfate transporter
Achondrogenesis I B	"	"
Atelosteogenesis, type II	"	"
3. *Type II collagenopathies*		
Achondrogenesis II (Langer–Saldino)	COL2A1	Type II collagen
Hypochondrogenesis	"	"
Kniest dysplasia	"	"
Spondyloepiphyseal dysplasia (SED) congenita	"	"
Spondyloepimetaphyseal dysplasia (SEMD) Strudwick type	"	"
SED with brachydactyly	"	"
Mild SED with premature-onset arthrosis	"	"
Stickler dysplasia (heterogeneous, some not linked to COL2A1)	"	"
4. *Type XI collagenopathies*		
Stickler dysplasia (heterogeneous)	COL11A1	Type XI collagen
Otospondylomegaepiphyseal dysplasia (OSMED)	COL11A2	"
5. *Multiple epiphyseal dysplasias and pseudoachondroplasia*		
Pseudoachondroplasia	COMP	Cartilage oligomeric matrix protein
Multiple epiphyseal dysplasia (MED; Fairbanks and Ribbing types)	"	"
Other MEDs	COL9A2	Type IX collagen
6. *Chondrodysplasia punctata (stippled epiphyses group)*		
Rhizomelic type	PEX 7	Peroxin-7
Zellweger syndrome	PEX 1,2,5,6	Peroxin 1,2,5,6
Conradi–Hünermann type	CPXD	
X-linked recessive type	CPXR	
Brachytelephalangic type E	ARSE	Arylsulfatase E
7. *Metaphyseal dysplasias*		
Jansen type	PTHR	PTHR/PTHRP
Schmid type	COL10A1	COL10 α chain
8. *Acromelic and acromesomelic dysplasias*		
Trichorhinophalangeal dysplasia, type I	TRPS1	
Trichorhinophalangeal dysplasia, type II (Langer–Giedion)	TRPS1 + EXT1	
Grebe dysplasia	CDMP1	Cartilage-derived morphogenic protein 1
Hunter–Thompson dysplasia	"	"
Brachydactyly type C	"	"
Pseudohypoparathyroidism (Albright hereditary osteodystrophy)	GNAS1	Guanine nucleotide binding protein of adenylate cyclase α-subunit
9. *Dysplasias with prominent membranous bone involvement*		
Cleidocranial dysplasia	CBFA1	Core-binding factor α_1-subunit
10. *Bent-bone dysplasia group*		
Campomelic dysplasia	SOX9	SRY-box 9
11. *Multiple dislocations with dysplasias*		
Larsen syndrome	LAR1	
12. *Dysostosis multiplex group*		
Mucopolysaccharidosis IH	IDA	α-l-Iduronidase
Mucopolysaccharidosis IS	"	"
Mucopolysaccharidosis II	IDS	Iduronidate-2-sulfatase
Mucopolysaccharidosis IIIA	HSS	Heparan sulfate sulfatase
Mucopolysaccharidosis IIID	GNS	N-Acetyl-glucosamine-6-sulfatase
Mucopolysaccharidosis IVA	GSLNS	Galactose-6-sulfatase
Mucopolysaccharidosis IVB	GLBI	β-Galactosidase

continued

TABLE 1. *Continued.*

Disorder	Gene	Protein
Mucopolysaccharidosis VI	ARSB	Arysulfatase B
Mucopolysaccharidosis VII	GUSB	β-Glucuronidase
Fucosidosis	FUCA	α-Fucosidase
α-Mannosidosis	MAN	α-Mannosidase
β-Mannosidosis	MANB	β-Mannosidase
Aspartylglucosaminuria	AgA	Aspartylglucosaminidase
GMI Gangliosidosis, several forms	GLB1	β-Galactosidase
Sialidosis, several forms	NEU	α-Neuraminidase
Sialic acid storage disease	SIASD	
Galactosialidosis, several forms	PPGB	β-Galactosidase–protective protein
Multiple sulfatase deficiency		Multiple sulfatases
Mucolipidosis II, III	GNPTA	N-Acetyl-glucosamine-phosphotransferase
13. *Dysplasias with decreased bone density*		
Osteogenesis imperfecta	COL1A1 & A2	Type I procollagen
14. *Dysplasias with defective mineralization*		
Hypophosphatasia	ALPL	Alkaline phosphatase
Hypophosphatemic rickets	PHEX	X-linked hypophosphatemia protein
Neonatal hyperparathyroidism	CASR	Calcium sensor
Transient neonatal hyperparathyroidism with hypocalciuric hypercalcemia	"	"
15. *Increased bone density without modification of bone shape*		
Osteopetrosis with renal tubular acidosis	CA2	Carbonic anhydrase II
Pycnodysostosis	CTSK	Cathepsin K
16. *Disorganized development of cartilaginous and fibrous components of the skeleton*		
Multiple cartilaginous exostoses	EXT1	Exostosin-1
Fibrous dysplasia (McCune–Albright and others)	GNAS1	Guanine nucleotide protein, α-subunit
17. *Patella dysplasias*		
Nail–patella dysplasia	NPS1	

Modified and reproduced from Lachman RS. International nomenclature and classification of the osteochondrodysplasias. *Pediatr Radiol* 1998;28:737–744, with permission.

and/or bone (see refs. 1, 7, and 8 for a review of the clinical nomenclature). Osteochondrodysplasias are, in turn, subdivided into several groups, some of which feature defects in the growth of tubular bones and/or the spine. These disorders are frequently referred to as chondrodysplasias (1). The region of the long bones that is most affected (epiphysis, metaphysis, or diaphysis) is the basis for the subclassifications of epiphyseal, metaphyseal, or diaphyseal dysplasia (1–3). When the vertebrae also are deformed, these conditions are grouped as spondyloepiphyseal dysplasia, and so on (Fig. 1).

Chondrodysplasias that feature primarily metaphyseal defects (metaphyseal dysplasia and spondylometaphyseal dysplasia) may be confused, from their radiographic appearance, with forms of rickets (Fig. 2). However, biochemical parameters of bone and mineral metabolism are typically normal, and the skeleton is generally well mineralized. Jansen syndrome, caused by mutations in the parathyroid hormone (PTH) receptor leading to hypercalcemia, is an interesting exception (5) (see Chapter 13). Indeed, the configuration of the metaphyseal defects can lead to accurate classification by the experienced radiologist. When abnormalities of the spine are present (Fig. 3), the correct diagnosis should be especially apparent.

Recent application of DNA-based technology led to impressive success at mapping the genes that cause skeletal dysplasias and is rapidly improving our understanding of their molecular/biochemical bases (5,6,9). Defects in a great variety of genes in these disorders reveal that many proteins are essential for human skeletal development (Table 1). Abnormalities in the type I, II, IX, and X collagen genes are now known to cause osteogenesis imperfecta, spondyloepiphyseal dysplasia, multiple epiphyseal dysplasia, and metaphyseal dysplasia (Schmid type), respectively (5,6). Cartilage oligomeric matrix protein gene mutations can be the basis for multiple epiphyseal dysplasia and pseudoachondroplasia. Fibroblast growth factor receptor-3 gene defects cause achondroplasia (5,6). The elastin and fibrillin genes are involved in Williams and Marfan syndromes, respectively (5). The number of "metabolic bone diseases" will continue to grow.

MUCOPOLYSACCHARIDOSES

The mucopolysaccharidoses are a group of inborn errors of metabolism that result from diminished activity of the lysosomal enzymes that degrade glycosaminoglycans (acid

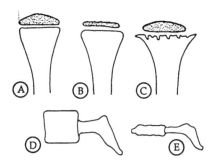

Involvement	Disease Category
A+D	Normal
B+D	Epiphyseal dysplasia
C+D	Metaphyseal dysplasia
B+E	Spondyloepiphyseal dysplasia
C+E	Spondylometaphyseal dysplasia
B+C+E	Spondyloepimetaphyseal dysplasia

FIG. 1. Chondrodysplasias. Classification based on radiographic involvement of long bones and vertebrae. (From Rimoin DL, Lachman RS. Chondrodysplasias. In: Rimoin DL, Conner JM, Pyeritz RE, eds. *Emery and Rimoin's principles and practice of medical genetics.* 3rd ed. London: Churchill Livingstone, 1996:2796.)

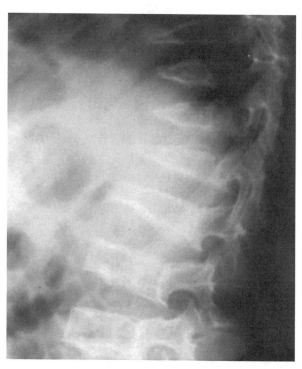

FIG. 3. Spondylometaphyseal dysplasia. Characteristic dysplastic changes at age 11 years are present in the vertebrae of the patient shown in Fig. 2 and establish a spondylometaphyseal rather than a metaphyseal dysplasia.

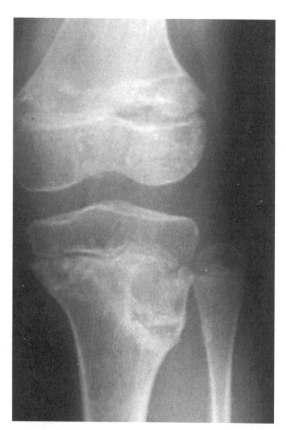

FIG. 2. Spondylometaphyseal dysplasia. The irregularity of the metaphyses in the knees of this 8½-year-old girl are sometimes mistaken for rickets.

mucopolysaccharides) (Table 1) (10,11). Accumulation of these complex carbohydrates within marrow cells leads to skeletal change that is generally referred to as dysostosis multiplex. However, the degree of severity and precise bony manifestations vary according to the specific disorder (1–4; see refs. 10 and 11 for detailed descriptions).

Patients with dysostosis multiplex share the following radiographic features: osteoporosis with coarsened trabeculae, macrocephaly, dyscephaly, a J-shaped sella turcica, oarshaped ribs, widened clavicles, oval or hook-shaped vertebral bodies, dysplasia of the capital femoral epiphyses, coxa valga, epiphyseal and metaphyseal dysplasia, proximal tapering of the second and fifth metacarpals, and dysplasia of long tubular bones (3,4).

REFERENCES

1. Rimoin DL, Lachman RS. Chondrodysplasias. In: Rimoin DL, Conner JM, Pyeritz RE, eds. *Emery and Rimoin's principles and practice of medical genetics.* 3rd ed. London: Churchill Livingstone, 1996:2779–2815.
2. Wynne-Davies R, Hall CM, Apley AG. *Atlas of skeletal dysplasias.* Edinburgh: Churchill Livingstone, 1985.
3. Resnick D, Niwayama G. *Diagnosis of bone and joint disorders.* 3rd ed. Philadelphia: WB Saunders, 1995.
4. Taybi H, Lachman RS. *Radiology of syndromes, metabolic disorders, and skeletal dysplasias.* 4th ed. St. Louis: Mosby, 1996.
5. McKusick VA. *Mendelian inheritance in man: a catalog of human genes and genetic disorders.* 12th ed. Baltimore: Johns Hopkins University Press, 1998.
6. Lachman RS. International nomenclature and classification of the osteochondrodysplasias. *Pediatr Radiol* 1998;28:737–744.
7. Rimoin DL, Lachman RS. Genetic disorders of the osseous skeleton.

In: *McKusick's heritable disorders of connective tissue.* 5th ed. St. Louis: CW Mosby, 1993:557–689.

8. Horton WA, Hecht JT. The chondrodysplasias. In: Royce PM, Steinmann B, eds. *Connective tissue and its heritable disorders.* New York: Wiley-Liss, 1993:641–675.

9. Horton WA. Molecular genetics of the human chondrodysplasias. *Eur J Hum Genet* 1995;3:357–373.

10. Leroy JG, Wiesmann U. Disorders of lysosomal enzymes. In: Royce PM, Steinmann B, eds. *Connective tissue and its heritable disorders.* New York: Wiley-Liss, 1993:613–639.

11. Neufeld EF, Muenzer J. The mucopolysaccharidoses. In: Scriver CR, Beaudet AL, Sly WS, Valle D, eds. *The metabolic and molecular bases of inherited disease.* 7th ed. New York: McGraw-Hill, 1995:2465–2494.

SECTION VIII

Acquired Disorders of Cartilage and Bone

Introduction

Michael P. Whyte, M.D.

Division of Bone and Mineral Diseases, Washington University School of Medicine at Barnes–Jewish Hospital, and Metabolic Research Unit, Shriners Hospital for Children, St. Louis, Missouri

Physicians who specialize in the care of patients with metabolic bone diseases encounter a considerable number and variety of acquired disorders of cartilage and bone. Among these conditions are skeletal neoplasms, problems that result from disruption of the vascular supply to the skeleton, and diseases that are characterized by proliferation or infiltration of the marrow space by specific types of cells. In certain metabolic bone diseases and some skeletal dysplasias, there is predisposition to neoplastic transformation (e.g., Paget disease, fibrous dysplasia), metabolic disturbances can cause skeletal ischemia (e.g., Cushing syndrome, storage diseases), and infiltrative marrow disorders may be associated with aberrant mineral homeostasis (e.g., sarcoidosis). This section provides an overview of some of the principal acquired disturbances of cartilage and bone.

74. Skeletal Neoplasms

Michael P. Whyte, M.D.

Division of Bone and Mineral Diseases, Washington University School of Medicine at Barnes–Jewish Hospital, and Metabolic Research Unit, Shriners Hospital for Children, St. Louis, Missouri

GENERAL CONSIDERATIONS

Among the acquired disorders of cartilage and bone are a variety of neoplasms. Some are malignant and cause considerable morbidity and can metastasize and kill. Others are benign, and some may heal spontaneously. Rarely, skeletal tumors behave as though they are transitional, with both benign and malignant characteristics. Diagnosis and treatment of bone tumors is a complex discipline. Only a brief overview is provided here. The reader should consider referring also to several detailed texts concerning aspects of this topic (1–7).

Histopathologic classification of skeletal neoplasms is based on the cell or tissue type from which they apparently originate (Table 1). The source of the tumor is usually revealed by the kind of tissue that the neoplastic cells make, such as osteoid or cartilage. However, in a few instances (e.g., giant-cell tumor of bone), the origin is less clear (1,6).

Biologic behavior of bone tumors also importantly influences their classification. Within the two major categories, benign and malignant, there are skeletal neoplasms with different degrees of aggressivity. Biologic behavior reflects the capacity of the tumor to exceed its natural barriers. Such barriers may include a tumor capsule (the shell of fibrous tissue or bone around the neoplasm), a reactive zone (composed in part of either fibrous tissue or bone that forms between the capsule and normal tissue), and any adjacent articular cartilage, cortical bone, or periosteum (1,6,7) (see later).

Skeletal neoplasms will be properly managed only if there is a thorough understanding of their clinical presentation and natural history, as well as use of current staging procedures, which often require histopathologic examination (1,6,8). Proper choice of therapy may include medical and/or surgical approaches (1–3,5,7,9,10). Optimal patient management requires multidisciplinary expertise (1–7). Improved radio-logic imaging studies, histopathologic methods, cytogenetic and molecular testing, surgical techniques, and chemotherapeutic regimens have all contributed to better survival and function of patients with skeletal sarcomas. Chemotherapy has improved the treatment of early metastatic deposits (11–14). Consequently, aggressive limb-salvaging procedures are now possible with survival rates that were previously achieved only by radical amputation (12,15–17).

BENIGN SKELETAL TUMORS

Benign skeletal tumors, with only rare exceptions, do not metastasize (18). Nevertheless, as a group, their biologic behavior can still be variable and may range from completely inactive to quite aggressive. Fortunately, the behavior can often be predicted by noting the clinical presentation and examining the radiologic features of the specific neoplasm (4,19,20); sometimes, histopathologic inspection is essential as well (1,6). Benign tumors can be classified generally as inactive, active, or aggressive (1,6,18).

Inactive benign bone tumors are sometimes called latent or static. They are encapsulated by mature fibrous tissue or by cortical bone–like material, and they do not expand or deform surrounding skeletal tissue. Each neoplasm will have only a minimal (if any) reactive zone, and their histopathologic appearance is that of a benign tumor with a low cell-to-matrix ratio, a well-differentiated matrix, and no cellular hyperchromasia, anaplasia, or pleomorphism. Inactive benign tumors are usually asymptomatic (1,6,18).

Active benign bone tumors can deform or destroy adjacent cortical bone or joint cartilage as they grow, but they do not metastasize. They are encapsulated within fibrous tissue, although a thin reactive zone can develop. These lesions generally cause mild symptoms but may lead to pathologic fractures (1,6,18).

TABLE 1. *Common skeletal neoplasms*

Tissue origin	Benign	Malignant
Osseous		Classic osteosarcoma
		Parosteal osteosarcoma
		Periosteal osteosarcoma
Cartilaginous	Enchondroma	Primary chondrosarcoma
	Exostosis	Secondary chondrosarcoma
Fibrous	Nonossifying fibroma	Fibrosarcoma
		Malignant fibrous histiocytoma
Reticuloendothelial		Ewing's sarcoma
		Multiple myeloma
Unknown	Giant-cell tumor in bone	

See references 1–5 for general reviews.

Aggressive benign bone tumors are not uncommon in children. They demonstrate invasive properties like those of low-grade malignancies. Their reactive zone forms a capsule or pseudocapsule that prevents the neoplasm itself from extending directly into normal tissue, but the tumor can resorb and destroy adjacent bone and spread to nearby skeletal compartments. Despite their aggressive behavior, the cytologic features are benign, including a well-differentiated matrix. These tumors cause symptoms and can result in pathologic fractures (1,6,18).

MALIGNANT SKELETAL TUMORS

Malignant skeletal tumors can metastasize. Nevertheless, as a group, their biologic behavior also varies considerably (1–3,5,7). Some grow slowly with a low probability of spreading, so that there is typically a long interval between the discovery of the primary neoplasm and the development and recognition of metastases. Others are very aggressive and not only cause rapid and extensive local tissue destruction, but also have a high incidence of metastases so that primary and metastatic lesions are frequently recognized together. The biologic behavior of malignant skeletal tumors can usually be predicted by their clinical, radiologic (4,19,20), and histopathologic features (1,5,6). Assessment of the histopathologic type and grade is the best predictor of biologic activity and is of paramount importance for successful treatment and accurate prognostication (see later) (1,5,6).

Low-grade sarcomas invade local tissues but grow slowly and have a low risk of metastasizing. They are usually asymptomatic and manifest as gradually growing masses. Nevertheless, the histopathologic features of malignancy are present, such as anaplasia, pleomorphism, and hyperchromasia, together with a few mitotic cells. The tumor capsule can be disrupted in many areas, and there may be an extensive reactive zone that forms a pseudocapsule and contains satellite tumor nodules, which slowly erode the various natural barriers. Over time and after repeatedly unsuccessful surgical excision with tumor recurrence, there is a risk of transformation to a high-grade sarcoma (1,5,6).

High-grade sarcomas readily extend beyond their reactive zone. They seem to have minimal pseudoencapsulation. Their margins are poorly demarcated. Metastases may appear in seemingly uninvolved areas of the same bone and often in the medullary canal. Extension to nearby tissues destroys cortical bone, joint capsules, and articular cartilage. These tumors show all of the histopathologic features that typify malignancy and produce a poorly differentiated (immature) matrix (1,5,6).

DIAGNOSIS OF SKELETAL TUMORS

A thorough history and complete physical examination are the foundation for successful diagnosis and management of skeletal neoplasms (21). The patient's age, presence or absence of predisposing conditions (e.g., Paget's bone disease), and anatomic site of the lesion provide important clues to the precise diagnosis (see later).

Radiologic studies should be selected both to help estab-lish the tumor type and to provide staging information that will be critical for choosing treatment and for understanding the patient's prognosis (4,22,23). The tumor stage reflects the neoplasm's location and extent, as well as its biologic activity or grade, and is based in part on the presence or absence of metastases (8). Radiographs establish the tumor location, often suggest the underlying histopathologic type (4,19,20), help to evaluate its extent, and guide the selection of additional staging studies. Clinical and radiologic examination is completed before biopsy or other surgical procedures (1,3,7,8,21).

Bone scanning helps to determine whether multiple areas of neoplasm are present and whether the extent of skeletal involvement exceeds that indicated by conventional radiographs. Avidity for radionuclide uptake generally reflects the tumor's biologic activity (19,20,22,23).

Computed tomography is very useful for precisely defining the anatomic extent of the primary lesion, detecting destruction of spongy or cortical bone, assessing compartmental changes, and locating neurovascular structures that may be impinged on by tumor or located near planned surgery (24). This technique also supplements conventional radiography for detecting pulmonary metastases.

Magnetic resonance imaging is especially helpful for defining tumor soft-tissue extension and for showing any disruption of the marrow space (23,25,26).

Angiography can help plan limb-salvage operations, because this procedure may reveal involvement of major neurovascular bundles (4).

Arthrography helps to demonstrate joint involvement and thus is useful for determining whether a cartilaginous tumor is of intraarticular or extraarticular origin (4).

Biopsy and histopathologic study are essential for successful staging and treatment of many skeletal neoplasms (1,2,27). Open (incisional) biopsy is typically the technique of choice if a malignant lesion is suspected, because it secures sufficient tissue for examination (1,2,27). However, this technique carries a greater risk of tumor contamination of uninvolved tissues (e.g., by dissecting hematoma) than does closed biopsy (28). Accordingly, open biopsy can potentially compromise a limb-salvage procedure because of added risk of local recurrence. Therefore, careful attention must be paid to where the incision for biopsy is made and to the surgical technique (1–3). Accessible benign tumors may be removed by incisional biopsy, as they are intracapsular, or with *en bloc* marginal incision (1–3).

INDIVIDUAL TYPES OF SKELETAL NEOPLASIA

Benign and Transitional Tumors

Benign skeletal neoplasms occasionally originate from marrow elements, but most often they are derived from cartilage or bone (29). Typically these tumors develop before skeletal maturation is complete or during the early adult years, and they are most common in areas of rapid bone growth and cellular metabolism (i.e., the epiphyses and metaphyses of the major long bones) (30). In some patients or families with specific heritable disorders, benign skeletal tumors (e.g., enchondromas or exostoses) are multiple and

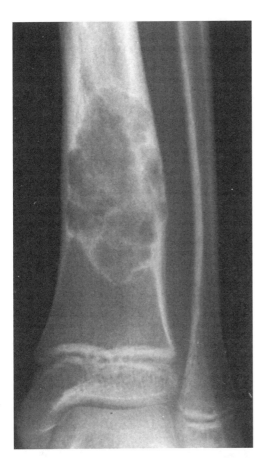

FIG. 1. Nonossifying fibroma. This 11-year-old boy has a typical, benign-appearing lesion of his distal left tibia. It is an ovoid, radiolucent, fibrous tumor located at the metadiaphyseal junction, is slightly expansile, and has a multiloculated appearance with regions of cortical scalloping and thinning.

have a significantly increased risk of malignant transformation (31,32). Most benign skeletal tumors, however, are solitary lesions and are associated with a good prognosis (29). The following paragraphs describe the principal types.

Nonossifying fibroma is the most common bone tumor (33,34). This lesion is often called a fibrous cortical defect. It is caused by a focal, developmental abnormality in periosteal bone formation that results in an area of failed ossification. Nonossifying fibromas most commonly occur in the metaphyses of the distal femur or distal tibia and are located eccentrically in or near the bony cortex (4,19,20). They are somewhat more prevalent in boys than in girls, develop in the older pediatric population, and are active lesions that enlarge throughout childhood yet typically do not cause symptoms. However, when more than 50% of the diameter of a long bone is involved, pathologic fracture can occur (33,34). Radiologic study may show a well-demarcated radiolucent zone with apparent trabecularization that results in a multilocular or even in a septated appearance (Fig. 1). Some cortical bone erosion may be present. The radiographic pattern can be considered diagnostic, and further staging is typically unnecessary (4,20,21). After puberty with skeletal maturation, nonossifying fibromas become inactive or latent and ultimately ossify. Surgical intervention is usually unneces-

sary unless pathologic fracture is a significant risk (35). Intracapsular curettage is effective, but bone grafting or other stabilizing techniques for fracture prevention or treatment may be required (33,34). Rarely, nonossifying fibromas cause oncogenic rickets (see Chapter 65).

Enchondroma is a benign and typically asymptomatic tumor of cartilage caused by focal disruption of endochondral bone formation. It can be considered a dysplasia of the central growth plate (18,36). Enchondromas appear as though they arise in the metaphysis and may eventually become incorporated into the diaphysis. Solitary lesions are usually noted in adolescence or in early adulthood. They most commonly involve small tubular bones of the hands or feet or the proximal humerus. However, several distinct disorders feature multiple enchondromas (enchondromatosis, Ollier's disease, and Maffucci syndrome). Fewer than 1% of asymptomatic solitary tumors undergo malignant transformation, but with enchondromatosis, the risk of malignant degeneration is estimated to be 10% (29,34).

Radiographs show a medullary, radiolucent lesion with a well-defined but only slightly thickened bony margin (Fig. 2) (4,19,20). This defect may enlarge slowly during its active

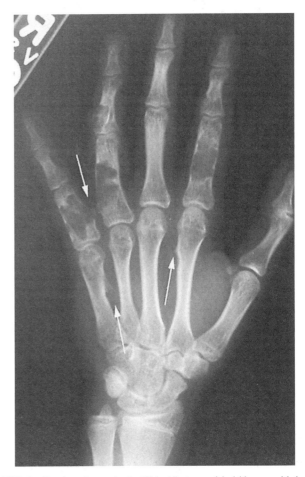

FIG. 2. Enchondromatosis. This 13-year-old girl has multiple, lucent, benign-appearing lesions of the phalanges. Each has produced expansion of the bone as well as cortical scalloping and thinning. Several periosteum-based chondromas show reactive bone formation at their margins *(arrows).*

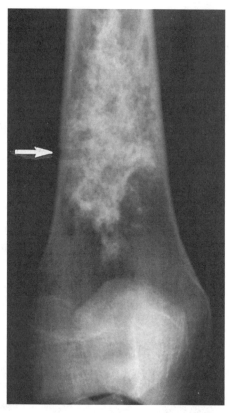

FIG. 3. Enchondroma. This 43-year-old woman has an extensively calcified lesion of the metadiaphyseal region of her distal femur. The calcification is amorphous and dense with little radiolucent component (*arrow* indicates a biopsy-needle track). This lesion is differentiated from a bone infarction, which typically has a dense, linearly marginated periphery.

phase in adolescence, but when the tumor becomes latent during the adult years, it calcifies to produce a diffusely punctate or stippled appearance (Fig. 3). In time, enchondromas become surrounded by dense reactive osseous tissue. Skeletal scintigraphy typically reflects the tumor's biologic activity and shows increased radioisotope uptake in the reactive zone (greatly increased uptake suggests malignant transformation). Accordingly, it is prudent to secure a baseline bone scan and radiographs for young adults with multiple enchondromas.

Biopsy is often not necessary, because the lesion's identity is revealed by characteristic radiography (4,19,20). Histopathologic examination may be required, however, to distinguish benign from low-grade malignant enchondromas. Here, the patient's age is an especially important consideration (36).

Solitary asymptomatic enchondromas are generally benign and require no treatment, although periodic follow-up is indicated. If they become symptomatic and begin to enlarge, careful surveillance is necessary (36). Imaging techniques may be helpful to search for evidence of malignancy (4,23,24). Surgical treatment would then be indicated.

Osteocartilaginous exostosis (osteochondroma) is a common dysplasia of cartilage involving the peripheral region of a growth plate (18,30,36). The lesion can arise in any

bone that derives from cartilage, but it usually occurs in a long bone. Typically either end of a femur, the proximal humerus or tibia, the pelvis, or a scapula is affected. Exostoses present as hard painful masses that are fixed to bone. They enlarge during childhood but become latent in adulthood. These lesions can irritate overlying soft tissues and may form a fluid-filled bursa. A painful and enlarging exostosis during adult life, especially in the pelvis or shoulder girdle, should suggest malignant transformation to a chondrosarcoma (30,32,36,37). Generally exostoses are solitary, but multiple hereditary exostoses is a well-characterized autosomal dominant entity that can result in significant angular deformity of the lower limbs, clubbing of the radius, and short stature (31).

Recently mutation within the EXT1 gene has been shown to cause this disorder (38,39). Radiographic study may show either a flat, sessile, or pedunculated metaphyseal bony lesion of variable density that is typically well defined and covered by a radiolucent cartilaginous cap (Fig. 4). A characteristic feature of an exostosis is the continuity of the tumor bone with metaphyseal bone (4,20,21). The diagnosis is rarely difficult. Following malignant transformation, there may be a soft-tissue mass on computed tomography or magnetic resonance imaging, and skeletal scintigraphy will demonstrate suddenly or considerably increased tracer uptake.

The cartilaginous cap of an exostosis appears histopathologically like a poorly organized growth plate. The trabecu-

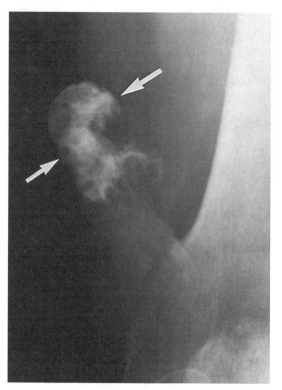

FIG. 4. Osteocartilaginous exostosis (osteochondroma). This 51-year-old woman has a typical pedunculated exostosis of her distal femur. The cortex and trabecular components of the exostosis are continuous with the host bone. Note how the exostosis slants away from the knee joint. The osteocartilaginous cap *(arrows)* is densely mineralized.

lae are not remodeled and thus contain cartilage cores (primary spongiosa), the histopathologic hallmark of osteopetrosis (see Chapter 70).

Excisional treatment of an active exostosis should include the cartilaginous cap and overlying perichondrium to minimize the risk of recurrence (1,3,7,36). There is about a 5% recurrence rate following marginal excision of a solitary lesion. Malignant degeneration occurs in fewer than 1% of solitary lesions, but the risk is almost 10% for multiple hereditary exostoses (31,32,36).

Giant-cell tumor of bone (osteoclastoma) is a common benign bone neoplasm. The cellular origin, however, is unknown (40–42). Men are more frequently affected than women, typically at age 20 to 40 years. These tumors cause chronic and deep pain that mimics an arthropathy. Pathologic fracture or effusion into the knee is a typical presentation. The epiphysis of a distal femur or proximal tibia is frequently affected. However, the distal radius, proximal humerus, distal tibia, and sacrum are also commonly involved. Often giant-cell tumors enlarge to occupy most of the epiphysis and portions of the adjacent metaphysis, and they can penetrate into subchondral bone and may even invade articular cartilage. In contrast to other benign skeletal neoplasms, they occasionally metastasize. Overexpression of the c-*myc* oncogene correlates with occurrence of metastasis (42). Accordingly, giant-cell tumors of bone are sometimes referred to as transitional neoplasms.

Radiologic studies show a relatively large lucent abnormality surrounded by an obvious reactive zone (4,20,21). The cortex can appear eroded from the endosteal surface (Fig. 5). A trabecular bone pattern may fill in the tumor cavity. Bone scanning may demonstrate decreased tracer uptake at the center of the lesion (the "doughnut" sign). Histopathologic examination shows numerous, scattered, multinucleated giant cells in a proliferative stroma; mitoses are occasionally present (1,6). The findings differ from the extraskeletal osteoclastomas recently characterized in exceptional patients with Paget bone disease (43).

Curettage (with bone grafting or use of cement) manages less advanced lesions. Recurrent or advanced tumors are removed with *en bloc* wide excision and reconstructive surgery.

Malignant Tumors

Multiple myeloma, the most common cancer of the skeleton, is a neoplasm of marrow origin (see also Chapter 35). However, a considerable variety of malignant tumors arise from bone, cartilage, fibrous tissue, histiocytes, and perhaps endothelial tissue in the skeleton (1,2,5,6). Malignant bone tumors typically cause skeletal pain that is noted especially at night. Accordingly, this symptom, particularly in adolescents or young adults, is reason for evaluation. The treatment of malignant bone tumors is complex and is primarily based on the tumor grade and staging (1,2,5,6). Only general comments are provided in this subsection in which the principal entities are discussed.

Multiple myeloma typically develops during middle age and affects many skeletal sites. Constitutional symptoms can include bone pain, fever, malaise, fatigue, and weight loss. Often, there is anemia, thrombocytopenia, and renal failure (44,45). Hypercalcemia, due to elaboration of osteoclast-activating factors (46), occurs in about 20% to 40% of patients (47). The diagnosis is made by examination of the bone marrow for plasmacytosis and demonstration of paraproteinemia by serum and urine immunoelectrophoresis (44). Infection with Kaposi's sarcoma–associated herpes virus may play a pathogenetic role (48).

Radiographic findings include classic, discrete, circular, osteolytic lesions, but generalized osteopenia is actually a more common presentation. Bone scintigraphy can seem unusual because of little tracer uptake in foci of osteolysis (4,19,20,22).

Myeloma is radiation sensitive and treatable by chemotherapy. Reossification of tumor sites can occur within several months of therapy. Prevention of pathologic fractures may require surgical stabilization (44). The primary mechanism of bone destruction is increased osteoclastic action (46). Bisphosphonate treatment has helped to reduce fracture and pain (49).

Osteosarcoma (osteogenic sarcoma) is the most common primary malignancy of the skeleton (1,7,50,51). There are about 1100 to 1500 new cases in the United States yearly. Typically, this cancer develops before age 30 years and is somewhat more common in male than in female patients. Although most of the tumors are the classic variety, additional variants include parosteal, periosteal, and telangiectatic types that have different presentations and prognoses (see later).

Classic osteosarcoma characteristically arises in the metaphysis of a long bone where there is the most rapid growth. It primarily affects teenagers. In about 50% of cases, these

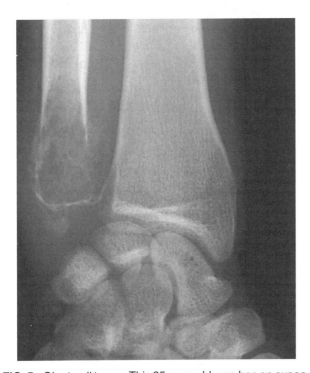

FIG. 5. Giant-cell tumor. This 25-year-old man has an expansile, destructive, lucent lesion of the distal ulna. The lesion extends to the end of the bone.

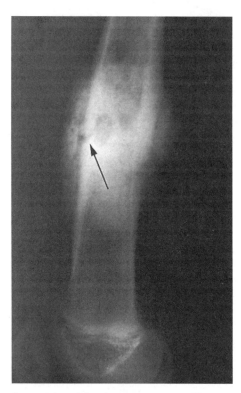

FIG. 6. Central (medullary) osteosarcoma. This 12-year-old boy has a sclerotic diaphyseal lesion that arose in the medullary cavity. It has penetrated the cortex and produced a densely mineralized mass surrounding the femur. Portions of the cortex appear to have been destroyed *(arrow)*, whereas other regions are thickened.

tumors develop near the knee in the distal femur or proximal tibia. Other commonly involved sites are the humerus, proximal femur and pelvis, but they can arise *de novo* anywhere in the skeleton. They also derive from malignant transformation of Paget's bone disease (Chapter 77) (52).

Typically an osteosarcoma presents as a tender bony mass. Pain is severe and unremitting. Pathologic fracture can occur. Osteosarcomas are aggressive neoplasms that readily penetrate metaphyseal cortical bone, and the majority have already infiltrated surrounding soft tissues at the time of diagnosis. At presentation, about 50% of affected adolescents show penetration of their growth plates with epiphyseal involvement, about 20% have metastases elsewhere in the cancerous bone, and in approximately 10% tumor has spread to lymph nodes or lung (50).

Radiologic study shows a destructive lesion that is composed of amorphous osseous tissue with poorly defined margins (4,19,20,53). Some osteosarcomas are predominantly osteoblastic and radiologically dense; others are predominantly osteolytic and radiolucent. Some have a mixed pattern (19,20). Cortical bone destruction is often apparent (Fig. 6). A characteristic "sunburst" configuration results from spicules of amorphous neoplastic osseous tissue that form perpendicular to the long axis of the affected bone. This is in contrast to the parallel or "onion skin" appearance of reactive periosteal new bone. Codman's triangle results from reaction and elevation of the periosteum that demarcates a

triangular area of cortical bone (Fig. 8). Bone scintigraphy shows intense uptake of tracer and may disclose more widespread disease than is indicated by conventional radiography (53). Computed tomography, magnetic resonance imaging, and angiography are helpful, as discussed previously. Microscopic examination typically shows a very malignant stroma that produces an amorphous and immature osteoid in a trabecular pattern (1–7).

Use of chemotherapy preoperatively (10,14,19,50) has significantly improved the prognosis for this malignancy and has allowed many osteosarcoma patients to be managed by limb-salvage procedures instead of radical amputation (7,9,17).

Parosteal osteosarcomas are juxtacortical (i.e., they develop between the bony cortex and the soft tissue as a surface neoplasm). Adolescents and young adults are most commonly affected by these slowly growing, low-grade tumors that typically occur as a fixed and painless mass posteriorly on the distal femur or medially on the proximal humerus. They are less aggressive than classic osteosarcomas and can be separated for a considerable length of time from the parent bone by a narrow radiolucent region of soft tissue. Eventually they may involve the underlying skeleton and degenerate into high-grade osteosarcomas (50).

Radiologic study typically reveals a densely ossified, broad-based, fusiform mass that seems to encircle the metaphyseal region of a long bone (Fig. 7) (4,19,20,53). Reactive tissue initially separates the neoplasm from the underly-

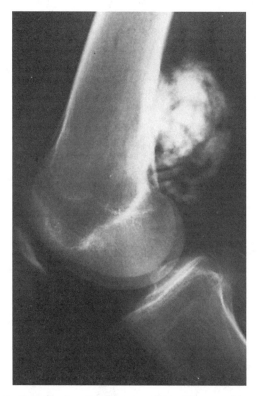

FIG. 7. Parosteal osteosarcoma. This 30-year-old woman has a very densely mineralized mass arising from the periosteal surface of the distal femoral metaphysis posteriorly. This tumor has lobular calcification and is attached to the femur by a broad pedicle.

ing bone that is destroyed once the tumor penetrates the normal cortex and the medullary canal becomes involved. Parosteal osteosarcomas have mature trabeculae with cement lines similar to those seen in Paget's disease (9); however, a low-grade malignant stroma is present. This tumor is often misdiagnosed as benign. Limb salvage with wide marginal excision is the usual treatment for less advanced disease. The prognosis is good. Chemotherapy is typically not used unless there has been dedifferentiation of the neoplasm (9,14,50).

Periosteal osteosarcoma often presents as a painless growing mass that extends from the surface of a bone into soft tissue (50). This is an uncommon variant of classic osteosarcoma that principally affects young adults. Radiologic study shows a poorly mineralized mass found primarily on a bone surface in an area of cortical erosion. The crater-like lesion has irregular margins and is associated with periosteal reaction (4,19,20). Penetration by this neoplasm through cortical bone into the medullary canal occurs more rapidly than with parosteal osteosarcoma. If this complication has occurred, the likelihood of pulmonary metastasis is greater, a feature that contributes to its poorer prognosis. Bone scintigraphy shows avid tracer uptake (53). Computed tomography reveals a mass that fills a shallow cortical bone defect but contains minimal calcification. Malignant mesenchymal stroma with neoplastic osteoid occurs in and around areas of mature cartilage (4,6,19,20).

Periosteal osteosarcoma is often treated with excision with a wide margin (46). Adjuvant chemotherapy is used when the tumor has regions of high-grade malignancy (11,14).

Chondrosarcoma occurs most often between ages 40 and 60 years, when this neoplasm develops as a primary tumor (36,54). In about 25% of patients, however, malignant transformation has occurred in a preexisting enchondroma or osteocartilaginous exostosis. Thus chondrosarcomas usually involve the pelvis, proximal femur, or shoulder girdle. Patients experience as the initial symptom a persistent dull ache that can mimic arthritis. Variants of the classic form of chondrosarcoma include a high-grade dedifferentiated neoplasm, an intermediate-grade clear-cell type, and a low-grade juxtacortical tumor. The particular designation depends on the histopathologic pattern and anatomic location (36,54).

Radiographs show a subtle radiolucent lesion that contains hazy or speckled calcification in a diffuse ''salt and pepper'' or ''popcorn'' pattern (4,19,20). Primary chondrosarcomas can develop either within the medullary canal or on the surface of a bone, where they can destroy the cortex and form a mass. On histopathologic examination, it can be difficult to demonstrate that high-grade tumors are cartilaginous in origin or that low-grade tumors are actually malignant (36,40).

Treatment of chondrosarcomas depends on the tumor stage. Limb amputation may be necessary for higher grade tumors. Adjuvant chemotherapy or radiation therapy has been disappointing (36).

Ewing sarcoma is a highly malignant neoplasm that arises from nonmesenchymal cells in the bone marrow (55–58). This cancer usually harbors a pathognomonic t(11:12) (q24;q12) translocation (59) and represents a form of primitive neuroectodermal tumor (53). It typically affects 10- to

15-year-old children and is more common in boys than in girls (1,55–58). Initial manifestations include an enlarging and tender soft-tissue swelling together with weight loss, malaise, fever, and lethargy. The erythrocyte sedimentation rate may be elevated, and there can be leukocytosis and anemia. The diaphysis of the femur is most commonly involved; alternatively, an ilium, tibia, fibula, or rib is affected. When this cancer occurs in the pelvis, it is usually found late and therefore has an especially poor prognosis (1,55–58).

Radiologic study typically reveals a diaphyseal lesion of patchy density that destroys cortical bone and frequently causes an onion-skin appearance of reactive periosteum (Fig. 8) (4,19,20). Bone scanning may show intense tracer uptake, which extends considerably beyond the radiographic abnormality.

Chemotherapy can be followed by wide excision or radiation therapy, depending on, among other factors, the anatomic site. Newer therapeutic approaches have reduced the incidence of pulmonary metastases and have markedly improved survival (1,60). Histologic response to preoperative chemotherapy and tumor size are important predictors of event-free survival (13).

Malignant fibrous histiocytoma occurs more frequently in soft tissues than in the skeleton and is less common than benign fibrous tumors (1,3,34). This cancer affects adults and often originates in Paget's bone disease or at the site

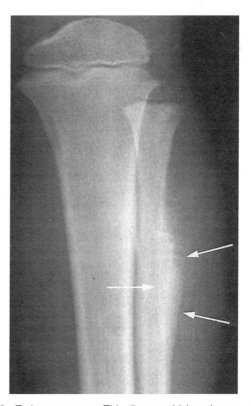

FIG. 8. Ewing sarcoma. This 5-year-old boy has a subtle permeative lesion of the proximal diaphysis of his fibula. The tumor is characterized by layered (onion-skin) periosteal reaction forming a Codman's triangle *(arrows)* and by sunburst new bone formation more proximally, which is characteristically perpendicular to the bone's long axis. A large soft-tissue mass is associated with the skeletal defects.

of a skeletal infarct. Typically this is an aggressive sarcoma that readily spreads within the lymphatics. Bone is infiltrated early on, and pathologic fracture is a common presenting manifestation.

Radiologic study reveals a poorly defined radiolucent lesion that causes cortical bone erosion (4,19,20). The histopathologic pattern is variable from area to area; extremely large and bizarre histiocytic cells are found in some sections, and undifferentiated cells that resemble histiocytic lymphoma are noted in others. Areas that contain fibrous tissue may suggest that the tumor is a fibrosarcoma. Special stains and electron microscopy can be required to establish the correct diagnosis (5,6,61). Staging studies direct the therapy, which may require radical resection or amputation and perhaps chemotherapy (1,36). The prognosis is guarded (34,61).

Fibrosarcoma is a painful neoplasm that typically arises in a major long bone of an adolescent or young adult (1–5,34). Radiologic study reveals a poorly defined and destructive lucent lesion in a metaphysis (4,19,20). Low-grade and high-grade fibrosarcomas have similar radiologic and histopathologic appearances. Accordingly, electron microscopy may be necessary to reveal the collagenous composition of the matrix of a high-grade tumor (6,34). Therapy depends on the staging results (1,3,5).

Metastatic bone tumors are considerably more common than primary skeletal malignancies (with a ratio of about 25:1) (1,4,5). Prostate, breast, thyroid, lung, and kidney cancers are the principal neoplasms that metastasize to bone. There is a predilection for deposition of malignant cells within blood-forming marrow spaces in the spine, ribs, skull, pelvis, and metaphyses of long bones (particularly the femur and humerus). In children, metastases within the skeleton usually reflect a neuroblastoma, leukemia, or Ewing sarcoma. In teenagers or young adults, lymphomas are the predominant source. After age 30 years, an adenocarcinoma is the likely primary. Osteoblastic metastases most commonly derive from carcinoma of the prostate or breast. Osteolytic metastases may come from the lung, thyroid, kidney, or gastrointestinal tract (4,19,21). In a significant number of patients, the primary site is not evident, and staging studies with biopsy are performed to explore the possibility of an intrinsic skeletal sarcoma (1–3,5,6).

REFERENCES

1. Dorfman HD, Czerniak B. *Bone tumors.* St Louis: Mosby-Year Book, 1997.
2. Levesque J. *Clinical guide to primary bone tumors.* Baltimore: Williams & Wilkins, 1998.
3. Simon M. *Surgery for bone and soft-tissue tumors.* Philadelphia: Lippincott-Raven Publishers, 1997.
4. Wilner D. *Wilner's radiology of bone tumors.* Philadelphia: WB Saunders, 1997.
5. Unni K, Dahlin DC. *Dahlin's bone tumors: general aspects and data on 11,087 cases.* 5th ed. Philadelphia: Lippincott-Raven, 1996.
6. Greenspan A, Remagen W. *Differential diagnosis of tumors and tumor-like lesions of bones and joints.* Philadelphia: Lippincott-Raven, 1998.
7. Simon MA, Springfield DS. *Surgery for bone and soft-tissue tumors.* Philadelphia: Lippincott-Raven, 1998.
8. Heare TC, Enneking WF, Heare MM. Staging techniques and biopsy of bone tumors. *Orthop Clin North Am* 1989;20:273–285.
9. Choong PF, Sim FH. Limb-sparing surgery for bone tumors: new developments. *Semin Oncol* 1997;13:64–69.
10. Biermann JS, Baker LH. The future of sarcoma treatment. *Semin Oncol* 1997;24:592–597.
11. Jaffe N. Chemotherapy for malignant bone tumors. *Orthop Clin North Am* 1989;20:487–503.
12. Sweetnam R. Malignant bone tumor management: 30 years of achievement. *Clin Orthop* 1989;247:67–73.
13. Wunder JS, Paulian G, Huvos AG, Heller G, Meyers PA, Healey JH. The histological response to chemotherapy as a predictor of the oncological outcome of operative treatment of Ewing sarcoma. *J Bone Joint Surg Am* 1998;80:1020–1033.
14. Bramwell VH. The role of chemotherapy in the management of non-metastatic operable extremity osteosarcoma. *Semin Oncol* 1997;24:561–571.
15. Nichter LS, Menendez LR. Reconstructive considerations for limb salvage surgery. *Orthop Clin North Am* 1993;24:511–521.
16. McDonald DJ. Limb-salvage surgery for treatment of sarcomas of the extremities. *Am J Roentgenol* 1994;163:509–513.
17. Langlais F, Tomeno B, eds. *Limb salvage: major reconstruction in oncologic and nontumoral conditions.* Berlin: Springer-Verlag, 1991.
18. Scarborough MT, Moreau G. Benign cartilage tumors. *Orthop Clin North Am* 1996;27:583–589.
19. Edeiken J, Dalinka M, Karasick D. *Edeiken's Roentgen diagnosis of diseases of bone.* 4th ed. Baltimore: Williams & Wilkins, 1990.
20. Resnick D, Niwayama G. *Diagnosis of bone and joint disorders.* 3rd ed. Philadelphia: WB Saunders, 1995.
21. Simon MA, Finn HA. Diagnostic strategy for bone and soft-tissue tumors. *J Bone Joint Surg Am* 1993;75:622–631.
22. Brown ML. Bone scintigraphy in benign and malignant tumors. *Radiol Clin North Am* 1993;31:731–738.
23. Murphy WA Jr. Imaging bone tumors in the 1990s. *Cancer* 1991;67:1169–1176.
24. Magid D. Two-dimensional and three-dimensional computed tomographic imaging in musculoskeletal tumors. *Radiol Clin North Am* 1993;31:426–447.
25. Berquist TM. Magnetic resonance imaging of primary skeletal neoplasms. *Radiol Clin North Am* 1993;31:411–424.
26. Redmond OM, Stack JP, Dervan PA, Hurson BJ, Carney DN, Ennis JT. Osteosarcoma: use of MR imaging and MR spectroscopy in clinical decision making. *Radiology* 1989;172:811–815.
27. Simon MA, Biermann JS. Biopsy of bone and soft-tissue lesions. *J Bone Joint Surg Am* 1993;75:616–621.
28. Schwartz HS, Spengler DM. Needle tract recurrences after closed biopsy for sarcoma: three cases and review of the literature. *Ann Surg Oncol* 1997;4:228–236.
29. Giudici MA, Moser RP Jr, Kransdorf MJ. Cartilaginous bone tumors. *Radiol Clin North Am* 1993;31:237–259.
30. Schubiner JM, Simon MA. Primary bone tumors in children. *Orthop Clin North Am* 1987;18:577–595.
31. Wicklund CL, Pauli RM, Johnston D, Hecht JT. Natural history study of hereditary multiple exostoses. *Am J Med Genet* 1995;55:43–46.
32. Ozaki T, Hillmann A, Blasius S, Link T, Winkelmann W. Multicentric malignant transformation of multiple exostoses. *Skeletal Radiol* 1998;27:233–236.
33. Hudson TM, Stiles RG, Monson DK. Fibrous lesions of bone. *Radiol Clin North Am* 1993;31:279–297.
34. Marks KE, Bauer TW. Fibrous tumors of bone. *Orthop Clin North Am* 1989;20:377–393.
35. Jee WH, Choe BY, Kang HS, et al. Nonossifying fibroma: characteristics at MR imaging with pathological correlation. *Radiology* 1998;209:197–202.
36. Greenspan A. Tumors of cartilage origin. *Orthop Clin North Am* 1989;20:347–366.
37. Merchan EC, Sanchez-Herrera S, Gonzalez JM. Secondary chondrosarcoma: four cases and review of the literature. *Acta Orthop Belg* 1993;59:76–80.
38. McCormick C, Leduc Y, Martindale D, et al. The putative tumour suppressor EXT1 alters the expression of cell-surface heparan sulfate. *Nat Genet* 1998;19:158–161.
39. Bridge JA, Nelson M, Orndal C, Bhatia P, Neff JR. Clonal karyotypic abnormalities of the hereditary multiple exostoses chromosomal loci 8q24.1 (EXT1) and 11p11-12 (EXT2) in patients with sporadic and hereditary osteochondromas. *Cancer* 1998;82:1657–1663.
40. Manaster BJ, Doyle AJ. Giant cell tumors of bone. *Radiol Clin North Am* 1993;31:299–323.

41. Richardson MJ, Dickinson IC. Giant cell tumor of bone. *Bull Hosp Joint Dis* 1998;57:6–10.
42. Gamberi G, Benassi MS, Bohling T, et al. Prognostic relevance of c-*myc* gene expression in giant-cell tumor of bone. *J Orthop Res* 1998;16:1–7.
43. Ziambaras K, Totty WA, Teitelbaum SL, Dierkes M, Whyte MP. Extraskeletal osteoclastomas responsive to dexamethasone treatment in Paget bone disease. *J Clin Endocrinol Metab* 1997;82:3826–3834.
44. Osserman EF, Merlini G, Butler VP Jr. Multiple myeloma and related plasma cell dyscrasias. *JAMA* 1987;258:2930–2937.
45. Lacy MQ, Gertz MA, Hanson CA, Inwards DJ, Kyle RA. Multiple myeloma associated with diffuse osteosclerotic bone lesions: a clinical entity distinct from osteosclerotic myeloma (POEMS syndrome). *Am J Hematol* 1997;56:288–293.
46. Roodman GD. Mechanisms of bone lesions in multiple myeloma and lymphoma. *Cancer* 1997;80:1557–1563.
47. Mundy GR. *Calcium homeostasis: hypercalcemia and hypocalcemia.* London: Martin Dunitz, 1989.
48. Berenson JR, Vescio RA, Said J. Multiple myeloma: the cells of origin--a two-way street. *Leukemia* 1998;12:121–127.
49. Bloomfield DJ. Should bisphosphonates be part of the standard therapy of patients with multiple myeloma or bone metastases from other cancers? An evidence-based review. *J Clin Oncol* 1998;16:1218–1225.
50. Meyers PA. Malignant bone tumors in children: osteosarcoma. *Hematol Oncol Clin North Am* 1987;1:655–665.
51. Meyers PA, Gorlick R. Osteosarcoma. *Pediatr Clin North Am* 1997;44:973–989.
52. Hadjipavlou A, Lander P, Srolovitz H, Enker IP. Malignant transformation in Paget disease of bone. *Cancer* 1992;70:2802–2808.
53. Fletcher BD. Imaging pediatric bone sarcomas: diagnosis and treatment-related issues. *Radiol Clin North Am* 1997;35:1477–1494.
54. Welkerling H, Dreyer T, Delling G. Morphological typing of chondrosarcoma: a study of 92 cases. *Virchows Arch A Pathol Anat Histopathol* 1991;418:419–425.
55. Horowitz ME, Tsokos MG, DeLaney TF. Ewing's sarcoma. *CA Cancer J Clin* 1992;42:300–320.
56. Eggli KD, Quiogue T, Moser RP Jr. Ewing's sarcoma. *Radiol Clin North Am* 1993;31:325–337.
57. Lawlor ER, Lim JF, Tao W, et al. The Ewing tumor family of peripheral primitive neuroectodermal tumors expresses human gastrin-releasing peptide. *Cancer Res* 1998;58:2469–2476.
58. Grier HE. The Ewing family of tumors: Ewing's sarcoma and primitive neuroectodermal tumors. *Pediatr Clin North Am* 1997;44:991–1004.
59. Maurici D, Perez-Atayde A, Grier HE, Baldini N, Serra M, Fletcher JA. Frequency and implications of chromosome 8 and 12 gains in Ewing sarcoma. *Cancer Genet Cytogenet* 1998;100:106–110.
60. Sandoval C, Meyer WH, Parham DM, et al. Outcome in 43 children presenting with metastatic Ewing sarcoma; the St. Jude Children's Research Hospital experience, 1962 to 1992. *Med Pediatr Oncol* 1996;26:180–185.
61. Womer RB. The cellular biology of bone tumors. *Clin Orthop* 1991;262:12–21.

75. Ischemic Bone Disease

Michael P. Whyte, M.D.

Division of Bone and Mineral Diseases, Washington University School of Medicine at Barnes–Jewish Hospital, and Metabolic Research Unit, Shriners Hospital for Children, St. Louis, Missouri

Regional interruption of blood flow to the skeleton causes this important acquired disorder of cartilage and bone (1–3). Ischemia, if sufficiently severe and prolonged, will kill osteoblasts and chondrocytes. Clinical problems arise if subsequent resorption of necrotic tissue during skeletal repair sufficiently compromises bone strength to cause fracture (4).

A change in skeletal density is the principal radiographic feature of ischemic bone disease (2,3). However, alterations may take several months to appear. Characteristic signs include crescent-shaped subchondral radiolucencies, patchy areas of sclerosis and lucency, bony collapse, and diaphyseal periostitis. Joint space is initially preserved despite the epiphyseal disease. A variety of conditions cause ischemic bone disease (Table 1), and a great number of clinical presentations occur based primarily on the affected skeletal site. Legg-Calvé-Perthes disease (LCPD) is discussed in some detail here, because it represents an archetypal form of ischemic bone disease. A few additional important clinical presentations are reviewed subsequently.

LEGG-CALVÉ-PERTHES DISEASE

Legg-Calvé-Perthes disease can be defined as idiopathic ischemic necrosis (osteonecrosis) of the capital femoral epiphysis in children (5–7). It is a common, complex, and controversial problem that affects boys more frequently than girls (4:1 to 5:1). Typically, LCPD presents between ages 2 and 12 years; the mean age at diagnosis is 7 years. When it manifests later in life, the term *adolescent ischemic necrosis* is used to indicate the poorer prognosis that also occurs when adults have ischemic bone disease (see later). Usually one hip is involved, but bilateral disease troubles about 20% of patients. Familial incidence varies from 1% to 20% (5–7).

Although the etiology of LCPD is unknown, the pathogen-

TABLE 1. *Causes of ischemic necrosis of cartilage and bone*

Endocrine/metabolic
  Glucocorticoid therapy
  Cushing syndrome
  Alcohol abuse
  Gout
  Osteomalacia
Storage diseases (e.g., Gaucher's disease)
Hemoglobinopathies (e.g., sickle cell disease)
Trauma (e.g., dislocation, fracture)
Dysbaric conditions
Collagen vascular disorders
Irradiation
Pancreatitis
Renal transplantation
Idiopathic, familial

From Edeiken J, Dalinka M, Karasick D. *Edeiken's roentgen diagnosis of diseases of bone.* 4th ed. Baltimore: Williams & Wilkins, 1990; and Resnick D, Niwayama G. *Diagnosis of bone and joint disorders.* 3rd ed. Philadelphia: WB Saunders, 1995.

esis is fairly well understood. Interruption of blood flow to the capital femoral epiphysis is the fundamental skeletal insult. However, ischemia at this site in children can occur from raised intracapsular pressure resulting from congenital or developmental abnormalities, episodes of synovitis, venous thrombosis, or perhaps increased blood viscosity (5–7). Most, if not all, of the capital femoral epiphysis is rendered ischemic. Consequently marrow cells, osteoblasts, and osteocytes may die. Endochondral ossification ceases temporarily because blood flow to chondrocytes in the growth plate is impaired. Articular cartilage, however, remains intact initially because it depends on synovial fluid for nourishment. Revascularization of necrosed areas then follows and proceeds from the periphery to the center of the epiphysis. New bone is deposited on the surface of subchondral cortical or central trabecular osseous debris. Subsequently the critical process of removal of necrotic bone begins, during which time the rate of bone resorption exceeds the rate of reparative new-bone formation. As a result, subchondral bone is weakened.

If there is no fracture in the area of reparative bone resorption, the child may remain asymptomatic and eventually heal. If, however, fracture occurs, there will be symptoms. Furthermore, trabecular bone collapse can cause a second episode of ischemia (5–7). Longitudinal growth of the proximal femur can be stunted, because the disrupted blood flow disturbs the physis and metaphysis. Premature closure of the growth plate may occur. As reossification of the epiphysis proceeds, the femoral head will remold its shape according to mechanical forces acting on it (2,3,5–7).

Children with LCPD typically limp, complain of pain in a knee or anterior thigh, and have limited mobility of the hip (especially with abduction or internal rotation). The Trendelenburg sign may be positive. If treatment is not successful, adduction and flexion contractures of the hip can develop, and thigh muscles may atrophy.

Laboratory investigation may show a slightly elevated erythrocyte sedimentation rate. Radiographic examination, which should include anteroposterior and frog lateral views for diagnosis and follow-up, often reveals a bone age that is 1 to 3 years delayed (2,3). Sequential studies typically demonstrate cessation of growth of the capital femoral epiphysis, resorption of necrotic bone, subchondral fracture, reossification and, finally, healing (Fig. 1). Magnetic resonance imaging (MRI) is helpful because signal-intensity patterns change with circulatory compromise, soft tissues as well as bone are visualized, and containment of the femoral head can be assessed (8).

The short-term prognosis for LCPD depends on the severity of femoral head deformity at the completion of the healing phase. The long-term outcome is conditioned by how much secondary degenerative osteoarthritis develops. In general, the more extensive the involvement of the capital femoral epiphysis, the worse the prognosis. Girls seem to have poorer outcomes than boys, because they tend to have greater involvement of the capital femoral epiphysis, and they mature earlier. Sexual maturation means less time for femoral head modeling before closure of the growth plates. Onset at age 2 to 6 years causes the least femoral head deformity; onset after age 10 years has a poor outcome (5–9).

Treatment for LCPD is directed principally by the orthopedic surgeon (10). Prevention of femoral head deformity is a major goal. Significant, not mild, distortion predisposes to osteoarthritis. Degenerative joint disease seems to be

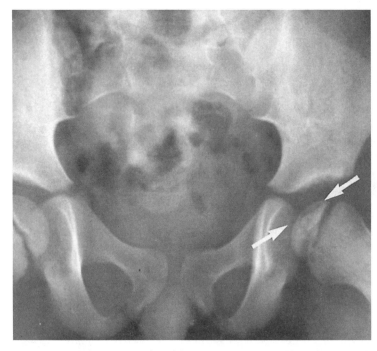
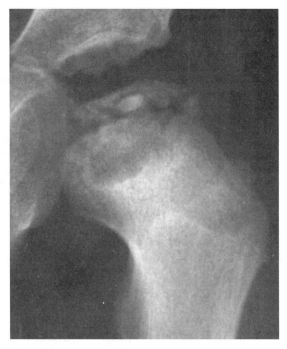

FIG. 1. Legg-Calvé-Perthes disease. **A:** The affected left capital femoral epiphysis of this 4-year-old boy is denser and smaller than the contralateral normal side. It shows a radiolucent area that forms the crescent sign *(arrows)* indicative of subchondral bone collapse. **B:** Seven months later, there is flattening of the capital femoral epiphysis with widening and irregularity of the femoral neck.

greatest for children who lose containment of the femoral head by the acetabulum. Hip subluxation and loss of motion from muscle spasm and contractures disproportionately increase mechanical stresses on some regions of the femoral head. One tries to improve the coverage of the femoral head by the acetabulum, thus allowing it to act as a mold during reparative reossification (5–7). Appropriate management may be observation alone, intermittent treatment of symptoms with periodic bed rest, stretching exercises to maintain hip range of motion, and early or late surgical prevention or correction of deformity (10,11). Bed rest does not seem to decrease compressive forces that may stimulate healing and bone modeling if properly distributed (5–7,10,11). Periodic radiographic follow-up is essential, and arthrography, bone scintigraphy, and especially MRI also can be useful (6,8). The long-term results of these treatments remain controversial. Whether containment is useful, and which method of achieving containment is best, are clinical questions that are being actively studied (5–7,10,11).

OTHER CLINICAL PRESENTATIONS

Numerous other presentations for ischemic bone disease manifest in children and adults (Table 2) (1–3). Symptoms result primarily from skeletal disintegration. The specific diagnosis, however, depends on the patient's age, the anatomic site, and the size of the area of bone where blood flow has been interrupted. LCPD is an excellent illustration

TABLE 2. *Common sites of osteochondrosis and ischemic necrosis of bone*

Adult skeleton
  Osteochondritis dissecans (König)
  Osteochondrosis of lunate (Kienböck)
  Fractured head of femur (Axhausen, Phemister)
  Proximal fragment of fractured carpal scaphoid
  Fractured head of humerus
  Fractured talus
  Osteonecrosis of the knee (spontaneous or idiopathic ischemic necrosis)
  Idiopathic ischemic necrosis of the femoral head
Developing skeleton
  Osteochondrosis of femoral head (Legg–Calvé–Perthes)
  Slipped femoral epiphysis
  Vertebral epiphysitis affecting secondary ossification centers (Scheuermann)
  Vertebral osteochondrosis of primary ossification centers (Calvé)
  Osteochondrosis of tibial tuberosity (Osgood–Schlatter)
  Osteochondrosis of tarsal scaphoid (Köhler)
  Osteochondrosis of medial tibial condyle (Blount)
  Osteochondrosis of primary ossification center of patella (Köhler) and of secondary ossification center (Sinding–Larsen)
  Osteochondrosis of os calcis (Sever)
  Osteochondrosis of head of second metatarsal (Freiberg) and of other metatarsals and metacarpals
  Osteochondrosis of the humeral capitellum (Panner)

From Edeiken J, Dalinka M, Karasic D, eds. *Edeiken's roentgen diagnosis of diseases of bone.* 4th ed. Baltimore: Williams & Wilkins, 1990.

that disruption of the microvasculature of the skeleton predisposes especially subchondral bone to infarction. However, several general mechanisms for vascular insufficiency may lead to ischemic bone disease, such as traumatic rupture, internal obstruction, or external pressure compromising blood flow. Arteries, veins, or sinusoids may be affected. The resulting ischemic bone disease has been referred to as ischemic, avascular, aseptic, or idiopathic necrosis (1–3). A considerable variety of conditions can cause ischemic bone disease (Table 1).

The pathogenesis of disrupted blood flow in ischemic bone disease is incompletely understood (1–3). For many types of nontraumatic ischemic necrosis, the predisposed sites of the skeleton seem to recapitulate the physiologic conversion of red marrow to fatty marrow with aging (2). This process occurs from distal to proximal in the appendicular skeleton. As the transition occurs, there is a decrease in marrow blood flow. Accordingly, disorders that increase the size and/or number of fat cells within critical areas of medullary space (e.g., alcohol abuse, Cushing syndrome) may ultimately compress sinusoids and infarct bone. However, fat embolization, hemorrhage, and abnormalities in the quality of susceptible bone tissue also may be pathogenetic factors in some types of traumatic or nontraumatic ischemic bone disease (2).

Radiographic features of ischemic bone disease depend on the amount of skeletal revascularization, reossification, and resorption of infarcted bone (2,3). Revascularization occurs within 6 to 8 weeks of the ischemic event and may cause trabecular bone resorption (radiolucent bands near necrotic areas). New bone formation then occurs on dead bone surfaces. Over months or years, dead bone may, or may not, be slowly resorbed. Osteosclerosis will occur if new bone encases dead bone and/or if there is bony collapse.

Histopathologic study is consistent with the pathogenesis that is suggested radiographically. It demonstrates that these various processes of skeletal death and repair are focal and may be occurring simultaneously (Fig. 2) (4).

Following infarction, necrotic bone does not change density for at least 10 days (2). Currently MRI is the most sensitive way to detect ischemic necrosis of the skeleton and therefore is particularly useful early on, although occasionally false negatives do occur (8,12,13). Bone scintigraphy with 99m-technetium diphosphonate, although not specific, also can detect osteonecrosis before radiographic changes are apparent (14,15). Before the process of revascularization, the infarcted area shows decreased radioisotope uptake; later increased tracer accumulation will occur. Computed tomography is especially helpful for detecting ischemic necrosis of the femoral head, because the bony structure centrally has an asterisk shape that is distorted by new-bone formation (16).

The various clinical presentations of ischemic bone disease (Table 2) are sometimes divided into two major anatomic categories: diaphysometaphyseal and epiphysometaphyseal (2).

Diaphysometaphyseal ischemia can be caused by dysbaric disorders, hemoglobinopathies, collagen vascular diseases, thromboembolic conditions, gout, storage disorders (e.g., Gaucher disease), acute or chronic pancreatitis, pheochromocytoma, and other conditions. Typically this category in-

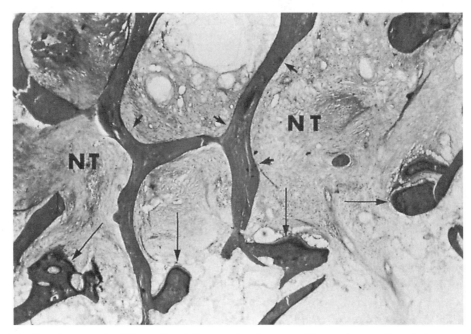

FIG. 2. Ischemic necrosis. This undecalcified section from an affected femoral head shows a typical area of dead bone *(arrows)* with a smooth acellular surface. A band of necrotic tissue (NT) is visible. Reparative bone formation is occurring in adjacent areas where darkly stained, newly synthesized osteoid is covered by osteoblasts *(arrowheads)* (Goldner stain; ×160).

volves large bones (especially the distal femur or proximal tibia), where radiographic changes extend into the metaphysis. Such lesions are often symmetric; however, the size of the involved areas can vary considerably. Small bones, however, may be affected, for example, in the hands and feet of infants with sickle cell anemia. New-bone deposition delineates infarcted bone especially well on radiographic study.

Epiphysometaphyseal infarcts can result from dysbaric conditions, sickle cell disease, Cushing syndrome, gout, trauma, storage problems, and other disorders. When the lesions are small, they are typically found in children or young adults and occur without a history of injury, although occult trauma may actually be important in their pathogenesis. Thrombosis, disease of arterial walls, or abnormalities within adjacent bone, such as those occurring in Gaucher disease or histiocytosis X (see Chapter 76), may cause this category of ischemic bone disease.

Osteochondrosis refers to atraumatic ischemic necrosis that typically affects a skeletal growth or ossification center (2). *Osteochondritis dissecans* describes a small epiphysometaphyseal infarct that can cause fracture immediately adjacent to a joint space. This lesion appears as a small, dense, button-like area of osseous tissue that is separated from the intact bone by a radiolucent band. This bone fragment can become loose and enter the joint, but it may also heal in place. Larger infarcts are often also idiopathic, occur frequently in adults, and typically involve the hip and the femoral condyles. Large areas of ischemic bone can collapse, thus flattening joint surfaces and destroying articular cartilage. Ultimately this complication will lead to osteoarthritis (Fig. 3). Very extensive epiphysometaphyseal infarction results from

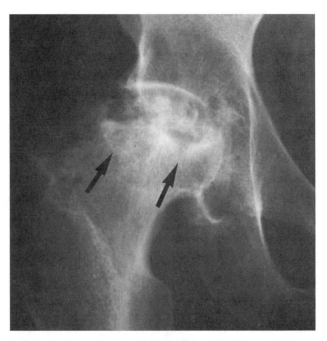

FIG. 3. Ischemic (avascular) necrosis. This 50-year-old man has advanced avascular necrosis of the femoral head. Note that much of the femoral head has been resorbed, causing collapse of the articular surface. The necrotic area is fragmented. A sclerotic zone of reparative tissue *(arrows)* indicates the interface between viable and necrotic tissues. The acetabular cartilage is focally thin. This finding indicates that he is developing secondary osteoarthritis.

trauma or systemic disease and frequently involves the femoral head [e.g., LCPD (2)].

Eponyms for specific presentations of osteochondrosis or ischemic necrosis of the skeleton are numerous (e.g., Blount disease, Scheuermann disease) and are widely used. However, classification according to the involved anatomic site is more informative. Table 2 matches the eponym with the affected skeletal region and helps to illustrate that the patient's age is an important factor for determining which areas of the skeleton are at risk (2).

Treatment of ischemic bone disease varies according to the site and size of the lesion and the patient's age. Conservative or surgical approaches may be appropriate (1,17,18).

REFERENCES

1. Mankin HJ. Nontraumatic necrosis of bone (osteonecrosis). *N Engl J Med* 1992;326:1473–1479.
2. Edeiken J, Dalinka M, Karasick D. *Edeiken's roentgen diagnosis of diseases of bone.* 4th ed. Baltimore: Williams & Wilkins, 1990.
3. Resnick D, Niwayama G. *Diagnosis of bone and joint disorders.* 3rd ed. Philadelphia: WB Saunders, 1995.
4. Plenk H Jr, Hofmann S, Eschberger J, et al. Histomorphology and bone morphometry of the bone marrow edema syndrome of the hip. *Clin Orthop* 1997;334:73–84.
5. Katz JE. *Legg-Calvé-Perthes disease.* New York: Praeger, 1984.
6. Conway JJ. A scintigraphic classification of Legg-Calvé-Perthes disease. *Semin Nucl Med* 1993;23:274–295.
7. Wenger DR, Ward WT, Herring JA. Current concepts review: Legg-Calvé-Perthes disease. *J Bone Joint Surg Am* 1991;73:778–788.
8. Lang P, Genant HK, Jergesen HE, Murray WR. Imaging of the hip joint: computed tomography versus magnetic resonance imaging. *Clin Orthop* 1992;274:135–153.
9. Mukherjee A, Fabry G. Evaluation of the prognostic indices in Legg-Calvé-Perthes disease: statistical analysis of 116 hips. *J Pediatr Orthop* 1990;10:153–158.
10. Herring JA. The treatment of Legg-Calvé-Perthes disease: a critical review of the literature. *J Bone Joint Surg Am* 1994;76:448–458.
11. Paterson DC, Leitch JM, Foster BK. Results of innominate osteotomy in the treatment of Legg-Calvé-Perthes disease. *Clin Orthop* 1991;266:96–103.
12. Mitchell MD, Kundel HL, Steinberg ME, Kressel HY, Alavi A, Axel L. Avascular necrosis of the hip: comparison of MR, CT, and scintigraphy. *Am J Roentgenol* 1986;147:67–71.
13. Mitchell DG, Rao VM, Dalinka MK, et al. Femoral head avascular necrosis: correlation of MR imaging, and clinical findings. *Radiology* 1987;162:709–715.
14. Bonnarens F, Hernandez A, D'Ambrosia RD. Bone scintigraphic changes in osteonecrosis of the femoral head. *Orthop Clin North Am* 1985;16:697–703.
15. Spencer JD, Maisey M. A prospective scintigraphic study of avascular necrosis of bone in renal transplant patients. *Clin Orthop* 1985;194:125–135.
16. Dihlmann W. CT analysis of the upper end of the femur: the asterisk sign and ischemic bone necrosis of the femoral head. *Skeletal Radiol* 1982;8:251–258.
17. Crenshaw AH. *Campbell's operative orthopaedics.* 8th ed. St. Louis: CV Mosby, 1992.
18. Smith SW, Fehring TK, Griffin WL, Beaver WB. Core decompression of the osteonecrotic femoral head. *J Bone Joint Surg Am* 1995;77:674–680.

76. Infiltrative Disorders of Bone

Michael P. Whyte, M.D.

Division of Bone and Mineral Diseases, Washington University School of Medicine at Barnes–Jewish Hospital, and Metabolic Research Unit, Shriners Hospital for Children, St. Louis, Missouri

Several important and interesting skeletal disorders feature excessive proliferation or infiltration of specific cell types within the marrow spaces. Reviewed briefly here are systemic mastocytosis and histiocytosis X.

SYSTEMIC MASTOCYTOSIS

Systemic mastocytosis is characterized by increased numbers of mast cells in the viscera, involving principally the liver, spleen, gastrointestinal tract, and lymph nodes (1–5). Additionally, the skin can contain numerous hyperpigmented macules that reflect dermal mast cell accumulation, a condition called *urticaria pigmentosa* (Fig. 1). Bone marrow is also typically involved, which may result in skeletal pathology.

Symptoms of systemic mastocytosis result primarily from release of mediator substances by the mast cells and include generalized pruritus, urticaria, flushing, episodic hypotension, diarrhea, weight loss, peptic ulcer, and syncope (1–5). With cutaneous involvement, histamine release occurs from stroking the skin, causing urtication (Darier's sign). Skeletal

problems develop relatively infrequently, but they include bone pain or tenderness from deformity resulting from fracture (1–9). Patients often succumb to a granulocytic neoplasm (1–3,10).

Radiographic abnormalities of the skeleton are common in systemic mastocytosis (about 70% of patients). The disturbances have been thoroughly characterized (11,12). Radiographs typically show diffuse, poorly demarcated, sclerotic and lucent areas where red marrow is present (i.e., in the axial skeleton; Fig. 2). However, circumscribed lesions can occur, especially in the skull and in the extremities. These focal findings may be mistaken for metastatic disease. Lytic areas are often small and have a surrounding rim of osteosclerosis.

Progression of the radiographic changes can occur as regional involvement becomes generalized (11,12). Focal bony changes may be absent despite extensive accumulation of mast cells in the skeleton. Generalized osteopenia (without focal bony abnormalities) also is a common presentation (6,7,9) but has a relatively benign prognosis (13). Bone scintigraphy helps detect involved skeletal areas (14) and can provide information regarding disease activity and prognosis

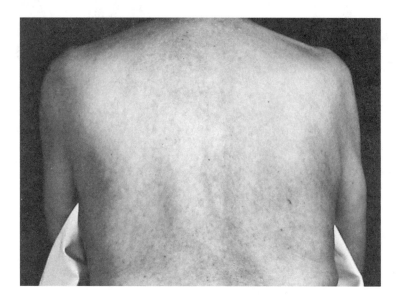

FIG. 1. Systemic mastocytosis. Numerous characteristic hyperpigmented macules (urticaria pigmentosa) are present on the back of this 61-year-old woman.

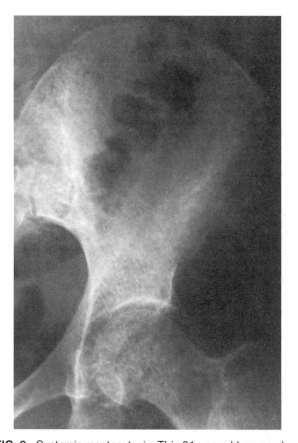

FIG. 2. Systemic mastocytosis. This 81-year-old woman has characteristic diffuse punctuate radiolucencies of her pelvis and hip that indicate a permeative process in the bone marrow.

(15). Reportedly, hip-bone density correlates positively with urinary excretion of the histamine metabolite, methylimidazoleacetic acid (16).

Histopathologic correlates of systemic mastocytosis in the skeleton also are well characterized (3,6,17,18). In fact, examination of undecalcified sections of bone can be an especially effective way to establish the diagnosis. Transiliac crest biopsy may be superior for this purpose to bone marrow aspiration or biopsy (6,17,18). Undecalcified sections of iliac crest show multiple nodules 150 to 450 μm in diameter that resemble granulomas. Within the granulomas are characteristic oval or spindle-shaped cells, eosinophils, lymphocytes, and plasma cells. The spindle-shaped cells resemble histiocytes or fibroblasts, but they contain granules that stain metachromatically and actually are a type of mast cell (Fig. 3). In addition, the marrow contains increased numbers of these mast cells individually or in small aggregates (6,17,18). Tetracycline-based histomorphometry shows that skeletal remodeling is rapid (17,18).

The etiology of systemic mastocytosis is unclear (1–5). Persistence of mast cell disease after bone marrow transplantation for an additional disorder suggests that a defective myeloid precursor cell is not the cause (19,20). The disorder appears to be a multitopic monoclonal proliferation of cytologically and/or functionally abnormal tissue mast cells (3). Some cases have mutation in the c-*kit* protooncogene (21).

The treatment of systemic mastocytosis is discussed in a number of articles (1–5,22–25). Severe bone pain from advanced bone disease has been reported to respond to radiotherapy (26). Intravenous pamidronate has controlled pain and improved bone density in early trials (27).

HISTIOCYTOSIS X

Histiocytosis X was the term coined in 1953 to unify what had been regarded as three distinct entities: Letterer–Siwe disease, Hand–Schüller–Christian disease, and eosinophilic

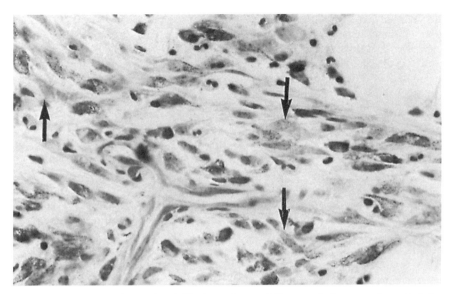

FIG. 3. Mast cell granuloma. A nondecalcified specimen of iliac crest shows a characteristic mast cell granuloma that contains numerous spindle-shaped mast cells *(arrows)*. (Toluidine blue stain; ×220.)

granuloma (28,29). The Langerhans cell has been recognized as the pathognomonic and linking feature, and the condition is now called Langerhans cell histiocytosis (28,29). Histiocytosis X seems to result from some poorly understood dysfunction of the immune system (28). It is an extremely heterogeneous condition. Nevertheless, the tripartite distinction for histiocytosis X continues to be used because of the generally different clinical courses and prognoses (28,29).

About 1200 cases of histiocytosis X are diagnosed yearly in the United States. Sex incidence is equal. Northern Europeans are affected more commonly than Hispanics, and the condition is rare in blacks. Many tissues and organs can be involved, including brain, lung, oropharynx, gastrointestinal tract, skin, and bone marrow. Diabetes insipidus is common in affected children and adults because of pituitary infiltration. Prognosis is age related; infants and the elderly have poorer outcomes. The signs and symptoms of the three principal clinical forms differ.

Letterer–Siwe disease presents between the ages of several weeks and 2 years with hepatosplenomegaly, lymphadenopathy, anemia, hemorrhagic tendency, fever, failure to grow, and skeletal lesions. It may end fatally after just several weeks (28,29).

Hand–Schüller–Christian disease is a chronic disorder that begins in early childhood, although symptoms may not manifest until the third decade (28,29). A classic triad of findings consists of exophthalmos, diabetes insipidus, and bony lesions. However, this presentation occurs in only 10% of cases. The most common skeletal manifestation is osteolytic lesions in the skull, with overlying soft-tissue nodules (Fig. 4) (30,31). Proptosis is associated with destruction of orbital bones. There may be spontaneous remissions and exacerbations. Soft-tissue nodules may remit without treatment.

Eosinophilic granuloma occurs most frequently in children between ages 3 and 10 years, and it is rare after age 15 years (28,29). A solitary and painful lesion in a flat bone

is the most common finding (30,31). There may be a soft-tissue mass. The calvarium is usually affected, although any bone can be involved. The prognosis is excellent, with monostotic lesions responding well to x-ray therapy or healing spontaneously.

The radiographic findings in the skeleton are similar in the three disorders (11,12,30,31). Single bony foci are most common. Nevertheless, multiple areas can be affected and show progressive enlargement. Individual lesions are well

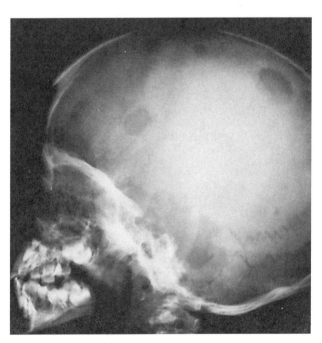

FIG. 4. Hand–Schüller–Christian disease. This 2 4/12-year-old boy has multiple, well-defined, beveled-edge, lucent lesions of the skull. Note the extensive destruction of the paranasal sinuses and at the base of the skull.

defined: "punched-out," osteolytic, and destructive with scalloped edges. They vary from a few millimeters to several centimeters in diameter. Fewer than half of these radiolucencies show marginal reactive osteosclerosis. Membranous bones as well as long bones can be affected. In the long bones, defects occur in the medullary canal where there is erosion of the endosteal cortex (commonly in the metaphyseal or epiphyseal regions). Periosteal reaction is frequent and produces a solid layer of new bone. In the skull, the bony tables can be eroded. Destruction of orbital bones may or may not be associated with exophthalmos. *Vertebra plana* (i.e., flattened vertebrae) can result from spinal involvement in young children. Radionuclide accumulation is poor during bone scanning (11,12). Biochemical parameters of mineral homeostasis are usually normal.

Histiocytosis X tends to be benign and self-limiting when there is no systemic involvement. Treatment for severe disease includes chemotherapy, radiation therapy, and immunotherapy (32). Methylprednisolone injected into lesions is an effective procedure (31). Central nervous system involvement is often treated with radiation therapy. Allogeneic bone marrow transplantation was reported to have been successful in a severe case with poor prognosis (33).

REFERENCES

1. Golkar L, Bernhard JD. Mastocytosis. *Lancet* 1997;10:1379–1385.
2. Valent P. Biology, classification and treatment of human mastocytosis. *Wiener Klin Wochenschr* 1996;108:385–397.
3. Horny HP, Ruck P, Krober S, Kaiserling E. Systemic mast cell disease (mastocytosis): general aspects and histopathological diagnosis. *Histol Histopathol* 1997;12:1081–1089.
4. Marone G, Spadaro G, Genovese A. Biology, diagnosis and therapy of mastocytosis. *Chem Immunol* 1995;62:1–21.
5. Genovese A, Spadaro G, Triggiani M, Marone G. Clinical advances in mastocytosis. *Int J Clin Lab Res* 1995;25:178–188.
6. Fallon MD, Whyte MP, Teitelbaum SL. Systemic mastocytosis associated with generalized osteopenia: histopathological characterization of the skeletal lesion using undecalcified bone from two patients. *Hum Pathol* 1981;12:813–820.
7. Harvey JA, Anderson HC, Borek D, Morris D, Lukert BP. Osteoporosis associated with mastocytosis confined to bone: report of two cases. *Bone* 1989;10:237–241.
8. Cook JV, Chandy J. Systemic mastocytosis affecting the skeletal system. *J Bone Joint Surg Br* 1989;71:536.
9. Lidor C, Frisch B, Gazit D, Gepstein R, Hallel T, Mekori YA. Osteoporosis as the sole presentation of bone marrow mastocytosis. *J Bone Miner Res* 1990;5:871–876.
10. Lawrence JB, Friedman BS, Travis WD, Chinchilli VM, Metcalfe DD, Gralnick HR. Hematologic manifestations of systemic mast cell disease: a prospective study of laboratory and morphologic features and their relation to prognosis. *Am J Med* 1991;91:612–624.
11. Edeiken J, Dalinka M, Karasick D. *Edeiken's roentgen diagnosis of diseases of bone.* 4th ed. Baltimore: Williams & Wilkins, 1990.
12. Resnick D, Niwayama G. *Diagnosis of bone and joint disorders.* 3rd ed. Philadelphia: WB Saunders, 1995.
13. Andrew SM, Freemont AJ. Skeletal mastocytosis. *J Clin Pathol* 1993;46:1033–1035.
14. Arrington ER, Eisenberg B, Hartshorne MF, Vela S, Dorin RI. Nuclear medicine imaging of systemic mastocytosis. *J Nucl Med* 1989;30:2046–2048.
15. Chen CC, Andrich MP, Mican JM, Metcalfe DD. A retrospective analysis of bone scan abnormalities in mastocytosis: correlation with disease category and prognosis. *J Nucl Med* 1994;35:1471–1475.
16. Johansson C, Roupe G, Lindstedt G, Mellstrom D. Bone density, bone markers and bone radiological features in mastocytosis. *Age Ageing* 1996;25:1–7.
17. de Gennes C, Kuntz D, de Vernejoul MC. Bone mastocytosis: a report of nine cases with a bone histomorphometric study. *Clin Orthop* 1991;279:281–291.
18. Chines A, Pacifici R, Avioli LV, Teitelbaum SL, Korenblat PE. Systemic mastocytosis presenting as osteoporosis: a clinical and histomorphometric study. *J Clin Endocrinol Metab* 1991;72:140–144.
19. Ronnov-Jessen D, Nielsen PL, Horn T. Persistence of systemic mastocytosis after allogeneic bone marrow transplantation in spite of complete remission of the associated myelodysplastic syndrome. *Bone Marrow Transplant* 1991;8:413–415.
20. Van Hoof A, Criel A, Louwagie A, Vanvuchelen J. Cutaneous mastocytosis after autologous bone marrow transplantation. *Bone Marrow Transplant* 1991;8:151–153.
21. Pignon JM. C-*kit* mutations and mast cell disorders: a model of activating mutations of growth factor receptors. *Hematol Cell Ther* 1997;39:114–116.
22. Gasior-Chrzan B, Falk ES. Systemic mastocytosis treated with histamine H_1 and H_2 receptor antagonists. *Dermatology* 1992;184:149–152.
23. Metcalfe DD. The treatment of mastocytosis: an overview. *J Invest Dermatol* 1991;96:55S–59S.
24. Póvoa P, Ducla-Soares J, Fernandes A, Palma-Carlos AG. A case of systemic mastocytosis: therapeutic efficacy of ketotifen. *J Intern Med* 1991;229:475–477.
25. Kluin-Nelemans HC, Jansen JH, Breukelman H, et al. Response to interferon alfa-2b in a patient with systemic mastocytosis. *N Engl J Med* 1992;326:619–623.
26. Johnstone PA, Mican JM, Metcalfe DD, DeLaney TF. Radiotherapy of refractory bone pain due to systemic mast cell disease. *Am J Clin Oncol* 1994;17:328–330.
27. Marshall A, Kavanagh RT, Crisp AJ. The effect of pamidronate on lumbar spine bone density and pain in osteoporosis secondary to systemic mastocytosis. *Br J Rheumatol* 1997;36:393–396.
28. Lam KY. Langerhans cell histiocytosis (histiocytosis X). *Postgrad Med J* 1997;73:391–394.
29. Nezelof C, Basset F. Langerhans cell histiocytosis research: past, present, and future. *Hematol Oncol Clin North Am* 1998;12:385–406.
30. Alexander JE, Seibert JJ, Berry DH, Glasier CM, Williamson SL, Murphy J. Prognostic factors for healing of bone lesions in histiocytosis X. *Pediatr Radiol* 1988;18:326–332.
31. Bollini G, Jouve JL, Gentet JC, Jacquemier M, Bouyala JM. Bone lesions in histiocytosis X. *J Pediatr Orthop* 1991;11:469–477.
32. Greenberger JS, Crocker AC, Vawter G, Jaffe N, Cassady JR. Results of treatment of 127 patients with systemic histiocytosis (Letterer-Siwe syndrome, Schüller-Christian syndrome and multifocal eosinophilic granuloma). *Medicine* 1981;60:311–388.
33. Ringdën O, Aohström L, Lönnqvist B, Boaryd I, Svedmyr E, Gahrton G. Allogeneic bone marrow transplantation in a patient with chemotherapy-resistant progressive histiocytosis X. *N Engl J Med* 1987;316:733–735.

SECTION IX

Paget's Disease

77. Paget's Disease of Bone

Ethel S. Siris, M.D.

Department of Medicine, Columbia University College of Physicians and Surgeons, and Metabolic Bone Diseases Program,
Columbia-Presbyterian Medical Center, New York, New York

Paget's disease of bone is a localized disorder of bone remodeling. The process is initiated by increases in osteoclast-mediated bone resorption, with subsequent compensatory increases in new-bone formation, resulting in a disorganized mosaic of woven and lamellar bone at affected skeletal sites. This structural change produces bone that is expanded in size, less compact, more vascular, and more susceptible to deformity or fracture than is normal bone (1). Clinical signs and symptoms will vary from one patient to the next depending on the number and location of affected skeletal sites, as well as on the rapidity of the abnormal bone turnover. It is believed that most patients are asymptomatic, but a substantial minority may experience a variety of symptoms, including bone pain, secondary arthritic problems, bone deformity, excessive warmth over bone from hypervascularity, and a variety of neurologic complications caused in most instances by compression of neural tissues adjacent to pagetic bone.

ETIOLOGY

The etiology of Paget's disease remains unknown. However, existing data from several different areas of investigation have provided some useful working hypotheses. First, Paget's disease appears to have a significant genetic component. Of patients with Paget's disease from several clinical series, 15% to 30% have positive family histories of the disorder (2). Genetic analyses of multiple affected kindreds support an autosomal dominant pattern of inheritance (3). In a study from Spain that used bone scans to identify the disease in relatives of diagnosed cases, 40% of the cases had a positive family history (4). Familial aggregation studies in a United States population (5) suggested that the risk of a first-degree relative of a pagetic subject developing the condition is 7 times greater than is the risk for someone who does not have an affected relative. Several studies have reported a possible linkage of Paget's disease to human leukocyte antigen (HLA), but these are inconclusive to date (6–9). Recently two studies reported a possible candidate gene for the disease on chromosome 18q (10,11) based on evaluation of large kindreds of affected patients. However, not all families studied possess this susceptibility locus, indicating that genetic heterogeneity is probable (11).

Ethnic and geographic clustering of Paget's disease also has been described, with the intriguing observation that the disorder is quite common in some parts of the world but relatively rare in others. Clinical observations indicate that the disease is most common in Europe, North America, Australia, and New Zealand. Studies surveying radiologists have computed prevalence rates in hospitalized patients older than 55 years in several European cities and found the highest percentages in England (4.6%) and France (2.4%), with other Western European countries reporting slightly lower prevalences (e.g., 0.7% to 1.7% in Ireland, 1.3% in

Spain and West Germany, and 0.5% in Italy and Greece) (12). There is a remarkable focus of Paget's disease in Lancashire, England, where 6.3% to 8.3% of people older than 55 years in several Lancashire towns had radiographs revealing Paget's disease (13).

Prevalence rates appear to decrease from north to south in Europe, except for the finding that Norway and Sweden have a particularly low rate (0.3%) (12). Few data are available from Eastern Europe, but Russian colleagues indicated that Paget's disease is not uncommon in that country. The disorder is seen in Australia and in New Zealand at rates of 3% to 4% (14). Paget's disease is distinctly rare in Asia, particularly in China, India, and Malaysia, although occasional cases of Indians living in the United States have been documented. Similar radiographic studies have described 0.01% to 0.02% prevalences in several areas of sub-Saharan Africa (14). In Israel the disease is seen predominantly in Jews (15) but was recently found to exist in Israeli Arabs as well. In Argentina the disease appears to be restricted to an area surrounding Buenos Aires and predominantly occurs in patients descended from European immigrants (16).

It is estimated, based on very few studies, that 2% to 3% of people older than 55 years living in the United States have Paget's disease. It is believed that most Americans with Paget's disease are white, of Anglo-Saxon or European descent. The disorder is described in African Americans, and most clinical series from hospitals in major American cities report having black patients (2,17).

There are also data that support a viral etiology for Paget's disease. It has been proposed that the changes in bone remodeling occur as a result of a viral infection of osteoclasts in pagetic bone. Inclusions that resemble viral nucleocapsids have been described in the nuclei and cytoplasm of osteoclasts at pagetic sites, but not in nonpagetic osteoclasts from the same patients or from normal subjects (18,19). The virus-like particles resemble members of the paramyxovirus family, but debate continues as to whether the putative virus is respiratory syncytial, measles, canine distemper, some mutation of one or more of these, or some other paramyxovirus. *In situ* hybridization studies have reported the detection of measles virus or canine distemper virus transcripts in pagetic osteoclasts (20,21). Studies of osteoclast precursors from Paget's disease patients show evidence of measles virus messenger ribonucleic acid (mRNA), including mutations of a specific region of the viral nucleocapsid gene (22). However, conflicting results have emerged from investigations using RNA extraction and polymerase chain reaction techniques, with some reporting the presence of viral RNA in pagetic bone and others failing to detect this (23,24).

Recently it has been shown that measles virus transcripts are present in both bone marrow mononuclear cells and a variety of peripheral blood cells from pagetic patients, including both osteoclast precursors and more primitive hematopoietic stem cells (25). The presence of osteoclast precursors expressing virus throughout the circulation seems to run counter to the finding that Paget's disease is a localized process. The recognition that increased concentrations of interleukin-6 are present in pagetic marrow plasma (26) suggests that cytokines in the marrow microenvironment may direct the differentiation of osteoclast precursors to limit the extent of pagetic transformation of bone to local sites once the initial lesion takes hold. Clearly more must be learned to understand the etiology of this disease, but the old hypothesis that the disorder results from a viral infection in a genetically susceptible host may in fact turn out to have some validity.

PATHOLOGY

Histopathologic Findings in Paget's Disease

The initiating lesion in Paget's disease is an increase in bone resorption. This occurs in association with an abnormality in the osteoclasts found at affected sites, as previously described. Pagetic osteoclasts are more numerous than normal and contain substantially more nuclei than do normal osteoclasts, with up to 100 nuclei per cell noted by some investigators. In response to the increase in bone resorption, numerous osteoblasts are recruited to pagetic sites where active and rapid new bone formation occurs. It is generally believed that the osteoblasts are intrinsically normal (27), but this is not proven conclusively.

In the earliest phases of Paget's disease, increased osteoclastic bone resorption dominates, a picture appreciated radiographically by an advancing lytic wedge or ''blade-of-grass'' lesion in a long bone or by osteoporosis circumscripta, as seen in the skull. At the level of the bone biopsy, the structurally abnormal osteoclasts are abundant. After this, there is a combination of increased resorption and relatively tightly coupled new-bone formation, produced by the large numbers of osteoblasts present at these sites. During this phase, and presumably because of the accelerated nature of the process, the new bone that is made is abnormal. Newly deposited collagen fibers are laid down in a haphazard rather than a linear fashion, creating more primitive woven bone. The woven-bone pattern is not specific for Paget's disease, but it does reflect a high rate of bone turnover. The end product is the so-called mosaic pattern of woven bone plus irregular sections of lamellar bone linked in a disorganized way by numerous cement lines representing the extent of previous areas of bone resorption. The bone marrow becomes infiltrated by excessive fibrous connective tissue and by an increased number of blood vessels, explaining the hypervascular state of the bone.

Bone matrix at pagetic sites is usually normally mineralized, and tetracycline labeling shows increased calcification rates. It is not unusual, however, to find areas of pagetic biopsies in which widened osteoid seams are apparent, perhaps reflecting inadequate calcium/phosphorus products in localized areas where rapid bone turnover heightens mineral demands.

In time, the hypercellularity at a locus of affected bone may diminish, leaving the end product of a sclerotic, pagetic mosaic without evidence of active bone turnover. This is so-called burned-out Paget's disease. Typically, all phases of the pagetic process can be seen at the same time at different sites in a particular subject.

Scanning electron microscopy affords an excellent view of the chaotic architectural changes that occur in pagetic bone and provides the visual imagery that makes comprehensible the loss of structural integrity. Figure 1 compares the appearances of normal and of pagetic bone by using this technique. Figure 2 demonstrates the mosaic pattern of disorganized bone in Paget's disease in most of the field, contrasted with a normal pattern of new-bone deposition following restoration of normal turnover with bisphosphonate therapy.

Biochemical Parameters of Paget's Disease

Increases in the urinary excretion of biomarkers of bone resorption [classically, total hydroxyproline has been measured, but more recently newer markers such as collagen cross-links and associated peptides are used (28)] reflect the primary lesion in Paget's disease, the increase in bone resorption. Increases in osteoblastic activity are associated with elevated levels of serum alkaline phosphatase. In untreated patients, the values of these two markers rise in proportion to each other, offering a reflection of the preserved coupling between resorption and formation. From the clinical perspective, the degree of elevation of these indices offers an approximation of the extent or severity of the abnormal bone turnover, with higher levels reflecting a more active, ongoing localized metabolic process. Interestingly, the patients with the highest alkaline phosphatase elevations (e.g., >10 times the upper limit of normal) typically have involvement of the skull as at least one site of the disorder. Active monostotic disease (other than skull) may have lower biochemical values than polyostotic disease. Lower values (e.g., <3 times the upper limit of normal) may reflect a lesser extent of involvement (i.e., fewer sites on bone scans or radiographs) or a burned-out form of Paget's disease, especially in a very elderly person known to have had extensive polyostotic disease in the past. However, minimal elevations in a patient with highly localized disease (e.g., the proximal tibia) may be associated with symptoms and clear progression of disease at the affected site over time. Indeed, a so-called ''normal'' alkaline phosphatase (e.g., a value a slightly less than the upper limit of normal for the assay) may not truly be normal for the pagetic patient. Today many would argue that to be confident that the value is normal (and the disease quiescent), a result in the middle of the normal range is required.

In addition to offering some estimate of the degree of abnormal bone turnover, the bone-resorption markers and alkaline phosphatase measurements are useful in observing the disorder over time and especially for monitoring the effects of treatment. With the potent new bisphosphonates that are capable of normalizing the biochemical markers (i.e., producing a remission of the bone-remodeling abnormality) in a majority of patients and bringing the markers to near normal in most others, the monitoring role has heightened importance. Urinary resorption markers such as the *N*-telopeptide of collagen or deoxypyridinoline may become

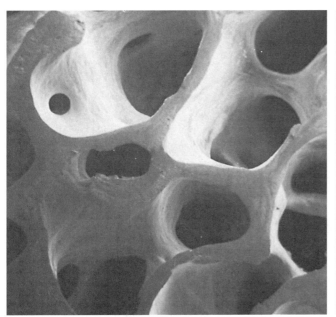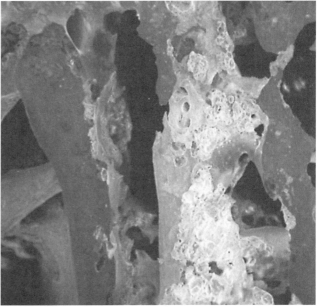

FIG. 1. Scanning electron microscope sections of normal bone *(left)* and pagetic bone *(right)*. Both samples were taken from the iliac crest. The normal bone shows the plates and marrow spaces to be well preserved, whereas the pagetic bone has totally lost this architectural appearance. Extensive pitting of the pagetic bone is apparent, due to dramatically increased osteoclastic bone resorption. (Photographs courtesy of Dr. David Dempster; reproduced from Siris ES, Canfield RE. Paget's disease of bone. In: Becker KL, ed. *Principles and practice of endocrinology and metabolism.* 2nd ed. Philadelphia: JB Lippincott, 1995:585–594, with permission.)

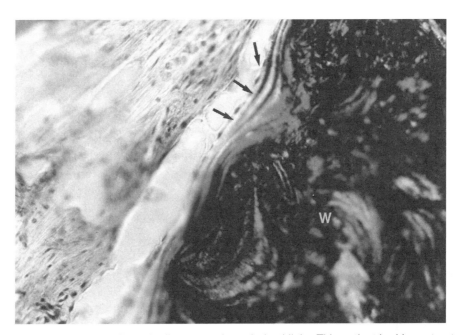

FIG. 2. Iliac crest bone with Paget's disease under polarized light. This patient had been treated with potent bisphosphonate therapy. Older bone is present in a pattern of woven bone *(W)*, but new-bone deposition after suppression of increased pagetic turnover shows a normal pattern of bone deposition *(arrows)*.

normal in days to a few weeks after bisphosphonate therapy is initiated. It is often most practical and the least expensive, however, to monitor serum alkaline phosphatase as the sole biochemical end point, with a baseline measure and subsequent follow-up tests at intervals appropriate for the therapy used (see later). If a patient has concomitant elevations of liver enzymes, a measurement of bone-specific alkaline phosphatase can be especially helpful. Serum osteocalcin, however, is not a useful measure in Paget's disease.

Serum calcium levels are typically normal in Paget's disease, but they may become elevated in two special situations. First, if a patient with active, usually extensive Paget's disease is immobilized, the loss of the weight-bearing stimulus to new-bone formation may transiently uncouple resorption and accretion, so that increasing hypercalciuria and hypercalcemia may occur. Alternatively, when a raised serum calcium is discovered in an otherwise healthy, ambulatory patient with Paget's disease, coexistent primary hyperparathyroidism may be the cause. Inasmuch as increased levels of parathyroid hormone (PTH) can drive the intrinsic pagetic remodeling abnormality to even higher levels of activity, correction of primary hyperparathyroidism in such cases is indicated.

Several investigators have commented on the 15% to 20% prevalence of secondary hyperparathyroidism (associated with normal levels of serum calcium) in Paget's disease, typically seen in patients with very high levels of serum alkaline phosphatase (29,30). The increase in PTH is believed to reflect the need to increase calcium availability to bone during phases of very active pagetic bone formation, particularly in subjects in whom dietary intake of calcium is inadequate. Secondary hyperparathyroidism and transient decreases in serum calcium also can occur in some patients being treated with potent bisphosphonates such as pamidronate, alendronate, or risedronate. This results from the effective and rapid suppression of bone resorption in the setting of ongoing new-bone formation (31). Later, as restoration of coupling occurs with time, PTH levels fall. The problem can be largely avoided by being certain that such patients are and remain calcium and vitamin D replete.

Elevations in serum uric acid and serum citrate have been described in Paget's disease and are of unclear clinical significance (1). Gout has been noted in this disorder, but it is uncertain whether it is more common in pagetic patients than in nonpagetic subjects. Hypercalciuria may occur in some patients with Paget's disease, presumably because of the increased bone resorption, and kidney stones are occasionally found as a consequence of this abnormality (1).

CLINICAL FEATURES

Paget's disease affects both men and women, with most series describing a slight male predominance. It is rarely observed to occur in individuals younger than age 25 years, it is thought to develop after the age of 40 in most instances, and it is most commonly diagnosed in people in their 50s. In a survey of over 800 selected patients, 600 of whom had symptoms, the average age at diagnosis was 58 years (32). It seems likely that many patients have the disorder for a period before any diagnosis is made, especially because it is often an incidental finding.

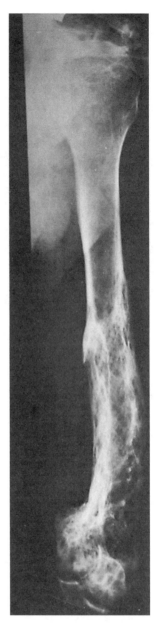

FIG. 3. Radiograph of a humerus showing typical pagetic change in the distal half, with cortical thickening, expansion, and mixed areas of lucency and sclerosis, contrasted with normal bone in the proximal half.

It is important to emphasize the localized nature of Paget's disease. It may be monostotic, affecting only a single bone or portion of a bone (Fig. 3), or may be polyostotic, involving two or more bones. Sites of disease are often asymmetric. A patient might have a pagetic right femur with a normal left, involvement of only half the pelvis, or involvement of several noncontiguous vertebral bodies. Clinical observation suggests that in most instances, sites affected with Paget's disease when the diagnosis is made are the only ones that will show pagetic change over time. Although progression of disease within a given bone may occur (Fig. 4), the sudden appearance of new sites of involvement years after the initial

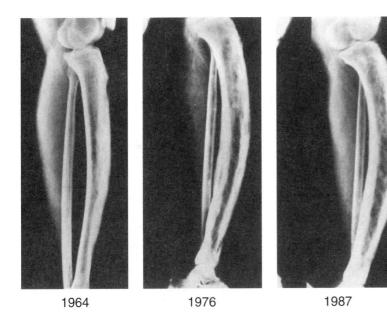

FIG. 4. This series of radiographs of a pagetic tibia demonstrates progression of pagetic change and bowing deformity in an untreated patient. This individual's Paget's disease was limited to the tibia and was associated with a serum alkaline phosphatase that was generally only mildly elevated to about twice the upper limit of normal. Note the distal progression of cortical thickening with time, as well as the worsening of the bowing deformity. (Reprinted from Siris ES, Feldman F. Clinical vignette: natural history of untreated Paget's disease of the tibia. *J Bone Miner Res* 1997;12:691–692, with permission.)

1964   1976   1987

diagnosis is uncommon. This information can be very reassuring for patients who often worry about extension of the disorder to new areas of the skeleton as they age.

The most common sites of involvement include the pelvis, femur, spine, skull, and tibia. The bones of the upper extremity, as well as the clavicles, scapulae, ribs, and facial bones, are less commonly involved, and the hands and feet are only rarely affected. It is generally believed that most patients with Paget's disease are asymptomatic and that the disorder is most often diagnosed when an elevated serum alkaline phosphatase is noted on routine screening or when a radiograph taken for an unrelated problem reveals typical skeletal changes. The development of symptoms or complications of Paget's disease is influenced by the particular areas of involvement, the interrelations between affected bone and adjacent structures, the extent of metabolic activity, and presence or absence of disease progression.

Signs and Symptoms

Bone pain from a site of pagetic involvement, experienced either at rest or with motion, is probably the most common symptom. The direct cause of the pain may be difficult to characterize and requires careful evaluation. Pagetic bone has an increased vascularity, leading to a warmth of the bone that some patients perceive as an unpleasant sensation. Small transverse lucencies along the expanded cortices of involved weight-bearing bones or advancing, lytic, blade-of-grass lesions sometimes cause pain. It is postulated that microfractures frequently occur in pagetic bone and can cause discomfort for a period of days to weeks.

A bowing deformity of the femur or tibia can lead to pain for several possible reasons. A bowed limb is typically shortened, resulting in specific gait abnormalities that can lead to abnormal mechanical stresses. Clinically severe secondary arthritis can occur at joints adjacent to pagetic bone, (e.g., the hip, knee, or ankle). The secondary gait problems

also may lead to arthritic changes on the contralateral nonpagetic side, particularly at the hip.

Back pain in pagetic patients is another difficult symptom to assess. Nonspecific aches and pains may emanate from enlarged pagetic vertebrae in some instances; vertebral compression fractures also may be seen. In the lumbar area, spinal stenosis with neural impingement may arise, producing radicular pain and possibly motor impairment. Degenerative changes in the spine may accompany pagetic changes, and it is useful for the clinician to determine which symptoms arise as a consequence of the pagetic process and which result from degenerative disease of nonpagetic vertebrae. Kyphosis may occur, or there may be a forward tilt of the upper back, particularly when a compression fracture or spinal stenosis is present. Treatment options will differ, depending on the basis of the symptoms. When Paget's disease affects the thoracic spine, there may rarely be syndromes of direct spinal cord compression with motor and sensory changes. Several cases of apparent direct cord compression with loss of neural function have now been documented to have resulted from a vascular steal syndrome, whereby hypervascular pagetic bone "steals" blood from the neural tissue (33).

Paget's disease of the skull, demonstrated radiographically in Fig. 5, may be asymptomatic, but common complaints in up to one third of patients with skull involvement may include an increase in head size with or without frontal bossing or deformity, or headache, sometimes described as a band-like tightening around the head. Hearing loss may occur as a result of isolated or combined conductive or neurosensory abnormalities; recent data suggest cochlear damage from pagetic involvement of the temporal bone is an important component (34). Cranial nerve palsies (such as in nerves II, VI, and VII) occur rarely. With extensive skull involvement, a softening of the base of the skull may produce platybasia, or flattening, with the development of basilar invagination, so that the odontoid process begins to extend upward as the skull sinks downward upon it. This

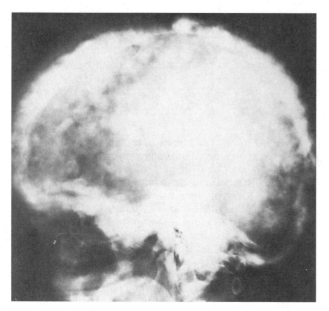

FIG. 5. Typical "cotton-wool" appearance of an enlarged pagetic skull with marked osteoblastic change. The patient had an increase in head size, and deafness.

feature can be appreciated by various radiographic measures including skull radiographs and computed tomography or magnetic resonance imaging scans. Although many patients with severe skull changes may have radiographic evidence of basilar invagination, a relatively small number develop a very serious complication, such as direct brainstem compression or an obstructive hydrocephalus and increased intracranial pressure caused by blockage of cerebrospinal fluid flow. Pagetic involvement of the facial bones may cause facial deformity, dental problems, and, rarely, narrowing of the airway. Mechanical changes of these types may lead to a nasal intonation when the patient is speaking.

Fracture through pagetic bone is an occasional and serious complication. These fractures may be either traumatic or pathologic, particularly involving long bones with active areas of advancing lytic disease; the most common involve the femoral shaft or subtrochanteric area (35). The increased vascularity of actively remodeling pagetic bone (i.e., with a moderately increased serum alkaline phosphatase) may lead to substantial blood loss in the presence of fractures due to trauma. Fractures also may occur in the presence of areas of malignant degeneration, a rare complication of Paget's disease. Far more common are the small fissure fractures along the convex surfaces of bowed lower extremities, which may be asymptomatic, stable, and persistent for years, but sometimes a more extensive transverse lucent area extends medially from the cortex and may lead to a clinical fracture with time. As described later, there are data indicating that blade-of-grass lytic areas as well as these larger transverse fractures may respond to antipagetic treatment and heal. These types of lesions warrant radiographic follow-up over time. Conversely, the smaller fissure fractures typically do not change with treatment and, in the absence of new pain, rarely require extensive radiographic monitoring.

In most cases, fracture through pagetic bone heals normally, although some groups have reported as high as a 10% rate of nonunion.

Neoplastic degeneration of pagetic bone is a relatively rare event, occurring with an incidence of less than 1%. This abnormality has a grave prognosis, typically manifesting itself as new pain at a pagetic site. The most common site of sarcomatous change appears to be the pelvis, with the femur and humerus next in frequency (36). Typically these lesions are osteolytic. The majority of the tumors are classified as osteogenic sarcomas, although both fibrosarcomas and chondrosarcomas are also seen. Current treatment regimens emphasize maximal resection of tumor mass and chemotherapy (or sometimes radiotherapy), but death from massive local extension of disease or from pulmonary metastases occurs in the majority of cases in 1 to 3 years.

Benign giant-cell tumors also may occur in bone affected by Paget's disease. These lesions may present as localized masses at the affected site. Radiographic evaluation may disclose lytic changes. Biopsy reveals clusters of large osteoclast-like cells, which some authors believe represent reparative granulomas (37). These tumors may show a remarkable sensitivity to glucocorticoids, so in many instances, the mass will shrink or even disappear after treatment with prednisone or dexamethasone (38).

DIAGNOSIS

When Paget's disease is suspected, the diagnostic evaluation should include a careful medical history and physical examination. The possibility of a positive family history and a symptom history should be ascertained. Gout, pseudogout, and arthritis are all possible complications of Paget's disease. Rarely patients with underlying intrinsic heart disease may develop congestive heart failure in the presence of severe Paget's disease. There are also reports suggesting that patients may have an increased incidence of calcific aortic disease (39). Angioid streaks are seen on funduscopic examination of the eye in some patients with polyostotic Paget's disease. The physical examination also should note the presence or absence of warmth, tenderness, or bone deformity in the skull, spine, pelvis, and extremities, as well as evidence of loss of range of motion at major joints or leg-length discrepancy.

Laboratory tests include measurement of serum alkaline phosphatase and in some cases a urinary marker of bone resorption, as described earlier. Radiographic studies (bone scans and conventional radiographs) complete the initial evaluation. Bone biopsy is not usually indicated, as the characteristic radiographic and laboratory findings are diagnostic in most instances.

Bone scans are the most sensitive means of identifying pagetic sites and are most useful for this purpose. Scans are nonspecific, however, and also can be positive in nonpagetic areas that have degenerative changes or, more ominously, may reflect metastatic disease. Plain radiographs of bones noted to be positive on the bone scan provide the most specific information, because the changes noted on the radiograph are usually characteristic to the point of being pathognomonic. Examples of these are shown in Figs. 3, 4, and

5. Enlargement or expansion of bone, cortical thickening, coarsening of trabecular markings, and typical lytic and sclerotic changes may be found. Radiographs also provide data on the status of the joints adjacent to involved sites, identify fissure fractures, indicate the degree to which lytic or sclerotic lesions predominate, and demonstrate the presence or absence of deformity or fracture.

Repeated scans or radiographs are usually unnecessary in observing patients over time, unless new symptoms develop or current symptoms become significantly worse. The possibility of an impending fracture or, rarely, of sarcomatous change should be borne in mind in these situations.

The characteristic radiographic and clinical features of Paget's disease usually eliminate problems with differential diagnosis. However, an older patient may occasionally present with severe bone pain, elevations of the serum alkaline phosphatase and urinary N-telopeptide or deoxypyridinoline, a positive bone scan, and less-than-characteristic radiographic areas of lytic or blastic change. Here the possibility of metastatic disease to bone or some other form of metabolic bone disease (e.g., osteomalacia with secondary hyperparathyroidism) must be considered. Old radiographs and laboratory tests are very helpful in this setting, as normal studies a year earlier would make a diagnosis of Paget's disease less likely. A similar dilemma occurs when someone with known and established Paget's disease develops multiple painful new sites; here, too, the likelihood of metastatic disease must be carefully considered, and bone biopsy for a tissue diagnosis may be indicated.

TREATMENT

Antipagetic Therapy

Specific antipagetic therapy consists of those agents capable of suppressing the activity of pagetic osteoclasts. Currently approved agents available by prescription in the United States include five bisphosphonate compounds: orally administered etidronate, tiludronate, alendronate, and risedronate and intravenously administered pamidronate; and parenterally administered calcitonin. Each of these is discussed later. Plicamycin, a cytotoxic anticancer agent approved for the management of hypercalcemia, has been used in the past (40) for refractory cases but has largely been replaced by potent newer bisphosphonates.

Between the mid-1970s and mid-1990s, the mainstays of therapy were calcitonin and etidronate. However, these agents should generally be replaced as the first lines of therapy by the newer bisphosphonates, all progressively more potent than either etidronate or calcitonin, offering the potential for greater disease suppression and frank remission (i.e., normalization of pagetic indices) for prolonged periods. In addition to the newer bisphosphonates mentioned earlier, clodronate, more potent than etidronate and available in several other countries, has been shown to be effective in Paget's disease (41). Olpadronate, neridronate, and ibandronate have significant activity as investigational agents in Paget's disease (42); zoledronate is the most potent bisphosphonate under investigation to date in this disease (43). Gallium nitrate, approved in the United States for the treatment of cancer hypercalcemia, also is being studied for efficacy in Paget's disease (44). Other symptomatic treatment for Paget's disease, including analgesics, antiinflammatory drugs, and selected orthopedic and neurosurgical interventions, also have roles in management.

Two logical indications for treatment of Paget's disease are to relieve symptoms and to prevent future complications. It has been clearly demonstrated that suppression of the pagetic process by any of the available agents can effectively ameliorate certain symptoms in the majority of patients. Symptoms such as bone aches or pain (probably the most common complaints of Paget's disease), excessive warmth over bone, headache due to skull involvement, low-back pain secondary to pagetic vertebral changes, and some syndromes of neural compression (e.g., radiculopathy and some examples of slowly progressive brainstem or spinal cord compression) are the most likely to be relieved. Pain due to a secondary arthritis from pagetic bone involving the spine, hip, knee, ankle, or shoulder may or may not respond to antipagetic treatment. Filling in of osteolytic blade-of-grass lesions in weight-bearing bones has been reported in some treated cases with either calcitonin or bisphosphonates. On the other hand, a bowed extremity or other bone deformity will not change after treatment, and deafness is unlikely to improve, although limited studies suggest that progression of hearing loss may be slowed (45).

A second indication for treatment is to prevent the development of late complications in those patients deemed to be at risk, based on their sites of involvement and evidence of active disease, as shown by elevated levels of bone-turnover markers. Admittedly, it has not been proved that suppression of pagetic bone turnover will prevent future complications. However, as shown in Fig. 2, there is a restoration of normal patterns of new-bone deposition in biopsy specimens after suppression of pagetic activity. It is also clear that active, untreated disease can continue to undergo a persistent degree of abnormal bone turnover for many years, with the possibility of severe bone deformity over time, as shown in Fig. 4. Indeed, substantial (e.g., 50%) but incomplete suppression of elevated indices of bone turnover with older therapies has been associated with disease progression (46); with bisphosphonates such as pamidronate, alendronate, and risedronate, however, indices become normal after treatment for extended periods in the majority of patients and approach normal in most of the rest.

Thus in the view of many investigators, the presence of asymptomatic but active disease (i.e., a serum alkaline phosphatase above normal) at sites where the potential for later problems or complications exists (e.g., weight-bearing bones, areas near major joints, vertebral bodies, extensively involved skull) is an indication for treatment. The need for treatment is particularly valid in patients who are younger, for whom many years of coexistence with the disorder are likely. However, even in the elderly, one can justify treatment if a degree of bone deformity is present that might create serious problems in the next few years.

Although controlled studies are not available to prove efficaciousness in this case, the use of antipagetic therapy before elective surgery on pagetic bone also is recommended. The goal here is to reduce the hypervascularity associated with moderately active disease (e.g., a threefold or more elevation in serum alkaline phosphatase) to reduce the amount of blood loss at operation.

Bisphosphonates

Etidronate

Etidronate was the first bisphosphonate to have been used clinically in the United States for Paget's disease (47,48) and was one of the two mainstays of therapy (with salmon calcitonin) for nearly 20 years. It is the least potent of the currently available bisphosphonate drugs. Etidronate is commercially available as Didronel (Procter and Gamble) in a 200- or 400-mg tablet. Although only a small percentage of the administered dose is absorbed, 5 mg/kg/day will provide a 50% lowering of biochemical indices and a reduction in symptoms in the majority of patients.

All bisphosphonates have the capacity to impair mineralization of newly forming bone if high enough doses are used. The dose of etidronate is limited by the fact that the doses that most effectively reduce the increased bone resorption can also impair mineralization, compelling the use of lower doses given for no longer than 6 months at a time. Thus the recommended regimen for the agent is 5 mg/kg/day (i.e., 400 mg in most patients, taken with a small amount of water mid-way in a 4-hour fast any time of day) for a 6-month period, followed by at least 6 months of no treatment. Many investigators in this area believe that etidronate is contraindicated in the presence of advancing lytic changes in a weight-bearing bone. Over several years of repeated 6-months-on, ≥6-months-off cycles, long-term benefit with maintenance of lower levels of pagetic biochemical activity has been observed in many patients, although others can become resistant to the agent after repeated courses. A failure to adhere to a cyclic low-dose regimen as described can induce bone pain and, occasionally, fracture due to focal osteomalacia secondary to mineralization problems from excessive etidronate. However, careful cyclic management is extremely well tolerated by the great majority of patients. Occasionally mild transient diarrhea may occur with etidronate, but this does not usually require more than a day or two of withholding the agent, after which it may be taken again. Rarely patients have some mild and transient achiness in bone after initiating therapy, which requires no intervention. More severe new pain in patients taking etidronate warrants stopping the drug and evaluating the patient before continuing therapy, to be certain that lytic disease or impending fracture (particularly in a weight-bearing extremity) has not been exacerbated.

Tiludronate

Tiludronate is about 10 times more potent than etidronate, and its use at effective doses is not associated with mineralization problems. Approved by the Food and Drug Administration (FDA) for Paget's disease in 1997, it is available as Skelid (Sanofi) in a 200-mg tablet. The recommended dosage is 400 mg daily for 3 months with a 3-month posttreatment observation period, after which the serum alkaline phosphatase is likely to have reached its nadir. This approach led to a normal serum alkaline phosphatase at the 6-month point in 24% to 35% of moderately affected subjects in clinical trials (49,50). It is generally very well tolerated, with a minority of patients experiencing mild upper gastrointestinal upset. It appears to offer the benefits of etidronate without the risk of mineralization problems in patients for whom this might be a concern (e.g., those with lytic disease in lower extremities) and half the total number of days of pills in a treatment course. As with etidronate, 400 mg should be taken with some water (in this case 6 to 8 oz) at least 2 hours away from food, and the patient should not lie down for the next 30 minutes. Patients also need to be calcium and vitamin D replete, but calcium supplements, like food, should not be taken within 2 hours of the tiludronate dose.

Tiludronate is a relatively new agent with few data regarding duration of efficacy. It is an attractive choice in patients with mild disease because it is well tolerated and requires only 3 months of active treatment. Patients who respond should have serum alkaline phosphatase measured at 3- to 4-month intervals and can be retreated when indices increase above normal or above a nadir level by 25% or more.

Pamidronate

Pamidronate is in the range of 100 times more potent than etidronate. With its availability in the mid-1990s, a new philosophy of and approach to management became available to the clinician. The greater potency of pamidronate (and of the newer agents, alendronate and risedronate) allows a majority of patients to experience a normalization of pagetic indices rather than only partial suppression, as is seen with calcitonin, etidronate, and (in most cases) tiludronate. Second, the effects may be longer lasting, so a limited course of treatment may provide many months of suppression. Third, all of the potent newer bisphosphonates have a much more favorable ratio of inhibition of bone resorption to inhibition of mineralization, so the threat of focal osteomalacia should be markedly reduced if not eliminated.

With pamidronate there is an opportunity to individualize the dosing regimen to the needs of the specific patient, and there really is no single best dose. Indeed, the literature is replete with numerous approaches (51,52), all of which seem to be effective. The package insert for pamidronate, available as Aredia (Novartis), recommends three daily infusions of 30 mg each, over a period of 4 hours each time, in 500 ml of normal saline or 5% dextrose in water. This is probably not a high enough dose to achieve normalization of indices for many patients. I find that patients with relatively mild disease may experience a substantial reduction of alkaline phosphatase to normal or near normal with a single 60-mg infusion given over a 3-hour period in 500 ml of 5% dextrose in water. Patients with more moderate to severe disease (e.g., serum alkaline phosphatase levels >3 to 4 times normal) may require multiple infusions of 60 to 90 mg infused as described and given on a once weekly or biweekly basis, primarily based on physician and patient convenience. Two to four 60-mg doses or three 90-mg doses may suffice in moderate disease (e.g., serum alkaline phosphatase in the range of 4 to 5 times normal). Total doses in the range of 300 to 500 mg may be required in some severe cases (serum alkaline phosphatase ≥10 to 20 times normal), given over a number of weeks.

Suppression of urinary markers can often be noted within a few days after an infusion, but the serum alkaline phosphatase may take up to 3 months to reach its nadir. For moderate to severe cases, giving three to four 60-mg doses and then reassessing at 3 months with the possibility of more treatment is a reasonable approach. A successful course of therapy can result in 1 year or more of continued disease suppression with markers of turnover at normal or near-normal levels. Side effects may include a low-grade fever the day after the first dose, flu-like symptoms in the first 24 hours after an infusion (decreasing in likelihood with repeated dosing), and the possibility of mild and transient hypocalcemia, hypophosphatemia, and lymphopenia. Venous irritation may arise, especially if an insufficient volume of fluid is used. It is desirable to provide oral calcium supplements at a dose of 500 mg, 2 or 3 times daily, and vitamin D, 400 to 800 U daily, to prevent or ameliorate a reduction in serum calcium and concomitant rise in PTH.

Overall, pamidronate offers the opportunity to titrate the dosage as required in the individual patient, with the possibility of normalization or near normalization of biochemical indices and the potential for substantial and prolonged reduction in disease progression in many patients. In my view, it is most useful in patients with mild disease, in whom a single infusion may afford long-term benefit in a very cost-effective manner, and in severe and refractory cases, in which delivery of drug by vein bypasses problems with oral absorption. The need for outpatient intravenous administration of multiple doses may be expensive and inconvenient in some cases. However, the rapid onset of symptomatic improvement and overall potency of the agent make it the drug of choice for cases with neurologic compression syndromes, for severe and painful lytic disease with or without impending fracture, and as a pretreatment of active Paget's disease before elective surgery to shrink the hypervascularity of the pagetic bone and decrease the amount of bleeding at operation. There has been one report of asymptomatic mineralization abnormalities with dosing in the usual clinical range (53), but this is not the general experience.

Alendronate

Approved by the FDA for the treatment of Paget's disease in the fall of 1995, alendronate, sold as Fosamax (Merck), is an orally administered aminobisphosphonate that is 700 times more potent than etidronate and is not associated with mineralization problems at therapeutically effective doses. In a study of 89 patients with moderate to severe disease who received 6 months of either alendronate, 40 mg daily, or etidronate, 400 mg per day, alendronate led to a normalized serum alkaline phosphatase in over 63% of subjects, compared with 17% for etidronate; overall, alendronate led to a mean fall in alkaline phosphatase of 79% compared with 44% with etidronate (54). Alendronate appeared to be as well tolerated as etidronate in this study, although symptoms of upper gastrointestinal discomfort or nausea, or the less common but more serious complication of esophageal ulceration, should be watched for at the 40-mg dose. Biopsies

from patients treated with alendronate revealed normal patterns of deposition of new bone (54,55) and radiologic improvement (55). The recommended dose is 40 mg daily for 6 months to be taken on arising in the morning with 8 oz of tap water. The patient is instructed not to take anything else by mouth (except more water) and not to lie down for at least 30 minutes after the dose. It is important with alendronate, as with pamidronate and tiludronate, that patients be replete in vitamin D and have a daily calcium intake of 1 to 1.5 g to avoid hypocalcemia early in the treatment course. Retreatment guidelines are incomplete until follow-up data on study patients become available, but several investigators have given a second 6-month course to previously treated patients once suppressed alkaline phosphatase values began to rise again, typically many months to a year or more after the end of the initial treatment, with good results.

Risedronate

More than 1000 times more potent than etidronate, risedronate is the newest available bisphosphonate, approved by the FDA for use in Paget's disease in 1998. Risedronate is available as Actonel (Procter and Gamble/Hoechst Marrion Roussel). Studies with risedronate have described the efficacy of a 30-mg dose given for 2 (56) or 3 (57) months to patients with moderately active disease. These short courses of therapy led to a nearly 80% reduction in serum alkaline phosphatase and normalization of indices of bone turnover in 50% to 70% of patients. Thus 30 mg can be given daily for 2 months, with a follow-up measurement of serum alkaline phosphatase 1 month later; if the value is not yet normal or near normal, a third or fourth month could be offered with a good likelihood of normalcy or near normalcy of indices thereafter, with a prolonged period of disease suppression. Once again, adequacy of calcium and vitamin D intake is important to avoid hypocalcemia. The 30-mg risedronate dose is taken with 8 oz of water on arising in the morning, with no other oral intake (except water) and no lying down for 30 minutes after the dose. In the clinical trials, the main side effects were mild upper gastrointestinal upset in 15% of patients; symptoms of esophageal irritation were not common in these clinical trials with the 30-mg dose but should be kept in mind by the physician until more data are available. A few cases of iritis were seen, something also reported rarely with pamidronate.

Calcitonin

The polypeptide hormone, salmon calcitonin, is available therapeutically as a synthetic formulation for parenteral administration. It, like human and other calcitonins, was first shown to be efficacious in Paget's disease more than 25 years ago (58,59). At present, the formulation approved for use in Paget's disease in the United States must be injected subcutaneously or intramuscularly. A nasal-spray formulation of salmon calcitonin, approved by the FDA for use in postmenopausal osteoporosis, is available although not specifically approved for treatment of Paget's disease.

Salmon calcitonin preparations for Paget's disease include Calcimar (Rhone Poulenc Rorer) and Miacalcin (Novartis), each available in a 400-U vial (2 ml). The usual starting dose is 100 U (0.5 ml), generally self-injected subcutaneously, initially on a daily basis. Symptomatic benefit may be apparent in a few weeks, and the biochemical benefit (typically about a 50% reduction from baseline in serum alkaline phosphatase) is usually seen after 3 to 6 months of treatment. After this period, many clinicians reduce the dose to 50 to 100 U every other day or 3 times weekly. Often, a dose of 50 U, 3 times weekly after the first few months of therapy, will maintain the achieved benefit. Patients with moderate to severe disease may require indefinite treatment to maintain a 50% reduction in the biochemical indices and symptomatic relief, but milder or monostotic disease may allow discontinuation of treatment for prolonged periods.

Escape from the efficacy of salmon calcitonin may sometimes occur after a variable period of benefit. In some cases this may be due to a postulated downregulation of receptors, but in other instances, it may be a consequence of the development of neutralizing antibodies to the salmon polypeptide (60). The main side effects of salmon calcitonin include, in a minority of patients, the development of nausea or queasiness, with or without flushing of the skin of the face and ears. These annoying side effects may last from a few minutes to several hours after each injection, although many patients can avoid them by experimenting with taking the agent at bedtime, with food, without food, and so on. Although these side effects are unpleasant, they do not appear to be serious or harmful, and most patients develop tolerance to them. Despite the requirement for parenteral administration, patients who experience benefit from calcitonin gladly tolerate the need for injection. However, it is apparent that newer bisphosphonates offer both greater effectiveness and ease of use, suggesting that this agent will be utilized in the future primarily by patients who do not tolerate oral or intravenous bisphosphonate therapy.

Intranasal calcitonin is available as Miacalcin Nasal Spray (Novartis). It appears to have a lower incidence of the side effects described earlier. The optimal dose in Paget's disease with the present formulation is not known, but anecdotal evidence suggests that in patients with mild disease, the 200-U single spray dose given daily may lower biochemical indices and relieve mild symptoms, such as increased warmth in a pagetic tibia.

Other Therapies

Analgesics and nonsteroidal antiinflammatory agents (NSAIDs) may be tried empirically with or without antipagetic therapy to relieve pain. Pagetic arthritis (i.e., osteoarthritis caused by deformed pagetic bone at a joint space) may cause periods of pain that are often helped by the NSAIDs.

Surgery on pagetic bone may be necessary in the setting of established or impending fracture. Elective joint replacement, although more complex with Paget's disease than with typical osteoarthritis, is often very successful in relieving refractory pain. Rarely osteotomy is performed to alter bowing deformity. Neurosurgical intervention is sometimes required in cases of spinal cord compression, spinal stenosis, or basilar invagination with neural compromise. Although medical management may be beneficial and adequate in some instances, all cases of serious neurologic compromise require immediate neurologic and neurosurgical consultation to allow the appropriate plan of management to be developed. As improved therapies emerge, long-term suppression of pagetic activity may have a preventive role in Paget's disease and may obviate the need for surgical management in many cases.

REFERENCES

1. Singer FR. *Paget's disease of bone.* New York: Plenum, 1977.
2. Siris ES, Canfield RE, Jacobs TP. Paget's disease of bone. *Bull N Y Acad Med* 1980;56:285–304.
3. McKusick VA. *Heritable disorders of connective tissue.* St. Louis: CV Mosby, 1972:718–723.
4. Morales-Piga AA, Rey-Rey JS, Corres-Gonzalez J, Garcia-Sagredo JM, Lopez-Abente G. Frequency and characteristics of familial aggregation of Paget's disease of bone. *J Bone Miner Res* 1995;10:663–670.
5. Siris ES, Ottman R, Flaster E, Kelsey JL. Familial aggregation of Paget's disease of bone. *J Bone Miner Res* 1991;6:495–500.
6. Tilyard MW, Gardner RJM, Milligan L, Cleary TA, Stewart RD. A possible linkage between familial Paget's disease and the HLA loci. *Aust N Z J Med* 1982;12:498–500.
7. Foldes J, Shamir S, Brautbar C, Schermann L, Menczel J. HLA-D antigens and Paget's disease of bone. *Clin Orthop* 1991;266:301–303.
8. Singer FR, Mills BG, Park MS, Takemura S, Terasaki PI. Increased HLA-DQw-1 antigen frequency in Paget's disease of bone. Proceedings of the 7th Annual Meeting of the American Society for Bone and Mineral Research. Washington, DC, 1985:8.
9. Singer FR, Siris ES, Knieriem A, Gjertson D, Terasaki PI. The HLA DRB1*1104 gene frequency is increased in Askenazi Jews with Paget's disease of bone. *J Bone Miner Res* 1996;11:S369.
10. Cody JD, Singer FR, Roodman GD, Otterund B, Lewis TB, Leppert M. Genetic linkage of Paget disease of bone to chromosome 18q. *Am J Hum Genet* 1997;61:1117–1122.
11. Haslam SI, Van Hul W, Morales-Piga A, et al. Paget's disease of bone: evidence for a susceptibility locus on chromosome 18q and for genetic heterogeneity. *J Bone Miner Res* 1998;13:911–917.
12. Barker DJ. The epidemiology of Paget's disease of bone. *Br Med Bull* 1984;40:396–400.
13. Barker DJP, Chamberlain AT, Guyer PB, Gardner MJ. Paget's disease of bone: the Lancashire focus. *Br Med J* 1980;280:1105–1107.
14. Barry HC. *Paget's disease of bone.* Edinburgh: E & S Livingstone, 1969.
15. Dolev E, Samuel R, Foldes J, Brickman M, Assia A, Liberman U. Some epidemiological aspects of Paget's disease in Israel. *Semin Arthritis Rheum* 1994;23:228.
16. Mautalen C, Pumarino H, Blanco MC, Gonzalez D, Ghiringhelli G, Fromm G. Paget's disease: the South American experience. *Semin Arthritis Rheum* 1994;23:226–227.
17. Guyer PB, Chamberlain AT. Paget's disease of bone in two American cities. *Br Med J* 1980;280:985.
18. Rebel A, Bregeon C, Basle M, Malkani K, Patezour A, Filmon R. Osteoclastic inclusions in Paget's disease of bone. *Rev Rhum Mal Osteoartic* 1942;42:637–641.
19. Mills BG, Singer FR. Nuclear inclusions in Paget's disease of bone. *Science* 1976;194:201–202.
20. Basle MF, Fournier JG, Rozenblatt S, Rebel A, Bouteille M. Measles virus mRNA detected in Paget's disease bone tissue by in situ hybridization. *J Gen Virol* 1986;67:907–913.
21. Gordon MT, Anderson DC, Sharpe PT. Canine distemper virus localized in bone cells of patients with Paget's disease. *Bone* 1991;12:195–201.
22. Reddy SV, Singer FR, Roodman GD. Bone marrow mononuclear cells from patients with Paget's disease contain measles virus nucleocapsid messenger ribonucleic acid that has mutations in a specific region of the sequence. *J Clin Endocrinol Metab* 1995;80:2108–2111.
23. Ralston SH, Digiovine FS, Gallacher SJ, Boyle IT, Duff GW. Failure

to detect paramyxovirus sequences in Paget's disease of bone using the polymerase chain reaction. *J Bone Miner Res* 1991;6:1243–1248.

24. Birch MA, Taylor W, Fraser WD, Ralston SH, Hart CA, Gallagher JA. Absence of paramyxovirus RNA in cultures of pagetic bone cells and in pagetic bone. *J Bone Miner Res* 1994;9:11–16.

25. Reddy SV, Singer FR, Mallette L, Roodman GD. Detection of measles virus nucleocapsid transcripts in circulating blood cells from patients with Paget's disease. *J Bone Miner Res* 1996;11:1602–1607.

26. Roodman GD, Kurihara N, Ohsaki Y, et al. Interleukin-6: a potential autocrine/paracrine factor in Paget's disease of bone. *J Clin Invest* 1992;89:46–52.

27. Rebel A, Basle M, Pouplard A, Malkani K. Filmon R, Lepatezour A. Bone tissue in Paget's disease of bone: ultrastructure and immunocytology. *Arthritis Rheum* 1980;23:1104–1114.

28. Uebelhart D, Ginetys E, Chapuy MC, Delmas PD. Urinary excretion of pyridinium crosslinks: a new marker of bone resorption in metabolic bone disease. *Bone Miner* 1990;8:87–96.

29. Meunier PJ, Coindre JM, Edouard CM, Arlot ME. Bone histomorphometry in Paget's disease: quantitative and dynamic analysis of pagetic and non-pagetic bone tissue. *Arthritis Rheum* 1980;23:1095–1103.

30. Siris ES, Clemens TP, McMahon D, Gordon AG, Jacobs TP, Canfield RE. Parathyroid function in Paget's disease of bone. *J Bone Miner Res* 1989;4:75–79.

31. Siris ES, Canfield RE. The parathyroids and Paget's disease of bone. In: Bilezikian J, Levine M, Marcus R, eds. *The parathyroids.* New York: Raven Press, 1994:823–828.

32. Siris ES. Indications for medical treatment of Paget's disease of bone. In: Singer FR, Wallach S, eds. *Paget's disease of bone: clinical assessment, present and future therapy.* New York: Elsevier, 1991:44–56.

33. Herzberg L, Bayliss E. Spinal cord syndrome due to non-compressive Paget's disease of bone: a spinal artery steal phenomenon reversible with calcitonin. *Lancet* 1980;2:13–15.

34. Monsell EM, Bone HG, Cody DD, et al. Hearing loss in Paget's disease of bone: evidence of auditory nerve integrity. *Am J Otol* 1995;16:27–33.

35. Barry HC. Orthopedic aspects of Paget's disease of bone. *Arthritis Rheum* 1980;23:1128–1130.

36. Wick MR, Siegal GP, Unni KK, McLeod RA, Greditzer HB. Sarcomas of bone complicating osteitis deformans (Paget's disease). *Am J Surg Pathol* 1981;5:47–59.

37. Upchurch KS, Simon LS, Schiller AL, Rosenthal DI, Campion EW, Krane SM. Giant cell reparative granulomas of Paget's disease of bone: a unique clinical entity. *Ann Intern Med* 1983;98:35–40.

38. Jacobs TP, Michelsen J, Polay J, D'Adamo AC, Canfield RE. Giant cell tumor in Paget's disease of bone: familial and geographic clustering. *Cancer* 1979;44:742–747.

39. Strickenberger SA, Schulman SP, Hutchins GM. Association of Paget's disease of bone with calcific aortic valve disease. *Am J Med* 1987;82:953–956.

40. Ryan WG, Schwartz TB, Perlia CP. Effects of mithramycin on Paget's disease of bone. *Ann Intern Med* 1969;70:549–557.

41. Delmas PD, Chapuy MC, Vignon E, et al. Long term effects of dichloromethylene diphosphonate in Paget's disease of bone. *J Clin Endocrinol Metab* 1982;54:837–844.

42. Fleisch H. *Bisphosphonates in bone disease.* 2nd ed. New York: Parthenon, 1995.

43. Arden-Cordone M, Siris ES, Lyles KW, et al. Antiresorptive effect of a single infusion of microgram quantities of zoledronate in Paget's disease of bone. *Calcif Tissue Int* 1997;60:415–418.

44. Bockman RS, Wilhelm F, Siris E, et al. A multicenter, prospective trial of gallium nitrate in patients with advanced Paget's disease of bone. *J Clin Endocrinol Metab* 1995;80:595–602.

45. El-Sammaa M, Linthicum FH, House HP, House JW. Calcitonin as treatment for hearing loss in Paget's disease. *Am J Otol* 1986;7:241–243.

46. Meunier PJ, Vignot E. Therapeutic strategy in Paget's disease of bone. *Bone* 1995;17:489S–491S.

47. Altman RD, Johnston CC, Khairi MRA, Wellman H, Serafini AN, Sankey RR. Influence of disodium etidronate on clinical and laboratory manifestations of Paget's disease of bone (osteitis deformans). *N Engl J Med* 1973;289:1379–1384.

48. Canfield R, Rosner W, Skinner J, et al. Diphosphonate therapy of Paget's disease of bone. *J Clin Endocrinol Metab* 1977;44:96–106.

49. Roux C, Gennari C, Farrerons J, et al. Comparative prospective, double-blind, multicenter study of the efficacy of tiludronate and etidronate in the treatment of Paget's disease of bone. *Arthritis Rheum* 1995;38:851–858.

50. McClung MR, Tou CPK, Goldstein NH, Picot C. Tiludronate therapy for Paget's disease of bone. *Bone* 1995;17:493S–496S.

51. Siris ES. Perspectives: a practical guide to the use of pamidronate in the treatment of Paget's disease. *J Bone Miner Res* 1994;9:303–304.

52. Harinck HI, Papapoulos SE, Blanksma HJ, Moolenaar AJ, Vermeij P, Bijvoet OL. Paget's disease of bone: early and late responses to three different modes of treatment with aminohydroxypropylidene bisphosphonate (APD). *Br Med J* 1987;295:1301–1305.

53. Adamson BB, Gallacher SJ, Byars J, Ralston SH, Boyle IT, Boyce BF. Mineralisation defects with pamidronate therapy for Paget's disease. *Lancet* 1993;342:1459–1460.

54. Siris E, Weinstein RS, Altman R, et al. Comparative study of alendronate vs. etidronate for the treatment of Paget's disease of bone. *J Clin Endocrinol Metab* 1996;81:961–967.

55. Reid IR, Nicholson GC, Weinstein RS, et al. Biochemical and radiologic improvement in Paget's disease of bone treated with alendronate: a randomized, placebo-controlled trial. *Am J Med* 1996;171:341–348.

56. Miller PD, Adachi JD, Brown JP, et al. Risedronate vs. etidronate: durable remission with only two months of 30 mg risedronate. *J Bone Miner Res* 1997;12:S270.

57. Siris ES, Chines AA, Altman RD, et al. Risedronate in the treatment of Paget's disease: an open-label, multicenter study. *J Bone Miner Res* 1998;13:1032–1038.

58. Woodhouse NJY, Bordier P, Fisher M, et al. Human calcitonin in the treatment of Paget's bone disease. *Lancet* 1971;1:1139–1143.

59. DeRose J, Singer F, Avramides A, et al. Response of Paget's disease to porcine and salmon calcitonins: effects of long term treatment. *Am J Med* 1974;56:858–866.

60. Singer FR, Ginger K. Resistance to calcitonin. In: Singer FR, Wallach S, eds. *Paget's disease of bone: clinical assessment, present and future therapy.* New York: Elsevier, 1991:75–85.

Extraskeletal (Ectopic) Calcification and Ossification

Introduction

Michael P. Whyte, M.D.

Division of Bone and Mineral Diseases, Washington University School of Medicine at Barnes–Jewish Hospital, and Metabolic Research Unit, Shriners Hospital for Children, St. Louis, Missouri

A significant number and variety of disorders cause extraskeletal deposition of calcium and phosphate (Table 1). In some, mineral is precipitated as amorphous calcium phosphate or as hydroxyapatite crystals; in others, bone tissue is formed. The pathogenesis of the ectopic mineralization in these conditions is generally ascribed to one of three mechanisms (Table 1). First, a supranormal "calcium/phosphate solubility product" in extracellular fluid can cause *metastatic* calcification. Alternatively, mineral may be deposited as *dystrophic* calcification into metabolically impaired or dead tissue despite normal serum levels of calcium and phosphate. Third, *ectopic* ossification or true bone formation occurs in a few disorders, for which the pathogenesis is poorly understood.

Discussed briefly in this section are these three mechanisms for extracellular calcification or ossification. Afterward, there follows a description of three principal disorders that illustrates each pathogenesis.

MECHANISMS FOR EXTRACELLULAR CALCIFICATION AND OSSIFICATION

Calcium and inorganic phosphate are normally present in serum or extracellular fluid at concentrations that form a "metastable" solution {i.e., their levels are too low for spontaneous precipitation but sufficiently great to cause hydroxyapatite $[Ca_{10}(PO_4)_6(OH)_2]$ formation once crystal nucleation has begun (1)}. Normally, the presence of a variety of inhibitors of mineralization, such as inorganic pyrophosphate, helps to prevent ectopic calcification from occurring in healthy tissues (2). The pathogenesis of metastatic and dystrophic calcification is partially understood at the cell level. The process typically involves mineral accumulation within matrix vesicles and sometimes within mitochondria (2). The pathogenesis of ectopic ossification is largely an enigma (see later).

Metastatic calcification is a risk if there is significant hypercalcemia or hyperphosphatemia (especially both) of any etiology (Table 1). In fact, therapy with phosphate supplements during mild hypercalcemia, or treatment with vitamin D or calcium during mild hyperphosphatemia, may trigger this problem (3).

Direct precipitation of mineral occurs when the calcium/phosphate solubility product in extracellular fluid is exceeded. A value of 75 for this parameter (milligrams/deciliter × milligrams/deciliter) is commonly taken as the level that, if surpassed, causes mineral precipitation. However, the critical value at which renal calcification might occur is not precisely defined and may vary with age (3). In adults, some

TABLE 1. *Disorders associated with extraskeletal calcification or ossification*

Metastatic calcification
  Hypercalcemia
    Milk-alkali syndrome
    Hypervitaminosis D
    Sarcoidosis
    Hyperparathyroidism
    Renal failure
  Hyperphosphatemia
    Tumoral calcinosis
    Hyperparathyroidism
    Pseudohypoparathyroidism
    Cell lysis after chemotherapy for leukemia
    Renal failure
Dystrophic calcification
  Calcinosis (universalis or circumscripta)
    Childhood dermatomyositis
    Scleroderma
    Systemic lupus erythematosus
  Posttraumatic
Ectopic ossification
  Myositis ossificans (posttraumatic)
    Burns
    Surgery
    Neurologic injury
  Fibrodysplasia (myositis) ossificans progressiva
  Progressive osseous heteroplasia

consider 70 to be the maximal safe value for the kidney. It is possible that children can tolerate a somewhat higher level, because they normally have higher serum phosphate levels compared with adults, but this is not well established (3). Mineral deposition can occur ectopically from hyperphosphatemia despite concomitant hypocalcemia.

The mineral that is deposited in metastatic calcification may be amorphous calcium phosphate initially, but hydroxyapatite is formed soon after (2). The pattern of deposition varies somewhat between hypercalcemia and hyperphosphatemia but occurs irrespective of the specific underlying condition or mechanism for the disturbed mineral homeostasis. There is a predilection for precipitation into certain tissues.

Hypercalcemia is typically associated with mineral deposits in the kidneys, lungs, and fundus of the stomach. In these "acid-secreting" organs or tissues, a local alkaline milieu may account for the calcium deposition. In addition, the media of large arteries, elastic tissue of the endocardium (especially the left atrium), conjunctiva, and periarticular soft tissues often are affected. However, the predisposition for these sites is not well understood. In the kidney, hypercalciuria may cause calcium phosphate casts to form within the tubule lumen or calculi to develop in the calyces or pelvis. Furthermore, calcium phosphate may precipitate in peritubular tissues. In the lung, calcification affects the alveolar walls and the pulmonary venous system. Wellestablished causes of metastatic calcification mediated by hypercalcemia include the milk-alkali syndrome, hypervitaminosis D, sarcoidosis, and hyperparathyroidism (Table 1).

Hyperphosphatemia of sufficient severity to cause metastatic calcification occurs with idiopathic hypoparathyroidism or pseudohypoparathyroidism and with the massive cell lysis (release of cellular phosphate) that can follow chemotherapy for leukemia (Table 1). Renal insufficiency is commonly associated with metastatic calcification—the mechanism may involve hyperphosphatemia, hypercalcemia, or both. Of interest, but unexplained, is the fact that ectopic calcification is more common in pseudohypoparathyroidism (type I) than in idiopathic hypoparathyroidism despite comparable elevations in serum phosphate levels. Furthermore, the location of ectopic calcification in pseudohypoparathyroidism and hypoparathyroidism (e.g., cerebral basal ganglion) is different from that which occurs from hypercalcemia. With hyperphosphatemia, calcification of periarticular subcutaneous tissues is characteristic and may be related to tissue trauma from the movement of joints (see later).

Dystrophic calcification occurs despite a normal serum calcium/phosphate solubility product. Injured tissue of any kind is predisposed to this type of extraskeletal calcification. Apparently such tissue can release material that has nucleating properties. One example of this phenomenon is the caseous lesion of tuberculosis. What local factor predisposes to the precipitation of calcium salts is unknown. Indeed, several mechanisms seem likely. It is clear that mineral precipitation into injured tissue is even more striking and more severe when either the calcium or phosphate level in extracellular fluid is increased. The deposited mineral, as for metastatic calcification, may be either amorphous calcium phosphate or crystalline hydroxyapatite.

The term *calcinosis* refers to an important type of dystrophic calcification that commonly occurs in (or under) the skin with connective tissue disorders—particularly dermatomyositis (discussed in this section), scleroderma, and systemic lupus erythematosus. Other etiologies for calcinosis include metastases and trauma that produces necrotic tissue. As the symptoms of the acute connective tissue disease and the inflammatory process in the subcutaneous tissues subside, painful masses of calcium phosphate appear under the skin. Calcinosis may involve a relatively localized area with small deposits in the skin and subcutaneous tissues, especially over the extensor aspects of the joints and the fingertips (*calcinosis circumscripta*); or it may be widespread and not only in the skin and subcutaneous tissues, but deeper in periarticular regions and areas of trauma as well (*calcinosis universalis*). The lesions of calcinosis are small or medium-sized hard nodules that can cause muscle atrophy and contractures.

Ectopic ossification is associated with two principal etiologies. It occurs with the fasciitis that follows neurologic injury, surgery, a burn, or trauma, in which it is called myositis ossificans. It occurs also as a principal feature of a separate, heritable entity—fibrodysplasia (myositis) ossificans progressiva—in which the pathogenesis is becoming understood (see Chapter 80). Some consider the primary reason for the ectopic bone formation in this latter condition to be a muscle abnormality (myositis ossificans progressiva), whereas others favor a connective tissue defect (fibrodysplasia ossificans progressiva). In these various conditions, "true" bone tissue is formed.

The bone is lamellar, actively remodeled by osteoblasts and osteoclasts, has haversian systems, and sometimes contains marrow. Apparently the injured or diseased tissue contains the necessary precursor cells and inductive signals to form osseous tissue.

Described in the following chapters are three conditions—tumoral calcinosis, dermatomyositis, and fibrodysplasia ossificans progressiva—that are principal examples of each type of ectopic mineralization.

REFERENCES

1. Fawthrop FW, Russell RGG. Ectopic calcification and ossification. In: Nordin BEC, Need AG, Morris HA, eds. *Metabolic bone and stone disease.* 3rd ed. Edinburgh: Churchill Livingstone, 1993:325–338.
2. Anderson HC. Calcific diseases: a concept. *Arch Pathol Lab Med* 1983;107:341–348.
3. Harrison HE, Harrison HC. *Disorders of calcium and phosphate metabolism in childhood and adolescence.* Philadelphia: WB Saunders, 1979:291–304.

78. Tumoral Calcinosis

Michael P. Whyte, M.D.

Division of Bone and Mineral Diseases, Washington University School of Medicine at Barnes–Jewish Hospital, and Metabolic Research Unit, Shriners Hospital for Children, St. Louis, Missouri

Tumoral calcinosis, first described in 1899, is a heritable disorder characterized by periarticular metastatic calcification (1). Mineral deposition manifests as soft-tissue masses around the major joints. Typically the hips and shoulders are affected, although additional joints can become involved (2). Visceral calcification does not occur, but segments of vasculature may contain mineral deposits (3). Hyperphosphatemia is a pathogenetic factor in many patients (4–6). The differential diagnosis includes periarticular metastatic calcification from hypercalcemia associated with renal failure, milk-alkali syndrome, sarcoidosis, and vitamin D intoxication.

CLINICAL PRESENTATION

Most patients in North America are black. About one third of cases are familial. Autosomal recessive inheritance is usually described, although autosomal dominant transmission also has been reported (1–3). There is no gender preference. Tumoral calcinosis often presents in childhood, but characteristic masses have been noted in infancy and in old age. Hyperphosphatemic patients are usually black, have a family history, manifest the disease before age 20 years, and have multiple lesions (5).

The soft-tissue tumors of ectopic calcification are typically painless and grow at variable rates (7). The major clinical complications of tumoral calcinosis are related to the metastatic calcifications that occur around joints and in skin, marrow, teeth, and blood vessels. After 1 or 2 years, the masses may be the size of an orange or grapefruit and weigh 1 kg or more. Often they are hard, lobulated, and firmly attached to deep fascia. Occasionally the swellings infiltrate into muscles and tendons (5). Because the deposits are extracapsular, joint range of motion is not impaired unless the tumors are particularly large. There can, however, be compression of adjacent neural structures. The lesions also can ulcerate the skin and form a sinus tract that drains a chalky fluid; this complication may lead to infection. Other potential secondary problems include anemia, low-grade fever, regional lymphadenopathy, splenomegaly, and amyloidosis. Some patients have features of *pseudoxanthoma elasticum* (i.e., skin and vascular calcifications and angioid streaks in the retina). A dental abnormality, featuring short bulbous roots and calcific deposits that often obliterate pulp chambers, is a characteristic finding (2,8). This is a life-long disorder.

RADIOGRAPHIC EXAMINATION

The tumors typically appear as large aggregations of irregular, densely calcified lobules that are confined to soft tissues (Fig. 1). Radiolucent fibrous septae account for the lobular appearance (9). Occasionally fluid layers are seen within the lobules. The joints *per se* are unaffected. Bone texture and

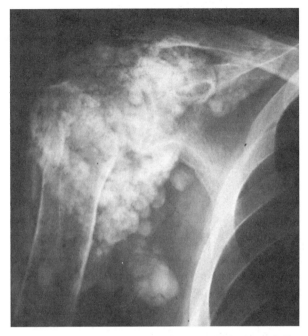

FIG. 1. Tumoral calcinosis. Lobular, periarticular calcifications are present at the right shoulder of this middle-aged man.

density also are unremarkable. Periarticular masses that are radiologically indistinguishable from those of tumoral calcinosis occur in chronic renal failure when mineral homeostasis is poorly controlled.

A "diaphysitis" has been recognized by using radiographs, computerized tomography (CT), or magnetic resonance imaging (MRI) in some cases of tumoral calcinosis. This finding may be confused with osteomyelitis or a neoplasm (10). New-bone formation occurs along the endosteal surface of the diaphysis, perhaps from calcific myelitis (7). When only calcific myelitis is present, CT and MRI a excellent tools for diagnosis (10). Bone scanning, howeve is the best method to detect and localize the calcified masse

LABORATORY FINDINGS

Serum calcium levels and alkaline phosphatase activit are usually normal. Hyperphosphatemia and increased seru calcitriol levels occur in some patients (5,11). The phospha transport maximum/glomerular filtration rate (TmP/GFF may be supranormal, but renal function is otherwise unr markable. Patients are in positive calcium/phosphate ba ance. Renal studies reflect both the ongoing calcium an phosphate retention, and some patients are frankly hypc calciuric. The chalky fluid found in lesions is predominantl hydroxyapatite (12,13).

HISTOPATHOLOGY

The masses of tumoral calcinosis are essentially foreign-body granuloma reactions that form multilocular, cystic structures (14). The early lesion may involve hemorrhage and histiocyte accumulation (14,15). There are ill-defined reactive-like perivascular solid cell nests admixed with mononuclear and iron-loaded macrophages, or well-organized variably sized fibrohistiocytic nodules embedded in a dense collagenous stroma (14). The cysts have tough connective tissue capsules, and their fibrous walls contain numerous foreign-body giant cells. Mature lesions are filled with calcareous material in a viscous milky fluid. Occasionally spicules of spongy bone and cartilage are found as well.

ETIOLOGY AND PATHOGENESIS

The genetic basis for tumoral calcinosis is unknown (1). The precise pathogenesis is poorly understood but may lie within the renal tubule cell. Increased renal reclamation of filtered phosphate seems to be an important pathogenetic factor (6). In hyperphosphatemic patients, enhanced renal tubular reabsorption of phosphate occurs independent of suppressed serum parathyroid hormone (PTH) levels (5,11). Deranged regulation of renal 25-hydroxyvitamin D, 1α-hydroxylase causes increased calcitriol synthesis. Consequently there is enhanced absorption of dietary calcium and suppression of serum PTH levels (5,11).

The masses may begin as calcific bursitis but then grow into adjacent fascial planes. Tissue damage with fat necrosis can be a pathogenetic factor (13).

TREATMENT

Surgical removal of subcutaneous calcified masses may be helpful if they are painful, interfere with function, or are cosmetically unacceptable. When excision of a tumor is complete, recurrence appears to be unlikely (16).

Radiation therapy and cortisone treatment have not been effective. Although it might seem that large apatite crystals would be refractory, dissolution of calcific tumors after aluminum hydroxide therapy (together with dietary phosphate and calcium deprivation) has been reported (4,17,18). Furthermore, reduction of phosphate levels in extracellular fluid could help to prevent re-formation of mineral deposits (4). Preliminary studies indicate that calcitonin therapy also may be efficacious by enhancing renal clearance of phosphate

(19). Acetazolamide together with aluminum hydroxide seemed to be helpful for one patient (20).

REFERENCES

1. McKusick VA. *Mendelian inheritance in man: a catalog of human genes and genetic disorders.* 12th ed. Baltimore: The Johns Hopkins University Press, 1998.
2. Lyles KW, Burkes EJ, Ellis GJ, et al. Genetic transmission of tumoral calcinosis: autosomal dominant with variable clinical expressivity. *J Clin Endocrinol Metab* 1985;60:1093–1096.
3. McGuinness FE. Hyperphosphataemic tumoral calcinosis in Bedouin Arabs: clinical and radiological features. *Clin Radiol* 1995;50:259–264.
4. Mozaffarian G, Lafferty FW, Pearson OH. Treatment of tumoral calcinosis with phosphorus deprivation. *Ann Intern Med* 1972;77:741–745.
5. Prince MJ, Schaefer PC, Goldsmith RS, Chausmer AB. Hyperphosphatemic tumoral calcinosis: association with elevation of serum 1,25-dihydroxy-cholecalciferol concentrations. *Ann Intern Med* 1982;96:586–591.
6. Smack D, Norton SA, Fitzpatrick JE. Proposal for a pathogenesis-based classification of tumoral calcinosis. *Int J Dermatol* 1996;35:265–271.
7. Narchi H. Hyperostosis with hyperphosphatemia: evidence of familial occurrence and association with tumoral calcinosis. *Pediatrics* 1997;99:745–748.
8. Burkes EJ Jr, Lyles KW, Dolan EA, Giammara B, Hanker J. Dental lesions in tumoral calcinosis. *Oral Pathol Med* 1991;20:222–227.
9. Steinbach LS, Johnston JO, Tepper EF, Honda GD, Martel W. Tumoral calcinosis: radiologic-pathologic correlation. *Skeletal Radiol* 1995;24:573–578.
10. Martinez S, Vogler JB, Harrelson JM, Lyles KW. Imaging of tumoral calcinosis: new observations. *Radiology* 1990;174:215–222.
11. Lyles KW, Halsey DL, Friedman NE, Lobaugh B. Correlations of serum concentrations of 1,25-dihydroxyvitamin D, phosphorus, and parathyroid hormone in tumoral calcinosis. *J Clin Endocrinol Metab* 1988;67:88–92.
12. Boskey AL, Vigorita VJ, Sencer O, Stuchin SA, Lane JM. Chemical, microscopic and ultrastructural characterization of mineral deposits in tumoral calcinosis. *Clin Orthop* 1983;178:258–270.
13. Kindbolm L-G, Gunterberg B. Tumoral calcinosis: an ultrastructural analysis and consideration of pathogenesis. *APMIS* 1988;96:368–376.
14. Pakasa NM, Kalengayi RM. Tumoral calcinosis: a clinicopathological study of 111 cases with emphasis on the earliest changes. *Histopathology* 1997;31:18–24.
15. Slavin RE, Wen J, Kumar WJ, Evans EB. Familial tumoral calcinosis: a clinical, histopathologic, and ultrastructural study with an analysis of its calcifying process and pathogenesis. *Am J Surg Pathol* 1993;17:788–802.
16. Noyez JF, Murphree SM, Chen K. Tumoral calcinosis, a clinical report of eleven cases. *Acta Orthop Belg* 1993;59:249–254.
17. Davies M, Clements MR, Mawer EB, Freemont AJ. Tumoral calcinosis: clinical and metabolic response to phosphorus deprivation. *Q J Med* 1987;242:493–503.
18. Gregosiewicz A, Warda E. Tumoral calcinosis: successful medical treatment. *J Bone Joint Surg Am* 1989;71:1244–1249.
19. Salvi A, Cerudelli B, Cimino A, Zuccato F, Giustina G. Phosphaturic action of calcitonin in pseudotumoral calcinosis [Letter]. *Horm Metab Res* 1983;15:260.
20. Yamaguchi T, Sugimoto T, Imai Y, Fukase M, Fujita T, Chihara K. Successful treatment of hyperphosphatemic tumoral calcinosis with long-term acetazolamide. *Bone* 1995;16:247S–250S.

79. Dermatomyositis

Michael P. Whyte, M.D.

Division of Bone and Mineral Diseases, Washington University School of Medicine at Barnes–Jewish Hospital, and Metabolic Research Unit, Shriners Hospital for Children, St. Louis, Missouri

Dermatomyositis is a multisystem connective tissue disorder caused by small-vessel vasculitis. Acute and chronic non-suppurative inflammation involves especially the skin and striated muscles. Dystrophic calcification often follows episodes of inflammation and can be severely debilitating (1–5).

CLINICAL PRESENTATION

There are more female than male patients and two peak ages of incidence: childhood (5 to 15 years) and adulthood (50 to 60 years). When the disorder manifests before age 16 years, it is called juvenile or childhood dermatomyositis (1–5). The adult form is associated with malignancy.

In juvenile dermatomyositis, the patient's sex and the age-of-onset of symptoms seem unrelated to the severity of calcinosis, although increased time to diagnosis and treatment worsen this complication (6). Calcification is generally noted 1 to 3 years after the disease onset and occurs in 25% to 50% of patients; however, calcinosis may predate the myopathy (7). Mineral deposits develop over a period of 1 to 3 years. In calcinosis universalis (see later), calcification occurs throughout the subcutaneous tissues, but primarily in periarticular regions or in areas that are subject to trauma (Fig. 1). In calcinosis circumscripta, the deposits are more localized and typically occur around joints. The ectopic mineralization can cause pain, ulcerate the skin, limit mobility, result in contractures, and predispose to abscess formation. Although the dystrophic calcification then typically remains stable, some spontaneous resolution has been reported, although not quantitated (1–5).

LABORATORY FINDINGS

Mineral metabolism in juvenile dermatomyositis has been studied (8). Hypercalcemia with hypercalciuria and hyperphosphaturia may occur, although these values are usually normal. Elevated levels of γ-carboxyglutamic acid have been found in the urine of children with dermatomyositis, especially if there is calcinosis (9).

RADIOGRAPHIC FINDINGS

In juvenile dermatomyositis, four types of dystrophic calcification occur (10):

1. Superficial masses (small circumscribed nodules or plaques) within the skin;
2. Deep discrete subcutaneous nodular masses (see Fig. 1) near joints that can impair movement (calcinosis circumscripta);
3. Deep, linear, sheet-like deposits within intramuscular fascial planes (calcinosis universalis); and
4. Lacy reticular subcutaneous deposits that encase the torso to form a generalized "exoskeleton."

Children with severe disease that is refractory to medical therapy seem to be especially prone to developing exoskeleton-like calcifications. The exoskeleton is in turn associated with severe calcinosis and poor physical function.

ETIOLOGY AND PATHOGENESIS

Juvenile dermatomyositis appears to be a form of complement-mediated microangiopathy (11). There seems to be an association with the HLA-DQA1*051 allele (12). The precise cause of the dystrophic calcification, however, is unknown. Immune deficiencies may predispose the patient to this complication (13). Calcinosis seems to occur in the majority of long-term survivors and may reflect a scarring process. This hypothesis is supported by the observation that mineral deposition seems to occur primarily in the muscles that were most severely affected during the acute phase of the disease. Electron microscopy shows that the calcification consists of hydroxyapatite crystals (14).

A variety of mechanisms have been considered for the dystrophic calcification, including release of alkaline phosphatase or discharge of free fatty acids from diseased muscle that, in turn, directly precipitate calcium or first bind acid mucopolysaccharides. Increased urinary levels of γ-carboxylated peptides suggest that calcium-binding proteins may be responsible for the mineral deposition.

TREATMENT

High-dose prednisone therapy soon after the onset of symptoms seems to be important for minimizing the risk of calcinosis and for ensuring good functional recovery (1,2,15,16). If the response is incomplete, consideration is given to additional immunosuppressive agents (2,4), including cyclosporine (17). Phosphate-binding antacid therapy may reverse the mineral deposition (18). In a small clinical trial, warfarin sodium treatment to decrease γ-carboxylation was not associated with changes in calcium or phosphorus excretion or in a reduction of calcinosis (19). Remarkable resolution of calcinosis universalis occurred in a young man treated with probenecid to improve renal handling of phosphate (20), and positive response to diltiazem has been described (21). Troublesome calcium deposits can be removed surgically.

PROGNOSIS

The clinical course of dermatomyositis in children is variable. Some have long-term relapsing or persistent disease, whereas others recover. When recovery is incomplete, there may be severe residual weakness, joint contractures, and calcinosis. The calcinosis may be the principal cause of long-term disability (1–5,20).

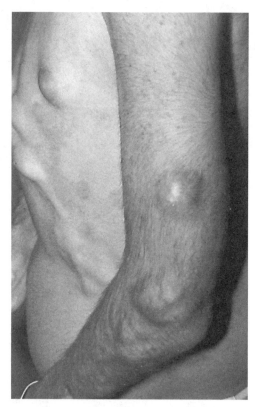 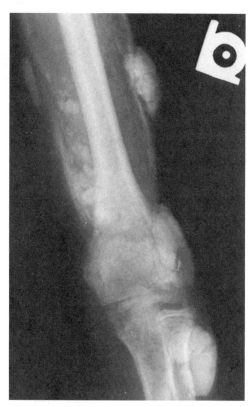

FIG. 1. *Calcinosis universalis* in childhood dermatomyositis. **A:** Characteristic subcutaneous nodules are apparent in the left arm and anterior chest wall of this 15-year-old boy. **B:** The nodules in this boy's arm are composed of dense lobular calcifications. In addition, the muscles of the upper arm are encased in a characteristic calcified sheath.

REFERENCES

1. Pachman LM. Juvenile dermatomyositis: pathophysiology and disease expression. *Pediatr Clin North Am* 1995;42:1071–1098.
2. Kaye SA, Isenberg DA. Treatment of polymyositis and dermatomyositis. *Br J Hosp Med* 1994;52:463–468.
3. Pachman LM. Juvenile dermatomyositis: new clues to diagnosis and pathogenesis. *Clin Exp Rheumatol* 1994;12(suppl 10):S69–S73.
4. Ansell BM. Juvenile dermatomyositis. *J Rheumatol Suppl* 1992; 33:60–62.
5. Olson JC. Juvenile dermatomyositis. *Dermatologica* 1992;11:57–64.
6. Pachman LM, Hayford JR, Chung A, et al. Juvenile dermatomyositis at diagnosis: clinical characteristics of 79 children. *J Rheumatol* 1998;25:1198–1204.
7. Wananukul S, Pongprasit P, Wattanakrai P. Calcinosis cutis presenting years before other clinical manifestations of juvenile dermatomyositis: report of two cases. *Australas J Dermatol* 1997;38:202–205.
8. Perez MD, Abrams SA, Koenning G, Stuff JE, O'Brien KO, Ellis KJ. Mineral metabolism in children with dermatomyositis. *J Rheumatol* 1994;21:2364–2369.
9. Lian JB, Pachman LM, Gundberg CM, Partridge REH, Maryjowski MC. Gamma-carboxyglutamate excretion and calcinosis in juvenile dermatomyositis. *Arthritis Rheum* 1982;25:1094–1100.
10. Blane CE, White SJ, Braunstein EM, Bowyer SL, Sullivan DB. Patterns of calcification in childhood dermatomyositis. *Am J Roentgenol* 1984;142:397–400.
11. Kissel JT, Mendell JR, Rammohan KW. Microvascular deposition of complement membrane attack complex in dermatomyositis. *N Engl J Med* 1986;314:329–334.
12. Reed AM, Pachman LM, Hayford J, Ober C. Immunogenetic studies in families of children with juvenile dermatomyositis. *J Rheumatol* 1998;25:1000–1002.
13. Moore EC, Cohen F, Douglas SD, Gutta V. Staphylococcal infections in childhood dermatomyositis: association with the development of calcinosis, raised IgE concentrations and granulocyte chemotactic defect. *Ann Rheum Dis* 1992;51:378–383.
14. Landis WJ. The strength of a calcified tissue depends in part on the molecular structure and organization of its constituent mineral crystals in their organic matrix. *Bone* 1995;16:533–544.
15. Bowyer SL, Blane CE, Sullivan DB, Cassidy JT. Childhood dermatomyositis: factors predicting functional outcome and development of dystrophic calcification. *J Pediatr* 1983;103:882–888.
16. DeSilva TN, Kress DW. Management of collagen vascular diseases in childhood. *Dermatol Clin* 1998;6:579–592.
17. Reiff A, Rawlings DJ, Shaham B, et al. Preliminary evidence for cyclosporin A as an alternative in the treatment of recalcitrant juvenile rheumatoid arthritis and juvenile dermatomyositis. *J Rheumatol* 1997;24:2436–2443.
18. Wang W-J, Lo W-L, Wong CK. Calcinosis cutis/juvenile dermatomyositis: remarkable response to aluminum hydroxide therapy [Letter]. *Arch Dermatol* 1988;124:1721–1722.
19. Moore SE, Jump AA, Smiley JD. Effect of warfarin sodium therapy on excretion of 4-carboxy-L-glutamic acid in scleroderma, dermatomyositis, and myositis ossificans progressiva. *Arthritis Rheum* 1986;29:344–351.
20. Eddy MC, Leelawattana R, McAlister WH, Whyte MP. Calcinosis universalis complicating juvenile dermatomyositis: resolution during probenecid therapy. *J Clin Endocrinol Metab* 1997;82:3536–3542.
21. Oliveri MB, Palermo R, Mautalen C, Hubscher O. Regression of calcinosis during diltiazem treatment in juvenile dermatomyositis. *J Rheumatol* 1996;23:2152–2155.

80. Fibrodysplasia (Myositis) Ossificans Progressiva

Frederick S. Kaplan, M.D., *Eileen M. Shore, Ph.D., and †Michael P. Whyte, M.D.

*Division of Molecular Orthopaedics and Metabolic Bone Diseases, Department of Orthopaedics; *Department of Orthopaedic Surgery, The University of Pennsylvania School of Medicine, Philadelphia, Pennsylvania; and †Division of Bone and Mineral Diseases, Washington University School of Medicine at Barnes–Jewish Hospital, and Metabolic Research Unit, Shriners Hospital for Children, St. Louis, Missouri*

Fibrodysplasia ossificans progressiva (FOP), also called myositis ossificans progressiva, is a rare heritable connective tissue disease characterized by (a) congenital malformation of the great toes, and (b) recurrent episodes of painful soft-tissue swelling that lead to heterotopic ossification (1–3).

Posttraumatic myositis ossificans, a different disorder, also features bone and cartilage formation within soft tissues. In this sporadic condition, injured sites may initially be painful, warm, and feel "doughy," but 4 to 6 weeks later, they contain mineralization that is apparent radiographically. Heterotopic ossification also may follow hip replacement and spinal cord injury.

FOP was first described in 1692; more than 600 cases have been reported (2). This disorder is among the rarest of human afflictions, with an estimated incidence of one per two million live births in Great Britain (2). Although white patients have been described most often, all races are affected (2). Autosomal dominant transmission with variable expressivity is established (4,5). However, reproductive fitness is low, and most cases are sporadic. Gonadal mosaicism seems to explain FOP isolated in sibships (6).

CLINICAL PRESENTATION

If the typical congenital skeletal malformations are recognized, FOP can be suspected at birth before soft-tissue lesions occur (1–3). The characteristic feature is short big toes caused by malformation (hallux valgus) of the cartilaginous anlage of the first metatarsal and proximal phalanx (Fig. 1). In some patients, the thumbs also are strikingly short. Synostosis and hypoplasia of the phalanges is typical (7). Nevertheless, the digital anomalies are not pathognomonic. FOP is usually diagnosed when soft-tissue swellings and radiographic evidence of heterotopic ossification are first noted (1–3).

The severity of FOP differs significantly among patients (8), although most become immobilized and confined to a wheelchair by the third decade of life (1,7,9). Typically, episodes of soft-tissue swelling begin during the first decade (10). Occasionally, the onset is as late as early adulthood. There are also reports of *in utero* involvement. Painful, tender, and rubbery soft-tissue lesions appear spontaneously or may seem to be precipitated by minor trauma including intramuscular injections (11). Swellings develop rapidly during the course of several days. Fever may occur during periods of induration and can erroneously suggest an infectious process (2,7). Typically, lesions affect the paraspinal muscles in the back or in the limb girdles and may persist for several months (12). Aponeuroses, fascia, tendons, ligaments, and connective tissue of voluntary muscles may be affected. Although some swellings may regress spontaneously, most mature through an endochondral pathway, en-

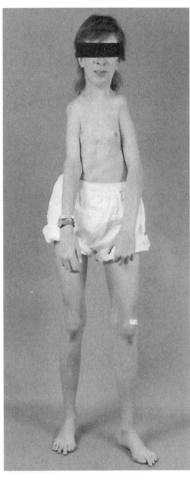

FIG. 1. Fibrodysplasia (myositis) ossificans progressiva. Severe underdevelopment of the chest has occurred from ectopic bone formation in the thorax of this 16-year-old boy. Also note the characteristic malformations of his great toes.

gendering true heterotopic bone (12). The episodes of induration recur with unpredictable frequency. Some patients seem to have periods of quiescent disease. However, once ossification develops, it is permanent.

Gradually, bony masses immobilize joints and cause contractures and deformity, particularly in the neck and shoulders. Ossification around the hips, typically present by the third decade of life, often prevents ambulation (9). Involvement of the muscles of mastication (frequently the outcome of injection of local anesthetic or overstretching of the jaw during dental procedures) can severely limit movement of the mandible and ultimately impair nutrition (13,14). Ankylosis of the spine and rib cage further restricts mobility and may imperil cardiopulmonary function (2,9,15). Scoliosis is

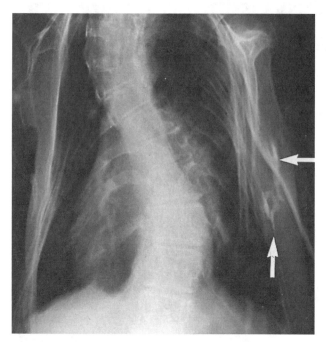

FIG. 2. At age 15 years, the thorax of the boy shown in Fig. 1 was markedly narrowed by ectopic bone within his chest wall *(arrows)*. Scoliosis also was present and contributed to restrictive lung disease that proved lethal 1 year later.

common and associated with heterotopic bone that asymmetrically connects the rib cage to the pelvis (Figs. 1 and 2) (16). Hypokyphosis results from ossification of the paravertebral musculature. Restrictive lung disease with predisposition to pneumonia may follow. However, the vocal muscles, diaphragm, extraocular muscles, heart, and smooth muscles are characteristically spared (2,7). Although secondary amenorrhea may develop, reproduction has occurred (2,5,7). Hearing impairment (beginning in late childhood or adolescence) and alopecia also manifest with increased frequency (1,2,7).

RADIOLOGIC FEATURES

Skeletal anomalies and soft-tissue ossification are the characteristic radiographic features of FOP (17). The principal malformations involve the great toe, although other anomalies of digits in the feet and hands may occur. Exostoses are frequent (2,7,12). A remarkable feature of FOP is progressive fusion of cervical vertebrae that may be confused with Klippel–Feil syndrome or Still's disease (2,7,17). The femoral necks may be broad yet short. However, the remainder of the skeleton is unremarkable (17).

Ectopic ossification in FOP progresses in several regular patterns or gradients (proximally before distally, axially before appendicularly, cranially before caudally, and dorsally before ventrally) (10). Paraspinal muscles are involved early in life, with subsequent spread to the shoulders and hips. The ankles, wrists, and jaw may be affected later.

Radiographic and bone-scan findings suggest normal modeling and remodeling of heterotopic bone (18). Fractures

are not increased but respond similarly in either the heterotopic or normotopic skeleton (19).

Bone scans are abnormal before ossification can be demonstrated by conventional radiography (18). Computerized tomography and magnetic resonance imaging of early lesions has been described (20).

LABORATORY FINDINGS

Routine biochemical studies of mineral metabolism are usually normal, although alkaline phosphatase activity in serum may be increased, especially during disease "flare-ups" (2,7,21).

HISTOPATHOLOGY

The earliest FOP lesion consists of significant aggregation of B and T lymphocytes in perivascular spaces of otherwise normal-appearing skeletal muscle (22). Subsequently, a nearly pure T-cell infiltrate is seen between edematous muscle fibers at the leading edge of an angiogenic fibroproliferative lesion, which is indistinguishable from *aggressive juvenile fibromatosis* (22,23). Misdiagnosis is common, but can be avoided simply by examining the patient's *toes*. Immunostaining with a monoclonal antibody against bone morphogenetic protein (BMP) 2/4 is intense in FOP lesions, but not in aggressive fibromatosis (23). Endochondral ossification is the major pathway for heterotopic bone formation (12). Mature osseous lesions have haversian systems. Cancellous bone can contain hematopoietic tissue.

ETIOLOGY AND PATHOGENESIS

The genetic defect causing FOP has not been mapped (4,5). Disregulation of BMP4 gene expression has been reported (24,25), but mutational screening and linkage-exclusion analysis indicate that the molecular defect lies elsewhere (26). Similarities between FOP and the decapentaplegic mutation of *Drosophila* may represent clues to FOP etiology and pathogenesis (27).

TREATMENT

There is no established medical treatment for FOP (1–3). The disorder's rarity, variable severity, and fluctuating clinical course pose substantial uncertainties when evaluating experimental therapies. Adrenocorticotropic hormone (ACTH), corticosteroids, binders of dietary calcium, intravenous infusion of ethylenediaminetetraacetic acid (EDTA), nonsteroidal antiinflammatory agents, radiotherapy, disodium etidronate, and warfarin are ineffective (1–3,28). Limited benefits have been reported using corticosteroids and disodium etidronate together during flare-ups, and by using isotretinoin to prevent disease activation (29,30). However, these impressions reflect uncontrolled studies. Accordingly, medical intervention is currently supportive. Nevertheless, physical therapy to maintain joint mobility may be harmful by provoking or exacerbating lesions (7). Surgical release of joint contractures is unsuccessful and risks new, trauma-induced heterotopic ossification (7). Removal of FOP lesions is often followed by significant recurrence. Osteotomy of ectopic bone to mobilize a joint is uniformly counterproductive because additional heterotopic ossification develops at the operative site. Spinal bracing is ineffective, and surgical intervention is associated with numerous complications (16). Dental therapy should preclude injection of local anesthetics and stretching of the jaw (2,13,14). In fact, newer dental techniques for focused administration of anesthetic are available. Guidelines for general anesthesia have been reported (13). Intramuscular injections should be avoided (11). Prevention of falls is crucial (31). Measures against recurrent pulmonary infections and the onset of cardiopulmonary complications of restrictive lung disease are important.

PROGNOSIS

Despite widespread heterotopic ossification and severe disability, some patients live productive lives into the seventh decade. Most, however, die earlier of pulmonary complications, including pneumonia, secondary to restricted ventilation from chest-wall involvement (2,7,15).

REFERENCES

1. Smith R. Fibrodysplasia (myositis) ossificans progressiva: clinical lessons from a rare disease. *Clin Orthop* 1998;346:7–14.
2. Connor JM. Fibrodysplasia ossificans progressiva. In: Royce PM, Steinmann B, eds. *Connective tissue and its heritable disorders.* New York: Wiley-Liss, 1993:603–611.
3. Beighton P. Fibrodysplasia ossificans progressiva. In: Beighton P, ed. *Heritable disorders of connective tissue.* St. Louis: Mosby, 1993:501–518.
4. McKusick VA. *Mendelian inheritance in man: a catalog of human genes and genetic disorders.* 12th ed. Baltimore: The Johns Hopkins University Press, 1998.
5. Delatycki M, Rogers JG. The genetics of fibrodysplasia ossificans progressiva. *Clin Orthop* 1998;346:15–18.
6. Janoff HB, Muenke M, Johnson LO, et al. Fibrodysplasia ossificans progressiva in two half-sisters: evidence for maternal mosaicism. *Am J Med Genet* 1996;61:320–324.
7. Connor JM, Evans DA. Fibrodysplasia ossificans progressiva: the clinical features and natural history of 34 patients. *J Bone Joint Surg Br* 1982;64:76–83.
8. Janoff HB, Tabas JA, Shore EM, et al. Mild expression of fibrodysplasia ossificans progressiva: a report of 3 cases. *J Rheumatol* 1995;22: 976–978.
9. Rocke DM, Zasloff M, Peeper J, Cohen RB, Kaplan FS. Age and joint-specific risk of initial heterotopic ossification in patients who have fibrodysplasia ossificans progressiva. *Clin Orthop* 1994;301:243–248.
10. Cohen RB, Hahn GV, Tabas JA, et al. The natural history of heterotopic ossification in patients who have fibrodysplasia ossificans progressiva: a study of 44 patients. *J Bone Joint Surg Am* 1993;75:215–219.
11. Lanchoney TF, Cohen RB, Rocke DM, Zasloff MA, Kaplan FS. Permanent heterotopic ossification at the injection site after diphtheria-teta-nus-pertussis immunizations in children who have fibrodysplasia ossificans progressiva. *J Pediatr* 1995;126:762–764.
12. Kaplan FS, Tabas JA, Gannon FH, Finkel G, Hahn GV, Zasloff MA. The histopathology of fibrodysplasia ossificans progressiva: an endochondral process. *J Bone Joint Surg Am* 1993;75:220–230.
13. Luchetti W, Cohen RB, Hahn GV, et al. Severe restriction in jaw movement after routine injection of local anesthetic in patients who have fibrodysplasia ossificans progressiva. *Oral Surg Oral Med Oral Pathol Oral Radiol Endod* 1996;81:21–25.
14. Janoff HB, Zasloff MA, Kaplan FS. Submandibular swelling in patients with fibrodysplasia ossificans progressiva. *Otolaryngol Head Neck Surg* 1996;114:599–604.
15. Kussmaul WG, Esmail AN, Sagar Y, Ross J, Gregory S, Kaplan FS. Pulmonary and cardiac function in advanced fibrodysplasia ossificans progressiva. *Clin Orthop* 1998;346:104–109.
16. Shah PB, Zasloff MA, Drummond D, Kaplan FS. Spinal deformity in patients who have fibrodysplasia ossificans progressiva. *J Bone Joint Surg Am* 1994;76:1442–1450.
17. Cremin B, Connor JM, Beighton P. The radiological spectrum of fibrodysplasia ossificans progressiva. *Clin Radiol* 1982;33:499–508.
18. Kaplan FS, Strear CM, Zasloff MA. Radiographic and scintigraphic features of modeling and remodeling in the heterotopic skeleton of patients who have fibrodysplasia ossificans progressiva. *Clin Orthop* 1994;304:238–247.
19. Einhorn TA, Kaplan FS. Traumatic fractures of heterotopic bone in patients who have fibrodysplasia ossificans progressiva: a report of 2 cases. *Clin Orthop* 1994;308:173–177.
20. Shirkhoda A, Armin AR, Bis KG, Makris J, Irwin RB, Shetty AN. MR imaging of myositis ossificans: variable patterns at different stages. *J Magn Reson Imaging* 1995;5:287–292.
21. Lutwak L. Myositis ossificans progressiva: mineral, metabolic, and radioactive calcium studies of the effects of hormones. *Am J Med* 1964;37:269–293.
22. Gannon FH, Valentine BA, Shore EM, Zasloff MA, Kaplan FS. Acute lymphocytic infiltration in an extremely early lesion of fibrodysplasia ossificans progressiva. *Clin Orthop* 1998;346:19–25.
23. Gannon FH, Kaplan FS, Olmsted E, Finkel GC, Zasloff MA, Shore E. Bone morphogenetic protein 2/4 in early fibromatous lesions of fibrodysplasia ossificans and aggressive juvenile fibromatosis. *Hum Pathol* 1997;28:339–343.
24. Shafritz AB, Shore EM, Gannon FH, et al. Overexpression of an osteogenic morphogen in fibrodysplasia ossificans progressiva. *N Engl J Med* 1996;335:555–561.
25. Lanchoney TF, Olmsted EA, Shore EM, et al. Characterization of bone morphogenetic protein 4 receptor in fibrodysplasia ossificans progressiva. *Clin Orthop* 1998;346:38–45.
26. Xu M, Shore EM. Mutational screening of the bone morphogenetic protein 4 gene in a family with fibrodysplasia ossificans progressiva. *Clin Orthop* 1998;346:53–58.
27. Kaplan FS, Tabas JA, Zasloff MA. Fibrodysplasia ossificans progressiva: a clue from the fly? *Calcif Tissue Int* 1990;47:117–125.
28. Moore SE, Jump AA, Smiley JD. Effect of warfarin sodium therapy on excretion of 4-carboxy-L-glutamic acid in scleroderma, dermatomyositis, and myositis ossificans progressiva. *Arthritis Rheum* 1986;29: 344–351.
29. Brantus JF, Meunier PJ. Effects of intravenous etidronate and oral corticosteroids in fibrodysplasia ossificans progressiva. *Clin Orthop* 1998;346:117–120.
30. Zasloff MA, Rocke DM, Crofford LJ, Hahn GV, Kaplan FS. Treatment of patients who have fibrodysplasia ossificans progressiva with isotretinoin. *Clin Orthop* 1998;346:121–129.
31. Glaser DL, Rocke DM, Kaplan FS. Catastrophic falls in patients who have fibrodysplasia ossificans progressiva. *Clin Orthop* 1998;346: 110–116.

SECTION XI

Nephrolithiasis

81. Nephrolithiasis

Fredric L. Coe, M.D. and *Joan H. Parks, M.B.A.

*Nephrology Section, Department of Medicine; and *Kidney Stone Program, The University of Chicago, Chicago, Illinois*

All kidney stones are aggregates of crystals mixed with a protein matrix, and all cause disease because of obstruction of urine flow in the renal collecting system, ureters, or urethra; bleeding; or local erosion into the kidney tissue. The common stone is calcium oxalate; this stone is small, recurrent, a cause of pain from passage and obstruction, and caused by metabolic disorders that mostly are treatable (1). Uric acid stones are uncommon (about 5% of all stones) and radiolucent but otherwise like calcium oxalate stones. Struvite stones, from infection, fill renal collecting systems, erode into the renal tissue, and cause obvious renal functional impairment. Cystine stones have only one cause, hereditary cystinuria. They grow large enough to fill the renal collecting system, begin in childhood, and can cause renal failure. Kidney stones are expensive, and it has been shown that it is cost effective to prevent them (1).

All stones need crystallographic analysis, by simple polarization microscopy, or x-ray diffraction when needed. Even if the first few stones are shown to contain uric acid, for example, the next may contain calcium oxalate or struvite. Radiographs are not helpful for identification except in the case of uric acid stones, which are lucent; the rest are similar, although some generalizations can be made: calcium oxalate stones resemble stars in the night sky, cystine stones are like eggs or staghorns and seem sculpted of a soft stone or wax, and struvite stones are mostly rugged, ringed staghorns that look like tree roots. We use flat plates to count stones; tomograms without prior radiocontrast injection are ideal but expensive. Laboratory evaluation is to detect causes, so measure 24-hour urine calcium, oxalate, uric acid, citrate, pH, volume, and creatinine to estimate completeness of collection. How many urine samples is best? One is certainly minimal; we favor three for better surety, and, if we found stones, we would measure four. Blood tests are for hypercalcemia; the rest is vague and unsure. Hormone measurements are never proper for initial evaluation; a parathyroid hormone (PTH) measurement is obtained for patients who are hypercalcemic.

CALCIUM STONES

Just as bone mineral forms when a supersaturated extracellular fluid contacts an appropriate nucleation site, kidney stones form when urine or, more probably, tubule fluid becomes highly supersaturated with a calcium salt such as calcium oxalate or a calcium phosphate phase. What distinguishes the two processes are the greater levels of supersaturation in urine compared with plasma, the presence in urine and tubule fluid of powerful inhibitors of the crystallization process, and the fact that calcium oxalate, not calcium phosphate, is the main constituent of stones. The causes of calcium stones can have other effects. They increase urine calcium or oxalate concentration; lower urine volume, so concentrations of all solutes increase; lower urine citrate, which normally forms a soluble salt with calcium and pre- vents crystallization; increase levels of molecules (uric acid in particular) that can promote calcium oxalate nucleation; or cause abnormally high urine pH, which promotes calcium phosphate crystallization, or low urine pH, which promotes uric acid crystallization.

Hypercalciuric States

Idiopathic hypercalciuria (IH) (2), the most common hypercalciuric state, occurs in families, affects both sexes equally, and has a pattern of horizontal and vertical transmission like that of a mendelian dominant trait. About 50% of patients with calcium oxalate stones have IH and are detected by a daily urine calcium excretion rate above the usual normal limits of 300 mg (for men) and 250 mg (for women); by normal serum calcium level; and by the absence of other hypercalciuric conditions such as sarcoidosis, vitamin D intoxication, immobilization, hyperthyroidism, glucocorticoid excess, rapidly progressive osteoporosis, Paget's disease, and Cushing's disease (3). Hypercalciuria increases urine calcium oxalate supersaturation (4), especially after eating. The mechanism of the hypercalciuria is surely intestinal calcium absorption at an abnormally high rate (5), and what controversy exists concerns the cause of the high absorption rate. The most satisfactory view is that 1,25-dihydroxyvitamin D or calcitriol levels in the serum are high as a primary defect; in eight studies, hypercalciuric patients had higher levels than normal subjects (6–13). The high calcitriol levels can increase calcium absorption and suppress PTH secretion, leading to reduced renal tubule calcium reabsorption. After eating, calcium will enter the blood at a more rapid rate than normal, and tubule reabsorption will be low, so serum calcium levels can remain near normal despite high absorption rates, and the calcium can be excreted rapidly into the urine. Alternative theories include a primary renal tubule leak of calcium and a primary increase in intestinal calcium absorption. Neither would explain the common pattern of low PTH (10) and high calcitriol levels, but they could account for hypercalciuria in some selected patients with high PTH levels or normal calcitriol levels.

In addition to hyperabsorption of calcium, hypercalciuric patients conserve calcium less well than normal people when given a low calcium intake in the range of 200 to 500 mg daily. In balance studies, when total calcium absorption can be measured, their urine calcium clearly exceeds net calcium absorption on such diets, meaning that bone mineral is being mobilized into the urine. The reason for their labile bone mineral stores may partly be an excessive action of calcitriol. When given to normal men, this hormone promotes the same behavior as seen among patients with infectious hepatitis, a loss of bone mineral during low-calcium diet (12,13). High levels of serum calcitriol are by no means universal among the patients, despite almost universal calcium hyperabsorption, suggesting that not only high serum levels but possibly also high levels of the calcitriol receptor could mediate excessive calcitriol effects. In rats bred for hypercalciuria, increased calcitriol receptor number is an established cause of increased calcitriol action (14).

Given the lability of bone mineral and the natural tendency of doctors to use low-calcium diets for treatment of hypercalciuria, one might expect reduced bone mineral density among IH patients, and to date five studies documented just this (15). In particular, the patients whose hypercalciuria persists during low-calcium diet show decisively low bone mineral densities, whereas those with normal or near-normal calcium retention during low-calcium diet (a minority) have normal bone mineral density. A clinical corollary of this finding must be caution concerning low-calcium diet as a treatment except among patients clearly able to respond to it with normal calcium conservation. Among patients otherwise prone to osteoporosis, low-calcium diet has an additional and obvious disadvantage. For these reasons, we favor its use in only very restricted circumstances (16).

Thiazide diuretic agents reduce urine calcium excretion, calcium oxalate supersaturation (17), and the rate of stone production (18). Thiazide affects the connecting segment of the nephron (19), increasing calcium reabsorption rate, and presumably reduces calcium excretion in patients by a direct renal action. The drugs reduce intestinal calcium absorption in patients who have severe hypercalciuria (20), but less than they lower urine calcium excretion, so calcium balance becomes more positive. Alternative treatments include low-calcium diet, sodium cellulose phosphate, and orthophosphate, all of which reduce intestinal calcium absorption. The long-term effects of reduced calcium absorption, especially from low-calcium diet, may include reduced bone mineral stores, because hypercalciuric patients do not reduce their urine calcium excretion rates to values as low as those in normal people when both are given a very low calcium intake (10). Men who are given calcitriol in excess but at a dose that does not increase serum calcium above normal (12,13) also fail to reduce urine calcium normally while eating a low-calcium diet.

Primary hyperparathyroidism causes hypercalciuria in about 5% of calcium stone formers (21); 85% have single enlarged glands, so-called adenoma; the rest have at least two enlarged glands, so-called hyperplasia (see Chapter 30). Serum calcium level is always increased, although the increase commonly is so mild that many values are needed to be sure hypercalcemia is present. Upper limits for our normal subjects are serum calcium levels of 10 mg/dL in women, and 10.1 mg/dL in men. Serum levels of at least half of our patients who have had curative surgery were all below 10.5 mg/dL (21). Urine calcium excretion is very high, despite the modest hypercalcemia, so a casual analysis can be misleading; extreme hypercalciuria and serum calcium levels of, for example, 10.1 to 10.3 mg/dL can lead one to think of idiopathic hypercalciuria, and probably account for misleading accounts of normocalcemic primary hyperparathyroidism (22–24), each of which, in retrospect, was almost certainly an instance of mild hypercalcemia.

Among patients who have had curative surgery, serum PTH levels have been elevated between 80% and 100% with a carboxyl terminal assay, and between 60% and 80% with amino terminal or mild molecule assays (21), so PTH assay is more confirmatory than a structural basis of diagnosis.

The best course is to establish whether hypercalcemia is present, and then to exclude other causes such as malignant tumors, sarcoidosis and other granulomatous diseases, vitamin D intoxication, thiazide use, lithium use, and the uncommon or rare disorders (21) (see Section IV). Familial hypocalciuric hypercalcemia is a mendelian dominant disorder, not a cause of stones, best diagnosed by family studies (21) (see Chapter 32). Low PTH levels are especially valuable to detect states of primary calcitriol excess (21). Serum calcitriol is increased in most patients (25–27) as a consequence of high PTH and low serum phosphorus level, and the calcitriol stimulates intestinal calcium absorption, causing most of the hypercalciuria. Bone mineral loss into the urine also occurs.

Treatment is surgical in patients with stone disease. Stone formation is greatly reduced, as urine calcium excretion decreases promptly. We follow up our patients to be sure that residual hypercalciuria is not present and that serum calcium levels remain normal.

Renal tubular acidosis (RTA) is ostensibly a cause of hypercalciuria (28), but we suspect that it is as often a consequence as a cause (see Chapter 67). The defect associated with stones is reduced ability to reduce urine pH; urine citrate excretion is very low, as a rule, and urine calcium is high. It is true that metabolic acidosis is a consequence of severe reductions of tubule ability to reduce pH, because a pH lower than that of blood is needed to titrate urine buffers with protons and to trap ammonia as ammonium ion, for excretion. Metabolic acidosis reduces urine citrate excretion and raises urine calcium, so one is tempted to consider the high pH, high urine calcium, and low urine pH as an expected clustering based on known physiology.

However, we (29) have found that alkali treatment, which should reduce urine calcium excretion, usually does not, although it may raise urine citrate excretion. Metabolic acidosis is not discernible in most patients. Early reports of RTA (30) included, as a majority, patients such as we have encountered, and labeled them as having incomplete RTA. In families, idiopathic hypercalciuria and RTA both appear (31), and the hypercalciuria of our patients usually responds to thiazide. We are inclined to believe that the hypercalciuria comes first and that nephrocalcinosis, perhaps hypercalciuria itself, damages collecting ducts and causes the incomplete RTA.

The patients form stones composed mainly of calcium phosphate salts. High urine pH increases urine levels of dissociated phosphate, which forms brushite calcium monohydrogen phosphate and apatite. The stones are larger than calcium oxalate stones, and they grow faster. Apart from sporadic and familial incomplete RTA, rare patients have complete RTA, usually inherited as an autosomal dominant trait. They have metabolic acidosis; their urine calcium excretions decrease with alkali treatment. Diamox (acetazolamide) reduces bicarbonate reabsorption by the proximal tubule and causes alkaline urine and stones. The urine is alkaline because the drug is given in multiple doses, so bicarbonate levels decrease, increase between doses, and decrease again as the bicarbonate is excreted. Inherited or acquired proximal RTA is a steady defect and causes neither stones nor alkaline urine. Hyperkalemic type 4 RTA resulting from obstruction, low renin or aldosterone secretion rates, or renal disease (32) causes an acid urine pH and not stones.

Hyperoxaluric States

Primary hyperoxaluria always comes from one of two hereditary enzyme defects that increase oxalate production (33). Oxalate is an end product, excreted only by the kidneys, which filter and secrete it (34). Urine oxalate excretion is above the usual normal limit of 40 mg daily (35), in the range of 80 to 120 mg. The oxalate crystallizes with calcium, causing stones that begin in childhood, and tubulointerstitial nephropathy, which leads to chronic renal failure. Renal tubular acidosis may be an early sign of nephropathy, causing an anion gap metabolic acidosis that increases the serum chloride level and lowers the bicarbonate level. Renal transplantation requires extensive dialytic preparation so that stored oxalate does not flood the graft and destroy it. Overproduction occurs from pyridoxine deficiency (in animals) and methoxyflurane anesthetic and occurs if one is so foolish or mistaken as to drink ethylene glycol (antifreeze) as a beverage. Treatment is with fluids, citrate (to reduce calcium ion levels), and pyridoxine, which may be helpful in low doses of 20 to 40 mg daily in some people. Others respond only to 300 to 400 mg daily, and some do not respond at all.

Enteric hyperoxaluria means that the colon absorbs oxalate excessively because small bowel malabsorption permits undigested fatty acids and bile acids to reach the colon epithelium and increase its permeability (36). Small-bowel resection, intestinal bypass for obesity, and small-bowel diseases such as Crohn's disease are common causes (37). Colectomy or ileostomy prevents the oxaluria. Urine oxalate is above normal, in the range of 75 to 150 mg daily. Urine citrate is low because of the alkali loss from the small bowel, and urine pH is low. Urine calcium usually is low, not high. Low-oxalate diet and low-fat diet reduce oxaluria; low fat reduces delivery of fatty acids to colon. Oral calcium, 1 to 4 g as calcium carbonate, taken with meals, crystallizes with oxalate in the gut lumen. Cholestyramine, 1 to 4 g with meals, adsorbs oxalate and also bile salts. The four treatments are synergistic and should be used together. Cholestyramine has important side effects of vitamin K depletion and reduced absorption of drugs.

In a way, dietary oxalate excess is an enteric oxaluria. Usual food culprits are nuts, pepper, chocolate, rhubarb, and spinach for a few devotees, and for the rest, mixtures of dark green vegetables and of fruits. Vitamin C in large doses may increase urine oxalate, and ascorbic acid itself may, in urine, break down to oxalic acid, giving a wrong impression of hyperoxaluria. Treatments are simply dietary.

Hyperuricosuric States

About 25% of calcium stone formers excrete more than 800 mg daily of uric acid (750 mg in women) and have no other apparent causes of their stones (38). Their urine pH is lower than the normal of 6.0, averaging 5.6 (39), so the uric acid can crystallize (40). Uric acid crystals can promote calcium oxalate crystallization (41) because they share structural features. Treatment with allopurinol reduced stone recurrence

in a prospective, controlled trial (42), and neither allopurinol nor its metabolites affect calcium oxalate crystallization. The hyperuricosuria results from high purine intake (43) from meats, and dietary treatment should be effective, although it has not been tested. We recommend reducing diet purine intake and reserving allopurinol for those who produce more stones, unless stone disease has been so severe that maximal certainty of treatment is desired despite the risk of drug side effects.

Low Urine Citrate

Women with stones excrete only 550 mg of citrate daily, compared with 750 mg daily for normal women (44). This decisive abnormality ought to increase the risk of stones because citrate forms a soluble calcium salt, and what calcium is in the salt is not free to combine with oxalic acid. Normal men excrete no more citrate than women with stones, and men who form stones excrete about the same amount of citrate, so low urine citrate in men is not so much an abnormality as it is a trait that explains why men are four out of every five people with stones. Any oral alkali can increase urine citrate. We prefer citrate to sodium bicarbonate for its longer duration of action, and we use 25 to 50 mEq, 2 or 3 times daily. Citrate treatment has been tested in one prospective controlled trial (45). Barcelo et al. (45) found that of the 38 patients who completed the 36-month trial, the stone-formation rate was lower in the treated than in the placebo group ($p < 0.001$) compared with that before treatment.

URIC ACID STONES

Mixed

About 12% of all calcium stones contain some uric acid (46), and patients who form the mixed stones from urine that is supersaturated with uric acid because its pH is below the normal level of 6.0. Hyperuricosuria also is common. The urine of mixed stone formers is like that of patients with hyperuricosuric calcium oxalate stones, and what distinguishes the two groups is simply that in one, uric acid is inferred as a promoter of calcium oxalate stones, and in the other, the uric acid crystals are seen in the stones themselves. Probably if all of the stones of the former group were studied, uric acid would be found in some; the distinction is not so intrinsic as it is based on accident of how patients are studied and the relative proportions of uric acid to calcium oxalate in their stones.

Treatment includes reduced diet purine for hyperuricosuria, oral alkali to raise urine pH to 6 or 6.5, and thiazide for hypercalciuria, which may occur in some patients. The hyperuricosuric calcium oxalate stone formers are defined by absence of hypercalciuria or other cause of stones, so thiazide is not usually needed or appropriate.

Pure

Only about 5% of stone formers produce pure uric acid stones. Their urine is very acid, with pH values below 5.3, which is the pK of uric acid, and frequently below 5.0. Uric acid solubility in urine is just below 100 mg/L, whereas the salts of monohydrogen urate are relatively much more soluble, so urine pH values near the pK raise uric acid supersaturation drastically by raising the fraction of the total urate that is fully protonated. For example, average normal men excrete 650 mg of uric acid in 1.2 L of urine (39), a concentration of 540 mg/L; at pK 6.0, less than 10% is undissociated, whereas at pH 5.3, 50% (270 mg/L) is undissociated (2.7 times above the solubility). Uric acid stones occur in people with gout and in others with familial uric acid stones. All have low urine pH, and the reason is unclear. Patients with ileostomy or who work in hot and dry places form scanty and acid urine and uric acid stones. Treatment is always alkali to raise urine pH to 6, and reduced purine intake or allopurinol for hyperuricosuria.

STRUVITE STONES

Only microorganisms that have urease enzyme can produce struvite stones, by hydrolyzing urine urea to carbon dioxide and ammonia, so urinary infection is the only clinical cause of these infection stones. Struvite forms as the ammonia raises local pH to above 9; phosphate is fully dissociated and combines with urine magnesium and ammonium ion. Carbonate apatite also is formed from the carbonate and calcium because of high pH, so pure struvite stones always contain both crystals. Mixed stones also contain calcium oxalate, which is not particularly favored to form under the same circumstances as struvite and denotes the combination of metabolic and infection stone in the same patient.

Mixed

We find that about one third of struvite stones are mixed; patients begin their stone careers with passage, and their prognosis for renal function and nephrectomy is excellent. Men are nearly one half of this group, and almost all men with struvite stones form mixed stones. Urine calcium excretion is above normal for the group in both sexes. Mean serum creatinine is normal. A few patients do have reduced creatinine clearance, which is rare among calcium stone formers (47).

Pure

More than half of this group are women. Stones are frequently staghorns that fill the renal collecting systems. Infection, bleeding, or flank pain, rather than stone passage, calls attention to the stones. Serum creatinine levels are above normal on average, creatinine clearance is low, and hypercalciuria is not usual. Thus struvite stones seem to be a primary problem, not a complication of metabolic stones.

Treatment

Mixed or pure, these infected stones are treated with removal. Current practice is percutaneous nephrolithotomy, if the stones are over 2 cm in diameter, followed by extracorporeal shock wave lithotripsy (ESWL) to fragment what is left, and then a second look with percutaneous nephrolithotomy to remove all debris. If stones are less than 2 cm in diameter, ESWL is an adequate monotherapy. Antibiotic agents are best used before and after removal to sterilize the urinary tract.

CYSTINE STONES

Cystine, lysine, ornithine, and citrulline share a common set of transporters in gut and kidney that can be deficient by heredity, as one of at least three autosomal recessive diseases (48). Only cystine causes disease, and only because it is insoluble enough to crystallize into stones. The stones begin in childhood, may be staghorns, and recur throughout life unless treated well.

The solubility of cystine in urine is about 1 mM and varies about twofold from person to person. Excretion rates in normal people and also in heterozygotes are micromolar, so neither forms cystine stones. In homozygous cystinuric people, excretion rates range from 1 to 15 mM daily, usual values being about 3 to 6 mM, so high fluid intake, of 3 to 6 L daily, is adequate for most people. Nocturia is mandatory because cystine is excreted constantly. Alkaline pH increases cystine solubility, but only above pH 7.4, and to raise urine pH above serum pH requires a high dose of alkali, enough to overbalance total daily acid production. Calcium phosphate stones could be fostered. Even so, alkali is generally recommended.

If water and alkali fail to prevent stones, add a drug that forms a soluble disulfide with cysteine, such as d-penicillamine (48). Cystine is itself the cysteine disulfide and is in equilibrium with cysteine; the drug forms its own cysteine disulfide and reduces free cysteine concentration, and cystine dissociates into cysteine. All available drugs cause allergic side effects such as skin rash and serum-sickness reactions and reduce smell and taste; the latter symptoms respond to zinc repletion. Tiopronin (Thiola), long in European use, is now also available in the United States.

REFERENCES

1. Parks JH, Coe FL. The financial effects of kidney stone prevention. *Kidney Int* 1996;50:1706–1712.
2. Coe FL, Parks JH, Moore EM. Familial idiopathic hypercalciuria. *N Engl J Med* 1979;300:337–340.
3. Coe FL, Parks JH. Familial (idiopathic) hypercalciuria. In: Coe FL, Parks JH, eds. *Nephrolithiasis: pathogenesis and treatment.* 2nd ed. Chicago: Yearbook Medical, 1988:108–138.
4. Weber DV, Coe FL, Parks JH, et al. Urinary saturation measurements in calcium nephrolithiasis. *Ann Intern Med* 1979;90:180–184.
5. Coe FL, Bushinsky DA. Pathophysiology of hypercalciuria. *Am J Physiol* 1984;247:F1–F13.
6. Haussler MR, Baylink J, Hughes MR, et al. The assay of 1,25-dihydroxy vitamin D₃: physiologic and pathologic modulation of circulating hormone levels. *Clin Endocrinol* 1976;5:151S–165S.
7. Kaplan RA, Haussler MR, Deftos LJ, et al. The role of 1-alpha,25-dihydroxyvitamin D in the mediation of intestinal hyperabsorption of calcium in primary hyperparathyroidism and absorptive hypercalciuria. *J Clin Invest* 1977;59:756–760.
8. Gray RW, Wilz DR, Caldas AE, et al. The importance of phosphate in regulating plasma 1,25 (OH)₂-vitamin D levels in humans: studies in healthy subjects, in calcium stone formers, and in patients with

primary hyperparathyroidism. *J Clin Endocrinol Metab* 1977;45: 299–306.

9. Shen FH, Baylink DJ, Neilsen RL. Increased serum 1,25-dihydroxyvitamin D in idiopathic hypercalciuria. *J Lab Clin Med* 1977;90:955–962.

10. Coe FL, Favus MJ, Crockett T, et al. Effects of low calcium diet on urine calcium excretion, parathyroid function and serum 1,25(OH)$_2$D$_3$ levels in patients with idiopathic hypercalciuria and in normal subjects. *Am J Med* 1982;72:25–31.

11. Broadus AE, Insogna KL, Lang R, et al. Evidence for disordered control of 1,25-dihydroxyvitamin D production in absorptive hypercalciuria. *N Engl J Med* 1984;311:73–80.

12. Adams ND, Gray RW, Lemann J Jr. The effects of oral CaCO$_3$ loading and dietary calcium deprivation on plasma 1,25-dihydroxyvitamin D concentrations in healthy adults. *J Clin Endocrinol Metab* 1979;48:1008–1016.

13. Maierhofer WJ, Lemann J Jr, Gray RW, et al. Dietary calcium and serum 1,25-(OH)$_2$-vitamin D concentrations as determinants of calcium balance in healthy men. *Kidney Int* 1984;26:752–759.

14. Coe L, Parks JH, Asplin JR. The pathogenesis and treatment of kidney stones, medical progress. *N Engl J Med* 1992;327:1141–1152.

15. Li XQ, Tembe V, Horwitz GM, Bushinsky DA, Favus MJ. Increased intestinal vitamin D receptor in genetic hypercalciuric rats: a cause of intestinal calcium reabsorption. *J Clin Invest* 1993;91:661–667.

16. Coe FL, Parks JH, Favus MJ. Diet and calcium: the end of an era? *Ann Intern Med* 1997;126:553–554.

17. Weber DV, Coe FL, Parks JH, et al. Urinary saturation measurements in calcium nephrolithiasis. *Ann Intern Med* 1979;90:180–184.

18. Coe FL. Treated and untreated recurrent calcium nephrolithiasis in patients with idiopathic hypercalciuria, hyperuricosuria, or no metabolic disorder. *Ann Intern Med* 1977;87:404–410.

19. Costanzo LS. Localization of diuretic action in microperfused rat distal tubules: Ca and Na transport. *Am J Physiol* 1985;248:F527–F535.

20. Coe FL, Parks JH, Bushinsky DA, Langman CV, Favus MJ. Chlorthalidone promotes mineral retention in patients with idiopathic hypercalciuria. *Kidney Int* 1988;33:1140–1146.

21. Coe FL, Parks JH. Primary hyperparathyroidism. In: Coe FL, Parks JH, eds. *Nephrolithiasis: pathogenesis and treatment.* 2nd ed. Chicago: Yearbook Medical, 1988:59–107.

22. Johnson RD, Conn JW. Hyperparathyroidism with a prolonged period of normocalcemia. *JAMA* 1969;210:2063–2066.

23. Yendt ER, Gagne RJA. Detection of primary hyperparathyroidism, with special reference to its occurrence in hypercalciuric females with normal or borderline serum calcium. *Can Med Assoc J* 1968;98: 331–336.

24. Wills MR, Pak CYC, Hammond WG, et al. Normocalcemic primary hyperparathyroidism. *Am J Med* 1979;47:384–391.

25. Broadus AE, Horst RL, Lang R, et al. The importance of circulating 1,25-dihydroxyvitamin D in the pathogenesis of hypercalciuria and renal-stone formation in primary hyperparathyroidism. *N Engl J Med* 1980;302:421–426.

26. Pak CYC, Nicar MJ, Peterson R, et al. A lack of unique pathophysiologic background for nephrolithiasis of primary hyperparathyroidism. *J Clin Endocrinol Metab* 1981;55:536–542.

27. LoCascio V, Adami S, Galvanini G, et al. Substrate-product relation of 1-hydroxylase activity in primary hyperparathyroidism. *N Engl J Med* 1985;313:1123–1130.

28. Transbol I, Gill JR, Lifschitz M, et al. Intestinal absorption and renal excretion of calcium in metabolic acidosis and alkalosis. *Acta Endocrinol* 1971;155(suppl):217.

29. Coe FL, Parks JH. Stone disease in distal renal tubular acidosis. *Ann Intern Med* 1980;93:6061.

30. Albright F, Burnett CH, Parson W, et al. Osteomalacia and late rickets: the various etiologies met in the United States with emphasis on that resulting from a specific form of renal acidosis, the therapeutic indications for each sub-group, and the relationship between osteomalacia and Milkmans syndrome. *Medicine (Baltimore)* 1946;25:399–479.

31. Buckalew VM Jr, Purvis ML, Shulman MG, et al. Hereditary renal tubular acidosis. *Medicine (Baltimore)* 1974;53:229–254.

32. Wrong O, Davies HEF. The excretion of acid in renal disease. *Q J Med* 1959;28:259–311.

33. Williams HE, Smith LH Jr. Disorders of oxalate metabolism. *Am J Med* 1968;45:715.

34. Hagler L, Herman RH. Oxalate metabolism. *Am J Clin Nutr* 1973; 26:758, 882, 1006, 1073, 1242.

35. Hodgkinson A, Wilkinson R. Plasma oxalate concentration and renal excretion of oxalate in man. *Clin Sci* 1974;46:61.

36. Kathpalia SC, Favus MJ, Coe FL. Evidence for size and change permselectivity of rat ascending colon: effects of ricinoleate and bile salts on oxalic acid and neutral sugar transport. *J Clin Invest* 1984;74:805–811.

37. Smith LH, Fromm H, Hoffman AF. Acquired hyperoxaluria, nephrolithiasis and intestinal disease. *N Engl J Med* 1972;286:1371.

38. Coe FL, Kavalich AG. Hypercalciuria and hyperuricosuria in patients with calcium nephrolithiasis. *N Engl J Med* 1974;291:1344.

39. Coe FL, Strauss AL, Tembe V, et al. Uric acid saturation in calcium nephrolithiasis. *Kidney Int* 1980;17:662–668.

40. Coe FL. Uric acid and calcium oxalate nephrolithiasis. *Kidney Int* 1983;24:392–403.

41. Deganello S, Coe FL. Epitaxy between uric acid and whewellite: experimental verification. *Am J Physiol* 1983;6:270–276.

42. Ettinger B, Tang A, Citron JT, et al. Randomized trial of allopurinol in the prevention of calcium oxalate calculi. *N Engl J Med* 1986;315:1386–1389.

43. Kavalich AG, Moran E, Coe FL. Dietary purine consumption by hyperuricosuric calcium oxalate kidney stone formers and normal subjects. *J Chronic Dis* 1976;29:745.

44. Parks JH, Coe FL. A urinary calcium-citrate index for the evaluation of nephrolithiasis. *Kidney Int* 1986;30:85–90.

45. Barcelo P, Wuhl O, Servitge E, Rousaund A, Pak CYC. Randomized double-blind study of potassium citrate in idiopathic hypocitraturic calcium nephrolithiasis. *J Urol* 1993;150:1761–1764.

46. Herring LC. Observations on the analysis of ten thousand urinary calculi. *J Urol* 1962;88:545–562.

47. Kristensen C, Parks JH, Lindheimer M, Coe FL. Reduced glomerular filtration rate, hypercalciuria and clinical morbidity in primary struvite nephrolithiasis. *Kidney Int* 1987;32:749–753.

48. Segal S, Thier SO. Cystinuria. In: Stanbury JB, Wyngaarden JB, Fredrickson DS, et al., eds. *The metabolic basis of inherited disease.* 5th ed. New York: McGraw-Hill, 1983:1774–1791.

82. Urologic Aspects of Nephrolithiasis Management

K. C. Saw, M.A., F.R.C.S. and *James E. Lingeman, M.D.

*Department of Endourology and Urolithiasis, *Methodist Hospital Institute for Kidney Stone Disease, Indianapolis, Indiana*

Technologic and technical improvements in extracorporeal shock wave lithotripsy (ESWL) (1), percutaneous nephrostolithotomy (PCNL) (2) and ureterorenoscopy (URS) (3) allow most symptomatic calculi to be removed with minimal morbidity, and these treatment modalities have largely replaced open surgery in the management of upper urinary tract calculi (4,5). The aims of modern stone management are to relieve symptoms, remove stones, avoid complications, prevent recurrence, and preserve renal function. When translated into clinical practice, this means to select the most appropriate technique(s) to achieve *maximal* stone clearance while *minimizing morbidity* to the patient (4,5). Important factors to consider in the choice of treatment modalities are those affecting treatment outcomes: the stone location, stone burden (size and number), stone composition, renal function, and the presence of infection or obstruction. Over the past decade, the outcomes produced, the limitations, advantages, and disadvantages of each treatment modality relative to one another have become clearer, and this overview provides a perspective regarding the current roles and indications for ESWL, PCNL, and URS. When dealing with patients with calculi, the use of a classification system is helpful (Table 1) and provides an organizational framework to think about these problems.

NONSTAGHORN RENAL CALCULI

Whereas most renal calculi can be successfully fragmented with most lithotripters, stone clearance is related to the amount of stone material requiring treatment (i.e., stone burden) and the location of the stones in the kidney (Fig. 1) (6). As the number and size of stones increases, the number of treatment sessions increases, the stone free rate decreases, and the need for ancillary procedures (e.g., ure-

TABLE 1. *Classification scheme for patients with urolithiasis*

Nonstaghorn renal calculi
Staghorn renal calculi
Special considerations
Lower-pole calculus
Renally impaired patient
Infection and obstruction
Horseshoe kidney
Ureteropelvic junction obstruction (UPJO)
Calyceal diverticulum
Ureteral calculi

teral stenting, ureteroscopy, percutaneous nephrostomy) increases (Fig. 2a) (7). The critical role of stone burden in the outcome expected with ESWL has been confirmed by numerous investigators (2,7,8). PCNL, although more invasive, does produce a significantly higher stone-free rate, lower retreatment rate, and need for ancillary procedures than does ESWL (Fig. 2b) (7). Based on the preceding observations, an NIH Consensus Conference (9) in 1988 concluded that renal stones smaller than 2 cm (which represent the great majority of cases) are generally effectively managed with ESWL, but stones larger than 2 cm should be approached initially with PCNL. However, certain stones that fragment with difficulty with ESWL [e.g., cystine, calcium oxalate monohydrate, and brushite (2,8,10,11)] may still be more appropriately managed with PCNL. In the future, radiologic features [e.g., radiodensity and stone outline (12), Hounsfield numbers on computed tomography (CT) scan (13,14)], may help to predict response to ESWL.

Another area that remains controversial is the management of lower-pole calyceal stones. Lower-pole calculi have a significantly lower clearance rate with ESWL than with

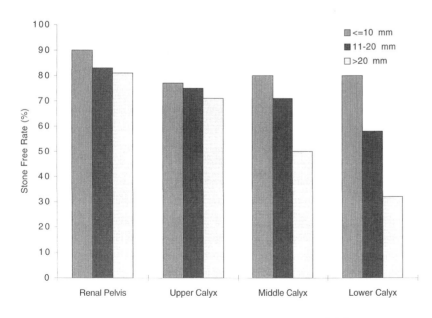

FIG. 1. Solitary renal calculi: stone-free rates with ESWL stratified by location and size. (From Lingeman JE. Lesson 28: update on ESWL. *AUA Update Series* 1995; 14:226–231.)

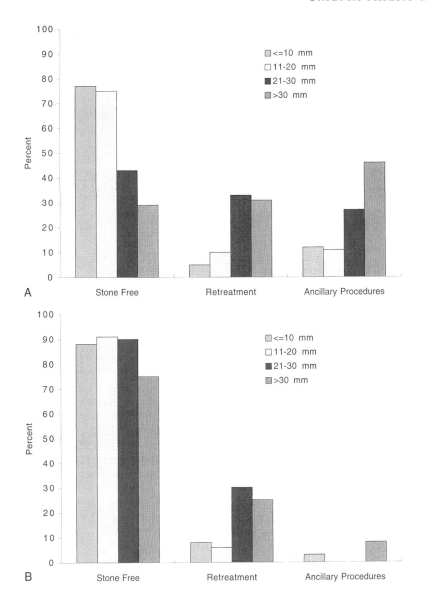

FIG. 2. A: Nonstaghorn calculi treatment with ESWL stratified by size. **B:** Nonstaghorn calculi treatment with PCNL stratified by size. (From Lingeman JE, Coury TA, Newman DM, et al. Comparison of results and morbidity of percutaneous nephrostolithotomy and extracorporeal shock wave lithotripsy. *J Urol* 1987;138:485–490.)

PCNL (2,15). Furthermore, residual fragments may regrow or become symptomatic and require intervention (16). Current experience suggests that only lower-pole calculi 10 mm or less achieve reasonable stone clearance after ESWL (Fig. 3) (15). Anatomic considerations may be particularly important when treating lower-pole stones (17). Certain anatomic features (simple collecting systems, large infundibulo–pelvic angle, short infundibular length, and wide infundibular diameter) (18–20) favor the passage of stone fragments. Recently renal stone fragmentation and extraction by using very small (7.5F) flexible ureteroscopes, in combination with Holmium:YAG laser, has become an increasingly viable option for calculi that do not or are not expected to respond well to ESWL (3,21,22). With sufficient technical expertise and appropriate instruments, most renal collecting systems, including the lower-pole calyces, can be reached transurethrally without prior ureteral dilatation, and stones can be successfully fragmented. However, as with ESWL, complete stone clearance remains problematic with the ureteroscopic approach, especially as stone burden increases.

STAGHORN RENAL CALCULI

Staghorn renal calculi are stones that fill a substantial portion of the renal collecting system. Typically, such stones will occupy the renal pelvis, and branches of the stone will extend into one or more of the calyces (4). Unfortunately, staghorn calculi vary greatly in size (Fig. 4), and there is no widely accepted way to express the amount of stone material represented by a staghorn calculus. As a result, stones of widely differing volumes are all referred to as *staghorns.* Our group has attempted to clarify this problem by promoting the use of stone surface area (8,23). Staghorn calculi most commonly represent the products of ureolysis (struvite and carbonate apatite), but cystine, uric acid, and calcium oxalate can also form staghorn calculi (2,4).

An untreated staghorn calculus is associated with a significant risk of renal loss and mortality (24,25). Infected staghorn calculi often harbor urea-splitting organisms deep within the interstices of the stone material, rendering sterilization of the urine impossible unless all the calculous mate-

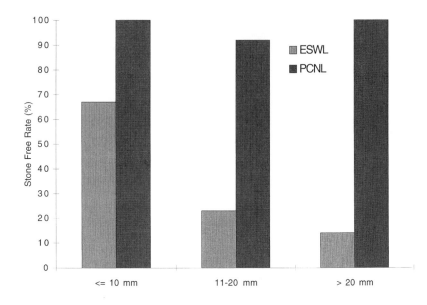

FIG. 3. Lower-pole calculi: Stone-free rates with ESWL and PCNL stratified by size. [From the Lower Pole Study Group. A prospective randomized trial of extracorporeal shock wave lithotripsy and percutaneous nephrostolithotomy for lower pole nephrolithiasis: initial results. *J Urol* (in press).]

rial is removed (4). Given the large stone burden represented by most staghorn calculi, PCNL is the treatment of choice (4,8). The combined use of rigid and flexible nephroscopes, supplemented when necessary by multiple access and secondary PCNL, have resulted in stone clearance comparable to that achieved with open surgery. Improved techniques and equipment have virtually eliminated the need for combination ESWL (sandwich) therapy (26). The results of PCNL, together with its lower morbidity (23), have enabled percutaneous techniques to supplant open surgery in the treatment of these often complex and difficult cases. The American Urological Association (AUA) Nephrolithiasis Clinical Guidelines Panel recommendations for managing staghorn calculi (4) are summarized in Table 2.

SPECIAL CONSIDERATIONS

The presence of certain features needs special consideration. The problem of lower-pole calculi was discussed earlier. When dealing with renally impaired patients with calculi, the aim is to preserve renal function. In these patients, although it may not be possible to achieve normal renal function results with stone removal, further deterioration of renal function may be averted, and this may help some patients avoid the need for dialysis (27). As stone clearance tends to be poorer and regrowth is likely in these poorly functioning kidneys, PCNL is preferable to ESWL. However, in the presence of a normal contralateral kidney, a poorly functioning kidney with large stone burden could reasonably be removed (4).

Infection within an obstructed kidney can result in rapid destruction of the kidney and urosepsis, an emergency situation best managed initially by relieving the obstruction with the insertion of a nephrostomy or ureteral stent. When the infection has been controlled, the stone can be removed by the most appropriate method. It also is important to relieve the obstruction at the same time as stone removal lest stone clearance be impeded or stones recur after removal.

A variety of congenital anomalies [e.g., horseshoe kidney,

ureteropelvic junction obstruction (UPJO), calyceal diverticulum] increase the risk of urolithiasis, probably as a result of obstruction and/or stasis.

Although ESWL may be used to treat renal calculi within horseshoe kidneys (28), the results of treatment are more sensitive to stone burden and location than are nonhorseshoe kidneys, reflecting the difficulty in both localizing and fragmenting calculi within horseshoe kidneys with ESWL and in eliminating gravel from these kidneys (29). PCNL, which provides significantly better results, is often preferred (29).

Obstruction distal to the stone remains a contraindication to ESWL. One third of patients with UPJOs have stones secondary to stasis, and the obstruction can be relieved by endopyelotomy at the time of PCNL. Endopyelotomy, the incision of the UPJO endoscopically, is successful in 64% to 95% of instances (30–32) and is easily combined with PCNL.

Calyceal diverticula are commonly complicated by the occurrence of renal calculi (33). Typically, the ostium connecting a calyceal diverticulum to the rest of the renal collecting system is tiny and, combined with lack of urine production, explains why few, if any, stones within calyceal diverticula can be successfully managed with ESWL (33,34). Stone-containing calyceal diverticuli are better managed via an endourologic approach (PCNL or URS) with or without concomitant fulguration of the diverticulum and/or dilatation of the calyceal neck (33).

URETERAL CALCULI

Most ureteral calculi are small (under 5 mm) and will pass spontaneously (4). However, when ureteral calculi are larger or symptoms intractable, virtually all can be managed with URS or ESWL. A recent trend in the management of ureteral calculi has been the increasing utilization of ESWL *in situ* (35), a technique that often requires minimal anesthesia. However, as ureteral calculi are more difficult to fragment than renal calculi of comparable size, retreatments or other ancillary procedures are necessary in about one third of

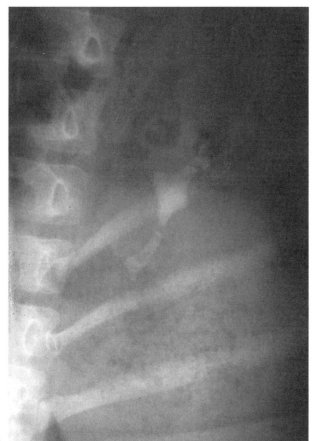

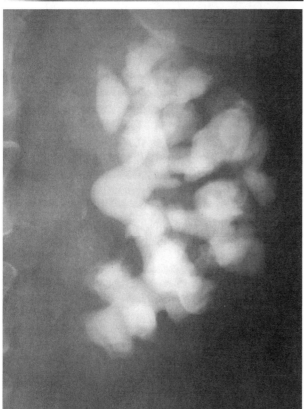

FIG. 4. A: Small staghorn calculus within a simple renal collecting system. **B:** Large complex staghorn calculus with a much larger stone burden.

TABLE 2. *American Urological Association Nephrolithiasis Clinical Guidelines Panel recommendations for managing staghorn calculi*

Standards
A newly diagnosed struvite staghorn calculus represents an indication for active treatment intervention. A policy of watchful waiting and observation is not in the best interest of the otherwise healthy patient with struvite staghorn calculi

Patients must be informed about the treatment modalities including the relative benefits and risks associated with each of these treatments

Guidelines
PCNL, followed by ESWL and/or repeated PCNL as warranted, should be utilized for most patients with struvite staghorn calculi, with PCNL being the first part of the combination therapy

ESWL monotherapy should not be used for most patients with struvite staghorn calculi as a first-line treatment choice

Open surgery (nephrolithotomy by any method) should not be used for most patients as a first-line treatment choice

Options
ESWL monotherapy and PCNL monotherapy are equally effective treatment choices for small (<500 mm^2) struvite staghorn calculi in collecting systems that are of normal or near-normal anatomy

Open surgery is an appropriate treatment alternative in unusual situations in which a staghorn calculus is not expected to be removable by a reasonable number of PCNL and/or ESWL procedures

For a patient with poorly functioning, stone-bearing kidney, nephrectomy is a reasonable treatment alternative.

Recommendations for treatment are made with three levels of flexibility, based primarily on the strength of the scientific evidence for estimating outcomes of interventions. A standard is defined as the least flexible of the three, a guideline is more flexible, and an option is the most flexible.

PCNL, percutaneous nephrostolithotomy; ESWL, extracorporeal shock wave lithotripsy. From Segura JW, Preminger GM, Assimos DG, et al. Nephrolithiasis Clinical Guidelines Panel Summary Report on the management of staghorn calculi [Special communication]. *J Urol* 1994; 151:1648–1651.

cases managed with ESWL *in situ* (Table 3) (5). Ultimately, approximately 80% to 85% of patients with ureteral calculi will become stone free with ESWL *in situ* (5), no matter where the location of the stone in the ureter.

URS, although slightly more invasive, achieves better stone clearance in the lower ureter (5). For calculi in the mid or upper ureter, URS with rigid instruments is less successful than ESWL *in situ* (5). However, in recent years, the advent of small flexible URS combined with laser lithotripsy has increased the effectiveness of URS for upper ureteral calculi (3,21,22,35). In addition, retrograde stone manipulation followed by ESWL and PCNL (alone or preceded by retrograde stone manipulation) also achieves excellent stone-free results (5,35). Therefore there are now several effective, minimally invasive approaches for the management of ureteral calculi, and the choice of treatment will

TABLE 3. *American Urological Association Ureteral Stones Clinical Guidelines Panel recommendations for managing ureteral stones*

General recommendations for all ureteral stones
  Standards
    A patient who has a ureteral stone (>0.5 cm in diameter) with a low probability of spontaneous passage must be informed about the existing active treatment modalities, including the relative benefits and risks associated with each modality. It is unacceptable to withhold certain treatments from the patient because of personal inexperience/unfamiliarity or local unavailability of equipment/expertise
  Guidelines
    Stones (<0.5 cm in diameter), especially in the distal ureter, may be expected to pass spontaneously and should be treated expectantly. However, difficulties in tolerating pain, multiple trips to the emergency room, or other factors may mandate treatment in a patient whose stone might otherwise be expected to pass
    Routine stenting to increase efficiency of fragmentation is not recommended as part of ESWL
Specific recommendations according to size and site of ureteral stone
  Stones ≤1 cm in the proximal ureter

Standards	Open surgery should not be first-line active treatment
Guidelines	ESWL is recommended as first-line treatment for most patients
Options	URS and PCNL are acceptable choices in situations when ESWL may not be appropriate or as salvage for failed ESWL

  Stones >1 cm in the proximal ureter

Guidelines	Open surgery should not be the first-line treatment
Options	ESWL, PCNL, and URS are all acceptable treatment choices. Open surgery may be appropriate for nonstandard cases and is an acceptable alternative as a salvage measure

  Stones ≤1 cm in the distal ureter

Standards	Open surgery should not be the first-line treatment
Guidelines	Blind basketing without fluoroscopy and guide wire cannot be encouraged
Options	ESWL and URS are acceptable treatment choices

  Stones >1 cm in the distal ureter

Standards	Blind basketing is not recommended as a treatment choice
Guidelines	Open surgery should not be the first-line treatment for most patients
Options	ESWL and URS are acceptable treatment choices

Recommendations for treatment are made with three levels of flexibility, based primarily on the strength of the scientific evidence for estimating outcomes of interventions. A standard is defined as the least flexible of the three, a guideline is more flexible, and an option is the most flexible.

ESWL, extracorporeal shock wave lithotripsy; PCNL, percutaneous nephrostolithotomy; URS, ureterorenoscopy. From Segura JW, Preminger GM, Assimos DG, et al. Ureteral Stones Clinical Guidelines Panel Summary Report on the management of ureteral calculi [Special communication]. *J Urol* 1997; 158:1915–1921.

depend to a large extent on patient preferences and local circumstances (i.e., the availability of a lithotripter, instruments, and expertise) (35).

SUMMARY

Whereas 80% to 85% of symptomatic urinary calculi are best managed initially with ESWL, it should be apparent that endourologic techniques retain significant roles in the management of urinary calculi. Patients with substantial stone burden or anatomic abnormalities are preferentially managed initially with PCNL. ESWL *in situ* for the management of ureteral calculi is increasingly popular, whereas URS, although more invasive, remains an effective alternative. In the current era, open surgery is rarely necessary.

REFERENCES

1. Lingeman JE. Extracorporeal shock wave lithotripsy: development, instrumentation and current status. *Urol Clin North Am* 1997;24: 185–211.
2. Wolf JS Jr, Clayman RV. Percutaneous nephrostolithotomy: what is its role in 1997? *Urol Clin North Am* 1997;24:43–58.
3. Conlin MJ, Marberger M, Bagley DH. Ureteroscopy, development and instrumentation. *Urol Clin North Am* 1997;24:25–42.
4. Segura JW, Preminger GM, Assimos DG, et al. Nephrolithiasis clinical guidelines panel summary report on the management of staghorn calculi [Special communication]. *J Urol* 1994;151:1648–1651.
5. Segura JW, Preminger GM, Assimos DG, et al. Ureteral stones clinical guidelines panel summary report on the management of ureteral calculi [Special communication]. *J Urol* 1997;158:1915–1921.
6. Lingeman JE. Lesson 28: update on ESWL. *AUA Update Series* 1995;14:226–231.
7. Lingeman JE, Coury TA, Newman DM, et al. Comparison of results and morbidity of percutaneous nephrostolithotomy and extracorporeal shock wave lithotripsy. *J Urol* 1987;138:485–490.
8. Lam HS, Lingeman JE, Barron M, et al. Staghorn calculi: analysis of treatment results between initial percutaneous nephrostolithotomy and extracorporeal shock wave lithotripsy monotherapy with reference to surface area. *J Urol* 1992;147:1219–1225.
9. NIH Consensus Conference. Prevention and treatment of kidney stones. *JAMA* 1988;260:977–981.
10. Klee LW, Brito CG, Lingeman JE. The clinical implications of brushite calculi. *J Urol* 1991;145:715–718.
11. Dretler SP, Polykoff G. Calcium oxalate stone morphology: fine tuning our therapeutic distinctions. *J Urol* 1996;155:828–833.
12. Bon D, Dore B, Irani J, Marroncle M, Aubert J. Radiographic prognostic criteria for extracorporeal shock-wave lithotripsy: a study of 485 patients. *Urology* 1996;48:556–561.
13. Wang YH, Grenabo L, Hedelin H, Petterson S, Wikholm G, Zachrisson BF. Analysis of stone fragility in vitro and in vivo with piezoelectric shock wave using the EDAP LT-01. *J Urol* 1993;149:699–702.
14. Mostafavi MR, Ernst RD, Saltzman B. Accurate determination of chemical composition of urinary calculi by spiral computerized tomography. *J Urol* 1998;159:673–675.
15. Lower Pole Study Group. A prospective randomized trial of extracorporeal shock wave lithotripsy and percutaneous nephrostolithotomy for lower pole nephrolithiasis: initial results. *J Urol* (in press).
16. Streem SB, Yost A, Mascha E. Clinical implications of clinically insignificant stone fragments after extracorporeal shock wave lithotripsy. *J Urol* 1996;155:1186–1190.
17. Sampaio FJB, Aragao AHM. Inferior pole collecting system anatomy: its probable role in extracorporeal shock wave lithotripsy. *J Urol* 1992;147:322–324.
18. Sabinis RB, Naik K, Patel SH, Desai MR, Bapat SD. Extracorporeal shock wave lithotripsy for lower calyceal stones: can clearance be predicted? *Br J Urol* 1997;80:853–857.
19. Elbahnasy AH, Shalhav AL, Hoenig DM, et al. Lower caliceal stone

clearance after shock wave lithotripsy or ureteroscopy: the impact of lower pole radiographic anatomy. *J Urol* 1998;159:676–682.

20. Sampaio FJB, D Anunciacó AL, Silva ECG. Comparative follow-up of patients with acute and obtuse infundibulum-pelvic angle submitted to extracorporeal shockwave lithotripsy for lower caliceal stones: preliminary report and proposed study design. *J Endourol* 1997;11: 157–161.

21. Gould DL. Holmium:YAG laser and its use in the treatment of urolithiasis: our first 160 cases. *J Endourol* 1998;12:23–26.

22. Grasso M. Experience with the holmium laser as an endoscopic lithotrite. *Urology* 1996;48:199–206.

23. Lam HS, Lingeman JE, Russo R, Chua GT. Stone surface area determination techniques: a unifying concept of staghorn stone burden assessment. *J Urol* 1992;148:1026–1029.

24. Blandy JP, Singh M. The case for a more aggressive approach to staghorn stones. *J Urol* 1976;115:505–506.

25. Rous SM, Turner WR. Retrospective study of 95 patients with staghorn calculus disease. *J Urol* 1977;118:902–904.

26. Lam HS, Lingeman JE, Mosbaugh PG, et al. Evolution of the technique of combination therapy for staghorn calculi: a decreasing role for extracorporeal shock wave lithotripsy. *J Urol* 1992;148:1058–1062.

27. Streem SB, Geisinger MA. Combination therapy for staghorn calculi in solitary kidneys: functional results with long-term follow-up. *J Urol* 1993;149:449–452.

28. Smith JE, Van Arsdalen KN, Hanno PM, Pollack HM. Extracorporeal shock wave lithotripsy treatment of calculi in horseshoe kidneys. *J Urol* 1989;142:683–686.

29. Esuvaranathan K, Tan EC, Tung KH, Foo KT. Stones in horseshoe kidneys: results of treatment by extracorporeal shock wave lithotripsy and endourology. *J Urol* 1991;146:1213–1215.

30. Oshinsky GS, Smith AD. Endopyelotomy. In: Smith AD, Badlani GH, Bagley DH, et al., eds. *Smith's textbook of endourology.* St. Louis: Quality Medical Publishing, 1996:1550–1557.

31. Motola JA, Badlani GH, Smith AD. Results of 212 consecutive endopyelotomies: an 8-year follow-up. *J Urol* 1993;149:453–456.

32. Van Cangh PJ, Nesa S, Galeon M, et al. Vessels around the ureteropelvic junction: significance and imaging by conventional radiology. *J Endourol* 1996;10:111–119.

33. Leveillee RJ, Hulbert JC. Treatment of caliceal diverticula and infundibular stenosis. In: Smith AD, Badlani GH, Bagley DH, et al., eds. *Smith's textbook of endourology.* St. Louis: Quality Medical Publishing, 1996:319–337.

34. Jones JA, Lingeman JE, Steidle CP. The roles of extracorporeal shock wave lithotripsy and percutaneous nephrostolithotomy in the management of pyelocaliceal diverticula. *J Urol* 1991;146:724–727.

35. Singal RK, Denstedt JD. Contemporary management of ureteral stones. *Urol Clin North Am* 1997;24:59–70.

SECTION XII

Dentistry

83. Development and Structure of Teeth and Periodontal Tissues

Sheila J. Jones, Ph.D. and Alan Boyde, Ph.D.

Department of Anatomy and Developmental Biology, University College London, London, England

NORMAL DENTAL DEVELOPMENT

Three of the five distinct types of mineralized tissues found in the human body, enamel, dentine, and cementum, occur only in teeth. As turnover in these tissues is nonexistent or minimal, they form a valuable, permanent record of conditions prevailing at their time of formation. Teeth form at special locations within the jaws mapped out by the overlapping of molecular signals common to many developmental processes (1). Combinations of homeobox genes in mesenchyme derived from the cranial neural crest are thought to control the types of teeth that form in different positions along the developing jaws (2). Sequential interactions at the interface between epithelium over the facial processes and the mesenchyme play a crucial role in tooth morphogenesis, the main signaling molecules being Shh, BMPs, FGF, and Wnt families (1).

The embryonic tooth germ passes through three morphologic stages, described as bud, cap, and bell, and has three main components, the enamel organ, the dental papilla, and the dental follicle. The epithelial enamel organ differentiates into a four-layered structure, within which the enamel knot appears to be the signaling center that regulates tooth shape (3). A complex sequence of epithelial–mesenchymal interactions results in a wave of differentiation, which starts at the eventual enamel–dentine junction underlying the cusp tips or incisal central mammelon and spreads away, eventually delineating the entire junction between the tissues as the tooth germ grows. The expression of secretory signal molecules varies continuously in the different cell types during tooth initiation and construction (4). Odontoblasts, which make dentine, are postmitotic cells that differentiate from mesenchymal cells of the dental papilla at the interface with the inner enamel epithelial cells of the enamel organ, which themselves differentiate into preameloblasts. Dentine formation triggers the preameloblasts to differentiate into ameloblasts, the cells that produce enamel (5). A bilayer of epithelial cells, the epithelial root sheath, extends from the enamel organ at the base of the developing crown to map out the dentine–cement junction and initiate the differentiation of the odontoblasts of the root. The third tissue type, cementum, is the product of both fibroblasts and cementoblasts, which differentiate from mesenchymal cells of the dental follicle adjacent to the dentine once epithelial cells of the root sheath have moved away from the interface. In human teeth, afibrillar cementum may form on the enamel surface close to the junction between the crown and the root if there are interruptions in the covering layer of epithelial cells once enamel formation has been completed. Within the developing tooth, a core of loose connective tissue remains and eventually forms the dental pulp.

The dental follicle, also derived from cells of the cranial neural crest, gives rise to three components of the periodontium: cementum, alveolar bone, and the intervening periodontal ligament. The tooth germs are partially enclosed by the developing alveolar bone—this is initially typical woven bone, formed by osteoblasts, with enclosed osteocytes, and is remodeled to accommodate the growing teeth by osteoclasts of hematopoietic origin. The follicle, a sac of loose connective tissue that separates the developing tooth from its bony crypt, is essential for eruption and will become the periodontal ligament on tooth eruption (6). This tissue contributes extrinsic collagen fibers to the cementum and alveolar bone, and its main cell type is the fibroblast.

NORMAL DENTAL STRUCTURE

Enamel

Enamel matrix is delicate when first secreted, at which time it is protected by the soft enamel organ. The mature, erupted enamel—the hardest of the hard tissues—is acellular and may contain 98% by weight or 96% by volume of an apatitic calcium phosphate of variable composition (7). The final strength of enamel partly derives from the dentine mold on which it grows. The junction between these tissues is ill defined and irregular on a microscopic scale, with tongues of dentine projecting into the enamel, crystals of unknown provenance at the common boundary, and many fine, short enamel tubules marking where ameloblast processes once contacted odontoblasts. Spindles, expanded continuations of dentine tubules within enamel, probably result from the envelopment of individual ameloblasts that died as amelogenesis commenced.

The extracellular proteinaceous matrix of developing enamel is secreted by ameloblasts, which are highly polarized, tall cells. Its main components are amelogenins, tissue-specific proteins rich in proline, leucine, histidine, and glutamyl residues (8). Other, nonacidic proteins include tuftelin and amelin (ameloblastin): the 3-D protein array is thought to control crystal growth (9). To achieve enamel's high degree of mineralization, much of its organic matrix is degraded by neutral metalloproteinases and serine proteases and removed, even while ameloblasts are still secretory. The crystals are initially very long and slender, and rich in carbonate, and then thicken with a concomitant decrease in carbonate content. In humans, relatively large amounts of mineral accumulate at early stages of development, and the enamel has a long postsecretory maturation period, during which it becomes hard.

The most notable feature of enamel is the organization of the crystals into enamel "prisms," about 6 μm across and up to several millimeters long, demarcated by a sharp change in crystal orientation (Fig. 1). Enamel crystals grow mainly with their long c-axes nearly parallel to each other,

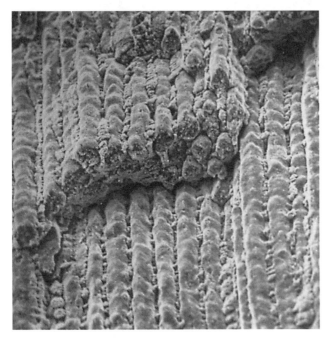

FIG. 1. Human enamel fractured to show the form of the prisms, which are about 6 μm across. SEM; field width, 82 μm.

and the larger sides of their flattened hexagonal cross sections parallel. Where the rate of formation is low, as in the superficial enamel, the secretory interface is nearly flat and there is little variation in the underlying crystal orientation. However, during most of enamel formation, the secretory (Tomes') process of each ameloblast is lodged in a pit at the interface. Enamel matrix is released between the pits, below a continuous belt of intercellular attachments, and at the pit wall/floor (10). The interpit phase is continuous and the crystals have their long axes perpendicular to the general plane of the developing enamel surface. In human enamel, the dividing lines of the prism junctions are incomplete, and the interlocking prisms are described as keyhole-shaped. The concentration of protein at the discontinuities in crystal orientation increases relatively during enamel maturation. Tufts and lamellae are other regions that finally contain less mineral and higher concentrations of enamel proteins.

As ameloblasts move away from the dentine, they travel in groups across the surface they make. This results in decussation of the enamel prisms, with zones of prisms with contrasting 3D courses forming the Hunter–Schreger bands. The sides of the prisms show varicosities (Fig. 1) with the same period as cross-striations in the prisms, that are thought to be due to circadian changes in the composition of the mineral component (10). A prominence of the cross-striations occurs at 7 to 10-day intervals (the regular striae of Retzius), and major life events, such as birth (the neonatal line), or severe illness during enamel formation, may be recorded as conspicuous incremental lines. At the finished enamel surface, perikymata or imbrication lines are outcrops of the internal growth layers. They grade from horizontal bands displaying pits alternating with smoother regions as more incisal or occlusal levels, to, near the neck of the tooth, small steps at the sharp boundary between the imbricating layers.

The unerupted crown is protected from resorption by a layer of cells termed the reduced enamel epithelium. This is lost once the tooth erupts. As the tooth wears during function, the surface features of the enamel become abraded, microcracks develop, particularly along developmental faults, and the chemistry of the mineral exposed to the oral environment changes.

Dentine

Dentine forms the bulk of the tooth and extends within both crown and root. It is a pale, creamy yellow color, in contrast to the much whiter, harder enamel. Dentine is tough and compliant, and its prime feature is its penetration by tubules that radiate out from the dental pulp to the periphery (Fig. 2). The peripheral, first-formed dentine is termed mantle dentine, and the inner, circumferential dentine. After differentiating from cells of the dental papilla, the odontoblasts retreat centripetally as a cone-shaped monolayer sheet, depositing a collagenous matrix of predentine and leaving lengthening cell processes with many side branches that remain in the tubules within the dentine (11). The curved paths that the cell bodies take are therefore recorded in the extracellular matrix. This is similar to that of bone, comprising type I collagen, acidic proteins, and proteoglycans. Two of the matrix proteins are thought to be unique: the highly phosphorylated dentine phosphoprotein, the predominant noncollagenous protein in dentine, and dentine sialoprotein (12)—these are products of the same gene: they bind to collagen and are postulated to control the initiation and growth of the apatite crystals. The predentine matrix matures and then mineralizes after a lag time of about 4 days (13). Dentine contains about 70% mineral (wet weight). Carbonate-rich calcium hydroxyapatite crystals form in relation to submicroscopic vesicles shed by the odontoblasts in

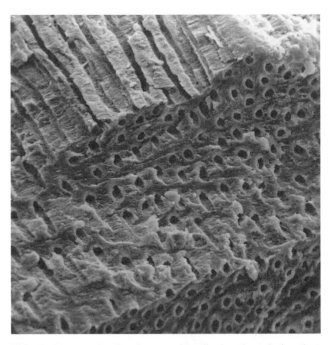

FIG. 2. Human dentine fractured to display the tubules that are about 2 μm across. SEM; field width, 88 μm.

the mantle layer, or at loci on collagen rich in noncollagenous proteins. Mineralization extends radially in the matrix, possibly by a process of secondary nucleation, forming regions of dentine known as calcospherites. These may fail to fuse, leaving unmineralized interglobular dentine between them. In a second, concurrent pattern of mineralization, crystals extend along the fine type I collagen fibrils, which lie in a feltwork parallel to the incremental planes. Peritubular dentine is deposited within the tubules, partially occluding them. It contains a negligible amount of collagen and mineralizes to a higher degree than the surrounding intertubular dentine.

Like enamel, dentine is deposited rhythmically, leaving lines marking daily and approximately weekly increments (14). Major life events, such as birth (the neonatal line) and illness or dietary deficiencies, are recorded as disturbances in the structure of the tissue forming at the time. Once eruption has occurred and root formation is complete, further dentine formation occurs as slowly deposited, regular secondary dentine or, irregularly, as a response of the pulp–dentine complex to attrition or disease. Nerves pass from the dental pulp between odontoblasts and extend into the dentine tubules for variable distances. Dentine is exquisitely painful if touched or subjected to large temperature or osmotic changes.

Like any other loose connective tissue, the dental pulp shows age changes, but these may include diffuse or local calcifications and the formation of dental stones. Occlusion of the dentine tubules with peritubular dentine extends coronally from the apex of the root; the resulting transparent dentine can be used as a guide to the age of the tooth.

Cementum

Cementum is a calcified connective tissue, which is deposited initially upon the newly mineralized dentine matrix of the root. Secretory proteins from the cells of the epithelial root sheath may be included in the first-formed matrix (15,16). Cementum is laid down centrifugally from the cement–dentine junction and is marked by incremental lines that are close together, continuous, and evenly spaced where apposition was slow, and patchy and irregular otherwise. The tissue is similar to bundle (Sharpey fiber) bone in that it incorporates extrinsic collagen fibers formed by fibroblasts (17): these fibers may be very closely packed, composing the whole tissue in slowly forming acellular cementum (18), or be separated from each other by intervening intrinsic collagen fibers, of cementoblast origin, which lie in the plane of the developing root surface (Fig. 3). Where cementum is deposited very rapidly, it is cellular, containing cementocytes, which resemble the osteocytes of bundle bone. In heavily remodeled root apices, there may be patches of cellular cementum without extrinsic fibers. Only in cementum containing intrinsic fibers is a well-defined region of unmineralized precementum, equivalent to osteoid, present at the surface of the tissue. The collagen of both the extrinsic and intrinsic fibers is type I. The main noncollagenous proteins of cementum identified so far (osteopontin, osteocalcin, bone sialoprotein, and α2HS-glycoprotein) do not distinguish it from other calcified tissues (19).

Cementum mineralization reflects the rate of formation and the composition of the matrix. In afibrillar coronal ce-

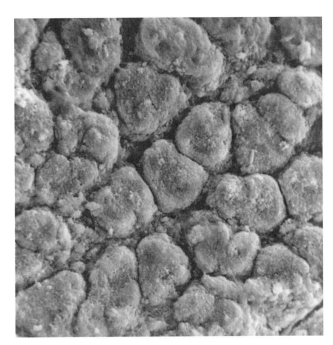

FIG. 3. Human cementum surface, made anorganic, showing mineralized ends of extrinsic fibers, about 6 μm diameter, separated by intrinsic fibers. SEM; field width, 30 μm.

mentum, the layer of noncollagenous proteins adsorbed onto the enamel surface mineralizes fully. Adjacent to the root dentine, an osteopontin-rich layer also becomes more highly mineralized than the neighboring tissues. The extrinsic fibers of slowly forming cementum mineralize completely, the advancing mineralized tidemark across the fibers being relatively flat and marking the border between cementum and the dental sac or periodontal ligament. This type of cementum is paler and more highly mineralized than dentine. Where only a small proportion of intrinsic fibers exists in acellular cementum, the extrinsic fibers lead the mineralization front. As the rate of deposition of cementum increases, and proportionately more intrinsic fibers are deposited, the likelihood increases that the extrinsic fibers will retain unmineralized cores. During periods of fast cellular cementogenesis, even the intrinsic fibers may retain unmineralized sections, and the mineralization front becomes irregular, with the extrinsic component lagging behind the intrinsic. This cementum type is the softest and least well mineralized of the calcified dental tissues. The mineralization front can be read to estimate the current rate of formation, and the degree of mineralization of the fibers within the tissue indicates past rates (17). The carbonate-rich apatite phase is similar to that of bone (Fig. 4).

INTERRELATIONS OF TEETH, PERIODONTAL TISSUES, AND ALVEOLAR BONE

Teeth are a highly specialized part of an integrated functional unit (see Fig. 5), the primary (but not sole) purpose of which is the mastication of food. Unique among the calcified tissues, enamel is exposed to the outer environment. As the tooth erupts, the alveolar bone is resorbed to allow its passage, its root develops, and the crown pierces the oral mucosa, which finally contributes to a tight ring seal of

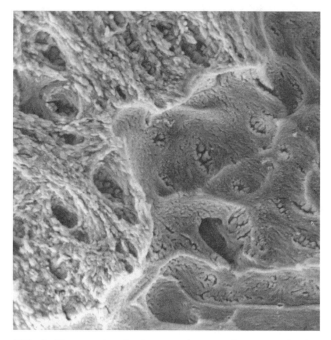

FIG. 4. Human alveolar bone surface made anorganic: the resorption lacunae reveal that the extrinsic (Sharpey's) fibers were only partly mineralized. The remainder of the surface was forming, as evidenced by incomplete mineralization of intrinsic and extrinsic fibers. SEM; field width, 110 μm.

epithelial cells on the enamel close to the junction of crown and root. The molecular signals controlling eruption are unknown (20). At emergence, the root of the tooth is not yet fully formed, and the pulpal aspect of the root end (apex) resembles a large closing cone. Root completion takes about a further 18 months in the deciduous teeth and up to 3 years in the permanent teeth. During root development, the follicle becomes organized into the periodontal ligament, which supports the tooth, provides nutrition and mechanosensation, and allows physiologic tooth movement. Through the groups of fibers of the periodontal ligament, functioning teeth are linked to each other, the gingiva, and the alveolar bone. On either side of the ligament, its principal fibers, composed of types I and III collagen, are incorporated within cementum

and bundle bone; within the ligament, there is constant adaptive remodeling of the fetal-like soft tissue.

Cementum in permanent teeth is little remodeled, but the surface of alveolar bone is continually resorbing and forming to allow the tooth to move in response to eruption, growth drift, or changing functional forces (6). Resorption of deciduous tooth roots begins shortly after their completion, appearing first and most extensively on the aspect adjacent to the successional tooth. Interspersed between resorptive bursts are occasional short periods of repair by cemento(osteo)blasts. Typical osteoclasts resorb both cementum and dentine and, in deciduous molars, a little enamel.

REFERENCES

1. Thesleff I, Sharpe P. Signalling networks regulating dental development. *Mech Dev* 1997;67:111–123.
2. Sharpe PT. Homeobox genes and orofacial development. *Connect Tissue Res* 1995;32:17–25.
3. Jernvall J, Åberg T, Kettunen P, Keranen S, Thesleff I. The life history of an embryonic signalling center: BMP-4 induces p21 and is associated with apoptosis in the tooth enamel knot. *Development* 1998;125: 161–169.
4. Åberg T, Wozney J, Thesleff I. Expression patterns of bone morphogenetic proteins (Bmps) in the developing mouse tooth suggests roles in morphogenesis and cell differentiation. *Dev Dyn* 1997;210:383–396.
5. Thesleff I, Åberg T. Tooth morphogenesis and the differentiation of ameloblasts. In: Chadwick D, Cardew G, eds. *Dental enamel.* (Ciba Foundation Symposium 205). Chichester: Wiley, 1997:1–17, 1997.
6. Marks SC, Schroeder HE. Tooth eruption: theories and facts. *Anat Rec* 1996;245:374–393.
7. Elliott JC. Structure, crystal chemistry and density of enamel apatites. In: Chadwick D, Cardew G, eds. *Dental enamel.* (Ciba Foundation Symposium 205). Chichester: Wiley, 1997:54–67.
8. Fincham AG, Simmer JP. Amelogenin proteins of developing dental enamel. In: Chadwick D, Cardew G, eds. *Dental enamel.* (Ciba Foundation Symposium 205). Chichester: Wiley, 1997:118–134.
9. Paine ML, Krebsbach PH, Chen LS, et al. Protein-to-protein interactions: criteria defining the assembly of the enamel organic matrix. *J Dent Res* 1998;77:496–502.
10. Boyde A. Microstructure of enamel. In: Chadwick D, Cardew G, eds. *Dental enamel.* (Ciba Foundation Symposium 205). Chichester: Wiley, 1997:18–31.
11. Sasaki T, Garant PR. Structure and organization of odontoblasts. *Anat Rec* 1996;245:235–249.
12. Butler WT, Ritchie HH, Bronckers AL. Extracellular matrix proteins of dentine. *Dental enamel.* (Ciba Foundation Symposium 205). Chichester: Wiley, 1997:107–115.
13. Linde A, Goldberg M. Dentinogenesis. *Crit Rev Oral Biol Med* 1993;4:679–728.
14. Dean MC, Scandrett AE. The relation between long-period incremental markings in dentine and daily cross-striations in enamel in human teeth. *Arch Oral Biol* 1996;41:233–241.
15. Snead ML. Enamel biology logodaedaly: getting to the root of the problem, or ''Who's on first. . .''. *J Bone Miner Res* 1996;11:899–904.
16. Bosshardt DD, Schroeder HE. Cementogenesis reviewed: a comparison between human premolars and rodent molars. *Anat Rec* 1996;245: 267–292.
17. Jones SJ. Cement. In: Osborn JW, ed. *Dental anatomy and embryology.* Boston: Blackwell Scientific, 1981:193–205, 286–294.
18. Groeneveld MC, van den Bos T, Everts V, Beertsen W. Formation of acellular root cementum: a new concept. In: Davidovitz Z, ed. *The biological mechanisms of tooth eruption, resorption and replacement by implants.* Boston: Harvard Society for the Advancement of Orthodontics, 1994:341–348.
19. McKee MD, Zalzal S, Nanci A. Extracellular matrix in tooth cementum and mantle dentin: localization of osteopontin and other noncollagenous proteins, plasma proteins and glycoconjugates by electron microscopy. *Anat Rec* 1996;245:293–312.
20. Wise GE, Lin F. The molecular biology of initiation of tooth eruption. *J Dent Res* 1995;74:303–306.

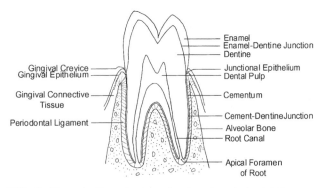

FIG. 5. Organization of mineralized and periodontal tissues in the erupted tooth.

84. Dental Manifestations of Disorders of Bone and Mineral Metabolism

Paul H. Krebsbach, D.D.S., Ph.D. and Peter J. Polverini, D.D.S., D.M.Sc.

Department of Oral Medicine/Pathology/Oncology, University of Michigan School of Dentistry, Ann Arbor, Michigan

ORAL MANIFESTATIONS OF GENETIC SKELETAL DISORDERS

Although development of the mammalian dentition differs substantially from that of the skeleton, the cells and the mineralized components share many features with those of bone. Oral changes can occur in response to disorders of mineral metabolism. The clinical presentation may vary from very mild asymptomatic changes to alterations that severely alter the form and function of craniofacial structures. This section provides a concise overview of the dental manifestations of selected disorders of bone and mineral metabolism.

Dentinogenesis Imperfecta

Developmental disorders of the dentition are often found concurrent with osteogenesis imperfecta (OI; see Chapter 72). Dental abnormalities have been described in several subtypes of OI, but are most prevalent in OI types IB, IC, and IVB (1). The diverse genetic and clinical presentations that define OI are also hallmarks of the changes observed in dentinogenesis imperfecta (DI). DI is an autosomal dominant inherited disorder that affects the development, structure, and function of dentin in both the primary and permanent dentitions. The dental defects associated with DI are specified as type I when they occur concurrent with OI, and type II, when only dental defects are observed. It has been reported that 10% to 50% of patients afflicted with OI also have DI. This assessment, however, may underestimate the true prevalence because mild forms of DI may require microscopic analysis for diagnosis (2). Type III DI, also known as the Brandywine type for a triracial isolate in Brandywine, Maryland, exhibits only dental defects and can vary in the clinical and radiographic presentation.

Clinically, the teeth of individuals with DI are characterized by an opalescent or amber-like appearance. The teeth are narrower at the cervical margins and thus exhibit a bulbous or bell-shaped crown. Other anomalies include fewer and irregular dentin tubules containing vesicles and abnormally thick collagen fibers (3). The structurally abnormal dentin may provide inadequate support for the overlying enamel. Although enamel is chemically and structurally normal in individuals with DI, the lack of support from dentin leads to fracturing and severe attrition of the teeth, a distinguishing clinical feature of DI. Radiographic analysis may aid in the diagnosis of DI. The short, conical roots and cervical constrictions are remarkable. In young individuals, the pulp chambers may appear normal, but with age, the overproduction of abnormal dentin leads to obliteration of the pulp. A notable radiographic exception is seen in type III DI, in which the pulp chambers and root canals are extraordinarily large.

Whereas most patients with OI have mutations in either the COL1A1 or COL1A2 genes that encode the subunits of type I collagen, the genetic defect causing DI has not been defined. The DI type II locus has been mapped to human chromosome 4q21-q23, a region that contains several genes associated with mineralized tissues. To date, several candidate genes including osteopontin and dentin matrix protein-1 have been excluded as causative genes (4,5). The dentin sialophosphoprotein gene, which contains coding information for both dentin sialoprotein and dentin phosphoprotein, also maps to human chromosome 4q and thus may be considered a candidate gene for DI type II because of their restricted tissue distribution and potential roles in biomineralization (6).

Dentin Dysplasia

Dentin dysplasia is an autosomal dominant disorder affecting dentin formation and, like DI, has been mapped to human chromosome 4q. Dental anomalies consistent with dentin dysplasia have been described in OI type IC. Therefore the candidate gene(s) for DI type II may also be candidates for dentin dysplasia. The clinical appearance of primary teeth is similar in patients with DI and dentin dysplasia. This similarity is lost, however, once the permanent teeth have erupted. With dentin dysplasia, the permanent teeth are normal in color, have short roots with "thistle-tube" pulp chambers, and contain pulp stones of irregular shape (7,8). The short roots often are associated with periapical radiolucencies that can lead to premature exfoliation of the teeth.

Osteopetrosis

The lack of appropriate bone resorption observed in osteopetrosis (see Chapter 70) has several implications in the craniofacial region. The jawbones are abnormally dense at the expense of cancellous bone, and these changes may affect normal tooth development. Because normal tooth eruption is dependent on resorption of alveolar bone surrounding the developing tooth germ, inadequate resorptive function in osteopetrosis may limit the eruptive mechanisms and place altered forces on the erupting teeth. Dental findings associated with osteopetrosis include congenitally absent teeth, unerupted and malformed teeth, delayed eruption, and enamel hypoplasia (9). There is a reduced calcium/phosphorous ratio in both enamel and dentin that may alter hydroxyapatite crystal formation and contribute to an increased caries index, as has been reported in several cases. Additionally, there are deviations in amino acid content, indicative of altered matrix composition (9). Perhaps the most serious dental complication of osteopetrosis is the propensity to develop osteomyelitis (10). Because the vascular supply to the jaws is compromised, avascular necrosis and infection after dental extractions may lead to osteomyelitis that is difficult to treat. Thus extraction of teeth must be performed as atraumatically as possible.

Mucopolysaccharidoses

The mucopolysaccharidoses (MPSs; see Chapter 73) are a family of related inherited diseases that are characterized by a deficiency in glycosaminoglycan catabolism. These disorders, classified MPS I through MPS VII, are distinguished from each other based on genetic, biochemical, and clinical analyses (1). Although heterogeneous, several craniofacial characteristics are similar between the different subgroups. The oral manifestations may include a short and broad mandible with abnormal condylar development and limited temporomandibular joint function. The teeth are often peg-shaped and exhibit increased interdental spacing, perhaps due to the frequently observed gingival hyperplasia and macroglossia. Some forms of MPS have abnormally thin enamel covering the clinical crowns and radiographic evidence of cystic lesions surrounding the molar teeth that contain excessive dermatan sulfate and collagen (11–14).

ORAL MANIFESTATIONS OF METABOLIC BONE DISEASES

Metabolic diseases of bone are disorders of bone remodeling that characteristically involve the entire skeleton and are often manifest in the oral cavity, which can lead to the diagnosis of the underlying systemic disease. Numerous studies suggest that subclinical derangements in calcium homeostasis and bone metabolism may also contribute to a variety of dental abnormalities including alveolar ridge resorption and periodontal bone loss in predisposed individuals. The significance of this spectrum of diseases and their overall impact on oral health and dental management are likely to increase as the elderly segment of the population increases in the coming decades (15).

Vitamin D Deficiency

In vitamin D–resistant rickets (see Chapter 63), the primary oral abnormality is similar to dentin dysplasia. Enamel is usually reported to be normal or hypoplastic. Patients also have delayed tooth eruption, and radiographically, teeth often display enlarged pulp chambers. Other salient radiographic findings include decreased alveolar bone density, thinning of bone trabeculae, loss of lamina dura, and retarded tooth calcification (16). In familial hypophosphatemia (see Chapter 45), dental findings are often the first clinically noticeable signs of the disease and resemble those seen in rickets and osteomalacia.

Hypophosphatasia

Hypophosphatasia (see Chapter 66) is characterized by defective mineralization of the skeletal and dental structures of the body and deficiencies in liver, bone, and kidney isoenzymes of alkaline phosphatase (17). The classic oral features of hypophosphatasia are premature tooth loss due to hypo-

plasia of cementum, large pulp spaces, late eruption of teeth, and delayed apical closure, especially of the permanent teeth. Bone loss is primarily horizontal, and in the adult form of the disease, there is often widespread dental caries.

Paget's Disease

Paget's disease, also known as osteitis deformans (see Chapter 77), a disorder of bone remodeling (18,19), is hallmarked by the presence of irregular islands of bone with prominent internal cement lines that create a mosaic pattern. In the craniofacial bones, radiographic lesions usually progress from irregular lytic lesions to areas of sclerosis that present with a distinctive cotton-wool appearance. Patients also may demonstrate alveolar ridge enlargement, poor denture adaptation, and separation of the teeth and hypercementosis. As the disease progresses, there may be extensive bone deformity with nerve compression and altered blood flow, conditions that can make tooth extraction problematic.

ORAL MANIFESTATIONS OF ACQUIRED DISORDERS

Benign Nonodontogenic Neoplasms of the Jaws

Benign fibroosseous lesions of the jaw are a heterogeneous group of disorders characterized by the replacement of normal trabecular bone and marrow with cellular fibrous connective tissue and a disorganized array of randomly oriented mineralized tissue. The most common group of lesions is known collectively as the cementoosseous dysplasias (20,21), so named because they contain spherical calcifications believed to be of cemental origin and randomly oriented mineralized structures resembling bone. Two other conditions included in this category are fibrous dysplasia and cherubism, which are of greater clinical significance because they tend to attain a larger size and have the potential for producing greater facial disfigurement and severe malocclusion. Among the cementoosseous dysplasias, the most common is a condition known as periapical cemental dysplasia. This asymptomatic lesion presents radiographically as a mixed radiolucent/radiopaque lesion that involves a single mandibular quadrant in middle-aged women. It is frequently encountered below the apices of the mandibular incisors. The involved teeth are vital, and no treatment is required. Florid cementoosseous dysplasia is a more extensive form of periapical cemental dysplasia that invariably involves multiple jaw quadrants. Fibrous dysplasia (see Chapter 71) is a self-limiting disorder that can affect single (monostotic) or multiple (polyostotic) bones. It begins as fibrous replacement of the medullary bone that progresses to woven bone and eventually to dense lamellar bone. The condition is commonly found in juveniles and young adults but can be encountered as an adult-onset form. Polyostotic fibrous dysplasia can occur as part of the McCune–Albright syndrome, in which it is associated with skin pigmentation and endocrinopathies. When it occurs in the absence of endocrine abnormalities, it is referred to as Jaffe syndrome. Recent studies suggest that the underlying defect in the McCune–Albright form of fibrous dysplasia may involve mutations in the Gs alpha gene, resulting in activation during maturation of precursor osteogenic cells to normal osteoblast cells (22). Cherubism is an autosomal dominant disorder that manifests as bilateral jaw enlargement primarily involving the mandibles of children.

Malignant Nonodontogenic Neoplasms of the Jaws

Osteosarcoma is the most common malignant neoplasm derived from bone cells, occurring in one of every 100,000 people (16). The peak incidence when it occurs in the jaws is approximately 10 years later than the peak incidence in the long bones. The radiographic appearance of osteosarcoma varies considerably depending on the histologic type. Osteosarcomas that produce large amount of mineralized bone-like tissue will present as large areas of radiopacity within a diffuse radiolucent background. A characteristic finding in jaw lesions is widening of the periodontal ligament in adjacent teeth. Although this finding is not unique to osteosarcoma, it is sufficiently consistent to be of diagnostic value. Occlusal radiographs also may reveal a sunburst pattern of radiopacity radiating from the periosteum and may be of assistance diagnostically.

REFERENCES

1. Gorlin RJ, Cohen MM Jr, Levin LS. *Syndromes of the head and neck.* Oxford Monographs on Medical Genetics. New York: Oxford University Press, 1990.
2. Waltimo J, Ojanotko-Harri A, Lukinmaa PL. Mild forms of dentinogenesis imperfecta in association with osteogenesis imperfecta as characterized by light and transmission electron microscopy. *J Oral Pathol Med* 1996;25:256–264.
3. Waltimo J. Hyperfibers and vesicles in dentin matrix in dentinogenesis imperfecta (DI) associated with osteogenesis imperfecta (OI). *J Oral Pathol Med* 1994;23:389–393.
4. Crosby AH, Edwards SJ, Murray JC, Dixon MJ. Genomic organization of the human osteopontin gene: exclusion of the locus from a causative role in the pathogenesis of dentinogenesis imperfecta type II. *Genomics* 1995;27:155–160.
5. Hirst KL, Simmons D, Feng J, Aplin H, Dixon MJ, MacDougall M. Elucidation of the sequence and the genomic organization of the human dentin matrix acidic phosphoprotein 1 (DMP1) gene: exclusion of the locus from a causative role in the pathogenesis of dentinogenesis imperfecta type II. *Genomics* 1997;42:38–45.
6. MacDougall M, Simmons D, Luan X, Nydegger J, Feng J, Gu TT. Dentin phosphoprotein and dentin sialoprotein are cleavage products expressed from a single transcript coded by a gene on human chromosome 4: dentin phosphoprotein DNA sequence determination. *J Biol Chem* 1997;272:835–842.
7. Giansanti JS, Allen JD. Dentin dysplasia, type II, or dentin dysplasia, coronal type. *Oral Surg Oral Med Oral Pathol* 1974;38:911–917.
8. Lukinmaa PL, Ranta H, Ranta K, Kaitila I, Hietanen J. Dental findings in osteogenesis imperfecta: II. Dysplastic and other developmental defects. *J Craniofac Genet Dev Biol* 1987;7:127–135.
9. Dick HM, Simpson WJ. Dental changes in osteopetrosis. *Oral Surg Oral Med Oral Pathol* 1972;34:408–416.
10. Dyson DP. Osteomyelitis of the jaws in Albers-Schonberg disease. *Br J Oral Surg* 1970;7:178–187.
11. Downs AT, Crisp T, Ferretti G. Hunter's syndrome and oral manifestations: a review. *Pediatr Dent* 1995;17:98–100.
12. Keith O, Scully C, Weidmann GM. Orofacial features of Scheie (Hurler-Scheie) syndrome (alpha-MD4l-iduronidase deficiency). *Oral Surg Oral Med Oral Pathol* 1990;70:70–74.
13. Kinirons MJ, Nelson J. Dental findings in mucopolysaccharidosis type IV A (Morquio's disease type A). *Oral Surg Oral Med Oral Pathol* 1990;70:176–179.
14. Smith KS, Hallett KB, Hall RK, Wardrop RW, Firth N. Mucopolysaccharidosis: MPS VI and associated delayed tooth eruption. *Int J Oral Maxillofac Surg* 1995;24:176–180.
15. Solt DB. The pathogenesis, oral manifestations, and implications for dentistry of metabolic bone disease. *Curr Opin Dent* 1991;1:783–791.
16. Neville BW, Damm DD, Allen CM. *Oral and maxillofacial pathology.* Philadelphia: WB Saunders, 1995.
17. Chapple IL. Hypophosphatasia: dental aspects and mode of inheritance. *J Clin Periodontol* 1993;20:615–622.
18. Carter LC. Paget's disease: important features for the general practitioner. *Comp Contin Edu Dent* 1991;11:662–669.
19. Merkow RL, Lane JM. Paget's disease of bone. *Orthop Clin North Am* 1990;21:171–189.
20. Sapp JP, Eversole LR, Wysocki GP. *Contemporary oral and maxillofacial surgery.* St. Louis: Mosby-Year Book, 1997.
21. Waldron CA. Fibro-osseous lesions of the jaws. *J Oral Maxillofac Surg* 1993;51:828–835.
22. Riminucci M, Fisher LW, Shenker A, Spiegel AM, Bianco P, Gehron Robey P. Fibrous dysplasia of bone in the McCune-Albright syndrome: abnormalities in bone formation. *Am J Pathol* 1997;151:1587–1600.

85. Periodontitis-Induced Alveolar Bone Loss and Its Treatment

Marjorie K. Jeffcoat, D.M.D.

Department of Periodontics, The University of Alabama at Birmingham School of Dentistry, Birmingham, Alabama

INTRODUCTION

Periodontitis is characterized by resorption of the alveolar bone (Fig. 1) as well as loss of the soft-tissue attachment to the tooth. Progressive periodontitis will result in continued alveolar bone loss and may result in tooth mobility, abscesses, and ultimately, tooth loss. Although the reported prevalence may vary according to the epidemiologic study design, the 1985 National Survey of Oral Health of United

States Adults indicated that 94% of female senior citizens examined demonstrated at least one site with at least 2-mm loss of attachment. The most recent NHANES study revealed that although 90% of persons 13 years or older had some loss of attachment, only 15% had clinical evidence of severe disease. The purpose of this chapter is to succinctly review current evidence supporting a role for modulators of the host response in reducing alveolar bone loss due to periodontitis.

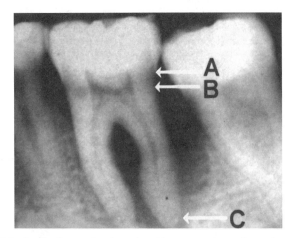

FIG. 1. Radiograph of tooth with severe bone loss due to periodontitis. **A:** Cemento–enamel junction. **B:** Approximate location of the alveolar crest in health. **C:** Location of the alveolar crest indicates severe bone resorption.

ETIOLOGY OF PERIODONTITIS

Periodontitis is initiated by bacterial pathogens in the dental plaque. Establishing a causative relation between a putative periodontopathic pathogen and periodontitis is not easy (1). The bacterial pathogen, *Actinobacillus actinomycetemcomitans (A.a.)*, is most clearly established for juvenile periodontitis. In adult periodontitis, a wide range of bacterial species has been implicated including *A.a., Porphyromonas gingivalis,* and *Bacteroides forsythus* (1). The development of periodontitis requires colonization of pathogenic bacteria in a susceptible host. For an excellent review of host factors involved in the pathogenesis of adult periodontitis, see Offenbacher, 1996 (2). This chapter focuses on those factors that may be altered with a resultant clinical benefit.

Inflammatory mediators play an important role in periodontal destruction. Prostaglandins are associated with bone loss *in vivo* and *in vitro*. In now-classic studies, Offenbacher et al. (3) demonstrated that high levels of gingival crevicular fluid prostaglandin E_2 (PGE_2) are associated with active progression of periodontitis. The role of cytokines also is of increasing interest. Interleukin-1 (IL-1) has been found in gingival crevicular fluid during inflammation, and levels decrease after periodontal treatment. In a recent study, Cavanaugh et al. (4) correlated gingival crevicular fluid levels of PGE_2 and IL-1 with bone loss that occurred around the teeth in the subsequent 6 months. Taken collectively, these two mediators could account for 78% of the bone resorption observed. Most recently, the search for genetic markers for susceptibility to oral disease has pointed to a specific genotype of the polymorphic IL-1 gene cluster being associated with severe periodontitis in nonsmokers, with an odds ratio of 18.9 for ages 40 to 60 years (5). IL-1β is of interest because the proinflammatory cytokines are key regulators of the host immune response to microbial infection, extracellular matrix catabolism, and bone resorption. Functionally, this polymorphism is associated with high levels of IL-1 production, and high levels of IL-1 have been associated with progressive periodontal breakdown (4).

CONVENTIONAL TREATMENT OF PERIODONTITIS AND ASSOCIATED BONE LOSS

The mainstay of periodontal treatment involves controlling plaque bacteria. Self-administered plaque control and scaling and root planing performed by the dental professional serve to reduce the mass of bacterial plaque. Furthermore, root planing and surgical procedures smooth off the root surfaces by removing decalcified cementum and bacterial components such as endotoxins. Periodontal surgery provides access to the roots for effective root planing and/or for regenerative pocket-reduction procedures. Plaque bacteria also may be controlled with topical antiseptic agents, which are available both over the counter and by prescription. These nonspecific agents are effective for the reduction of plaque and gingivitis, but their effect on periodontitis has not been determined. To date, antibiotics, especially tetracycline and metronidazole, have been most successful in controlling or eradicating the *A.a.* of juvenile periodontitis. Although a wide range of systemic antibiotics (including tetracyclines, penicillins, metronidazole, clindamycin, and erythromycins) have been tested in adult periodontitis, the results are mixed (6). It is currently believed that the varied results in treating adult periodontitis with antibiotics may be because plaque is a biofilm, thereby limiting the efficacy of the antibiotics.

Slowing Alveolar Bone Loss by Decreasing Cyclooxygenase Metabolites

Recent studies have begun to address agents that control the host's contribution to the establishment of periodontitis. Tetracyclines have been shown to inhibit collagenase independent of their antibacterial effects (7). Our understanding of the role of mediators such as PGE_2 in periodontal disease is leading to new strategies for the treatment of periodontitis. In the early 1970s, investigators reported that inflamed gingiva from patients with periodontal diseases had significantly higher levels of PGE_2 than those in control patients. When such gingiva are cultured, the media resorbs bone *in vitro,* and this bone loss may be blocked by indomethacin. In a pioneering study, Offenbacher (3) later demonstrated that patients undergoing active periodontal destruction had higher gingival crevicular fluid PGE_2 levels than either healthy patients or patients with quiescent periodontitis (3). Beginning in the early 1980s, controlled studies in animals demonstrated the efficacy of nonsteroidal antiinflammatory drugs in slowing bone loss due to periodontitis (summarized in Table 1). In the absence of adequate plaque control, beagle dogs develop plaque, calculus, periodontal pockets, and alveolar bone loss that can eventually lead to tooth loss. Thus the beagle dog with naturally occurring periodontitis provides an excellent model for the study of agents that may slow alveolar bone loss. The nonsteroidal antiinflammatory agents flurbiprofen (8) and ibuprofen (9) significantly slowed the progression of bone loss relative to placebo in naturally occurring periodontal disease in beagles. Furthermore, gingival crevicular fluid levels of both PGE_2 and thromboxane were shown to decrease with flurbiprofen and ibuprofen treatment (10). Results of using the monkey ligature model

TABLE 1. *Studies of NSAIDs for the reduction of alveolar bone loss in animal models*

Model	Treatment period	Number of animals	Bone loss in placebo group	Bone loss in test group(s)	Comments	Authors
Beagles, natural periodontitis	6 months	12	4.38% of root length	0.78% of root length	p < 0.01	Williams (1985)
Beagles, natural periodontitis	6 months	22	6.42%	3.0% (4.0 mg ibuprofen) 1.8% (4.0 mg-sustained release ibuprofen) No significant difference for 0.4 mg ibuprofen)	Significant decreases in GCF PGE$_2$, TxB2 with treatment	Williams (1988) Offenbacher (1992)
Beagles, natural periodontitis	6 months	16	6.0% of root length	1.02% (0.02 mg/kg flurbiprofen) No significant difference for 1.0 mg/kg indomethacin	Significant decreases in GCF PGE$_2$, TxB2 with treatment	Offenbacher (1992) Williams (1987, 1988)
Beagles, natural periodontitis	6 months	12	6.42%	2.04% for topical flurbiprofen	Significant decreases in GCF PGE$_2$, TxB2 with treatment	Williams (1988) Offenbacher (1992)
Rhesus monkeys/ligated teeth to induce periodontitis	6 months	32			Significant reduction in alveolar bone loss and dose dependent inhibition of PGE$_2$ and Txb$_2$ with flurbiprofen	Offenbacher (1987, 1989)
Rhesus monkeys/ligated teeth to induce periodontitis	6 months	8 per group	1.40 mm loss	0.78 mm GAIN ketoprofen 1% cream	Suppression of GCF PGE$_2$ and LTB4 with treatment	Li (1996)
Cynomologus monkeys/ligated teeth and application of P. gingivalis to induce periodontitis	20 weeks	18	Bone loss in all sites	Bone loss in 67% of ibuprofen treated and 44% of meclofenamic acid treated animals		Kornman (1990)

for induced periodontitis also were supportive of the concept. In this model, a ligature, usually of silk suture material, is tied around the teeth to promote plaque accumulation and speed periodontal destruction. Some laboratories also apply putative periodontopathic bacteria (such as *P. gingivalis*) to the ligature to enhance further the rate of destruction. A slowing of the progression of periodontitis relative to placebo was observed in studies using flurbiprofen (11), ibuprofen, and meclofenamic acid (12). The ligature model also was used to demonstrate that topically applied ketoprofen cream also slows the progression of bone loss in periodontitis (13). A dose-dependent suppression of gingival crevicular fluid PGE$_2$ and thromboxane was observed in this model with flurbiprofen treatment (14). As a result of the success of the animal studies, double-blind placebo-controlled randomized clinical trials studying the efficacy of nonsteroidal antiinflammatory drugs to slow bone loss due to periodontitis were initiated. Technology, such as digital subtraction radiography, made it possible to detect small changes in bone support that have occurred over the course of a study with a standardized radiographic protocol, allowing an investigator to determine whether a drug is successful in reducing the progression of alveolar bone loss in a relatively short study period. Multicenter studies have shown that digital subtraction radiography is sensitive and specific in detecting bony changes as small as 1 mg, and that the quantitative methods estimate the size of the change in bone mass with a correlation better than 90% (15). Composite results from separate randomized double-blind studies using flurbiprofen. naproxen, meclofenamic acid, and topical ketorolac are shown in Table 2 (16–18). All nonsteroidal antiinflammatory drugs had a significant effect on slowing the progression of periodontitis.

Slowing Alveolar Bone Loss by Decreasing Collagenase and Osteoclastic Activity

Another approach to treating the bone loss in periodontitis is to exploit mechanisms and treatment established for osteoporosis. Common mechanisms may be involved in oral bone loss and osteoporosis (see Chapter 47). This hypothesis has begun to be explored with studies of alendronate. This bisphosphonate belongs to a class of drugs called bisphosphonates, which are synthetic analogues of pyrophosphate

TABLE 2. *Clinical studies of NSAIDs for the reduction of alveolar bone loss*

Disease	Length of study	Number of patients	Bone loss in placebo group	Bone loss in test group	Comments	Authors
Adult periodontitis	2 months	15	.11 mm loss	.13 mm gain with 50 mg bid flurbiprofen	$p < 0.02$	Jeffcoat (1988)
Rapidly progressive periodontitis	3 months	15	.14 mm loss	.27 mm gain with 500 mg bid naproxen	$p < 0.001$	Jeffcoat (1991)
Adult periodontitis	2 years	56	6% of root length over 2 years	4.08% over 2 years with 50 mg bid flurbiprofen	$p < 0.01$ at 12 mo	Williams (1989)
Rapidly progressive periodontitis	6 months	22	.42 mm loss	0.07 mm gain with 50 mg meclomen 0.20 mm gain with 100 mg bid meclomen	$p < 0.001$	Reddy (1993)
Adult periodontitis	6 months	55	0.63 mm loss	0.10 mm loss in 50 mg bid flurbiprofen group 0.20 mm gain in ketorolac rinse (1%) bid group	$p < 0.01$ significant decreases in PGE_2 in flurbiprofen and ketorolac rinse groups	Jeffcoat (1995)

that bind to the hydroxyapatite, and they act as specific inhibitors of osteoclast-mediated bone resorption. Alendronate used in the treatment of osteoporosis in postmenopausal women resulted in significant increases in bone mineral density. The results of an animal and a pilot clinical study for the treatment of alveolar bone loss are summarized in Table 3. Brunsvold et al. (19) and Reddy et al. (20) observed a bone sparing effect of alendronate by using ligature models for induced periodontitis in monkeys and dogs, respectively.

In a pilot study of patients with periodontitis, subjects who received placebo in addition to conventional scaling and root planing were at more than twice the risk for loss of alveolar bone height and density when compared with subjects receiving 20 mg/day alendronate and root planing (21). These results indicate that use of current and yet-to-be-developed therapies for the treatment of osteoporosis may provide new methods for dealing with the oral bone loss associated with periodontitis.

TABLE 3. *Studies of alendronate for the reduction of alveolar bone loss*

Type of study	Disease or model	Length of study	Number of subjects	Results	Author
Animal	Cynomolgous monkeys with ligature induced periodontitis	16 weeks	27	0.05 mg/kg alendronate significantly reduced progression of periodontitis as measured by bone density changes	Brunsvold (1992)
Animal	Beagles with ligature induced periodontitis	6 months	16	1.4 mm loss placebo group 0.20 mm loss in the alendronate group (3.0 mg/kg weekly)	Reddy (1995)
Human	Adult periodontitis	9 months	35	Relative risk of progressive bone loss is 0.45 in patients treated with 20 mg alendronate compared with placebo	Jeffcoat (1996)

REFERENCES

1. Zambon J. Periodontal diseases: microbial factors. *Ann Periodontol* 1996;1:879–925.
2. Offenbacher S. Periodontal diseases: pathogenesis. *Ann Periodontol* 1996;1:821–878.
3. Offenbacher S, Odle BM, Van Dyke TE. The use of crevicular fluid prostaglandin E_2 levels as a predictor of periodontal attachment loss. *J Periodontal Res* 1986;21:101–112.
4. Cavanaugh PF Jr, Meredith MP, Buchanan W, Doyle MJ, Reddy MS, Jeffcoat MK. Coordinate production of PGE_2 and IL-1 beta in the gingival crevicular fluid of adults with periodontitis: its relationship to alveolar bone loss and disruption by twice daily treatment with ketorolac tromethamine oral rinse. *J Periodontal Res* 1998;33:75–82.
5. Kornman KS, Crane A, Wang HY, et al. The interleukin-1 genotype as a severity factor in adult periodontal disease. *J Clin Periodontol* 1997;24:72–77.
6. Drisko CH. Non-surgical pocket therapy: pharmacotherapeutics. *Ann Periodontol* 1996;1:491–566.
7. Golub LM, Ciancio S, Ramamurthy NS, Leung M, McNamara TF. Low dose doxycycline therapy: effect on gingival and crevicular fluid collagenase activity in humans. *J Periodontal Res* 1990;25:321–330.
8. Williams RC, Jeffcoat MK, Kaplan ML, Goldhaber P, Johnson HG, Wechter WJ. Flurbiprofen: a potent inhibitor of alveolar bone loss in beagles. *Science* 1985;227:640–642.
9. Williams RC, Jeffcoat MK, Howell TH, et al. Ibuprofen: an inhibitor of alveolar bone resorption in beagles. *J Periodontal Res* 1988;23:225–229.
10. Offenbacher S, Williams RC, Jeffcoat MK, et al. Effects of NSAIDs on beagle crevicular cyclooxygenase metabolites and periodontal bone loss. *J Periodontal Res* 1992;27:207–213.
11. Offenbacher S, Braswell LD, Loos AS, et al. Effects of flurbiprofen on the progression of periodontitis in *Macaca mulatta*. *J Periodontal Res* 1987;22:473–481.
12. Kornman KS, Blodgett RF, Brunsvold M, Holt SC. Effects of topical applications of meclofenamic acid and ibuprofen on bone loss, subgingival microbiota and gingival PMN response in the primate *Macaca fascicularis*. *J Periodontal Res* 1990;25:300–307.
13. Li KL, Vogel R, Jeffcoat MK, et al. The effect of ketoprofen creams on periodontal disease in rhesus monkeys. *J Periodontal Res* 1996;3:525–532.
14. Offenbacher S, Odle BM, Braswell LD, et al. Changes in cyclooxygenase metabolites in experimental periodontitis in *Macaca mulatta*. *J Periodontal Res* 1989;24:63–74.
15. Jeffcoat MK, Reddy MS, Magnusson I, et al. Efficacy of quantitative digital subtraction radiography using radiographs exposed in a multicenter trial. *J Periodontal Res* 1996;31:157–160.
16. Williams RC, Jeffcoat MK, Howell TH, et al. Altering the progression of human alveolar bone loss with the non-steroidal anti-inflammatory drug flurbiprofen. *J Periodontol* 1989;60:485–490.
17. Reddy MS, Palcanis KG, Barnett ML, Haigh S, Charles CH, Jeffcoat MK. Efficacy of meclofenamate sodium in the treatment of rapidly progressive periodontitis. *J Clin Periodontol* 1993;20:635–640.
18. Jeffcoat MK, Reddy MS, Haigh S, et al. A comparison of topical ketorolac, systemic flurbiprofen, and placebo for the inhibition of bone loss in adult periodontitis. *J Periodontol* 1995;66:329–338.
19. Brunsvold MA, Chaves ES, Kornman KS, Aufdemorte TB, Wood R. Effects of a bisphosphonate on experimental periodontitis in monkeys. *J Periodontol* 1992;63:825–830.
20. Reddy MS, Weatherford TW III, Smith CA, West BD, Jeffcoat MK, Jacks TM. Alendronate treatment of naturally occurring periodontitis in beagles. *J Periodontol* 1995;66:211–217.
21. Jeffcoat MK, Reddy MS. Alveolar bone loss and osteoporosis: evidence for a common mode of therapy using the bisphosphonate alendronate. In: Davidovitch Z, Norton L, eds. *The biologic mechanism of tooth resorption and replacement by implants*. Boston: Harvard Society for the Advancement of Orthodontics, 1996:365–373.

86. Bioengineering of Oral Tissues

Martha J. Somerman, D.D.S., Ph.D. and *Jeffrey O. Hollinger, D.D.S., Ph.D.

*Department of Periodontics/Prevention/Geriatrics, University of Michigan School of Dentistry, and Department of Pharmacology, University of Michigan School of Medicine, Ann Arbor, Michigan; and *Department of Surgery, Division of Plastic and Reconstructive Surgery, Oregon Health Sciences University, Portland, Oregon*

Traditional and fundamental approaches for dentists who treat deficiencies of oral tissues are based on repair. For example, treatment for dental caries requires removal of the decayed tooth structure followed by restoration with either a metallic or nonmetallic dental material. Although dental restoration does not regenerate tissue, bioengineering and tissue regeneration are emerging as new treatment modalities. We define regeneration as a series of cellular, molecular, and matrix elements dynamically interacting to renew form and function to a deficient biologic structure. The restored structure should be identical in form, physiology, and function to the original. Contemporary bioengineering technology does not yet offer sufficient sophistication to allow for complete regeneration of tooth–periodontal ligament–alveolar bone complex. Regeneration of enamel, cementum, and periodontal ligament may be possible; however, regeneration of dentin and bone of the orofacial complex (e.g., mandible, maxilla) is highly feasible now.

OROFACIAL BONE

Whereas the elements of oral–facial bone are common with other bone in the body, the functional and physiological challenges are not. Oral–facial bone is confronted constantly with biofunctional demands from swallowing and mastication, as well as the pernicious potential for destruction from oral microorganisms. Bioengineering regenerative therapies for oral–facial bone may include combinations or individual elements of cells, matrices, and signaling molecules.

Bioengineered Devices: Requirements

A Source of Osteogenic Progenitors

An essential component is recruitment, or site-directed delivery of cells that will become osteoblasts. Site-directed delivery refers to the introduction of cells (bone or bone marrow derived), from another site or after *ex vivo* expansion, directly into the tissue to be restored.

Delivery System

This component must thwart soft-tissue prolapse, may enable cell delivery, may direct cell and tissue ingress (e.g., guided tissue regeneration; GTR), and permits cell anchorage and localization of cells and signaling factors. These functional roles promote restoration of form and function. Candidate delivery systems may include polymers such as type I collagen and biodegradable polymers such as poly(α-hydroxy acids) (1). In addition, calcium phosphate–based materials have established a notable record for bone regeneration and may be good candidates to deliver cells and factors.

Signaling Molecules

It is now well recognized that a suite of bone morphogenetic proteins (BMPs) direct body patterning during embryogenesis (e.g., limb development), tissue and organ formation, and during bone regeneration (2–5) (also see Chapter 3). It is the capacity of BMPs, such as BMP-2 and BMP-7, to promote conversion of undifferentiated mesenchymal cells into osteoblasts (6,7) that is a key focus of bioengineering bone-regenerative therapies.

BMP-mediated strategies to regenerate bone require a delivery system to localize and sustain BMP action. A delivery system is more than a transit vehicle; it delivers, localizes, sustains, and provides initial extracellular matrix cues to support the dynamic progression of orofacial tissue renewal. Furthermore, BMP action also may depend on responsive osteoblastic progenitor cells (OPCs) (8), and there must be a sufficient quantity of these cells whose response(s) will produce the desired outcome: restoring form and function to bone. Coadministration of OPCs could minimize the therapeutic dose of BMPs and augment a locally responsive cell stock that would differentiate into osteoblasts. Furthermore, local BMPs may be enhanced by genetically bolstering the capacity of OPCs to express this molecule. This novel approach to local BMP regulation by OPCs could be accomplished with a plasmid expression vector containing a BMP gene (Fig. 1). An additional option could involve osteoblast-specific factor 2 (Osf2), which activates the osteocalcin tran-

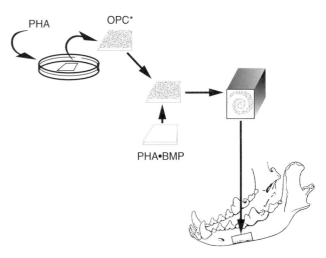

FIG. 2. Poly(α-hydroxy acid) (PHA) and osteoprogenitor cells (OPCs) are augmented with a PHA–bone morphogenetic protein (BMP) substructure that is conveniently shaped by the surgeon for insertion into the orofacial defect. In the example depicted in the figure, the experimental formulation was used to regenerate a component of the inferior border of the mandible of a dog.

scriptional promoter region. Studies by Ducy et al. (9) revealed that Osf2 causes osteoblast differentiation of nonosteoblastic cells, and it is postulated that Osf2 may trigger mesenchymal stem cells to differentiate into osteoblasts during the developmental (or perhaps even regenerative) processes (9,10).

A Potential Strategy

An option to exploit the strengths of cell therapy, BMP(s), and a poly(α-hydroxy acid) delivery system is illustrated in Figs. 1 and 2.

PERIODONTAL TISSUES

Left untreated, periodontal disease results in destruction of periodontal tissues including cementum, bone, and the periodontal ligament (PDL), followed by subsequent tooth loss. Increased research efforts focused on understanding periodontal disease at the cellular, molecular, and clinical level have resulted in improved modalities for arresting disease progression. Moreover, substantial evidence exists indicating that restoration of lost periodontal tissues (i.e., bone, cementum, and a functional PDL) is a feasible treatment approach for selected situations (11,12). This recognition has resulted in an increased number of products available to the clinician for use in attempts to regenerate periodontal tissues; however, there is a need to improve the predictability of regenerative procedures.

Current Therapies

Clinical procedures used to promote periodontal regeneration are based on several concepts including (a) that a mature

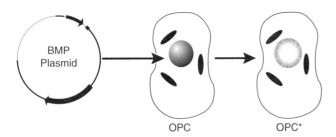

FIG. 1. The bone morphogenetic protein (BMP) engineered plasmid is incorporated into the osteoprogenitor cell (OPC). The OPC has been genetically altered to enhance BMP expression (OPC).

periodontium contains cells that when triggered appropriately, have the potential to reform tissues with characteristics of tissues lost to disease or to injury (13); (b) that factors promoting cell proliferation and/or cell differentiation, or with osteoinductive or osteoconductive properties, may serve as triggers for the regenerative process (14); c) that use of implanted tissue barriers or other matrix materials may facilitate selective cellular repopulation of the root surface (GTR) (12); and (d) that epithelial–mesenchymal signaling may promote both development and regeneration of periodontal tissues (15).

Current materials available include barrier membranes, both nonresorbable, such as expanded polytetrafluoroethylene (ePTFE) membranes and resorbable, such as collagen, polylactide acid (PLA) and polyglycolide acid (PGA). The objective of GTR is to exclude the epithelial and gingival corium from the root surface during wound healing in view of the fact that these tissues inhibit regeneration of periodontal tissues. Other products available include bone or bone-like substitutes (calcium sulfate, hydroxyapatite, and ceramic materials) used in attempts to trigger cell differentiation. Most recently, an enamel-like product (amelogenin) has been marketed, based on the principle that epithelial–mesenchymal interactions may be important both for development and for regeneration of periodontal tissues (16) (see Fig. 3).

New Therapies

Critical to improving the predictability of regenerative therapies is a greater understanding of cellular and molecular events required to restore periodontal tissues and designing appropriate delivery systems. Studies are under way to identify factors present during development of tissues that may also act to trigger cell activity as needed to regenerate tissues (12,14); to establish the role of BMPs and growth factors (e.g., PDGF/IGF) by using *in vitro* and *in vivo* models (14,17,18); to examine novel delivery systems with which presentation of factors/cells to the local site can be regulated; and to develop strategies for use of gene therapies (14,19). With active research in the field of periodontal regeneration, the likelihood for developing more predictable treatments to regenerate periodontal tissues is high.

ENAMEL

Enamel differs from the other mineralized tissues such as bone, dentin, and cementum because of the ectodermal origin of the cells that make it, the ameloblasts. Furthermore, its mineralized matrix does not contain collagen, and virtually the entire organic matrix is removed during maturation. To date, three specific enamel matrix proteins have been cloned (amelogenins, tuftelin, and ameloblastin). Although the exact role of these proteins has yet to be defined, current data suggest that enamel matrix protein interactions regulate enamel mineral crystallite formation (20,21).

Current Therapies

Methods currently used for treating defective enamel include, first, removal of the diseased structure, as needed,

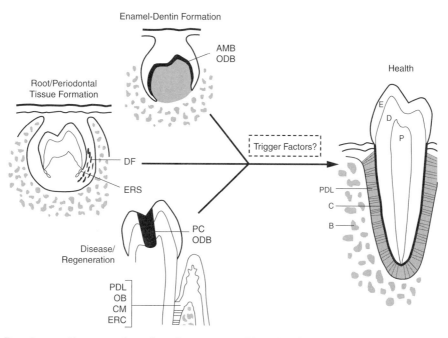

FIG. 3. Development/regeneration of tooth structures. Note that factors identified as having a role in formation of specific tissues also may function in regeneration of these tissues. AMB, ameloblasts; ODB, odontoblasts; DF, dental follicle cells; ERS, epithelial root sheath; PC, pulp cells; PDL, periodontal ligament (cells); OB, osteoblasts; CM, cementoblasts; ERC, epithelial rest cells; E, enamel; D, dentin; P, pulp; C, cementum; B, bone.

followed by restorative procedures, such as a crown for large defects to amalgam, glass ionomers, composite resins, and so on, for less destructive lesions. In addition, materials containing fluoride and other agents having remineralization properties are used prophylactically to prevent decay from recurring and also in an attempt to promote remineralization of small lesions. Sealants also are used in prophylactic procedures to prevent decay within teeth having fissure-like structures (e.g., molars).

New Therapies

Investigations directed at understanding the properties of ameloblasts and of associated proteins will provide the knowledge necessary for designing natural enamel matrix. Such matrices may serve as restorative materials as well as agents to use in attempts to regenerate mineralized tissues. In terms of preventive therapies, areas of ongoing research include those directed at developing vaccines to prevent dental caries.

DENTIN

Dentin acts to protect vital tissues within the pulp region (see Fig. 3). During development, cells responsible for promoting dentin formation are the odontoblasts. In addition, existing evidence suggests that pulp cells in mature tissues, when triggered appropriately, can differentiate into cells having the capacity to function as odontoblasts [i.e., promote mineralized tissue formation (22)]. The several types of dentin include primary and secondary dentin formed during tooth development, and tertiary dentin, which refers to dentin formed after maturation. Types of tertiary dentin include reparative dentin and reactionary dentin. By definition, reparative dentin refers to formation of tertiary dentin through activation of new odontoblasts, whereas reactionary dentin is formation of tertiary dentin by remaining functional odontoblasts.

Current Therapies

Destruction of dentin due to caries or injury can be extensive, resulting in damage to pulp tissues and acute pain for patients. Current treatment modalities including pulp capping with an hydroxyapatite-like material in an attempt to reform mineralized tissue in less severe injuries, with removal of pulp tissue (root canal–endodontic therapy) when there is more extensive damage. Removal of pulp tissue results in brittle teeth that then require surface replacement materials (e.g., crowns) to protect the weakened tooth structure. Tooth extraction is an option in selected situations.

New Directions

The accumulating data indicating that BMPs have the potential to induce mineral tissue formation, subsequent to pulp exposure (22), have resulted in increased efforts focused on determining whether such proteins or other dentin proteins, in appropriate delivery systems, have therapeutic potential. In addition, new materials may serve a role in decreasing root sensitivity, in treatment of root fractures, and in sealing off apical lesions, as needed.

REFERENCES

1. Hollinger J, Jamiolkowski D, Shalaby S. Bone repair and a unique class of biodegradable polymers: the poly(α-esters). In: Hollinger JO, ed. *Biomedical applications of synthetic biodegradable polymers.* Boca Raton: CRC Press, 1995:197–222.
2. Kingsley DM. The TGF-beta superfamily: new members, new receptors, and new genetic tests of function in different organisms. *Genes Dev* 1994;8:133–146.
3. Kaplan FS, Shore EM. Bone morphogenetic proteins and c-*fos*: early signals in endochondral bone formation. *Bone* 1996;19:13–22.
4. Storm EE, Huynh TV, Copeland NG, Jenkins NA, Kingsley DM, Lee S. Limb alterations in brachypodism mice due to mutations in a new member of the TGF-beta superfamily. *Nature* 1994;368:639–643.
5. Tickle C. On making a skeleton. *Nature* 1994;368:587–588.
6. Thies RS, Bauduy M, Ashton BA, Kurtzberg L, Wozney JM, Rosen V. Recombinant human bone morphogenetic protein-2 induces osteoblastic differentiation in W-20-17 stromal cells. *Endocrinology* 1992;130:1318–1324.
7. Yamaguchi A, Ishizuya T, Kintou N, et al. Effects of BMP-2, BMP-4, and BMP-6 on osteoblastic differentiation of bone marrow-derived stromal cell lines, ST2 and MC3T3-G2/PA6. *Biochem Biophys Res Commun* 1996;220:366–371.
8. Rosen V, Thies S. The BMP proteins in bone formation and repair. *Trends Genet* 1992;8:97–102.
9. Ducy P, Zhang R, Geoffroy V, Ridall A, Karsenty G. Osf2/Cbfa1: a transcriptional activator of osteoblast differentiation. *Cell* 1997;89: 747–754.
10. Rodan G, Harada S-I. The missing bone. *Cell* 1997;89:677–680.
11. Pitaru S, McCulloch CAG, Narayanan SA. Cellular origins and differentiation control mechanisms during periodontal development and wound healing. *J Periodontal Res* 1994;29:81–94.
12. Somerman MJ, Wang H-L, MacNeil RL. Promise and uncertainty in regeneration of oral tissues: craniofacial growth series 34. In: McNamara JA Jr, Trotman CA, eds. *Distraction osteogenesis and tissue engineering.* Ann Arbor: University of Michigan, Center for Human Growth & Development, 1998:199–224.
13. Melcher AH. On the repair potential of periodontal tissues. *J Periodontol* 1976;47:256–260.
14. McCauley LK, Somerman MJ. Biological modifiers in periodontal regeneration. *Dental Clin North Am* 1998;42:361–387.
15. Maas R, Bei M. The genetic control of early tooth development. *Crit Rev Oral Biol Med* 1997;8:4–39.
16. Lindhe J, ed. Emdogain: a biological approach to periodontal regeneration. *J Clin Periodontol* 1997;24:657–714.
17. Giannobile WV, Ryan S, Shih M-S, Su DL, Kaplan PL, Chan TCK. Recombinant human osteogenic protein-1 (OP-1) stimulates periodontal wound healing in class III furcation defects. *J Periodontol* 1998;69:129–137.
18. D'Errico JA, MacNeil RL, Takata T, Berry JE, Strayhorn CL, Somerman MJ. Expression of bone associated markers by tooth root lining cells, in situ and in vitro. *Bone* 1997;20:117–126.
19. Giannobile WV, Pomahac B, Eriksson E. Gene transfer to periodontal wounds. *J Dental Res* 1998;77:302.
20. Paine ML, Krebsbach PH, Chen LS, et al. Protein-to-protein interactions: criteria defining the assembly of the enamel organic matrix. *J Dental Res* 1998;77:496–502.
21. Deutsch D, Dafni L, Palmon A, Hekmati M, Young MF, Fisher LW. Enamel mineralization and amelogenesis imperfecta. In: Chadwick DJ, Cardew G, eds. *Dental enamel.* Chichester: John Wiley and Sons, 1997:135–155.
22. Charette MF, Rutherford RB. Regeneration of dentin. In: Lanza R, Langer R, Chick W, eds. *Principles of tissue engineering.* San Diego, CA: RG Landes Company, Texas & Academic Press, 1997:727–734.

Section **XIII**

Appendix

i. Growth Charts for Males and Females

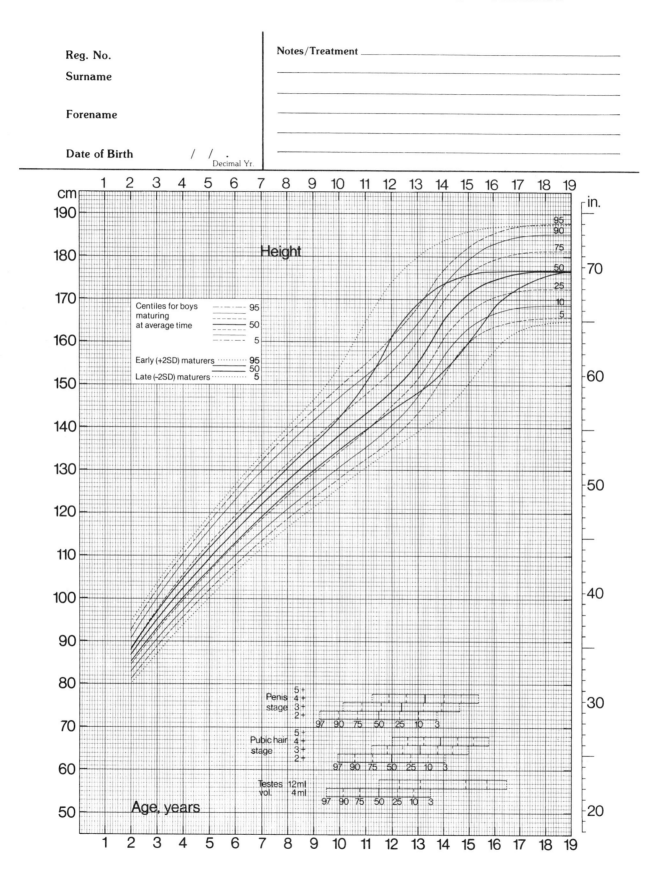

Reg. No.

Surname

Forename

Date of Birth   /   /   .
                    Decimal Yr.

Notes/Treatment

Reg. No.

Surname

Forename

Date of Birth　　/　/　.
Decimal Yr.

Notes/Treatment

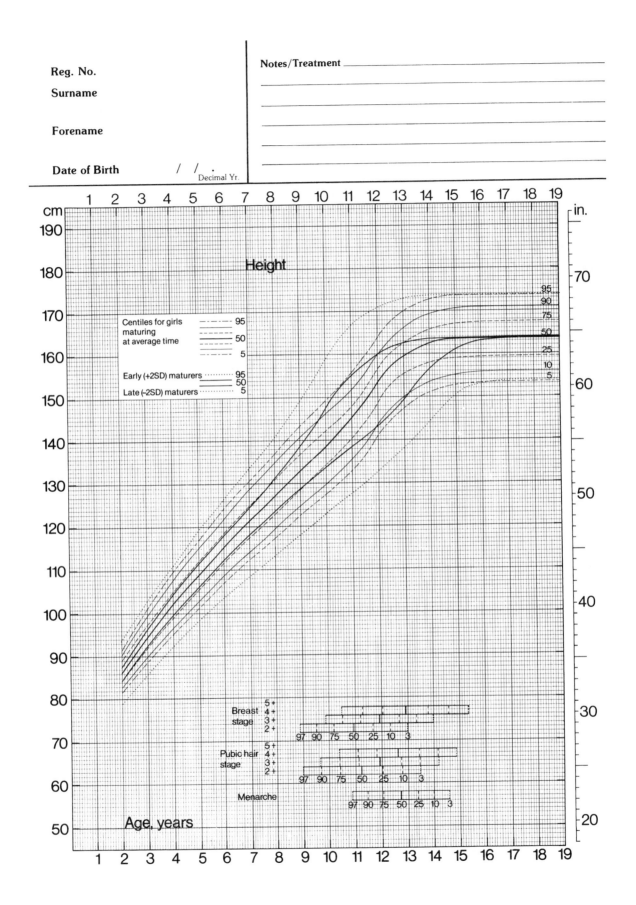

Height

Centiles for girls
maturing
at average time —·— 95
——— 50
——— 5

Early (+2SD) maturers ········· 95
——— 50
Late (–2SD) maturers ········· 5

Breast stage 5+ 4+ 3+ 2+

97 90 75 50 25 10 3

Pubic hair stage 5+ 4+ 3+ 2+

97 90 75 50 25 10 3

Menarche

97 90 75 50 25 10 3

Age, years

ii. Ossification Centers

Age-at-appearance percentiles for major postnatal ossification centers

	Percentiles					
	Boys			Girls		
Ossification center	5th	50th	95th	5th	50th	95th
Head of humerus	37g	2w	4m	37g	2w	3m3
Proximal epiphysis of tibia	34g	2w	5w	34g	1w	2w
Coracoid process of scapula	37g	2w	4m2	37g	2w	5m
Cuboid of tarsus	37g	3w	3m3	37g	3w	2m
Capitate of carpus	—	3m	7m	—	2m	7m
Hamate of carpus	2w	3m3	10m	2w	2m1	7m
Capitulum of humerus	3w	4m	13m	3w	3m	9m1
Head of femur	3w	4m1	7m3	2w	4m	7m2
Third cuneiform of tarsus	3w	5m2	19m	—	2m3	14m3
Greater tubercle of humerus	3m	10m	2y4	2m2	6m1	13m3
Primary center, middle segment of 5th toe	—	12m2	3y10	—	9m	2y1
Distal epiphysis of radius	6m2	12m1	2y4	4m3	10m	20m2
Epiphysis, distal segment of 1st toe	8m2	12m3	2y1	4m3	9m2	20m1
Epiphysis, middle segment of 4th toe	5m	14m3	2y11	5m	11m	3y
Epiphysis, proximal segment of 3rd finger	9m1	16m2	2y5	5m	10m1	19m2
Epiphysis, middle segment of 3rd toe	5m	17m	4y3	2m3	12m1	2y6
Epiphysis, proximal segment of 2nd finger	9m2	17m	2y2	5m	10m2	19m2
Epiphysis, proximal segment of 4th finger	9m3	18m	2y5	5m	11m	20m
Epiphysis, distal segment of 1st finger	9m	17m1	2y8	5m	12m	20m3
Epiphysis, proximal segment of 3rd toe	11m	19m	2y6	6m1	12m3	22m3
Epiphysis of 2nd metacarpal	11m1	19m2	2y10	7m3	13m	20m1
Epiphysis, proximal segment of 4th toe	11m2	19m3	2y8	7m2	15m	2y1
Epiphysis, proximal segment of 2nd toe	11m3	21m	2y8	7m3	14m2	2y1
Epiphysis of 3rd metacarpal	11m2	21m2	3y	8m	13m2	23m1
Epiphysis, proximal segment of 5th finger	12m	22m1	2y10	8m	14m2	2y1
Epiphysis, middle segment of 3rd finger	12m1	2y	3y4	7m3	15m2	2y4
Epiphysis of 4th metacarpal	13m	2y	3y7	9m	15m2	2y2
Epiphysis, middle segment of 2nd toe	10m3	2y1	4y1	6m	14m1	2y3
Epiphysis, middle segment of 4th finger	12m	2y1	3y3	7m3	15m	2y5
Epiphysis of 5th metacarpal	15m1	2y2	3y10	10m2	16m2	2y4
First cuneiform of tarsus	10m3	2y2	3y9	6m	17m1	2y10
Epiphysis of 1st metatarsal	16m3	2y2	3y1	11m3	19m	2y3
Epiphysis, middle segment of 2nd finger	15m3	2y2	3y4	8m	17m2	2y7
Epiphysis, proximal segment of 1st toe	17m2	2y4	3y4	10m3	18m3	2y5
Epiphysis, distal segment of 3rd finger	15m3	2y5	3y9	8m3	17m3	2y8
Triquetrium of carpus	6m	2y5	5y6	3m2	20m2	3y9
Epiphysis, distal segment of 4th finger	16m2	2y5	3y9	8m3	18m1	2y10
Epiphysis, proximal segment of 5th toe	18m2	2y6	3y8	11m3	20m3	2y8
Epiphysis of 1st metacarpal	17m2	2y7	4y4	11m	19m1	2y8
Second cuneiform of tarsus	14m2	2y8	4y3	9m3	21m3	3y
Epiphysis of 2nd metatarsal	23m1	2y10	4y4	14m3	2y2	3y5
Greater trochanter of femur	23m	3y	4y4	11m2	22m1	3y
Epiphysis, proximal segment of 1st finger	22m1	3y	4y7	11m1	20m2	2y10
Navicular of tarsus	13m2	3y	5y5	9m1	23m1	3y7
Epiphysis, distal segment of 2nd finger	21m3	3y2	5y	12m3	2y6	3y4
Epiphysis, distal segment of 5th finger	2y1	3y4	5y	12m	23m2	3y6
Epiphysis, middle segment of 5th finger	23m1	3y5	5y10	10m3	23m3	3y7
Proximal epiphysis of fibula	22m2	3y6	5y3	16m	2y7	3y11
Epiphysis of 3rd metatarsal	2y4	3y6	5y	17m1	2y6	3y8
Epiphysis, distal segment of 5th toe	2y4	3y11	6y4	14m1	2y4	4y1
Patella of knee	2y6	4y	6y	17m3	2y6	4y
Epiphysis of 4th metatarsal	2y11	4y	5y9	21m1	2y10	4y1
Lunate of carpus	18m2	4y1	6y9	13m	2y8	5y8
Epiphysis, distal segment of 3rd toe	3y	4y4	6y2	16m2	2y9	4y1
Epiphysis of 5th metatarsal	3y1	4y5	6y4	2y1	3y3	4y11

continued

Age-at-appearance percentiles for major postnatal ossification centers   (Continued)

Ossification center	Percentiles					
	Boys			Girls		
	5th	50th	95th	5th	50th	95th
Epiphysis, distal segment of 4th toe	2y11	4y5	6y5	16m2	2y7	4y1
Epiphysis, distal segment of 2nd toe	3y3	4y8	6y9	18m	2y11	4y6
Capitulum of radius	3y	5y3	8y	2y3	3y11	6y3
Scaphoid of carpus	3y7	5y8	7y10	2y4	4y11	6y
Greater multangular of carpus	3y7	5y11	9y	23m1	4y1	6y4
Lesser multangular of carpus	3y1	6y3	8y6	2y5	4y2	6y
Medial epicondyle of humerus	4y3	6y3	8y5	2y1	3y5	5y1
Distal epiphysis of ulna	5y3	7y1	9y1	3y4	5y5	7y8
Epiphysis of calcaneus	5y2	7y7	9y7	3y7	5y5	7y4
Olecranon of ulna	7y9	9y8	11y11	5y8	8y	9y11
Lateral epicondyle of humerus	9y3	11y3	13y8	7y2	9y3	11y3
Tubercle of tibia	9y11	11y10	13y5	7y11	10y3	11y10
Adductor sesamoid of 1st finger	11y	12y9	14y8	8y8	10y9	12y8
Acetabulum	11y11	13y7	15y4	9y7	11y6	13y5
Acromion	12y2	13y9	15y6	10y4	11y11	13y10
Epiphysis, iliac crest of hip	12y	14y	15y11	10y10	12y10	15y4
Accessory epiphysis, coracoid process of scapula	12y9	14y4	16y4	10y5	12y3	14y5
Ischial tuberosity	13y7	15y3	17y1	11y9	13y11	16y

From Garn SM, Rohmann CG, Silverman FN. Radiographic standards for postnatal ossification and tooth calcification. *Med Radiogr Photogr* 1967;43:45–66.

g, gestational week; w, week; m, month; y, year. The number following m or y refers to the next smaller time unit (e.g., 9y4 = 9 years 4 months).

iii. Dental Ossification Centers

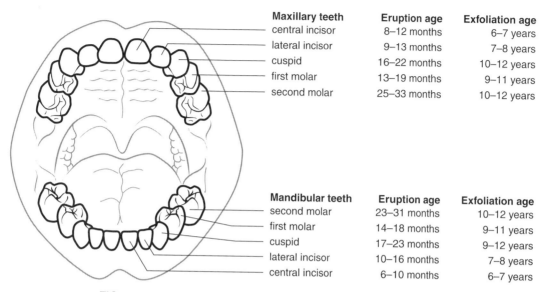

Maxillary teeth	Eruption age	Exfoliation age
central incisor	8–12 months	6–7 years
lateral incisor	9–13 months	7–8 years
cuspid	16–22 months	10–12 years
first molar	13–19 months	9–11 years
second molar	25–33 months	10–12 years

Mandibular teeth	Eruption age	Exfoliation age
second molar	23–31 months	10–12 years
first molar	14–18 months	9–11 years
cuspid	17–23 months	9–12 years
lateral incisor	10–16 months	7–8 years
central incisor	6–10 months	6–7 years

FIG. 1. Normal eruption and exfoliation ages for the primary teeth.

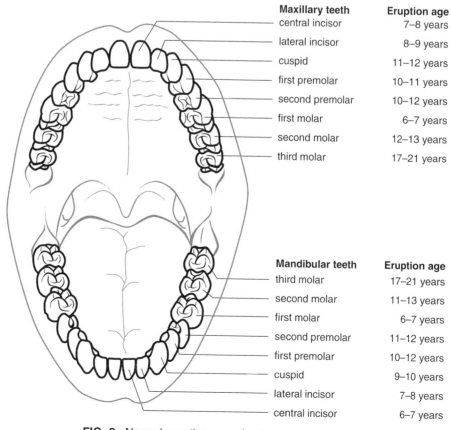

Maxillary teeth	Eruption age
central incisor	7–8 years
lateral incisor	8–9 years
cuspid	11–12 years
first premolar	10–11 years
second premolar	10–12 years
first molar	6–7 years
second molar	12–13 years
third molar	17–21 years

Mandibular teeth	Eruption age
third molar	17–21 years
second molar	11–13 years
first molar	6–7 years
second premolar	11–12 years
first premolar	10–12 years
cuspid	9–10 years
lateral incisor	7–8 years
central incisor	6–7 years

FIG. 2. Normal eruption ages for the permanent teeth.

475

iv. Laboratory Values of Importance for Calcium Metabolism and Metabolic Bone Disease

Laboratory values of importance for calcium metabolism and metabolic bone disease[a]

Test	Source of specimen	Reference population	Reference range	Reference range (SI units)
Calcium, ionized	Serum or plasma	Cord	5.5 ± 0.3 mg/dL	1.37 ± 0.07 mmol/L
		Newborn		
		3–24 h	4.3–5.1 mg/dL	1.07–1.27 mmol/L
		24–48 h	4.0–4.7 mg/dL	1.00–1.17 mmol/L
		Adult	4.48–4.92 mg/dL	1.12–1.23 mmol/L
		>60 yr		1.13–1.30 mmol/L
Calcium, total	Serum[b]	Child	8.8–10.8 mg/dL	2.2–2.7 mmol/L
	Urine	Adult	8.4–10.2 mg/dL	2.1–2.55 mmol/L
		Ca^{2+} in diet		
		Free Ca^{2+}	5–40 mg/dL	0.13–1.0 mmol/d
		Low to average	50–150 mg/dL	1.25–3.8 mmol/d
		Average (20 mmol/d)	100–300 mg/dL	2.1–7.5 mmol/d
Magnesium	Feces	Average 0.64 g/d		16 mmol/d
	Serum	1.3–2.1 mEq/d (higher in women during menses)		0.65–1.05 mmol/d
	Urine, 24-h	6.0–100 mEq/d		3.0–5.0 mmol/d
Phosphatase, acid				
Prostatic (RIA)	Serum	<3.0 ng/mL		<3.0 μg/L
Roy, Brower, and Hayden, 37 C		0.11–0.60 U/L		0.11–0.60 U/L
Phosphatase, alkaline				
p-Nitrophenyl phosphate, carbonate buffer, 30 C	Serum	Infant		50–165 U/L
		Child		20–150 U/L
		Adult		20–70 U/L
		>60 yr		30–75 U/L
Bowers and McComb, 30 C IFCC, 30 C	Serum	Male		30–90 U/L
		Female		20–80 U/L
Bone-specific alkaline phosphatase				
Hybritech/Beckman Coulter, Inc. IRMA, ELISA	Serum	Male	6.9–20.1 ng/mL	
		Female		
		Premenopausal	4.6–14.3 ng/mL	
		Postmenopausal	7.3–22.4 ng/mL	
Metra Biosystems, ELISA	Serum	Male	15.0–41.3 U/L	
		Female		
		Premenopausal	11.6–29.6 U/L	
Phosphorus, inorganic	Serum	Cord	3.7–8.1 mg/dL	1.2–2.6 nmol/L
		Child	4.5–5.5 mg/dL	1.45–1.78 nmol/L
		Thereafter	2.7–4.5 mg/dL	0.87–1.45 nmol/L
		>60 year		
		Male	2.3–3.7 mg/dL	0.74–1.2 nmol/L
		Female	2.8–4.1 mg/dL	0.9–1.3 nmol/L
	Urine	Adult on diet containing 0.9–1.5 g P and 10 mg Ca/kg <1.0 g/d		On diet containing 29–48 mmol P and 0.25 mmol Ca/kg: <32 mmol/d
		Unrestricted diet 0.4–1.3 g/d		Unrestricted diet: 13–42 mmol/d
Tubular reabsorption of phosphate	Urine, 4-h (0800–1200 h), and serum		82–95%	Fraction reabsorbed: 0.82–0.95
Vitamin A				
Quest Diagnostics/ Nichols Institute	Serum	Pediatric		
		1–6 yr	20–43 μg/dl	
		7–12 yr	26–49 μg/dl	
		13–19 yr	26–72 μg/dl	
		Adult >19 yr	38–98 μg/dl	
Mayo Medical Labs	Serum	Retinol	360–1200 μg/L	
		Retinyl esters	≤10 μg/L	

continued

Laboratory values of importance for calcium metabolism and metabolic bone disease[a] (Continued)

Test	Source of specimen	Reference population	Reference range	Reference range (SI units)
Vitamin D$_3$, 25 hydroxy				
Mayo Medical Labs	Serum	Summer (total):	15–80 ng/mL	37–200 nmol/L
		Winter (total):	14–42 ng/mL	
RIA, DiaSorin	Serum/Plasma	Adults	9.0–37.6 ng/mL	35–105 nmol/L
			(mean, 23.0 ng/mL)	
Vitamin D$_3$, 1,25 dihydroxy				
Mayo Medical Labs	Serum	Adults	25–45 pg/ml	12–46 μmol/L
			15–60 pg/ml	
RIA, DiaSorin	Serum/Plasma	Adults	15.9–55.6 pg/mL	
			(mean, 35.7 pg/mL)	
Calcitonin[c]				
Quest Diagnostics/ Nichols Institute two-site ICMA*	Serum	Basal		
		Male	≤8 pg/mL	
		Female	≤4 pg/mL	
		Pentagastrin/Ca		
		Male	10–491 pg/mL	
		Female	≤70 pg/mL	
CIS Bio international two-site IRMA	Serum	Basal		
		Male	<10 pg/mL	
		Female	<10 pg/mL	
		Pentagastrin		
		Male	<30 pg/mL	
		Female	<30 pg/mL	
Mayo Medical Labs	Plasma	Basal		
		Male	<19 pg/mL	
		Female	<14 pg/mL	
		Pentagastrin		
		Male	<110 pg/mL	
		Female	<30 pg/mL	
RIA, DiaSorin	Serum	Adult	0–95 pg/mL	
			(mean, 47 pg/mL)	
Parathyroid hormone (intact)[c]				
Mayo Medical Labs	Serum	Basal		1.0–5.2 pmol/L
Quest Diagnostics/ Nichols Institute	Serum	Basal	10–65 pg/ml	
IRMA, DiaSorin	Serum/Plasma		13–54 pg/mL	
			(mean, 26 pg/mL)	
Osteocalcin[c]				
Quest Diagnostics/ Nichols Institute	Serum	Male	8.0–52.0 ng/mL	
		Female		
CIS Bio international		Premenopausal	5.8–41.0 ng/mL	
		Postmenopausal	8.0–56.0 ng/mL	
Mayo Medical labs CIA	Serum	Male		
		20–50 yr	2–15 ng/mL	
		51–70 yr	2–10 ng/mL	
		Female		
		20–50 yr	2–15 ng/mL	
		51–80 yr	6–22 ng/mL	
IRMA, DiaSorin	Serum	Male	3.2–12.2 ng/mL	
			(mean, 6.25 ng/mL)	
		Female	2.7–11.5 ng/mL	
			(mean, 5.58 ng/mL)	
ELISA, Metra Biosystems	Serum	Male	3.4–8.6 ng/mL	
		Female	3.8–10.0 ng/mL	
ELISA, N-Mid, Osteometer BioTech A/S	Serum/Plasma	Male	23.2 ± 7.2 ng/mL	
		Female		
		Premenopausal	17.7 ± 6.4 ng/mL	
		Postmenopausal	28.9 ± 9.7 ng/mL	
IRMA, N-Mid, Osteometer BioTech A/S	Serum/Plasma	Male	23.0 ± 9.7 ng/mL	
		Female		
		Premenopausal	18.4 ± 8.9 ng/mL	
		Postmenopausal	29.9 ± 11.5 ng/mL	

continued

Laboratory values of importance for calcium metabolism and metabolic bone disease[a]   (Continued)

Test	Source of specimen	Reference population	Reference range	Reference range (SI units)
PTHrP[c]				
Quest Diagnostics/ Nichols Institute	Serum	Basal		<1.3 pmol/L
IRMA, DiaSorin	Plasma	Adults		<1.5 pmol/L
Collagen cross-links				
Free deoxypyridino- line (DPD)				
Metra Biosystems, ELISA	Urine	Male		2.3–5.4 nmol/mmol creatinine
		Female Premenopausal		3.0–7.4 nmol/mmol creatinine
Free pyridinoline (Pyd)				
Metra Biosystems, ELISA	Urine	Male		12.8–25.6 nmol/ mmol creatinine
		Female		16.0–37.0 nmol/ mmol creatinine
	Serum	Male		1.59 ± 0.38 nmol/L
		Female		1.55 ± 0.26 nmol/L
C-telopeptide (CTx)				
Osteometer Biotech A/S, ELISA	Urine	Male		207 ± 128 μg/mmol creatinine
		Female Premenopausal		220 ± 128 μg/mmol creatinine
		Postmenopausal		363 ± 160 (μg/mmol creatinine
Osteometer Biotech A/S, RIA	Urine	Male		290 ± 120 μg/mmol creatinine
		Female Premenopausal		227 ± 90 μg/mmol creatinine
		Postmenopausal		429 ± 225 μg/mmol creatinine
N-telopeptide (NTx)				
Ostex International, ELISA	Urine	Male		3–63 nM BCE/mM creatinine
		Female Premenopausal		5–65 nM BCE/mM creatinine
		Postmenopausal		17–188 nM BCE/ mM creatinine
Ostex International, ELISA	Serum	Male		5.4–24.2 nM BCE
		Female Premenopausal		6.2–19.0 nM BCE
		Postmenopausal		8.1–38.7 nM BCE

ELISA, enzyme-linked immunosorbent assay; RIA, radioimmunoassay; IRMA, immunoradiometric assay; IFCC, International Federation of Clinical Chemistry; BCE, bone collagen equivalents.

* Immunochemiluminescent assay

[a] Selected laboratory values in this table were kindly compiled by Barry C. Kress, Ph.D., Hybritech Incorporated, a subsidiary of Beckman Coulter, Inc., San Diego, CA. Every effort was made to include values from all known companies for the various categories.

[b] Divide by 2 to get mEq/L. The total serum calcium can be corrected for alterations in the serum protein concentration by the following formula: Corrected total serum calcium (mg/dL) = observed total serum calcium + [(the normal mean albumin concentration − the observed albumin concentration) × 0.8]. In most situations, the normal mean albumin concentration equations 4 g/dL.

[c] The normal values listed include commercial assays. These are listed not to provide an endorsement for these assays, but because they are representative of values available for daily clinical use. It is likely that normal values in other research or commercial assays will vary to some extent; where ± values are given, the mean plus or minus one standard deviation is given.

v. Formulary of Drugs Commonly Used in Treatment of Mineral Disorders

Formulary of drugs commonly used in treatment of mineral disorders[a]

Drug	Application in treatment of bone and mineral disorders	Dosage (adult)[b]	Rx Cat[c]	Notes[d]
Hormones and analogs				
1. Calcitonin				
Human (Cibacalcin) i.m. or s.c. (0.5-mg vials)	Paget's disease	0.25–0.5 mg i.m. or s.c.; q24h	Rx	
Salmon (Calcimar, Miacalcin) i.m. or s.c. (100, 200 IU/mL) (s.c. preferred)	Paget's disease, osteoporosis, hypercalcemia	50–100 IU, i.m. or s.c.; qod or qd for Paget's or osteoporosis; 4–6 IU/kg i.m. or s.c.; qid for hypercalcemia	Rx	Modestly effective and short-lived in treatment of hypercalcemia
Nasal spray (200 IU/spray)	Osteoporosis	200 IU nasal qd	Rx	
2. Estrogens				
Estinyl estradiol p.o. (0.02, 0.05, 0.5 mg)	Postmenopausal osteoporosis (prevention and treatment)	0.02–0.05 mg; qd 3/4 wk	Rx	To reduce risk of endometrial cancer, estrogens can be cycled with a progesterone during last 7–10 days or given concurrent with a progestin throughout the cycle (less breakthrough bleeding). In women who have not had a hysterectomy, a progesterone should be used with the estrogen and does not appear to alter the skeletal effectiveness of estrogen.
17β estradiol (Estrace), p.o. (0.5, 1, 2 mg)		0.5 mg qd	Rx	
Transderm patch (Estraderm)		0.05–0.1 mg 2x/wk	Rx	
Conjugated equine estrogens (Premarin), p.o. (0.3, 0.625, 0.9, 1.25, 2.5 mg)		0.625–1.25 mg qd 3/4 wk	Rx	0.3 mg conjugated equine estrogens (CEE) with calcium also may be effective
Esterified estrogens (Estratab) p.o. (0.3, 0.625, 2.5)		0.3–1.25 mg qd		
Estropipate (Ortho-Est .625) p.o. (0.75, 1.5 mg)		0.75 mg qd		
Conjugated equine estrogen with medroxyprogesterone acetate (MPA)				
(Premphase)		0.625 mg estrogen qd on days 1–14 and 0.625 mg estrogen with 5 mg MPA qd on days 15–28		
(Prempro)		0.625 mg estrogen with 2.5 or 5 mg MPA qd		
3. Selective estrogen-receptor modulators (SERMs)				
Raloxifene (Evista)	Postmenopausal osteoporosis (prevention)	60 mg qd	Rx	Aggravates hot flashes. Decrease endometrial and breast cancer
4. Glucocorticoids				
Prednisone (Deltasone), p.o. (2.5, 5, 10, 20, 50 mg)	Hypercalcemia due to sarcoidosis, vitamin D intoxication, and certain malignancies such as multiple myeloma and related lymphoproliferative disorders	10–60 mg; qd	Rx	Long-term use results in osteoporosis and adrenal suppression. Other glucocorticoids with minimal mineralocorticoid activity can be used

continued

479

Formulary of drugs commonly used in treatment of mineral disorders[a] (Continued)

Drug	Application in treatment of bone and mineral disorders	Dosage (adult)[b]	Rx Cat[c]	Notes[d]
5. Parathyroid hormone Human 1–34 (Parathor), i.v. (200 U/vial)	Diagnosis of pseudohypoparathyroidism	200 U; over 10-min infusion	Rx	The use of PTH to treat osteoporosis is being evaluated
6. Testosterone Testosterone cypionate Testosterone enanthate Transdermal patch	Male hypogonadism	200–300 mg i.m. q2–3 wk 200–300 mg i.m. q2–3 wk	Rx	
Testoderm		4–6 mg scrotal patch q24 hr	Rx	
Testoderm TTS Androderm		5-mg body patch Two 2.5-mg patches q24 hr	Rx Rx	
7. Vitamin D preparations Cholecalciferol or D_3, p.o. (125, 250, 400 U, often in combination with calcium)	Nutritional vitamin D deficiency, osteoporosis, malabsorption, hypoparathyroidism, refractory rickets	400–1000 U; as dietary supplement	OTC	D_2 (or D_3) has been shown to reduce fractures and increase BMD in elderly women at 400–1000 U doses
Ergocalciferol or D_2 (Calciferol), p.o. (8000 U/ml drops; 25,000, 50,000 U tabs)		25,000–100,000 U; 3×/wk to qd	Rx	
Calcifediol or 25 (OH) D_3 (Calderol), (20, 50 mg)	Malabsorption, renal osteodystrophy	20–50 μg; 3×/wk to qd	Rx	25 (OH) D_3 may be useful in treatment for steroid-induced osteoporosis
Calcitriol or 1,25 (OH)$_2$ D_3 (Rocaltrol), p.o. (0.25, 0.5 μg); (Calcijex), i.v. (1 or 2 μg/ml)	Renal osteodystrophy, hypoparathyroidism, refractory rickets	0.25–1.0 μg; qd to b.i.d.	Rx	Role of calcitriol in treatment of osteoporosis, psoriasis, and certain malignancies is being evaluated, primarily with new analogs
Dihydrotachysterol (DHT), p.o. (0.125, 0.2, 0.4 mg)	Renal osteodystrophy, hypoparathyroidism	0.2–1.0 mg; qd	Rx	
Bisphosphonates **1. Etidronate** (Didronel), p.o. (200, 400 mg); i.v. (300 mg/6 ml vial)	Paget's disease, heterotopic ossification, hypercalcemia of malignancy	p.o., 5 mg/kg, qd for 6/12 mo for Paget's disease; 20 mg/kg, qd 1 mo before to 3 mo after total hip replacement; 10/20 mg/kg, qd for 3 mo after spinal cord injury for heterotopic ossification. i.v., 7.5 mg/kg, qd for 3 d, given in 250–500 ml normal saline for hypercalcemia of malignancy 5 mg qd for osteoporosis prevention.	Rx	Etidronate is a first-generation bisphosphonate. High doses may cause a mineralization disorder not seen with newer bisphosphonates
2. Alendronate (Fosamax), p.o. (5, 10, 40 mg)	Osteoporosis prevention and treatment, Paget's disease	5 mg qd for osteoporosis prevention; 10 mg qd for osteoporosis treatment; 40 mg qd for Paget's disease	Rx	Ingest 30 min before breakfast with 1 glass water; remain upright. Esophagitis is a risk
3. Pamidronate (Aredia), i.v. (30–90 mg/10 ml)	Hypercalcemia of malignancy, Paget's disease	60–90 mg given as a single i.v. infusion over 24 h for hypercalcemia of malignancy; 4-h infusions also effective for 30- or 60-mg doses. 30-mg doses over 4 h on 3 consecutive days for a total of 90 mg for Paget's disease	Rx	
4. Risedronate (Actonal)	Paget's disease	30 mg qd for 2 mo	Rx	
5. Tiludronate (Skelid)	Paget's disease	400 mg qd for 3 mo	Rx	

continued

Formulary of drugs commonly used in treatment of mineral disorders[a] *(Continued)*

Drug	Application in treatment of bone and mineral disorders	Dosage (adult)[b]	Rx Cat[c]	Notes[d]
Minerals				
1. **Bicarbonate, sodium,** p.o. (325, 527, 650 mg)	Chronic metabolic acidosis leading to bone disease	Must be titrated for each patient	Rx, OTC	
2. **Calcium preparations**				
Calcium carbonate (40% Ca), p.o. (500, 650 mg)	Hypocalcemia (if symptomatic should be treated i.v.), osteoporosis, rickets, osteomalacia, chronic renal failure, hypoparathyroidism, malabsorption, enteric oxaluria	p.o., 400–2000 mg elemental Ca in divided doses; qd	OTC	Calcium carbonate is the preferred form because it has the highest percentage of calcium and is the least expensive, although calcium citrate may be somewhat better absorbed. In normal subjects, the solubility of the calcium salt has not been shown to affect its absorption from the intestine. In achlorhydric subjects, $CaCO_3$ should be given with meals
Calcium citrate (21% Ca), p.o. (950–1500 mg)				
Calcium chloride (36% Ca), i.v. (100% solution)				
Calcium bionate (6.5% Ca), p.o. (1.8 g in 5 ml)				
Calcium gluconate (9% Ca), p.o. (500, 600, 1000 mg), i.v. (10% solution, 0.465 mEq/ml)		i.v., 2–20 ml 10% calcium gluconate over several hours	Rx	Calcium gluconate is the preferred i.v. form because, unlike calcium chloride, it does not burn
Calcium lactate (13% Ca), p.o. (325, 650 mg)				
Calcium phosphate, dibasic (23% Ca), p.o. (486 mg)				
Tricalcium phosphate (39% Ca) p.o. (300, 600 mg)				
3. **Magnesium preparations**				
Magnesium oxide (Mag-Ox, Uro-Mag), p.o. (84.5, 241.3 mg Mg)	Hypomagnesemia	240–480 mg elemental Mg; qd	OTC	Low magnesium often coexists with low calcium in alcoholics and malabsorbers. Also found in many antacids and vitamin formulations
4. **Phosphate preparations**				
Neutra-Phos, p.o. (250 mg P, 278 mg K, 164 mg Na)	Hypophosphatemia, vitamin-D–resistant rickets, hypercalcemia, hypercalciuria	p.o., 1–3 g in divided doses; qd	Rx, OTC	
Neutra-Phos-K, p.o. (250 mg P, 556 mg K)				
Fleet Phospha-Soda, p.o. (815 mg P, 760 mg Na in 5 ml)				
In-Phos, i.v. (1 g P in 40 ml)		i.v., 1.5 g over 6–8 h		i.v., phosphorus is seldom necessary and can be toxic if infusion is too rapid
Hyper-Phos-K, i.v. (1 g P in 15 ml)				
Diuretics				
1. **Thiazides**				
Hydrochlorothiazide, p.o. (25, 50, 100 mg)	Hypercalciuria, nephrolithiasis	25–50 mg; qd or b.i.d.	Rx	Other thiazides may also be effective but are less commonly used for this purpose. These uses are not FDA approved
Chlorthalidone, p.o. (25, 50 mg)				

continued

Formulary of drugs commonly used in treatment of mineral disorders[a] (Continued).

Drug	Application in treatment of bone and mineral disorders	Dosage (adult)[b]	Rx Cat[c]	Notes[d]
2. Loop diuretics Furosemide, p.o. (20, 40, 80 mg), i.v. (10 mg/ml)	Hypercalcemia; if symptomatic, use i.v.	p.o., 20–80 mg, q6h as necessary i.v., 20–80 mg over several minutes, repeat as necessary	Rx	Ethacrynic acid may also be effective but is less commonly used for this purpose. These uses are not FDA approved
Miscellaneous **1. Mitramycin or plicamycin** (Mithracin), i.v. (2.5 mg/vial)	Hypercalcemia of malignancy	25 μg/kg in 1 L D5W or normal saline over 4–6 hr	Rx	Has been used in treatment of severe Paget's disease, but toxicity makes it treatment of last resort for this purpose, and it has not been approved by the FDA for this purpose

BMD, bone mineral density; FDA, Food and Drug Administration; PTH, parathyroid hormone.

[a] This table is not intended to be an official guideline. See PDR or package insert for more complete information. Selected information kindly provided by Daniel D. Bikle, M.D., Ph.D., Professor, Departments of Medicine and Dermatology, University of California, San Francisco, and Co-Director Special Diagnostic and Treatment Unit, Department of Medicine, Veterans Affairs Medical Center, San Francisco, California.

[b] qd, every day; qod, every other day; b.i.d., twice a day; t.i.d., 3 times a day; q.i.d., 4 times a day; s.c., subcutaneously; i.m., intramuscularly; p.o., orally; i.v., intravenously; IU, International Units.

[c] Rx Cat, prescription category: Rx, prescriptions required; OTC, over-the-counter preparations available.

[d] Where comments are not specifically aligned with preparations or their dosages, they apply to all preparations listed in that column.

vi. Bone Density Reference Data

The following data were provided by the manufacturer of Hologic QDR systems. They are listed for the 5-year age increments for which they are available with mean ±2 standard deviations (95% confidence interval).

For more information, contact Hologic Inc., 590 Lincoln Street, Waltham, MA 02451.

TABLE 1. *Normal bone mineral density (BMD) values for reference population U.S. white female*

Age (yr)	L1–L4 AP spine	L2–L4 AP spine	L2–L4 lateral spine	Femoral neck	Femur total	⅓ radius	Whole body
20	1.019 ± 0.220	1.051 ± 0.220	0.820 ± 0.168	0.849 ± 0.222	0.942 ± 0.244	0.694 ± 0.120	1.102 ± 0.174
25	1.040 ± 0.220	1.072 ± 0.220	0.813 ± 0.168	0.849 ± 0.222	0.942 ± 0.244	0.691 ± 0.120	1.095 ± 0.174
30	1.047 ± 0.220	1.079 ± 0.220	0.803 ± 0.168	0.840 ± 0.222	0.939 ± 0.244	0.687 ± 0.120	1.087 ± 0.174
35	1.041 ± 0.220	1.073 ± 0.220	0.789 ± 0.168	0.831 ± 0.222	0.933 ± 0.244	0.681 ± 0.120	1.077 ± 0.174
40	1.024 ± 0.220	1.056 ± 0.220	0.770 ± 0.168	0.817 ± 0.222	0.922 ± 0.244	0.673 ± 0.120	1.065 ± 0.174
45	0.997 ± 0.220	1.030 ± 0.220	0.746 ± 0.168	0.803 ± 0.222	0.907 ± 0.244	0.663 ± 0.120	1.051 ± 0.174
50	0.967 ± 0.220	0.997 ± 0.220	0.716 ± 0.168	0.768 ± 0.222	0.886 ± 0.244	0.651 ± 0.120	1.036 ± 0.174
55	0.930 ± 0.220	0.960 ± 0.220	0.680 ± 0.168	0.732 ± 0.222	0.860 ± 0.244	0.636 ± 0.120	1.020 ± 0.174
60	0.892 ± 0.220	0.920 ± 0.220	0.636 ± 0.168	0.707 ± 0.222	0.827 ± 0.244	0.617 ± 0.120	1.002 ± 0.174
65	0.854 ± 0.220	0.878 ± 0.220	0.584 ± 0.168	0.682 ± 0.222	0.793 ± 0.244	0.595 ± 0.120	0.982 ± 0.174
70	0.815 ± 0.220	0.840 ± 0.220	0.523 ± 0.168	0.650 ± 0.222	0.759 ± 0.244	0.570 ± 0.120	0.961 ± 0.174
75	0.784 ± 0.220	0.805 ± 0.220	0.453 ± 0.168	0.618 ± 0.222	0.725 ± 0.244	0.541 ± 0.120	0.938 ± 0.174
80	0.752 ± 0.220	0.754 ± 0.220	0.373 ± 0.168	0.594 ± 0.222	0.691 ± 0.244	0.507 ± 0.120	0.914 ± 0.174
85	0.731 ± 0.220	NA	0.283 ± 0.168	0.569 ± 0.222	0.657 ± 0.244	0.470 ± 0.120	0.888 ± 0.174

TABLE 2. *Normal BMD values for reference population U.S. white male*

Age (yr)	L1–L4 AP spine	L2–L4 AP spine	Femoral neck	Femur total	⅓ Radius
20	1.091 ± 0.220	1.115 ± 0.220	0.930 ± 0.272	1.033 ± 0.302	0.817 ± 0.053
25	1.091 ± 0.220	1.115 ± 0.220	0.930 ± 0.272	1.033 ± 0.302	0.816 ± 0.302
30	1.091 ± 0.220	1.115 ± 0.220	0.907 ± 0.272	1.023 ± 0.302	0.813 ± 0.302
35	1.091 ± 0.220	1.115 ± 0.220	0.885 ± 0.272	1.014 ± 0.302	0.810 ± 0.302
40	1.079 ± 0.220	1.115 ± 0.220	0.865 ± 0.272	1.004 ± 0.302	0.806 ± 0.302
45	1.068 ± 0.220	1.091 ± 0.220	0.845 ± 0.272	0.995 ± 0.302	0.800 ± 0.302
50	1.053 ± 0.220	1.076 ± 0.220	0.829 ± 0.272	0.985 ± 0.302	0.793 ± 0.302
55	1.038 ± 0.220	1.061 ± 0.220	0.814 ± 0.272	0.975 ± 0.302	0.784 ± 0.302
60	1.023 ± 0.220	1.045 ± 0.220	0.802 ± 0.272	0.966 ± 0.302	0.773 ± 0.302
65	1.008 ± 0.220	1.030 ± 0.220	0.790 ± 0.272	0.957 ± 0.302	0.761 ± 0.302
70	0.993 ± 0.220	1.015 ± 0.220	0.769 ± 0.272	0.933 ± 0.302	0.747 ± 0.302
75	0.978 ± 0.220	.999 ± 0.220	0.749 ± 0.272	0.910 ± 0.302	0.730 ± 0.302
80	0.963 ± 0.220	.984 ± 0.220	0.723 ± 0.272	0.876 ± 0.302	0.711 ± 0.302
85	0.947 ± 0.220	.968 ± 0.220	0.698 ± 0.272	0.842 ± 0.302	0.690 ± 0.302

The following data were provided by the manufacturer of Lunar DPX and Expert systems. They are listed for the 10-year age increments for which they are available with mean ±2 standard deviations (95% confidence interval).

For more information, contact Lunar Corporation, 313 Beltline Highway, Madison, WI 53713.

TABLE 3. *Normal BMD for total body regions for U.S./Europe female reference population*

Age (yr)	L2–L4 AP spine	Femoral neck	Femur total	Pelvis	Forearm radius	Total body
20–29	1.196 ± 0.24	0.996 ± 0.24	1.006 ± 0.24	1.078 ± 0.20	0.70 ± 0.14	1.120 ± 0.16
30–39	1.210 ± 0.24	0.972 ± 0.24	0.997 ± 0.24	1.115 ± 0.20	0.71 ± 0.14	1.141 ± 0.16
40–49	1.180 ± 0.24	0.948 ± 0.24	0.982 ± 0.24	1.100 ± 0.20	0.70 ± 0.14	1.123 ± 0.16
50–59	1.102 ± 0.24	0.887 ± 0.24	0.935 ± 0.24	1.057 ± 0.20	0.66 ± 0.14	1.086 ± 0.16
60–69	1.015 ± 0.24	0.813 ± 0.24	0.871 ± 0.24	1.015 ± 0.20	0.58 ± 0.14	1.030 ± 0.16
70–79	0.993 ± 0.24	0.763 ± 0.24	0.811 ± 0.24	0.942 ± 0.20	0.53 ± 0.14	0.998 ± 0.16

TABLE 4. *Normal BMD for total body regions for U.S./Europe male reference population*

Age (yr)	L2–L4 AP spine	Femoral neck	Femur total	Pelvis	Forearm radius	Total body
20–29	1.241 ± 0.24	1.098 ± 0.26	1.105 ± 0.26	1.218 ± 0.20	0.79 ± 0.14	1.234 ± 0.16
30–39	1.215 ± 0.24	1.045 ± 0.26	1.071 ± 0.26	1.204 ± 0.20	0.82 ± 0.14	1.215 ± 0.16
40–49	1.180 ± 0.24	0.984 ± 0.26	1.042 ± 0.26	1.196 ± 0.20	0.82 ± 0.14	1.210 ± 0.16
50–59	1.145 ± 0.24	0.956 ± 0.26	1.029 ± 0.26	1.196 ± 0.20	0.78 ± 0.14	1.232 ± 0.16
60–69	1.157 ± 0.24	0.909 ± 0.26	1.000 ± 0.26	1.164 ± 0.20	0.77 ± 0.14	1.203 ± 0.16
70–79	1.173 ± 0.24	0.876 ± 0.26	0.961 ± 0.26	1.126 ± 0.20	0.74 ± 0.14	1.177 ± 0.16

The following data were provided by the manufacturer of Norland pDEXA, Excell, Eclipse, XR-36, and ApolloDXA systems. They are listed for the 10-year age increments for which they are available with mean ±2 standard deviations (95% confidence interval).

For more information, contact Norland Medical Systems Inc., W6340 Hackbarth Road, Fort Atkinson, WI 53538.

TABLE 5. *Normal BMD values for reference population U.S. female*

Age (yr)	L2–L4 AP spine	Femoral[a] neck	Distal radius and ulna[b]	Proximal radius and ulna[b]	Heel[c]
20	1.164 ± 0.324	1.018 ± 0.242	0.35 ± 0.1004	0.818 ± 0.1258	0.6382 ± 0.24
50	1.05 ± 0.324	0.91 ± 0.242	0.343 ± 0.1142	0.838 ± 0.1714	—
60	—	—	0.304 ± 0.119	—	—
70	—	—	0.265 ± 0.094	0.623 ± 0.2018	—
90	0.814 ± 0.324	0.569 ± 0.242	—	—	—
95	—	—	0.252 ± 0.092	0.557 ± 0.1898	

[a] Excell, Eclipse, and XR-36 systems.
[b] pDEXA system.
[c] Apollo DXA system.

TABLE 6. *Normal BMD values for reference population U.S. male*

Age (yr)	L2–L4 AP spine	Femoral neck	Distal radius and ulna[b]	Proximal radius and ulna[b]	Heel[c]
20	1.109 ± 0.334	1.015 ± 0.242	0.45 ± 0.1348	0.991 ± 0.1782	0.739 ± 0.2154
40			0.468 ± 0.1348	—	—
60			—	0.959 ± 0.1782	—
80	0.947 ± 0.334	0.711 ± 0.242	—	—	—
90			0.366 ± 0.1348	0.782 ± 0.1782	

[a] Excell, Eclipse, and XR-36 systems.
[b] pDEXA system.
[c] Apollo DXA system.

Subject Index